Operative Orthopedics of the Upper Extremity

Notice

Operative Orthopedics of the Upper Extremity

Edited By

David J. Slutsky, MD

Assistant Professor of Orthopedics
Harbor-UCLA Medical Center
The Hand and Wrist Institute
Torrance, California

McGraw Hill Education | Medical

New York Chicago San Francisco Athens London Madrid
Mexico City Milan New Delhi Singapore Sydney Toronto

Operative Orthopedics of the Upper Extremity

1 2 3 4 5 6 7 8 9 0 CTP/CTP 19 18 17 16 15 14

ISBN 978-0-07-178927-1
MHID 0-07-178927-8

This book was set in Minion Pro by Thomson Digital.
The editors were Brian Belval and Christie Naglieri.
The production supervisor was Catherine Saggese.
Project management was provided by Ritu Joon, Thomson Digital.
The cover was designed by Anthony Landi.
China Translation & Printing Services, Ltd. was printer and binder.

Library of Congress Cataloging-in-Publication Data

Operative orthopedics : upper extremity / edited by David J. Slutsky.
p. ; cm.
Includes bibliographical references.
ISBN 978-0-07-178927-1 (print book : alk. paper) — ISBN 0-07-178927-8 (print book : alk. paper) — ISBN 978-0-07-178928-8 (ebook)
I. Slutsky, David J., editor of compilation.
[DNLM: 1. Upper Extremity—surgery. 2. Orthopedic Procedures. WE 805]
RD557
617.5'7—dc23

2013022623

This book is dedicated to my mother Rose Slutsky who is the glue that has held us all together and the guiding light in our lives who gave us the motivation and courage to achieve our dreams. We love you Mom.

CONTENTS

CONTRIBUTORS

Jeffrey S. Abrams, MD
Clinical Professor
Attending Surgeon
Department of Surgery
Seton Hall University School of Graduate Medicine
University Medical Center of Princeton at Plainsboro
Plainsboro, New Jersey
Chapter 48: Shoulder Arthroscopy: Treatment of Subacromial Impingement, Rotator Cuff Tears, and Superior Labral Anterior and Posterior Tears

Julie E. Adams, MD
Assistant Professor of Orthopaedic Surgery
Department of Orthopaedic Surgery
University of Minnesota
Minneapolis, Minnesota
Chapter 38: Elbow Arthroscopy

George S. Athwal, MD, FRCSC
Associate Professor
Roth | McFarlane Hand and Upper Limb Centre
University of Western Ontario
London, Ontario, Canada
Chapter 37: Simple Elbow Dislocations—A Practical Guide

Andrea Atzei, MD
Consultant Hand Surgeon
Fenice HSRT Hand Surgery and Rehabilitation Team
Centro di Medicina, Treviso, Italy and Policlinico San Giorgio
Pordenone, Italy
Chapter 32: DRUJ Arthroscopy

James Richard Bailey, MD
Orthopaedic Surgeon, Instructor of Surgery
Department of Orthopaedic Surgery
Department of Surgery
Naval Hospital Bremerton, School of Medicine, Uniformed Services University of Health Sciences (USUHS)
Bremerton, Washington
Chapter 51: Pectoralis Major Tendon Repair

Gregory I. Bain, MBBS, FRACS, FA(Ortho) A, PhD
Associate Professor
Department of Orthopaedics and Trauma, and Discipline of Anatomy and Pathology
University of Adelaide
Royal Adelaide Hospital
Modbury Public Hospital
North Adelaide, Australia
Chapter 41A: Tendon Repairs About the Elbow—Part A: Distal Biceps Tendon Ruptures
Chapter 41B: Tendon Repairs About the Elbow—Part B: Triceps Tendon Rupture

Michael S. Bednar, MD
Chief, Professor
Hand Surgery
Department of Orthopaedic Surgery and Rehabilitation
Stritch School of Medicine
Loyola University—Chicago
Maywood, Illinois
Chapter 5: Nonunions and Malunions of the Metacarpals and Phalanges

Jayme Augusto Bertelli, MD, PhD
Professor of Neurosurgery
Center of Biological and Health Sciences
Department of Orthopedic Surgery
University of Southern Santa Catarina (Unisul)
Governador Celso Ramos Hospital
Tubarão, Santa Catarina, Brazil
Florianópolis, Santa Catarina, Brazil
Chapter 54: Accessory to Suprascapular and Radial to Axillary Nerve Transfers for Shoulder Reconstruction with Brachial Plexus Lesions

Alex Lluch Bergadà, MD
Associated Professor of Orthopaedic Surgery
Hand Unit
Institute Kaplan
Valld'Hebron Hospital
UniversitatAutònoma de Barcelona
Barcelona, Spain
Chapter 17: Carpal Instability—Scapholunate, Lunotriquetral, and Midcarpal

Anders Björkman, MD, PhD
Associate professor and Senior Consultant
Departments of Clinical Sciences Malmö—Hand Surgery
Lund University
Malmö, Sweden
Chapter 8: Principles of Nerve Repair

David M. Brogan, MD
Resident Physician
Department of Orthopedic Surgery
Mayo Clinic
Rochester, Minnesota
Chapter 31: Distal Ulnar Head and Neck Fractures

Kyle Caswell, DO
Shoulder Service
The Carrell Clinic
Dallas, Texas
Chapter 46: Fractures of the Shoulder Girdle: Humeral Shaft, Humeral Head, Scapula and Glenoid, and Clavicle

Angela Cheng, MD
Assistant Professor
Division of Plastic Surgery
Department of Surgery
Emory University
Atlanta, Georgia
Chapter 52: Soft Tissue Coverage of the Shoulder

Saeed A. Chowdhry, MD
Plastic Surgery Fellow
Department of Surgery
University of Louisville
Louisville, Kentucky
Chapter 11: Flexor Tendon Repair and Reconstruction

Kevin C. Chung, MD, MS
Professor of Surgery
Assistant Dean for Faculty Affairs
Section of Plastic Surgery
The University of Michigan Health System
Ann Arbor, Michigan
Chapter 6A: Metacarpophalangeal Joint and Proximal Interphalangeal Joint Arthroplasty
Chapter 6B: Metacarpophalangeal and Interphalangeal Joint Fusions

Nathan Coleman, MD
Resident
Department of Orthopaedics and Sports Medicine
University of Washington Medical Center
Seattle, Washington
Chapter 19: Scaphoid Fractures and Nonunions

Lars B. Dahlin, MD, PhD
Professor and Senior Consultant
Departments of Clinical Sciences Malmö—Hand Surgery
Lund University
Skåne University Hospital
Malmö, Sweden
Chapter 8: Principles of Nerve Repair

Umer Dasti, MD
Resident
Department of Surgery
Division of Orthopaedic Surgery
Seton Hall University School of Graduate Medicine
Orange, New Jersey
Chapter 48: Shoulder Arthroscopy: Treatment of Subacromial Impingement, Rotator Cuff Tears, and Superior Labral Anterior and Posterior Tears

David G. Dennison, MD
Consultant
Department of Orthopedic Surgery
Mayo Clinic
Rochester, Minnesota
Chapter 31: Distal Ulnar Head and Neck Fractures

Christian Dumontier, MD
Professor
Department of Plastic, Reconstructive and Esthetic Surgery, Hand Surgery
Hôpital St Roch
Nice, France
Chapter 29: Radiocarpal Dislocation

Christopher J. Dy, MD, MPH
Chief Resident
Hand and Upper Extremity Surgery
Hospital for Special Surgery
New York, New York
Chapter 12: Extensor Tendon Injuries in the Hand: Acute and Chronic

Kevin Eng, MBBS, FRACS
Upper Limb and Hand Fellow
Department of Orthopaedics and Trauma
Royal Adelaide Hospital
Modbury Public Hospital
North Adelaide, Australia
Chapter 41A: Tendon Repairs About the Elbow—Part A: Distal Biceps Tendon Ruptures
Chapter 41B: Tendon Repairs About the Elbow—Part B: Triceps Tendon Rupture

Ida K. Fox, MD
Assistant Professor of Plastic Surgery
Division of Plastic Surgery
Department of Surgery
Washington University School of Medicine
Saint Louis, Missouri
Chapter 10: Sensory Nerve Transfers

Rachel M. Frank, MD
Resident
Department of Orthopaedic Surgery
Rush University Medical Center
Chicago, Illinois
Chapter 51: Pectoralis Major Tendon Repair

Marc Garcia-Elias, MD, PhD
Institute Kaplan
Barcelona, Spain
Chapter 17: Carpal Instability—Scapholunate, Lunotriquetral, and Midcarpal

Günter Germann, MD, PhD
Professor for Plastic and Hand Surgery
Medical Director—ETHIANUM
ETHIANUM—Clinic for Plastic and Reconstructive Surgery
Aesthetic and Preventive Medicine at Heidelberg University Hospital
Germany
Chapter 23: Soft Tissue Coverage of the Carpus

Marcos Flávio Ghizoni, MD, MSc
Professor of Neurosurgery
Center of Biological and Health Sciences
University of Southern Santa Catarina (Unisul)
Tubarão, Santa Catarina, Brazil
Chapter 54: Accessory to Suprascapular and Radial to Axillary Nerve Transfers for Shoulder Reconstruction with Brachial Plexus Lesions

Gertrude Gradl, MD
Attending Surgeon
Department of Trauma and Reconstructive Surgery
University Hospital Aachen
Aachen, Germany
Chapter 28: Malunion and Nonunion of the Distal Radius

Michael R. Hausman, MD
Lippmann Professor of Orthopedic Surgery
Vice-Chair
Chief, Hand and Elbow Service
Department of Orthopedic Surgery
Mount Sinai Medical Center
New York, New York
Chapter 36: Fractures of the Elbow

Kathryn A. Heim, MD
Hand & Upper Extremity Surgery Fellow
Department of Orthopaedic Surgery
University of Pittsburgh Medical Center
Pittsburgh, Pennsylvania
Chapter 15: Kienböck Disease

Guillaume Herzberg, MD, PhD
Professor of Orthopaedic Surgery
Orthopaedic Upper Limb Surgery Unit
Edouard Herriot Hospital Claude Bernard University of Lyon
Lyon, France
Chapter 21: Acute Perilunate Dislocations and Fracture–Dislocations
Chapter 50: Latissimus Dorsi Tendon Transfer for Massive Irreparable Rotator Cuff Tears

PC Ho, MBBS, FRCS(Edinburgh), FHKAM(Orthopedic Surgery), FHKCOS
Consultant, Clinical Professor (Honorary)
Department of Orthopaedics and Traumatology
Prince of Wales Hospital
Chinese University of Hong Kong
Hong Kong
Chapter 14: Hand and Finger Replantation

Jerry Huang, MD
Assistant Professor
Department of Orthopaedics and Sports Medicine
University of Washington Medical Center
Seattle, Washington
Chapter 19: Scaphoid Fractures and Nonunions

Peter JL Jebson, MD
Associate Professor
Instructor
Department of Orthopaedic Surgery
Michigan State University College of Human Medicine
Grand Rapids Medical Education Partners
Condit and Jebson
Grand Rapids, Michigan
Chapter 2: Periarticular Fractures of the Metacarpals and Phalanges

David B. Jones, Jr., MD
Hand Surgery Fellow
Division of Hand Surgery
Mayo Clinic, Rochester, Minnesota
Rochester, Minnesota
Chapter 16: Preiser Disease

Jesse B. Jupiter, MD
Hansjorg Wyss/AO Professor
Department of Orthopaedic Surgery
Harvard Medical School
Boston, Massachusetts
Chapter 28: Malunion and Nonunion of the Distal Radius

Lara Just-Kovac, MD
Resident for Plastic Surgery
Department of Plastic-, Hand- and Reconstructive Surgery
BG-Trauma Center Frankfurt am Main
Germany
Chapter 22: Salvage Procedures for the Wrist

John Kadzielski, MD
MGH Orthopaedic Hand and Upper Extremity Service
Massachusetts General Hospital
Boston, Massachusetts
Chapter 35: Forearm Fractures

Stephen Kennedy, MD
Assistant Professor
Orthopaedics and Sports Medicine
University of Washington Medical Center
Seattle, Washington
Chapter 19: Scaphoid Fractures and Nonunions

Graham JW King, MD, MSc, FRCSC
Director
Roth | McFarlane Hand and Upper Limb Centre
Professor
Departments of Surgery, Medical Biophysics and Biomedical Engineering
St. Joseph's Health Centre, Western University
London, Ontario, Canada
Chapter 40: Elbow Arthroplasty

Melissa Klausmeyer, MD
Clinical Fellow
Private Practice and Hospital Mutua Montañesa
Instituto de Cirugía Plástica y de la Mano
Santander, Spain
Chapter 27: Arthroscopic Treatment of Distal Radius Fractures

Brian J. Klika, MD
Resident Physician
Department of Orthopedic Surgery
Mayo Clinic
Rochester, Minnesota
Chapter 31: Distal Ulnar Head and Neck Fractures

Daniel T. Kokmeyer, MD
Fellow
The Indiana Hand to Shoulder Center
Indianapolis, Indiana
Chapter 2: Periarticular Fractures of the Metacarpals and Phalanges

Philippe Kopylov, MD, PhD
Senior Consultant
Hand Unit
Department of Orthopedics
Lund University Hospital
Lund, Sweden
Chapter 34A: Partial Head Distal Radioulnar Joint Implants

Evan Kowalski, BS
Research Associate
Section of Plastic Surgery
University of Michigan Health System
Ann Arbor, Michigan
Chapter 6A: Metacarpophalangeal Joint and Proximal Interphalangeal Joint Arthroplasty

Sumant "Butch" Krishnan, MD
Director
The Shoulder Center
Baylor University Medical Center
Dallas, Texas
Chapter 46: Fractures of the Shoulder Girdle: Humeral Shaft, Humeral Head, Scapula and Glenoid, and Clavicle

Shawn M. Kutnik, MD
Hand and Upper Extremity Surgery
Premier Care Orthopedics
Saint Louis, Missouri
Chapter 36: Fractures of the Elbow

Michael A.C. Lapner, MD, FRCSC
Department of Surgery
University of Alberta
Edmonton OR London
Ontario, Canada
Chapter 37: Simple Elbow Dislocations—A Practical Guide

Meredith Larsen, MD
Department of Orthopaedic Surgery and Rehabilitation
Stritch School of Medicine
Loyola University - Chicago
Maywood, Illinois
Chapter 5: Nonunions and Malunions of the Metacarpals and Phalanges

Steve K. Lee, MD
Associate Professor of Orthopaedic Surgery
Hand, Upper Extremity, and Microsurgery
Hospital for Special Surgery, Weill Cornell Medical College
New York, New York
Chapter 12: Extensor Tendon Injuries in the Hand: Acute and Chronic

David M. Lichtman, MD
Professor and Chairman
Department of Orthopaedic Surgery
University of North Texas Health Science Center and John Peter Smith Hospital
Fort Worth, Texas
Chapter 15: Kienböck Disease

Riccardo Luchetti, MD
Consultant Hand Surgeon
Rimini Hand Surgery and Rehabilitation Center
Rimini, Italy
Chapter 32: DRUJ Arthroscopy

Susan E. Mackinnon, MD
Shoenberg Professor and Chief of Plastic Surgery
Division of Plastic Surgery
Department of Surgery
Washington University School of Medicine
Saint Louis, Missouri
Chapter 10: Sensory Nerve Transfers

Timothy R. McAdams, MD
Associate Professor
Department of Orthopaedic Surgery
Stanford University
Redwood City, California
Chapter 53: Nerve Entrapments—Quadrilateral Space, Supraspinatus Nerve Entrapment

Frank McCormick, MD
Attending Physician
Department of Orthopaedic Surgery
Holy Cross Orthopaedic Institute
Ft. Lauderdale, Florida
Chapter 51: Pectoralis Major Tendon Repair

Lucas S. McDonald, MD, MPH&TM
Staff Surgeon, Assistant Professor
Department of Orthopaedic Surgery
Naval Medical Center San Diego,
Uniformed Services University of the Health Sciences
San Diego, California
Chapter 47: Shoulder Dislocation: Anterior, Posterior, Multidirectional

John W. McNeil II, BA
Medical Student
Department of Orthopaedic Surgery
Naval Medical Center San Diego
San Diego, California
Chapter 51: Pectoralis Major Tendon Repair

Elliot S. Mendelsohn, MD
Chief Resident
Department of Orthopaedic Surgery
Harbor-UCLA Medical Center
Torrance, California
Chapter 55: Management of Traumatic Bone Loss in the Hand

Greg Merrell, MD
Indiana Hand to Shoulder Center
Indianapolis, Indiana
Chapter 3: Dislocations of the Thumb and Fingers

Todd C. Moen, MD
Shoulder Service
The Carrell Clinic
Dallas, Texas
Chapter 46: Fractures of the Shoulder Girdle: Humeral Shaft, Humeral Head, Scapula and Glenoid, and Clavicle

Steven L. Moran, MD
Professor of Orthopedics and Plastic Surgery
Division of Hand Surgery
Mayo Clinic, Rochester, Minnesota
Rochester, Minnesota
Chapter 16: Preiser Disease

Soheil Najibi, MD, PhD
Director of Pelvis and Acetabular Trauma
Department of Orthopaedic Surgery
Harbor-UCLA Medical Center
Torrance, California
Chapter 55: Management of Traumatic Bone Loss in the Hand

Toshiyasu Nakamura, MD, PhD
Assistant Professor
Department of Orthopaedic Surgery
School of Medicine, Keio University,Tokyo
Tokyo, Japan
Chapter 30: Causes and Management of Acute and Chronic Distal Radioulnar Joint Instability

Timothy R. Niacaris, MD, PhD
Assistant Professor
Department of Orthopaedic Surgery
University of North Texas Health Science Center
Chief of Hand Surgery - John Peter Smith Health Network
Fort Worth, Texas
Chapter 15: Kienböck Disease

Michael J. O'Brien, MD
Associate Professor of Orthopaedic Surgery
Department of Orthopaedic Surgery
Tulane University
New Orleans, Louisiana
Chapter 39: Arthroscopic and Open Management of Instability of the Elbow

Kagan Ozer, MD
Clinical Associate Professor
Department of Orthopedic Surgery
The University of Michigan Health System
Ann Arbor, Michigan
Chapter 6B: Metacarpophalangeal and Interphalangeal Joint Fusions

Collier S. Pace, MD
Resident
Division of Plastic Surgery
Medical College of Virginia
Richmond, Virginia
Chapter 25: Distal Anterior Interosseous Nerve Transfer for Intrinsic Reanimation

Loukia K. Papatheodorou, MD
Hand & Upper Extremity Surgery
Allegheny General Hospital
Pittsburgh, Pennsylvania
Chapter 33: Salvage Procedures of the DRUJ

Francisco del Piñal, MD, PhD
Surgeon
Private Practice and Hospital Mutua Montañesa
Instituto de Cirugía Plástica y de la Mano
Santander, Spain
Chapter 27: Arthroscopic Treatment of Distal Radius Fractures

Matthew T. Provencher, MD
Chief of Sports Medicine and Surgery
Associate Professor of Surgery
Department of Orthopaedic Surgery
Massachusetts General Hospital
Harvard Medical School
Boston, Massachusetts
Chapter 47: Shoulder Dislocation: Anterior, Posterior, Multidirectional
Chapter 51: Pectoralis Major Tendon Repair

David C. Ring, MD, PhD
Director of Research
MGH Orthopaedic Hand and Upper Extremity Service
Massachusetts General Hospital
Boston, Massachusetts
Chapter 35: Forearm Fractures

Marco Rizzo, MD
Professor of Orthopedics
Division of Hand Surgery
Mayo Clinic, Rochester, Minnesota
Rochester, Minnesota
Chapter 16: Preiser Disease

Lauren Rosenblatt, BS
Research Assistant
Hand and Upper Extremity Surgery
Hospital for Special Surgery
New York, New York
Chapter 12: Extensor Tendon Injuries in the Hand: Acute and Chronic

Rudy Kovachevich, MD
Hand Surgery Associates, P.C.
Denver, Colorado
Chapter 3: Dislocations of the Thumb and Fingers

Philippe Saffar, MD
Hand and Orthopedic Surgeon
Institut Francais De Chirurgie De La Main
Paris, France
Chapter 29: Radiocarpal Dislocation

Michel Saint-Cyr, MD, FRCS
Professor of Plastic Surgery
Department of Plastic Surgery
Mayo Clinic
Rochester, Minnesota
Chapter 52: Soft Tissue Coverage of the Shoulder

Michael Sauerbier, MD, PhD
Chair, Professor
Department for Plastic, Hand and Reconstructive Surgery
Hand Trauma Center -BG-Trauma Center Frankfurt am Main
Frankfurt am Main, Germany
Chapter 22: Salvage Procedures for the Wrist

Felix H. Savoie, III, MD
Professor of Orthopaedic Surgery
Department of Orthopaedic Surgery
Tulane University
New Orleans, Louisiana
Chapter 39: Arthroscopic and Open Management of Instability of the Elbow

Morne Scheepers, MD
Department of Orthopaedics and Trauma
Modbury Public Hospital
Modbury, Australia
Chapter 41B: Tendon Repairs About the Elbow—Part B: Triceps Tendon Rupture

Frances Sharpe, MD
Adjunct assistant clinical professor USC Keck School of Medicine
Department of Orthopedics
Southern California Permanente Medical Group and University of Southern California Keck School of Medicine/Los Angeles County Medical Center
Fontana, California
Chapter 42A: Soft Tissue Coverage of the Elbow
Chapter 42B: Vascularized Free Fibula Bone Graft for Upper Extremity Reconstruction
Chapter 44: Nerve Transfer for Restoration of Elbow Flexion: The Modified Oberlin Procedure

Juan P. Simone, MD
Reconstructive Upper Extremity Fellow
Department of Orthopedic Surgery
Mayo Clinic
Rochester, Minnesota
Chapter 49: Shoulder Arthroplasty: Humeral Head Replacement, Total Shoulder and Reverse Total Shoulder Replacement

David J. Slutsky, MD
Assistant Professor of Orthopedics
Harbor-UCLA Medical Center
The Hand and Wrist Institute
Torrance, California
Chapter 4: Small Joint Arthroscopy
Chapter 7: Thumb Arthroplasty and Arthrodesis
Chapter 9: Nerve Repair and Reconstruction: Elbow to Fingertips
Chapter 13: Soft Tissue Coverage of the Hand
Chapter 18: Wrist Arthroscopy
Chapter 20: Pedicled Vascularized Bone Grafts for Scaphoid Nonunion
Chapter 24: Nerve Compression Syndromes at the Wrist
Chapter 26: Management of Distal Radius Fractures
Chapter 34B: Distal Radioulnar Joint Implants
Chapter 43: Nerve Compression Syndromes at the Elbow
Chapter 44: Nerve Transfer for Restoration of Elbow Flexion: The Modified Oberlin Procedure
Chapter 45: Nerve Transfers to Restore Wrist and Finger Extension
Chapter 55: Management of Traumatic Bone Loss in the Hand

Dean G. Sotereanos, MD
Professor
Department of Orthopaedic Surgery
Hand & Upper Extremity Surgery
Drexel University, School of Medicine
Allegheny General Hospital
Pittsburgh, Pennsylvania
Chapter 33: Salvage Procedures of the DRUJ

John W. Sperling, MD
Professor of Orthopedic Surgery
Department of Orthopedic Surgery
Mayo Clinic
Rochester, Minnesota
Chapter 49: Shoulder Arthroplasty: Humeral Head Replacement, Total Shoulder and Reverse Total Shoulder Replacement

Scott P. Steinmann, MD
Professor of Orthopedic Surgery
Department of Orthopedic Surgery
Mayo Clinic
Rochester, Minnesota
Chapter 38: Elbow Arthroscopy

Peter J. Stern, MD
Hill Professor and Chairman
Department of Orthopaedic Surgery
University of Cincinnati College of Medicine
Cincinnati, Ohio
Chapter 1: Metacarpal and Phalangeal Shaft Fractures

Milan Stevanovic, MD
Professor of Orthopedics and Surgery
Department of Orthopedic
University of Southern California Keck School of Medicine
Los Angeles County Medical Center
Los Angeles, California
Chapter 42A: Soft Tissue Coverage of the Elbow
Chapter 42B: Vascularized Free Fibula Bone Graft for Upper Extremity Reconstruction
Chapter 44: Nerve Transfer for Restoration of Elbow Flexion: The Modified Oberlin Procedure

Cristiano Paulo Tacca, MD
Consultant Hand Surgeon
Department of Orthopedic Surgery
Governador Celso Ramos Hospital
Florianópolis, Santa Catarina, Brazil
Chapter 54: Accessory to Suprascapular and Radial to Axillary Nerve Transfers for Shoulder Reconstruction with Brachial Plexus Lesions

Niels Thomsen, MD, PhD
Senior Consultant
Departments of Clinical Sciences Malmö—Hand Surgery
Lund University
Malmö, Sweden
Chapter 8: Principles of Nerve Repair

Suraj S. Trivedi, MD
Battalion Surgeon
3rd Marine Division, 3rd Battalion, 12th Marines
Okinawa, Japan
Chapter 47: Shoulder Dislocation: Anterior, Posterior, Multidirectional

WL Tse, MBChB, MRCS, FRCSEd(Orth), FHKAM(Orthopedic Surgery), FHKCOS
Associate Consultant
Department of Orthopaedics and Traumatology
Prince of Wales Hospital
Chinese University of Hong Kong
Hong Kong
Chapter 14: Hand and Finger Replantation

Magnus Tägil, MD, PhD
Professor
Hand Unit
Department of Orthopedics
Lund University Hospital
Lund, Sweden
Chapter 34A: Partial Head Distal Radioulnar Joint Implants

Lindley B. Wall, MD
Assistant Professor
Department of Orthopaedic Surgery
Washington University
St. Louis, Missouri
Chapter 1: Metacarpal and Phalangeal Shaft Fractures

Robert A. Waltz, MD
LCDR MC USN
Department of Orthopaedics
Naval Health Clinic New England
Newport, State: Rhode Island
Chapter 51: Pectoralis Major Tendon Repair

Keming Wang, MD
Attending Physician
Department of Plastic Surgery
Plastic Surgery Hospital of Peking Union Medical College
Beijing, China
Chapter 6A: Metacarpophalangeal Joint and Proximal Interphalangeal Joint Arthroplasty

Bradon J. Wilhelmi, MD, FACS
Chief and Professor Plastic Surgery
Plastic Surgery Residency Program Director
Department of Surgery
University of Louisville
Louisville, Kentucky
Chapter 11: Flexor Tendon Repair and Reconstruction

Clara WY Wong, MBChB, MRCS, FRCSEd(Orth), FHKAM(Orthopedic Surgery), FHKCOS
Associate Consultant
Department of Orthopaedics and Traumatology
Prince of Wales Hospital
Chinese University of Hong Kong
Hong Kong
Chapter 14: Hand and Finger Replantation

Michael B. Wood, MD
Professor
Department of Orthopedic Surgery
Mayo Medical School
Rochester, Minnesota
Chapter 25: Distal Anterior Interosseous Nerve Transfer for Intrinsic Reanimation

Craig Wright, MD
Resident
Department of Surgery, Division of Orthopaedic Surgery
Seton Hall University School of Graduate Medicine
Orange, New Jersey
Chapter 48: Shoulder Arthroscopy: Treatment of Subacromial Impingement, Rotator Cuff Tears, and Superior Labral Anterior and Posterior Tears

Andrew Yee, BS
Research Associate
Division of Plastic Surgery
Department of Surgery
Washington University School of Medicine
Saint Louis, Missouri
Chapter 10: Sensory Nerve Transfers

PREFACE

This book covers the gamut of treatment for injuries and disorders of the upper extremity from the shoulder to fingertips. It is organized both by level and by anatomic structure. For example, when one is treating an injury of the wrist, repair or reconstruction of each individual component is comprehensively covered, starting with bone, joint, and ligament to nerve, tendon, and soft tissue. For those injuries which are nonreconstructible each section is followed by a chapter on suitable salvage procedures. In this manner the book offers a one-stop comprehensive guide for the treatment of each segment of the upper extremity.

This book is intended to serve as a user's manual for both the entry-level upper extremity surgeon as well as the experienced operator. The methodology and the practical aspects of each procedure are stressed along with myriad pearls and tips, oftentimes from the originators of the technique.

I am indebted to the contributors without whom this book would not exist and I am indebted to each and every one of the authors for all of their efforts and personal sacrifice that they have expended to educate their peers. I am also indebted to Brian Belval, senior editor of clinical medicine at McGraw-Hill, for allowing me to move forward with this project as well as Christie Naglieri, the senior project development editor, who worked tirelessly to chase down all of the manuscript files and put this project together. It was a real joy working with many of the pioneers and innovators in upper extremity surgery and I hope the reader experiences the same.

David J. Slutsky MD.

I

HAND

1

Metacarpal and Phalangeal Shaft Fractures

Lindley B. Wall, MD
Peter J. Stern, MD

BACKGROUND

Metacarpal and phalangeal fractures are common.[1] While most of these fractures can be treated nonoperatively, there has been a recent trend toward operative fixation because of improved implant design, fixation techniques, implant materials, ease of fluoroscopic imaging, and postoperative rehabilitation.[2] Surgical intervention also allows for early mobilization that may minimize stiffness and hence accelerate a return to full function.

METACARPAL SHAFT FRACTURES

Metacarpal shaft fractures commonly occur from a fall or direct blow to the hand. They most frequently occur in males between the ages of 10 and 40 years, and border digits are the most commonly involved.

Patients present with painful and restricted motion and have difficulty making a fist. There is dorsal swelling, ecchymosis, and tenderness over the fractured metacarpal(s). A dorsal prominence, particularly with displaced shaft fractures, may also be appreciated. Digit rotation should also be assessed by the following techniques: digital scissoring on synchronous active digital flexion, visualization of fingernail orientation, or the tenodesis effect with wrist flexion and extension.

All patients suspected of having a metacarpal fracture should undergo a radiographic assessment. The recommended views include a posterior–anterior, lateral, and an oblique view of the hand. A Brewerton view, which is an anterior-to-posterior view with the metacarpophalangeal (MCP) joints flexed to 60°, can be obtained to assess if there is any metacarpal head involvement. CT examination is usually unnecessary.

Indications

There are multiple indications for the operative treatment of shaft fractures. Open fractures and those with rotational deformity (digital overlap or scissoring) are clear indications. Strauch et al[3] showed that metacarpal shortening creates an extensor lag, and for every 2 mm of shortening, there is a 7° lag. Thus, it is generally accepted that greater than 5 mm of shortening may result in a noticeable extensor lag and operative fixation is indicated. Transverse metacarpal shaft fractures generally deform with an apex dorsal angulation. The amount of acceptable angulation is greater in the ring and small fingers due to the greater degree of compensatory motion at their carpometacarpal (CMC) joints. The reported cutoff for acceptable angulation is 10° in the index and middle metacarpal, 20° to 30° in the ring, and 30° to 40° in the small metacarpal.[4,5] Pseudoclawing (MCP hyperextension and proximal interphalangeal [PIP] joint flexion on active finger extension) can also occur with shaft fractures and is a relative indication for fixation in selected patients. Classically, it has been taught that multiple shaft fractures are a surgical indication, yet the amount of displacement and instability of the fractures should be assessed before immediate fixation.

Most periarticular fractures involving the MP joint require internal fixation. These are more difficult to treat due to the smaller fracture fragments and risk of articular impingement with an implant.

Contraindications

Unstable soft tissue coverage and active infection are contraindications to internal fixation and favor temporary external fixation.

Nonoperative Treatment

CLOSED REDUCTION AND CASTING

All isolated shaft fractures should be considered for closed reduction and casting. If an acceptable reduction is obtained and can be maintained by a cast, this is the treatment of choice. Tavassoli et al[6] showed that the type of cast and position of the digits were not critical for maintenance of reduction or range of motion or grip strength. However, classical teaching dictates immobilization in the intrinsic plus position (MCP joints at 70° flexion and PIP joint extension) to minimize the risk of an MCP joint contracture due to shortening of the collateral ligaments. We continue cast immobilization for 3 to 4 weeks, and then place the patient's hand in a removable splint for an additional 2 weeks while initiating active range of motion.

To obtain a reduction, the Jahss maneuver can be utilized to reduce the apex dorsal deformity.[7] This involves flexing the MCP joint and the PIP joint to 90°, and using the proximal phalanx as a reduction tool applying a dorsally directed force onto the distal fracture fragment of the metacarpal while simultaneously exerting downward pressure on the proximal segment of the fractured metacarpal.

Surgical Treatment

When closed reduction and immobilization are inadequate for fracture stabilization, operative intervention should be implemented.

There are many methods of fracture fixation. The most appropriate fixation technique is dependent primarily on the fracture pattern, which includes transverse, oblique, spiral, and comminuted fractures.

There are several advantages to Kirschner wire (K-wire) fixation. They are readily available, inexpensive, and versatile. They are easy to insert with a simple power driver, and there is minimal soft tissue disruption especially when they are placed percutaneously. Disadvantages include the fact that K-wires are less rigid than screw or plate fixation, they may loosen with time, and they may also distract the fracture site during placement. Early mobilization may be difficult with pins placed percutaneously as they can interfere with splinting and therapy. Lastly, and most importantly, they place the patient at risk of pin tract infections (Fig. 1-1). Botte et al reported an 18% complication rate in their series.[8]

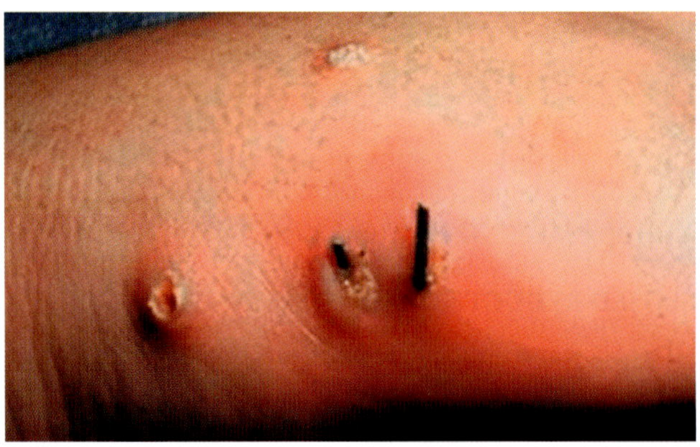

FIGURE 1-1 Pin site infection.

CLOSED REDUCTION AND PINNING

Fractures that can be reduced by closed methods, but are unstable and not amenable to casting alone, can be treated with supplemental percutaneous K-wire fixation. The size of the K-wire is dependent on the size of the metacarpal, ranging from 0.7 to 1.6 mm. While the Jahss maneuver can be utilized for reduction prior to pin fixation, another reduction tool is a pointed tenaculum that can be used to manipulate the ends of the fractured metacarpal prior to K-wire placement.

The K-wires can be placed in many different configurations including multiple transmetacarpal wires (at least 2 wires above the fracture and 1 below) into the adjacent metacarpal (Fig. 1-2), crossing pins (Fig. 1-3), and stacked intramedullary wires (Fig. 1-4). While transverse cross-pins assist with rotational control and shortening, cross-pins are not favored for transverse fractures because the fracture can potentially be distracted. Also, transverse pins can contribute to interosseous adhesions because they pass through the intermetacarpal space.

K-wires can also be used for intramedullary fixation. Of note, there are also small intramedullary rods designed specifically for metacarpal fractures. This type of fixation can consist of 1 single, large K-wire (1.6 mm) or Steinmann pin placed down the shaft of the metacarpal (Fig. 1-4) or multiple stacked intramedullary K-wires as in the bouquet technique (Fig. 1-5). Intramedullary fixation is not recommended for oblique fractures or for comminuted fractures because it cannot control fracture shortening, but is ideally suited for transverse fractures because it can maintain the metacarpal length. However, it still can be difficult to maintain rotational control. This can be addressed using multiple prebent intramedullary K-wires, which assist in rotational control through 3-point fixation. Disadvantages include pin migration and fracture distraction.

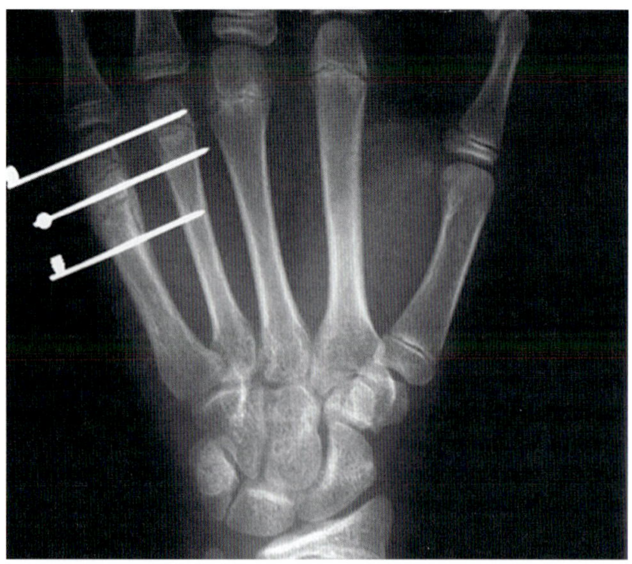

FIGURE 1-2 Transversing K-wires.

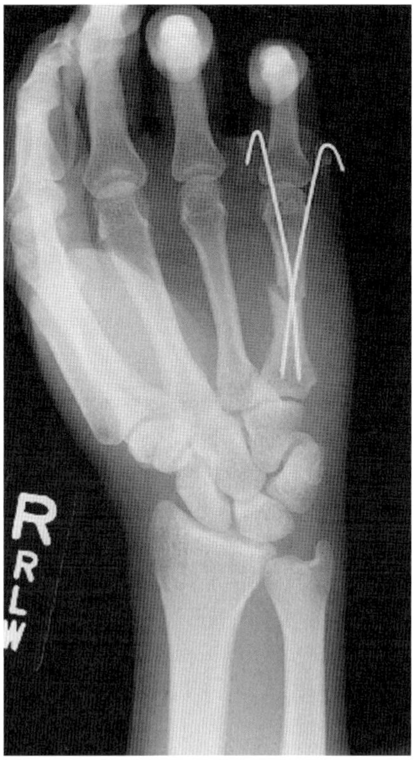

FIGURE 1-3 Cross-pinning fixation.

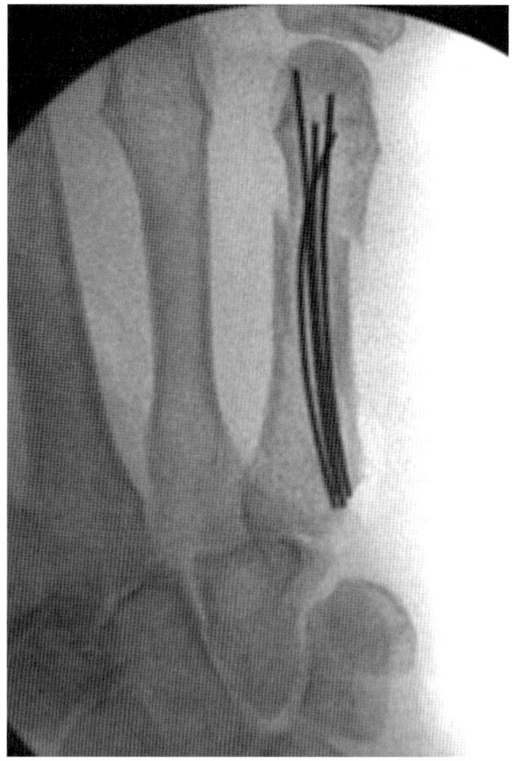

FIGURE 1-5 Bouquet fixation.

OPEN REDUCTION

Some metacarpal shaft fractures cannot be reduced with closed methods and open reduction is necessary. Many times this is the result of interposed soft tissues. Metacarpal shaft fractures are exposed through a dorsal longitudinal adjacent to a fractured metacarpal (to minimize adhesions between the skin and underlying bone). If all 4 metacarpals are fractured, the incisions should be placed between the index and middle metacarpals and ring and small metacarpals.

Periarticular fractures can be stabilized with low-profile locking plates or the older minicondylar blade plates. Metacarpal base fractures can be treated with temporary joint spanning plate fixation or intramedullary fixation crossing the CMC joint with small proximal fragments.

Pinning and Intramedullary K-wire Fixation. K-wire fixation and intramedullary fixation should still be considered following an open reduction.

Cerclage Wiring. Cerclage fixation with 24-gauge wire can be used to supplement pin fixation and provide compression, especially for long oblique and spiral fractures. The addition of a cerclage wire in combination with K-wire stabilization greatly improves the fracture stability[9,10] and the incidence of fracture healing (Fig. 1-6).

Screw Fixation. Screw fixation has both advantages and disadvantages. Screws provide an anatomic, stable construct that permits early mobilization. It also minimizes hardware prominence especially when compared with plate and screw constructs. Unfortunately this type of fixation is applicable for very specific fracture types and there is a low margin for error with reduction and fixation.

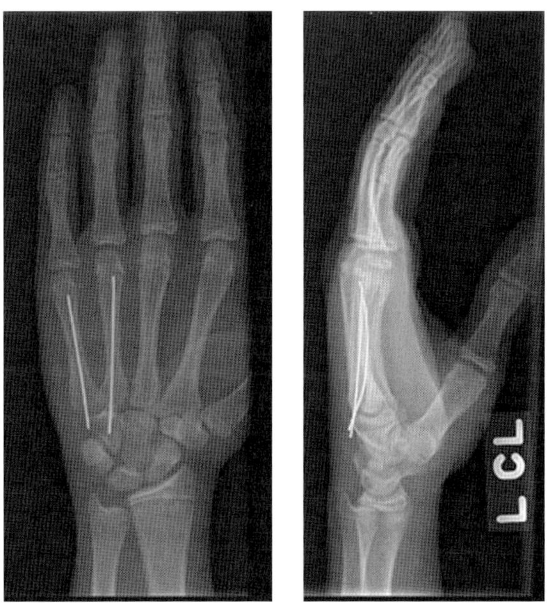

FIGURE 1-4 Intramedullary K-wire fixation.

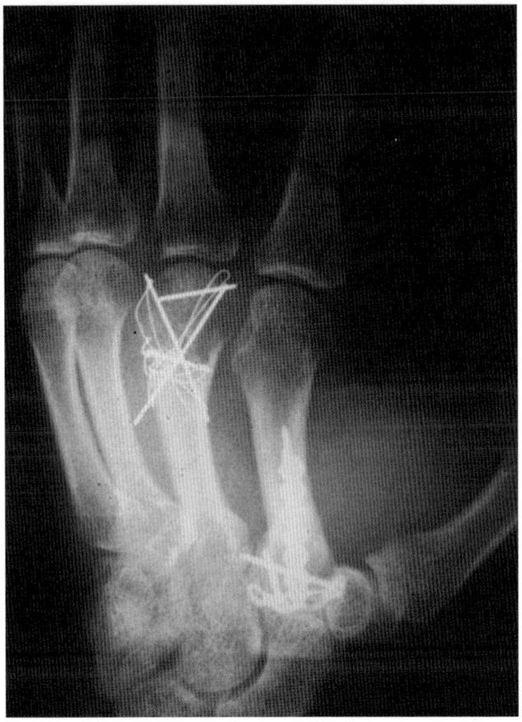

FIGURE 1-6 K-wire and cerclage wire combination fixation. (Copyright David J. Slutsky, MD.)

Screw fixation is ideal for long oblique or spiral fractures (Fig. 1-7). At least two 2.4 or 2.0 mm screws (4 cortices), and ideally 3, should be used. At a minimum, the fracture length must be equal to 2 diameters (preferably 3 diameters) of the metacarpal to prevent screw cutout. Screws placed at 90° to the fracture provide the most fracture site compression, whereas screws placed parallel to the metacarpal long axis are the most efficient at resisting shortening; hence, a combination of screws in different planes is used. The screws are countersunk to reduce the irritation and adhesions to extensor tendons.

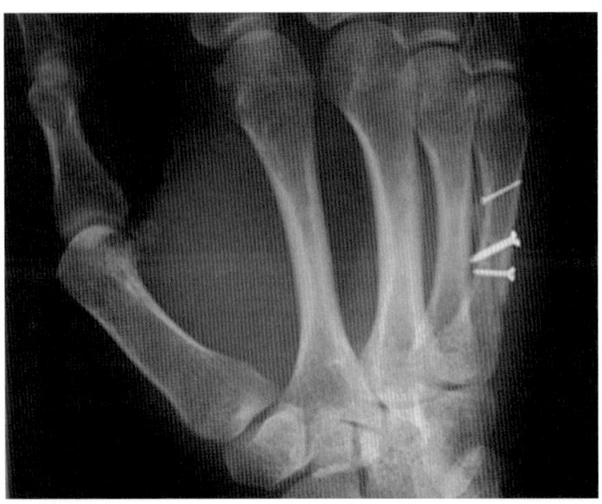

FIGURE 1-7 Screw fixation.

Plate and Screw Fixation. Plate and screw fixation can be used for the majority of fracture configurations. It is recommended to engage at least 6 cortices (ie, 3 bicortical screws) above and below the fracture for fixation (Fig. 1-8). The size of plate ranges from 2.0 to 2.7 mm depending on the size of the metacarpal. Both stainless steel and titanium implants, with and without locking technology, are available.

Plate fixation provides rigid fixation and maintains metacarpal length. It can be used as a neutralization plate following an anatomic reduction and also for highly comminuted fractures in bridge plate fashion. The greatest advantage following plate fixation is the ability to start the patients on early wrist and finger mobilization, but lifting is restricted to a few pounds for the initial 4 to 6 weeks.

Plate fixation has disadvantages. Extensive soft tissue stripping is required that can lead to adhesions and finger contractures. Plates are also higher profile than other types of fixation and can cause extensor tendon irritation or adhesions, which may require implant removal. Removal is not recommended before 6 months.

External Fixation. External fixators can be used for comminuted fractures, open fractures, and infected fractures. They can be applied with minimal soft tissue disruption and minimal periosteal stripping, while preserving the metacarpal blood supply. Two bicortical pins are inserted proximal and distal to the fracture site. The disadvantages include the fact that the fixators are cumbersome and disliked by patients, there is a risk of pin tract infections, and the construct provides flexible rather than rigid fixation. One advantage, however, is that it can be removed in the office.

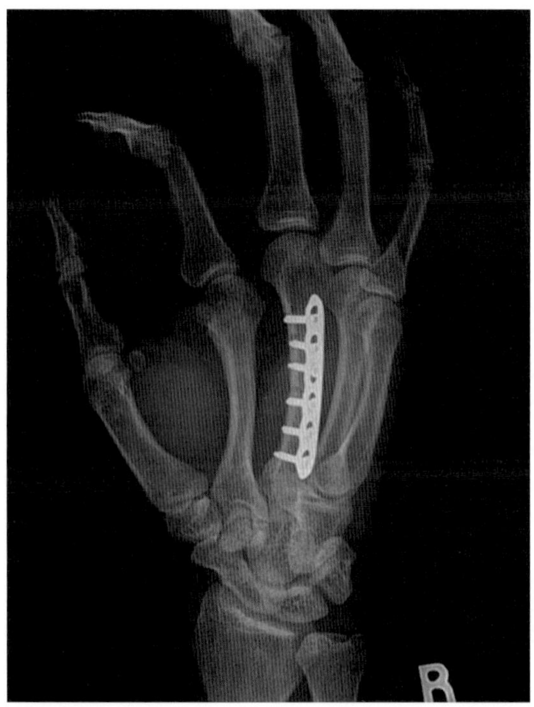

FIGURE 1-8 Plate and screw fixation.

Outcomes

Al-Qattan reviewed the results in 36 patients with metacarpal shaft fractures with a mean age of 31 years (range, 12-52 years) who were treated with interosseous loop wire fixation and immediate postoperative mobilization.[11] There were 26 transverse and 10 oblique/spiral fractures treated with cerclage loop and a volar plaster splint for 3 weeks, while allowing immediate finger motion. After a mean follow-up of 8 weeks, 34/36 patients had regained full range of motion of the fingers, with a total arc of motion of 260°.[11] The 2 patients with less than normal motion, lacking 15° and 10° total motion, were the 2 oldest patients in the series (ages 52 and 53 years). Our preference is to use cerclage wires in addition to K-wire fixation as described by Greene et al.[12] These authors reported the results of composite wiring in 33 patients with 33 metacarpal fractures treated using various configurations of K-wire fixation and stainless steel wire sutures, followed by active motion within 1 week of surgery. The patients achieved a final mean total active motion (TAM) of 256° (standard deviation 13.4) (normal TAM 260°).

Acceptable outcomes can also be obtained in periarticular fractures that are treated with stable fixation and early motion. Omakawa et al[13] reviewed 51 patients with periarticular fractures with metaphyseal comminution and intra-articular split or depression in 22 hands. The average age was 38 years (range, 14-63), and the average follow-up was 1 year. The final range of TAM (%TAM) was excellent (85% of the uninjured hand) for 26, good (70%-84%) for 17, fair (50%-69%) for 5, and poor (49%) for 3. Postoperative complications occurred in 5 patients, including fracture redisplacement in 2, a collapse or absorption of the condylar head in 2, and superficial infection due to hardware exposure in 1. Plates were removed in 30 cases, and additional surgery was required in 20 cases.

Zhang et al reviewed 265 patients with 302 MCP periarticular fractures, with a mean age of 32.5 years (range, 17-59 years).[14] A "T"-shaped plate, double-row plate, or a condylar plate was used for A2, A3, C1, and C2 type fractures. Screws alone were used for B type fractures. Active and passive flexion and extension exercises were begun at day 3 post operation. At an average follow-up of 4.6 months (range, 4-24 months) there were 113 excellent, 136 good, and 53 poor results using the TAM criteria. The average PROM of MP joint was 82.3° ± 4.7° and the average QuickDASH score 17.4.

Intramedullary fixation also allows for good results, a low nonunion rate,[4,15] and good postoperative motion.[4] Kelsch and Ulrich analyzed the clinical results of 35 patients with fifth metacarpal neck fractures that had been treated with closed reduction and at least 2 intramedullary K-wires. At a median follow-up of 1.1 years 34/35 patients achieved normal motion, with a 15° extension lag and malrotation in 1 patient.[15] More recently, Orbay and Touhami reported on the results of 110 metacarpal fractures, a combination of neck and shaft fractures, treated with intramedullary fixation, using a custom-designed 1.1- or 1.6-mm flexible intramedullary nail (Hand Innovations, Miami, Florida), 34 locked and 76 nonlocked, which were inserted antegrade through a small stab incision in the metacarpal base, and removed after 4 to 6 weeks. At an average follow-up time of 18 weeks (range, 12-68 weeks) they reported a 100% union rate with a TAM of 239° in the nonlocked group and 244° in the locked group. There was hardware irritation in 4 patients, penetration of the MP joint in 3 patients, and 2 delayed unions.[4]

Our preference is to use the least invasive method of fixation of metacarpal shaft fractures, thus limiting soft tissue disruption and periosteal stripping.

Complications

Plate fixation has a higher complication rate than other fixation techniques.[16] However, this may be because plate fixation is used in more complex fracture patterns, such as a comminuted fracture, where it is ideal of maintaining reduction and bone length. Fusetti et al reported complications in 28/157 metacarpal fractures treated with plate fixation between 1993 and 1999 with 1 or more complications including difficulty with fracture healing (12 patients), stiffness (8 patients), plate loosening or breakage (7 patients), complex regional pain syndrome (2 patients), and deep infection (1 patient). It must be acknowledged that older bulky implants contributed to the poor outcomes.[16] Interestingly, when plate fixation (14 patients) was compared with the Hand Innovations intramedullary nail by Ozer et al (38 patients) for both midshaft and distal third metacarpal fractures, it was found that there was no statistical difference between the final postoperative TAM between the 2 groups.[17] Plate fixation did show an advantage over intramedullary fixation with regards to final displacement; there was postoperative displacement in 5 patients in the IMN group, and no displacement with plate fixation.

PHALANGEAL SHAFT FRACTURES

Phalangeal shaft fractures present with pain, swelling, and localized tenderness over the traumatized digit. Additionally, rotational or angular deformity and shortening may be present.

Radiographs should include 3 views: posteroanterior (PA), splay lateral, and 45° oblique views.

Distal Phalanx Fractures

Shaft fractures of the distal phalanx can be either transverse or longitudinal and are usually the result of a crushing injury. These fractures are usually stabilized by the surrounding soft tissues and simply require immobilization to heal. If the fractures are displaced, they may be treated with longitudinal percutaneous pin fixation. In the presence of an open fracture, a nail bed injury is nearly always present and must be repaired.

Middle and Proximal Phalanx Fractures

Middle and proximal phalanx fractures can be transverse, spiral, oblique, or comminuted. Transverse fractures of the proximal phalanx usually angulate apex palmar secondary to pull the interossei on the proximal fragment (Fig. 1-9) and may also angulate in the coronal plane. Transverse fractures through the base of the proximal phalanx can be difficult to assess radiographically and multiple views may be necessary. Oblique and spiral fractures characteristically produce malrotation and may also angulate in the coronal plane. Comminuted fractures shorten and are usually quite unstable.

CLOSED REDUCTION AND CASTING

If there is no rotational deformity or shortening, these fractures can often be treated with closed reduction and immobilization with a cast or splint for 4 weeks in the intrinsic plus position. This is followed by a removable splint for an additional 2 weeks and protected finger motion.

CLOSED REDUCTION AND PINNING

Closed reduction and percutaneous pinning can be used to maintain the reduction of an unstable phalanx fracture that minimizes soft tissue disruption and stripping of the periosteum at the fracture site. Middle phalanx fractures can be reduced and held with percutaneously placed reduction clamps or by manipulation of the fragments with the K-wire during fixation. Most middle phalanx fractures can be stabilized with 2 to 3 K-wires placed in a crossed pattern for transverse fractures and placed perpendicular to the fracture plane for spiral and oblique fractures.

Transverse proximal phalanx fractures are reduced by flexing both the MCP and PIP joints to 90°. This position allows for either antegrade or retrograde placement of the K-wires. When placing pins retrograde, the starting point is the retrocondylar fossa of the head of the proximal phalanx. For more proximal shaft fractures, antegrade fixation can be utilized. One method of antegrade pinning is 2 cross-pins with a starting point on either side of the base of the proximal phalanx (Fig. 1-10). The other method is a transarticular approach; the MCP joint is flexed and a K-wire is placed centrally into the metacarpal head through the joint and down the shaft of the proximal phalanx (Fig. 1-11). Pins should be removed at 3 to 4 weeks. Then the digit should be protected for an additional 2 to 3 weeks with buddy taping while the fracture consolidates, but range of motion is initiated to minimize stiffness. Both percutaneous transarticular and cross-pinning are reasonable choices for transverse metaphyseal fractures; unfortunately, both can produce complications, especially stiffness.[18]

OPEN REDUCTION

When closed methods are insufficient to obtain fracture reduction, it may be necessary to perform an open reduction

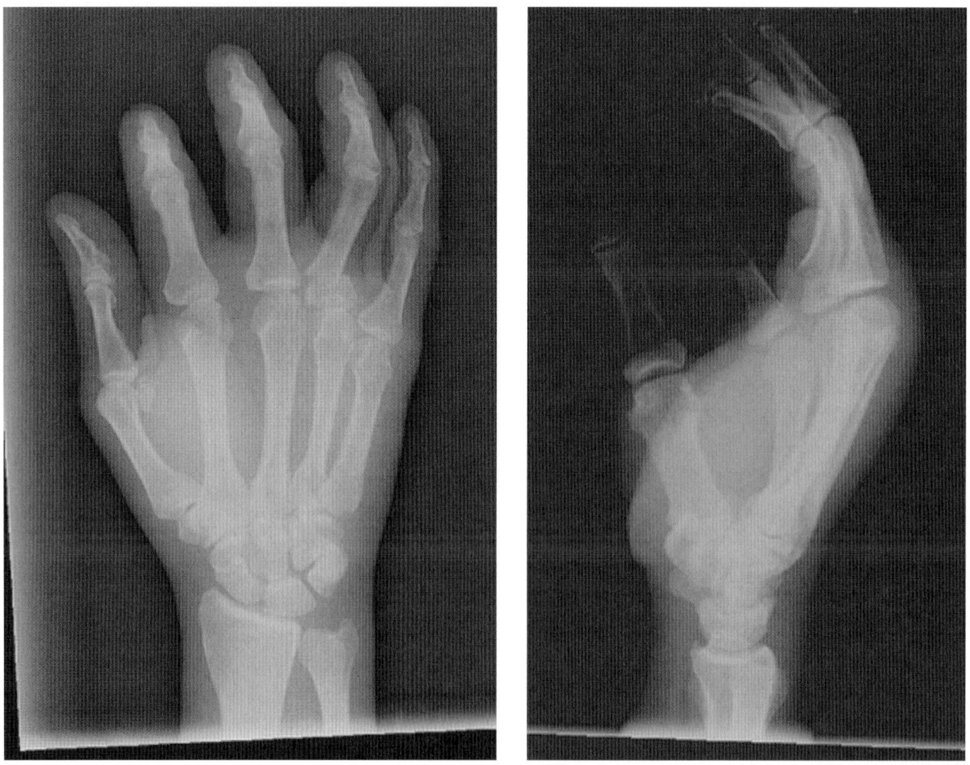

FIGURE 1-9 Proximal phalanx base fracture with angulation.

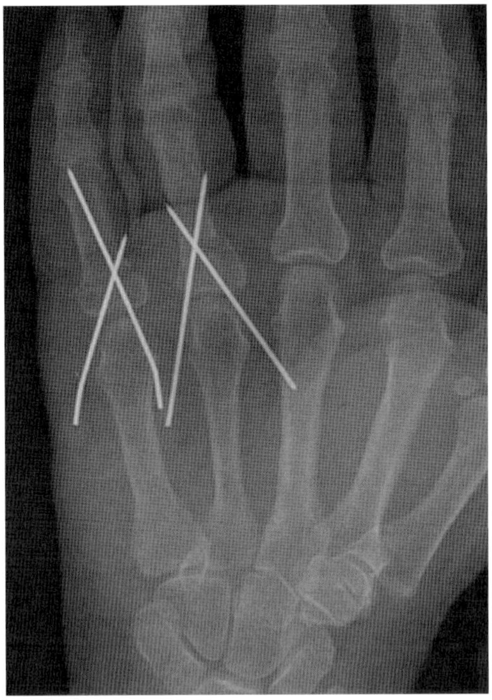

FIGURE 1-10 Proximal phalanx base fracture fixation with cross K-wires.

with internal fixation. Similar to metacarpal shaft fractures, many fixation methods can be utilized, including K-wire, cerclage wires, screw fixation, plate and screw constructs, and external fixation. The advantages and disadvantages for these fixation techniques are the same as described with metacarpal shaft fixation.

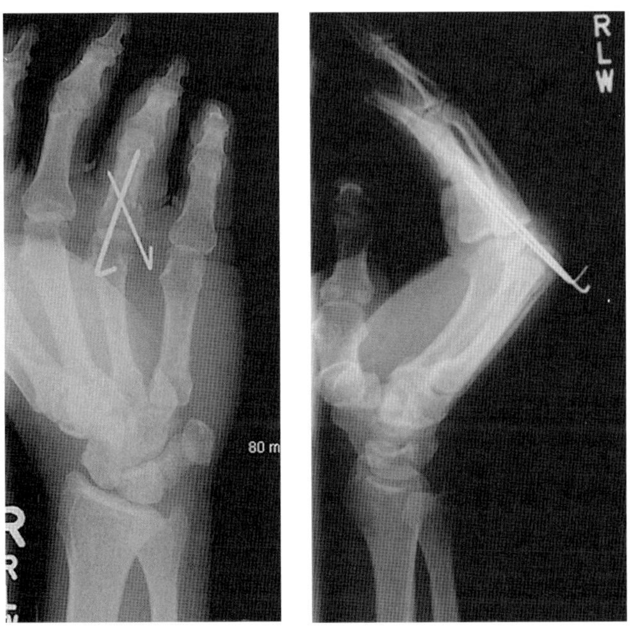

FIGURE 1-11 Proximal phalanx base fracture fixation with transarticular K-wires.

There are 2 surgical approaches for the treatment of these fractures: a dorsal and a midaxial incision. A dorsal extensor splitting approach can be utilized for proximal phalanx fixation, with care to maintain integrity of the central slip of the dorsal apparatus. It has been argued that this can cause increased scarring of the dorsal apparatus. For middle phalanx fractures, when a dorsal approach is made, the transverse retinacular ligament is divided longitudinally at its insertion into the extensor mechanism, and the tendon can be retracted either radially or ulnarly. A midaxial approach can also be used for both phalanges. With this approach, it is recommended to excise the lateral band on the side of exposure to improve the visualization and prevent postoperative scarring.

Most phalanx fractures can be treated with K-wire fixation that can be used for majority of fracture patterns. K-wires can be placed in a crossed configuration for transverse fractures, in parallel for long oblique or spiral fractures, or intramedullary for transverse or short oblique fractures (Fig. 1-12). Unfortunately K-wires do not provide rigid fixation and must be supplemented with a splint or cast. This can contribute to tendon scarring and stiffness. The addition of cerclage wiring with pin fixation increases the strength of the construct. This method is recommended for transverse fractures and in digital replantation.[9,10] Cerclage wires are also often used in isolation with replantation of the digits because of their low profile (Fig. 1-13).

Screw fixation is ideal for unstable oblique or spiral fractures (Fig. 1-14). It controls rotation and shortening and does not distract the fracture during insertion, as can happen with crossed K-wire fixation of transverse fractures. We recommend 2 to 3 screws (2.0 or 1.5 mm for the proximal phalanx and 1.5 or 1.3 mm for the middle phalanx).

We use plate and screw fixation of phalanx fractures infrequently. This construct provides stable anatomic fixation and allows early mobilization, but is fraught with complications, most notably stiffness and scarring.[19] We recommend lateral placement of a plate to minimize extensor tendon adhesions

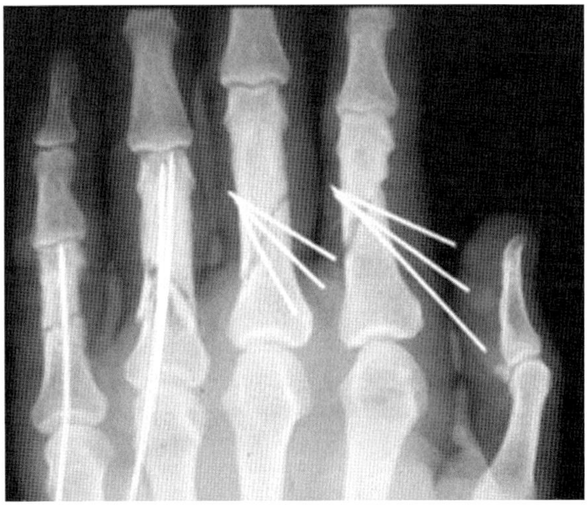

FIGURE 1-12 K-wire fixation of phalanx fractures.

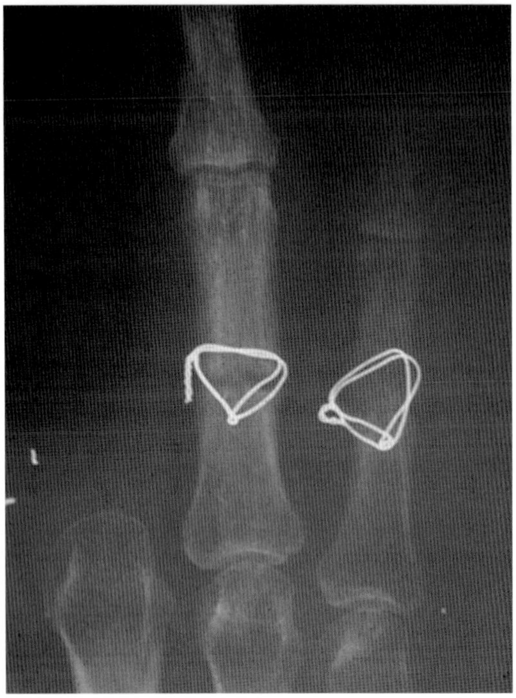

FIGURE 1-13 Cerclage wire used for digit replantation. (Copyright David J. Slutsky, MD.)

and stiffness (Fig. 1-15). One biomechanical study suggests that lateral plate placement can result in less PIP joint contracture than dorsal application, but this has not been proven clinically.[20]

External fixation is indicated for highly unstable open fractures with a compromised soft tissue envelope and extreme comminution.

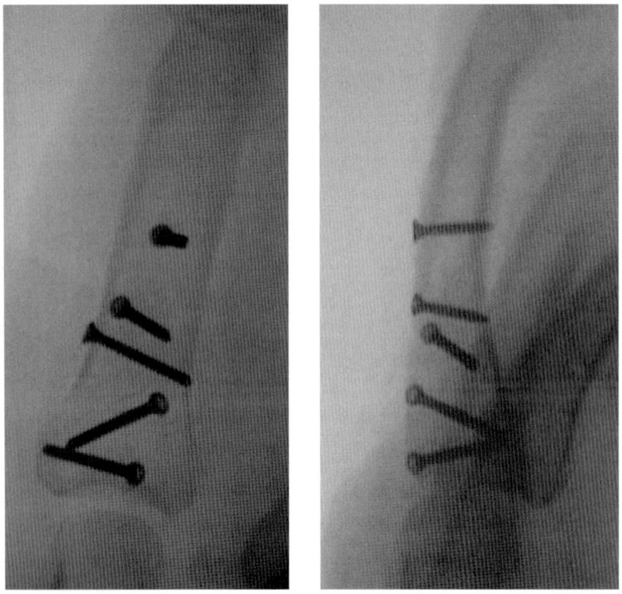

FIGURE 1-14 Screw fixation of phalanx fracture. (Copyright David J. Slutsky, MD.)

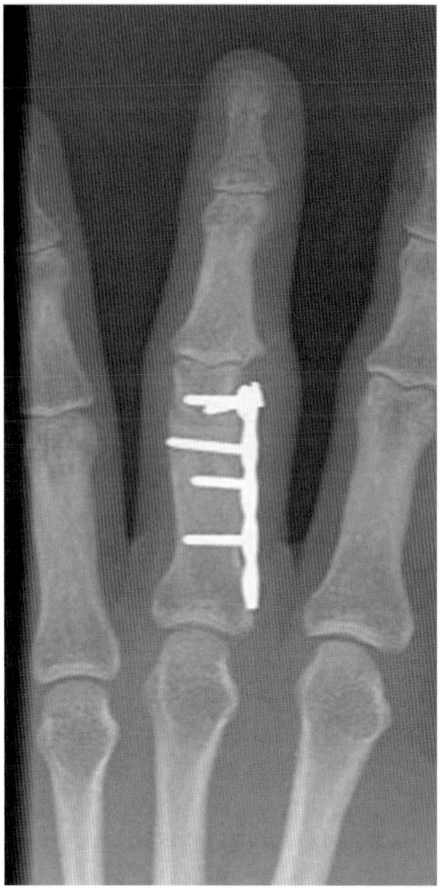

FIGURE 1-15 Lateral plate placement for phalanx fracture.

Complications

As with metacarpal shaft fractures, phalanx shaft fracture complications are noteworthy, the most common being stiffness, resulting from the injury itself, immobilization, and surgical intervention. Other complications include infection, malrotation, angulation, shortening, nonunion, extensor mechanism failure, and flexor tendon adhesions.

Outcomes

Many reports have been published concerning the outcomes of phalanx fracture treatment. Treatment after closed reduction and immobilization produces satisfactory functional results when mobilization was begun within the first 4 weeks, ranging 75% to 80% of a normal motion arc versus 66% when fracture immobilization was greater than 4 weeks.[21] To avoid stiffness following hand fractures, Borgeskov emphasized early motion, which produced good functional results in 68% of 483 metacarpal and phalanx fractures.[22]

Closed reduction and percutaneous pin fixation is the mainstay of treatment and produces very good results. Belsky et al[23] reported on proximal phalanx fractures located at different levels treated with percutaneous pin fixation and early range of motion of the PIP joint. They reported good to excellent results in 90% of the fractures. Green and Anderson[24] also reported good results after treatment of proximal phalanx fractures, achieving full range of motion in 18 of 22 patients with 26 oblique fractures. Cerclage wire stabilization can also produce satisfactory results. Pehlivan et al[25] treated 20 patients with unstable phalanx fractures and reported very good results, obtaining 92% range of motion in proximal phalanxes and 76% in middle.

Screw fixation has been shown to produce good results for phalanx shaft fractures. Horton et al[26] compared screw fixation with closed pin fixation in proximal phalanx shaft fractures and found the techniques to produce equivalent outcomes.

Lastly, plate and screw fixation has been shown to have a relatively high complication level by Page and Stern.[19] They reported considerable postoperative stiffness and a grave prognosis in patients with open fractures. More recently, they reviewed their experience with 50 unstable proximal phalanx fractures, which were defined as angulation greater than 5° to 10° in the coronal plane and greater than 20° in the sagittal plane, that were treated with either closed reduction and percutaneous transarticular pinning through the metacarpal head (25 patients) or cross-pinning through the base of the proximal phalanx (25 patients).[18] The mean TAM for the transarticular group and cross-pinning group was 201° and 198°. The arc of MCP motion was 0° to 79° versus 3° to 81°, PIP joint 11° to 83° versus 7° to 79°, and DIP joint 4° to 54° versus 2° to 51°. Almost half of the patients in each group had a PIP flexion loss of more than 20° (average, 27°) and almost one third of patients in both groups had a fixed PIP flexion contracture of greater than 15°. There were more secondary procedures in the transarticular group[6] than in the cross-pinning group.[2] There was, however, no statistical significance between groups in any of the outcome parameters used. Pun et al also had mediocre results, with 26% good, 33% fair, and 41% poor results after treatment of unstable phalanx fractures with plate fixation.[27] It has been shown that poor outcomes result not only from the severity of the injury but also from technical errors with application of these small plate constructs.[28,29]

REFERENCES

1. Kelsey JL, Pastides H, Kreiger N, et al. *Upper Extremity Disorders: A Survey of Their Frequency and Cost in the United States*. St. Louis: CV Mosby; 1980.
2. Stern PJ. Management of fractures of the hand over the last 25 years. *J Hand Surg Am*. 2000;25:817–823.
3. Strauch RJ, Rosenwasser MP, Lunt JG. Metacarpal shaft fractures: the effect of shortening on the extensor tendon mechanism. *J Hand Surg Am*. 1998;23:519–523.
4. Orbay JL, Touhami A. The treatment of unstable metacarpal and phalangeal shaft fractures with flexible nonlocking and locking intramedullary nails. *Hand Clin*. 2006;22:279–286.
5. Henry MH. Fractures of the proximal phalanx and metacarpals in the hand: preferred methods of stabilization. *J Am Acad Orthop Surg*. 2008;16:586–595.
6. Tavassoli J, Ruland RT, Hogan CJ, Cannon DL. Three cast techniques for the treatment of extra-articular metacarpal fractures: comparison of short-term outcomes and final fracture alignments. *J Bone Joint Surg Am*. 2005;87:2196–2201.
7. Jahss SA. Fractures of the metacarpals: a new method of reduction and immobilization. *J Bone Joint Surg Am*. 1938;20:178–186.
8. Botte MJ, Davis JL, Rose BA, et al. Complications of smooth pin fixation of fractures and dislocations in the hand and wrist. *Clin Orthop Relat Res*. 1992;276:194–201.
9. Gingass RP, Fehring B, Matloub H. Intraosseous wiring of complex hand fractures. *Plast Reconstr Surg*. 1980;66:383–394.
10. Lister G. Intraosseous wiring of the digital skeleton. *J Hand Surg Br*. 1990;15:291–294.
11. Al-Qattan MM. Metacarpal shaft fractures of the fingers: treatment with interosseous loop wire fixation and immediate postoperative finger mobilization in a wrist splint. *J Hand Surg Br*. 2006;31:377–382.
12. Greene TL, Noellert RC, Belsole RJ, Simpson LA. Composite wiring of metacarpal and phalangeal fractures. *J Hand Surg Am*. 1989;14:665–669.
13. Omakawa S, Fujitani R, Dohi Y, Okawa T, Yajima H. Prospective outcomes of comminuted periarticular metacarpal and phalangeal fractures treated using a titanium plate system. *J Hand Surg Am*. 2008;33:857–863.
14. Zhang B, Zhang YZ, Shao XZ, et al. Application of AO miniplate and screw in the treatment of metacarpophalangeal joint periarticular fractures. *Zhonghua Yi Xue Za Zhi*. 2012;92:188–191.
15. Kelsch G, Ulrich C. Intramedullary k-wire fixation of metacarpal fractures. *Arch Orthop Trauma Surg*. 2004;124(8):523–526.
16. Fusetti C, Meyer H, Borisch N, et al. Complications of plate fixation in metacarpal fractures. *J Trauma*. 202;52:535–539.
17. Ozer K, Gillani S, Williams A, Peterson SL, Morgan S. Comparison of intramedullary nailing versus plate-screw fixation of extra-articular metacarpal fractures. *J Hand Surg Am*. 2008;33:1724–1731.
18. Faruqui S, Stern PJ, Kiefhaber TR. Percutaneous pinning of fractures in the proximal third of the proximal phalanx: complications and outcomes. *J Hand Surg Am*. 2012;37:1342–1348.
19. Page SM, Stern PJ. Complications and range of motion following plate fixation of metacarpal and phalangeal fractures. *J Hand Surg Am*. 1998;23:827–832.
20. Nunley JA, Kloen P. Biomechanical and functional testing of plate fixation devices for proximal phalangeal fractures. *J Hand Surg Am*. 1991;16:991–998.
21. Strickland JW, Steichen JB, Kleinman WB, et al. Phalangeal fractures: factors influencing digital performance. *Orthop Rev*. 1982;11:39–50.
22. Borgeskov S. Conservative therapy for fractures of the phalanges and metacarpals. *Acta Chir Scand*. 1967;133:123–130.
23. Belsky MR, Eaton RG, Lane LB. Closed reduction and internal fixation of proximal phalangeal fractures. *J Hand Surg Am*. 1984;9:725–729.
24. Green DP, Anderson JR. Closed reduction and percutaneous pin fixation of fractured phalanges. *J Bone Joint Surg Am*. 1973;55:1651–1654.
25. Pehlivan O, Kiral A, Solakoglu C, et al. Tension band wiring of unstable transverse fractures of the proximal and middle phalanges of the hand. *J Hand Surg Br*. 2004;29:130–134.
26. Horton TC, Hatton M, Davis TR. A prospective randomized controlled study of fixation of long oblique and spiral shaft fractures of the proximal phalanx: closed reduction and percutaneous Kirschner wiring versus open reduction and lag screw fixation. *J Hand Surg Br*. 2003;28:5–9.
27. Pun WK, Chow SP, So YC, et al. Unstable phalangeal fractures: treatment by A.O. screw and plate fixation. *J Hand Surg Am*. 1991;16: 113–117.
28. Buchler U, Fischer T. Use of a minicondylar plate for metacarpal and phalangeal periarticular injuries. *Clin Orthop Relat Res*. 1987;214: 53–58.
29. Ouellette EA, Freeland AE. Use of the minicondylar plate in metacarpal and phalangeal fractures. *Clin Orthop Relat Res*. 1996;327: 38–46.

2

Periarticular Fractures of the Metacarpals and Phalanges

Peter JL Jebson, MD
Daniel T. Kokmeyer, MD

INTRODUCTION

Fractures of the phalanges and metacarpals are very common, accounting for approximately 10% of all fractures overall. Minimally or nondisplaced fractures with good clinical alignment are amenable to nonoperative treatment. However, unstable and/or displaced fractures require operative management primarily because of the development of a malunion and its deleterious effects on hand function. Although there are several different periarticular fracture patterns involving the metacarpals and phalanges, certain types are more commonly encountered than others (Fig. 2-1). Despite the treatment goal of restoring normal finger and hand function, there is no consensus on the preferred operative approach for any particular injury pattern. The technique selected is based on many factors including fracture pattern, location, associated soft tissue injury, closed versus open injury, surgeon experience, and patient factors such as age, occupation, medical comorbidities, and ability to comply with postoperative rehabilitation. Economic factors have become more important with implant cost and reimbursement influencing implant selection. The "optimal" fixation technique provides stable fixation with minimal soft tissue damage, scar formation, and stiffness with early mobilization if feasible.

INDICATIONS

Operative treatment is recommended for an open or unacceptably angulated or inherently unstable fracture, or in those patients who have failed nonoperative treatment. Although the amount of acceptable angulation or displacement varies with the fracture pattern, clinical malrotation with finger overlap or divergence or a mechanical block to motion demands operative treatment. The ideal candidate is a healthy, compliant, and motivated individual with good bone quality and a stable soft tissue envelope. Although smoking is not a contraindication to surgery, and there is no good evidence that it is associated with a poor outcome following operative management of an acute hand fracture, we always educate the patient as to its deleterious effects and encourage him or her to stop immediately.[1] Operative treatment may be performed on all age groups. Some fractures are more commonly encountered in certain populations such as the "boxer's fracture" in the dominant hand of the young ill tempered male. Patients with preexisting joint stiffness or arthritis have a difficult time postoperatively recovering motion, thus compromising their eventual outcome. Open highly contaminated injuries require urgent operative treatment. Simple, low-energy open fractures may be treated with intravenous antibiotics and irrigation and debridement in the emergency room followed by delayed surgical treatment. Closed injuries are usually fixed within 7 to 10 days post injury. Waiting more than 3 weeks before surgical treatment may make percutaneous techniques less feasible and open reduction more likely because of fracture healing. Prior to surgery, I inform the patient of the importance of limb elevation to reduce edema, minimize scarring, and make palpation of anatomic landmarks for percutaneous pinning easier. Preoperative use of a compression glove can also be helpful.

CONTRAINDICATIONS

An absolute contraindication to operative management of a periarticular fracture of the metacarpals and phalanges is a confirmed allergy to the selected implant, although this is extremely rare. Relative contraindications include an inability to comply with postoperative instructions and rehabilitation, an active wound infection, significant comorbidities with a high perioperative risk of serious complications, and poor bone quality, although the development of locking implants has proven beneficial in treating this subpopulation.

SURGICAL TECHNIQUE

Surgery is usually performed in the operating theater, although some fractures may be amenable to wrist block anesthesia and closed reduction and percutaneous pinning

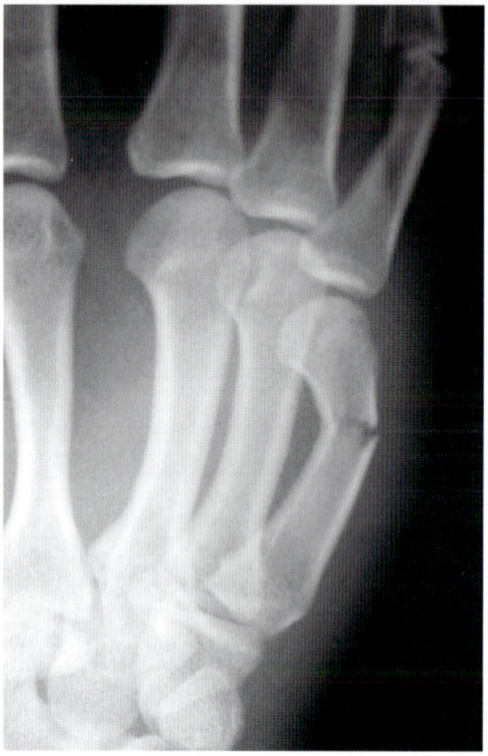

FIGURE 2-1 Fracture of the small metacarpal neck ("boxer's type").

(CRPP) in an office procedure suite if image intensification is available. The patient is positioned supine with the affected extremity placed on a radiolucent hand table. A padded pneumatic brachial tourniquet is applied. Surgery may be performed under regional or general anesthesia. Practical tips include the following: a good assistant is invaluable; always use image intensification; the surgeon must be versatile and well versed in various percutaneous and open fixation techniques; have all necessary implants available; an impervious drape can be helpful for removing other fingers from the operative field[2] (Fig. 2-2); for CRPP, I apply

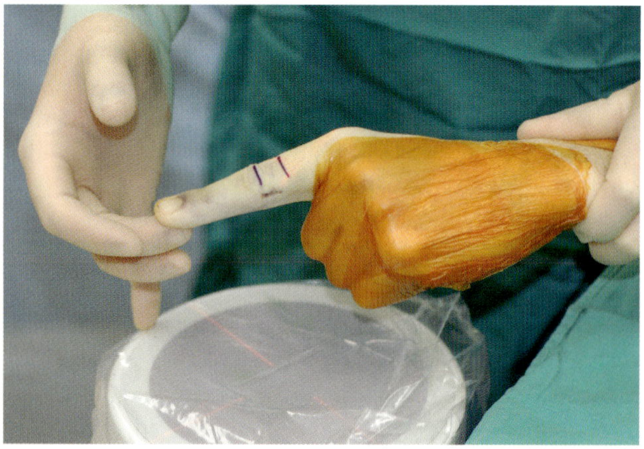

FIGURE 2-2 Ioban is placed around the uninvolved fingers during CRPP to improve visualization and efficiency.

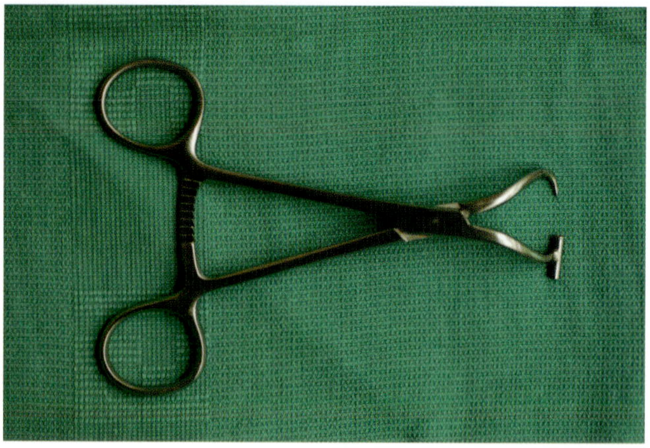

FIGURE 2-3 Reduction clamp with an attached drill guide.

the K-wire manually under image intensification to find the correct starting position and then I insert it into the wire driver before pinning; I make a small stab incision and use a drill guide during pinning to protect adjacent structures if necessary; I bury all K-wires beneath the skin to reduce the chance of infection; for CRPP, I use a reduction pin clamp (Fig. 2-3) that simultaneously stabilizes the reduced fracture while guiding wire insertion; if using intramedullary (IM) pinning/nailing, scrutinize the radiographs carefully for a narrow medullary canal/isthmus that may prohibit implant insertion; provisional fracture reduction is best achieved with a reduction clamp placed such that it does not subsequently interfere with implant placement; external fixation is useful for temporary stabilization in complex comminuted contaminated wounds prior to definitive fixation and soft tissue management; I do not use bioabsorbable implants as they lose strength with time and result in an excessive inflammatory response; locking low-profile plates are indicated for bone loss, comminution, and osteoporotic bone; always confirm rotational alignment after CRPP or ORIF and compare with the opposite side if necessary; always confirm that there is no mechanical block or tendon impingement following implant insertion.

Metacarpal Base

Short oblique or transverse fractures of the central metacarpal bases are best stabilized with low-profile dorsal plate and screw fixation and immediate mobilization. A dorsal longitudinal approach is used. For noncomminuted transverse fractures, anatomic reduction with compression plating and 4 cortices of fixation in both the proximal and distal fragments is recommended. Fractures with metaphyseal comminution or osteopenia require fixation with a locking plate and screw construct (Fig. 2-4). Short oblique fractures may be fixed with a lag screw combined with a dorsal neutralization plate. Base fractures involving the border metacarpals are amenable to CRPP. I typically use a minimum of two 0.045 smooth K-wires.

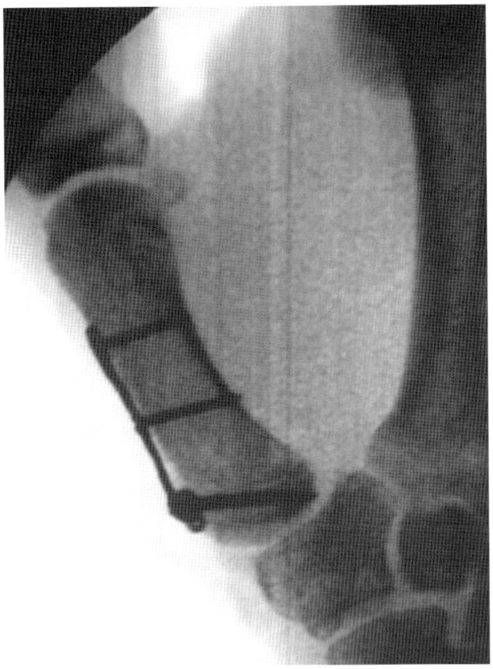

FIGURE 2-4 ORIF of an unstable extra-articular fracture of the thumb metacarpal base.

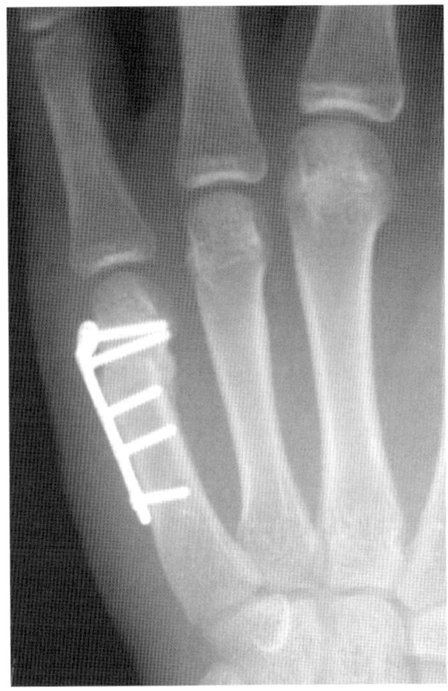

FIGURE 2-5 Small metacarpal neck fracture treated with ORIF using a precontoured locking plate (Stryker, Kalamazoo, Michigan).

Metacarpal Neck

Stabilization may be achieved with CRPP or ORIF. I prefer CRPP as ORIF is associated with capsular scarring, extensor tendon adhesions, and stiffness. Precontoured locking low-profile plates have been designed for use with small finger metacarpal neck fractures ("boxer's fracture") (Fig. 2-5). ORIF with interfragmentary screws alone may also be used (Fig. 2-6). However, the indications and benefits compared with CRPP have not been clearly defined. There are several methods for achieving CRPP of a metacarpal neck fracture. I use collateral recess pinning for central metacarpal neck fractures and for border fractures with a narrow medullary canal where bouquet pinning cannot be achieved.[3] Regardless of the technique chosen, a satisfactory closed reduction must be achievable. For metacarpal recess pinning, a 0.045 smooth K-wire is inserted by hand onto the radial or ulnar collateral recess as the metacarpophalangeal (MCP) joint is held in flexion. The starting position is more distal and volar than one thinks. Image intensification is used to confirm correct positioning during wire insertion. The fracture is held in a reduced position as the wire is advanced down the medullary cavity into the base. The second wire is similarly placed in the opposite recess. Bouquet pinning, or antegrade IM nailing, is particularly useful for index and small metacarpal neck fractures (Fig. 2-7). A small longitudinal incision is made over the radial aspect of the index or ulnar aspect of the small metacarpal base. The entry site is at the metaphysis which is identified using fluoroscopy. The canal is entered with a 3 mm drill bit or small awl. A 0.045 K-wire is prepared by cutting off the sharp tip, bending the last 5 mm into a gentle curve, and gently bending the wire along its length. The wire is inserted and advanced down the IM canal, with fluoroscopy assistance, and across the reduced fracture with a T-handle chuck or large needle holder. Additional 0.045 and/or 0.035 wires are similarly inserted to achieve "fill"

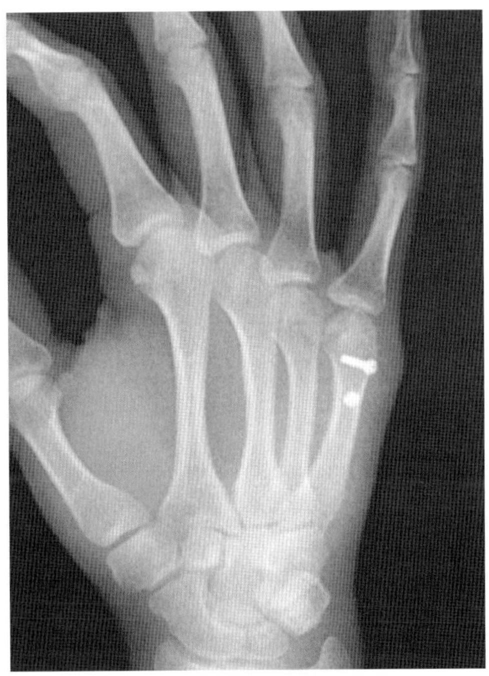

FIGURE 2-6 ORIF of a small metacarpal neck fracture using interfragmentary screws.

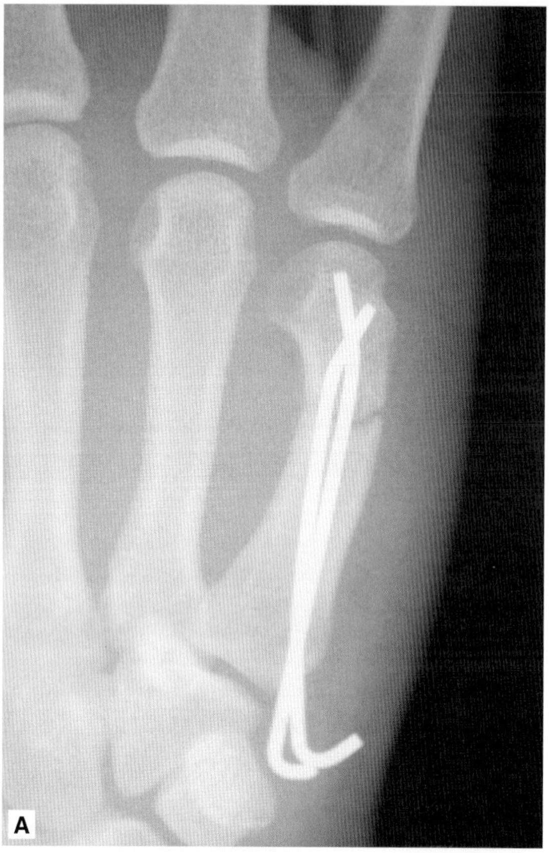

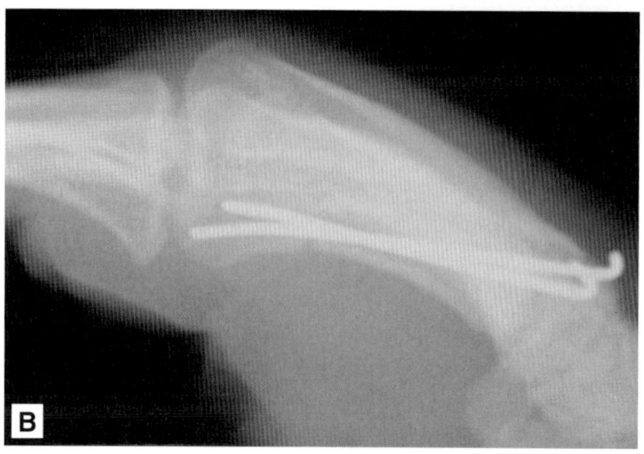

FIGURE 2-7 **A.** Anteroposterior (AP) view of a displaced small metacarpal neck fracture treated with IM nailing. **B.** Lateral view.

of the canal and purchase in the subchondral bone of the metacarpal head. Choose appropriately-sized wires to permit insertion of a minimum of 2 wires for rotational control. The proximal ends of the wires are then bent, cut, and rotated away from the adjacent tendons and dorsal sensory nerve branches. Alternatively, a commercial system can be used that provides an awl with a preloaded IM "nail" (DePuySynthes, Warsaw, Indiana). Other CRPP techniques for border metacarpal neck fractures include parallel transverse pinning into the adjacent metacarpal or a combination of a longitudinal collateral ligament recess pin with a transverse pin. Regardless of the technique used, careful examination must be performed following fixation to confirm an acceptable reduction and avoid malrotation.

Proximal Phalanx Base

The decision to proceed with CRPP or ORIF is based on the ability to obtain an intraoperative satisfactory closed reduction. ORIF is reserved for irreducible fractures or those fractures that cannot be satisfactorily reduced by closed methods. ORIF is associated with implant prominence, extensor tendon adhesions, scarring, and loss of motion. For these reasons, I prefer CRPP whenever possible. ORIF can be accomplished with dorsal or midaxial plate and screw fixation, lag screw fixation alone (oblique fracture pattern), or interosseous wiring. I prefer the broad exposure afforded by a dorsal curvilinear incision. The proximal phalanx can be approached midaxially or dorsally. The approach is determined by the fracture location. The dorsal approach is better suited for proximal fractures and the midaxial approach is preferred for more distal fractures. If a midaxial approach is used, a portion of the lateral band is excised and the extensor digitorum communis (EDC) tendon is reflected. Alternatively, the tendon is split at the midline followed by extraperiosteal dissection and reflection. Metaphyseal transverse, short oblique, and comminuted fractures are stabilized with a low-profile dorsal T plate or 2 smaller plates placed orthogonally (Fig. 2-8). For dorsal or orthogonal plates, avoid placing too long of a screw with subsequent irritation of the flexor tendons. If rigid fixation is achieved, immediate mobilization is essential to minimize scarring. CRPP is ideal for transverse metaphyseal fractures.[4] There are 2 possible techniques: transarticular (across the MCP joint) and extra-articular cross-pinning. For the transarticular technique, a closed reduction is achieved with the MCP joints in flexion as 2 smooth 0.045 K-wires are inserted through

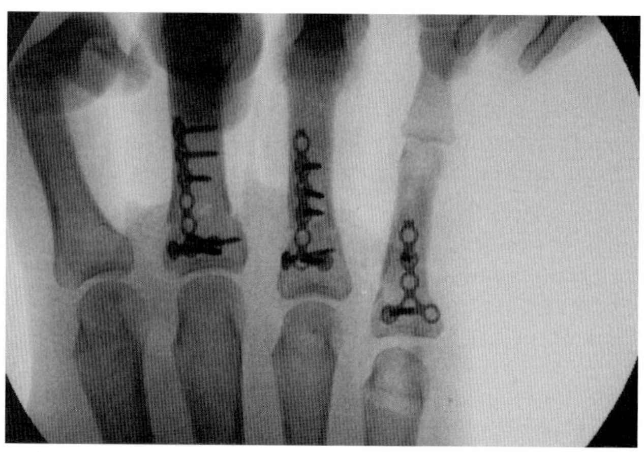

FIGURE 2-8 Unstable multiple proximal phalanx fractures following a crush injury. The fractures could not be satisfactorily reduced and stabilized with CRPP. Low-profile plates were placed dorsally.

the metacarpal head into the proximal phalanx distally. The extra-articular technique involves the same closed reduction method followed by manual wire placement on either side of the MCP head, thus avoiding the extensor apparatus, into the proximal phalanx condyle followed by power-assisted insertion to achieve crossing distal to the fracture site. Distraction of the fracture should be avoided. If CRPP is used for a short oblique fracture, percutaneous placement of 1 or more small reduction clamps to stabilize the fracture is advisable. For CRPP of all phalangeal fractures, I use the midaxial line as a guide and apply my clamp dorsal to it because the phalanx itself lies predominantly dorsally. Image intensification is always used and fixation is only accomplished *after* a satisfactory reduction is confirmed.

Proximal Phalanx Neck

I prefer CRPP with crossed K-wires inserted in retrograde fashion for very distal neck fractures. Usually 0.045 K-wires are used, although 0.035 wires may be necessary for the small finger. The bouquet technique is used for more proximal metadiaphyseal fractures and involves the "stacking" of several K-wires inserted in a proximal to distal (antegrade) direction into the subchondral bone of the phalangeal head. ORIF is associated with extensor tendon adhesions and stiffness. If performed, a low-profile plate is used and can be placed dorsally or midaxially. If the plate is placed dorsally, avoid overly long screws distally that may occlude the retrocondylar recess and limit proximal interphalangeal joint (PIPJ) flexion. Because of the metaphyseal flare, contouring of a standard straight plate for midaxial placement can be challenging. Alternatively, a blade plate can be used, but correct positioning and insertion is technically challenging.

Middle Phalanx Base

CRPP is used for transverse or short oblique fractures. Antegrade crossed K-wire fixation is used for transverse fractures, whereas oblique fractures are reduced and stabilized with a reduction clamp followed by insertion of a minimum of 2 K-wires across the fracture site through the opposite cortex. ORIF is rarely used and is limited by the central slip that should not be detached. If plate and screw fixation are necessary, the plate may be placed directly on top of the central slip attachment or midaxially.

Middle Phalanx Neck

The techniques used for neck fractures of the proximal phalanx may be applied to the middle phalanx. CRPP using retrograde crossed K-wires or longitudinal IM wires inserted through the distal phalanx and across the distal interphalangeal joint (DIPJ) is preferred to ORIF (Fig. 2-9). If ORIF is used, the EDC terminal slip must be preserved (Fig. 2-10).

Potential Pitfalls

Several potential pitfalls can be encountered with operative management of periarticular metacarpal or phalangeal fractures. Regardless of the fixation technique used, the surgeon must recognize and avoid malalignment, particularly malrotation associated with displaced unstable and/or comminuted fractures. After fixation I routinely assess clinical alignment by passively flexing and extending the wrist and observing the normal finger cascade and alignment (Fig. 2-11). Multiple attempts at wire insertion during CRPP should be avoided as it compromises wire purchase and can lead to loosening, wire migration, infection, and/or loss of reduction. This is particularly important in patients with poor-quality bone. Wires should be placed manually followed by power-assisted insertion and avoidance of injury to the adjacent tendons and neurovascular structures. Reduction clamps should be placed carefully to avoid impeding subsequent wire insertion. Careful attention should be paid to the diameter of the IM canal, particularly the isthmus if CRPP or bouquet pinning is used. Surprisingly, the ring metacarpal shaft is often the narrowest of all of the metacarpals. We routinely leave K-wires below the skin as we believe this reduces the chances of a pin tract infection. Postoperative rehabilitation under the supervision of a hand therapist is extremely important. Emphasis should be on immediate limb elevation and edema control. The decision to begin immediate versus delayed motion and what joints are mobilized is dependent on patient factors, particularly compliance, and the quality of fixation as determined by the surgeon intraoperatively.

COMPLICATIONS

The most common complication overall is loss of motion. Careful soft tissue handling, use of low-profile implants, early mobilization, and elimination of edema are important to optimize patient outcome. Immobilization of phalangeal fractures beyond 3 weeks should be avoided.[5] Malunion is relatively common and is usually the result of an inadequate closed reduction, loss of fixation, or poor surgical technique. Accurate assessment of alignment intraoperatively is critical and should be routinely performed in the management of all hand fractures. Delayed union can occur in patients with an infection or such comorbidities as peripheral vascular disease, immunosuppression, diabetes, and/or smoking. Fortunately, nonunion is rare and is usually also encountered in the aforementioned patient population. Treatment involves revision surgery, consisting of ORIF with autogenous bone grafting. Infection can occur following an open fracture or with exposed K-wires. K-wires left above the skin should be cleaned regularly. We prefer twice-a-day diligent cleaning with a hydrogen peroxide–soaked cotton-tipped applicator. If a pin tract infection occurs, antibiotics are required; loose pins should be removed and any deep infection such as osteomyelitis or pyathrosis should be treated with wound exploration, debridement, and antibiotics. Cold

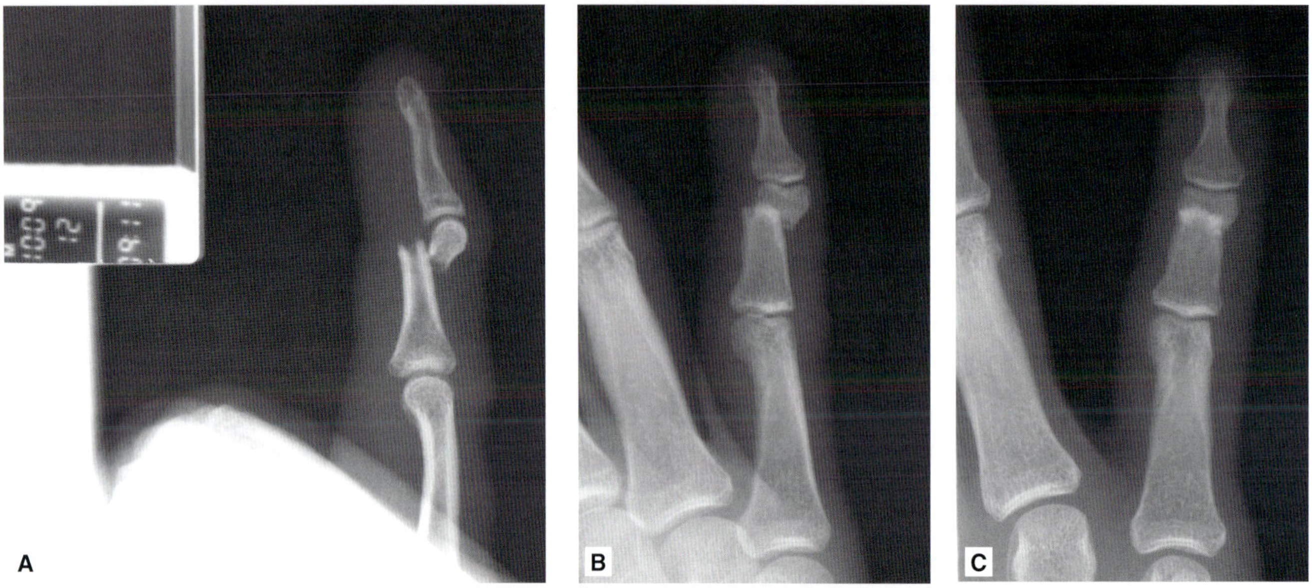

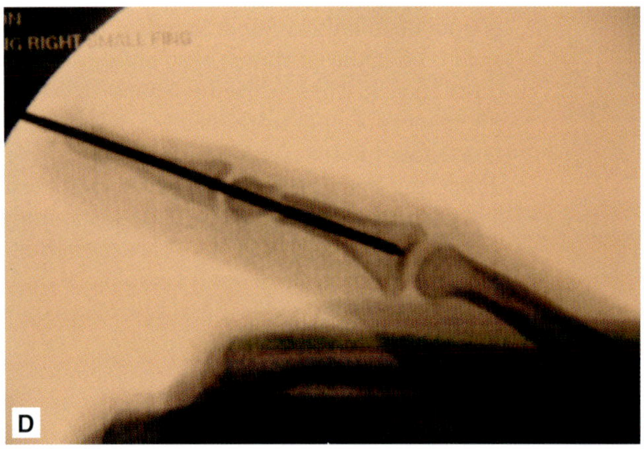

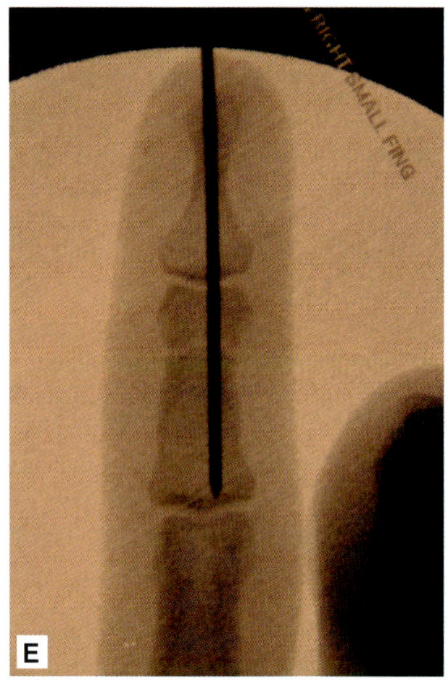

FIGURE 2-9 Lateral (**A**) and oblique (**B**) and AP (**C**) views of a displaced fracture of the middle phalanx neck treated with closed reduction and IM nailing with a longitudinal K-wire (**D** and **E**).

intolerance or pain associated with a retained implant is very common in our experience. Some patients are helped with implant removal after radiographic evidence of healing. Posttraumatic refracture can also occur following K-wire removal. Complex regional pain syndrome (CRPS) is a condition with a characteristic constellation of complaints and clinical findings. A high index of suspicion with early recognition and initiation of appropriate treatment is essential.

OUTCOMES

There is no technique that has been proven to be superior for the fixation of periarticular fractures of the metacarpals and phalanges. For extra-articular metacarpal fractures, Ozer et al demonstrated no differences in the clinical outcome between IM nailing and dorsal plating.[6] Although operative time was shorter with IM nailing, the incidences of loss of reduction, wire penetration into the MCP joint, and secondary surgery for hardware removal were higher.

For fractures of the small MCP neck, Wong et al demonstrated that there was no difference in pain, total active range of motion (TAM), or grip strength when transverse pinning was compared with IM nailing.[7] In a prospective randomized trial Winter et al noted a better outcome in those patients who underwent antegrade bouquet pinning versus transverse pinning.[8] Schadel-Hopfner et al demonstrated better clinical results following antegrade IM nailing compared with retrograde crossed pinning, although there was no difference in the DASH score.[9] Sletten et al assessed the

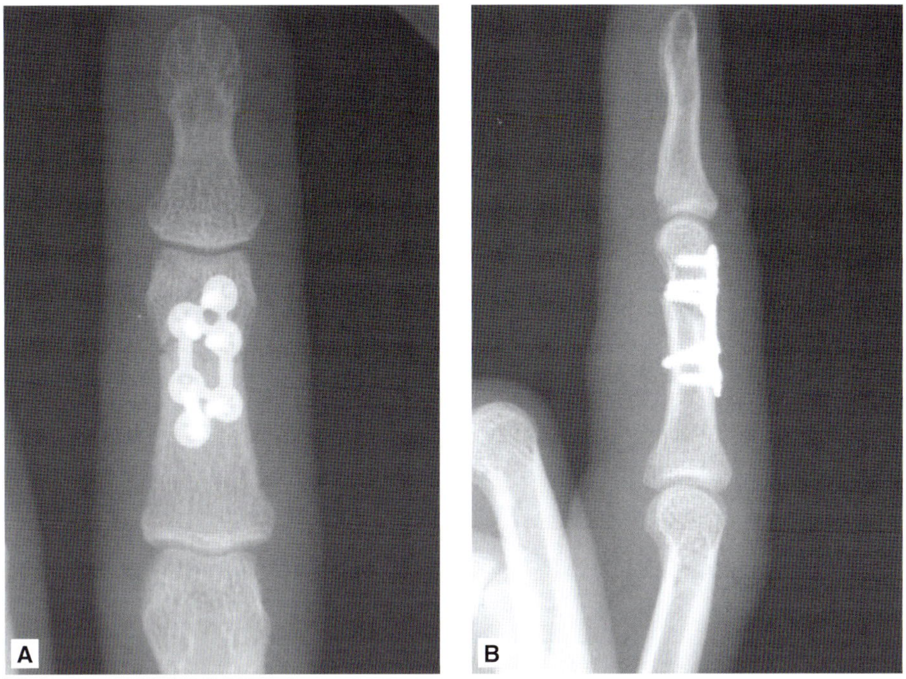

FIGURE 2-10 **A** and **B.** ORIF of a middle phalanx neck fracture.

results of transverse or IM nailing in patients with an isolated fracture of the ring or small metacarpal neck or shaft.[10] They noted no difference in outcome between the 2 techniques. However, there was an 18% incidence of superficial pin infection, all with transverse pinning with the wires left exposed, leading them to recommend leaving all K-wires beneath the skin. In addition, 16% of patients had impaired sensation at the pin site entrance, 29% of patients complained of cold intolerance, and 10% had other complications including 2 patients with posttraumatic refracture of the same metacarpal within 2 months postoperatively following bouquet pinning and 3 patients with a fracture of the small metacarpal through one of the pinholes following transverse pinning of a ring metacarpal fracture.

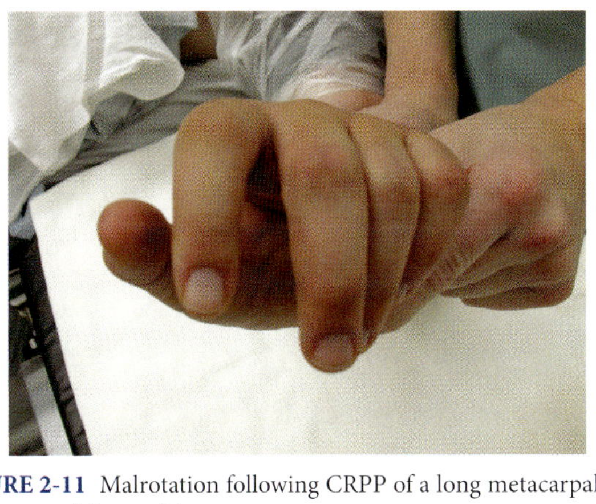

FIGURE 2-11 Malrotation following CRPP of a long metacarpal neck fracture requiring revision surgery.

Percutaneous fixation of proximal phalanx fractures has been associated with satisfactory clinical results. Joshi reported a 90% satisfaction rate in 53 patients with 62 proximal phalanx fractures treated with closed reduction and extra-articular percutaneous pinning.[11] Green and Anderson retrospectively assessed 26 fractures in 21 patients treated with the same technique.[12] All but 3 of the 21 patients regained full motion. Belsky et al reported their experience with closed reduction and transarticular percutaneous pinning in 100 proximal phalangeal fractures.[13] Approximately 90% achieved excellent or good results, with 61% achieving a TAM of 215° or more. Hornbach and Cohen also reported excellent results using transarticular pinning.[14] In a retrospective review of 12 cases, they noted an average TAM of 265° with 1 PIP joint flexion contracture and 1 rotational deformity. Complications and unsatisfactory outcomes are well recognized with both pinning techniques. Elmaraghy et al reported the results in 24 patients with 35 fractures who underwent transarticular pinning.[15] One-third of the fingers developed a PIP joint flexion contracture that averaged 18°. Secondary procedures were performed in 6 patients. A loss of reduction with rotational deformity occurred in 4 fingers and 1 developed a nonunion. Recently Faruqui et al retrospectively assessed the complications and outcomes for both pinning techniques in a series of 50 patients.[16] There were no statistically significant differences between the groups for any of the outcome parameters. However, an alarming overall complication rate was noted in both groups: 56% in the transarticular group and 48% in the cross-pinning group. Approximately half of the patients in each group had a PIP joint flexion loss greater than 20° (average, 27°). Nearly one-third of patients in both groups had a fixed PIP joint flexion contracture greater than 15°. There were more secondary procedures required in the transarticular group than in the cross-pinning group.

REFERENCES

1. Wei DH, Strauch RJ. Smoking and hand surgery. *J Hand Surg Am.* 2013;38:176–179.
2. Verma MK, Bradley J, Jebson PJL. The Ioban drape: a simple method to improve finger surgery safety and efficiency. *Tech Hand Upper Ext Surg.* 2012;16(4):202–203.
3. Foucher G. "Bouquet" osteosynthesis in metacarpal neck fractures: a series of 66 patients. *J Hand Surg Am.* 1995;20:86–90.
4. Crofoot CD, Saing M, Raphael J. Intrafocal pinning for juxtaarticular phalanx fractures. *Tech Hand Upper Ext Surg.* 2005;9:164–168.
5. Strickland JW, Steichen JB, Kleinman WB. Phalangeal fractures: factors influencing digital performance. *Orthop Rev.* 1982;11:39–50.
6. Ozer K, Gillani S, Williams A, Peterson SL, Morgan S. Comparison of intramedullary nailing versus plate-screw fixation of extra-articular metacarpal fractures. *J Hand Surg Am.* 2008;33(10):1724–1731.
7. Wong TC, Ip FK, Yeung SH. Comparison between percutaneous transverse fixation and intramedullary K-wires in treating closed fractures of the metacarpal neck of the little finger. *J Hand Surg Br.* 2006;31:61–65.
8. Winter M, Blaguer T, Bessiere C, Carles M, Lebreton E. Surgical treatment of the boxer's fracture: transverse pinning versus intramedullary pinning. *J Hand Surg Eur.* 2007;32:709–713.
9. Schadel-Hopfner M, Wild M, Windolf J, Linhart W. Antegrade intramedullary splinting or percutaneous retrograde crossed pinning for displaced neck fractures of the fifth metacarpal? *Arch Orthop Trauma Surg.* 2007;127:435–440.
10. Sletten IN, Nordsletten L, Husby T, Odegaard RA, Hellund JC, Kvernmo HD. Isolated extra-articular neck and shaft fractures of the 4th and 5th metacarpals: a comparison of transverse and bouquet (intra-medullary) pinning in 67 patients. *J Hand Surg Eur.* 2012;37(5):387–395.
11. Joshi BB. Percutaneous internal fixation of fractures of the proximal phalanges. *Hand.* 1976;8:85–92.
12. Green DP, Anderson JR. Closed reduction and percutaneous pin fixation of fractured phalanges. *J Bone Joint Surg Am.* 1973;55A:1651–1652.
13. Belsky MR, Eaton RG, Lane LB. Closed reduction and internal fixation of proximal phalangeal fractures. *J Hand Surg Am.* 1984;9A:725–729.
14. Hornbach EE, Cohen MS. Closed reduction and percutaneous pinning of fractures of the proximal phalanx. *J Hand Surg Br.* 2001;26B:45–49.
15. Elmaraghy MW, Elmaraghy AW, Richards RS, Chinchalkar SJ, Turner R, Roth JH. Transmetacarpal intramedullary K-wire fixation of proximal phalangeal fractures. *Ann Plast Surg.* 1998;41:125–130.
16. Faruqui S, Stern PJ, Kiefhaber TR. Percutaneous pinning of fractures in the proximal third of the proximal phalanx: complications and outcomes. *J Hand Surg Am.* 2012;37(7):1342–1348.

Dislocations of the Thumb and Fingers

3

Rudy Kovachevich, MD
Greg Merrell, MD

INTRODUCTION

Traumatic dislocations of small joints of the thumb and fingers are rare but challenging injuries. Early recognition of these injuries, prompt joint reduction, and maintenance of articular congruency are important goals needed to minimize shear forces on the affected articular cartilage and subsequent posttraumatic arthritis. This chapter will outline the anatomy, general considerations, treatment, and outcomes of pure ligamentous dislocations of the small joints involving the hand.

CARPOMETACARPAL (CMC) JOINT

Finger CMC Joint

ANATOMY

The index and long finger metacarpals form the central portion of the transverse metacarpal arch and are stable, with less than 5° of motion. In contrast, on the ulnar portion of the arch, the fourth and fifth metacarpals demonstrate 15° of motion in the ring and up to 25° to 30° in the small finger.[1] The mobility of the fourth and fifth rays, combined with that of the first ray, allows the transverse metacarpal arch to adapt as required to grip objects of different size. The strong dorsal, volar, and interosseous ligamentous support of these joints is reinforced by the broad insertions of the wrist flexors and extensors. The fifth CMC joint is also reinforced by the pisometacarpal ligament, an extension of the flexor carpi ulnaris insertion. The numerous periarticular soft tissue attachments at the CMC joint level explain why CMC fracture–dislocations are more common than pure ligamentous dislocations.

GENERAL CONSIDERATIONS

Dislocations of the finger CMC joints are usually high-energy injuries and therefore careful evaluation for other occult injuries is warranted (Fig. 3-1). The motor branch of the ulnar nerve lies below the fifth CMC and its function needs to be evaluated in either a volar or dorsal fifth CMC dislocation. Although volar dislocations have been reported, the overwhelming majority of these injuries are dorsal. The mechanism of injury consists of a longitudinal force to the dorsal metacarpal heads causing simultaneous flexion and longitudinal compression. As the metacarpal head is forced volarly, the base is driven dorsally.

The increased mobility on the ulnar aspect of the hand predisposes it to a greater frequency of injury, with the fifth CMC joint most commonly involved. Isolated dislocations or fracture–dislocations of the remaining CMC joints are less common. Making the diagnosis with PA and lateral plain radiographs can be difficult and may require additional views, such as the 30° pronated oblique view, in which the fifth CMC joint is projected in profile to demonstrate displacement. On a PA radiograph in a noninjured hand, Hodgson and Shewring described drawing "metacarpal cascade lines" down the central axis of the finger metacarpals and noted they should converge on the radial shaft approximately 2 cm proximal to the radiocarpal joint. In the setting of dislocation, the lines will instead diverge and this method was found to have 94% sensitivity in their series (Fig. 3-2).[2] Clinically, CMC dislocations viewed down the axis of the hand will typically show a rotational and abducted divergence of the digit (Fig. 3-3).

TREATMENT/SURGICAL TECHNIQUE

The traditional treatment of acute injuries consists of closed reduction and percutaneous Kirschner wire fixation (CRPP) and is usually successful if performed within 24 to 48 hours of injury. Splint/cast immobilization for inherently stable injuries and open reduction internal fixation (ORIF) for irreducible dislocations secondary to tendon interposition have been reported. Late-presenting injuries typically require ORIF or arthrodesis. Due to the posttraumatic arthritis changes within the fifth CMC joint, some recommend interposition arthroplasty to preserve some motion with modest results.[3]

The technique of CRPP involves restoration of anatomic length to the shortened and dislocated metacarpals through

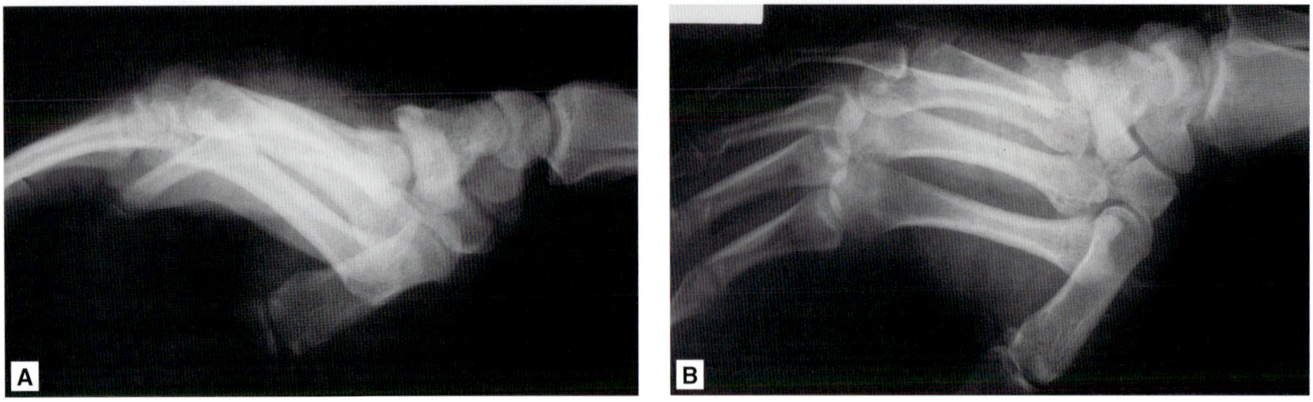

FIGURE 3-1 **A** and **B.** Multiple CMC dislocations. (Copyright David J. Slutsky, MD, 2012.)

the use of a local nerve block anesthesia, the combined application of longitudinal traction (weighted finger traps), and direct upward pressure on the metacarpal bases. After adequate reduction, percutaneous fixation is achieved with a 0.062 K-wire placed obliquely across the base of the metacarpal into the carpus with a second K-wire placed transversely from the unstable metacarpals into the adjacent stable metacarpals (Fig. 3-4). Placement of K-wires should err on the dorsal aspect of the joint, as penetration of the volar cortex by 1.5 mm can injure the motor branch of the ulnar nerve. The pins should remain in place for 4 to 6 weeks with immediate MP and interphalangeal (IP) joint motion encouraged. Another technique described that is beneficial in cases with multiple CMC dislocations is retrograde intramedullary metacarpal K-wire placement across a reduced CMC joint.[4] In this technique the MP joint is held in 60° of flexion, which draws the sagittal band distal to the metacarpal head placing the collateral ligaments under tension. The Kirschner wire is then introduced into the radial or ulnar collateral recess to avoid penetrating the extensor tendon. Open reduction techniques are the same as those for CRPP with the open portion of the procedure being used strictly for reduction purposes.

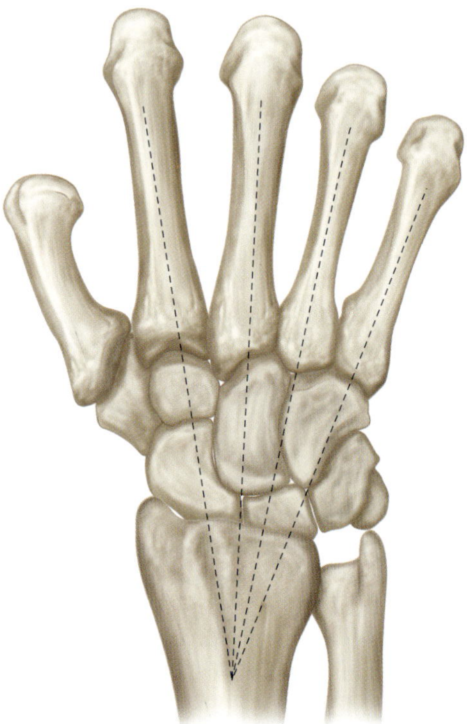

FIGURE 3-2 Radiographic convergence for normal CMC joints.

OUTCOMES/COMPLICATIONS

Frick et al[5] performed a retrospective study of 100 CMC dislocations. The most common mechanism was due to a punch (56%). In half the cases, lesions were located only within the fifth ray. Carpal or metacarpal fractures were associated in 88%. Sixty were treated with closed reduction and percutaneous pinning, and 40 by open reduction and internal fixation. At a mean follow-up of 5 months 68 joints remained reduced radiographically. Unsatisfactory reductions were mainly associated with closed reduction and percutaneous pinning, prompting the authors to recommend open treatment routinely. At the final follow-up, 81% of the patients were pain-free and had recovered complete range of motion. In 16% of patients, pain was only present during gripping.

Thumb CMC Joint

ANATOMY

The articular surfaces of the TMC joint resemble 2 reciprocally opposed saddles whose transverse axes are perpendicular. The concavoconvex joint geometry produces a minimal level of inherent stability, with the joint capsule and ligamentous structures producing the primary stability. The keys to TMC function and stability are the beak of the thumb metacarpal, the recess in the trapezium (adjacent to the volar beak ligament) into which the volar beak inserts, and the dorsal ligament complex.[6] These anatomic keys permit screw-home torque rotation in the final phase of opposition, creating stability for pinch and grasping activities.

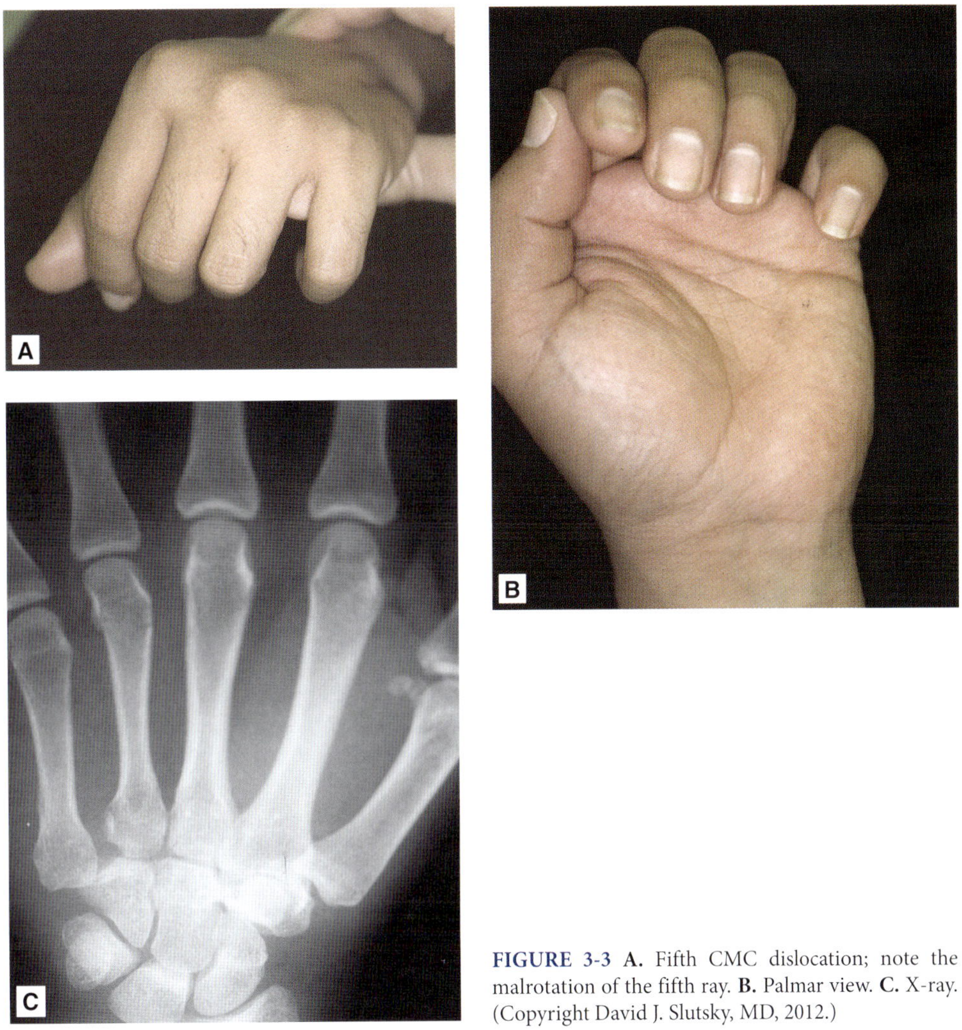

FIGURE 3-3 **A.** Fifth CMC dislocation; note the malrotation of the fifth ray. **B.** Palmar view. **C.** X-ray. (Copyright David J. Slutsky, MD, 2012.)

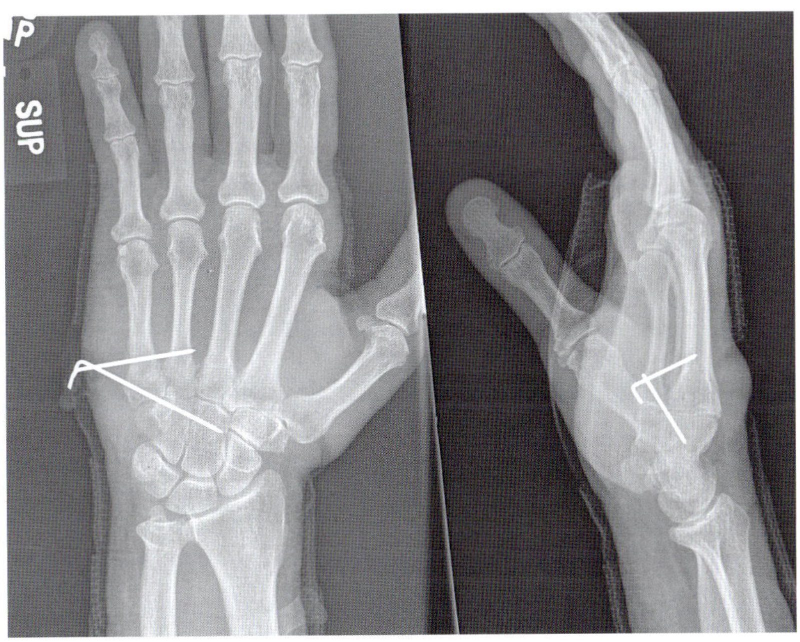

FIGURE 3-4 CMC dislocations reduced and pinned. (Copyright Gregory A. Merrell, MD, 2012.)

The critical ligamentous structure stabilizing the TMC joint has been debated. Originally, the volar beak ligament (also known as the anterior oblique ligament or palmar beak ligament) was attributed as the most important structure.[7] It arises from the volar beak of the thumb metacarpal and has its insertion on the trapezium. Subsequent cadaveric and clinical studies have refuted this theory and shown it to be lax during the screw-home torque phase of opposition. The dorsal ligament complex, composed of the dorsal radial ligament and the posterior oblique ligaments, is the largest, thickest, and strongest ligament stabilizing the TMC joint in power pinch and grasp.[8,9] The ligament complex arises from the tubercle of the trapezium and inserts onto the radial aspect of the thumb metacarpal base near the insertion site of the abductor pollicis longus (APL) tendon. Cadaveric and biomechanical studies have shown that loss of ligament integrity produces gross instability at the TMC joint.

GENERAL CONSIDERATIONS

Similar to the finger CMC joints, pure traumatic dislocations of the trapeziometacarpal joint are rare when compared with fracture–dislocations. All reported trapeziometacarpal dislocations have been dorsal. The mechanism of injury is thought to occur through axial loading of a flexed thumb metacarpal, which drives the metacarpal base in a dorsal direction. In the pure dislocation of the TMC joint the critically important dorsal ligament necessarily ruptures and must be treated. The diagnosis is confirmed by observing joint space widening or dorsoradial shifting of the metacarpal using standard posteroanterior and true lateral radiographs. This imaging is also important to rule out a Bennett fracture–dislocation as well as existing pathological changes within the TMC joint.

TREATMENT/SURGICAL TECHNIQUE

Treatment options vary from closed reduction and thumb spica cast immobilization to open reduction and dorsal ligament repair or reconstruction. Controversy exists as to the best treatment algorithm. Patients with acute posttraumatic pain in the TMC joint without gross instability or radiographic subluxation can be considered to have partial ligament tears and be treated with long opponens splint, thumb spica splint, or cast immobilization for a minimum of 6 weeks. The thumb should be positioned in palmar abduction and extension with the thumb unable to oppose the surrounding digits to minimize axial compression on the first ray. Documented dislocations with adequate reduction may also be treated with immobilization and close follow-up. Closed reduction and percutaneous 0.045-in Kirschner wire fixation is typically required in reducible dislocations to provide sufficient stability for ligament healing. One to 2 percutaneous wires are used: 1 driven in a retrograde direction obliquely across the TMC joint with the metacarpal held in palmar abduction and extension and a second across the first metacarpal base into the index metacarpal, if needed. With continued instability or incongruity after closed joint reduction, open reduction and ligamentous repair versus reconstruction is indicated.

Open reduction of the thumb CMC joint begins with exposure of the joint through a modified Wagner approach with care taken to protect the volar branch of the superficial radial artery, palmar cutaneous branch of the median nerve, and branches of the lateral antebrachial cutaneous and superficial radial nerves. The thenar musculature is then elevated subperiosteally, exposing the underlying volar radial capsule. The joint is then reduced and any interposed tissue extricated. At this point, the decision between repair and reconstruction must be undertaken. Open repair of the critical dorsal ligament complex occurs after reduction of the volar thumb metacarpal beak into the trapezial recess in full passive screw-home torque opposition and transfixation of the thumb metacarpal shaft to the index metacarpal shaft with a 0.045-in K-wire. At this point, repair through bone tunnels or suture anchors can be undertaken.[10] If the injury is diagnosed late or that of the dorsal ligamentous complex is irreparable, then reconstruction is recommended. Reconstruction techniques typically involve using a portion of the flexor carpi radialis (FCR) tendon as a reinforcement weave. The TMC tenodesis described by Eaton and Littler[7] is performed by creating a bone tunnel in the base of the thumb metacarpal in a sagittal plane perpendicular to the thumbnail. The radial half of the FCR is harvested beginning 6 to 8 cm proximal to its insertion site on the index metacarpal and the transected proximal end is passed through the thumb metacarpal bone tunnel in the volar base of the metacarpal to emerge dorsally. With the metacarpal held reduced with Kirschner wire fixation as above, the tendon is sutured to the dorsal periosteum to set the construct tension. The remaining tendon is placed deep to the APL tendon and around or through the remaining intact FCR tendon and finally reflected radially to be sutured to a remnant of the joint capsule or to the APL insertion. Immobilization and Kirschner wire fixation are continued for 4 weeks, after which time gentle progressive motion is started.

OUTCOMES

Both nonsurgical and percutaneous techniques have shown acceptable results in the literature as long as reduction is maintained.[11-14] Other authors have recommended dorsal ligament complex repair[9] or reconstruction,[15] stating that additional ligament treatment is required in these injuries for good outcomes. Simonian and Trumble[15] treated 8 patients with an average age of 25 years (range, 18-36 years) (group A) with a closed reduction and pinning. The average follow-up period was 49 months (range, 25-74 months). Four patients were noted to have recurrent subluxation, based on findings on nonstress radiographs with 3 of these requiring a revision using an FCR tendon weave reconstruction. One patient required a TMC fusion for OA. Nine patients (group B) underwent early ligamentous reconstruction. The average follow-up period was 49 months (range, 25-74 months). Eight patients reported no pain while working, and 1 patient complained of occasional discomfort. The functional variables affected most in both groups were thumb abduction, which was decreased by 10%, and pinch strength, which was decreased by 13%, in group B, as compared with 20% and 19%, respectively, for the patients in group A. Radiographically, the joint space was slightly narrowed (Eaton stage II) in 3 cases in group B; however, these were asymptomatic. In group A, 5 patients demonstrated degenerative changes of the CMC joint (3 Eaton stage II, 2 stage III), and 3 patients were symptomatic after treatment.

METACARPOPHALANGEAL (MCP) JOINT

Finger MCP Joint

ANATOMY

Traumatic dislocations of the MCP joint are relatively rare secondary to the inherent joint stability from intrinsic ligamentous structures, the supporting flexor and extensor tendon systems, and their relatively protected position at the base of the fingers. The metacarpal head is asymmetric in the coronal and sagittal planes with the head narrowed dorsally and the ulnar aspect of articular surface hypoplastic compared with the radial side. Therefore, the MP joints are most vulnerable to dorsal and ulnarly directed forces and are more stable in flexion than extension secondary to the cam effect created by the nonspherical metacarpal head shape. The joint capsule extends from the metacarpal neck to the base of the proximal phalanx and is reinforced dorsally by the loose insertion of the common extensor tendon, volarly by the volar plate, and on the sides by the collateral ligaments.

GENERAL CONSIDERATIONS

MCP joint dislocations can be classified as simple or complex or by the direction of displacement. Simple dislocations refer to joint subluxations where the volar plate is draped over the metacarpal head, present with a locked hyperextension posture of 60° to 80°, and can be easily reducible without open surgical procedures. Radiographic evaluation confirms the dorsal subluxation of the proximal phalanx with finger hyperextension. In contrast, complex dislocations are considered complete and imply the need for open reduction secondary to volar plate interposition within the joint or a buttonholed metacarpal head through the palmar structures (Fig. 3-5).[16] The clinical presentation reveals an MCP joint held in slight hyperextension with the digit deviated toward its adjacent central digit (Fig. 3-6). Palmarly, the skin may be puckered with a prominent metacarpal head and dorsally, a defect can be palpated. Radiographs may reveal joint space widening or associated fractures of the metacarpal head.

Dorsal dislocations are more common than volar dislocations. The index finger is most frequently involved, followed by the thumb and small finger, with central digit

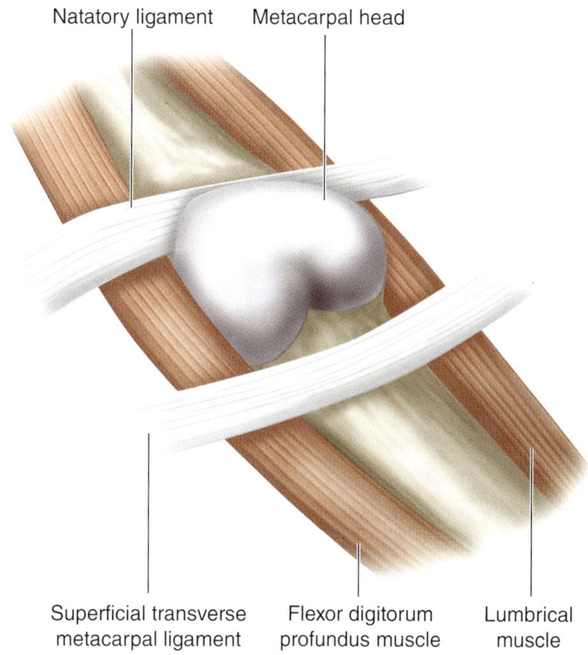

FIGURE 3-5 Buttonholing of metacarpal head in dorsal MP dislocation.

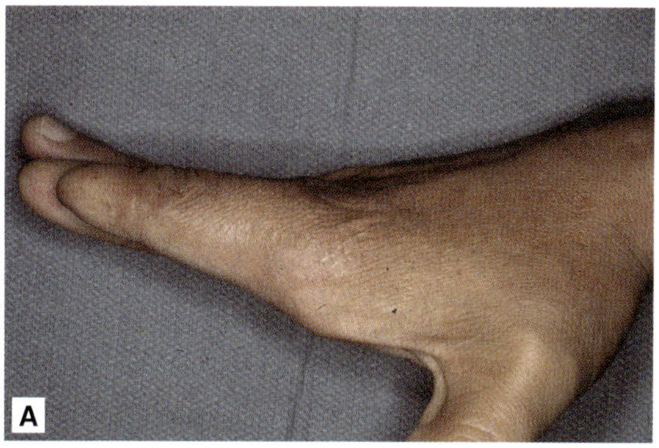

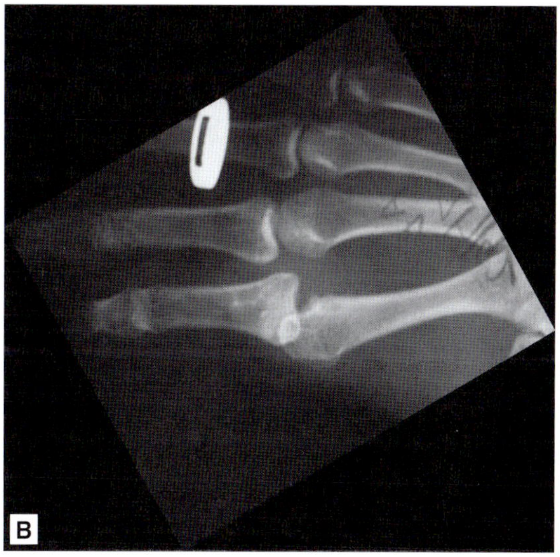

FIGURE 3-6 **A.** A 1-year-old MP joint dislocation. **B.** AP x-ray. (Copyright David J. Slutsky, MD, 2012.)

dislocations rarely occurring in isolation without concomitant dislocation of a border digit. The mechanism of injury typically involves a fall onto an outstretched hand causing forced hyperextension of the MCP joint. Volar dislocations, exceedingly uncommon, can occur through a hyperflexion or hyperextension mechanism, and are usually complex in nature. Interposition of dorsal capsule, distal volar plate, collateral ligament, and junctura tendinum in a border digit have been implicated in irreducibility.[17–19]

TREATMENT/SURGICAL TECHNIQUE

The reduction maneuvers used when dealing with dorsal MCP dislocations are extremely important. Simple dislocations in which either hyperextension or traction manipulation is employed can transform a simple lesion to a complex one by drawing the volar plate into the joint and blocking a successful closed reduction. Proper technique entails flexion of the wrist to relax the flexor tendons while applying a distal and volarly directed force onto the proximal phalanx base. This allows the proximal phalanx and the attached volar plate to slide volarly over the metacarpal head. Dorsal simple dislocations are typically stable after closed reduction and early range of motion is encouraged with the use of dorsal extension-blocking splint use to prevent MCP joint hyperextension. Volar dislocation reduction maneuver is similar, except the MCP joint is flexed with gentle pressure applied to the volar surface of the proximal phalanx as it is brought into extension.

Complex dorsal dislocations and irreducible volar dislocations can be approached dorsally, volarly, or in combination. The dorsal approach, popularized by Becton et al,[20] describes a straight longitudinal split through skin, extensor mechanism, and joint capsule to access the joint and extricate the interposed volar plate. A freer elevator can be inserted pushing the volar plate out of the way and gently levering the reduction into position. Proponents note easier access to the interposed volar plate, the ability to treat associated metacarpal head fractures, and a decreased risk of neurovascular injury. In contrast, a volar approach described by Kaplan[16] involves exposure through an oblique palmar incision overlying the involved metacarpal head. A modification by McLaughlin[18] involved an extension of the incision into the finger through a midlateral approach. Care must be taken during the skin incision because the metacarpal head is displaced directly beneath the subcutaneous tissues and the neurovascular bundles may be tented over the metacarpal and are at risk of injury. Despite this risk, the volar approach provides excellent visualization of any entrapped structures and provides access to extricate and repair them accordingly. Reduction is also aided by release of the A1 pulley, which relaxes the tension on the flexor tendon unit that can entrap the metacarpal head like a noose. Release of the natatory ligament, superficial transverse metacarpal ligament, and volar plate may also be needed. Post reduction, the involved joint is immobilized in approximately 30° of flexion for 2 weeks, after which time active ROM is started with use of a 10° dorsal extension-blocking splint for an additional 4 weeks.

OUTCOMES/COMPLICATIONS

There have not been any recent series on outcomes after MCP dislocation and the majority of literature consists of small case series that focus on surgical approaches and mechanism of injury. However, with concentric reduction obtained, patients can expect to regain the majority of their preinjury ROM within 4 to 6 weeks.[21] Timely open treatment of irreducible MCP dislocations is an important factor in obtaining a successful outcome. Joint stiffness is the primary complication seen after this type of injury secondary to prolonged immobilization, late reduction, or severe adjacent soft tissue injury. Failure of diagnosis with prolonged dislocation and repeated attempts at closed reduction or traumatic open reduction may also lead to early degenerative arthritic changes within the MCP joint or osteonecrosis of the metacarpal head. As stated above, digital neurovascular bundle injury secondary to its superficial tenting over the displaced metacarpal head can lead to division during volar surgical exposure. Premature physeal closure has also been reported in the pediatric population.

Thumb MCP Joint

ANATOMY

The thumb MCP joint is similar anatomically to that of the fingers. However, the shape of the articular surface differs in that it is more hinge-like than multiaxial, with a primary arc of motion in the flexion/extension plane. The surrounding ligamentous, capsular, intrinsic musculature, and extrinsic tendon structures help to stabilize the joint, which has little intrinsic stability due to a relatively large radius of curvature of the proximal phalanx base. The radius of curvature of the metacarpal head itself, however, is highly variable and because of this the thumb MP joint has the most variation in range of motion of any joint in the human body.[22]

GENERAL CONSIDERATIONS

The thumb MCP joint is second only to the index finger in frequency of dislocation of MCP joints. Most dislocations are dorsal with a hyperextension mechanism of injury (Fig. 3-7), which leads to volar plate, capsule, and variable collateral ligament ruptures. Reduction is mechanically blocked most commonly by the volar plate, but can also be limited by the flexor pollicis longus (FPL) tendon. Similar to the finger MCP joint, a noose-like phenomenon may occur with the ulnarly displaced FPL and the radially displaced thenar intrinsic tendons, which along with possible interposition of the thumb sesamoids may lead to a complex, irreducible dislocation. Volar dislocations, in contrast, are uncommon and have a higher likelihood of requiring open reduction. Tissue interposition in a volar dislocation usually consists of dorsal capsule, volar plate, or incarcerated extensor tendons.[23–25]

Thumb MP joint dorsal dislocations are usually easy to diagnose secondary to the gross deformity that they cause.

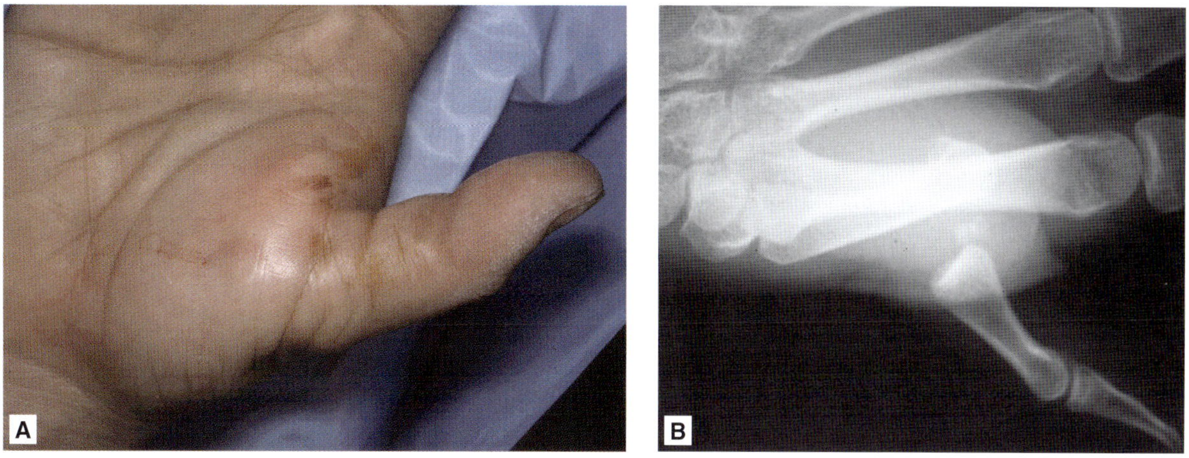

FIGURE 3-7 **A.** Thumb MP dislocation. **B.** AP x-ray. (Copyright David J. Slutsky, MD, 2012.)

The proximal phalanx is hyperextended and the metacarpal adducted. Radiographic examination may show phalanx hyperextension, but also may show bayonet apposition of the phalanx to the metacarpal. Dorsal subluxation of the thumb MP joint can also occur, which presents with a less severe hyperextension deformity or a "locked" joint that is unable to flex. This entity is thought to be secondary to entrapment of the radial condyle of the metacarpal through the radial aspect of the volar plate.

TREATMENT/SURGICAL TECHNIQUE

The closed reduction maneuver described above for finger MCP joints can also be used to treat thumb MCP joint dislocations with an increased likelihood of success. Again, simple longitudinal traction maneuvers should be avoided and the metacarpal should be placed in a flexed and adducted position to relax the volar "noose" around the metacarpal head, with digital pressure on the base of the phalanx and slight hyperextension to slide it over the metacarpal head. The digit is immobilized in a dorsal extension-blocking splint in 10° more than the point of instability and extended 10° per week. Post reduction, it is also important to determine if any associated collateral ligament injury is present as this would necessitate longer immobilization. In dorsal subluxations, closed reduction can be attempted with local joint insufflation and a volar-directed, twisting force on the proximal phalanx on the metacarpal head. Volar dislocations are reduced in a similar manner to dorsal dislocations with joint hyperflexion and manual dorsal direct pressure placed on the volar base of the proximal phalanx. There is a higher risk of associated collateral ligament injury in volar dislocations and may require prolonged immobilization. Signs of irreducibility in volar dislocations have been found to be lack of a palpable EPL in initial examination, radial or ulnar displacement of the EPL or EPB, interposed sesamoids on x-ray, or paradoxical MCP joint flexion and IP extension with attempted MCP extension.[26]

If open reduction is required secondary to interposed palmar structures, dorsal, volar, and lateral approaches have been described. In an acute injury, a limited dorsal incision can be used to insert a freer elevator into the joint to assist with extrication of interposed soft tissue structures over the metacarpal head and reduction. A chevron volar approach may be necessary to extricate incarcerated structures as these injuries can be surprisingly recalcitrant to a simple reduction. Supplemental Kirschner wire fixation may be used as indicated.

OUTCOMES/COMPLICATIONS

Patients should be advised they will likely have a stable joint after closed or open reduction. Collateral ligament injury may require prolonged immobilization and may lead to joint stiffness. Due to the requirement of joint stability at the thumb MP joint, it is important to immobilize these injuries properly to obtain stability even at the expense of range of motion. It is especially important to limit forceful joint extension while the volar plate is healing during the initial 6 to 8 weeks post injury.

PROXIMAL INTERPHALANGEAL JOINT

Anatomy

The proximal interphalangeal (PIP) joint is a bicondylar joint that functions as a hinge. It confers stability from its congruous articular surface, proper and accessory collateral ligaments, and the volar plate. The stability provided by the osseous structures is easily appreciated when dealing with fracture–dislocations. The collateral ligaments arise from a concave fossa on the lateral aspect of the proximal phalanx condyles and pass obliquely and volarly to their insertions on the middle phalanx. The proper and accessory ligaments are anatomically confluent at their origin but insert at the base of the volar one-third of the middle phalanx and volar plate, respectively. The volar plate forms the floor of the joint and completes a box-like configuration that strongly resists PIP displacement and provides excellent inherent stability.

General Considerations

PIP joint injuries are very common in the hand and produce a spectrum of severity ranging from a simple sprain to comminuted fracture–dislocations. Determining the level of ligamentous, osseous, and articular involvement is important and requires careful clinical and radiographic assessment. Whether dealing with an isolated joint dislocation or one involving an associated fracture, the main determinant of treatment is the ability to achieve and maintain concentric reduction with active motion. However, it is important to keep in mind that the poor tolerance of the PIP joint to prolonged immobilization requires a prompt diagnosis, rational treatment plan, and early active protected ROM.

Clinically, functional stability can often be evaluated with a digital block and 2-phase active and passive stability testing.[27] Radiographically, posteroanterior and true lateral views of the digit itself must be obtained to adequately evaluate the joint surface for articular injury and congruency. Subtle residual subluxation or incongruency can be identified by looking for the "V" sign (Fig. 3-8).

The PIP joint can dislocate in 1 of 3 directions: dorsal, lateral, or volar. Dorsal dislocations are common and typically occur through a hyperextension mechanism combined with a degree of longitudinal compression. They present either with a hyperextension deformity with the joint surfaces still touching or in bayonet apposition. A small avulsion fracture of the middle phalanx base is common with dorsal hyperextension dislocations and should not alter treatment. Lateral PIP dislocations occur frequently in the PIP joint and indicate rupture of 1 collateral ligament and at least partial avulsion of the volar plate from the middle phalanx. Ligamentous laxity >20° on full extension stress testing indicates complete proper and accessory collateral ligament disruption and at least 1 additional secondary stabilizer.[28]

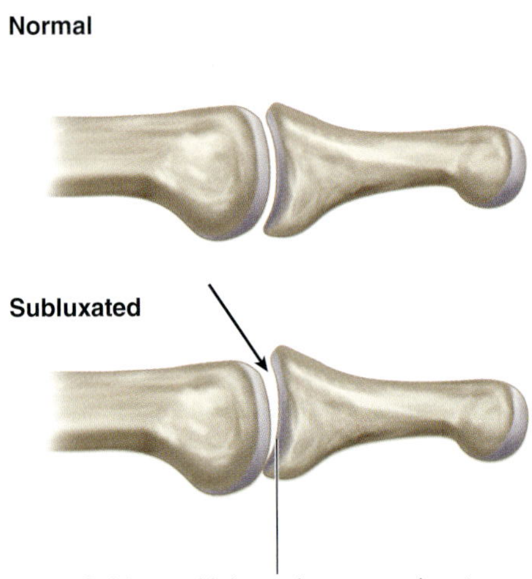

FIGURE 3-8 Subtle residual subluxation or incongruency can be identified by looking for the "V" sign.

Volar dislocations, in contrast, are rare injuries and may involve pure translatory displacement (volar dislocation) or an associated rotatory component (volar rotatory subluxation). Distinguishing between these 2 entities is critical. When a volar translatory dislocation occurs, the central slip invariably ruptures with variable injury to the collateral ligaments and volar plate (Fig. 3-9). In volar rotatory subluxation, as the middle phalanx displaces volarly, the involved condyle herniates through the extensor mechanism, usually between the central slip and ipsilateral lateral band, and can become entrapped.

Treatment/Surgical Technique

Dorsal dislocations are usually able to be successfully reduced closed with the use of digital block local anesthesia.

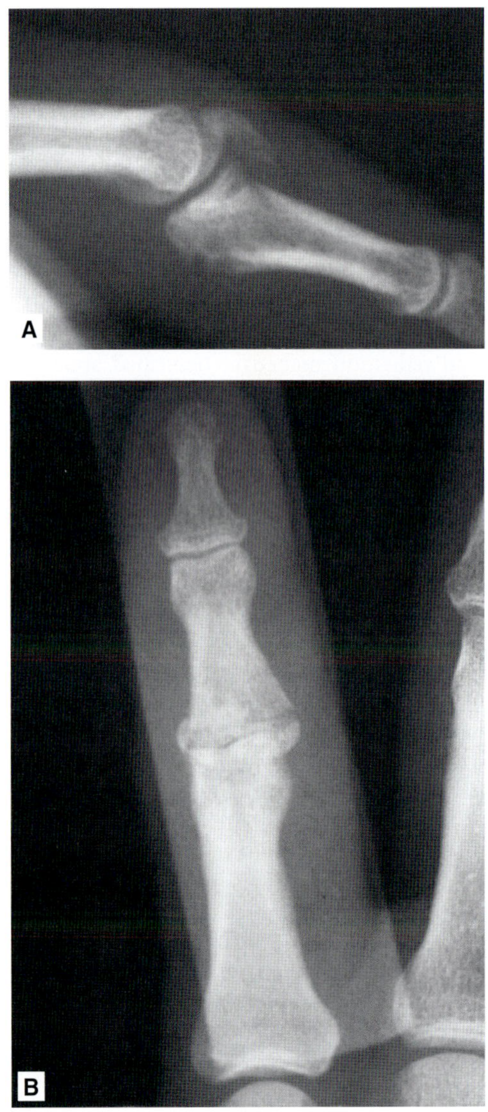

FIGURE 3-9 A and **B.** Central slip injury with volar PIP dislocation. (Copyright David J. Slutsky, MD, 2012.)

Irreducible dislocations secondary to interposed volar plate are quite rare. In hyperextension deformities, reduction consists of manual manipulation using a volar flexion-directed force. Bayonet apposition requires an extension force applied to the middle phalanx, followed by a volar flexion force directing the phalanx base over the metacarpal head. Similar to the MCP joint dislocations, pure longitudinal traction reduction can lead to an irreducible dislocation and should be avoided. A stable joint after reduction should begin immediate ROM with protective buddy taping. Residual instability can be treated with progressive extension block splinting starting at 10° more flexion than the point of instability with a goal of discontinuing the splint within 3 weeks or with dorsal block pinning (Fig. 3-10). The requirement of flexion >30° to maintain reduction requires operative repair or dynamic skeletal traction (Fig. 3-11).

Lateral dislocations, with few exceptions, reduce spontaneously or easily by closed means and will heal with controlled early motion and buddy-tape protection for 3 weeks. Volar dislocations are typically easily reduced under digital block anesthesia with a dorsal extension-directed force to translate the middle phalanx base over the proximal phalanx head. Volar rotatory dislocation treatment is controversial, with numerous authors advocating open reduction and extensor mechanism repair.[29,30] However, closed reduction should be attempted and open reduction performed only after failure of the former. The majority of volar rotatory dislocations can be reduced with gentle longitudinal traction, flexion of the MP and PIP joints to relax the volarly displaced lateral band, and a rotatory motion to disengage the condyle from the lateral band. Postreduction full active extension is usually possible secondary to the contralateral

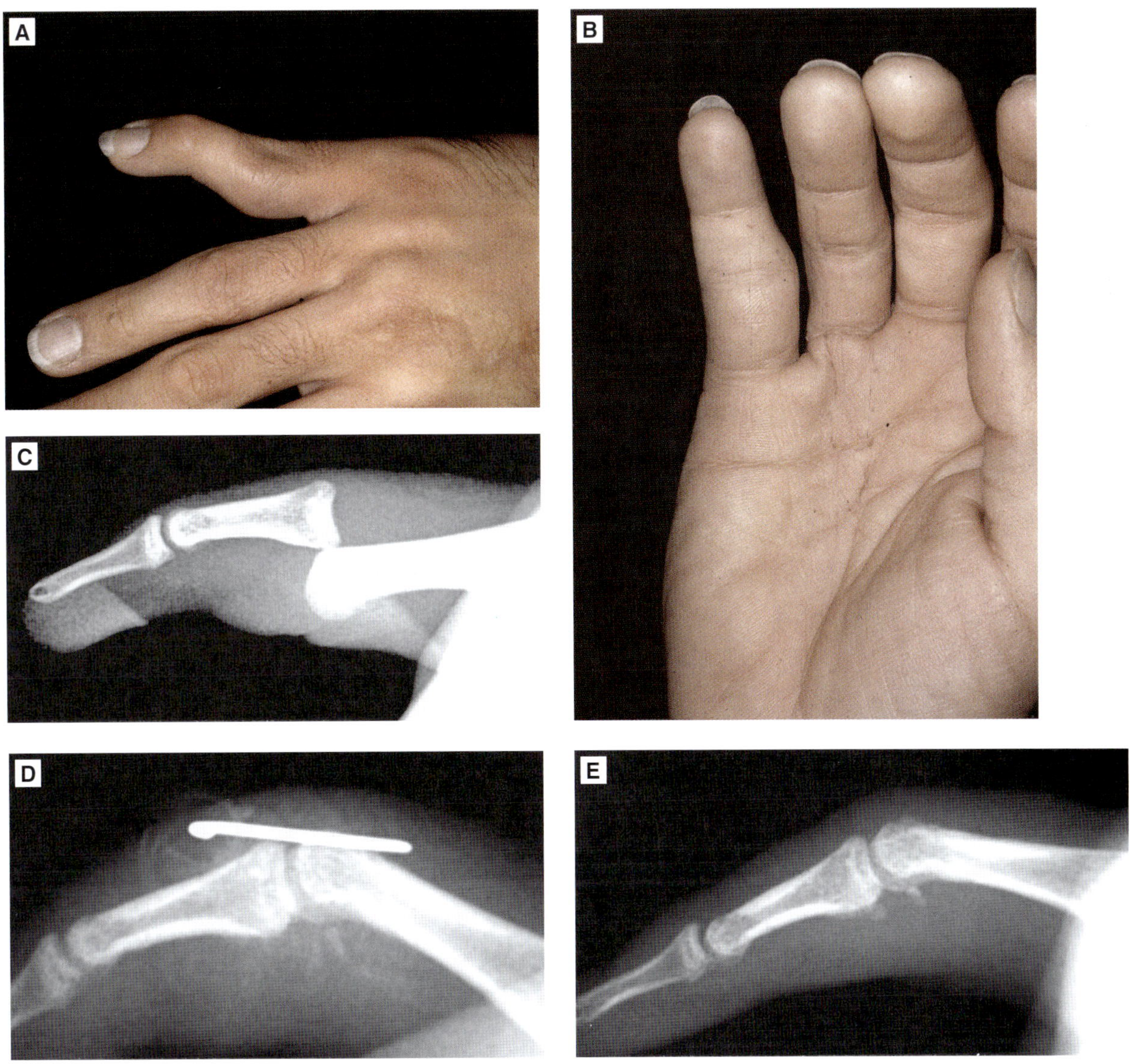

FIGURE 3-10 **A.** Dorsal PIP dislocation, clinical appearance. **B.** Palmar view. **C.** Lateral x-ray. **D.** Dorsal block pinning. **E.** Final result. (Copyright David J. Slutsky, MD, 2012.)

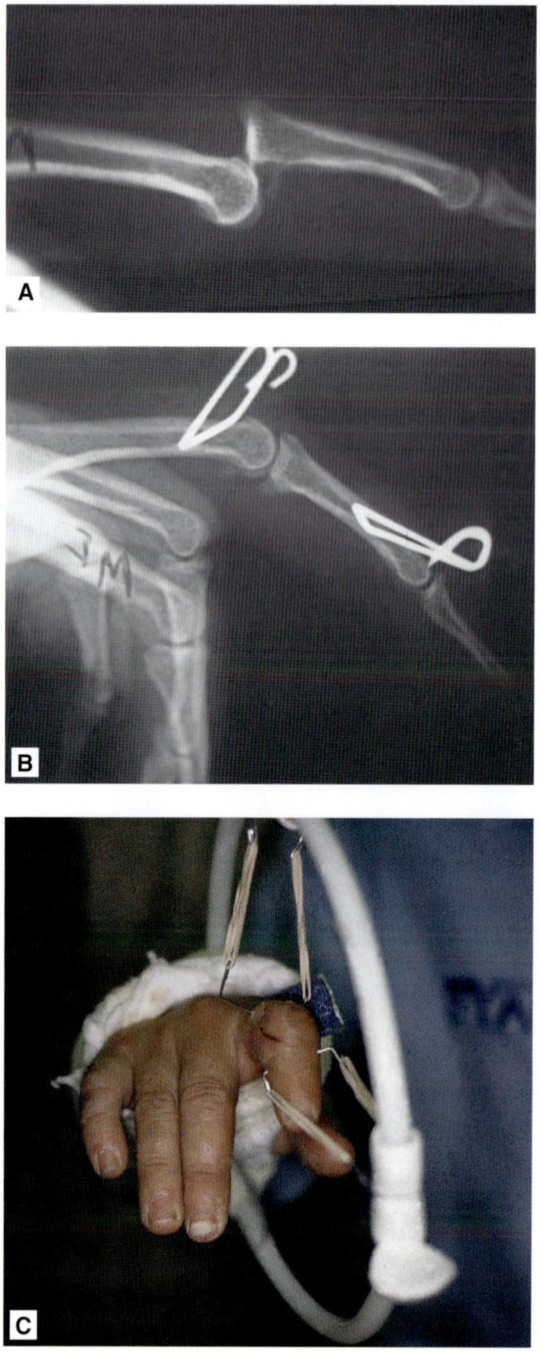

FIGURE 3-11 **A.** Dorsal PIP dislocation. **B.** Reduced with dynamic digital traction. **C.** Clinical photograph. (Copyright David J. Slutsky, MD, 2012.)

lateral band and a portion of the central slip remaining intact. Those volar rotatory dislocations that are unable to be reduced closed require open reduction through a dorsal incision on the side of ligamentous disruption under digital or wrist local anesthetic block. The entrapped lateral band is freed from the joint and reduction typically can then easily be performed. The lateral band can then be either repaired or excised depending on the degree of injury. Stable joints in both volar dislocation scenarios, with active extension, can be immediately mobilized with buddy taping similar to their dorsal counterparts. If extension is unable to be maintained, the patient is treated similar to an acute boutonniere with full-time extension splinting for 6 weeks.

Open treatment of dorsal and volar dislocations can typically be performed through a midaxial approach (or dual midaxial if needed) to extricate any interposed tissues impeding reduction.

Vigilance by either the surgeon or an experienced therapist is required to treat any PIP dislocation with respect to contracture or partial central slip injury. Because digit comfort is often in a flexed position or treatment requires a period of flexion, missed central slip injuries or persistent contracture are common. Diligence in examination and vigorous therapy can overcome these issues in most cases.

Outcomes/Complications

In pure ligamentous PIP joint dislocations, postinjury stiffness is the most common complication that occurs. Residual instability is quite rare in this situation, in stark contrast to this being the chief issue in fracture–dislocations. Patients should be counseled to expect a permanently enlarged joint and a prolonged recovery period (up to 18 months) of occasional pain and stiffness. Average arc of motion around 80° with 10° of extensor lag is common.[31] Residual stiffness and loss of motion not responsive to aggressive hand therapy and splinting would be a candidate for open joint capsulectomy and collateral ligament release.

Arora et al[32] reviewed 50 patients who had sustained dorsal PIP joint dislocations who were randomized to cast immobilization (group A) versus dorsal block splinting and early motion (group B). In group A, 9 patients showed a normal range of motion, whereas a limitation of extension of 10° or more was seen in 16 patients. All PIP joints were clinically stable. In group B, only 2 of 25 patients showed a limitation of extension of 10° or more, whereas 23 patients showed a normal range of motion. Instability of 1 collateral ligament was seen in 2 cases.

DISTAL INTERPHALANGEAL JOINT

Finger DIP and Thumb IP Joints

ANATOMY

The distal interphalangeal (DIP) and thumb IP joints, similar to the PIP joint, are bicondylar and function as a hinge. They confer stability from their congruous articular surface, proper and accessory collateral ligaments, and the volar plate. Compared with its PIP joint counterpart, the DIP/IP joint has increased stability secondary to the shorter lever arm of the distal phalanx and adjacent insertions of the flexor digitorum profundus and terminal extensor tendons.

GENERAL CONSIDERATIONS

Dislocations of the finger DIP or thumb IP joints without tendon rupture are rare and typically occur dorsal or lateral. They are typically reducible. Inability to obtain reduction is thought to occur secondary to interposed volar plate, osteochondral fracture fragment, sesamoid bone, or the middle phalanx condyle buttonholing through the FDP, extensor tendon, or volar plate.[33–38] Volarly directed injuries are commonly fracture–dislocations with associated fractures of the dorsal articular surface. Injuries involving these joints require a high level of suspicion for skin compromise and open traumatic volar transverse arthrotomy secondary to the tight surrounding skin envelope.

TREATMENT/SURGICAL TECHNIQUE

Most DIP or IP joint dislocations can be reduced in a closed fashion under digital block local anesthesia. Dorsal reduction consists of longitudinal traction with a simultaneous volarly directed force and joint flexion. Stable reductions may begin immediate ROM. The rare unstable dorsal dislocation should be immobilized for 2 to 3 weeks in a 20° extension-block splint or a percutaneous 0.035-in Kirschner wire used to stabilize the joint for 3 to 4 weeks. Lateral dislocations and dorsal dislocations with complete collateral ligament injuries, in addition, should be protected from lateral stress for 4 to 6 weeks. Similarly, volar dislocations should be treated as mallet injuries with full-time extension splinting for a duration of 6 weeks ± percutaneous transarticular K-wire pinning.

Open reduction of these injuries is typically needed in the above rare irreducible dislocations, open injuries, as well as in patients with delayed presentations (greater than 3 weeks). Exposure consists of a transverse dorsal incision at the level of the DIP joint crease with surgical removal of offending anatomic structures by placement of a freer elevator into the joint. Care must be taken to protect the terminal extensor tendon or extensor pollicis longus tendon. Evaluation for possible small osteochondral or chondral injury should also be performed at the time of reduction.

OUTCOMES/COMPLICATIONS

The most common complication that occurs after DIP or IP joint dislocations is stiffness. After open surgery, unique complications that occur include impaired wound healing and tip hypersensitivity. These have to do with disruption of the longitudinal venous channels supplying the narrow skin flap between the incision and the dorsal nail fold and damage to the accompanying distal branches of the dorsal digital nerves and subsequent small neuroma formations, respectively.

REFERENCES

1. El-shennawy M, Nakamura K, Patterson RM, Viegas SF. Three-dimensional kinematic analysis of the second through fifth carpometacarpal joints. *J Hand Surg Am.* 2001;26A:1030–1035.
2. Hodgson PD, Shewring DJ. The "metacarpal cascade lines"; use in the diagnosis of dislocations of the carpometacarpal joints. *J Hand Surg Eur Vol.* 2007;32E:277–281.
3. Gainor BJ, Stark HH, Ashworth CR, Zemel NP, Rickard TA. Tendon arthroplasty of the fifth carpometacarpal joint for treatment of post-traumatic arthritis. *J Hand Surg Am.* 1991;16A:520–524.
4. Kleinman WB, Grantham SA. Multiple volar carpometacarpal joint dislocations: case report of traumatic volar dislocation of the medial four carpometacarpal joints in a child and review of the literature. *J Hand Surg Am.* 1978;3A:377–382.
5. Frick L, Mezzadri G, Yzem I, Plotard F, Herzberg G. Acute carpometacarpal joint dislocation of the long fingers: study of 100 cases. *Chir Main.* 2011;30:333–339.
6. Edmunds JO. Concepts of the anatomy of the thumb trapeziometacarpal joint. *J Hand Surg Am.* 2011;36A:170–182.
7. Eaton RG, Littler JW. Ligament reconstruction for the painful thumb carpometacarpal joint. *J Bone Joint Surg Am.* 1973;55A:1655–1666.
8. Strauch RJ, Behrman MJ, Rosenwasser MP. Acute dislocation of the carpometacarpal joint of the thumb: an anatomic and cadaver study. *J Hand Surg Am.* 1994;19A:93–98.
9. Edmunds JO. Traumatic dislocations and instability of the trapeziometacarpal joint of the thumb. *Hand Clin.* 2006;22:365–392.
10. Okita G, Anayama S, Sato N, Haro H. Surgical reconstruction using suture anchor for dislocation of the carpometacarpal joint of the thumb: a case report. *Arch Orthop Trauma Surg.* 2011;131:225–228.
11. Uchida S, Sakai A, Okazaki Y, Okimoto N, Nakamura T. Closed reduction and immobilization for traumatic isolated dislocation of the carpometacarpal joint of the thumb in rugby football players. Two case reports. *Am J Sports Med.* 2001;29:242–244.
12. Khan AM, Ryan MG, Teplitz GA. Bilateral carpometacarpal dislocations of the thumb. *Am J Orthop.* 2003;32:38–41.
13. Watt N, Hooper G. Dislocation of the trapezoi-metacarpal joint. *J Hand Surg Br.* 1987;12B:242–245.
14. Bosmans B, Verhofstad HJ, Gosens T. Traumatic thumb carpometacarpal joint dislocations. *J Hand Surg Am.* 2008;33A:438–441.
15. Simonian PT, Trumble TE. Traumatic dislocation of the thumb carpometacarpal joint: early ligamentous reconstruction versus closed reduction and pinning. *J Hand Surg Am.* 1996;21A:802–806.
16. Kaplan EB. Dorsal dislocation of the metacarpophalangeal joint of the index finger. *J Bone Joint Surg Am.* 1957;39A:1081–1086.
17. Green DP, Terry GC. Complex dislocation of the metacarpophalangeal joint: correlative pathological anatomy. *J Bone Joint Surg Am.* 1973;55A:1480–1486.
18. McLaughlin HL. Complex "locked" dislocation of the metacarpophalangeal joints. *J Trauma.* 1965;5:683–688.
19. Patel MR, Bassini L. Irreducible palmar metacarpophalangeal joint dislocation due to junctura tendinum interposition: a case report and review of the literature. *J Hand Surg Am.* 2000;25A:166–172.
20. Becton JL, Christian JD Jr, Goodwin HN, Jackson JG III. A simplified technique for treating the complex dislocation of the index metacarpophalangeal joint. *J Bone Joint Surg Am.* 1975;57A:698–700.
21. Barry K, McGee H, Curtin J. Complex dislocation of the metacarpophalangeal joint of the index finger: a comparison of the surgical approaches. *J Hand Surg Br.* 1988;13B:466–468.
22. Shaw J, Morris MA. The range of motion of the metacarpophalangeal joint of the thumb and its relationship to injury. *J Hand Surg Br.* 1992;17A:164–166.
23. Moneim MS. Volar dislocations of the metacarpophalangeal joint. Pathological anatomy and report of two cases. *Clin Orthop.* 1983;176:186–189.
24. Gunther SF, Zielinski CJ. Irreducible palmar dislocation of the proximal phalanx of the thumb—case report. *J Hand Surg Am.* 1982;7A:515–517.
25. Miyamoto M, Hirayama T, Uchida M. Volar dislocation of the metacarpophalangeal joint of the thumb. *J Hand Surg Br.* 1986;11B:51–54.
26. Beck JD, Klena JC. Closed reduction and treatment of 2 volar thumb metacarpophalangeal dislocations: report of 2 cases. *J Hand Surg Am.* 2011;36A:665–669.
27. Eaton RG, Littler JW. Joint injuries and their sequelae. *Clin Plast Surg.* 1976;3:85–98.
28. Kiefhaber TR, Stern PJ, Grood ES. Lateral stability of the proximal interphalangeal joint. *J Hand Surg Am.* 1986;11A:661–669.
29. Grant IR. Irreducible rotational anterior dislocation of the proximal interphalangeal joint. *J Hand Surg Br.* 1993;18B:648–651.

30. Posner MA, Wilenski M. Irreducible volar dislocation of the proximal interphalangeal joint of a finger caused by interposition of an intact central slip: a case report. *J Bone Joint Surg Am.* 1978;60A: 133–134.
31. Peimer CA, Sullivan DJ, Wild DR. Palmar dislocation of the proximal interphalangeal joint. *J Hand Surg Am.* 1984;9A:39–48.
32. Arora R, Lutz M, Fritz D, Zimmermann R, Gabl M, Pechlaner S. Dorsolateral dislocation of the proximal interphalangeal joint: closed reduction and early active motion or static splinting; a retrospective study. *Arch Orthop Trauma Surg.* 2004;124:486–488.
33. Failla JM. Irreducible thumb interphalangeal joint dislocation due to a sesamoid and palmar plate: a case report. *J Hand Surg Am.* 1995;20A:490–491.
34. Sabapathy SR, Bose VC, Rex C. Irreducible dislocation of the interphalangeal joint of the thumb due to sesamoid bone interposition: a case report. *J Hand Surg Am.* 1995;20:487–489.
35. Ghobadi F, Anapolle DM. Irreducible distal interphalangeal joint dislocation of the finger: a new cause. *J Hand Surg Am.* 1994;19A:196–198.
36. Palmer AK, Linscheid RL. Irreducible dorsal dislocation of the distal interphalangeal joint of the finger. *J Hand Surg Am.* 1977;2A:406–408.
37. Salamon PB, Gelberman RH. Irreducible dislocation of the interphalangeal joint of the thumb: report of three cases. *J Bone Joint Surg Am.* 1978;60A:400–401.
38. Stripling WD. Displaced intra-articular osteochondral fracture—cause for irreducible dislocation of the distal interphalangeal joint. *J Hand Surg Am.* 1982;7A:77–78.

4

Small Joint Arthroscopy

David J. Slutsky, MD

METACARPOPHALANGEAL JOINT ARTHROSCOPY

The metacarpophalangeal (MP) joint is ideally suited for arthroscopic evaluation. The MP joint represents a single compartment; the bony and tendinous landmarks are easy to identify and the neurovascular structures are remote from the portals; hence, there is a short learning curve. It is mostly used for synovectomy and loose body removal, but it has some applications following trauma as well.

Indications

INFLAMMATORY ARTHRITIS

MP joint arthroscopy is useful in evaluating the status of the articular cartilage as well as synovial proliferation, especially in rheumatoid arthritis (Fig. 4-1). A synovial biopsy and synovectomy can be performed without the need for arthrotomy. Sekiya et al[1] described their experience with an arthroscopic synovectomy in 45 finger joints (18 MP joints, 26 proximal interphalangeal joints) and 1 interphalangeal thumb joint in 23 rheumatoid patients using a 1.5-mm scope. They could not access the palmar recess, but there was resolution of the joint space swelling in the short term with no postoperative complications.

ACUTE ULNAR COLLATERAL LIGAMENT INJURY OF THE THUMB

Although arthroscopic reduction of a complete ulnar collateral ligament (UCL) tear of the thumb MP joint was first described by Ryu and Fagan in 1995,[2] it has not achieved widespread use. They used MP arthroscopy to both identify and aid in reducing the Stener lesion by flipping the torn proximal UCL from its position dorsal to the adductor aponeurosis back into the joint so that it could heal primarily with the distal torn end after thumb spica cast immobilization for 4 weeks.

REDUCTION OF MP JOINT FRACTURES

MP arthroscopy has applications in the treatment of some simple articular fractures of the metacarpal (MC) head and the proximal phalangeal base. The fracture fragments are directly visualized, reduced with a probe, and held with percutaneous pin fixation (Fig. 4-2A-D).

POSTTRAUMATIC VOLAR PLATE ADHESIONS

Choi et al described painful volar plate adhesions of the thumb MP joint in 15 patients, which were demonstrated by an intraoperative arthrogram.[3] Congruent joint flexion was accomplished after a synovectomy and release of the volar plate adhesions using a Freer elevator.

REMOVAL OF LOOSE BODIES

Loose bodies are commonly seen in patients with inflammatory arthritis or in cases with posttraumatic cartilage damage and can result in painful locking. The loose bodies are frequently lodged in the radial and ulnar synovial recesses.

Contraindications

Irreducible extensor tendon dislocation or subluxation is a relative contraindication due to the risk of tendon damage during portal placement. Similarly, an unstable joint or poor soft tissue coverage that precludes the use of finger trap traction is a contraindication.

Surgical Technique

The patient is placed supine with the arm abducted on an arm board, under tourniquet control, using general or regional anesthesia. A sterile finger trap is applied to the finger or thumb and 10 lb of traction is applied using a traction tower or overhead traction. A dorsal radial and a dorsal ulnar portal are used. They are established on either side of the central

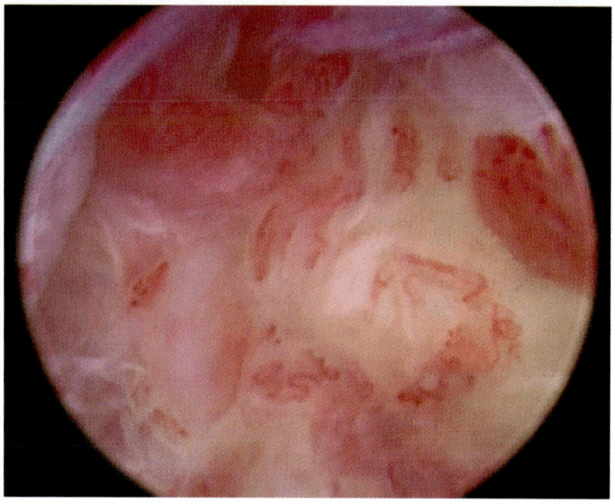

FIGURE 4-1 Arthroscopic view of MP joint synovitis.

extensor tendon by first identifying the joint space with a 22-gauge needle, followed by joint distension with saline and a superficial skin incision (Fig. 4-3). Fluoroscopy can aid this step in difficult cases. Careful wound spread technique is used since there is no internervous plane. Tenotomy scissors are used to dissect through the sagittal band fibers and dorsal capsule between the extensor tendon and the collateral ligaments, which arise from the palpable tubercles at the base of the proximal phalanx. A 1.9- or 2.7-mm 30° small joint arthroscope is then inserted in 1 portal and a 3-mm hook probe in the other portal, which are interchanged as necessary. A pressure bag is often needed for fluid inflow through the arthroscope. The collateral ligaments can be visualized, running obliquely from the MC head to the base of the proximal phalanx (Fig. 4-4). The volar plate can be partially seen palmar to the MC head. The volar recess is hidden from view but can be reached with a probe or Freer elevator when

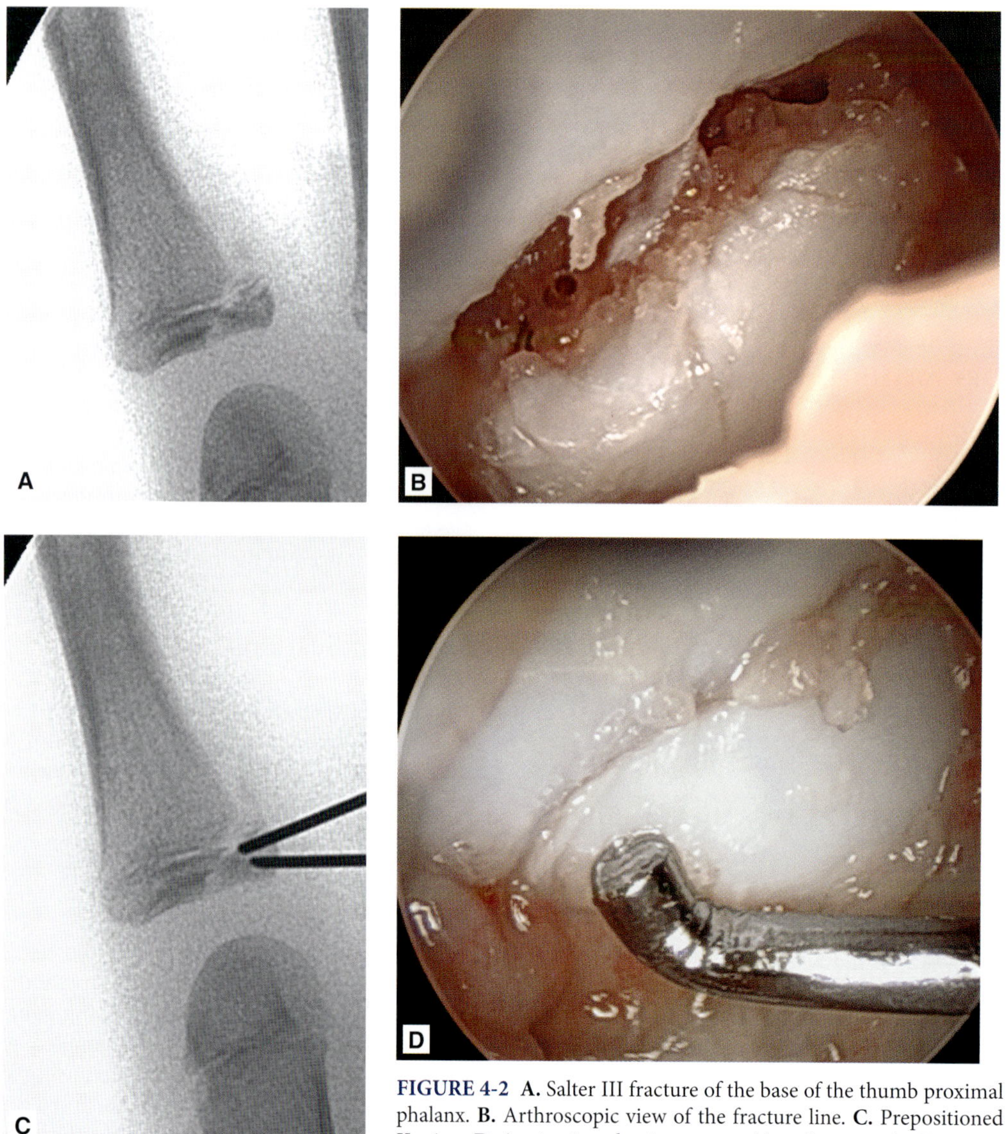

FIGURE 4-2 **A.** Salter III fracture of the base of the thumb proximal phalanx. **B.** Arthroscopic view of the fracture line. **C.** Prepositioned K-wires. **D.** Anatomic reduction captured by advancing the K-wires.

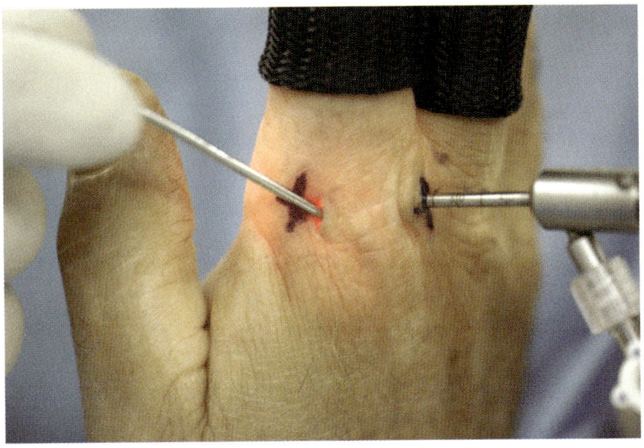

FIGURE 4-3 Clinical photo of MP joint arthroscopy with the scope in the ulnar portal and probe in the radial portal.

releasing adhesions between the volar plate and the MC head. The radial, ulnar, and dorsal synovial recesses can be visualized when searching for loose bodies or when performing a synovectomy. Small chondral defects can be drilled to stimulate fibrocartilage formation. Following the procedure, the portals are sutured and a bulky dressing or splint is applied.

Complications

Since the joint capsule is relatively thin, the skin, neurovascular bundles and tendons are especially at risk during thermal shrinkage. Choi et al reported 1 case of flexor pollicis longus rupture 3 weeks after thermal shrinkage of the volar plate.[3] The risk can be minimized by maintaining an adequate fluid inflow, short duration bursts, and use of the minimal wattage. Articular cartilage damage is also a risk due to the small joint volume; hence, instrumentation must be gentle.

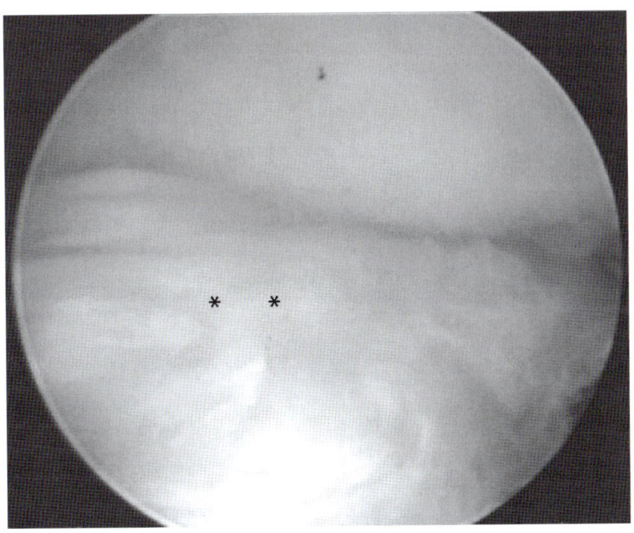

FIGURE 4-4 View of the ulnar collateral ligament (*).

TRAPEZIOMETACARPAL ARTHROSCOPY

Ligament Anatomy/Biomechanics

Imaeda et al dissected the trapeziometacarpal (TM) joint of 30 cadaver specimens and described the anatomy and properties of 3 major ligaments.[4] Bettinger et al revisited this and further described 16 ligaments stabilizing the TM joint.[5] Only those ligaments that can be seen from an arthroscopic perspective will be discussed.

The anterior oblique ligament (AOL) is a 2-part ligament that consists of a superficial portion and an intra-articular deep portion (Fig. 4-5). The superficial anterior oblique ligament (sAOL) is a broad, loose, and curtain-like capsular ligament that is immediately deep to the thenar musculature, which overlies the volar aspect of the TM joint. The ligament originates 0.5 mm proximal to the articular surface at the volar tubercle of the trapezium and inserts broadly over the volar-ulnar tubercle of the thumb MC base, 2 mm distal to the volar styloid process. The sAOL is lax throughout most of the TM range of motion and becomes taut at the extremes of thumb pronation and extension. In a biomechanical study of 17 cadaver hands, Colman et al[6] found that the superficial portion of the ligament plays only a minor role in joint stability, does not prevent dorsal MC subluxation, and limits the joint's motion only in pronation.

The deep anterior oblique ligament (dAOL), formerly known as the volar beak ligament, is an intra-articular ligament that lies deep to the sAOL. It originates from the volar central apex of the trapezium, ulnar to the ulnar edge of the trapezial ridge, and inserts into the articular margin ulnar to the volar styloid process (volar beak) of the thumb MC base. The dAOL becomes taut with increasing thumb abduction,

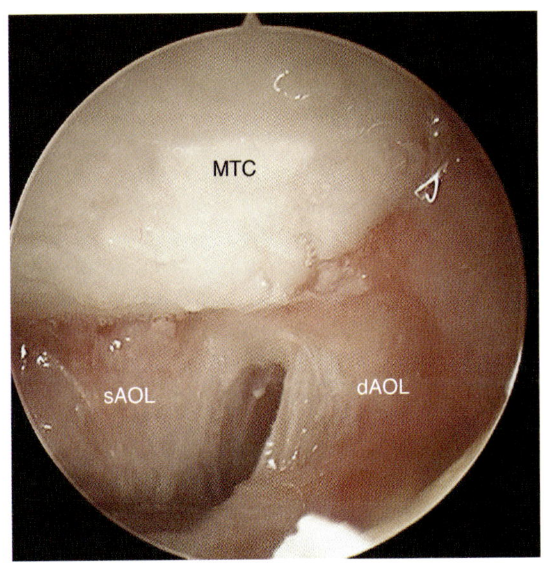

FIGURE 4-5 Superficial (sAOL) and deep (dAOL) anterior oblique ligament seen from the 1-U portal. MTC, metacarpal base.

pronation, and extension. Colman et al[6] found the intra-articular dAOL to be a major stabilizer of the joint. Since it is the closest ligament to the center of the joint, it acts as a pivot point to guide the MC during the pronation that occurs as a part of thumb opposition. Its intra-articular fibers run obliquely from distal ulnar to proximal radial; thus, this ligament is positioned to prevent an ulnar shift of the MC that would tighten the oblique fibers, whereas a radial shift would slacken them. The sulcus between the sAOL and dAOL can often be palpated with an arthroscopic probe.

The UCL is an extracapsular ligament that is slightly ulnar to and superficial to the sAOL. It originates from the flexor retinaculum, and then runs obliquely from a palmar proximal position and attaches to the palmar-ulnar tubercle of the first MC base. It is taut in extension, abduction, and pronation and also helps prevent volar subluxation of the MC base. Arthroscopically, it is identified by its oblique fibers running ulnar to the AOL.

The dorsal aspect of the thumb is covered by 2 main ligaments. The posterior oblique ligament (POL) is an intracapsular ligament that originates from a fan-shaped base on the dorsoulnar side of the trapezium. It runs obliquely to insert into the dorsoulnar aspect and palmar-ulnar tubercle of the first MC base. This ligament is taut at the extremes of abduction, opposition, and supination that prevents ulnar translation of the thumb MC base during opposition and abduction.

The dorsoradial ligament (DRL) is the shortest, thickest, and widest ligament that spans the joint. The DRL is a fan-shaped capsular ligament, located immediately radial to the POL, that arises from the dorsoradial tubercle of the trapezium and has a broad insertion into the dorsal base of the thumb MC. It is believed to be the most important stabilizer that resists dorsal translation of the thumb MC base and is a checkrein against radial subluxation. In a biomechanical study by Bettinger et al[7] the ultimate load to failure of the DRL (205.5 ± 60.2 N) was significantly greater than the other ligaments, which they believed was due to the size and bulk of the ligament. The stiffness for the DRL (78.3 ± 21.9 N/mm) was significantly higher than for the AOL (24.1 ± 13.3 N/mm) and therefore likely to be the most significant restraint to lateral dislocation. The AOL demonstrated the least stiffness and the greatest hysteresis and was thought to be a poor stabilizer of the TMC joint. A recent histochemical study by Hagert et al showed that the dorsal ligaments, including the DRC, DRL, and POL, had a statistically significant greater degree of innervation than both the AOL and the UCL.[8] They believe that this is consistent with their role as primary stabilizers of the TM joint.

Edmunds emphasizes the point that in the static resting position, the prominent volar beak of the thumb MC is disengaged from its recess in the trapezium, the TM joint space is relatively large, and both the volar beak ligament and the dorsal ligament complex are lax. In the final phase of opposition during either active or passive screw home torque rotation, the dorsal ligament complex tightens, the volar beak ligament becomes even more lax and redundant, the TM joint is compressed, and the volar beak of the thumb MC is tightly compressed into its recess area in the trapezium. This dynamic force couple changes the TM joint from incongruity to congruity and from laxity to rigid stability. It changes a normally lax TM joint into a stable TM joint to support the powerful forces on the thumb in power pinch and grasp.[9] If the dorsal ligament complex is cut or torn (as occurs in a pure TM dislocation), gross instability of the TM joint results, and the joint dislocates, even if the volar beak ligament is intact.

Ladd et al performed a recent comparative study of the arthroscopic and gross anatomy of the ligaments of the thumb CMC joint.[10] They found that the volar ligaments including the superficial and deep AOL ligaments and UCL varied in their location and caliber, whereas the dorsal ligaments including the POL and DRL were highly consistent. They further subdivided the UCL into the UCL and dorsal trapeziometacarpal ligament (DTM-1). The UCL is a complementary, volar counterpart of the DTM-1 that was previously misidentified as being the POL (Fig. 4-6). They found the DRL actually consisted of the dorsal radial ligament and the dorsal central ligament (DCL). The DCL is radial to the 1-U portal and lies deep to the extensor pollicis brevis (EPB). The DRL is radial to the DCL (Fig. 4-7).

Trapeziometacarpal Joint Portals

STANDARD PORTALS

Menon initially presented his work on arthroscopy of the TM joint as a meeting exhibit in 1994.[11] He then published his experience with the arthroscopic management of TM arthritis in 1996.[12] He described 2 working portals, a volar portal

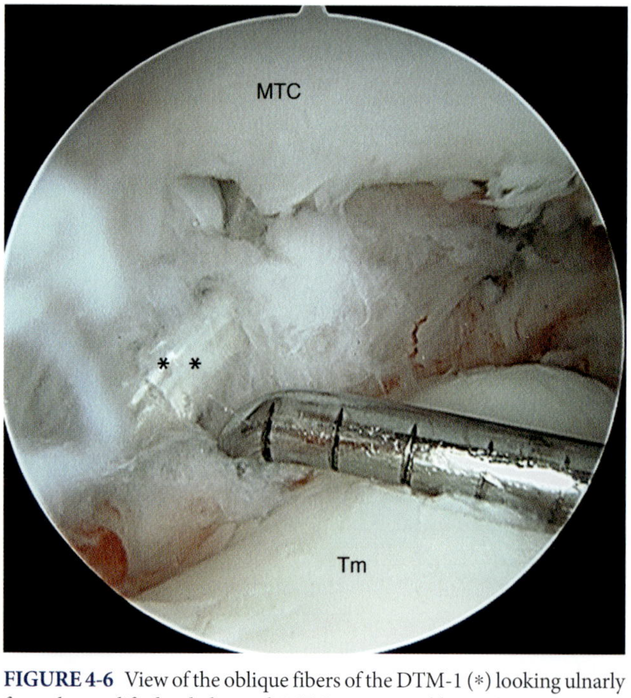

FIGURE 4-6 View of the oblique fibers of the DTM-1 (*) looking ulnarly from the modified radial portal. MTC, metacarpal base; Tm, trapezium.

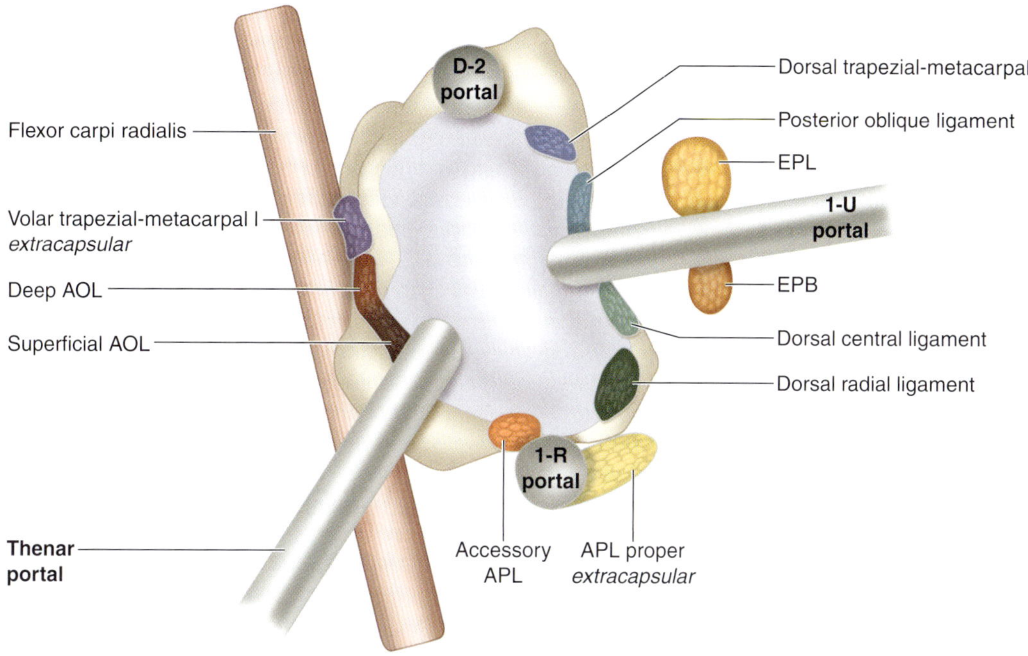

FIGURE 4-7 Diagram of the arthroscopic cross-sectional ligamentous anatomy and portal positions. AOL, anterior oblique ligament; APL, abductor pollicis longus; EPB, extensor pollicis brevis; EPL, extensor pollicis longus. (After Zhang, et al. *J Wrist Surg*. 2012.)

just radial to the abductor pollicis longus (APL) tendon and a dorsal portal that is just ulnar to the APL along the line of the joint. Berger independently developed his technique for arthroscopic evaluation of the first carpometacarpal joint that he first presented as an instructional course in 1995. He then published his clinical work in 1997. He named the volar radial portal (RP) the 1-R portal and the dorsal ulnar portal the 1-U.[13] He defined the term dorsal as being in the plane of the thumb nail and volar in the plane of the distal pulp. Radial and ulnar referred to the thumb when its nail is parallel to the finger nails with the thumb supinated and radially abducted. He noted that the plane of the 1-R portal passes through the nonligamentous capsule just lateral to the AOL. The plane of the 1-U portal that is just posterior and ulnar to the EPB passes between or through DRL and POL. This portal provides views of the AOL and the UCL. Both portals are along the radial border of the thumb, which makes it difficult to assess the lateral side of the joint. The POL is ulnar and adjacent to the portal. There is no true internervous plane since branches of the superficial radial nerve (SRN) surround the field and are at risk for injury with improper technique. The radial artery courses immediately posterior and ulnar to the arthroscopic field. Ropars et al dissected 30 forearms and recorded the distances for the 3 branches of the SRN to the 1-R, 1-U, and a distal–dorsal (D-2) accessory portal (see below).[14] The SRN typically has a major volar branch (SR1) and a major dorsal branch that subdivides into a volar (SR2) and a dorsal (SR3) branch. SR1 generally parallels the first extensor compartment, whereas SR2 crosses the first web space. In 24 cases (80%), when the 1-R portal was established radial (volar) to the SR3 branch, the mean distance was 4.8 mm (0-8). In 6 cases (20%) when the 1-R portal was inserted ulnar (dorsal) to the SR3 branch, the distance was less than 2 mm. The SR3 was always remote from the 1-U portal at a mean 13 mm (7-22). The D-2 portal was very close to the SR2 at a mean distance of 1.7 mm (0-6).

MODIFIED RADIAL PORTAL

Orellana and Chow described a modified RP for improving the radial view of the TMJ.[15] The RP is located just distal to the oblique ridge of the trapezium following a line along the radial border of the flexor carpi radialis (FCR) tendon rather than the APL. In an anatomic study of 6 cadaver arms, the SRN was located a mean of 6.3 mm (4-8 mm) from the 1-U portal and 7.8 mm (4-12 mm) from the RP. The radial artery passed within 2.7 mm (2-3.5 mm) of the 1-U portal and 10 and 15 mm from the RP. To establish the RP, the scope is placed in the 1-U portal. The light source is pointed to the RP that lies just radial to the AOL. A 22-gauge needle is inserted just distal to the ridge of the trapezium. The skin is incised followed by blunt dissection through the capsule and insertion of the trocar and cannula, and then the arthroscope.

THENAR PORTAL

A thenar portal was subsequently described by Walsh et al.[16] This portal is placed by illuminating the thenar eminence with the arthroscope in the 1-U portal, and then inserting a 22-gauge needle through the bulk of the thenar muscles at the level of the TM joint, approximately 90° from the 1-U portal. This portal is straddled by the UCL and allows preferential views of the ulnar recess and the ulnar tubercle of the trapezium. They measured the distances of the surrounding neurovascular structures to 3 portals in a cadaver study of 7 limbs. The mean distance from SR2 was 11.6 ± 1.0 mm for the 1-U, 25.7 ± 1.2 mm for the 1-R, and 33.7 ± 1.68 mm for the thenar portal. The mean distance from SR3 was 12.9 ± 1.1 mm for the 1-U, 7.4 ± 1.3 mm for the 1-R, and 19.07 ± 1.17 mm for the thenar portal. The mean distance from the radial artery was 13.3 ± 1.1 mm for the 1-U, 20.7 ± 0.9 mm for the 1-R, and 29.4 ± 1.15 mm for the thenar portal. The motor branch of the median nerve was an average of 23.0 ± 1.6 mm from the thenar portal. There were no neurovascular complications from use of this portal in a recent small series of 11 patients, although transient scar tenderness was noted.[17]

DISTAL-DORSAL PORTAL

Access to medial osteophytes may sometimes be difficult; hence, I have found the use of a D-2 accessory portal to be of some value.[18] Its main utility is that it allows one to look down on the trapezium rather than across it, which facilitates resection of medial osteophytes. This accessory portal allows views of the dorsal capsule with rotation of the scope and facilitates triangulation of the instrumentation. It is situated in the dorsal aspect of the first web space. An anatomic study of 5 cadaver hands revealed that the D-2 portal surface landmark is ulnar to the extensor pollicis longus (EPL) tendon and 1 cm distal to V-shaped cleft at the juncture of the index and thumb MC bases. The portal lies just distal to the dorsal intermetacarpal ligament (DIML). The DIML is an extracapsular ligament that originates from the dorsoradial aspect of the index MC radial to the extensor carpi radialis longus insertion. It inserts onto the palmar-ulnar tubercle of the base of the thumb MC along with the POL and UCL. A trocar placed through the D-2 portal was found to pass through the first dorsal interosseous muscle and penetrate the DIML, entering the joint either through or between the UCL and POL. Branches of the SRN passed within 3.2 mm (range 1-5 mm), the radial artery was 3.8 mm away (range 3-5 mm), the first dorsal metacarpal artery (FDMA) within 2.8 mm (2-4 mm), and the cephalic vein was within 2.8 mm (1-5 mm) of this portal. On average, the D-2 portal was 17.2 mm from the 1-U portal (12-20 mm). There is no true safe zone for the D-2 portal, with branches of the SRN or the FDMA or one of its branches coming within 1 mm of the portal. Hugging the ulnar border of the thumb MC and moving 1 cm distal to the thumb/index MC juncture increases the space between the portal and the radial artery. Careful wound spread technique is of paramount importance when establishing this portal.

ARTHROSCOPIC TREATMENT FOR TRAPEZIOMETACARPAL OA

Eaton and Littler described a radiographic staging classification of TM OA.[19] Stage I comprises normal articular surfaces without joint space narrowing or sclerosis. There is less than one-third subluxation of the MC base. Stage II reveals mild joint space narrowing, mild sclerosis, or osteophytes <2 mm in diameter. Instability is evident on stress views with >1/3 subluxation. The STT joint is normal. In stage III, there is significant joint space narrowing, subchondral sclerosis, and peripheral osteophytes >2 mm in diameter but a normal STT joint. In stage IV, there is pantrapezial OA with narrowing, sclerosis, and osteophytes involving both the TM and STT joints. Badia proposed a more specific classification based on the arthroscopic changes.[20] Stage I included intact articular cartilage, stage II included eburnation on the ulnar one-third of the MC base and central trapezium, and stage III comprised widespread full-thickness cartilage loss on both surfaces.

Indications

The main indication for surgery is basilar thumb pain that is unresponsive to conservative treatment. This typically includes a trial of splinting with a forearm- or palmar-based thumb spica splint, NSAIDs, and activity modification. A TM joint cortisone injection may be used as a temporizing procedure. Although it is well known that the x-ray findings do not always correlate with the clinical symptoms, they are nevertheless instrumental in determining which patients may be appropriate candidates for an arthroscopic resection. As a general rule, any patient who is an appropriate candidate for a hemiresection arthroplasty of the TM joint would also be suitable for an arthroscopic hemitrapeziectomy. This would typically include patients in Eaton stage II and III with unremitting pain despite appropriate conservative measures. This form of treatment does not preclude an open trapeziectomy and/or ligament reconstruction at a later date as a salvage procedure for failed arthroscopic surgery. The presence of Eaton stage IV disease is a relative contraindication to a hemitrapeziectomy, although a small series on successful arthroscopic resection arthroplasty for combined carpometacarpal and scaphotrapeziotrapezoid OA has been recently published.[21] Any significant lateral subluxation of the thumb MC base will not be corrected without some type of ligament reconstruction or capsular shrinkage, and may compromise the long-term result if not corrected. Conventional teaching has stated that MP joint hyperextension must also be corrected to prevent recurrent TM subluxation, although this notion has been recently challenged.[22]

Contraindications

This would include any general contraindication to thumb arthroscopy including distortion of the anatomy due to swelling, unstable or friable skin that would preclude the use of traction, and recent infection. Ehlers-Danlos syndrome is a relative contraindication for this procedure, although a successful arthroscopic tendon arthroplasty has been reported.[23]

Surgical Technique

The patient is positioned supine on the operating table with the arm extended on a hand table. The thumb is suspended by finger traps with 10 to 15 lb of countertraction, which forces the wrist into ulnar deviation. The relevant landmarks are outlined including the proximal and dorsal edge of the thumb MC base, the tendons of the APL and the EPL, and the radial artery in the snuff box. The procedure is performed with a tourniquet elevated to 250 mm Hg. Saline inflow irrigation is provided through the arthroscope and a small joint pump or pressure bag. I prefer using a 2.7-mm 30° angled scope with a camera attachment, although others prefer a smaller 1.9-mm scope. A 3-mm hook probe is needed for palpation of intracarpal structures. A motorized shaver is needed for debridement. A diathermy unit is required if a capsular shrinkage is contemplated. Intraoperative fluoroscopy is employed to assess the adequacy of bone resection and for locating the portals as needed.

To establish the 1-R portal, the thumb MC base is palpated and the joint is identified with a 22-gauge needle just radial to the APL, followed by joint distension with saline. A superficial skin incision is made followed by wound spread technique with tenotomy scissors. The capsule is pierced and a cannula and a blunt trocar are inserted, followed by the arthroscope. An identical procedure is used to establish the 1-U portal, just ulnar to the EPB tendon, followed by insertion of a 3-mm hook probe. The portals are interchangeably used to systematically inspect the joint, which is facilitated by use of a 2.0-mm full radius resector.

The D-2 portal is used to increase the distance for instrument triangulation and to facilitate resection of any medial osteophytes. To establish the D-2 portal, the intersection of the base of the index and thumb MC is identified just distal and ulnar to the EPL tendon. A 22-gauge needle is inserted 1 cm distal to this juncture and angled in a proximal, radial, and palmar direction, hugging the thumb MC while viewing from either the 1-R or 1-U portal. A small skin incision is made and tenotomy scissors are used to spread the soft tissue and pierce the joint capsule. This is followed by insertion of a blunt trocar and cannula and then the arthroscope or alternatively a hook probe, motorized shaver, or 2.9-mm burr. The modified RP is identified with a 22-gauge needle, distal to the oblique ridge of the trapezium following a line along the radial border of the FCR tendon (Fig. 4-8A and B).

ARTHROSCOPIC DEBRIDEMENT AND CAPSULAR SHRINKAGE

The essence of arthroscopic capsular shrinkage is akin to that of an AOL reconstruction. It relies on thermal heating of the collagenous fibers in the surrounding ligaments and capsule, followed by a period of joint immobilization in a reduced position. A motorized shaver is used to debride any synovitis and to expose the capsular ligaments. A diathermy probe is then employed to paint the AOL taking care to leave bands of tissue in between. The probe is kept away from the joint surfaces to prevent cartilage necrosis and the outflow fluid temperature can be monitored to prevent overheating. Use of an 18-gauge needle in an accessory portal enhances fluid circulation.

ARTHROSCOPIC PARTIAL OR COMPLETE TRAPEZIECTOMY WITHOUT TENDON INTERPOSITION

The 1-R and 1-U portals are established as described. The AOL is identified and preserved. After joint debridement, a 2.9-mm burr is applied in a to-and-fro manner to resect 3 to 4 mm of the distal trapezium. The diameter of the burr along with fluoroscopy provides a gauge as to the amount of bony resection. A larger 3.5-mm burr may be substituted as the space between the MC base and distal trapezium enlarges. After the bony resection is complete, the thumb may be immobilized in a pronated and abducted position (Fig. 4-9A-D). If there is lateral subluxation of the MC base, thermal shrinkage of the AOL can be performed at this time.

ARTHROSCOPIC PARTIAL OR COMPLETE TRAPEZIECTOMY WITH INTERPOSITION

After a partial or complete resection of the trapezium, autogenous tendon graft such as the palmaris longus, one half of the FCR, or a slip of the APL is harvested through multiple transverse incisions. Landstrom recently reported a technique for harvesting an accessory slip of the APL by enlarging the 1-R portal.[24] Alternatively, some other form of interposition material can be substituted. An absorbable suture is placed in the leading end of the tendon graft and swedged onto a large curved needle, which is used to pass the graft through the joint. The needle is passed through the 1-U portal and brought out through the volar capsule and bulk of the thenar eminence. Traction on the suture pulls the graft into the joint. The remaining graft is packed in with forceps and the portals are closed. The thumb is K-wired in abduction for 4 weeks.

The thumb is immobilized in abduction by cast or splint for 4 weeks following any of these procedures. The use of a temporary TM joint K-wire is based on surgeon's preference, and is removed at 4 weeks. Thumb abduction and extension are instituted, followed by adduction and opposition after 6 weeks. Strengthening ensues once motion has been restored. The rehabilitation protocol is modified as necessary if concomitant surgery on the MP joint has been performed.

Outcomes

Menon reported his results on performing a partial arthroscopic resection of the trapezium and an interposition arthroplasty in 31 patients (33 hands).[12] The mean age was 59 years (48-81 years) with an average follow-up of 37.6 months (24-48 months). Gortex was used in 19 patients and autogenous tendon or allograft in 14. Complete pain relief was obtained in 25 patients/hands (75.7%). Three patients had mild pain (4 hands) and 4 patients had persistent pain

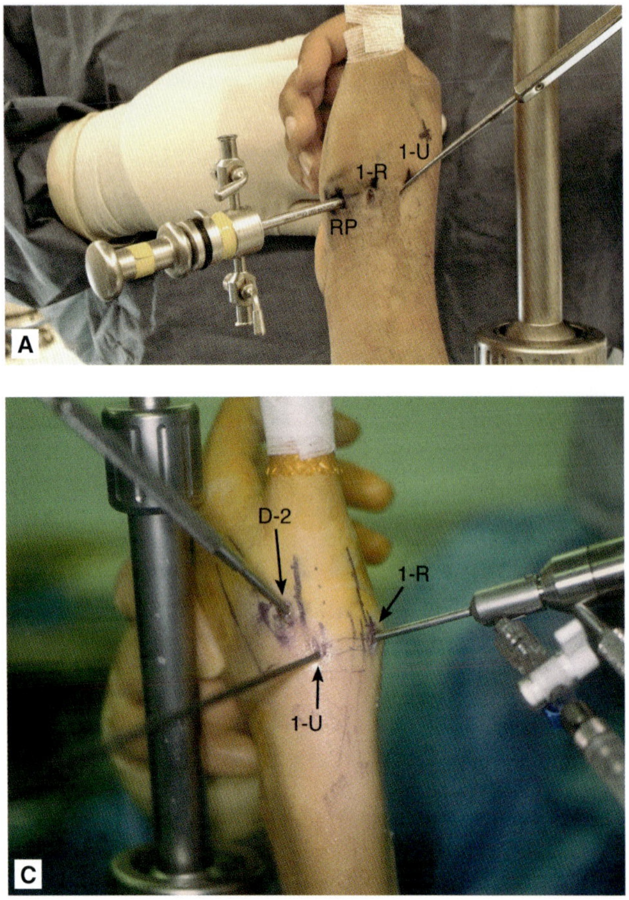

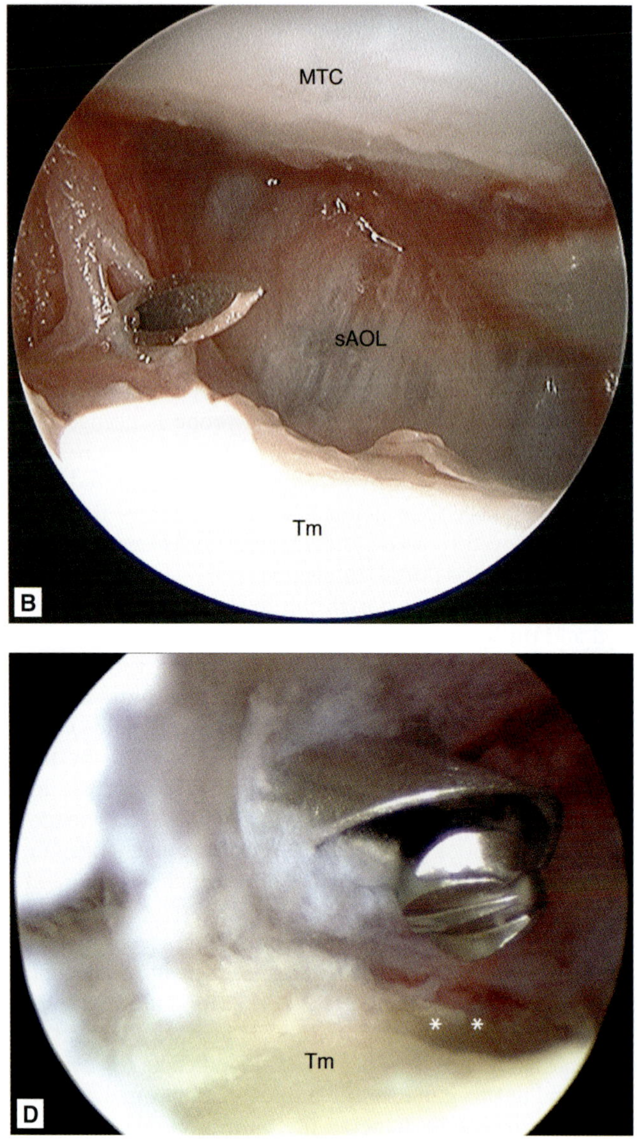

FIGURE 4-8 **A.** Clinical photo of the scope in the radial portal (RP) and the probe in the 1-U. **B.** View from the 1-R portal of a needle in the radial portal. MTC, metacarpal base; sAOL, superficial anterior oblique ligament; Tm, trapezium. **C.** Relative positions of the portals from the radial aspect of the wrist. **D.** View from the 1-U portal of a burr in the D-2 portal resecting a medial osteophyte (*). Tm, trapezium.

that required conversion to an open trapeziectomy and ligament reconstruction. All patients maintained their preoperative motion. Pinch strength improved from 6 psi preoperatively to 11.1 psi postoperatively. Because of osteolysis in 3 patients/4 hands, the use of Gortex as an interpositional substance was not recommended.

Furia published his experience with arthroscopic debridement and synovectomy of the TM joint in 23 patients with Eaton stage I and II OA as compared with a control group of 21 patients treated with nonoperative measures.[25] The pretreatment mean VAS were 7.7 in the operative group and 7.5 in the control group and the DASH scores were 55.6 and 54.4, respectively. At the 1-year follow-up the mean VAS were 2.7 in the operative group and 7.3 in the control group and the DASH scores were 26 and 53.1, respectively. The mean pinch strength for the surgical and control groups was 6.2 ± 1.3 and 4.9 ± 1.1 kg.

Hofmeister et al reviewed the long-term results in 18 patients following an arthroscopic hemitrapeziectomy, thermal capsular shrinkage, and temporary K-wire fixation.[26] At an average follow-up of 7.6 years they noted a subjective improvement in pain, pinch activities, strength, and range of motion in all patients. No patient required further surgery on their thumb. No patient had a positive TM test or any laxity by examination. The total thumb range of motion decreased by 20%, but all patients could oppose to the fifth finger. Grip strength remained unchanged, key pinch improved from 8 to 11 lb, and tip pinch improved from 4 to 5 lb. Radiographs showed a MC subsidence of 1.8 mm (0-4 mm). Four complications were noted: 2 cases of dorsal radial nerve neuritis, 1 rupture of the flexor pollicis longus, and 1 case of a prolonged hematoma.

Edwards and Ramsey reported similar findings.[27] They prospectively evaluated 23 patients with Eaton stage III OA

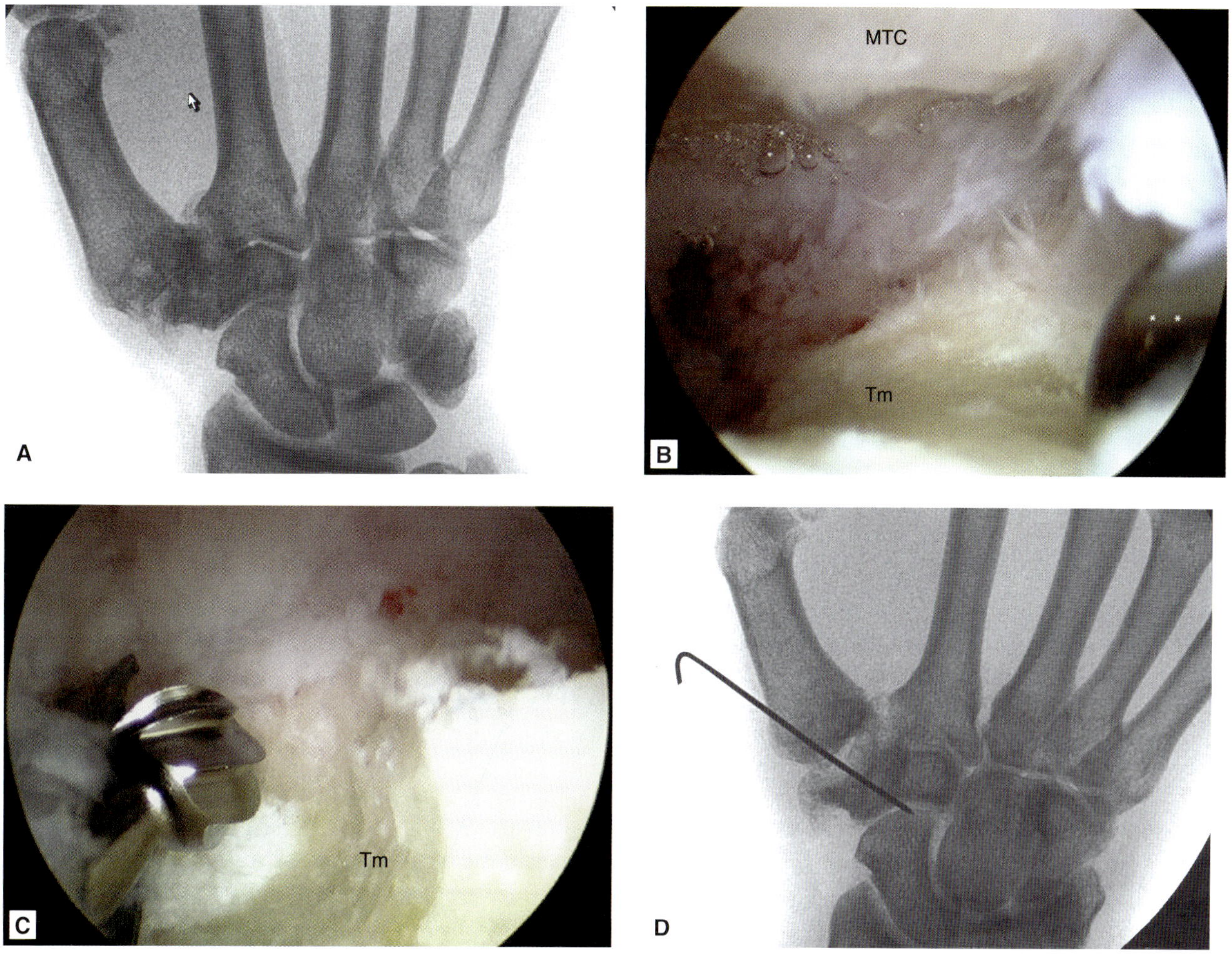

FIGURE 4-9 **A.** AP view of advanced TM OA. **B.** Arthroscopic view from the 1-U portal. Note how the trapezium (Tm) is devoid of all cartilage. MTC, metacarpal base. **C.** Partial resection of the trapezium. **D.** Completed hemitrapeziectomy.

at a minimum follow-up of 4 years, who were treated with an arthroscopic hemitrapeziectomy and thermal capsular shrinkage, without interposition, plus K-wire fixation for 3 to 4 weeks. At 3 months postoperatively the average DASH score improved from 61 to 10 and pain scores decreased from 8.3 to 1.5. Grip and key pinch strength improved to 6.8 and 1.9 kg, respectively, and the wrist and finger motion were unchanged. Proximal migration of the first MC averaged 3 mm and translation decreased from 30% to 10%. These findings remained unchanged at 4 years or more. Pegoli et al performed an arthroscopic hemitrapeziectomy and tendon interposition using the palmaris longus tendon in 16 patients with stage I and II disease.[28] At 12 months, there were 6 excellent, 6 good, 3 fair, and 1 poor result using the modified Mayo score. Adams et al treated 17 patients with an arthroscopic debridement and interposition arthroplasty for stage II and III disease, using a folded acellular dermal matrix allograft.[29] The average age was 61.7 (range 47-86) and the follow-up averaged 17 (range, 6-39) months. Eighty-eight percent of the patients reported no pain, or only occasional pain, on activities with an average pain score of 1.125 out of 10. The average grip strength was 18.3 kg versus 22.6 kg preoperatively and the average pinch strength was 4.0 kg versus 4.8 kg. Only 2 patients had limited range of motion, as assessed by the palm flat test and the ability to oppose the thumb to the fifth MC head. None of the patients required revision surgery and there were no instances of graft reaction.

Arthroscopic Treatment of Metacarpal Base Fractures

FIRST METACARPAL BASE

The Bennett fracture refers to an intra-articular fracture separating the volar-ulnar aspect of the MC base, separating it from the remaining thumb MC. It is thought to be caused by an axial load on a partially flexed MC. The volar-ulnar fragment is held in place by the AOL while the APL, EPB, and EPL pull the shaft fragment in a dorsal, radial, and proximal direction along with some supination. Nonoperative treatment has been associated with a bad outcome since external immobilization alone cannot control the radial subluxation. Open or percutaneous reduction and fixation have become the standard of treatment. Fracture reduction requires palmar abduction of the thumb and pronation of the MC base that tensions the dorsal ligament complex. Direct pressure on the MC base may also be needed. Thumb extension causes fracture displacement. There are no published long-term, large prospective randomized outcome studies, but many authors consider ≤2 mm of intra-articular incongruity to be acceptable. A Rolando fracture is a Y- or T-pattern fracture that includes the volar-ulnar Bennett fragment in addition to a dorsal radial fragment. This fracture pattern is more difficult to treat and has a worse prognosis than the Bennett fracture. It often requires an open reduction, but the fracture is occasionally amenable to percutaneous techniques.

Arthroscopy allows one to assess the articular reduction and to assess for any hardware penetration. The use of standard radiographs and fluoroscopy leads to an underestimation of the degree of articular incongruity. In a recent study in 8 fresh-frozen cadaveric hands, Capo et al artificially created a Bennett fracture and then performed a closed reduction and pinning.[30] Under fluoroscopic examination, the measured fracture step-off and displacement were less than 1.5 mm in all specimens. Standard x-rays demonstrated an average displacement of 0 mm on the AP view, a 0.1-mm gap on the lateral view, and an articular step-off of 1.1 mm. A direct examination of the joint surface however showed an average displacement of 3.1 mm, an average articular gap of 0.9 mm, and an average step-off of 2.1 mm.

Surgical Technique

The methodology and portals are similar to that described above. Thumb traction tends to place it in some abduction and pronation that often provisionally reduces the fracture in the proximal/distal plane, but the fracture fragments are malrotated since the MC shaft fragment is extended and supinated. I prefer to perform this procedure without constant fluid irrigation since it is less complicated and views of the articular surface and ligaments are superior. Intermittent irrigation is used as needed by attaching a 10-cm^3 saline-filled syringe to the inflow portal and using a full radius resector for suction and debridement of hematoma. Blunt elevators and curettes can be used, but a dental pick is useful for both fracture manipulation and reduction. The D-2 portal is useful for fracture reduction using a Freer elevator, especially if the fracture is 3 to 4 weeks old. Two 0.45-mm K-wires are prepositioned at the MC base but not crossing the fracture site. They can be used to manipulate the main shaft fragment into pronation and abduction while holding the volar-ulnar fragment reduced with the tip of the dental pick. Once an acceptable reduction has been achieved, it is captured by driving the K-wires across the fracture line (Fig. 4-10A-D). One K-wire is usually insufficient to control rotation. If percutaneous cannulated screw fixation is used, one must be careful to avoid entering the CMC joint of the thumb/index MC articulation with the tip of the screw. In case of a Rolando fracture, cross-pinning the distracted thumb MC to the index MC can maintain the reduction of the comminuted shaft fragments (Fig. 4-11A-D). Articular pinning may also be necessary. A thumb spica splint is used for 4 to 6 weeks followed by K-wire removal and range of motion exercises.

FIFTH METACARPAL BASE

The same techniques for arthroscopy of the first carpometacarpal joint can be applied to fracture–dislocations involving the fifth CMC joint. This is one situation where arthroscopy is definitely of benefit since the articular fracture fragment is often volar and difficult to visualize and reduce from a dorsal approach.

ANATOMY/PATHOMECHANICS

Nakamura et al studied 80 cadaver arms and described the carpometacarpal joint in detail.[31] Two distinct dorsal ligaments were identified that attached to the dorsal aspect of the fifth MC. One of these extended from the ulnar base of the fifth MC to the hamate (fifth MC ulnar-side base–hamate ligament) and the other from the radial base of the fifth MC to the hamate and sometimes to the fourth MC ulnar base (fourth MC ulnar-side base–fifth MC radial-side base ligament). There was an intermetacarpal ligament that attached the radial base of the fifth MC to the ulnar base of the fourth MC. There was 1 volar ligament that attached to the fifth MC base and extended either to the hook of the hamate or to the ulnar base of the fourth MC. There were no intra-articular ligaments except for 1 ligament that was located between the third/fourth MC and the capitate/hamate.

Dzwierzynski et al also studied the intermetacarpal ligament anatomy.[32] They noted that the alignment of the interosseous ligaments between the fourth and fifth MCs differed from the ligament alignment between the second–third and third–fourth MCs, which allows a greater degree of motion in the fifth CMC joint (approximately 25° of flexion/extension) as compared with the fourth CMC joint (approximately 15°). They also observed that when these MCs flex at the CMC joints, as in grasping, the dorsal interosseous ligament tightens and the anterior interosseous ligament relaxes. When the MCs extend at the CMC joints, the anterior ligament tightens and the posterior ligament relaxes, which retains a rigid interconnection between the bones.

An axial load to the fourth and fifth MC heads secondary to a clenched fist blow is often cited as the most common mechanism of injury of a fracture–dislocation of the fifth carpometacarpal joint. In 1 clinical study, the authors postulated that flexion during impact results in a dorsal dislocation of the small finger MC base, dorsal CMC ligament disruption, and oftentimes a hamate dorsal rim fracture.[33] Yoshida et al attempted to reproduce the mechanism of injury in a cadaver

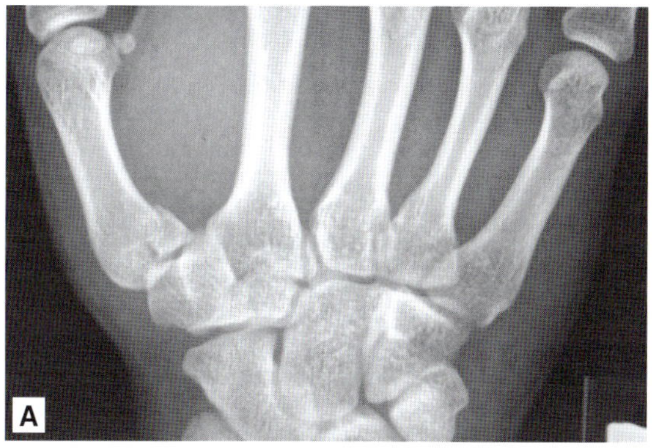

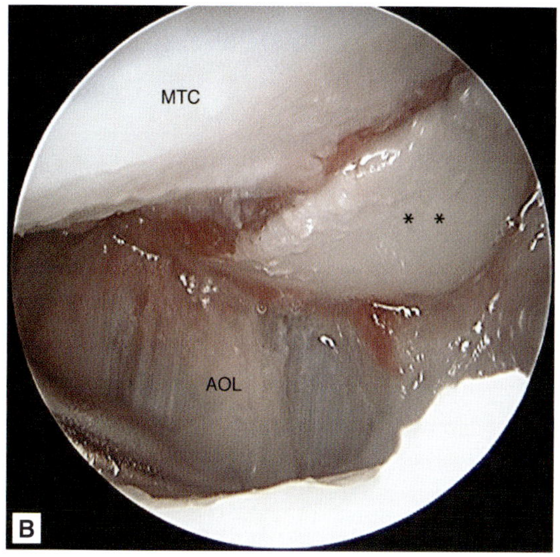

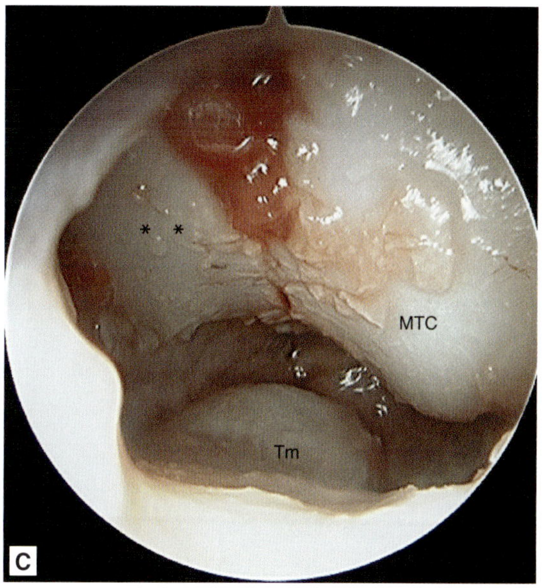

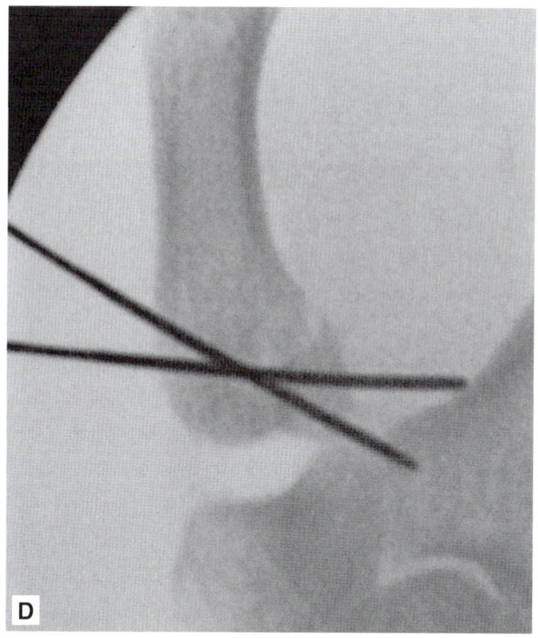

FIGURE 4-10 **A.** AP fluoroscopic view of a Bennett fracture. **B.** Arthroscopic view from the 1-U portal shows some persistent displacement of the volar-ulnar fragment (*). AOL, anterior oblique ligament; MTC, metacarpal shaft. **C.** Anatomic reduction of the articular surface viewed from the modified radial portal. **D.** AP fluoroscopic view following K-wire fixation.

study by dropping an 8-kg weight from various heights onto the fourth and fifth MC heads in a specially designed jig.[34] The hand was placed in the clenched fist position with the ring CMC joint in 20° of flexion, the small CMC joint in 30° of flexion, and the wrist in 20° of extension. A dorsal hamate fracture occurred in 45% of the specimens, whereas a fracture of the volar aspect of the ring and of small finger MC base were present in 40% and 20% of the specimens, respectively. The small MC volar base fracture fragment remained attached to the ring MC ulnar-side base–small MC radial-side base ligament.

IMAGING

Anteroposterior and lateral radiographs do not allow for an accurate assessment since the ring and small CMC joints are obscured by overlap of the hamate on the MC bases. Cain et al noted that a 45° pronation oblique view allowed for a good assessment of injuries to both the ring and small CMC joints.[33] Occasionally a 15° pronation oblique projection is required to assess damage to the dorsal portion of the small finger CMC joint.[34]

Surgical Technique

The patient is positioned supine on the operating table with the arm extended on a hand table. The small and ring fingers are suspended by finger traps with 10 to 15 lb of countertraction. In general, a 2.7-mm 30° angled scope along with a camera attachment is used, although a 1.9-mm scope can be substituted. A 3-mm hook probe is needed for palpation

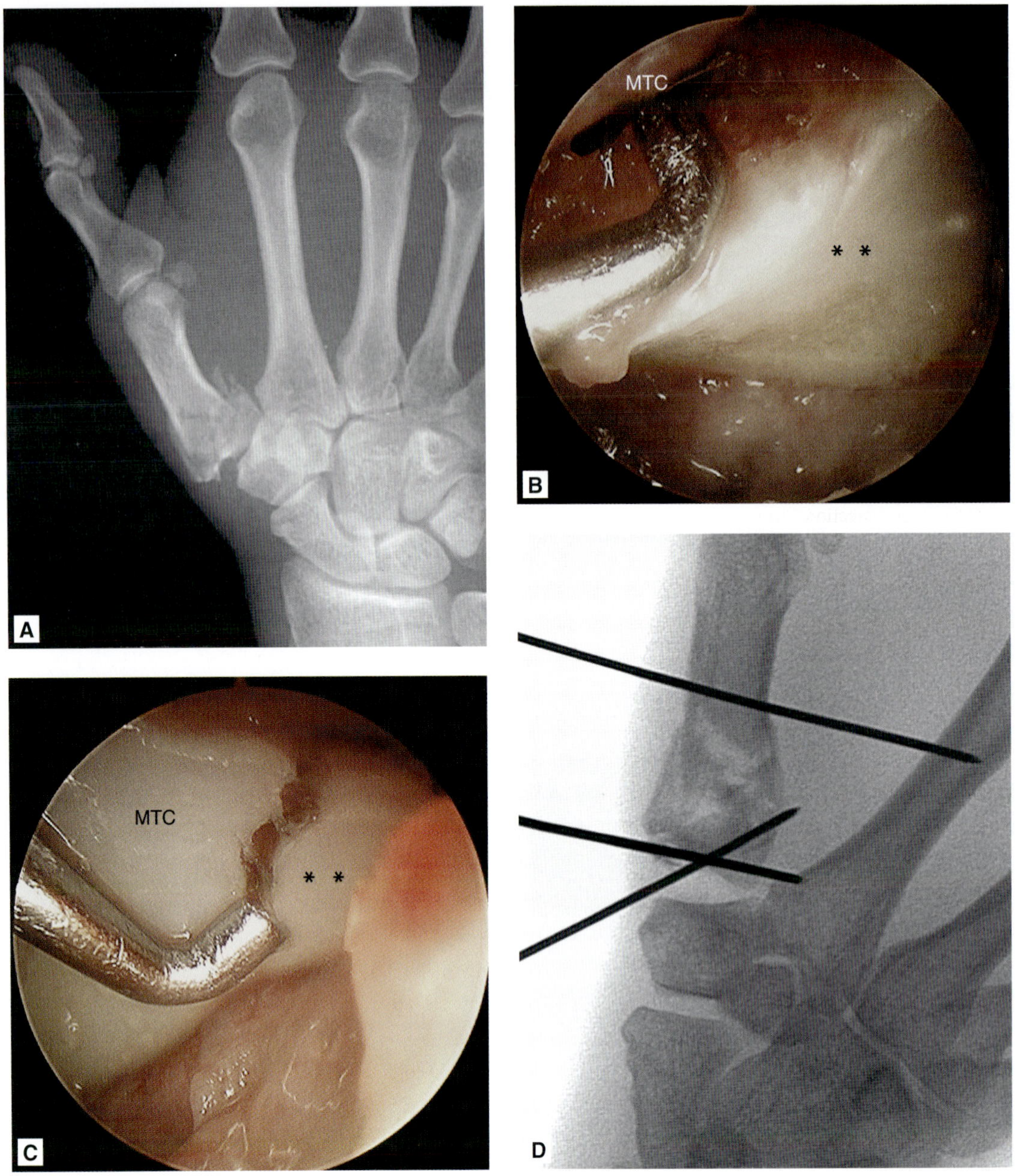

FIGURE 4-11 **A.** AP x-ray of a Rolando fracture. **B.** Arthroscopic view of the volar fracture line through the 1-U portal. **C.** Reduction of volar-ulnar fragment (*). MTC, metacarpal shaft. **D.** The radial articular fragment is reduced with ligamentotaxis by K-wiring the distracted thumb metacarpal to the index metacarpal.

of intracarpal structures. A motorized 2.9-mm full radius resector is needed for debridement of hematoma as well as small curettes and a dental hook for manipulation of the fracture fragments. The procedure is done under fluoroscopic control. The relevant landmarks are outlined including the proximal and dorsal edge of the fifth MC base, the ECU tendon, and, if possible, the extensor tendons to the small and ring fingers. The procedure is performed with a tourniquet elevated to 250 mm Hg. It is my preference to use a dry technique with intermittent saline irrigation through the scope using a 10-cm^3 syringe and suction using the full radius resector as previously described. Two main portals are used (Fig. 4-12A and B). There is an ulnar portal or fifth metacarpohamate portal (5-MH) that is located between the fifth MC ulnar-side base–hamate ligament and the extensor digiti quinti tendon, at the level of CMC joint. The RP, or the fourth metacarpohamate portal (4-MH), is just radial to the fourth MC ulnar-side base–hamate ligament extensor tendon to the ring finger. Each joint is localized with a 22-gauge needle followed by injection of 2 cm^3 of saline. This step may be facilitated by fluoroscopy. A small transverse skin incision is made followed by wound spread technique with tenotomy

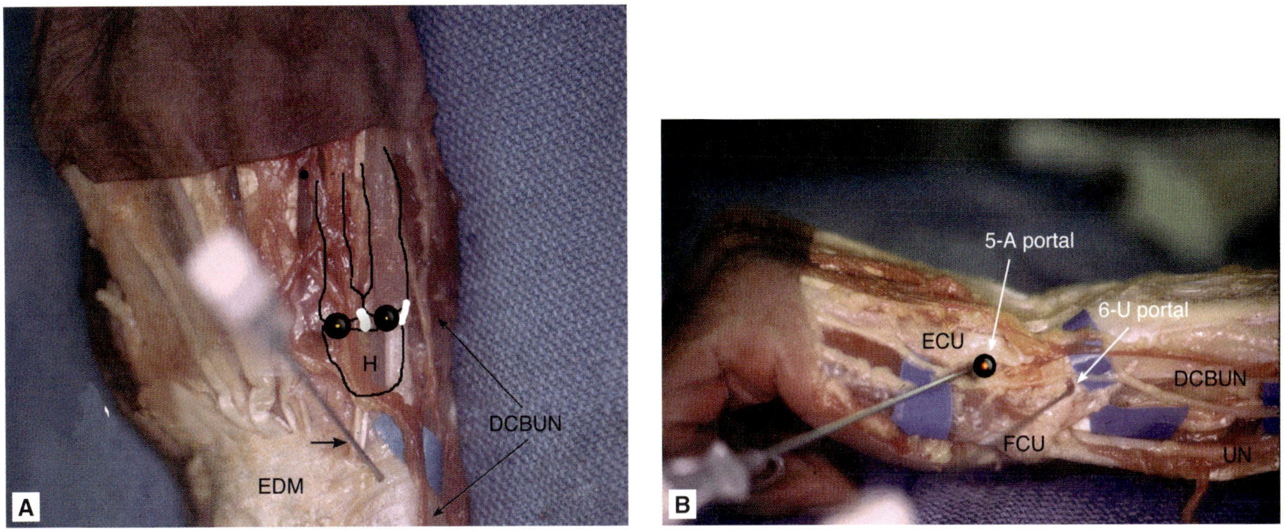

FIGURE 4-12 **A.** Cadaver dissection demonstrating the position of the 2 dorsal arthroscopy portals at the base of the fourth and fifth metacarpal bases (radio buttons) in relation to the metacarpohamate ligaments (in white). DCBUN, dorsal cutaneous branch of the ulnar nerve; EDM, extensor digiti minimi; H, hamate. **B.** Lateral view demonstrating the relative position of the 5-A (accessory) portal that is located at the level of the fifth CMC joint, volar to the extensor carpi ulnaris (ECU). FCU, flexor carpi ulnaris; UN, ulnar nerve.

scissors. The capsule is pierced and a cannula and a blunt trocar are inserted, followed by the arthroscope. The portals are interchangeably used to systematically inspect the joint, which is facilitated by judicious use of a 2.9-mm resector. An accessory portal (5-A) can facilitate triangulation and is located along the ulnar base of the fifth MC just dorsal to the hypothenar muscles and approximately 1 cm distal to the 6-U wrist arthroscopy portal. There is no internervous plane and injury to the dorsal cutaneous branch of the ulnar nerve is a risk with all of these portals; hence, careful wound spread technique is mandatory. The dorsal subluxation of the fifth MC base can be reduced by inserting a Freer elevator through the 5-MH portal at the base of the fifth MC (Fig. 4-13A-G). The 4-MH portal is established as described followed by insertion of the blunt trocar and cannula, and then the arthroscope. A 2.9-mm full radius resector is inserted through the 5-MH portal and interchanged with a curette for debridement of the fracture debris. The 4-MH can be used as the viewing portal with the 5-MH as the working portal. A 0.045-mm K-wire can be inserted into the volar articular fragment and the MC base and used to manipulate the fragments. The volar articular fragment often remains attached to the fourth MTC base through an intact intermetacarpal ligament. This prevents displacement of the volar articular fragment, similar to the Bennett fracture fragment that remains attached to the first intermetacarpal ligament. A useful maneuver is to pull the volar articular fragment dorsally with the dental pick while pushing volarly on the MC base to reduce the fracture gap. Prepositioned K-wires inserted in both of the fracture fragments are then advanced to capture the reduction. It is often necessary to cross-pin the fifth CMC joint to the hamate or capitate for 4 to 6 weeks to prevent recurrent dorsal subluxation.

Postoperatively, the small and ring fingers are immobilized in a finger spica splint for 4 weeks followed by protected finger motion. If the fixation is stable, passive and active MP joint flexion can be instituted early on. The K-wires are removed at 6 weeks. Strengthening ensues once motion has been restored. Clenched fist striking, and contact and ball sports are allowed at 12 weeks but may be permitted sooner if a playing cast or orthosis is used.

Complications

Potential complications of this procedure include injury to the DCBUN that cloak the operative field. Direct or indirect extensor tendon injury or postoperative extensor tendon adhesions can be minimized by careful operative technique during the establishment of the portals and insertion of the K-wires and by the institution of early finger motion. Iatrogenic articular damage can be minimized by using small joint instruments and joint distraction. Recurrent dorsal subluxation of the fifth MC base can be minimized by temporary K-wire fixation of the fifth CMC joint to allow ligamentous healing as well as internal fixation of any significant-sized dorsal hamate rim fractures. The use of arthroscopy provides a magnified view of the fracture line as well as the ability to directly visualize the quality of the articular reduction. Akin to other joints, however, an anatomic reduction of the articular surface is desirable, but there are no data to establish that this results in improved clinical outcomes. Long-term follow-up is unavailable as yet; hence, this procedure should be viewed as a useful adjunctive technique in the treatment of a fracture–dislocation of the fifth carpometacarpal joint, but it is unlikely to supplant the more time-tested open procedures.

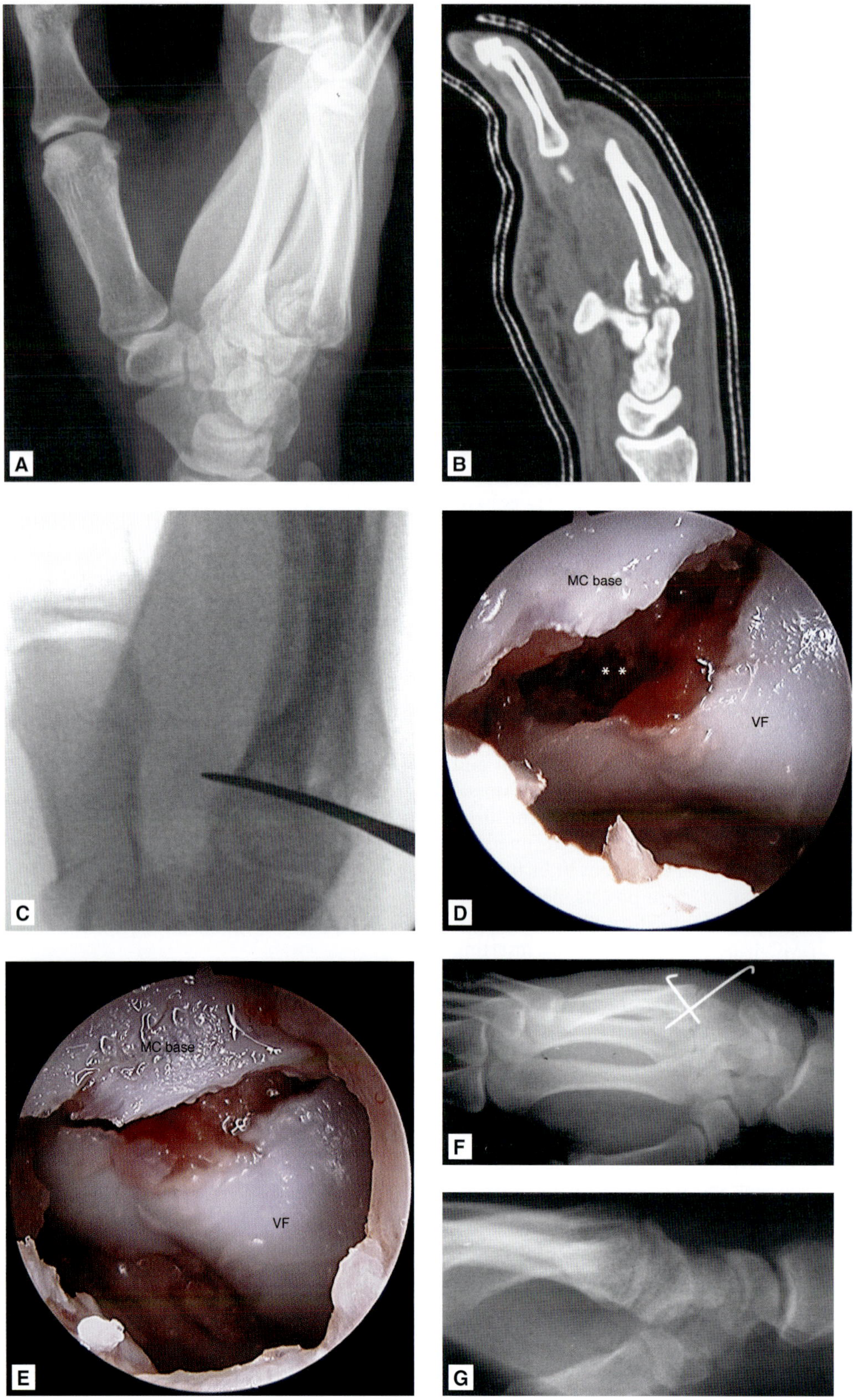

FIGURE 4-13 **A.** Lateral view of a fracture–dislocation of the fifth metacarpal CMC joint as a comminuted dorsal. **B.** Lateral CT scan demonstrating the volar articular fragment. **C.** Percutaneous insertion of a Freer elevator. **D.** View of the volar articular fragment (VF) of the fifth metacarpal base with the scope in the 4-MH portal demonstrating the fracture gap. MC base, dorsal metacarpal base. **E.** Reduction of the fracture gap. **F.** 15° pronation oblique view highlighting the reduction of the dorsal subluxation of the fifth metacarpal base. **G.** Lateral view at 6 weeks after K-wire removal showing an anatomic union of the fracture fragments.

SCAPHOTRAPEZIAL JOINT ARTHROSCOPY

Scaphotrapeziotrapezoidal Joint Portal Anatomy

STT-U PORTAL

Bowers and Whipple have described a scaphotrapezial joint (STT-U) portal that they used to aid arthroscopic resections of the distal scaphoid with STT OA. They used this portal in conjunction with the MCR. The STT-U portal is located in line with the midshaft axis of the index MC, just ulnar to the EPL.[35] Entry into this portal requires traction on the index finger. Leaving the EPL to the radial side of the STT portal protects the radial artery in the snuffbox from injury.

STT-R PORTAL

A RP for STT arthroscopy (STT-R) has been described.[36] This portal is radial to the APL tendon at the level of the STT joint. Access to the joint is eased by use of a 1.9-mm 30° angled arthroscope. Cadaver dissections demonstrated that maintaining a position palmar and radial to the APL tendon at the STT joint level avoids the radial artery by a mean of 8.8 mm (range 6-10 mm). As with the 1-/,2 portal, branches of the SRN virtually surround the arthroscopic field; hence, blunt dissection of the capsule and knowledge of the regional anatomy are essential. Ashwood et al used a portal that was radial to the EPL tendon along with the MCR for arthroscopic debridement of isolated STT OA.[37] They recommended a 1.5-cm skin incision to enable safe blunt dissection.

STT-P PORTAL

Baré et al described another accessory palmar portal (STT-P) based on a dissection of 10 cadaver arms.[38] They identified a safe portal of entry that was midway between the radial styloid and the base of the first MC, 3 mm ulnar to the APL tendon and 6 mm radial to the scaphoid tubercle. The trocar is inserted into the STT joint aiming toward the base of the fifth MC while holding the thumb in extension and adduction. This portal lay 7.6 mm (5-11 mm) from the radial artery, 6.5 mm (4-11 mm) from the superficial branch of the radial artery, and 11.6 mm (3-20 mm) from the closest radial sensory nerve branch.

Surgical Technique for an Arthroscopic Distal Scaphoid Resection

The patient is positioned supine under general anesthesia with the arm abducted, under tourniquet control. The thumb is suspended by finger traps with 10 lb of countertraction. I prefer to use a 2.7-mm 30° angled scope along with a camera attachment, although a 1.9-mm scope may be substituted until after the space has been partially decompressed. A 3-mm hook probe is needed for palpation. If there is the clinical suspicion of a coexisting scapholunate instability as manifested by radial-sided wrist pain and a positive Watson test, a standard wrist arthroscopy is performed and any scapholunate ligament pathology is addressed. It is common to enter the TM joint by mistake; hence, patience and gentle persistence are requisite. Intraoperative fluoroscopy is employed to assess the adequacy of bone resection and for locating the portals as needed. The STT-U portal is localized by finding the STT joint with a 22-gauge needle just ulnar to the EPL tendon, in line with the index MC. Two cubic centimeters of saline is injected followed by a small skin incision to aid in locating the joint and to inflate the joint that lessens the risk of chondral injury during insertion of the instruments. More recently, however, I perform the initial joint inspection without fluid in many instances. Tenotomy scissors are used to spread the soft tissues and pierce the capsule, and then a cannula and a blunt trocar are inserted, followed by the arthroscope. An identical procedure is used to establish the STT-P portal that is identified roughly 3 mm ulnar to the APL tendon and 6 mm radial to the scaphoid tubercle (Fig. 4-14A-D). Portal placement can be aided by advancing the scope through the STT-U portal, across the joint until it lights up the capsular interval. The angle between the 2 portals is 130° that improves triangulation. Both portals are interchangeable for viewing and for instrumentation.

The joint debridement is debrided using a combination of a full radius resector and a thermal probe. Once any residual articular cartilage has been removed, a 2.9-mm burr is applied to the distal scaphoid in a to-and-fro manner. The bony resection is limited to 3 to 4 mm in an attempt to preserve the insertion of the scaphotrapezial ligaments and to lessen the risk of a symptomatic DISI deformity. The diameter of the burr, along with fluoroscopy, provides a gauge as to the amount of bony resection. When there is coexisting TM OA, a double arthroscopic resection can be performed.

Complications

An inadequate excision of the distal scaphoid articular surface can lead to residual scaphotrapezial impingement and persistent pain. For this reason, many authors recommend excision of one-fourth of the distal scaphoid. Radial artery injury in the snuffbox is a risk as well as trauma to the SRN branches that can result in a symptomatic neuroma formation. The development of a dorsal midcarpal instability may lead to persistent wrist pain due to painful dorsal subluxation of the capitate (Fig. 4-9A-D).[9] This is particularly frequent among patients whose STT osteoarthritis has been caused by a chronic inflammatory process, such as chondrocalcinosis or rheumatoid arthritis, in whom the carpus was already malaligned before excision of the distal scaphoid.[39] Another possible complication, in cases where a pyrocarbon implant has been used as spacer, is a dislocation of the implant. The most usual direction of the subluxation is toward the anteromedial corner of the joint, where it is likely to impinge against the FCR tendon,

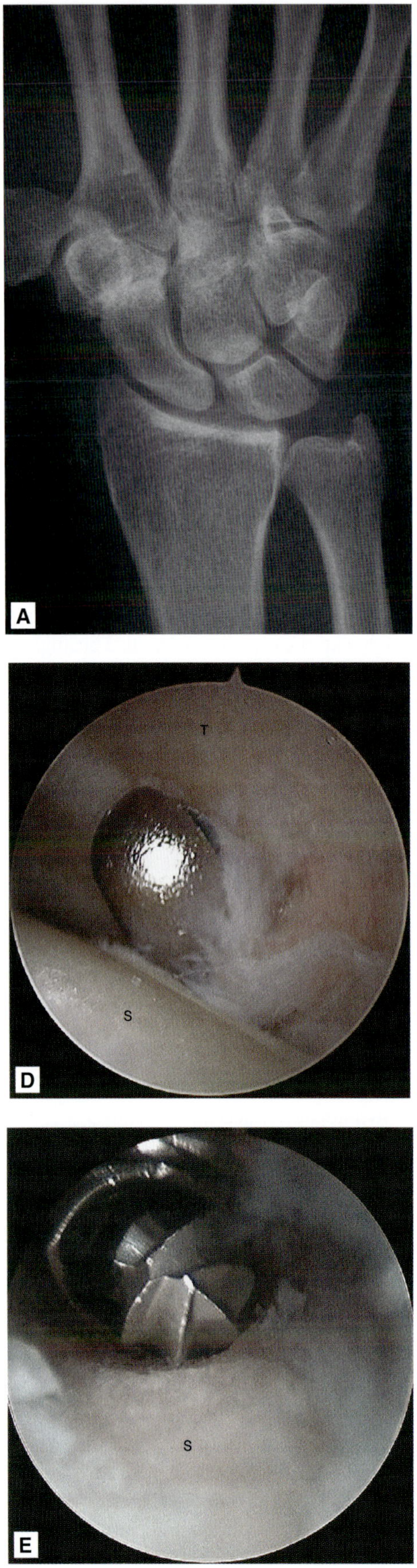

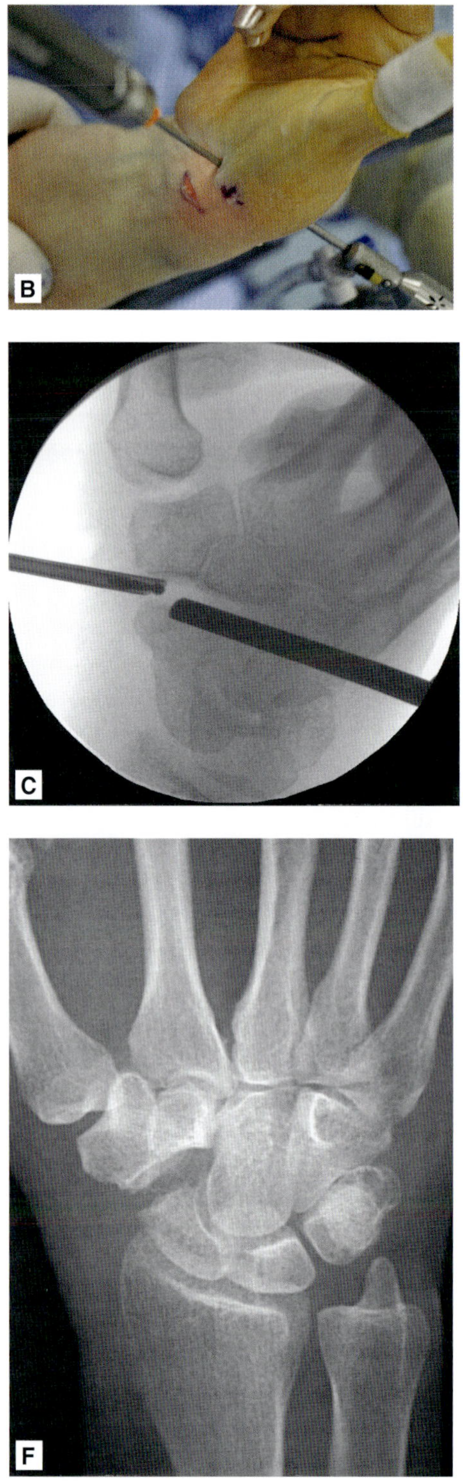

FIGURE 4-14 A. AP x-ray revealing narrowing of the STT joint and sclerosis. **B.** Insertion of an arthroscopic shaver in the STT-P portal with the scope in the STT-U portal. **C.** Fluoroscopic view. **D.** View from the STT-U portal with a resector in the STT-P portal. Note the marked loss of cartilage on the scaphoid (S) and proximal trapezium (T). **E.** A 2.9-mm burr is used to resect the distal scaphoid (S) down to cancellous bone. **F.** Postoperative x-ray.

or toward the anterolateral aspect of the scaphoid where it will irritate the SRN branches and may cause pain. In 1 series, subluxation of the implant was due to an inadequate resection of the distal pole that left a medial bone "wall" responsible for inadequate insertion of the implant.[40]

Outcomes

Ashwood et al reported their results with arthroscopic debridement of the scaphotrapezial joint without distal resection in 10 consecutive patients.[37] Good or excellent subjective results were achieved in 9 patients at final review at an average of 36 months (12-65 months). All patients showed a reduction in visual analogue pain scores, which improved from a mean of 86 to 14 points. The mean Green and O'Brien wrist scores improved from 63 to 91. Tham and Dagge performed an arthroscopic resection of the distal scaphoid and tendon interposition for isolated STT OA in 7 patients (average age 58 years).[41] At a mean follow-up of 13.3 months (7-21 months), 5 patients described no pain or mild intermittent activity-related pain. The preoperative average VAS of 7.4 improved to a postoperative average of 0.2. There was no change in wrist motion and the mean grip strength increased from 12 to 26 kg and key pinch strength from 4 to 7.6 kg. There were 2 failures due to persistent pain resulting from an inadequate resection of the distal scaphoid. Radiographically, there were no cases of worsening of the radiolunate angle. Cobb et al recently reported a series of 34 patients who underwent a combined arthroscopic resection arthroplasty for stage IV disease, with interposition of acellular allograft skin (GraftJacket, Wright Medical, Arlington, Tennessee) in 23 cases.[21] At a minimum of 1-year follow-up, the pain score had diminished from a mean of 7 to 1, the DASH scores had improved from a mean of 51 to 19, and the key pinch increased by a mean 1.3 kg. There were no apparent differences between interposition and resection arthroplasty, but the numbers are too small to draw firm conclusions. Radiographs to rule out a secondary DISI posture and long-term outcomes were not as yet available.

Most of the data on the use of pyrocarbon spacers come from Europe since they are not FDA approved in North America. Pequignot et al[42] inserted a discoid pyrocarbon implant (STPI®, Bioprofile-Tornier, Grenoble, France) following an open distal scaphoid excision in 15 patients (mean age 65 years) for the treatment of STT OA. At a mean follow-up of 4 years (range, 1-8 years) the VAS improved from an average of 8.5 to 2. There was a minimal loss of radial deviation (<10°) and extension (<15°). Grip strength was similar to the normal side and there was a slight decrease in pinch strength (0.8 kg). There were no implant dislocations and no instances of a DISI deformity. Similarly favorable results were reported in another small series of 10 patients each with short-term follow-ups of 2 to 35 months, following an open or combined open/arthroscopic approach.[43]

Da Rin and Mathoulin performed arthroscopic resections of 2 to 3 mm of the distal pole of the scaphoid for isolated STT OA in 26 women.[40] Thirteen patients had an open insertion of a pyrolytic carbon STT spacer (average age 62 years) and 13 had no interposition (average age 58 years). The longest follow-up was 4 years. The Green and O'Brien score improved from an average of 50 preoperatively to 90 postoperatively in patients without the spacer and pinch increased from 5 to 15 kg, which compared favorably with the spacer.

REFERENCES

1. Sekiya I, Kobayashi M, Okamoto H, et al. Arthroscopic synovectomy of the metacarpophalangeal and proximal interphalangeal joints. *Tech Hand Up Extrem Surg.* 2008;12:221–225.
2. Ryu J, Fagan R. Arthroscopic treatment of acute complete thumb metacarpophalangeal ulnar collateral ligament tears. *J Hand Surg Am.* 1995;20:1037–1042.
3. Choi AK, Chow EC, Ho PC, et al. Metacarpophalangeal joint arthroscopy: indications revisited. *Hand Clin.* 2011;27:369–382.
4. Imaeda T, An KN, Cooney WP 3rd, et al. Anatomy of trapeziometacarpal ligaments. *J Hand Surg Am.* 1993;18:226–231.
5. Bettinger PC, Linscheid RL, Berger RA, et al. An anatomic study of the stabilizing ligaments of the trapezium and trapeziometacarpal joint. *J Hand Surg Am.* 1999;24:786–798.
6. Colman M, Mass DP, Draganich LF. Effects of the deep anterior oblique and dorsoradial ligaments on trapeziometacarpal joint stability. *J Hand Surg Am.* 2007;32:310–317.
7. Bettinger PC, Smutz WP, Linscheid RL, et al. Material properties of the trapezial and trapeziometacarpal ligaments. *J Hand Surg Am.* 2000;25:1085–1095.
8. Hagert E, Lee J, Ladd AL. Innervation patterns of thumb trapeziometacarpal joint ligaments. *J Hand Surg Am.* 2012;37:706–714.e1.
9. Edmunds JO. Current concepts of the anatomy of the thumb trapeziometacarpal joint. *J Hand Surg Am.* 2011;36:170–182.
10. Ladd AL, Lee J, Hagert E. Macroscopic and microscopic analysis of the thumb carpometacarpal ligaments: a cadaveric study of ligament anatomy and histology. *J Bone Joint Surg Am.* 2012;94(16):1468–1477.
11. Menon J. Arthroscopic management of trapeziometacarpal joint arthritis of the thumb. *Arthroscopy.* 1996;12:581–587.
12. Menon J. Arthroscopic evaluation of the first carpometacarpal joint. *J Hand Surg Am.* 1998;23:757.
13. Berger RA. A technique for arthroscopic evaluation of the first carpometacarpal joint. *J Hand Surg Am.* 1997;22:1077–1080.
14. Ropars M, Fontaine I, Morandi X, et al. Preserving the superficial branch of the radial nerve during carpometacarpal and metacarpophalangeal joint arthroscopy: an anatomical study. *Surg Radiol Anat.* 2010;32:271–276.
15. Orellana MA, Chow JC. Arthroscopic visualization of the thumb carpometacarpal joint: introduction and evaluation of a new radial portal. *Arthroscopy.* 2003;19:583–591.
16. Walsh DM, Howe TE, Johnson MI, et al. Transcutaneous electrical nerve stimulation for acute pain. *Cochrane Database Syst Rev.* 2009;(2):CD006142.
17. Tsujii M, Satonaka H, Hori K, Uemura T, Sudo A. Evaluation for usefulness and complication of thenar portal and standard portal in arthroscopic surgery of thumb trapeziometacarpal joint. In: American Society for Surgery of the Hand Annual Meeting; September 9, 2011.
18. Slutsky DJ. The use of a dorsal-distal portal in trapeziometacarpal arthroscopy. *Arthroscopy.* 2007;23:1244.e1–e4.
19. Eaton RG, Littler JW. Ligament reconstruction for the painful thumb carpometacarpal joint. *J Bone Joint Surg Am.* 1973;55:1655–1666.
20. Badia A. Trapeziometacarpal arthroscopy: a classification and treatment algorithm. *Hand Clin.* 2006;22:153–163.
21. Cobb T, Sterbank P, Lemke J. Arthroscopic resection arthroplasty for treatment of combined carpometacarpal and scaphotrapeziotrapezoid (pantrapezial) arthritis. *J Hand Surg Am.* 2011;36:413–419.
22. Poulter RJ, Davis TR. Management of hyperextension of the metacarpophalangeal joint in association with trapeziometacarpal joint osteoarthritis. *J Hand Surg Eur.* 2011;36:280–284.

23. Badia A, Riano F, Young LC. Bilateral arthroscopic tendon interposition arthroplasty of the thumb carpometacarpal joint in a patient with Ehlers-Danlos syndrome: a case report. *J Hand Surg Am*. 2005;30:673–676.
24. Landstrom JT. Radial portal tendon harvest and interposition in arthroscopic treatment of thumb basilar joint osteoarthritis. *J Hand Surg Am*. 2008;33:442–445.
25. Furia JP. Arthroscopic debridement and synovectomy for treating basal joint arthritis. *Arthroscopy*. 2010;26:34–40.
26. Hofmeister EP, Leak RS, Culp RW, et al. Arthroscopic hemitrapeziectomy for first carpometacarpal arthritis: results at 7-year follow-up. *Hand (N Y)*. 2009;4:24–28.
27. Edwards SG, Ramsey PN. Prospective outcomes of stage III thumb carpometacarpal arthritis treated with arthroscopic hemitrapeziectomy and thermal capsular modification without interposition. *J Hand Surg Am*. 2010;35:566–571.
28. Pegoli L, Parolo C, Ogawa T, et al. Arthroscopic evaluation and treatment by tendon interpositional arthroplasty of first carpometacarpal joint arthritis. *Hand Surg*. 2007;12:35–39.
29. Adams JE, Merten SM, Steinmann SP. Arthroscopic interposition arthroplasty of the first carpometacarpal joint. *J Hand Surg Eur*. 2007;32:268–274.
30. Capo JT, Kinchelow T, Orillaza NS, et al. Accuracy of fluoroscopy in closed reduction and percutaneous fixation of simulated Bennett's fracture. *J Hand Surg Am*. 2009;34:637–641.
31. Nakamura K, Patterson RM, Viegas SF. The ligament and skeletal anatomy of the second through fifth carpometacarpal joints and adjacent structures. *J Hand Surg Am*. 2001;26:1016–1029.
32. Dzwierzynski WW, Matloub HS, Yan JG, et al. Anatomy of the intermetacarpal ligaments of the carpometacarpal joints of the fingers. *J Hand Surg Am*. 1997;22:931–934.
33. Cain JE Jr, Shepler TR, Wilson MR. Hamatometacarpal fracture-dislocation: classification and treatment. *J Hand Surg Am*. 1987;12:762–767.
34. Yoshida R, Shah MA, Patterson RM, et al. Anatomy and pathomechanics of ring and small finger carpometacarpal joint injuries. *J Hand Surg Am*. 2003;28:1035–1043.
35. Bowers WH, Whipple T. Arthroscopic anatomy of the wrist. In: McGinty J, ed. *Operative Arthroscopy*. New York: Raven Press; 1991:613–623.
36. Carro LP, Golano P, Farinas O, et al. The radial portal for scaphotrapeziotrapezoid arthroscopy. *Arthroscopy*. 2003;19:547–553.
37. Ashwood N, Bain GI, Fogg Q. Results of arthroscopic debridement for isolated scaphotrapeziotrapezoid arthritis. *J Hand Surg Am*. 2003;28:729–732.
38. Baré J, Graham AJ, Tham SK. Scaphotrapezial joint arthroscopy: a palmar portal. *J Hand Surg Am*. 2003;28:605–609.
39. Garcia-Elias M, Lluch A. Partial excision of scaphoid: is it ever indicated? *Hand Clin*. 2001;17:687–695, x.
40. Da Rin F, Mathoulin C. Arthroscopic treatment of osteoarthritis of scaphotrapezotrapezoid joint. *Chir Main*. 2006;25(suppl 1):S254–S258.
41. Tham SK, Dagge B. Arthroscopic resection of distal scaphoid and tendon interposition for isolated scaphotrapezial trapezoid arthritis. In: Slutsky DJ, ed. *Principles and Practice of Wrist Surgery*. Philadelphia, PA: Elsevier Inc; 2010.
42. Pequignot JP, D'Asnieres de Veigy L, Allieu Y. Arthroplasty for scaphotrapeziotrapezoidal arthrosis using a pyrolytic carbon implant. Preliminary results. *Chir Main*. 2005;24:148–152.
43. Low AK, Edmunds IA. Isolated scaphotrapeziotrapezoid osteoarthritis: preliminary results of treatment using a pyrocarbon implant. *Hand Surg*. 2007;12:73–77.

5

Nonunions and Malunions of the Metacarpals and Phalanges

Meredith Larsen, MD
Michael S. Bednar, MD

RATIONALE AND BASIC SCIENCE PERTINENT TO THE PROCEDURE

Nonunions of the Metacarpals and Phalanges

Nonunion is a rare complication after metacarpal or phalangeal fractures. Its incidence has been reported at 0.7% in the metacarpal shaft[1] and 0.2% in the phalanges and metacarpals.[2] Nonunions tend to occur in association with more severe injury, including infection, nerve damage, or substantial bone or soft tissue loss.[3]

Jupiter et al defined delayed union and nonunion as those metacarpal and phalangeal fractures that fail to demonstrate clinical and radiographic signs of healing within 4 months from injury.[3] In their review of 100 consecutive phalangeal (finger and toe) fractures, Smith and Rider described radiographic healing occurring up to 14 months after injury.[4] These authors found the average time to radiographic union was 5 months, whereas clinical healing was evident in just one-fourth of that time. Based on the variability of radiographic healing, they concluded that a fracture should not be deemed a nonunion until 12 months from injury.[4] Clinical indicators of nonunion include gross fracture instability or hardware failure (in cases of operative treatment). Persistent pain, however, is a less reliable sign as it may originate from other etiologies such as stiffness or nerve injury.

An atrophic nonunion of the metacarpal or phalanx is more common than a hypertrophic nonunion, and demonstrates little or no callus at the fracture site.[3,5] Atrophic nonunion occurs in the setting of infection, bone loss, or with operative treatment that leaves the fracture site distracted, dysvascular, or with inadequate stability (Fig. 5-1). Treatment includes debridement of infection or interposed fibrous tissue from the nonunion site, bone grafting of areas of bone loss, and stable fixation. Jupiter et al reported 100% union rates in 17 metacarpal and phalangeal nonunions treated with plate and screw or K-wire fixation. The K-wire group, on average, lost motion postoperatively while the digits treated with lag screws and plate fixation demonstrated gains in motion. These authors felt the benefits of rigid fixation included the ability to perform a concomitant tenolysis and arthrolysis, and allowed for early postoperative range of motion.[3]

Infected nonunions are treated with debridement of the soft tissues and fracture site, as well as intravenous antibiotics. Bony length and alignment can be maintained with an external fixator, bone cement, or a K-wire spacer during this time. When the nonunion site is free of infection, definitive bone grafting and internal fixation can be undertaken.[5]

Hypertrophic nonunion reflects insufficient fracture stability secondary to inadequate immobilization, poor fracture fixation, or soft tissue interposition at the fracture site (Fig. 5-2). Attempts at bone healing are indicated by the presence of fracture callus. Rigid stabilization with lag screws or compression plating is essential to foster bony union. The use of bone graft is not always necessary.[6]

Treatment aimed at achieving bony union is appropriate for digits that will be functional after bony healing. Amputation may be preferred for a nonunion where there is permanent sensory loss of the involved finger, chronic infection, severe joint contracture, or poor soft tissue coverage. Such a nonunion may cause stiffness at adjacent digits and jeopardize the overall hand function.[3,5] Arthrodesis may be appropriate for intra-articular and periarticular nonunions complicated by severe joint stiffness that is unlikely to improve even after obtaining bony union. Arthrodesis necessitates debridement of the nonunion site, removal of articular cartilage from the adjacent joint, and fixation that crosses both the nonunion site and the joint. Bone grafting may or may not be necessary.[5] Fixation options include K-wires, intraosseous wiring, or plate and screws. Nonunions of the distal phalanx, especially the tuft, can be asymptomatic and may not require treatment.

Indications

Operative treatment of metacarpal or phalangeal nonunions is appropriate for digits in which dexterity or hand function can realistically be improved, that is, those with intact flexor

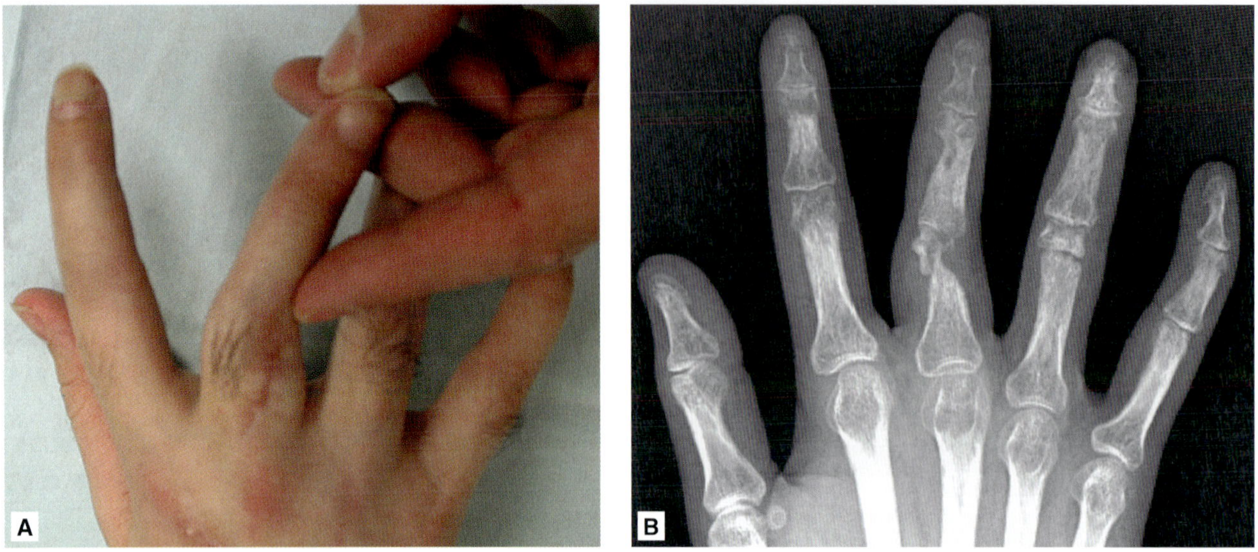

FIGURE 5-1 Atrophic nonunion. **A.** Grossly unstable digit. **B.** Radiographs demonstrate lack of bony consolidation at the middle finger proximal phalanx after open fracture complicated by osteomyelitis. (A and B from Balaram AK, Bednar MS. Complications after the fractures of metacarpal and phalanges. *Hand Clin*. 2010;26:169–177, with permission. Copyright Elsevier.)

and extensor tendons and intact neurovascular structures. The risks and benefits of surgery, as well as the patient's functional goals, must be carefully considered. Candidates must be medically fit to undergo surgery and be willing to comply with postoperative therapy.[5,7]

Surgical repair of a nonunion may occur when both clinical exam and radiographs point toward a diagnosis of nonunion.

Contraindications

Absolute contraindications to surgical treatment include those patients who are unable or unwilling to comply with an aggressive postoperative therapy program, especially when capsulotomy or tenolysis is planned. Amputation or arthrodesis may be the preferred treatment for a nonunion

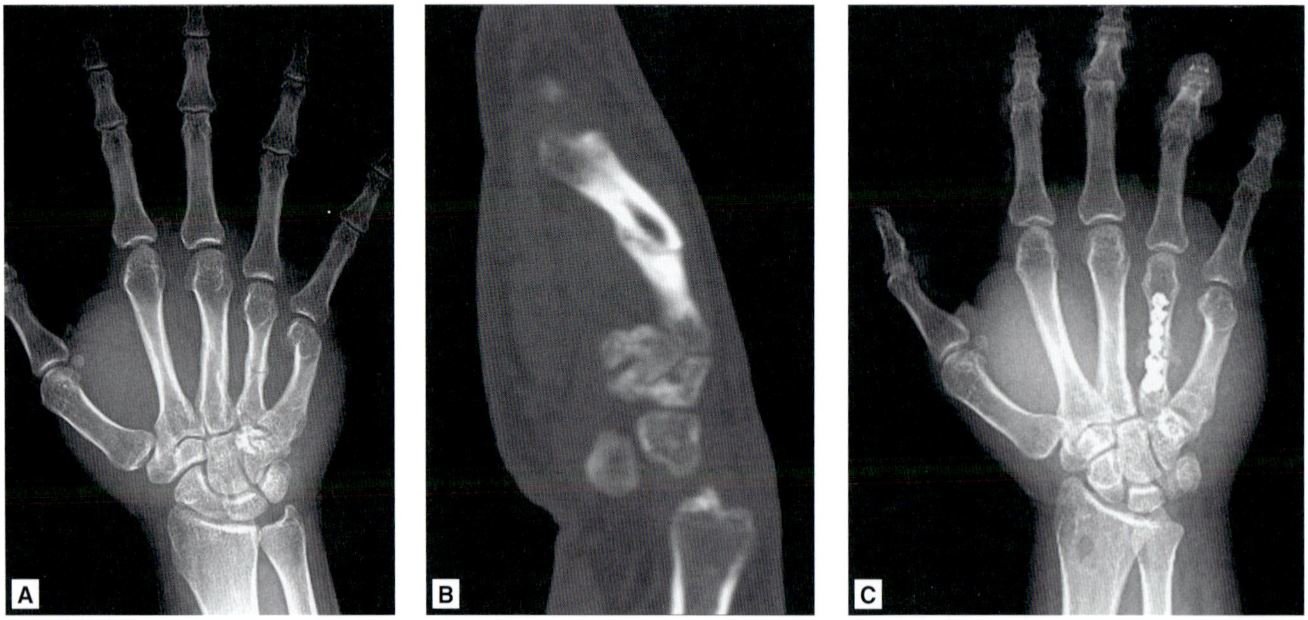

FIGURE 5-2 Hypertrophic nonunion. **A.** Radiograph taken 3 months after ring finger metacarpal shaft fracture. Little fracture site callus is present. **B.** CT scan demonstrating metacarpal nonunion. **C.** Treatment consisted of nonunion debridement and rigid internal fixation with plate and screws. (A–C from Balaram AK, Bednar MS. Complications after the fractures of metacarpal and phalanges. *Hand Clin*. 2010;26:169–177, with permission. Copyright Elsevier.)

with severe contracture or arthrosis when bony union alone is not expected to improve the function of the digit or hand. Infected nonunions must be adequately debrided and free from infection prior to definitive fixation.

Surgical Technique

The patient is positioned supine with the upper extremity on a hand table, and placed under a general anesthesia. A well-padded, nonsterile tourniquet is placed high in the axilla. Intraoperative imaging is essential for bony fixation. A mini C-arm fluoroscopy unit is draped sterile and utilized from the axillary side of the hand table.

ATROPHIC NONUNIONS

An atrophic nonunion with bone loss at the level of the metacarpal or the proximal end of proximal phalanx can be approached from a dorsal midline skin incision over the nonunion site. Full thickness skin flaps are created and the extensor tendon is retracted to the side for the metacarpal nonunion, or is split longitudinally and retracted radially and ulnarly in the approach to the proximal phalangeal nonunion. The periosteum is incised and elevated, and the nonunion site is debrided of fibrous tissue or infection with a curette and dental pick. Nonunion site cultures are obtained, and then intraoperative antibiotics may be administered. Bony loss is grafted with autogenous cancellous bone from the distal radius or iliac crest. A 1.0-mL tuberculin syringe can be used to compress the cancellous bone into a semisolid core to fill bony defects.[5] Rigid plating is performed with 6 cortices of fixation on either side of the nonunion. An MP and/or PIP joint capsulotomy and extensor and/or flexor tenolysis are performed if necessary.[3,6] The periosteum is closed over the plate with an absorbable suture, the extensor tendon is repaired, and the overlying skin is closed with a nonabsorbable suture.

Repair of nonunions of the distal half of the proximal phalanx is undertaken from a midaxial skin incision extending from the PIP joint flexion crease to the distal metacarpophalangeal (MCP) flexion crease. The subcutaneous tissues are elevated, with care taken to identify and retract the digital neurovascular bundle palmarly. The oblique fibers of the lateral band are retracted dorsally to expose the nonunion. The periosteum is elevated and the nonunion site is cultured, bone grafted, and stabilized as described above. At the level of the middle phalanx, a midaxial skin incision extending from the DIP to the PIP flexion crease is utilized. After the subcutaneous tissues are elevated and the digital neurovascular bundle is retracted, the transverse retinacular ligament is divided along the midaxial line, while protecting the underlying collateral ligament with a dental pick. The dorsal aspect of the transverse retinacular ligament and the lateral band are elevated dorsally and the palmar retinacular ligament is tagged with suture and retracted in a palmar direction for access to the nonunion site. After the nonunion is repaired, the transverse retinacular ligament is reapproximated prior to wound closure.

An infected nonunion requires surgical debridement of all devitalized bone and soft tissue, as well as intravenous antibiotic treatment. Areas of bone loss can be held out to length with an external fixator, bone cement, or a K-wire spacer until definitive fixation. Bone grafting and bony fixation with a plate and screws should take place once all infection is eradicated.

HYPERTROPHIC NONUNIONS

Plate and screw stabilization for hypertrophic nonunions of the metacarpal or proximal half of the proximal phalanx is performed through a dorsal approach, whereas repair of distal proximal phalangeal and middle phalangeal nonunions is approached through a midaxial incision. In this case, the nonunion is debrided with a dental pick and curette only to the extent that a reduction can be obtained, and is then compressed with a plate and screw construct with 6 cortices of fixation on either side of the nonunion. Bone grafting is not necessary. The periosteum is closed over the plate, if possible, with absorbable suture and the tendon is repaired with a nonabsorbable suture. The skin is closed with a nonabsorbable suture. Generally, the implant used should be 1 size larger than that used for acute fracture fixation (eg, a 2.0-mm instead of a 1.5-mm implant for the proximal phalanx) and remain in place indefinitely unless tendon or soft tissue irritation occurs.[5] Periarticular nonunions may be best treated with a T-shaped locking plate or condylar blade plate. Metacarpal and phalangeal nonunions may also be stabilized with K-wires, but there is a higher risk of failure with nonrigid fixation. Interosseous wires may increase the rigidity of the construct.

Complications

Outcomes of a nonunion repair include joint stiffness and contracture, infection, K-wire loosening or migration, intraosseous wire breakage, and plate-associated tendon irritation. Subsequent surgery may be necessary for plate removal, tenolysis, or capsulotomy.[3,7]

Outcomes

Few reports on outcomes of the treatment of metacarpal and phalangeal nonunions have been published. The series of Jupiter et al[3] from 1985 consisted of 25 delayed unions and nonunions, of which 15 were associated with crush, machine-related, or gunshot injury mechanisms. Thirteen injuries were open, and 13 had an associated tendon, soft tissue, or nerve injury. Bony union was obtained in all cases, but those nonunions treated with K-wires demonstrated a loss of motion and limited digital function. Of the 7 nonunions treated with lag screws and plates, 3 also underwent acapsulotomy and tenolysis; the average postoperative gains in motion were limited realizing that larger and bulkier implants were used and nonlocking implants were not available.

RATIONALE AND BASIC SCIENCE PERTINENT TO THE PROCEDURE

Malunions of the Metacarpals

Malunion is the most common complication after a metacarpal or phalangeal fracture.[6] The musculotendinous forces acting on the fracture fragments result in reproducible patterns of metacarpal and phalangeal deformity, including shortening, malrotation, and angulation in the sagittal and coronal planes. Such deformity may cause aesthetic as well as functional problems for the patient.

SHORTENING

Spiral and oblique fractures of the metacarpal shaft can result in shortening at the fracture site due to the intrinsic and extrinsic flexor forces acting on the distal fracture fragment. For every 2 mm of metacarpal shortening, an average 7° MCP joint extensor lag[8] and 8% loss of grip strength results.[8,9] However, the MCP joint hyperextends approximately 20°, and may compensate for metacarpal shortening up to 6 mm to achieve near-neutral MCP joint extension with little or no functional deficit or physical deformity.[8] Malunion with greater amounts of shortening may require open reduction and internal fixation with or without bone grafting for deformity correction and to regain metacarpal length.

ANGULAR DEFORMITY

Transverse and short oblique fractures of the metacarpal shaft and neck typically angulate with an apex dorsal deformity. Fractures closer to the midshaft produce greater angular deformity and are more likely to result in a metacarpal head palpable in the palm. Sagittal plane angulation of 10° to 15° in the index and middle metacarpals and 30° to 40° in the ring and small metacarpals is permissible, allowing normal digital function.[7] These functional ranges result from small amounts of carpometacarpal joint motion in the flexion–extension plane of the ring and small digits that compensate for the effects of the angular deformity at the fracture site. Deformity beyond this can be addressed with an opening or closing wedge osteotomy. An opening wedge osteotomy with cancellous bone graft is used for metacarpals with substantial shortening to restore bony anatomy.[10] Closing wedge osteotomies produce bony apposition with limited amounts of shortening, and correction of the angulation recoups some of the lost metacarpal length. Fixation of the osteotomy can be secured with a dorsal plate and screw construct with 4 cortices of fixation on each side of the fracture.

ROTATIONAL DEFORMITY

Metacarpal malrotation commonly results after spiral or oblique fractures. The cosmetic deformity can be prominent and is poorly tolerated as the entire digit is affected distal to the point of the malunion. Ten degrees of rotational deformity has been shown to result in 2 cm of digital overlap at the fingertips.[11] Deformity consisting of both rotational and angular components must be corrected at the fracture site, whereas pure rotational deformity can also be addressed at the metacarpal base. Weckesser first described a transverse osteotomy through the metaphyseal metacarpal base to derotate metacarpal and proximal phalangeal malunions.[12] This transverse osteotomy can correct 18° to 19° malrotation in the index, middle, and ring metacarpals and 20° to 30° in the small metacarpal. The degree of deformity correction is limited by the deep transverse metacarpal ligament.[13] The osteotomy is secured with a plate and screws. Alternatively, a step-cut osteotomy through the metacarpal shaft provides 8.6 mm of rotational deviation of the fingertip for each 1 mm strip of dorsal cortex removed.[11] This osteotomy produces ample bony contact for healing and can be fixed with lag screws to allow for early range of motion.[11,14]

Malunions of the Phalanges

ANGULAR DEFORMITY

An apex palmar angulation typically results after a proximal phalanx fracture. The lumbricals flex the proximal fracture fragment and the central slip of the extensor tendon extends the distal fragment, creating the characteristic deformity. Angulation with shortening can cause functional deficits, as each millimeter of proximal phalangeal shortening leads to a 12° extensor lag at the PIP joint.[15] In addition to an extensor lag and flexion contracture, palmar angulation greater than 25° to 30° limits PIP flexion.[16] Such malunions can be treated by an opening wedge osteotomy, bone grafting, and K-wire or plate fixation.[17] A closing wedge osteotomy may also be employed, utilizing the intact dorsal periosteum as a hinge. The osteotomy is stabilized with a dorsally or laterally placed plate. Coronal plane angulation may result in overlap of adjacent digits, which is not well tolerated.[18] Varus or valgus angulation should be corrected along with any other concomitant plane of deformity, often with a laterally based opening or closing wedge osteotomy (Fig. 5-3).

Middle phalangeal fractures angulate palmarly or dorsally depending on the location of the fracture with respect to the central slip of the extensor tendon and the insertion of the flexor digitorum superficialis tendon. Distal third fractures tend to result in apex palmar deformity, whereas proximal third fractures angulate dorsally.[19]

Most distal phalanx fractures are nondisplaced, as both the terminal slip of the extensor tendon and flexor digitorum profundus tendons insert on the distal aspect of the phalanx. The nail plate acts as an external splint for these fractures. Only those that are substantially displaced and unstable benefit

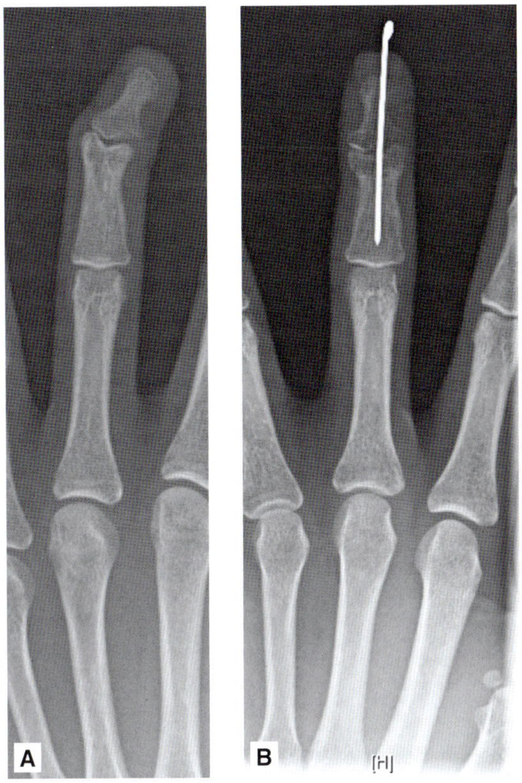

FIGURE 5-3 Intra-articular malunion of the middle finger distal interphalangeal joint. A. Varus angulation is appreciated at both the middle phalangeal condyle and the distal phalanx. B. Treatment with staged closing wedge osteotomies of the middle and distal phalanges.

from operative fixation to prevent a future nail deformity. The pediatric physeal fracture with a nail bed injury must be opened so the nail matrix trapped in the fracture site can be removed and the physis can be reduced to prevent physeal and nail deformity. The distal phalanx and DIP joint are pinned percutaneously if the fracture is unstable (Fig. 5-4).

SHORTENING

Shortening occurs with short oblique, long spiral, or comminuted fractures. Maintenance of fracture position after a closed reduction is difficult. Shortening alone is not an indication for operative treatment due to the potential complications of surgery, but shortening with angulation or malrotation may benefit from an opening wedge osteotomy with bone graft.[7] A shortened proximal phalanx fracture can result in a spike of bone that impinges on PIP joint flexion. This spike can simply be resected (Fig. 5-5).[6]

ROTATIONAL DEFORMITY

Rotational deformity of the phalanges can result after an oblique or spiral fracture and, as with the metacarpals, is poorly tolerated. Any overlap of the digits or lack of digital convergence toward the scaphoid tubercle while the patient makes a fist may indicate a rotational deformity. Malrotation can be missed if the digits are examined in the extended position, although the plane of the fingertip can determine if there is abnormal pronation or supination. An osteotomy can be performed either at the fracture site (Fig. 5-6) or at the base of the metacarpal using a transverse or modified step-cut osteotomy. The transverse osteotomy is technically easier and avoids violating the extensor tendon at the proximal phalanx level, but limited amounts of correction can be obtained.

Intra-articular Malunions

Unreduced intra-articular condyle fractures of the metacarpal and phalanx can cause deformity, joint stiffness, and pain, and may eventually culminate in posttraumatic arthritis. The treatment of intra-articular malunions remains challenging. The reconstructive options include an intra- or juxta-articular osteotomy. Young patients without signs of joint degeneration may benefit from an intra-articular osteotomy, to

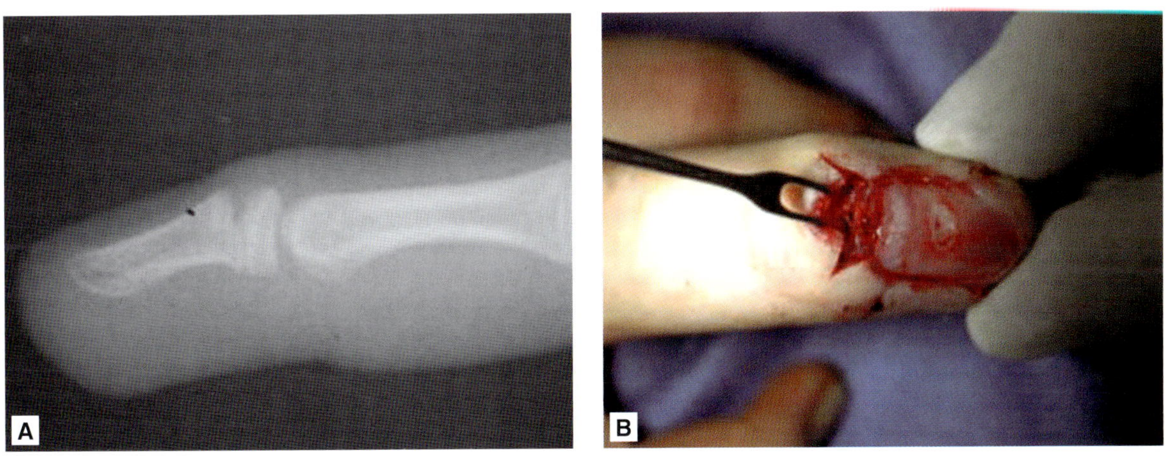

FIGURE 5-4 Adolescent Seymour fracture. A. Lateral radiograph demonstrated a physeal fracture. B. Open treatment revealed that the nail bed was interposed in the physis as well as a full thickness nail bed burn from nail plate trephination at the time of initial treatment.

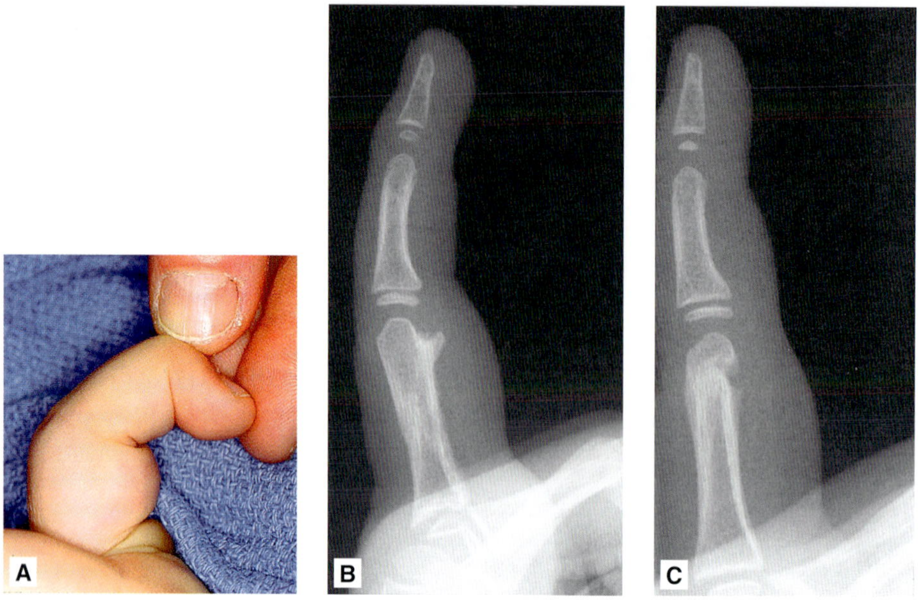

FIGURE 5-5 Middle finger proximal phalanx fracture that healed in a shortened position. **A** and **B.** The resulting volar bony spike of the proximal fragment limited PIP joint flexion. **C.** Resection of the bony spike restored full flexion.

reduce the articular surface and restore alignment (Fig. 5-7). Less commonly, these malunions occur in the sagittal plane (Fig. 5-8). An intra-articular osteotomy is technically difficult, and is ideally performed before the fracture has completely healed.[5] The osteotomy is most easily undertaken when the fracture line is visible, bone quality is good, and fracture fragments are amenable to stable fixation and early range of motion.[7,20] For a late osteotomy, Teoh et al described a condylar advancement osteotomy for mature unicondylar malunions of the proximal and middle phalanges. A wedge

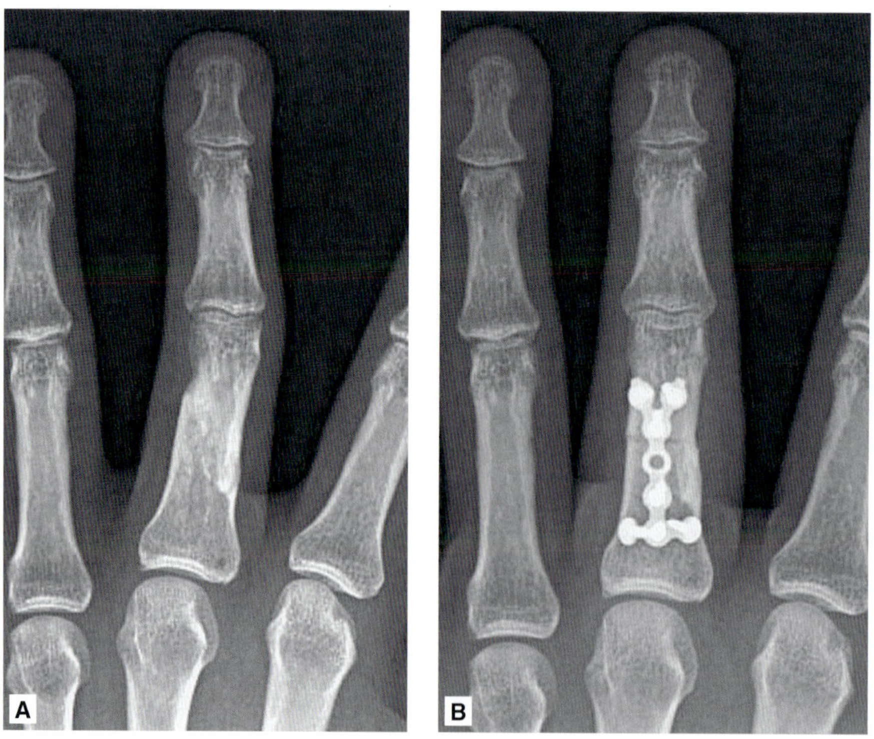

FIGURE 5-6 Rotational and angular deformity of the proximal phalanx. **A.** Radiograph demonstrating malunion with malrotation and varus angulation. **B.** Treatment with a dual-plane osteotomy and rigid internal fixation.

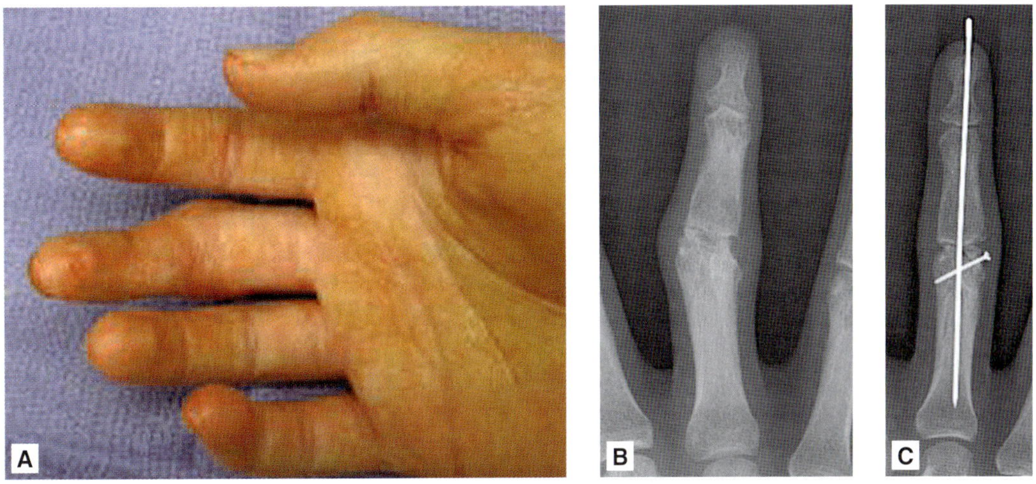

FIGURE 5-7 Intra-articular malunion of the proximal phalanx condyle. **A.** Deviation and rotation of the digit. **B.** Radiograph demonstrating the valgus deformity of the malunion. **C.** Open treatment with intra-articular osteotomy with screw and K-wire fixation to restore articular joint congruity.

of intercondylar callus is resected, followed by an osteotomy and advancement of the larger bony fragment including the malunited condyle to obtain articular congruity. This approach creates an articular bone block that is easier to realign and secure with screws.[21]

Extra-articular osteotomies correct angular and rotational deformity but do not address articular incongruity, which may leave the patient with pain and joint stiffness.[22] Interphalangeal joints with degenerative changes are less likely to benefit from an intra-articular osteotomy and may be better suited for arthrodesis.[20] The PIP and DIP joints of the fingers and IP and MCP joints of the thumb tolerate fusion well and provide satisfactory function.[23] A hemihamate osteochondral graft is also a viable treatment option for restoring PIP motion.[24]

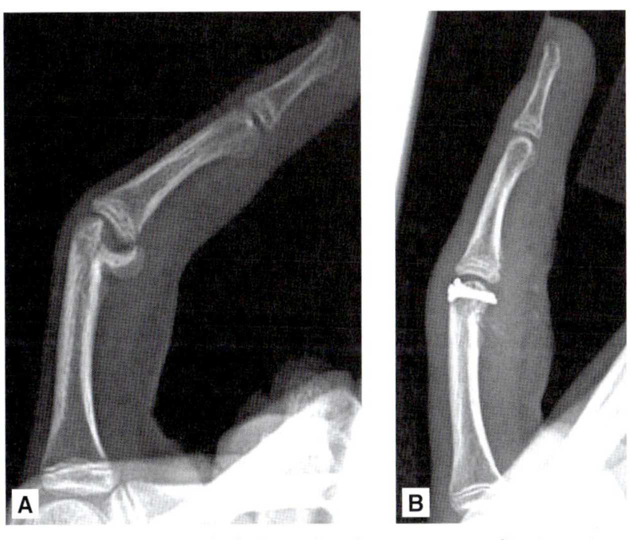

FIGURE 5-8 Proximal phalangeal malunion in a pediatric patient. **A.** Lateral radiograph demonstrating the sagittal plane malunion. **B.** Treatment with open reduction and internal fixation.

Indications

Surgical correction of a metacarpal or phalangeal malunion is appropriate for patients where digital dexterity or hand function can be realistically improved. Indications may include pain from a prominent metacarpal head, pseudoclawing, and malrotation of the fingertip greater than 10°. The risks and benefits of surgery, as well as the patient's functional goals, must be considered. Patients must be medically fit for surgery and be willing to comply with postoperative therapy.[5,7]

The timing of surgical correction for malunion shapes the treatment strategy and outcome. The osteotomy is indicated as soon as it is evident that the malunion is responsible for a functional deficit. Early intervention, before the fracture is completely healed (up to 10 weeks after injury), may allow for a takedown of immature callus to restore the original fracture site that allows for an anatomic reduction. Correction during this time period is also often prior to the development of tendon adhesions and joint contracture.[5,10] If stiffness is present or an osteotomy is not feasible early on, correction should be undertaken in a delayed fashion (at or after 3 months), when digital range of motion has plateaued after a trial of formal hand therapy.[10] Intra-articular malunions are optimally addressed when the fracture plane is visible and bone quality is adequate for solid fixation. This should take place within 4 to 6 months from injury so that damage to the articular cartilage is minimized.[25] A juxta-articular osteotomy may be performed on a late basis.[10,20]

Contraindications

Patients who are unable or unwilling to comply with an aggressive postoperative therapy program, especially when capsulotomy or tenolysis is planned, should not undergo surgical correction.

In most cases, an osteotomy should be performed only after the digital motion has plateaued. Phalangeal shortening alone is rarely an indication for a corrective osteotomy due to the risk of tendon adhesion and adjacent joint stiffness. A multiplanar deformity that includes a loss of phalangeal length is an indication for a corrective osteotomy and bone grafting to restore the bony length.[7]

Surgical Technique

The patient is positioned supine with the upper extremity on a hand table, and placed under a general anesthesia. A well-padded, nonsterile tourniquet is placed high in the axilla. A mini C-arm fluoroscopy unit is draped sterile and brought in from the axillary side of the hand table.

OPENING WEDGE OSTEOTOMY FOR SAGITTAL PLANE DEFORMITY OF THE METACARPAL AND PHALANX

Preoperative planning is critical to determine the size of the opening wedge to correct the deformity. On the lateral radiograph of an apex palmar deformity, a line is drawn parallel to the long axis of the proximal fragment and a second line is drawn parallel to the long axis of the distal fragment. Another line is drawn parallel to each of the first 2 lines. The intersection of the second 2 lines delineates the angle of the bony opening wedge to be created.[18]

A 1- to 2-cm dorsal longitudinal midline skin incision is centered over the malunion site and full thickness skin flaps are raised. Extensor tendon adhesions are lysed during the dissection. The extensor tendon is retracted to the side of the metacarpal or split in line with its fibers over the proximal phalanx. The underlying periosteum is reflected from the malunion site. The proposed bone cut is marked perpendicular to the long axis of the distal fragment. Smooth 0.045-in K-wires are placed perpendicular to the long axis of the proximal and distal fragments in a dorsal to palmar direction, at a distance from the osteotomy site. A near-complete transverse osteotomy is made parallel to the distal K-wire at the apex of the deformity from dorsal to palmar with an oscillating saw. The kerf of the saw blade should be less than 1.0 mm to minimize excessive bone resection.[17,26] The saw must be used with care to prevent a tendon injury. The palmar cortex and periosteum are left intact and the osteotomy is completed with an osteotome. The K-wires are aligned until they are parallel, creating a palmar, wedge-shaped gap in which cancellous bone graft from the distal radius or iliac crest is matched to fill the defect. The osteotomy is fixed in place with 1 or two 0.045-in smooth K-wires in an oblique fashion and the extensor tendon is repaired with nonabsorbable suture. After 3 weeks of immobilization, the K-wires are removed and active and passive finger motion is begun.

Alternatively, a dorsal miniplate may be utilized with 3 points of fixation on each side of the osteotomy. Fixation with plate and screws must be meticulous since as little as 1-mm offset in screw hole placement can lead to 10° of rotation.[10] The periosteum should be closed over the plate with absorbable suture. Locking plates should be considered for bone loss or osteopenic bone.[7] A stable plate and screw construct enables active and passive motion to begin 2 to 3 days postoperatively.

CLOSING WEDGE OSTEOTOMY FOR SAGITTAL PLANE DEFORMITY OF THE METACARPAL AND PHALANX

Preoperative planning is essential. On the lateral radiograph, a line is drawn perpendicular to both the proximal and distal joint lines. The angle formed by the intersection of these lines represents the size of the closing wedge.

A dorsal longitudinal midline skin incision is centered over the malunion site. Full thickness skin flaps are created and an extensor tenolysis is performed if needed. The extensor tendon is split in line with its fibers (over the phalanx) or retracted to the side (over the metacarpal) and the periosteum is dissected from the malunion site. Smooth 0.045-in K-wires are placed in the proximal and distal fragments in a dorsal to volar direction, parallel to the respective joint lines, to serve as reference points. The first osteotomy is a near-complete transverse osteotomy made perpendicular to joint line of the larger bone fragment with an oscillating saw,[26] leaving the palmar cortex and periosteum intact. A second near-complete osteotomy is made perpendicular to the distal joint line, with the far edge of the osteotomy ending at the tip of the first bone cut to create a wedge of bone. The resection is completed with an osteotome and the bone wedge is removed. The K-wires are brought together until the bony edges are opposed and the deformity is corrected. The osteotomy is fixed in place with 1 or 2 obliquely oriented 0.045-in smooth K-wires. The extensor tendon is repaired. The digit is immobilized for 3 weeks, and then the K-wires are removed and passive and active finger motion is begun. Fixation may also be undertaken with a dorsal compression miniplate. Loosely fixing the plate to the bone with a single screw and rotating it out of the way prior to the osteotomy simplifies the plate fixation. Three points of fixation are obtained on each side of the osteotomy. The periosteum is closed over the plate with absorbable suture, if possible. Plate and screw fixation allows postoperative finger motion to begin within 2 to 3 days. Typically, a 2.0-mm straight plate is used for the metacarpal and a 1.5-mm plate for the proximal phalanx.[18,26]

TRANSVERSE OSTEOTOMY FOR ROTATIONAL DEFORMITY OF THE METACARPAL AND PHALANX

A dorsal longitudinal skin incision is made over the metacarpal, extending 5 cm distal to the CMC joint. Full thickness skin flaps are raised, the extensor tendon paratenon is preserved, and the tendon is retracted to the side. The periosteum is dissected off the bone in line with the skin incision. A 2.0- or 2.4-mm T plate is sized and contoured to the metacarpal base. The osteotomy site is marked at the metaphyseal base. The holes in the horizontal portion of the plate are positioned over the metacarpal base so that at least 3 holes in the plate lie distal to the osteotomy site. These metacarpal base holes and the first hole distal to the osteotomy site are predrilled unicortically. An oscillating saw is used to make a transverse osteotomy at the proposed site. A 0.054-in K-wire is placed in the drill hole distal to the osteotomy to rotate the distal fragment. Optimal derotation is achieved when the patient's digits converge toward the scaphoid tuberosity with passive finger flexion. A second K-wire is passed transversely through an adjacent metacarpal into the distal fragment to hold the reduction. The first K-wire is removed and the T plate is fixed to the metacarpal base at the predrilled holes. The most proximal shaft screw is drilled and filled with a unicortical screw in a compression mode. The transverse K-wire is removed and the remaining 2 distal screws are placed. An absorbable suture is used to close the periosteum over the plate and the extensor tendon is anatomically repositioned. The skin is closed with a nonabsorbable suture and the digit is immobilized. Active finger motion is begun within 2 to 3 days after surgery with protective splinting for 3 weeks.[27]

MODIFIED STEP-CUT OSTEOTOMY FOR METACARPAL AND PHALANGEAL ROTATIONAL DEFORMITY

The metacarpal step-cut osteotomy is ideal because it affords precise correction, control of the bony fragments, a large surface area for healing, and minimal fixation with lag screws.[14] Using a step-cut allows the metacarpal to be cut by 2 hemitransverse cuts spaced 2 to 3 cm apart. The deformity is corrected through resection of a dorsal wedge of bone that connects these hemitransverse cuts. Before the surgical procedure, the amount of rotational deformity is measured. The deformity is largest at the midpoint of finger flexion and decreases as the finger moves into a fully flexed position. At the maximal point of deformity, the degree of rotation is estimated compared with the normal position of the finger. This measurement is used to determine the amount of dorsal bone resection needed for correction, with the guideline that 2 mm of resection achieves a 20° or 2-cm correction at the fingertip. The direction of the transverse step-cuts is marked on the skin before incision to help visualize the position of the cuts. A dorsal longitudinal incision is made over the metacarpal shaft of the affected finger. The extensor tendon is retracted and periosteum over the metacarpal shaft is opened longitudinally. An oscillating saw is used to make a hemitransverse cut in the proximal and distal diaphysis. Because the proximal segment of the metacarpal is fixed by ligamentous attachments to the carpus, the distal segment is rotated to achieve the correction. The distal hemitransverse cut is made in the direction of the deformity. The cuts are placed on opposite sides of the shaft, as determined by the direction of derotation, approximately 2.5 cm apart. Two parallel, dorsal longitudinal cuts are made to remove a strip of bone, leaving the volar cortex intact. The dorsal cortical gap is reduced with a pointed reduction forceps, cracking the volar cortex while keeping the periosteum intact. The digital rotation is checked with passive flexion and extension of the wrist and metacarpal joint, using the tenodesis effect on the digits. A wider strip of dorsal cortex sometimes needs to be taken to achieve full correction. Fixation is achieved with 1.5- or 2.0-mm lag screws placed in an interfragmentary manner. Digital motion is started the day after surgery, with protective splinting for comfort for 3 weeks.

INTRA-ARTICULAR OSTEOTOMY FOR MALUNION OF THE METACARPAL AND PHALANX

A dorsal longitudinal skin incision is employed, retracting the extensor tendon over the metacarpal or splitting the tendon over the phalanx. The fracture site is identified and exposed with a dental pick, Freer elevator, or small osteotome, while preserving the collateral ligaments and joint capsule. Immature callus is removed, the articular fragments are mobilized, and the joint surface is realigned. Provisional reduction is held with K-wires and fragments are fixed with intraosseous wires, K-wires, screws, or a minicondylar blade plate. A concomitant capsulotomy and tenolysis may also be performed to improve digital motion. The extensor tendon is repaired with nonabsorbable suture and the skin is closed. The digit is immobilized and K-wires are removed after 3 weeks. Solid fixation with plate and screws allows for early active range of motion.

A condylar advancement osteotomy can be used to correct a phalangeal condylar malunion. A longitudinal dorsal midline skin incision is made and the extensor tendon is split in the midline. The joint is flexed to facilitate visualization. A longitudinal midline phalangeal osteotomy is made with an oscillating saw, starting at the articular surface and extending 1 to 1.5 cm proximally. A second, transverse osteotomy is made at the distal end of the longitudinal osteotomy to create a box-shaped bony fragment that incorporates the malunited condyle. A wedge of bone lying between the osteotomy edge and the intra-articular extent of the fracture is removed from this fragment with a burr or osteotome. This additional resection corrects the malrotation and allows the bony block to lie flush against the shaft when it is advanced distally to restore the articular congruity. K-wires hold the reduction while two 1.5-mm interfragmentary screws are used to fix the bony block to the shaft. Care must be taken with the soft tissue handling to minimize the risk of avascular necrosis of the condyle. A capsulotomy may improve the passive motion. The extensor tendon is repaired and the skin is closed with a nonabsorbable suture. The digit is immobilized and early active finger range of motion is begun on the second postoperative day.[21]

Complications

Complications include infection, joint stiffness, K-wire loosening or migration, incomplete or loss of correction, and the need for additional surgery for tenolysis, implant removal, or refracture.[7,18] Risks of juxta- and intra-articular osteotomy also include collateral ligament injury and avascular necrosis of the metacarpal head.[18,25]

Outcomes

Gollamudi and Jones[22] obtained good and excellent results in 5 patients who underwent 6 metacarpal derotational osteotomies. They achieved an excellent result in 1 and fair results in 4 phalangeal malunions treated with phalangeal osteotomy fixed with intraosseous wiring. Three of the latter were intra-articular malunions treated with an extra-articular osteotomy. Jawa et al[14] reviewed 12 patients with a mean age of 32 years (range, 14-55 years) with a scissoring deformity due to a malunion who were treated with a derotational step-cut osteotomy. The average duration of follow-up was 25 months (range, 4-68 months). Seven original fractures involved the metacarpal and 5 involved the proximal phalanx. Seven of the 12 patients had their initial fractures managed surgically and 7 patients had limited range of motion before the procedure. All of the osteotomies united. All patients maintained or improved their total active motion after the osteotomy. The average preoperative total active motion of the involved digit was 214°, whereas the average postoperative total active motion was 251°. Five patients had full total active motion before the osteotomy that was unchanged by the procedure. Three patients who had limited preoperative motion regained full motion after the osteotomy. Four patients did not have full motion after treatment owing to preoperative stiffness. One patient did not achieve full deformity correction, but had acceptable alignment postoperatively with approximately 5° of rotatory malalignment. Light[20] treated 6 intra-articular PIP joint malunions with intra-articular osteotomy between 6 weeks and 1 year after injury. He demonstrated substantial gains in motion in 5 digits and a 100% bony union rate, and all patients experienced postoperative pain relief. Büchler et al[10] reviewed the results of corrective osteotomies performed in 59 phalangeal multiplanar malunions with a concomitant capsulotomy and tenolysis in half of the cases. They demonstrated a satisfactory correction in 76% of patients with net gains in motion in 89%. There were no nonunions.

REFERENCES

1. Barton NJ. Fractures of the shafts of the phalanges of the hand. *Hand.* 1979;11:119–133.
2. Borgeskov S. Conservative therapy for fractures of the phalanges and metacarpals. *Acta Chir Scand.* 1967;133:123–130.
3. Jupiter JB, Koniuch MP, Smith RJ. The management of delayed union and nonunion of the metacarpals and phalanges. *J Hand Surg Am.* 1985;10A:457–466.
4. Smith FL, Rider DL. A study of the healing of one hundred consecutive phalangeal fractures. *J Bone Joint Surg Am.* 1935;17A:91–109.
5. Ring D. Malunion and nonunion of the metacarpals and phalanges. *Instr Course Lect.* 2006;55:121–128.
6. Green DP. Complications of phalangeal and metacarpal fractures. *Hand Clin.* 1986;2:307–328.
7. Day CS, Stern PJ. Fractures of the metacarpals and phalanges. In: Wolfe SW, Hotchkiss RN, Pederson WC, Kozin SH, eds. *Green's Operative Hand Surgery.* 6th ed. Philadelphia: Elsevier Churchill Livingstone; 2011:239–290.
8. Strauch RJ, Rosenwasser MP, Lunt JG. Metacarpal shaft fractures: the effect of shortening on the extensor tendon mechanism. *J Hand Surg Am.* 1998;23A:519–523.
9. Meunier MJ, Hentzen E, Ryan M, Shin AY, Lieber RL. Predicted effects of metacarpal shortening on interosseous muscle function. *J Hand Surg Am.* 2004;29A:689–693.
10. Büchler U, Gupta A, Ruf S. Corrective osteotomy for post-traumatic malunion of the phalanges in the hand. *J Hand Surg Br.* 1996;21B: 33–42.
11. Manktelow RT, Mahoney JL. Step osteotomy: a precise rotation osteotomy to correct scissoring deformities of the fingers. *Plast Reconstr Surg.* 1981;68:571–576.
12. Weckesser EC. Rotational osteotomy of the metacarpal for overlapping fingers. *J Bone Joint Surg Am.* 1965;47A:751–756.
13. Gross MS, Gelberman RH. Metacarpal rotational osteotomy. *J Hand Surg Am.* 1985;10A:105–108.
14. Jawa A, Zucchini M, Lauri G, Jupiter J. Modified step-cut osteotomy for metacarpal and phalangeal rotational deformity. *J Hand Surg Am.* 2009;34A:335–340.
15. Vahey JW, Wegner DA, Hastings H 3rd. Effect of proximal phalangeal fracture deformity on extensor tendon function. *J Hand Surg Am.* 1998;23A:673–681.
16. Coonrad RW, Pohlman MH. Impacted fractures in the proximal portion of the proximal phalanx of the finger. *J Bone Joint Surg Am.* 1969;51A:1291–1296.
17. Froimson AI. Osteotomy for digital deformity. *J Hand Surg Am.* 1981;6A:585–589.
18. Freeland AE, Lindley SG. Malunions of the finger metacarpals and phalanges. *Hand Clin.* 2006;22:341–355.
19. Kozin SH, Thoder JJ, Lieberman G. Operative treatment of metacarpal and phalangeal shaft fractures. *J Am Acad Orthop Surg.* 2000;8:111–121.
20. Light TR. Salvage of intraarticular malunions of the hand and wrist: the role of realignment osteotomy. *Clin Orthop.* 1987;214:130–135.
21. Teoh LC, Yong FC, Chong KC. Condylar advancement osteotomy for correcting condylar malunion of the finger. *J Hand Surg Br.* 2002;27B:31–35.
22. Gollamudi S, Jones WA. Corrective osteotomy of malunited fractures of phalanges and metacarpals. *J Hand Surg Br.* 2000;25B:439–441.
23. Light TR, Bednar MS. Management of intra-articular fractures of the metacarpophalangeal joint. *Hand Clin.* 1994;10:303–314.
24. Calfee RP, Kiefhaber TR, Sommerkamp TG, Stern PJ. Hemi-hamate arthroplasty provides functional reconstruction of acute and chronic proximal interphalangeal fracture–dislocations. *J Hand Surg Am.* 2009;34A:1232–1241.
25. Duncan KH, Jupiter JB. Intraarticular osteotomy for malunion of metacarpal head fractures. *J Hand Surg Am.* 1989;14A:888–893.
26. Trumble T, Gilbert M. In situ osteotomy for extra-articular malunion of the proximal phalanx. *J Hand Surg Am.* 1998;23A:821–826.
27. Bindra RR, Burke FD. Metacarpal osteotomy for correction of acquired phalangeal rotational deformity. *J Hand Surg Am.* 2009;34A:1895–1899.

Metacarpophalangeal Joint and Proximal Interphalangeal Joint Arthroplasty

Keming Wang, MD
Evan Kowalski, BS
Kevin C. Chung, MD, MS

6A

INTRODUCTION

Metacarpophalangeal (MCP) joint and proximal interphalangeal (PIP) joint arthroplasty are common surgical treatments for patients suffering from joint pain, stiffness, and deformity. Rheumatoid arthritis, with a reported prevalence of 1% in the US population,[1] commonly requires MCP and PIP arthroplasty. Osteoarthritis has an overall prevalence of 3% to 7% in US adults,[2] and PIP joint arthroplasty may be indicated if the appropriate conditions are met. MCP joint arthroplasty, on the other hand, is rarely applied in osteoarthritis because MCP joint osteoarthritis is uncommon.

Osteoarthritis is a localized disorder, characterized by a deterioration of the articular cartilage that leads to a progressive structural and functional loss at the joint. As this deterioration occurs, the subchondral bone responds to the changes and attempts to limit the damage via endochondral ossification and the formation of osteophytes at the peripheral joint surface. The joints of the hand most commonly affected by osteoarthritis are the distal interphalangeal joints (35% of osteoarthritic subjects) and the carpometacarpal joint of the thumb (21% of osteoarthritic subjects).[3] In addition, 50% of patients with DIP involvement also have PIP joint involvement,[4] whereas MCP joint involvement is rare in osteoarthritis.

Rheumatoid arthritis is a systemic disease affecting the synovial tissue of the joints, which destroys the articular cartilage, invades the subchondral bone, and stretches the supporting flexor and extensor tendons. Unlike osteoarthritis, reparative changes are rare during the progression of rheumatoid arthritis. In addition, involvement of 1 joint can affect the balance of the flexor and extensor forces across adjacent joints, resulting in a disruption of the normal architecture of the hand and wrist. Typically, the wrist is the earliest and most frequent site of involvement in RA, in addition to the MCP and PIP joints.

In the MCP joint of the fingers, an arthroplasty is generally preferred over a joint effusion to preserve motion. The surgical options available for treatment in the PIP joints are dependent on the fingers affected. In the little and ring fingers, where motion is very important for power grip, implant arthroplasty is preferred. In contrast, in the index and middle fingers an arthrodesis is preferred as they are used mostly for chuck pinch, and there is a higher risk of implant dislocation or fracture.[5] In situations where PIP motion is desirable, however, an arthroplasty may be performed.[6]

METACARPOPHALANGEAL JOINT AND PROXIMAL INTERPHALANGEAL JOINT ARTHROPLASTY IN PATIENTS WITH OSTEOARTHRITIS

Rationale and Basic Science Pertinent to the Procedure

The typical physical findings of the osteoarthritic hand may reveal Heberden and Bouchard nodes located at the DIP and PIP joint, respectively. Early radiographic findings are characterized by joint space narrowing and osteophyte formation.[7] More advanced stages include a broadening at the base of the phalanx, increased density of the bone ends, and irregularities at the joint surfaces.[8] It should be noted that symptom severity does not always correlate with the radiographic findings, so MCP and PIP joint arthroplasty should be based on the patients' complaints and symptom severity.[7]

Pyrolytic carbon implant designs consist of modular proximal and distal components that require minimal bone resection while preserving the collateral ligaments, which makes them well suited for MCP and PIP joint arthroplasty in osteoarthritis.[9–12] Unconstrained implants,[11,13] however, are not appropriate for unstable joints. One long-term study demonstrated good patient outcomes[14] with a 16-year survival rate of 84%. A more recent paper, however, demonstrated high complication rates ranging from 37.5% to 42.9%.[15]

Indications

Indications for MCP and PIP joint arthroplasty for patients with osteoarthritis include pain at rest, loss of strength, and morning stiffness following a trial of failed conservative treatment with medication, activity modification, splinting, and intrasteroid injections.

Contraindications

Contraindications include inadequate soft-tissue coverage and recent joint infection.

Surgical Technique

The procedure is done under fluoroscopic control with the patient under regional anesthesia, in the supine position using a tourniquet inflated to 250 mm Hg. Instrumentation includes a starter awl, an oscillating saw, and an oblique osteotomy guide in addition to the instrumentation accompanying the implant system.

MCP JOINT ARTHROPLASTY

A dorsal "lazy S"–shaped incision is made over the MCP joint for a single joint arthroplasty. The radial sagittal band is incised to expose the MCP joint, and any osteophytes are excised after resecting the metacarpal head.

The starter awl is inserted into the metacarpal head to enlarge the medullary canal. The prepared canal should be parallel to the long axis of the metacarpal bone and from one-half to two-thirds of the metacarpal bone length. The proximal osteotomy guide with a 27.5° palmarly angled slot is then placed on an alignment awl, and an oscillating saw is used to resect the metacarpal head with the MCP joint held in flexion (Fig. 6A-1A). The osteotomy should be performed 1.5 mm distal to the origin of the collateral ligaments at the metacarpal head in order to preserve the ligaments. A partial cut is made through the dorsal cortex, and then the osteotomy guide and alignment awl are removed before completing the osteotomy of the metacarpal head.

A starter awl is then used to enlarge the medullary canal at the base of the proximal phalanx. As in the metacarpal bone, the starter awl can be advanced from one-half to two-thirds of the length of the proximal phalanx. A 5° dorsally angled osteotomy is performed using the osteotomy guide at the base of the proximal phalanx (Fig. 6A-1B). A series of broaches are then used in consecutive order to enlarge the medullary canal and provide the appropriate amount of space for the implant. The trial implant is inserted to be sure it fits well into the defect. The permanent implant tends to be slightly larger than the trial implant, and should be press-fit gently into the canal.

Once the implant has been placed, the joint capsule and radial sagittal band are repaired with absorbable sutures, after which time the tourniquet is deflated and bipolar

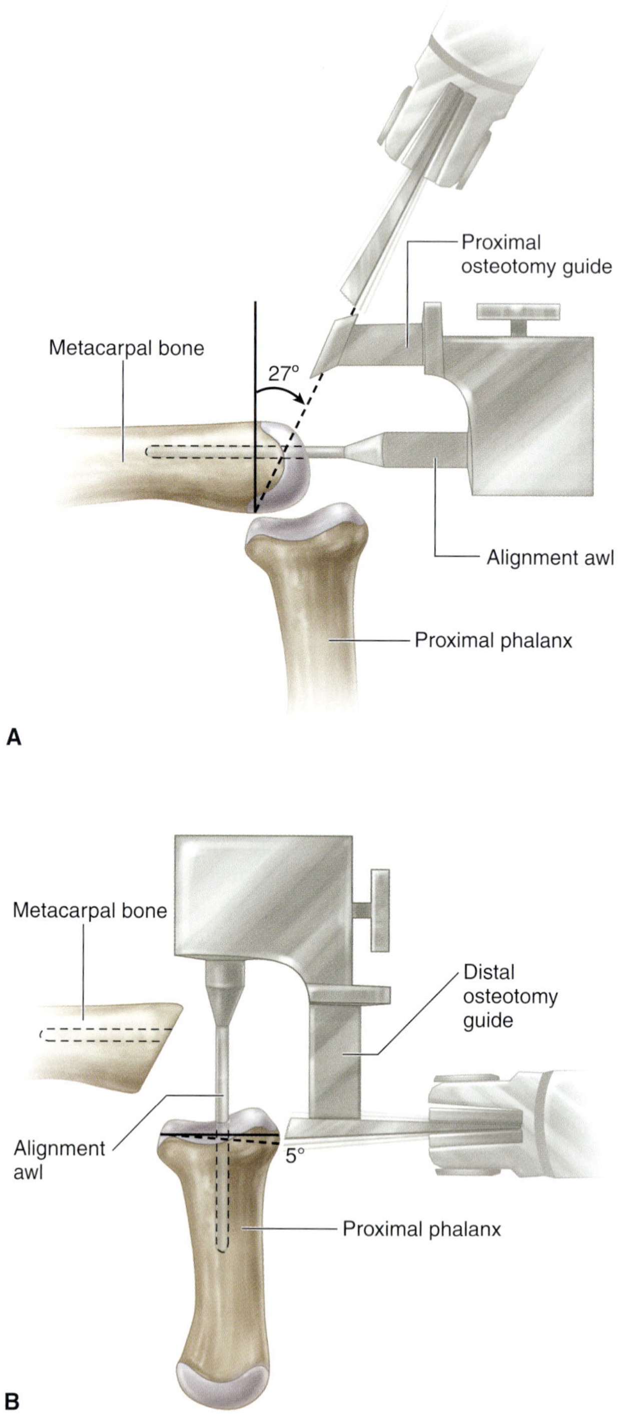

FIGURE 6A-1 **A.** An osteotomy guide tilted at 27.5° distally is placed on an alignment awl, and an oscillating saw is then used to remove the metacarpal head. **B.** An oscillating saw is utilized to perform an osteotomy at the base of the proximal phalanx.

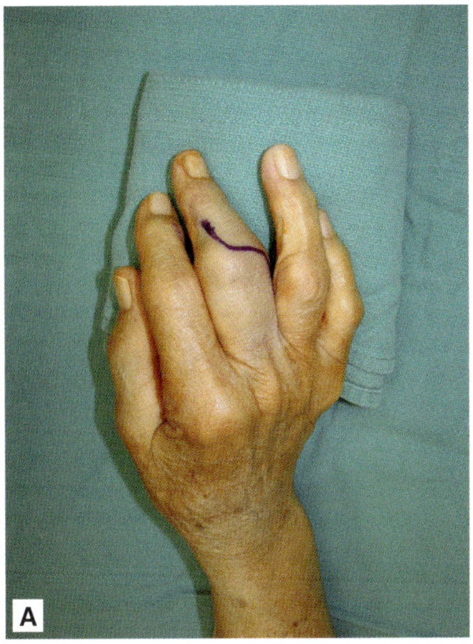

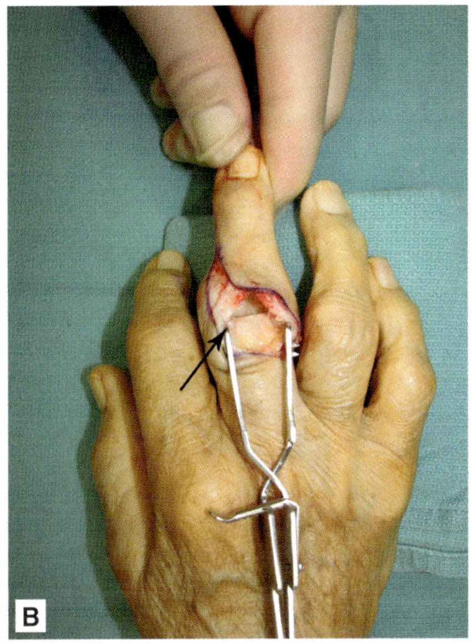

FIGURE 6A-2 **A.** During PIP joint arthroplasty for osteoarthritis, a lazy S-shaped incision provides wide exposure of the joint. **B.** The head of the proximal phalanx is resected just 1 to 2 mm distal to the collateral ligaments (shown by arrow).

electrocautery is used to achieve hemostasis. The incisions are closed with interrupted absorbable sutures in the dermis and interrupted horizontal mattress nylon sutures to approximate the skin. Following the procedure, the joint should be kept in extension with a well-padded plaster splint for 6 weeks followed by progressive mobilization.

PIP JOINT ARTHROPLASTY

For PIP joint arthroplasty, we prefer a dorsal approach using a lazy S-shaped incision to provide wide exposure of the joint (Fig. 6A-2A). A tendon-splitting incision is used to expose the PIP joint, because it allows for a side-to-side tendon closure and potentially avoids a PIP extension lag by preserving the central slip attachment. We have modified the procedure by resecting the head of the proximal phalanx at the flare, which provides a superior exposure to the medullary cavity for broaching, and have found this to be much more efficient than to place the starter awl over the tight, arthritic PIP joint. An oscillating saw is used to resect the head of the proximal phalanx just 1 to 2 mm distal to the collateral ligaments (Fig. 6A-2B). A series of broaches are then used as described previously to enlarge the medullary canal. A 60° oblique cutting guide is used to complete a volar oblique osteotomy, which fits the anatomic condylar design of the implant (Fig. 6A-3A and B).

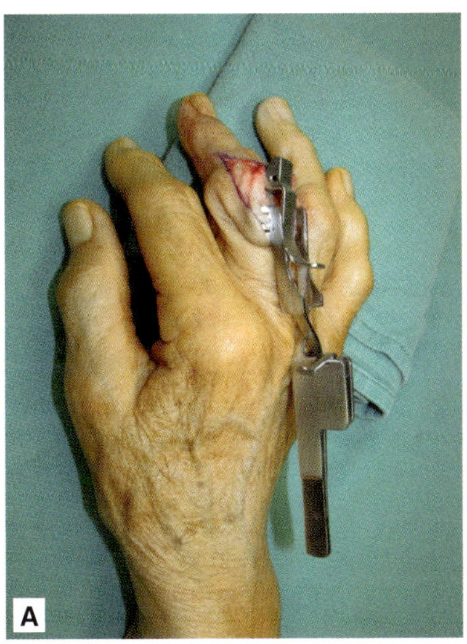

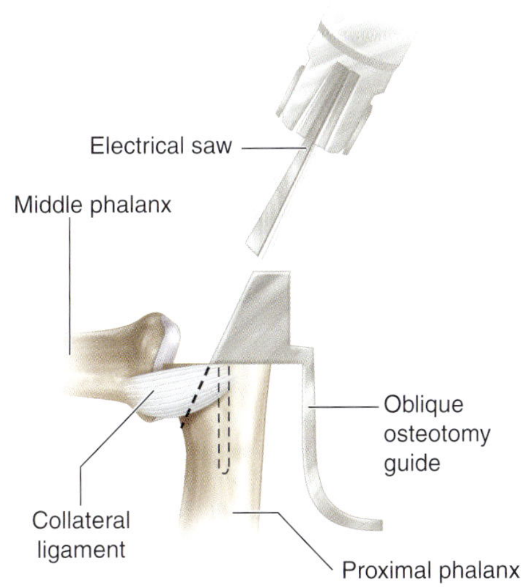

FIGURE 6A-3 **A.** The oblique cutting guide is seen inserted into the medullary canal at the head of the proximal phalanx. **B.** The oblique cutting guide is set at 60° and directs an oscillating saw to complete a volar oblique osteotomy that will shape the proximal phalanx to fit the implant.

To prepare the middle phalanx for the implant, a small oval bur is initially used to enlarge the medullary canal. A sequential series of broaches is then used to expand the medullary canal to the appropriate size for the implant without any bony resection. The size of the implant in the middle phalanx dictates the size of the proximal implant. For example, a #20 implant for the middle phalanx can match with a #20 or a #30 implant for the proximal phalanx. Typically, the middle phalangeal bone is quite hard, which makes broaching difficult, and a smaller implant is more appropriate, whereas the proximal phalanx has a more generous medullary cavity capable of accommodating an implant that is 1 size larger. One can mismatch an implant that is 1 size larger for the PIP joint, whereas for the MCP joint, no mismatch is permitted. A trial implant is used as a model to make sure the correct implant size is used, and once the proper size is selected, the implant is inserted into the medullary canals of the proximal and middle phalanx and gently tapped into place. The extensor tendon is then sutured in a side-to-side fashion, followed by closure of the skin, and the finger is splinted in extension. Figure 6A-4A and B shows the implant postoperatively at 2 months.

- It is important to preserve the collateral ligaments.
- Dorsal and palmar stability and the position of the implant should be checked fluoroscopically prior to closure.
- Any osteophytes and ridges must be completely removed. An osteophyte as small as 1 mm can prevent full seating of the implant.

Some authors recommend silicone implant arthroplasty for OA,[16,17] but we favor pyrolytic carbon implant arthroplasty because these patients generally have competent ligaments and adequate capsular support that help to prevent implant dislocation.

Complications

Extensor tendon rupture and chronic pain after MCP joint arthroplasty, requiring implant removal, have been reported.[10] Implant fracture in the proximal phalanx may also occur.[18,19] Ono et al documented that 62% of pyrolytic carbon implants had radiographic loosening at 44-month follow-up, whereas 33% had joint subluxation. Most of these complications occurred in the index and middle fingers.[5]

Outcomes

There is a paucity of studies on the use of pyrolytic MCP arthroplasty for OA. Parker et al reviewed 17 pyrolytic MPJ replacements in 15 patients with an average age of 55 years (range, 21-77 years). The preoperative average MPJ flexion was from 21° to 66°. At an average follow-up of 17 months (range, 3-42 months) the analog pain score decreased from 75.2 to 8.5 of 100. The postoperative average motion arc increased from 15° to 73° of flexion with an MCP extension lag decrease of 28%. This represented an increase in

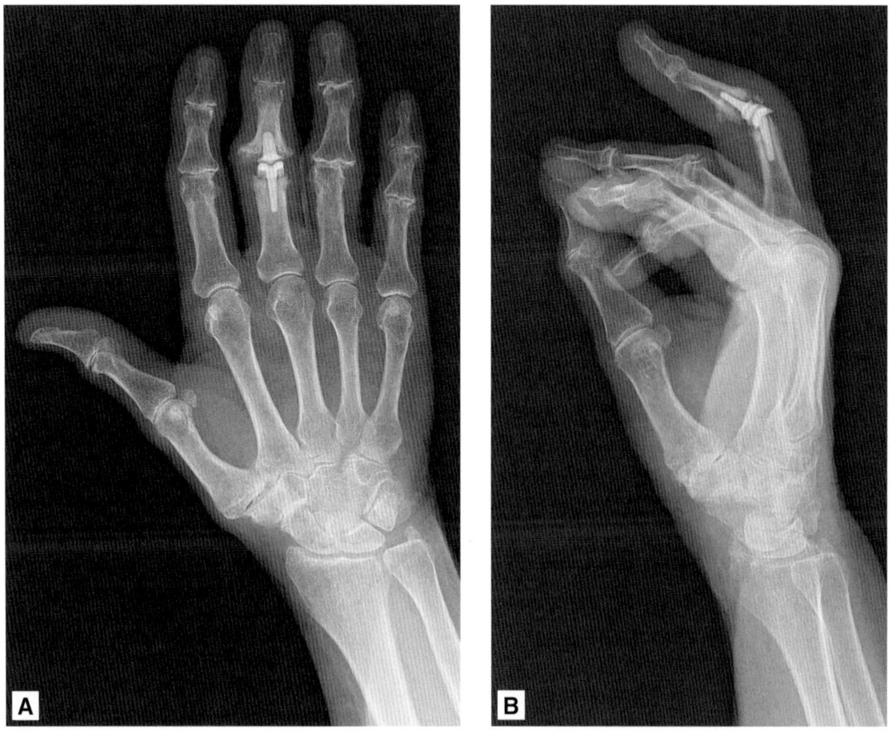

FIGURE 6A-4 A. PA radiograph of patient with pyrolytic pyrocarbon implant in the middle finger for osteoarthritis at 2 months postoperative. **B.** Lateral radiograph of the same patient at 2 months postoperative.

MCP motion arc from 44° to 58° that was not statistically significant.[10,11]

Rettig et al reviewed 12 patients with an average age of 62 years (range, 48-79 years) following 13 silicone MCP joint implant arthroplasties for idiopathic osteoarthritis.[17] At an average follow-up of 40 months (range, 9-132 months), 9 patients (10 implants) reported greater than 75% functional improvement. MPJ flexion averaged 53° preoperatively and 59° at the final follow-up. Six patients gained between 5° and 40° arc of MCP motion, but 6 patients lost between 2° and 15° arc of motion. The average radioulnar deviation was 6°. The average pinch strength for the group was 3.83 kg (range, 1.35-7.88 kg), and the average grip strength was 21.6 kg (range, 10.8-33.3 kg) on the operated hand as compared with 24.75 kg (range, 15.75-33.75 kg) for the contralateral hand.

Mashhadi et al analyzed the results of 24 pyrolytic PIP joints in 19 hands of 16 patients and reported a 10° improvement in the mean active range of motion at a mean follow-up of 48 months.[15] We reviewed our experience in 13 patients who underwent 21 PIP pyrocarbon implants. At a mean follow-up of 44 months, there was no statistical improvement in grip strength, key pinch strength, and active arc of motion, but all domains of the Michigan Hand Outcomes Questionnaire showed improvement, especially pain and satisfaction. There were, however, 10 complications in 9 joints.[5]

Tuttle and Stern reviewed 18 pyrolytic PIP arthroplasties in 8 women aged 62 years (range, 52-71) with severe OA, at an average follow-up of 13 months (range, 6-30).[20] The average preoperative ROM was 10° to 63°, and the average postoperative ROM was 18° to 71°, with increased motion in 9 joints and decreased motion in 9 joints. All joints were stable laterally, but the x-rays showed 2 cases of loosening at 4 months. Complications included 8 squeaky joints, 5 joint contractures, and 2 dislocations. Pain was relieved completely in 8 joints, with a VAS of 3.6 out of 10 for 8 patients. Although there was residual deformity in 4 joints, patients believed that 15 of 16 joints had improved in appearance.

METACARPOPHALANGEAL JOINT AND PROXIMAL INTERPHALANGEAL JOINT SILICONE IMPLANT ARTHROPLASTY IN PATIENTS WITH RHEUMATOID ARTHRITIS

Rationale and Basic Science Pertinent to the Procedure

In MCP joint and PIP joint arthroplasty for rheumatoid arthritis, silicone implants are indicated because these linked implants provide greater stability than pyrocarbon implants from the deforming forces and weak ligament support common with this type of arthritis.[21] The more proximal joints should always be treated before the distal joints, because deformities in the proximal joints affect the position of the distal joints.[7] The wrist deformity should be corrected before the MCP joints because a persistent wrist deformity will result in early recurrence of ulnar deviation at the MCP joints.

Indications

Indications for MCP joint arthroplasty include ulnar deviation and volar subluxation at the MCP joint resulting in stiffness and pain, as well as a decreased arc of motion of 40° or less, coupled with poor function of the fingers.[22] Indications for PIP joint arthroplasty include an established swan neck deformity and limited PIP joint motion with joint destruction.

Contraindications

Contraindications for both the MCP and PIP joints include infection or bone loss in the joint, or an absence of adequate soft-tissue coverage of the joint. For the MCP joint, arthroplasty should exclude patients who are able to achieve an active arc of motion greater than 60°, because arthroplasty may not always improve the arc of motion beyond this arc postoperatively.[22] An arthroplasty is not recommended in patients with a boutonniere deformity, since a large amount of bone must be resected to properly seat the implant, resulting in the destruction of the collateral ligaments, leading to decreased stability.[23] When severe joint involvement exists at both the MCP and PIP joints, it is recommended to perform arthroplasty for the MCP joint and arthrodesis for the PIP joint to provide the highest level of stability and functionality.

Surgical Technique

MCP JOINT ARTHROPLASTY

For a single joint replacement, a dorsal "lazy S"–shaped incision is made over the MCP joint. For multiple joint replacements, a dorsal transverse incision is performed over the head of the metacarpals, with careful preservation of the longitudinal dorsal veins (Fig. 6A-5A). The ulnarly deviated extensor tendon is identified, and the radial sagittal band is incised to expose the MCP joint. A synovectomy is performed. The metacarpal heads are exposed and resected transversely at the metacarpal neck level using an oscillating saw distal to the origin of the collateral ligament (Fig. 6A-5B). Any contracted ulnar lateral bands are released. An awl is then used to enlarge the medullary canal at the base of the proximal phalanx (Fig. 6A-6).

The canal is enlarged using consecutively larger broaches (Fig. 6A-7). Two drill holes are made with a 0.035-in Kirschner wire on the radial side of the metacarpal bone, and 3/0 nonabsorbable braided sutures are placed through the 2 holes. A trial implant was inserted and adequate stability was assessed. The final implant is then inserted using a

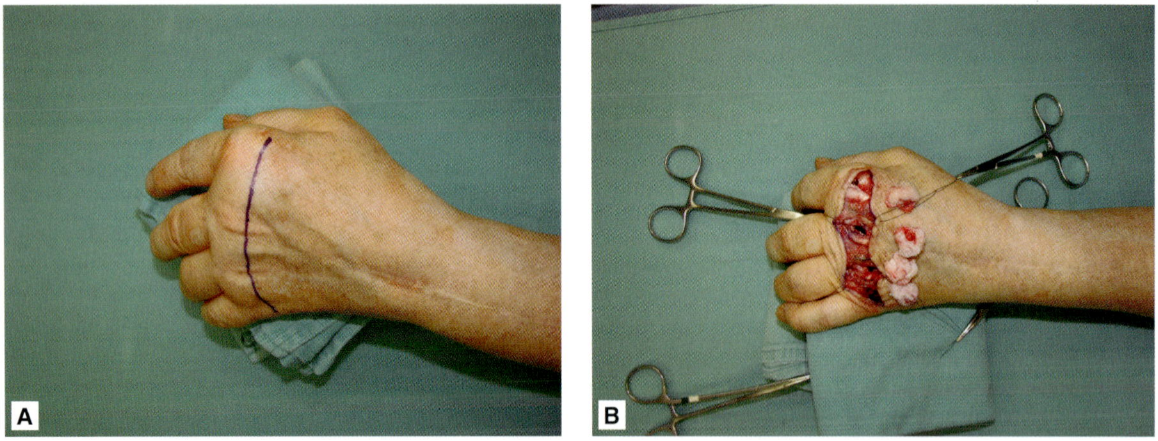

FIGURE 6A-5 **A.** For MCP joint arthroplasty in RA patients, a dorsal transverse incision is made over the head of the metacarpals. **B.** Following exposure of the metacarpal heads, they are cut in a transverse fashion distal to the collateral ligaments. Care must be taken not to damage the collateral ligaments due to their proximity to the osteotomy site.

no touch technique. After the implant is inserted, the radially placed 3/0 sutures are used to reattach the radial collateral ligament to the metacarpal bone (Fig. 6A-8A-C). If necessary, the ulnar sagittal band is released to centralize the tendon over the metacarpal head. Once all of the ligamentous structures and tendons are reattached and the incision closed, the MP joint should be splinted in extension for 6 weeks using a dorsal outrigger, but PIP and DIP flexion is allowed. The 6-week postoperative radiographs are displayed in Figure 6A-9.

PIP JOINT ARTHROPLASTY

Incision Placement and Dissection. The incision and surgical approach to this procedure are the same as those of PIP joint arthroplasty for osteoarthritis. In contrast to pyrocarbon arthroplasty, no alignment guide is required during osteotomy of the proximal phalanx for PIP silicone implant arthroplasty. Only the distal aspect of the proximal phalanx requires resection, and an awl is sufficient to make a trough in the middle phalanx due to the softened bone in RA patients. When broaching the medullary cavities of the proximal and middle phalanx, it is possible to perforate the cortex because the bones in RA patients are particularly soft. To avoid this complication, be sure to properly identify the medullary canal, and perform the broaching as carefully as possible.

Similar to an MCP joint silicone implant arthroplasty, 2 drill holes are made with a 0.035-in Kirschner wire in the

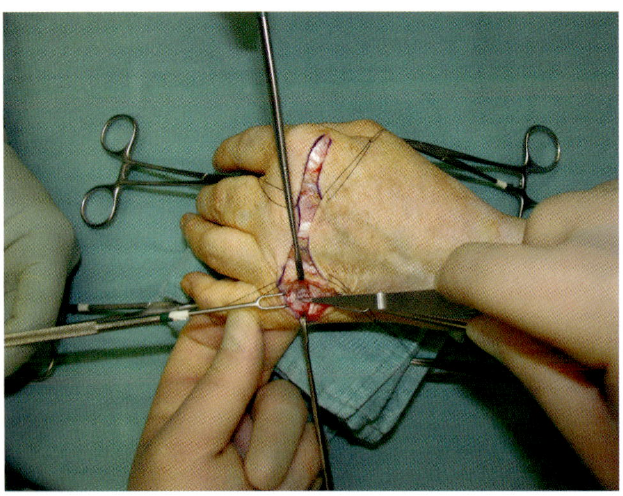

FIGURE 6A-6 To establish a medullary canal at the base of the proximal phalanx, a starter awl creates the initial puncture providing a starting point for a series of broaches to sequentially enlarge the canal to fit the implant.

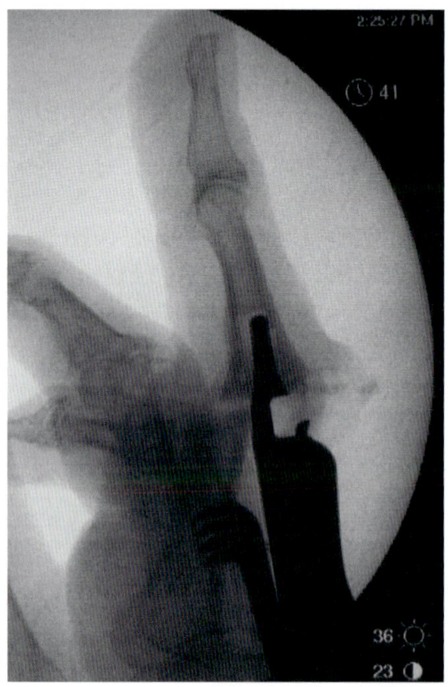

FIGURE 6A-7 Broaches are used to enlarge the medullary canal to the appropriate size.

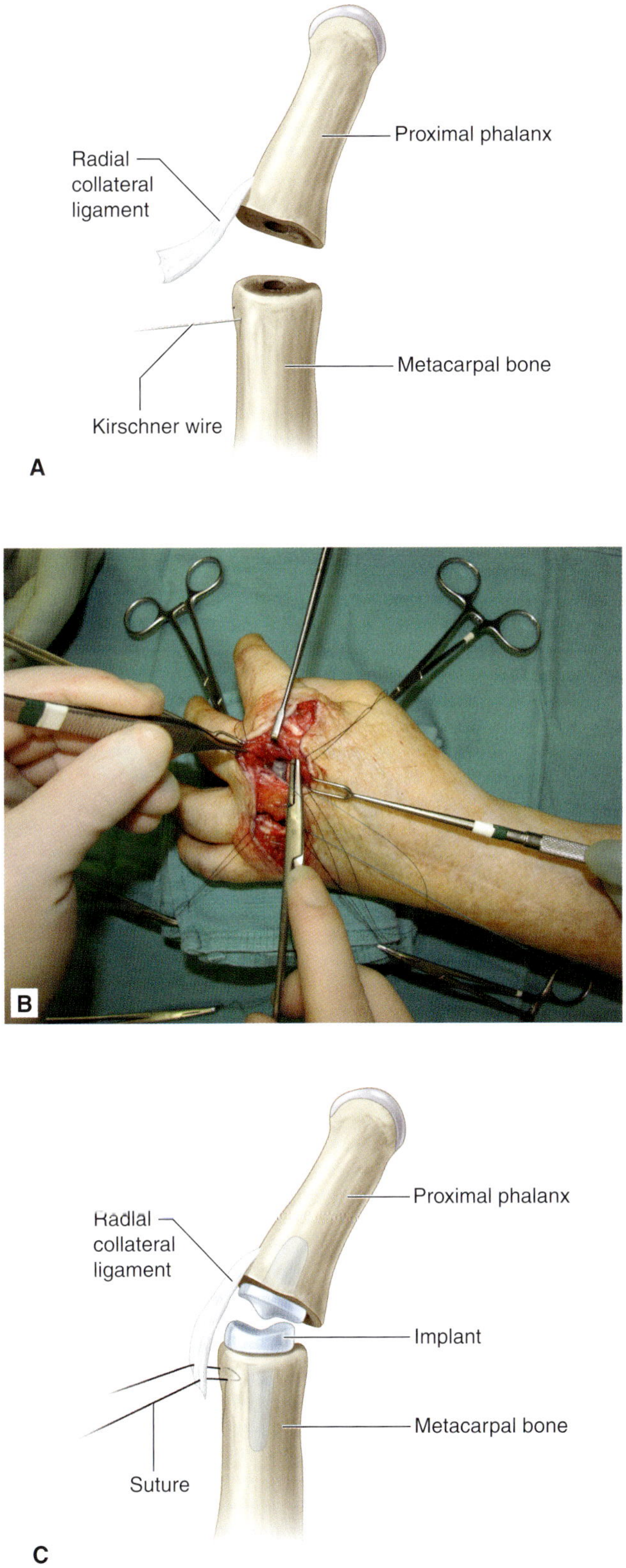

FIGURE 6A-8 **A.** Before inserting the implant, 2 drill holes are made with 0.035-in Kirschner wire on the radial side of the metacarpal, and 3-0 braided sutures are then placed into the drill holes to imbricate the radial collateral ligaments. **B.** Implant insertion. **C.** The radially placed 3-0 sutures are used to reattach the radial collateral ligament to the metacarpal bone.

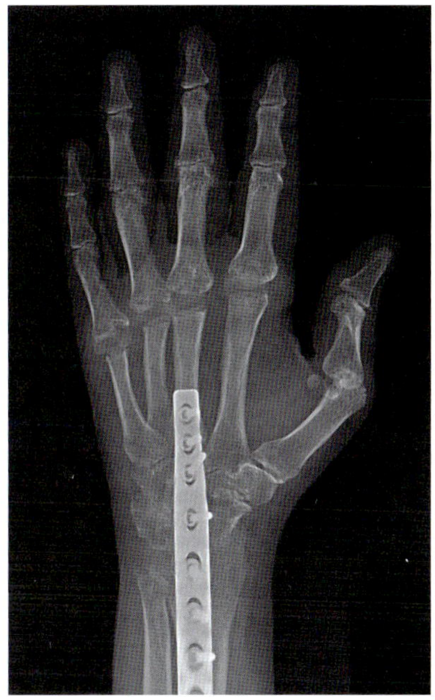

FIGURE 6A-9 A patient treated with silicone implant metacarpophalangeal arthroplasty for rheumatoid arthritis at 6 weeks postoperative.

proximal phalanx and 3/0 nonabsorbable braided sutures are placed through the 2 holes to later repair the collateral ligaments before inserting the implant, if the joint is unstable.

In most cases, the ulnar lateral bands are relaxed after sufficient metacarpal head removal and do not need to be released.

It is our preference to perform a PIP joint fusion in the index finger for superior stability for strong pinch, whereas in arthroplasty it is preferred in the ring and little fingers. The surgical treatment must be evaluated on a case-by-case basis to determine the option that will most appropriately address the needs of each individual patient.

Complications

Destructive changes to the bone surrounding the joints are the most frequently reported complications associated with silicone implant arthroplasty.[24] Additional complications include implant fractures, failure to control ulnar drift, and the gradual loss of motion in the long term. Postoperative infections, although rare, require implant removal and the use of intravenous antibiotics. Takigawa et al found that implant fracture, occurring in 11 out of 70 implants, is the most common complication associated with PIP joint silicone implant arthroplasty[25] at an average follow-up period of 6.5 years.

Outcomes

We reviewed 46 patients with a mean age of 60 years with rheumatoid arthritis following an MCP silicone arthroplasty at a 2-year follow-up. The patients showed an improvement in the ulnar drift from an average of 62° preoperatively to 9° postoperatively.[26] The grip strength, key, tip, and palmar pinch strength did not change from the baseline and were found to have no correlation with patient satisfaction.[26] The extensor lag improved from 63° to 25° and the ulnar drift improved from 37° to 15° and both were significantly correlated with patient satisfaction. The MCP arc of motion improved from 21° to 34°.

Takigawa et al reviewed 48 patients at a mean follow-up of 8 years (range, 21-19.2 years) following a silicone PIP arthroplasty: 13 of these patients had RA.[25] The average preoperative ROM was 26° and 19° at the final follow-up. The RA patients had poorer results than OA with respect to pain relief and motion.

Trail et al reviewed the records and radiographs of 381 patients with rheumatoid arthritis who had undergone 1336 silastic MP joint replacements.[27] At 17 years, 63% were still in place, although there was x-ray evidence of fracture in two-thirds of the implants. Factors that correlated with an improved survival included soft-tissue balancing, crossed intrinsic transfer, and realignment of the wrist. Surgery to the thumb and PIP joint had a deleterious effect. The use of grommets did not protect the implant from fracture.

REFERENCES

1. Lawrence RC, Felson DT, Helmick CG, et al. Estimates of the prevalence of arthritis and other rheumatic conditions in the United States. Part II. *Arthritis Rheum*. 2008;58:26–35.
2. Fumagalli M, Sarzi-Puttini P, Atzeni F. Hand osteoarthritis. *Semin Arthritis Rheum*. 2005;34:47–52.
3. Kalichman L, Hernandez-Molina G. Hand osteoarthritis: an epidemiological perspective. *Semin Arthritis Rheum*. 2010;39:465–476.
4. Beasley J. Osteoarthritis and rheumatoid arthritis: conservative therapeutic management. *J Hand Ther*. 2012;25:163–172.
5. Ono S, Shauver MJ, Chang KW, Chung KC. Outcomes of pyrolytic carbon arthroplasty for the proximal interphalangeal joint at 44 months' mean follow-up. *Plast Reconstr Surg*. 2012;129:1139–1150.
6. Schwartz DA, Peimer CA. Distal interphalangeal joint implant arthroplasty in a musician. *J Hand Ther*. 1998;11:49–52.
7. Kozlow JH, Chung KC. Current concepts in the surgical management of rheumatoid and osteoarthritic hands and wrists. *Hand Clin*. 2011;27:31–41.
8. Swanson AB, de Groot Swanson G. Osteoarthritis in the hand. *Clin Rheum Dis*. 1985;11:393–420.
9. Bravo CJ, Rizzo M, Hormel KB, Beckenbaugh RD. Pyrolytic carbon proximal interphalangeal joint arthroplasty: results with minimum two-year follow-up evaluation. *J Hand Surg Am*. 2007;32:1–11.
10. Parker WL, Rizzo M, Moran SL, Hormel KB, Beckenbaugh RD. Preliminary results of nonconstrained pyrolytic carbon arthroplasty for metacarpophalangeal joint arthritis. *J Hand Surg Am*. 2007;32:1496–1505.
11. Parker W, Moran SL, Hormel KB, Rizzo M, Beckenbaugh RD. Nonrheumatoid metacarpophalangeal joint arthritis. Unconstrained pyrolytic carbon implants: indications, technique, and outcomes. *Hand Clin*. 2006;22:183–193.
12. Watts AC, Hearnden AJ, Trail IA, Hayton MJ, Nuttall D, Stanley JK. Pyrocarbon proximal interphalangeal joint arthroplasty: minimum two-year follow-up. *J Hand Surg Am*. 2012;37:882–888.
13. Nunley RM, Boyer MI, Goldfarb CA. Pyrolytic carbon arthroplasty for posttraumatic arthritis of the proximal interphalangeal joint. *J Hand Surg Am*. 2006;31:1468–1474.
14. Cook SD, Beckenbaugh RD, Redondo J, Popich LS, Klawitter JJ, Linscheid RL. Long-term follow-up of pyrolytic carbon metacarpophalangeal implants. *J Bone Joint Surg Am*. 1999;81:635–648.
15. Mashhadi SA, Chandrasekharan L, Pickford MA. Pyrolytic carbon arthroplasty for the proximal interphalangeal joint: results after minimum 3 years of follow-up. *J Hand Surg Eur*. 2012;37:501–505.
16. Stahlenbrecher A, Hoch J. Proximal interphalangeal joint silicone arthroplasty—comparison of Swanson and NeuFlex implants using a new evaluation score. *Handchir Mikrochir Plast Chir*. 2009;41:156–165.
17. Rettig LA, Luca L, Murphy MS. Silicone implant arthroplasty in patients with idiopathic osteoarthritis of the metacarpophalangeal joint. *J Hand Surg Am*. 2005;30:667–672.
18. Syed MA, Smith A, Benjamin-Laing H. Pyrocarbon implant fracture after metacarpophalangeal joint arthroplasty: an unusual cause for early revision. *J Hand Surg Eur*. 2010;35:505–506.
19. Young L, Chojnowski A. Fracture of the proximal phalanx pyrocarbon implant after metacarpophalangeal arthroplasty. *J Hand Surg Eur*. 2011;36:157–158.
20. Tuttle HG, Stern PJ. Pyrolytic carbon proximal interphalangeal joint resurfacing arthroplasty. *J Hand Surg Am*. 2006;31:930–939.
21. Chung KC, Kotsis SV. Outcomes of hand surgery in the patient with rheumatoid arthritis. *Curr Opin Rheumatol*. 2010;22:336–341.
22. Abboud JA, Beredjiklian PK, Bozentka DJ. Metacarpophalangeal joint arthroplasty in rheumatoid arthritis. *J Am Acad Orthop Surg*. 2003;11:184–191.
23. Chung KC, Pushman AG. Current concepts in the management of the rheumatoid hand. *J Hand Surg Am*. 2011;36:736–747 [quiz 47].
24. Foliart DE. Swanson silicone finger joint implants: a review of the literature regarding long-term complications. *J Hand Surg Am*. 1995;20:445–449.
25. Takigawa S, Meletiou S, Sauerbier M, Cooney WP. Long-term assessment of Swanson implant arthroplasty in the proximal interphalangeal joint of the hand. *J Hand Surg Am*. 2004;29:785–795.
26. Waljee JF, Chung KC. Objective functional outcomes and patient satisfaction after silicone metacarpophalangeal arthroplasty for rheumatoid arthritis. *J Hand Surg Am*. 2012;37:47–54.
27. Trail IA, Martin JA, Nuttall D, Stanley JK. Seventeen-year survivorship analysis of silastic metacarpophalangeal joint replacement. *J Bone Joint Surg Br*. 2004;86:1002–1006.

6B

Metacarpophalangeal and Interphalangeal Joint Fusions

Kagan Ozer, MD
Kevin C. Chung, MD, MS

RATIONALE AND BASIC SCIENCE PERTINENT TO THE PROCEDURE

The stability and function of the small joints in the hand rely on articular congruity, musculotendinous balance, integrity of ligaments, and the capsular structures, especially the volar plate.[1–3] Fusion of the small joints is usually indicated if those structures are irreparably damaged or arthroplasty has failed.

In terms of hand function, fusion of a single joint usually does not interfere with the normal activities of daily living. Woodworth et al recently studied the impact of proximal interphalangeal (PIP) joint fusion on the overall function of the hand[4] using 15 healthy subjects who had their PIP joint held in 40° of flexion in all 4 fingers to simulate fusion. Although 1 of the 2 activities of daily living that involved a power grasp showed a significant increase in metacarpophalangeal (MCP) flexion or abduction, there was no overall significant increase in MCP joint motion in the power grasp category. When compared with an unrestricted hand, none of the activities of daily living requiring power grasp were perceived to be more difficult when the PIP joint was constrained. In contrast, precision handling tasks did show an increased MCP flexion, but because 7 of the 9 tasks involved precision handling, these results may only indicate a greater sense of perceived disability than the actual amount of impairment caused by the splinting. In search of an ideal position for interphalangeal joint fusion, Domalain et al studied the kinematics of precision pinch at various positions of the index finger PIP joint on 11 healthy subjects.[5] They concluded that a PIP joint fusion at 40° to 50° leads to a more natural precision pinch posture, but restricts grip span and reduces pinch precision. In our clinical practice, we determine the ideal fusion angle based on a patient's needs. Particularly in the MCP joint, splinting the affected joint in various positions prior to surgery can help a patient to decide the ideal position for optimal function.

The need for a finger MCP fusion is quite rare. The arc of motion of the fingers is initiated at the MCP joint and its fusion can cause substantial impairment. However, in severe trauma when the bone stock cannot support an implant, MCP joint fusion may be necessary. The general rule is to fuse the MCP joint at 25° for the index finger, increasing the amount of flexion by 5° increments from the radial to ulnar direction, fusing the small finger MCP joint at 40°. For the PIP joint, the index finger should be fused at 40°, increasing the amount of flexion by 5° from the radial to ulnar direction while fusing the small joint PIP at 55°. For the distal interphalangeal (DIP) joint, the ideal position of fusion is 0° to 5° throughout all of the digits.[6–8]

INDICATIONS

Candidates for a MCP or a PIP joint fusion are patients with a failed arthroplasty or those with substantial bone and/or soft tissue loss resulting in joint instability, pain, or deformity. Depending on the injury characteristics and conditions of the soft tissues, the procedure can be performed in the acute setting or at a later date, with no real time limits. In addition, a small joint fusion can be performed in any age group, making this a versatile treatment option. However, the risks and benefits of alternative treatment strategies should be weighed against the advantages and limitations of fusion, particularly in the case of the MCP joint. Although fusions of the PIP and DIP joints provide satisfactory pain relief and function, fusion of the MCP joint is not as well tolerated from a functional standpoint. In fact, small joint fusions are better tolerated from a distal to proximal direction, fusion usually being the first choice for degenerative conditions at the DIP joint.

CONTRAINDICATIONS

Unlike small joint arthroplasties, there seems to be no absolute contraindication to performing a small joint fusion. However, many relative contraindications exist:

- Significant bone and soft tissue loss with neurovascular injury following trauma involving a single digit
- Inadequate potential to heal the fusion site due to chronic illness (renal failure, poor nutritional status) or poor circulation
- Limited range of motion in the adjacent joints and decreased total active motion of the finger

SURGICAL TECHNIQUE

The procedure is performed under tourniquet control with the patient in a supine position. We prefer a regional block for the surgery. A straight longitudinal, a zigzag, or a lazy-S incision is made over the dorsal aspect of the joint. The extensor apparatus is split longitudinally, and the joint surfaces are exposed. The preparation of the articular surfaces to provide cancellous-to-cancellous bone contact without excessive bone shortening is of the utmost importance. For the articular surface, 1 of 2 surface preparation techniques is commonly used: the cup and cone technique or the flat-surface technique. The cup and cone technique provides a larger contact surface area with perhaps less stability, but with the freedom to make fine adjustments. This is in contrast to chevron-type cuts that provide increased stability but that require extreme precision and have less tolerance for error.

The available methods of fixation are numerous, and include K-wires, intraosseous wire loops, compression screws, and plate and screw techniques. The simplest and most commonly used methods are the crossed Kirschner wire technique and the axial Kirschner wire combined with an oblique Kirschner wire configuration.[9,10] In these methods, the pins are inserted percutaneously leaving the bent ends out of the skin. We prefer the use of 0.045-in K-wires for the MP and PIP joints and 0.035-in K-wires for the DIP joints. Cross K-wires are used in order to prevent a rotational deformity, especially in the case of cup and cone arthrodesis.

90-90 intraosseous wiring with 26-gauge surgical steel wire (Fig. 6B-1) is another common method of fusion.[11,12] After the articular surfaces are prepared, a 0.035-in Kirschner wire is used to drill parallel orthogonal holes in a dorsal to volar direction and in a radial to ulnar direction, approximately 3 to 4 mm on either side of the fusion site. We prefer to use a 20-gauge needle to facilitate the passage of 26-gauge surgical steel wire that is formed into a loop around the arthrodesis site. Once both wires are passed, they are tightened, and buried to prevent soft tissue irritation. Although this is a simple technique providing stable fixation, it requires greater soft tissue stripping and exposure than similar techniques.

Another popular method involves the use of K-wires and cerclage wires together to form a tension band construct.[13–16] Unlike cross K-wire fixation, in this technique the K-wires are buried in bone (Fig. 6B-2). From a biomechanical standpoint, this method provides the most stable anteroposterior and bending torsion strength than other methods involving K-wire and cerclage wires.[17] Care is taken to ensure that the interosseous wire is placed dorsal to the midlateral line to provide compression of the fusion site.

Fusion can also be achieved using 2.0- or 2.7-mm compression screws for the MCP and PIP joints, and 1.5- or 2.0-mm compression screws for the DIP joint. Screws are

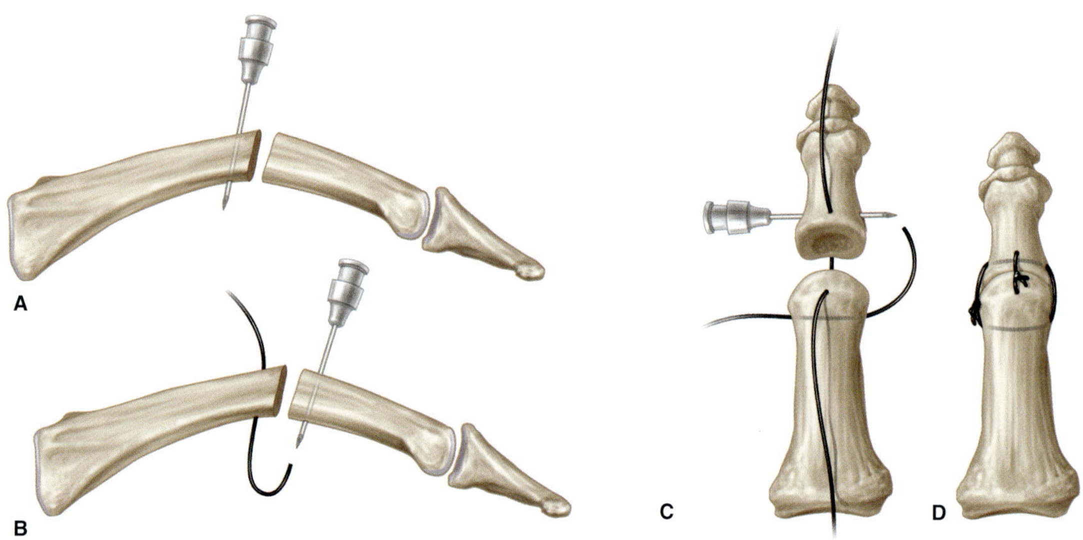

FIGURE 6B-1 Intraosseous wiring. **A.** The articular surfaces are prepared parallel at a desired angle using an oscillating saw. **B.** Using a 0.035-in K-wire, 2 parallel holes are created 3 to 4 mm away from the proximal and distal bone ends at the osteotomy site. With the aid of a 20-gauge needle, a 26-gauge surgical steel wire is passed through these holes. **C.** This procedure is repeated for another orthogonal wire. **D.** Once both wires are passed, they are twisted and tightened.

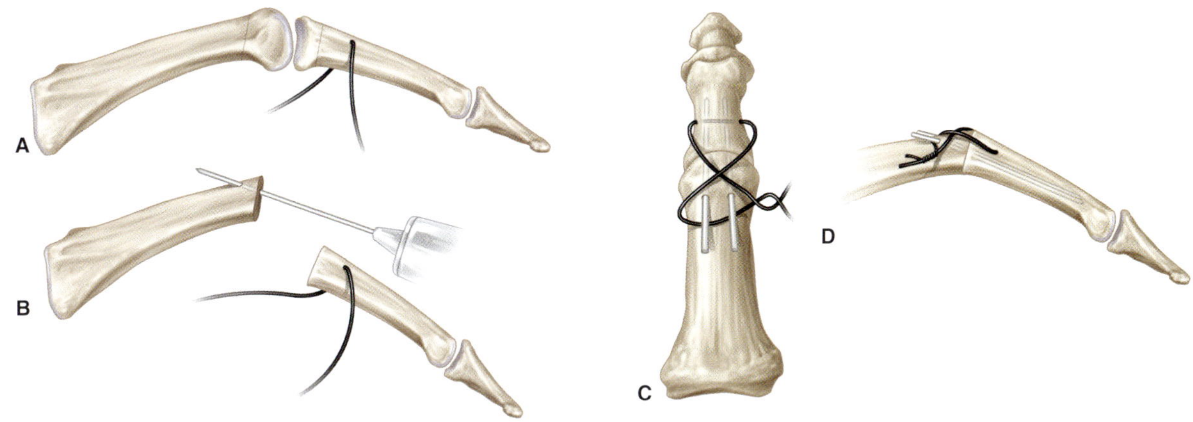

FIGURE 6B-2 Tension band wiring. The main principle of tension band wiring is to convert the distracting force to a compressive force. **A.** First, the articular surfaces are prepared parallel at a desired angle using an oscillating saw. Next, a transverse hole is drilled, 8 to 10 mm distal to the osteotomy site using 0.035-in K-wire. **B.** A 26-gauge surgical steel wire is then passed through these holes. Two parallel 0.035-in K-wires are then passed through the proximal phalanx in a retrograde fashion. **C.** Once the articular surfaces have been adapted, both K-wires are advanced to the distal fragment and stopped at a point engaging the far cortex. Cerclage wire is then wrapped around 2 K-wires in a figure-of-8 fashion, twisted, and tightened. **D.** The tips of both K-wires and the cerclage wire are bent and buried into the proximal cortex.

placed either into the medullary canal of the distal fragment or obliquely across the joint.[18,19] We prefer to use screws in the DIP joint due to the simplicity of the technique and high patient satisfaction rate. However, because of the small size and the curved nature of the distal phalanx, precision is of utmost importance to ensure that the screw is placed entirely within the distal phalanx (Fig. 6B-3).

In addition to the techniques previously described, plate fixation has been used for MCP and PIP joint fusion.[15,20,21] This requires a more extensile approach and is especially indicated in cases with segmental bone loss when the plate can bridge the defect and restore length prior to cortical bone graft insertion into the defect (Fig. 6B-4). We use a pre-bent 1.5- to 2.7-mm plate with a minimum of 3 bicortical

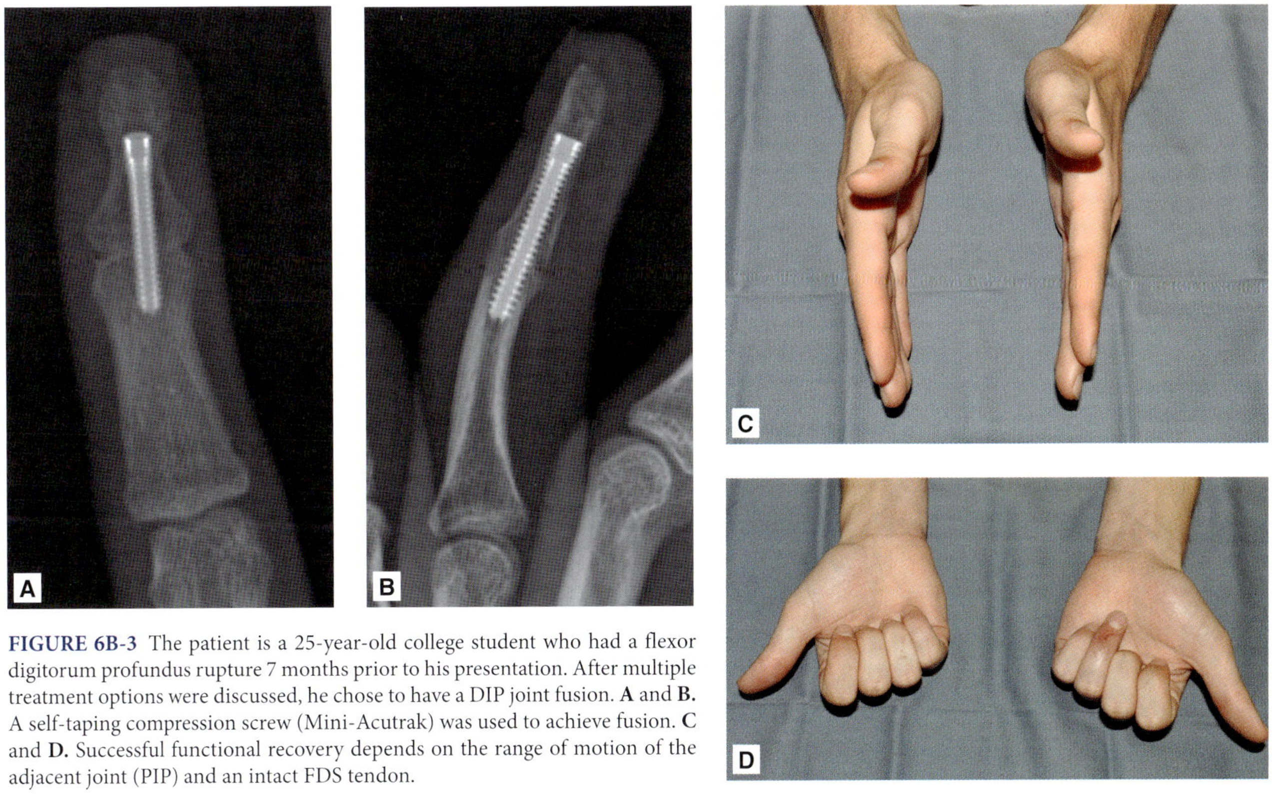

FIGURE 6B-3 The patient is a 25-year-old college student who had a flexor digitorum profundus rupture 7 months prior to his presentation. After multiple treatment options were discussed, he chose to have a DIP joint fusion. **A** and **B.** A self-taping compression screw (Mini-Acutrak) was used to achieve fusion. **C** and **D.** Successful functional recovery depends on the range of motion of the adjacent joint (PIP) and an intact FDS tendon.

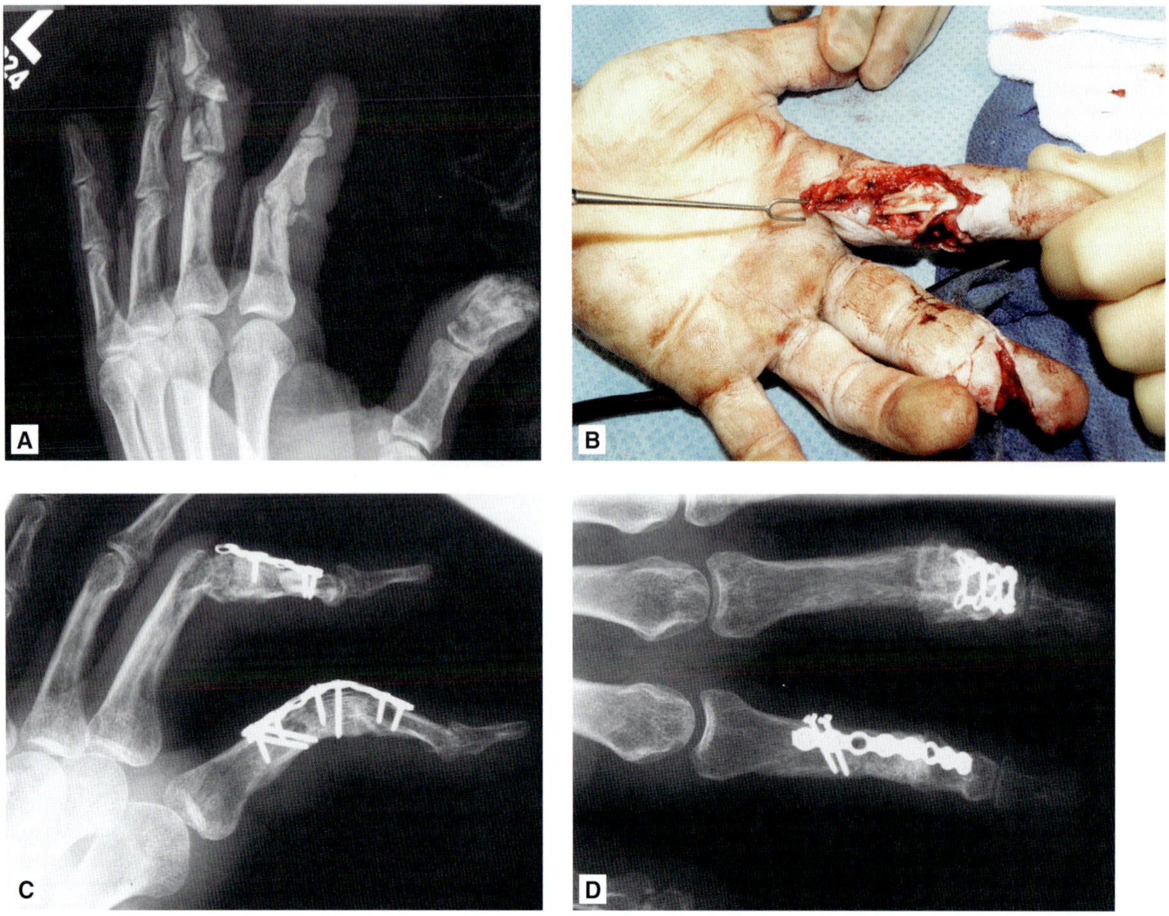

FIGURE 6B-4 A 45-year-old construction worker presented with a crush injury to multiple digits sustaining open fractures to his thumb, index, and long digits. **A** and **B.** His index finger PIP joint suffered a severe crush injury, tendon laceration, and bone loss. **C** and **D.** Following repair of his tendon, we used an intercalary bone graft with a plate to fuse the index finger PIP joint in order to provide satisfactory lateral stability. Six months following surgery, the bone graft was completely incorporated resulting in stable fusion.

screws on each side of the arthrodesis site. Finally, the use of various external fixation devices has also been described for fusion of the MP and PIP joints, particularly in cases of bone or soft tissue loss, infection, and a failed prior arthrodesis.[22,23]

The extensor apparatus is closed using a running 4.0 Monocryl suture. The patient is immobilized in a bulky dressing with a protective plaster splint. Postoperative splinting is continued until bony union is achieved.

Pitfalls of Fixation

The use of K-wires to achieve fusion is not only technically simple but also cost-effective. Despite these advantages, it carries the risk of pin-track infection and loss of fixation. When using compression screws, good bone quality is usually required to achieve effective compression. The screw head should be buried well into the bone to avoid prominent hardware and potential secondary surgeries. Although plate and screw fixation provides superior stability, it requires extensive soft tissue dissection and often another surgery for the removal of the hardware and tenolysis. With recent advances in external fixation devices, union rates are comparable to other techniques, with an increased risk of stiffness in adjacent joints and pin-track infection.

OUTCOMES AND COMPLICATIONS

In general, the "time to union" ranges from 6 to 12 weeks, regardless of the method of fixation and the joint (Table 6B-1). Although the majority of reports consist of case series, a few studies compare the outcomes of various methods of fixation. In a review of 181 DIP joint fusions, Stern and Fulton reported a 20% major complication rate (nonunion, malunion, deep infection, or osteomyelitis) and a 16% minor complication rate (skin necrosis, cold intolerance, PIP joint stiffness, paresthesias, superficial wound infection, or prominent hardware).[18] The nonunion rate was found to be similar in all methods of fixation. Leibovic and Strickland reviewed 224 PIP fusions fixed with 1 of the 4 methods of fixation.[15] They reported a 14% nonunion rate, with the highest seen

TABLE 6B-1: A Review of Case Series Published to Date

Author	Joint	Method of Fixation	Nonunion (*n*)	Time to Union
Ayres et al[24]	PIP	Herbert screw	2% (1/51)	—
Braun and Rhoades[25]	MP–IP	External fixator	0% (0/31)	8
Brutus et al[26]	DIP	Compression screw	11% (4/27)	8-10
Buchler and Aikin[21]	PIP	Plate + bone graft	8% (23/25)	—
Burton et al[27]	PIP	K-wire	0.6% (1/171)	8
Carroll and Hill[28]	IP	C&C, K-wire	4% (22/635)	10
Granowitz and Vainio[29]	PIP	Crossed K-wire	0% (0/122)	7
Hogh and Jensen[30]	IP	K-wire and cerclage	7% (3/45)	8
Ijsselstein et al[13]	MP–PIP	K-wire	15% (9/60)	6
		Tension band wire	5% (7/143)	—
Katzman et al[31]	PIP–DIP	Herbert screw	0% (0/51)	8
Khuri[14]	MP–PIP	Tension band wire	0% (0/15)	7
Leibovic and Strickland[15]	MP–PIP–DIP	K wire	16% (16/99)	10
		Tension band wire	5%(3/69)	11
		Herbert screw	0% (0/35)	9
		Plate	0% (0/4)	12
Lister[11]	IP	Interosseous wire	10% (5/53)	10
McGlynn et al[9]	PIP–DIP	C&C, K-wire	0% (1/103)	8
Moberg and Hendrickson[32]	IP	Bone peg	6% (9/150)	6
Seitz et al[23]	MP–PIP–DIP	External fixator	5% (1/20)	6
Stern and Fulton[18]	DIP	K-wire	12% (13/111)	—
		Interossesous wire	12% (5/43)	—
		Herbert screw	11% (3/27)	—
Stern et al[16]	MP and PIP	Tension band wire	3% (9/290)	—
Teoh et al[19]	IP	Compression screw	4% (22/23)	8.2
Watson and Shaffer[10]	IP	K-wire	21% (11/40)	10
Wright and McMurty[20]	MP–PIP	Plate	2% (2/74)	—

in patients who had psoriatic arthritis, an intermediate rate in rheumatoid arthritis, and a lower rate in acute trauma and posttraumatic reconstruction. It is interesting to note that the incidence of nonunion appeared nonexistent in osteoarthritis. In terms of the method of fixation, the highest nonunion rate was seen following the use of Kirschner wires, followed by the use of tension band wires, and lowest incidence was seen using Herbert screws. These results suggest that methods that compress the fusion site are superior to other techniques. Host factors, particularly the quality of bone, also play an important role in achieving a successful outcome.

REFERENCES

1. Minami A, An KN, Cooney WP 3rd, et al. Ligament stability of the metacarpophalangeal joint: a biomechanical study. *J Hand Surg Am.* 1985;10:255–260.
2. Minamikawa Y, Horii E, Amadio PC, et al. Stability and constraint of the proximal interphalangeal joint. *J Hand Surg Am.* 1993;18:198–204.
3. Tamai K, Ryu J, An KN, et al. Three-dimensional geometric analysis of the metacarpophalangeal joint. *J Hand Surg Am.* 1988;13:521–529.
4. Woodworth JA, McCullough MB, Grosland NM, Adams BD. Impact of simulated proximal interphalangeal arthrodeses of all fingers on hand function. *J Hand Surg Am.* 2006;31(6):940–946.
5. Domalain M, Evans PJ, Seitz WH Jr, Li ZM. Influence of index finger proximal interphalangeal joint arthrodesis on precision pinch kinematics. *J Hand Surg Am.* 2011;36(12):1944–1949.
6. Buck-Gramcko D. Compression arthrodesis of joints in the hand. In: Tubiana R, ed. *The Hand.* Vol. 2. Philadelphia: WB Saunders; 1985:703–706.
7. Tubiana R. Arthrodesis of the fingers. In: Tubiana R, ed. *The Hand.* Vol. 2. Philadelphia: WB Saunders; 1985:698–702.
8. Amadio PC, Shin AY. Arthrodesis and arthroplasty of the small joints of the hand. In: Green D, ed. *Operative Hand Surgery.* Philadelphia: Elsevier; 2011:389–406.
9. McGlynn JT, Smith RA, Bogumill GP. Arthrodesis of small joints of the hand: a rapid and effective technique. *J Hand Surg Am.* 1988;13:595–599.
10. Watson HK, Shaffer SR. Concave-convex arthrodesis in joints of the hand. *Plast Reconstr Surg.* 1970;46:368–371.
11. Lister G. Intraosseous wiring of the digital skeleton. *J Hand Surg Am.* 1978;3:427–435.
12. Vanik RK, Weber RC, Matloub HS, et al. The comparative strengths of internal fixation techniques. *J Hand Surg Am.* 1984;9:216–221.
13. Ijsselstein CB, van Egmond DB, Hovius SER, et al. Results of small joint arthrodesis: comparison of Kirschner wire fixation with tension band wire technique. *J Hand Surg Am.* 1992;17:952–956.
14. Khuri SM. Tension band arthrodesis in the hand. *J Hand Surg Am.* 1986;11:41–45.
15. Leibovic SJ, Strickland JW. Arthrodesis of the proximal interphalangeal joint of the finger: comparison of the use of the Herbert screw with other fixation methods. *J Hand Surg Am.* 1994;19:181–188.
16. Stern PJ, Gates NT, Jones TB. Tension band arthrodesis of small joints in the hand. *J Hand Surg Am.* 1993;18:194–197.
17. Kovach JC, Werner FW, Palmer AK, et al. Biomechanical analysis of internal fixation techniques for proximal interphalangeal joint arthrodesis. *J Hand Surg Am.* 1986;11:562–566.
18. Stern PJ, Fulton DB. Distal interphalangeal joint arthrodesis: an analysis of complications. *J Hand Surg Am.* 1992;6:1139–1145.
19. Teoh LC, Yeo SJ, Singh I. Interphalangeal joint arthrodesis with oblique placement of an AO lag screw. *J Hand Surg Br.* 1994;19:208–211.

20. Wright CS, McMurtry RY. AO arthrodesis in the hand. *J Hand Surg Am.* 1983;8:932–935.
21. Buchler U, Aikin MA. Arthrodesis of the proximal interphalangeal joint by solid bone grafting and plate fixation in extensive injuries to the dorsal aspect of the finger. *J Hand Surg Am.* 1988;13:589–594.
22. Bishop AT. Small joint arthrodesis. *Hand Clin.* 1993;9:683–689.
23. Seitz WH, Sellman DC, Scarcella JB, et al. Compression arthrodesis of the small joints of the hand. *Clin Orthop Relat Res.* 1994;304: 116–121.
24. Ayres JR, Goldstrohm GL, Miller GJ, et al. Proximal interphalangeal joint arthrodesis with the Herbert screw. *J Hand Surg Am.* 1988;13:600–603.
25. Braun RM, Rhoades C. Dynamic compression for small bone arthrodesis. *J Hand Surg Am.* 1985;10:340–343.
26. Brutus JP, Palmer AK, Mosher JF, Harley BJ, Loftus JB. Use of a headless compressive screw for distal interphalangeal joint arthrodesis in digits: clinical outcome and review of complications. *J Hand Surg Am.* 2006;31A:85–89.
27. Burton RI, Margles SW, Lunseth PA. Small-joint arthrodesis in the hand. *J Hand Surg Am.* 1986;11:678–682.
28. Carroll RE, Hill NA. Small joint arthrodesis in hand reconstruction. *J Bone Joint Surg Am.* 1969;51:1219–1221.
29. Granowitz S, Vainio K. Proximal interphalangeal joint arthrodesis in rheumatoid arthritis: a follow-up study of 122 operations. *Acta Orthop Scand.* 1966;37:301–310.
30. Hogh J, Jensen P. Compression-arthrodesis of finger joints using Kirschner wires and cerclage. *Hand.* 1982;14:149–152.
31. Katzman SS, Gibeault JD, Dickson K, et al. Use of a Herbert screw for interphalangeal joint arthrodesis. *Clin Orthop Relat Res.* 1993;296:127–132.
32. Moberg E, Hendrickson B. Technique for digital arthrodesis: a study of 150 cases. *Acta Chir Scand.* 1960;18:331–338.

7

Thumb Arthroplasty and Arthrodesis

David J. Slutsky, MD

INTRODUCTION

Osteoarthritis commonly involves the thumb. In a large radiographic study of over 3000 patients between the ages of 40 and >80, 35% demonstrated involvement of the trapeziometacarpal (TM) joint, with a higher prevalence in women of 15% versus 7% for men.[1] Osteoarthritis is not merely a wear and tear or age-related phenomenon, but it is a common disease of articular cartilage that becomes more prevalent with advancing age. The biomechanical loads are of importance. In a biomechanical study, Cooney and Chao demonstrated that a pinch force of 1 kg at the thumb tip was amplified to 3.68 kg at the interphalangeal (IP) joint, 6.61 kg at the MCP joint, and up to 13.42 kg at the TM joint. The typical joint compression forces averaged 3 kg of force at the IP joint, 5.4 kg at the metacarpophalangeal joint, and 12.0 kg at the TM joint during simple pinch. Compression forces of as much as 120 kg may occur at the TM joint during strong grasp.[2] The alterations in the contact forces that may occur after injury or surgery to the TM joint due to ligamentous insufficiency can lead to even higher forces that can accentuate the wear on the articular cartilage. This chapter will focus on OA affecting the thumb IP, the MP, and the TM joints.

INTERPHALANGEAL JOINT

The mainstay of treatment consists of activity modification with the use of assistive devices and removable static IP joint splints. NSAIDs and selected cortisone injections are often beneficial provided medical monitoring is instituted with chronic use. Save for historical reports,[3] implant arthroplasty for the IP joint is not common.

Surgical Indications

With unrelieved pain or disabling joint instability an IP joint fusion is the procedure of choice. Marked joint instability that impairs pinching is another common indication. There is no specific age range, although it is preferable if the growth plates are closed. This is a salvage procedure that can be done at any time. The techniques are straightforward. Most consist of a dorsal capsulotomy followed by removal of the joint surfaces and immobilization of the joint with percutaneous K-wires or a headless compression screw.

Contraindications

This would include a history of recent infection and unstable soft tissue coverage. Marked bone loss is a relative contraindication.

Surgical Technique for IPJ Arthrodesis

A longitudinal or S-shaped incision is made centered over the IP joint. The extensor mechanism and dorsal capsule are divided in the midline, keeping the tissue planes separate for soft tissue closure over any exposed hardware. The collateral ligaments are released by sliding a scalpel blade underneath the insertion of the ligament on the neck of the proximal phalanx and cutting upwards to prevent injury to the neurovascular bundles. It is my preference to use a cup and cone arthrodesis that allows one to adjust the amount of rotation and varus/valgus without increasing the risk of joint incongruity. The joint can be fused in neutral or 15° to 25° of flexion. A rongeur is used to gently remove any cartilage remnants on the head of the proximal phalanx while preserving the normal convexity of the condyles since the metaphyseal bone is often quite soft that can lead to excessive bone removal. The cartilage and subchondral bone are removed from the base of the distal phalanx matching the curve of the head of the proximal phalanx and preserving a circumferential rim of cortical bone. Two convergent double-ended 0.035- or 0.045-in K-wires are advanced in a retrograde fashion through the base of the distal phalanx and out through the thumb tip. Ideally the K-wires should be placed immediately underneath the nail plate. The joint surfaces are then manually compressed in the desired degree of rotation and in neutral angulation or mild flexion while the K-wires are advanced down the intramedullary canal of the proximal phalanx, until

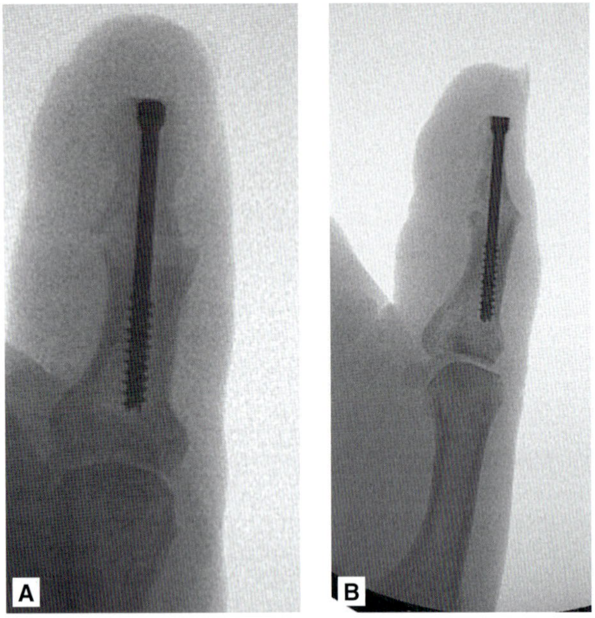

FIGURE 7-1 **A.** AP view of a chevron osteotomy and IP fusion with a headless screw. **B.** Note screw head is well buried in the intramedullary canal of the distal phalanx.

they abut the cortex or subchondral bone plate of the phalangeal base. The K-wire position is checked fluoroscopically and adjusted as necessary. Any defects at the fusion site can be packed with local bone graft or bone substitute. The capsule and extensor mechanism are closed in layers followed by tourniquet release and skin closure. When a headless screw is used, the joint is fused in neutral to prevent screw cutout and to permit adequate insertion down the intramedullary canal of the proximal phalanx (Fig. 7-1A and B). One of the K-wires is used as a guidewire to allow screw insertion in a retrograde fashion through the distal pulp. Postoperatively the IP joint is immobilized for 6 to 8 weeks until there are radiographic signs of union at which time a home program of gradual strengthening is instituted.

Complications

Infection can occur, especially with exposed K-wires. Nonunion is possible due to the small surface area for fusion. Malunion or malrotation can occur with loss of fixation. Due to the small canal size care is required during screw fixation to prevent screw cutout in the distal phalanx or interference with the nail matrix that can lead to a nail deformity. The screw head should be buried in the distal tuft to prevent tenderness with tip pinch while insuring there are adequate numbers of screw threads (at least 4) crossing the fusion site.

Outcomes

Most series are concerned mostly with the results of DIP arthrodesis and include but a few cases of thumb IPJ arthrodesis. Sieber and Segmuller however reported a series of 32 IP joint fusions using a figure-of-8 tension band wire and 2 crossed K-wires.[4] They adapted the angle of fusion based on the patient needs: for instrument grip the IP joint was fused in 5° to 10° of flexion, while for precision grip a larger angle of 20° to 30° was preferred. They believed tactile gnosis was best preserved when pronation of 5° to 10° and slight ulnar deviation of 5° of the distal phalanx in relation to the proximal phalanx was achieved. They also switched from an H-shaped incision to a fork-shaped incision to better preserve distal sensation. Stern and Fulton reviewed 131 patients (61 with OA) who underwent a distal joint fusion, 37 of whom had an IP joint fusion. Techniques included crossed K-wires with and without cerclage wires or Herbert screws, but the breakdown by joint was not listed. There were 4/37 IPJ nonunions as compared with 17/144 DIP nonunions. Time to union was not specified by joint but averaged 9 weeks for K-wires, 7.5 weeks with cerclage wires, and 10 weeks with screws. There were 2 thumb infections versus 4 finger infections. Clearly, the data are lacking to recommend one type of fixation method over another with IP joint OA; hence, surgeon preference largely dictates the technique.

METACARPOPHALANGEAL JOINT

The MP joint can be adequately splinted using a custom palmar-based thumb spica splint. NSAIDs and activity modification with avoidance of repetitive pinching exercises will provide adequate pain control in many cases. One or 2 selected cortisone injections can provide temporary relief but should not be used as a chronic form of treatment.

Surgical Indications

Symptomatic primary osteoarthritis that has not responded to conservative treatment is an indication for surgery. Symptomatic posttraumatic OA following an intra-articular fracture or from a chronic radial or ulnar collateral ligament tear is an additional indication for surgery. An MP joint hyperextension deformity of more than 30° that can be associated with TM OA may require a fusion.

Contraindications

Similar to the IPJ, these would include a history of recent infection and unstable soft tissue coverage. Marked bone loss can more easily be managed with intercalary bone graft and plate fixation (Fig. 7-2A and B).

MP Joint Arthroplasty

Thumb MP arthroplasty for OA is not commonly performed. Swanson popularized the use of silastic arthroplasty using a silicone dioxide elastomer, which was used as

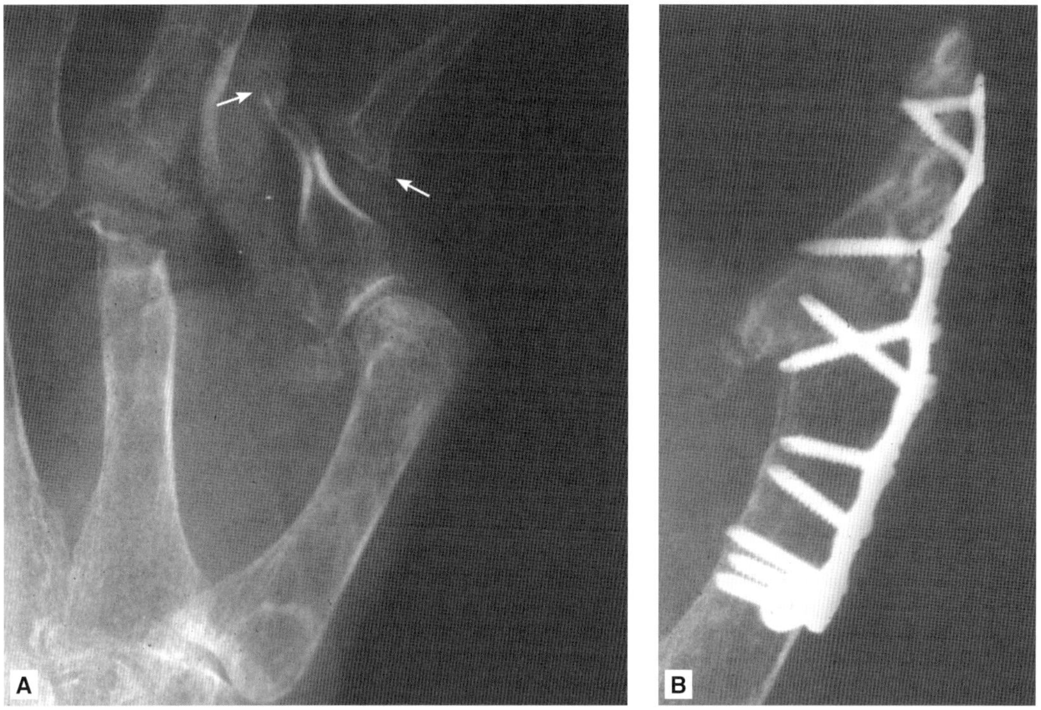

FIGURE 7-2 **A.** Marked instability of the IP joint that is no longer articulating with the head of the proximal phalanx (arrows). **B.** Combined fusion of the IP and MP joint using a 1.5-mm plate.

an elastic spacer for the treatment of rheumatoid arthritis. A requirement for this procedure was stable collateral ligaments. They have a longer life in low joint loading situations; hence, they are rarely used for thumb MP osteoarthritis. In 1981, Beckenbaugh and Steffee reported their experience with a 2-part metal and polyethylene prosthesis that were snap locked together.[5] Their series included 8/42 MP joint replacements in patients with MP OA. Due to the limited arc of motion (16°) and equal functional and esthetic outcomes as compared with an MP fusion this prosthesis was largely abandoned. Pyrocarbon implants are currently in vogue for treatment of MP OA in the finger joints, but studies on their use in the thumb MP joint are lacking.

Surgical Technique of an MP Fusion

The most popular form of treatment for painful MP joint OA or instability is an arthrodesis. There are a number of options including K-wire fixation (Fig. 7-3), with and without adjuvant tension band fixation, screw, and plate fixation. According to Inglis et al the MP joint of the thumb should be fused in approximately 15° of flexion, along with mild pronation and abduction of the proximal phalanx to facilitate tip pinch with the fingers.[6]

Most procedures begin with a straight or S-shaped incision centered over the MP joint, followed by a midline incision through the extensor hood and capsule. A cup and cone technique is my preference similar to the IP joint, with the thumb flexed approximately 15°. With severe deformity or

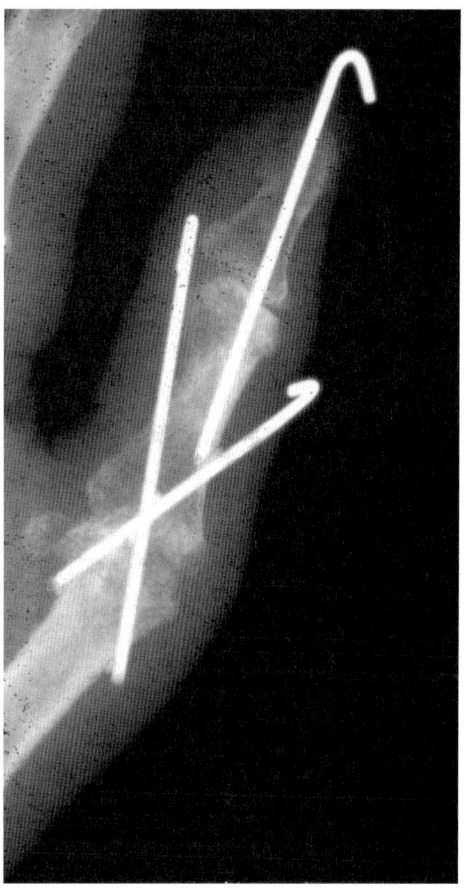

FIGURE 7-3 MP joint fusion with crossed K-wires.

bone loss, matching bone cuts can be made, but it is more difficult to achieve congruity at the fusion site if the MP joint is placed in flexion. The articular cartilage and subchondral bone are removed preserving the matching convexity/concavity of the joint surfaces. The joint is held in mild flexion and 2 convergent 0.035- or 0.045-in Kirschner wires are inserted through the dorsal neck of the thumb metacarpal neck and advanced distantly down the intramedullary canal of the proximal phalanx to the subchondral bone at the IP joint or alternatively engaging the palmar cortex at the midportion of the proximal phalanx. A transverse bone tunnel is made dorsal to the neutral axis at least 5 mm from the fusion site with a 0.045-in K-wire to prevent cutout. A 22-gauge wire strand is passed through the bone tunnel, looped in a figure-of-8 fashion over the longitudinal pins, and simultaneously twisted on the radial and ulnar sides just until the point of deformation of the twisted loop is seen. The K-wires are then withdrawn 5 mm, bent 90° using a needle holder and suction tip, and then tamped back into place capturing the tension band loop with the hooked ends, which are buried in bone (Fig. 7-4A-C). Bone graft substitute can be used to fill any gaps at the fusion site. All sharp metal

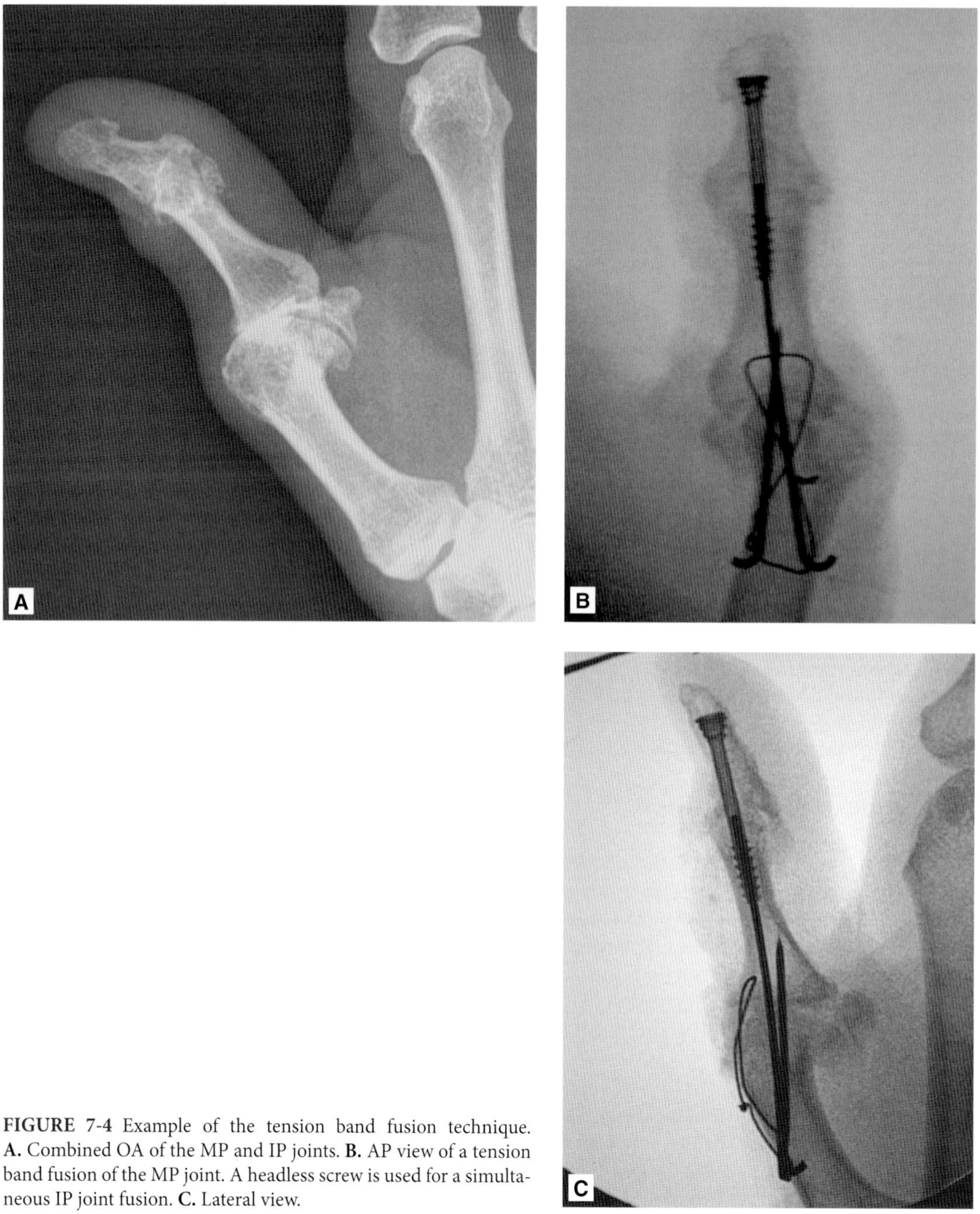

FIGURE 7-4 Example of the tension band fusion technique. **A.** Combined OA of the MP and IP joints. **B.** AP view of a tension band fusion of the MP joint. A headless screw is used for a simultaneous IP joint fusion. **C.** Lateral view.

ends are trimmed and the capsule is closed over the exposed hardware. The extensor mechanism and skin are sutured followed by a thumb spica splint for 6 to 8 weeks or until there is radiographic evidence of fusion.

One large-diameter or 2 smaller-diameter headless screws can be used in lieu of K-wire fixation provided there is adequate bone stock. A dorsally applied 1.5- to 2.0-mm plate can be used in cases with bone loss or for revision surgery.

Complications

Akin to the IP joint, infection and nonunion are possible complications. Malunion or malrotation can occur but can be compensated for by motion at the TM joint. Injuries to the branches of the superficial radial nerve can result in a painful neuroma.

Outcomes

Stanley et al reviewed 42 cases of MP arthrodesis using a chevron arthrodesis. Most of the cases were for inflammatory arthritis with an 83% patient satisfaction rate. Seven patents had continued pain or instability.[7] Schmidt et al used a cup and cone technique using a 3.0-mm cannulated AO screw and threaded washer in 26 patients.[8] The indications included instability (12), osteoarthritis (6), inflammatory arthritis (7), and paralytic boutonniere (1). Twenty-five of 26 joints went on to fusion at an average time of 10 weeks. There were no infections and no need for hardware removal. Bicknell et al performed a retrospective review of an interesting method of MP fusion used by Roth.[9] This consisted of bone excision creating 2 flat surfaces followed by use of a single 0.062-in K-wire inserted in a retrograde manner across the IP and MP joints with the MP in 10° of flexion and neutral deviation. The average age of the 28 patients was 49 ± 17 years. The indications included instability (9), inflammatory arthritis (18), OA (5), trauma (5), and skeletal dysplasia (1). The patients were casted for 4 weeks and splinted until there was radiographic union followed by pin removal at an average of 78 ± 32 days. Older patients took longer to unite, 209 days in 1 case! Although the mean DASH score was 28 ± 24, dexterity, hand function, and pinch were not significantly different from the opposite side and patient satisfaction was high. There were 3 complications consisting of pin loosening (1) and superficial infection (2). Twenty-five patients (89%) were able to return to their previous occupations. There were no radiographic malunions or nonunions.

TRAPEZIOMETACARPAL JOINT

The radiographic evaluation of the thumb carpometacarpal joint includes a true anteroposterior view, which is performed by placing the forearm in maximum pronation with the dorsal aspect of the thumb resting on the x-ray table and a true lateral view. A radial stress view of the thumb can be performed by asking the patient to push the radial borders of their thumbs together. This can demonstrate the degree of joint laxity by the amount of lateral subluxation of the metacarpal base. Eaton and Littler described a radiographic staging classification of TM OA that is in wide use.[10] Stage I comprises normal articular surfaces without joint space narrowing or sclerosis. There is less than one-third subluxation of the metacarpal base. Stage II reveals mild joint space narrowing, mild sclerosis, or osteophytes <2 mm in diameter. Instability is evident on stress views with >1/3 subluxation. The scaphotrapeziotrapezoidal (STT) joint is normal. In stage III there is significant joint space narrowing, subchondral sclerosis, and peripheral osteophytes >2 mm in diameter but a normal STT joint. In stage IV there is pantrapezial OA with narrowing, sclerosis, and osteophytes involving both the TM and STT joints. Similar to other joints, the radiographic severity of osteoarthritic changes at the TM joint does not correlate with the severity of clinical symptoms. The main thrust of treatment is pain management. A trial of activity modification and splinting should in general be undertaken in any patient prior to any surgical consideration. This involves avoidance of any repetitive pinching or grasping activities and the use of assistive devices as needed. Therapy may be useful for retaining range motion and augmenting thumb stability, whereas strengthening exercises are generally avoided while the patient has pain. NSAIDs are commonly used in addition to a limited number of selected cortisone injections in the TM joint for flare-ups or persistent pain that is unresponsive to conservative measures. Hyaluronic acid injections are still investigational but do not appear to be superior to steroid injections. The use of splints can provide pain relief and help enforce activity modification. In general, a forearm-based thumb spica splint with the thumb held in palmar abduction can be used on a full-time basis until the pain has been controlled and then intermittently as needed. Whether the IP joint is immobilized is largely dependent on patient and surgeon preference. A palmar-based thumb spica splint that immobilizes the TM joint by abducting the thumb can provide pain relief and may be more functional.

Surgical Indications

There are myriad techniques for the open treatment of TM osteoarthritis. There has been a stepwise evolution in these procedures over time that has created a bewildering number of surgical choices. It is therefore instructive to discuss these options in light of the stage of the disease. In the early stages the treatment options have included a volar ligament reconstruction without bony resection or an extension osteotomy of the thumb metacarpal. In more advanced stages various authors have advocated for a partial or complete trapezium excision with or without ligament reconstruction and with or without either tendon or an artificial interposition substance. Joint resurfacing arthroplasty or total joint replacement will not be specifically discussed due to the paucity of nonindustry-related long-term clinical data on the treatment of TM osteoarthritis.

STAGE I TO II DISEASE

Volar Ligament Reconstruction. This procedure is mostly indicated in patients with painful symptomatic laxity of the TM joint or stage I disease. The joint surfaces are typically normal, but there may be TM synovitis. An incision is made along the radial border of the thumb metacarpal curving proximally to the radial border of the FCR tendon preserving any sensory nerve branches. The thenar muscles are elevated from the metacarpal along with an exposure of the TM and STT joints. A volar to dorsal drill hole of progressively larger diameters is created using a cannulated 3.0-mm drill guide across the metacarpal base parallel to the TM joint and perpendicular to the metacarpal long axis. The TM joint is reduced and can be temporarily pinned in abduction with a 0.045-in K-wire. The FCR tendon is identified in the proximal extent of the incision. A number of small transverse incisions are made proximally along the course of the tendon up to its musculotendinous junction. The tendon is then split into a radial and ulnar half at the wrist incision and a 26-gauge wire loop is used to split the tendon proximally by grasping the loop with a needle holder and then pulling the wire proximally through each transverse incision. Since the FCR tendon rotates 180° as it courses distally, the ulnar half of the FCR is released at the musculotendinous junction since it lies radially at the wrist incision. The volar portion of the transverse carpal ligament is split and the superficial communicating branch of the radial artery is either retracted or ligated and divided. If there is an associated carpal tunnel syndrome, dividing the dorsal leaf of the transverse carpal ligament that forms the floor of the FCR sheath will decompress the carpal canal. The FCR graft is then pulled into the TM incision, while preserving its attachment onto the base of the index metacarpal. A suture retriever is used to pass the free end of the FCR graft through the drill hole from volar to dorsal, where it is sutured to the periosteum with a 3-0 nonabsorbable suture. The remaining end of the graft is passed through the abductor pollicis longus tendon insertion and across the volar capsule and sutured at both places. The tendon graft is then looped around the remaining FCR tendon and sutured to itself. The thenar muscles are repaired and the K-wire is removed. The thumb is immobilized in a spica splint or cast for 4 weeks followed by mobilization and strengthening.

Outcomes. Eaton et al had 1 of the largest long-term series, reviewing 50 patients with an average follow-up of 7 years.[11] Intractable pain was the primary indication for surgery. Ninety-five percent of the patients with stage I or II disease achieved good or excellent pain relief. All stage I cases and 82% of stage II cases showed no x-ray evidence of osteoarthritis up to 13 years postoperatively. Only 74% of patients with stage III and IV disease achieved good or excellent results. Lane and Henley included some of these patients in their review of 37 thumbs in 35 patients with an average follow-up of 5.2 years (range, 1-17 years).[12] Sixty-seven percent had excellent results and 30% had good results with almost universal partial or complete pain relief. All patients had a stable TM joint and an improvement in pinch strength. There was no clinical or x-ray evidence of osteoarthritis in any patient at the final follow-up.

Thumb Metacarpal Extension Osteotomy. Pellegrini et al demonstrated in a biomechanical study that the volar contact area of the TM joint was unloaded and shifted more dorsally as long as the location of the OA did not extend more dorsal than the midpoint of the trapezium, which provides the rationale for this procedure.[13] It is indicated in symptomatic Eaton stage I and II disease both for pain relief and to restore thumb stability. A 3-cm dorsal incision is made from the base of the thumb metacarpal moving distally. Sensory nerve branches are protected and retracted. A subperiosteal dissection is performed and a dorsally based 30° wedge of bone is resected 1 cm distal to the metacarpal base. The wedge of bone is removed and the distal metacarpal is extended to close the wedge, and then the osteotomy is held in place with K-wires, staples, or a plate.

Outcomes. There are no large series on this procedure. Tomaino prospectively evaluated 12 patients treated with an extension osteotomy with an average follow-up of 2.1 years (range, 6-46 months). Eleven patients were satisfied with the outcome and the grip and pinch strength increased by an average of 8.5 and 3 kg, respectively.[14] Parker et al reviewed Amadio's experience with 8 patients treated with this procedure with stage I (3 patients), stage II (3 patients), and stage III (2 patients) TM osteoarthritis at a mean follow-up of 9 years (range, 6-13 years).[15] The average lateral pinch strength was 5 kg or 129%, oppositional pinch strength 3 kg or 103%, and grip strength 19 kg or 108% of the opposite side. There was no radiographic progression of the arthritis in 5 of the 8 patients. Gwynne-Jones et al reviewed the results of thumb extension osteotomies without internal fixation in 28 patients with a mean age 54 years (range, 30-69 years).[16] At a mean follow-up of 34 months (range, 12-73 months) 21 patients with 22 procedures had good or excellent results, 2 had fair, and 1 had a poor result. Three patients required further surgery for persistent pain. Key pinch, pulp pinch, and tripod pinch were 22% to 32% lower, but there was no decrease in grip strength. The Michigan Hand Outcomes Questionnaire scores increased by an average of 28 points (range, 1-56), with a significant improvement in pain (44 points), activities of daily living (41 points), and satisfaction (35 points).

STAGE II TO IV DISEASE

Ligament Reconstruction Interposition (LRTI) Arthroplasty. This procedure described by Burton and Pellegrini in 1986 is typically used for more advanced stage II and III disease.[17] An 8-cm dorsoradial incision is made along the radial border of the thumb metacarpal curving down to the FCR tendon at the wrist. Branches of the superficial radial nerve and radial artery are identified and protected throughout the procedure. A longitudinal incision is made through the TM joint capsule. An oscillating saw is used to remove the base of the thumb metacarpal and the medullary canal is enlarged with a curette. A trapeziectomy is then performed by inserting a 0.62-in K-wire to act as a joystick by sequentially elevating soft tissue restraints until the trapezium can be removed in 1 piece. Alternatively the trapezium can be osteotomized into 4 sections and removed piecemeal while taking care to avoid injury to the FCR tendon that is in the volar depths of the wound. Caution is needed to prevent injury to the radial artery in the snuffbox that is just proximal to the STT joint. A 6-mm bony window is made with a power burr along the dorsal aspect of the thumb metacarpal 1 cm distal to the base (Fig. 7-5A-I).

One half of the FCR tendon is harvested and pulled into the thumb incision as described above. Some authors prefer to use the entire FCR, without any apparent deleterious effects. The free end of the tendon slip is passed into the

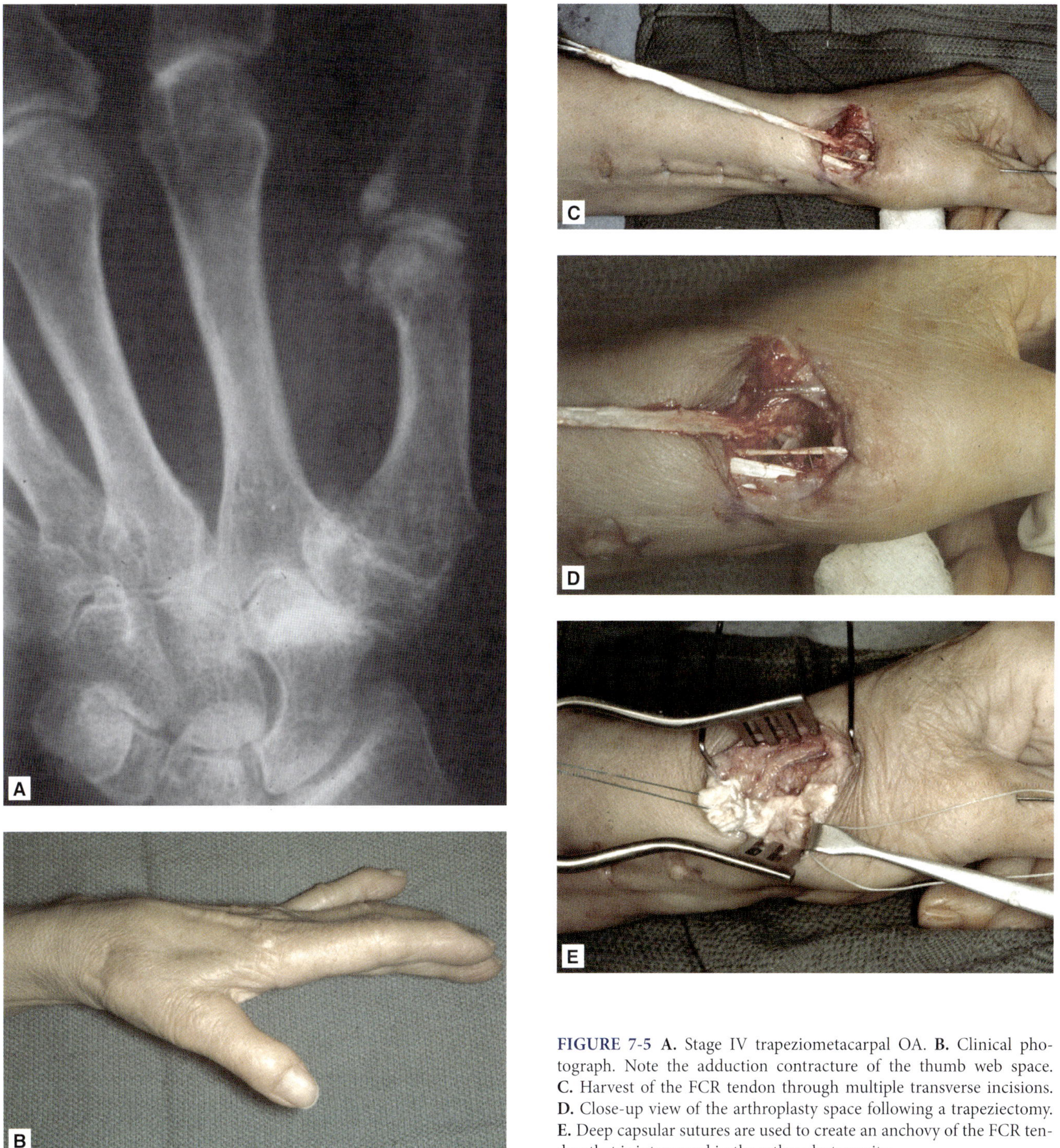

FIGURE 7-5 **A.** Stage IV trapeziometacarpal OA. **B.** Clinical photograph. Note the adduction contracture of the thumb web space. **C.** Harvest of the FCR tendon through multiple transverse incisions. **D.** Close-up view of the arthroplasty space following a trapeziectomy. **E.** Deep capsular sutures are used to create an anchovy of the FCR tendon that is interposed in the arthroplasty cavity.

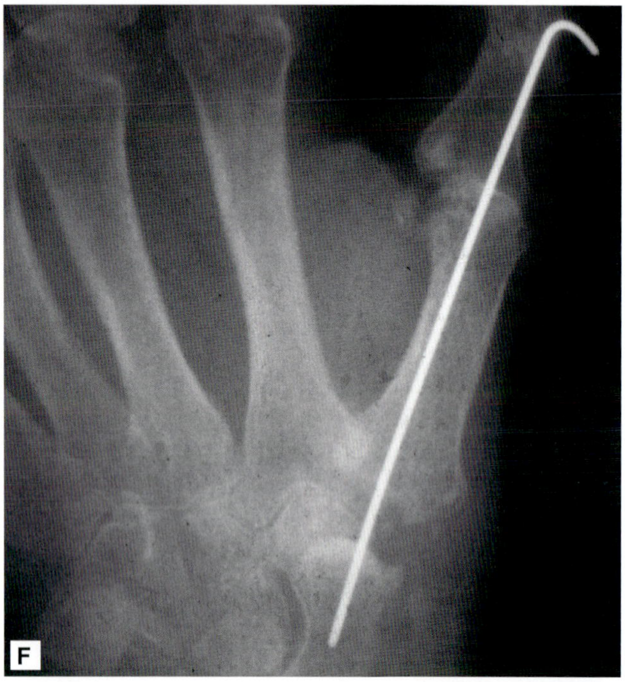

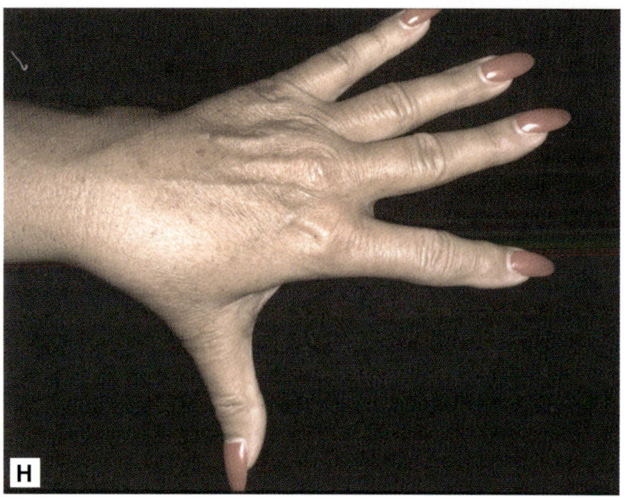

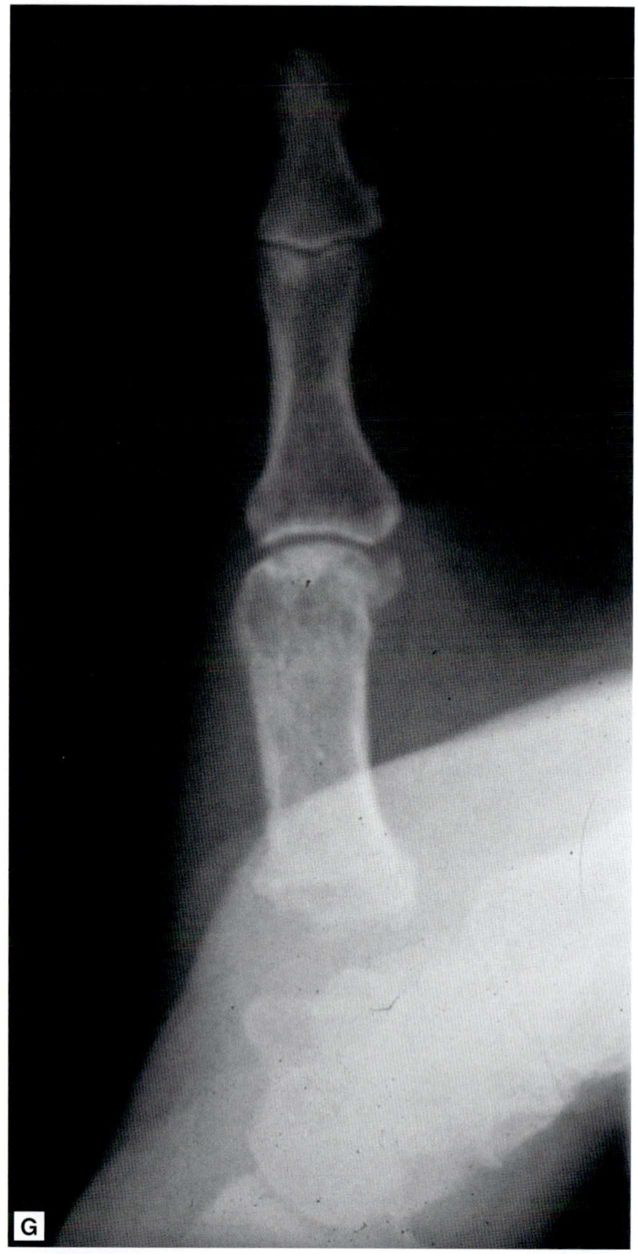

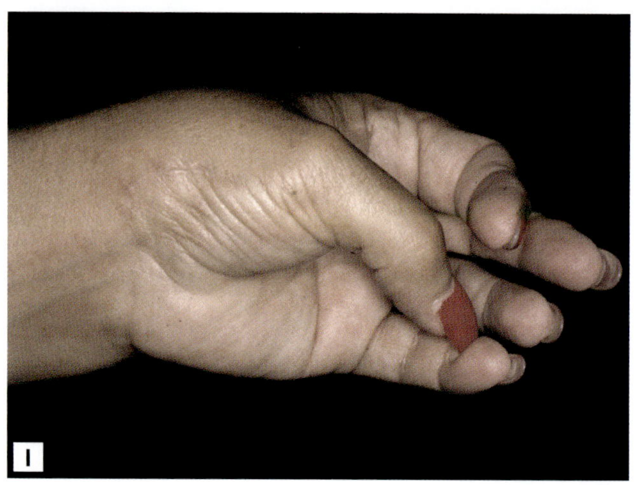

FIGURE 7-5 (*Continued*) **F.** Immediate postoperative photo demonstrating K-wire fixation of the arthroplasty site with the thumb metacarpal base distracted to the level of the index CMC joint. **G.** Maintenance of the arthroplasty space at 4 months. **H.** Postoperative photo at 4 months demonstrating widening of the thumb web space. **I.** Note the restored thumb opposition.

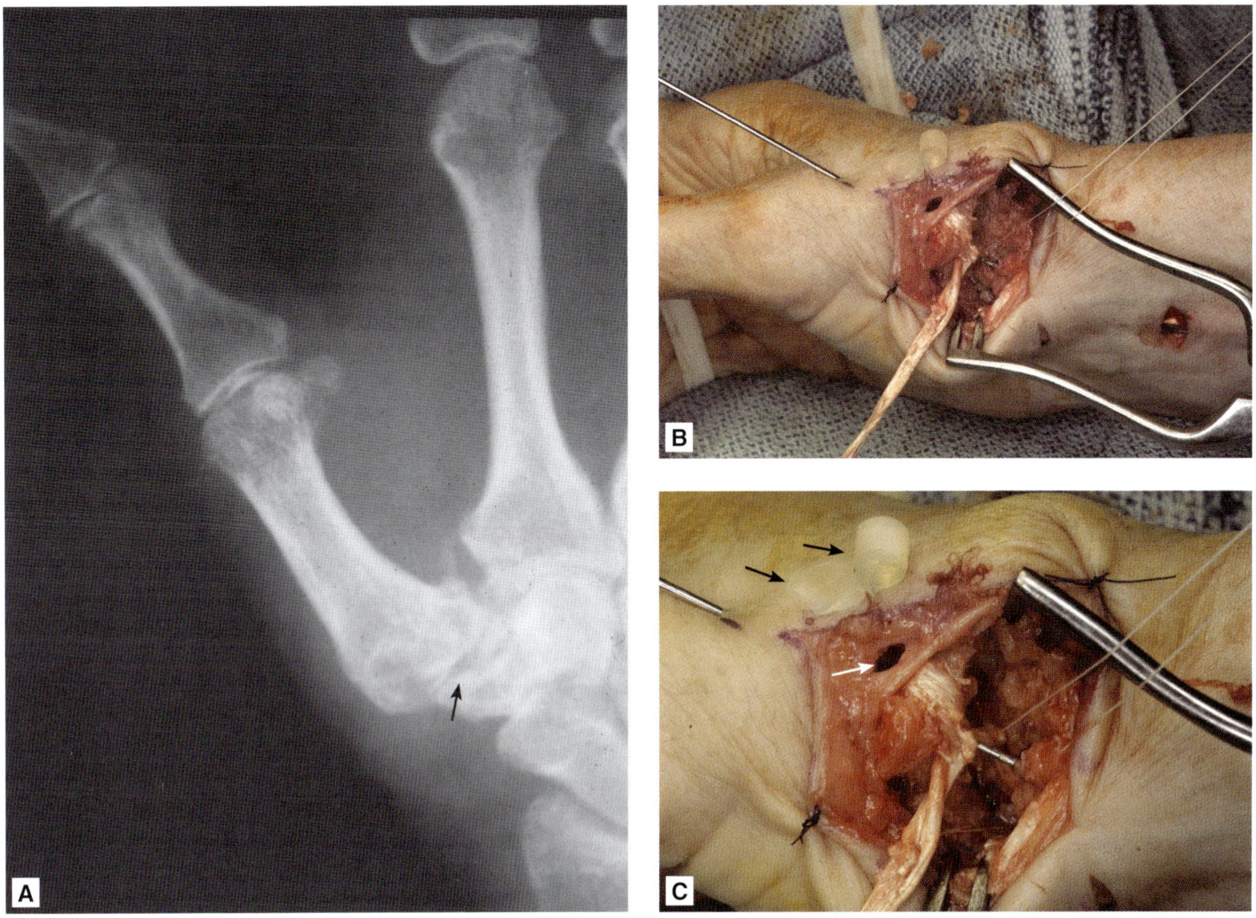

FIGURE 7-6 **A.** Recurrent basilar thumb pain at 5 years following a partial trapeziectomy and insertion of a silicone spacer (arrow). **B.** Removal of the silicone prosthesis and trapeziectomy. **C.** Close-up demonstrating the fragmented silicone prosthesis (black arrows) and the FCR tendon exiting from a lateral cortical window (white arrow) and wrapped around the metacarpal base.

medullary canal of the thumb metacarpal and out the dorsal cortical window, where it is sutured to the periosteum. It is then looped around the metacarpal base and sutured to itself while longitudinal traction is applied until the metacarpal base is even with the index CMC joint (Fig. 7-6A-C). Proper tensioning of the FCR graft helps prevent proximal migration and radial subluxation of the thumb. An optional percutaneous 0.045-in K-wire can be inserted through the metacarpal base and into the distal scaphoid with the thumb in abduction to maintain the arthroplasty space, according to surgeon preference. Two 2-0 nonabsorbable sutures are then placed in the deep volar capsular. One of the sutures is left attached to the deep capsule and threaded through the distal end of the FCR tendon slip to create an anchovy interposition, which is then tied down to the capsule. The remaining deep suture is used to repair the capsule over the anchovy in a vest over pants fashion. In the original surgical description, the extensor pollicis brevis is released from its insertion and tenodesed to the metacarpal shaft proximal to the metacarpophalangeal joint to eliminate the hyperextension moment acting on the proximal phalanx. The subcutaneous tissue and skin are closed in layers and a thumb spica splint is applied. Postoperatively a thumb spica splint is maintained until 4 weeks at which time any K-wires are removed and thumb abduction and extension exercises are instituted. Opposition is started at 6 weeks followed by progressive strengthening exercises.

Variants of the LRTI have included the following: tendon interposition alone, ligament reconstruction alone, a partial or complete trapeziectomy with tendon interposition but no ligament reconstruction, a limited trapeziectomy with tendon interposition and volar ligament reconstruction, a trapezial resection suspension plasty using the abductor pollicis longus tendon, and a partial trapeziectomy with implantation of a synthetic biological implant. A double interposition resurfacing arthroplasty was described for stage IV disease and involves a TM joint and STT joint resection and interposition.[18]

Trapeziectomy. This procedure is used in stage III and IV disease. A simple trapeziectomy has been complicated by metacarpal subsidence that can theoretically weaken the pinch strength and in extreme cases lead to metacarpal scaphoid impingement (Fig. 7-7A and B). This procedure has largely been supplanted by a hematoma distraction arthroplasty that consists of a trapeziectomy and temporary

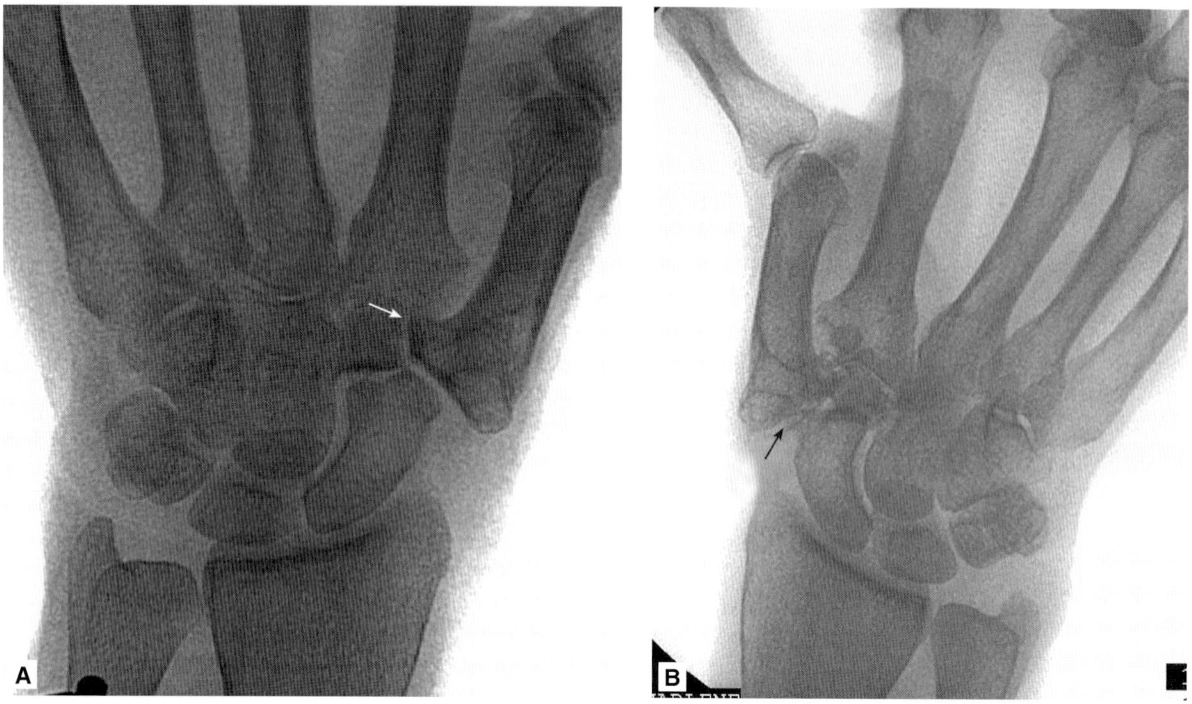

FIGURE 7-7 **A.** Marked subsidence following a trapeziectomy. Note the osteophyte formation at the metacarpal-trapezoid articulation (arrow). **B.** Subsidence with impingement of the metacarpal base and distal scaphoid (arrow).

distraction pinning of the thumb metacarpal. This procedure relies on the development of a stable pseudarthrosis that develops from the ingrowth of fibrous tissue that replaces the initial hematoma. The trapeziectomy is performed as described above. The thumb is then grasped and held in a position of wide palmar abduction, slight opposition, and distraction and 1 or two 0.062-in percutaneous K-wires are inserted from the base of the thumb metacarpal in a transverse orientation into the base of the index metacarpal or the trapezoid. Pinning the thumb metacarpal base to the index for 5 to 6 weeks is integral to the procedure, but tendon interposition or reconstruction of the TM joint capsule is not.

Complications. These include scar tenderness, tendon adhesion or rupture, injury to the superficial radial nerve branches or palmar cutaneous branch of the median nerve, or complex regional pain syndrome. K-wire infection can occur, especially when it is exposed. Metacarpal subsidence is a frequent occurrence but does not necessarily affect the outcome unless there is metacarpal–distal scaphoid impingement.

Outcomes. Froimson described the use of a rolled-up tendon anchovy for an interposition arthroplasty in 1970.[19] Although he reported pain relief in 80 procedures and 72 patients, the long-term follow-up showed a 30% reduction in pinch strength in addition to a 50% decrease in the arthroplasty space. Eaton and Littler introduced the concept of a beak ligament reconstruction in 1973.[10] Although they removed osteophytes if any, no trapeziectomy was performed. They reported that all the patients with stage II disease and 63% with stage III disease had excellent results at 1 year. They subsequently modified their procedure by adding a resection of the second metacarpal base and distal trapezium with 92% good or excellent results reported in 1985.[20] In 1986 Burton and Pellegrini published their technique of an LRTI.[17] They used one half of the FCR tendon to reconstruct the volar oblique ligament combined with a partial or complete trapeziectomy and interposition of the remaining tendon as an anchovy. In a retrospective series of 25 thumbs treated with an LRTI and hemitrapeziectomy (stage II and III), or complete trapeziectomy (stage IV, pantrapezial disease) at an average follow-up of 2 years, 92% of the patients had excellent pain relief and an average increase in pinch and grip strength of 19% (Fig. 7-8).

De Smet et al compared the outcomes of 22 patients who underwent a trapeziectomy, and 34 patients were treated with an LRTI at a follow-up of 26 to 34 months.[21] They found that the trapezial arthroplasty space was better maintained in the LRTI group with a loss of height of only 32% at the latest follow up as compared with a 57.5% decrease in height in the trapeziectomy group. Despite this finding there was no statistically significant difference for pain relief, patient satisfaction, DASH score, or grip strengths, but the key pinch strength was correlated with the amount of metacarpal subsidence.

Gray and Meals[22] believed that the poor results following a simple trapeziectomy that was reported by Gervis in 1949[23] could be improved by adding K-wire immobilization of the thumb in a distracted position for 5 to 6 weeks to allow the postoperative hematoma to organize, and the surrounding capsular remnants to consolidate to sufficiently anchor the metacarpal base. They reported their results with

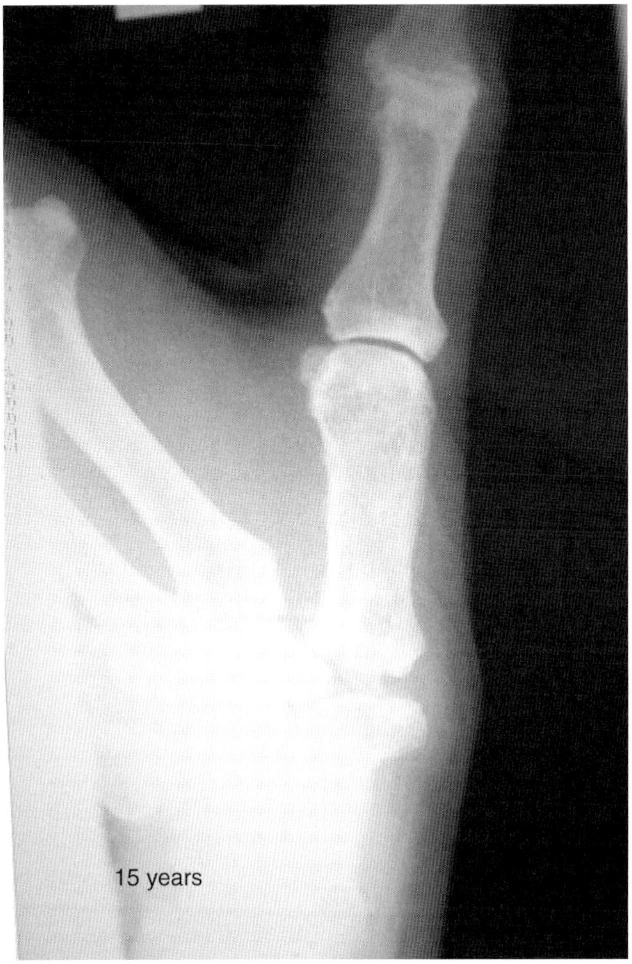

FIGURE 7-8 Asymptomatic patient at 15 years post LRTI demonstrating some subsidence but maintenance of an arthroplasty space.

this procedure in 22 patients with an average follow-up of 88 months. Eighteen patients were pain free, 21 of 22 thumbs adducted fully into the plane of the palm, and 21 of 22 opposed to the small finger metacarpal head. There was an average of 21% increase in grip strength and tip pinch strength, and an 11% increase in key pinch strength over preoperative values. They did note, however, that there was more metacarpal subsidence as compared with a more formal ligament reconstruction, but this did not correlate with outcomes.

Salem and Davis performed randomized prospective study of 99 patients (114 thumbs) comparing 59 procedures with a trapeziectomy without a ligament reconstruction, soft tissue interposition, or temporary Kirschner wire fixation in 59 cases and an LRTI in 55 cases.[24] At a mean follow-up of 6.2 years (range, 4.2-8.1), they found no significant differences between the 2 treatments in any subjective or objective outcome measure. The patients treated with an isolated trapeziectomy had an average DASH score of 31 and mean key pinch of 3.7 kg as compared with the LRTI group with a mean DASH score of 30 and mean key pinch of 4.1 kg.

Gangopadhyay et al performed a prospective, randomized controlled study on 174 patients with TM osteoarthritis who were randomized to a simple trapeziectomy, trapeziectomy with palmaris longus (PL) interposition, or trapeziectomy with ligament reconstruction and tendon interposition using one half of the FCR tendon.[25] K-wire fixation was used for 6 weeks in all patients. At a mean of 6 years (range, 5-18 years) patients had no pain or pain with an after use, but there were no restrictions in the trapeziectomy and LRTI groups. Although some patients in the PL interposition group had limitation with activity, there was no statistical difference between the groups. There was no difference in the ability to perform activities such as writing, turning a key, opening a screw-top jar, handling coins, and knitting, nor any significant difference between pinch and grip nor thumb opposition among the 3 groups. They concluded that the outcomes of these 3 variations of trapeziectomy were very similar and that although the use of additional soft tissue procedures was not detrimental, they were not necessary and excision of the trapezium remained the most important part of the surgery.

Wajon et al performed a meta-analysis of the Cochrane database of 7 studies with 384 patients having stage II or III disease who had undergone a trapeziectomy, trapeziectomy with interpositional arthroplasty, trapeziectomy with ligament reconstruction, trapeziectomy with LRTI, and joint replacement.[26] No procedure demonstrated any superiority over another in terms of pain, function, range of motion, or strength. However, participants who underwent trapeziectomy had 16% fewer adverse effects ($P \leq .001$).

Associated MP Joint Hyperextension. MP joint hyperextension often accompanies advanced TM osteoarthritis that produces a dorsal subluxation stress at the TM joint arthroplasty site and may lead to recurrent subluxation. Correction of this MP hyperextension reverses the metacarpal collapse and improves the force transmission along the thumb ray. If there is MP joint OA, an MP joint fusion is indicated. In cases of a mild MP joint hyperextension of 20° to 30°, Eaton and Floyd have recommended transferring the EPB to the base of the thumb metacarpal, which eliminates the extension force on the MP joint and augments abduction of the thumb metacarpal.[27] The joint is pinned or casted in flexion for 4 weeks postoperatively. For MP joint hyperextension of 30° or more, an MP joint volar capsulodesis or a sesamoidesis is added. In their series of MP capsulodesis of 13 patients with an average follow-up of 39 months, 10 patients had complete correction of the MP hyperextension deformity with 9 excellent results, 3 good results, and 1 fair result.

Poulter and Davis[28] reviewed 297 thumbs with painful TM osteoarthritis. Preoperatively 101 had no hyperextension of the MP joint, and 168 had a hyperextension deformity of 30° or less of whom 157 received no treatment. Twenty-eight patients had hyperextension >30°, 8 of whom were not treated. Nine were treated by temporary insertion of a Kirschner wire, 6 by MP fusion, 5 by sesamoidesis with a lag screw, and 11 by palmar capsulodesis using a bone anchor. At a 1-year follow-up, there was no progression in the deformity and there were no significant differences in the pain levels and key and tip pinch strengths between the thumbs without preoperative MP hyperextension and those with untreated hyperextension ≤30°. All 5 cases of sesamoidesis with a screw were successful, but 3 patients required a screw removal. In the 11 patients with hyperextension >30° treated with a capsulodesis using a bone anchor, the deformity was reduced from a preoperative mean of 48° (range, 35°-70°) to 16° (range, 0°-35°). There were no significant differences in the pain levels and key and tip pinch strengths between the untreated hyperextension group and those treated with a bone anchor capsulodesis. Temporary insertion of a Kirschner wire did not result in improvement in the hyperextension deformity or clinical outcome.

Trapeziometacarpal Fusion. TM fusion has been advocated for patients with stage II and III disease with strong functional demands such as manual laborers and patients younger than 40 years with posttraumatic osteoarthritis since it provides a stable thumb ray with no risk of instability. The TM joint is exposed and the joint surfaces are denuded of cartilage and subchondral bone to create 2 parallel surfaces. The thumb is positioned in 35° to 45° of palmar abduction and 20° to 30° of radial abduction and pronation so that the thumb pulp rests on the radial aspect of the index finger middle phalanx in mild opposition. K-wire, staple, or plate fixation can be used (Fig. 7-9). In cases of revision or if there is bone loss with a small trapezial remnant, a minicondylar blade plate is ideal. A short arm thumb spica cast is used for 6 weeks, followed by a splint until there are signs of fusion.

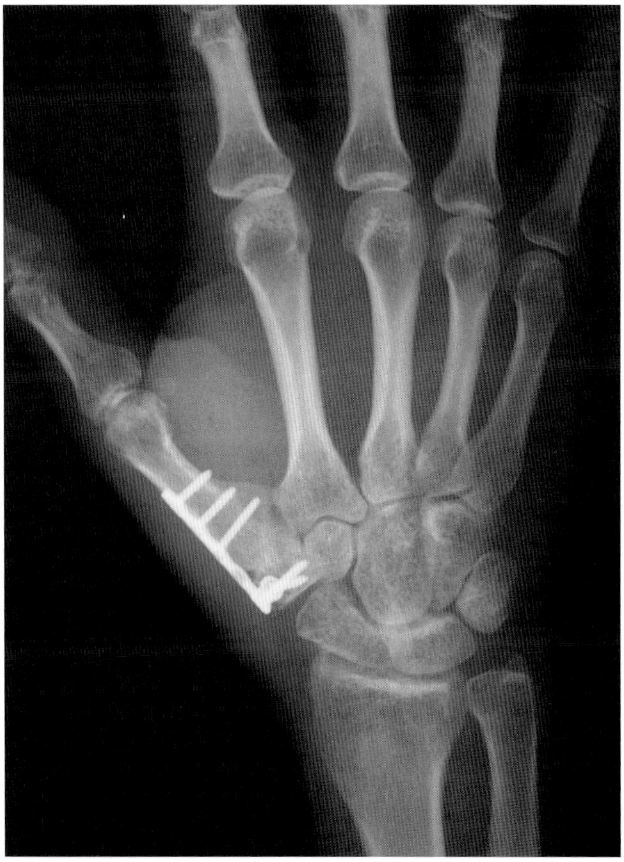

FIGURE 7-9 Trapeziometacarpal fusion using a laterally applied plate.

Complications. Forseth and Stern reviewed 19 patients who underwent a TM arthrodesis with plate and screw fixation.[29] At an average follow-up of 40 months there were 2 painful nonunions and 6 hardware malpositions most frequently associated with a screw in the trapeziotrapezoid joint. Seven arthrodeses had a second procedure, most commonly hardware removal. In 59 patients treated with K-wire fixation there were 4 nonunions and 2 required a secondary procedure.

Outcomes. Rizzo et al examined the Mayo clinic experience of TM fusion for OA in 114 patients/126 thumbs at an average follow-up of 11.2 years (range, 3-28 years).[30] The average patient age was 57 years (range, 32-77). Supplemental bone graft was used in 90 thumbs. There were 17 nonunions, 9 of them requiring reoperation. The appositional pinch increased to 5.9 kg versus 3.0 kg preoperatively, oppositional pinch 5.4 kg versus 2.7 kg, and grip strengths 23 kg versus 14 kg. The average pain score decreased to 0.4 versus 6.6 preoperatively (*P* <.01). Thirty-nine patients developed radiographic signs of STT OA, but only 8 patients were symptomatic. MP joint OA occurred in 16 patients, but no additional treatment was needed.

There are many published case series that examined the results of these disparate procedures. Taylor et al performed a retrospective study of 83 patients with TM joint osteoarthritis who were treated with a TM fusion (36), trapeziectomy with and without ligament reconstruction (25), or a silastic replacement (22).[31] The follow-up ranged from 1 to 5 years. There was a higher rate of complications and reoperation in the fusion group but otherwise no significant differences in terms of patient satisfaction, range of movement, and tip and key pinch.

Raven et al reviewed 54 patients (74 thumbs) with TM OA who were treated with a trapeziectomy (18 thumbs), trapeziectomy with tendon interposition (17 thumbs), or TM arthrodesis (28 thumbs). The average follow-up was 13 years for the resection group, 8 years for the trapeziectomy group, and 9 years for the arthrodesis group. Patients in the trapeziectomy group had significantly less pain and better radial abduction as compared with the arthrodesis group. There was no difference among the 3 groups in grip and tip pinch strength. None of the patients in the trapeziectomy group needed a reoperation, 1 patient in the resection arthroplasty group had a reoperation, and 22 patients in the arthrodesis group had 1 or more reoperations for hardware removal or because of a complication.

REFERENCES

1. Wilder FV, Barrett JP, Farina EJ. Joint-specific prevalence of osteoarthritis of the hand. *Osteoarthritis Cartilage*. 2006;14:953–957.
2. Cooney WP 3rd, Chao EY. Biomechanical analysis of static forces in the thumb during hand function. *J Bone Joint Surg Am*. 1977;59:27–36.

3. Wilgis EF. Distal interphalangeal joint silicone interpositional arthroplasty of the hand. *Clin Orthop Relat Res*. 1997:38–41.
4. Sieber HP, Segmuller G. Arthrodesis of the interphalangeal joint of the thumb: indication, technic, results. *Handchir Mikrochir Plast Chir*. 1983;15:11–16.
5. Beckenbaugh RB, Steffee A. Total joint arthroplasty for the metacarpophalangeal joint of the thumb—a preliminary report. *J Bone Joint Surg Am*. 1981;4:295–297.
6. Inglis AE, Hamlin C, Sengelmann RP, et al. Reconstruction of the metacarpophalangeal joint of the thumb in rheumatoid arthritis. *J Bone Joint Surg Am*. 1972;54:704–712.
7. Stanley JK, Smith EJ, Muirhead AG. Arthrodesis of the metacarpophalangeal joint of the thumb: a review of 42 cases. *J Hand Surg Br*. 1989;14:291–293.
8. Schmidt CC, Zimmer SM, Boles SD. Arthrodesis of the thumb metacarpophalangeal joint using a cannulated screw and threaded washer. *J Hand Surg Am*. 2004;29:1044–1050.
9. Bicknell RT, MacDermid J, Roth JH. Assessment of thumb metacarpophalangeal joint arthrodesis using a single longitudinal K-wire. *J Hand Surg Am*. 2007;32:677–684.
10. Eaton RG, Littler JW. Ligament reconstruction for the painful thumb carpometacarpal joint. *J Bone Joint Surg Am*. 1973;55:1655–1666.
11. Eaton RG, Lane LB, Littler JW, et al. Ligament reconstruction for the painful thumb carpometacarpal joint: a long-term assessment. *J Hand Surg Am*. 1984;9:692–699.
12. Lane LB, Henley DH. Ligament reconstruction of the painful, unstable, nonarthritic thumb carpometacarpal joint. *J Hand Surg Am*. 2001;26:686–691.
13. Pellegrini VD Jr, Parentis M, Judkins A, et al. Extension metacarpal osteotomy in the treatment of trapeziometacarpal osteoarthritis: a biomechanical study. *J Hand Surg Am*. 1996;21:16–23.
14. Tomaino MM. Treatment of Eaton stage I trapeziometacarpal disease with thumb metacarpal extension osteotomy. *J Hand Surg Am*. 2000;25:1100–1106.
15. Parker WL, Linscheid RL, Amadio PC. Long-term outcomes of first metacarpal extension osteotomy in the treatment of carpal–metacarpal osteoarthritis. *J Hand Surg Am*. 2008;33:1737–1743.
16. Gwynne-Jones DP, Penny ID, Sewell SA, et al. Basal thumb metacarpal osteotomy for trapeziometacarpal osteoarthritis. *J Orthop Surg (Hong Kong)*. 2006;14:58–63.
17. Burton RI, Pellegrini VD Jr. Surgical management of basal joint arthritis of the thumb. Part II. Ligament reconstruction with tendon interposition arthroplasty. *J Hand Surg Am*. 1986;11:324–332.
18. Barron OA, Eaton RG. Save the trapezium: double interposition arthroplasty for the treatment of stage IV disease of the basal joint. *J Hand Surg Am*. 1998;23:196–204.
19. Froimson AI. Tendon arthroplasty of the trapeziometacarpal joint. *Clin Orthop Relat Res*. 1970;70:191–199.
20. Eaton RG, Glickel SZ, Littler JW. Tendon interposition arthroplasty for degenerative arthritis of the trapeziometacarpal joint of the thumb. *J Hand Surg Am*. 1985;10:645–654.
21. De Smet L, Sioen W, Spaepen D, et al. Treatment of basal joint arthritis of the thumb: trapeziectomy with or without tendon interposition/ligament reconstruction. *Hand Surg*. 2004;9:5–9.
22. Gray KV, Meals RA. Hematoma and distraction arthroplasty for thumb basal joint osteoarthritis: minimum 6.5-year follow-up evaluation. *J Hand Surg Am*. 2007;32:23–29.
23. Gervis WH. Excision of the trapezium for osteoarthritis of the trapezio-metacarpal joint. *J Bone Joint Surg Br*. 1949;31B:537–539 [illust].
24. Salem H, Davis TR. Six year outcome excision of the trapezium for trapeziometacarpal joint osteoarthritis: is it improved by ligament reconstruction and temporary Kirschner wire insertion? *J Hand Surg Eur*. 2012;37:211–219.
25. Gangopadhyay S, McKenna H, Burke FD, et al. Five- to 18-year follow-up for treatment of trapeziometacarpal osteoarthritis: a prospective comparison of excision, tendon interposition, and ligament reconstruction and tendon interposition. *J Hand Surg Am*. 2012;37:411–417.
26. Wajon A, Ada L, Edmunds I. Surgery for thumb (trapeziometacarpal joint) osteoarthritis. *Cochrane Database Syst Rev*. 2005:CD004631.
27. Eaton RG, Floyd WE 3rd. Thumb metacarpophalangeal capsulodesis: an adjunct procedure to basal joint arthroplasty for collapse deformity of the first ray. *J Hand Surg Am*. 1988;13:449–453.
28. Poulter RJ, Davis TR. Management of hyperextension of the metacarpophalangeal joint in association with trapeziometacarpal joint osteoarthritis. *J Hand Surg Eur*. 2011;36:280–284.
29. Forseth MJ, Stern PJ. Complications of trapeziometacarpal arthrodesis using plate and screw fixation. *J Hand Surg Am*. 2003;28:342–345.
30. Rizzo M, Moran SL, Shin AY. Long-term outcomes of trapeziometacarpal arthrodesis in the management of trapeziometacarpal arthritis. *J Hand Surg Am*. 2009;34:20–26.
31. Taylor EJ, Desari K, D'Arcy JC, et al. A comparison of fusion, trapeziectomy and silastic replacement for the treatment of osteoarthritis of the trapeziometacarpal joint. *J Hand Surg Br*. 2005;30:45–49.

8

Principles of Nerve Repair

Lars B. Dahlin, MD, PhD
Niels Thomsen, MD, PhD
Anders Björkman, MD, PhD

INTRODUCTION

Rational and Basic Science

Although nerve injuries and disorders have a relatively low frequency, as compared with other injuries, their impact on the injured individual may be substantial. Even an injury to a digital nerve in the hand, which is the most frequently severed peripheral nerve, may reduce hand function and dexterity in spite of the limited size of skin area innervation by the digital nerve.[1] A median or ulnar nerve injury have an even stronger impact on the individual's life due to the sensory and motor dysfunction after such injuries.[2] Thus, repair and reconstruction of injured nerve trunks are crucial to restore hand function in the affected patient.

The age of the patient is an important determinant of outcome. Sensory function is often permanently disturbed if the injured patient has passed puberty.[3,4] The age of the patients may also determine the time needed to return to work.[5] There are also other factors that may determine outcome after nerve injuries, such as a slow outgrowth of axons, the misdirection of the outgrowing nerve fibers at the site of injury, the sensory nerve cell death in dorsal root ganglia and the extensive changes in the central nervous system induced after a nerve injury.[6,7] In spite of intensive research, there is no clinically available technique to increase the rate and to improve the accuracy of axonal outgrowth, but sensory nerve cell death may be possible to prevent by pharmacological substances as an adjunct to surgery.[8] The central nervous system has a tremendous ability to continuously modulate its organization as a response to activity, behavior, skill acquisition, and injury, a phenomenon often referred to as plasticity.[7,9,10] This plasticity can be used to create new treatment strategies after nerve repair and reconstruction.[11] Specific factors related to the patient's cognitive capacity, such as verbal learning and visuospatial logic capacity, are also correlated to return of functional sensibility after median and ulnar nerve injuries.[12] In addition, patient-related factors, such as sense of coherence, motivation, and coping strategies, to improve outcome are also relevant in this context.[13] Other factors beyond the influence by the surgeon are the type of nerve, as well as the level and the type of injury (eg, the severity), where the level of injury and the type of injured nerve are particularly important for motor recovery.[14] It is generally believed that there is a better recovery of motor function after a median than after an ulnar nerve.[14,15]

However, there are 2 factors that the surgeons definitely can attend to—performance of a proper nerve repair or reconstruction and to perform the procedure with appropriate timing. The latter view is based on the knowledge of the cellular and molecular processes, by which the neuron and Schwann cells orchestrate survival and provide optimal conditions for the axons to extend from their cell bodies after nerve injury and repair,[16] which points toward the advantage of early repair after nerve injury. The injured neurons must reconstitute their damaged membrane as well as redistribute and manufacture their production of substances with the purpose of survival, growth, and formation of new synapses, where the outgrowing axons have to face a more mature and complex environment than during development,[16,17] an environment which may be even more complex in the central nervous system.[18] Delayed nerve repairs often impair the nerve regeneration process. The extent of axonal outgrowth correlates positively to presence of molecular substances important for survival and outgrowth,[19] and negatively to occurrence of apoptotic Schwann cells.[20,21] In addition, outgrowing axons may also directly influence the activation, proliferation, and apoptosis of Schwann cells,[21,22] indicating a close interaction between axons and Schwann cells. In this context, the behavior of the motor and sensory neurons in the spinal cord and in dorsal root ganglia, respectively, is also relevant for the timing of nerve repair.[19,23] The possibility to introduce pharmacological intervention as a neuroprotective procedure, as an adjunct to surgical repair, is also time dependent.[24] Thus, there are a variety of factors that influence outcome of nerve injury and repair, where symptoms, such as motor and sensory dysfunction, allodynia, neuropathic pain, as well as cold intolerance, may have a substantial impact on the affected patient.

INDICATIONS

The crucial issue in all types of hand injuries is to make a correct diagnosis by a proper examination of motor and sensory function distally to the suspected level of injury. After listening to the patient's history, judgment of the patient's tentative other injuries, and inspection of the wound, the motor and sensory function of the affected nerve distal to the site of injury is carefully assessed. Weakness or any atrophy of individual muscles is evaluated to get an impression if the nerve is injured, partially or completely. Assessment of the patient's ability to feel pain (eg, applied by small forceps) in the skin area innervated by the specific nerve, evaluation of subjective sensation (eg, monofilament test), measuring the 2-point discrimination (2-PD), judgment of sudomotor function, and detection of any Tinel sign are methods in the diagnostic arsenal to monitor sensory function.

Decision making of surgery and exploration requires an experienced surgeon. Generally, there is no limit at what age nerve repair can be performed at wrist level or in the hand, but the results are poorer in older age groups. Data indicate that patients older than 40 years have a significantly poorer recovery of sensation than younger patients[25,26] as well as higher costs for treatment.[1] However, it should be emphasized that a nerve repair or reconstruction procedure even in a patient at high age may reduce the formation of neuroma and therefore the possibility of tentative neuropathic pain.

TIMING OF NERVE REPAIR OR RECONSTRUCTION

As a general rule, nerve trunks should be repaired as soon as possible and an immediate repair is preferable within the first 48 hours, a statement that has support by neurobiological data. However, repair can be done at later time points, practically and preferably within 2 to 3 weeks after the injury, since nerve injuries with wounds that happened more than 48 hours earlier may be more securely explored and repaired or reconstructed after the wound has completely healed. If there is a longer delay than 3 weeks, the delayed nerve repair procedure may actually be a nerve reconstruction procedure requiring a nerve graft. The upper time limit, where a nerve reconstruction procedure is not recommended, cannot be stated with certainty, but the cellular and molecular processes in neurons and Schwann cells, induced by the injury, deteriorate over time.

If a sharp transection of the nerve is present, an immediate exploration, revision, and nerve repair or reconstruction, depending on the status of the nerve, are advisable. If there is an open wound and a crushed nerve is found with continuity, the wound is revised and closed if the surgeon believes that the nerve regeneration can proceed across the site of injury. In such situations, it is mandatory to follow any signs of regeneration and reinnervation by regularly examining Tinel sign or return of muscle function—that is, active surveillance—and hopefully nerve function will return. However, nerve repair or reconstruction procedures are recommended only if the wound is tidy and a macroscopic nerve discontinuity is found. On the other hand, if a contaminated wound is present, single or repeated revisions are performed and delayed nerve repair or reconstruction is done at a time when there is no risk for postoperative infection.

A particular problem is closed traction injuries of nerve trunks. Depending on the amount and character of the trauma the principle of active surveillance can be applied in such cases. If no functional recovery is seen, the nerve should be explored. However, if there are indications to explore and repair other tissues in the hand or fingers (eg, fractures) at an early stage, one should consider also exploring a dysfunctional nerve trunk to avoid an unnecessary delay in repair or reconstruction. A further problem is open wounds in connection with gunshot or blast injuries, where nerve repair or reconstruction can immediately be done if there is a tidy wound and the necrotic part of the injured nerve can be resected with certainty. If the latter is not possible and particularly if the wound is impregnated with foreign bodies, debris, and bacteria, which is the most common situation, a delayed nerve repair or most probably a nerve reconstruction has to be done as soon as the local wound conditions allow such procedures.

Neurography or an electromyography can be a valuable diagnostic aid to establish the diagnosis or to identify injured parts of a nerve preoperatively and postoperatively. However, it may take up to 4 weeks after injury before clear signs of nerve degeneration and denervation activity in muscles can be detected. Nevertheless, the clinical examination is more important and electrophysiological examination should not delay exploration, since timing of nerve repair and reconstruction is important.

CONTRAINDICATIONS

Generally, there are no contraindications for exploration of nerve injuries if the patient's general medical health allows surgery, although nerve regeneration can be impaired if the patient has some kind of neuropathy. An individual judgment should be made of the patients, and the factors pointed out to influence the outcome should be considered, as well as the potential risks and benefits from surgery. Contraindications for nerve repair or reconstruction are mainly related to the condition of the wound, with the potential risk of an iatrogenic infection, or the bed for a nerve graft may not have an optimal condition. In such cases appropriate reconstruction procedures, such as application of different flaps to cover sensitive tissues, for example, bone, tendons, and vessels, may create a more viable environment for future nerve grafting. Such procedures should be done after a careful debridement to remove any nonviable and necrotic tissue from the contaminated wound before one can consider doing any further nerve repair or reconstruction. In specific situations even multiple debridements may be necessary followed by appropriate soft-tissue coverage of the area before nerve repair or reconstruction is considered. Preferably, nerve reconstruction should be done within 3 weeks after injury, a time span when scarred parts of the peripheral nerve trunks can easily be defined and resected.

SURGICAL TECHNIQUE

The patient is placed in a supine position with the arm abducted. The hand is positioned properly on the arm table allowing the specific nerve to be explored. The procedures can be performed in general anesthesia or, preferably, in an axillary plexus block with a tourniquet applied around the upper arm (eg, inflated 80-100 mm Hg above the systolic pressure). Thus, the nerve, and any additional injuries to other tissues, such as tendons and blood vessels, can be explored and repaired. However, if there surely is only a single digital nerve injury in the finger, one may consider just a finger block with a finger tourniquet applied.

Conventional preoperative preparations, as in all type of hand surgery, with scrubbing and skin cleansing of the arm are done. Preoperative antibiotics are prescribed if necessary, preferably to protect against *Staphylococcus aureus*, for example, cloxacillin or clindamycin, or, if severely untidy (eg, outdoor injury), another strategy may be needed (eg, combination of sulfamethoxazole and trimethoprim). It is strongly recommended to liberally use swabs for bacterial cultures from the wound and to discuss strategy of antibiotic treatment with appropriate expertise.

Microsurgical instruments and the use of loop magnification or a microscope are advisable to use for the surgeon, who should have proper microsurgical training and technical skills. Conventional incisions in the hand or around the wrist are combined with the wound to explore the main nerve trunk, that is, the median nerve, the ulnar nerve, or the radial nerve, with their common digital nerve or digital nerve branches (Fig. 8-1). The tissues are dissected with an atraumatic approach avoiding damage to the surrounding and nervous tissue. The dissection and repair should be done stepwise.

The injured nerve trunk is longitudinally dissected and the nerve ends are identified. Necrotic parts of the proximal and distal nerve ends are resected, preferably by use of fresh surgical blades. The fascicular pattern of the nerve trunk can thereby be visualized. After the initial *preparation* of the nerve ends, these structures are now approximated, which should be done without any tension. It is possible to mobilize the proximal and distal nerve ends to facilitate the *approximation*. However, this should be made with caution since stretching of the nerve trunk may reduce the intraneural blood flow, thereby causing apoptosis and impaired activation of Schwann cells.[27] Such cellular events lead to deterioration of nerve regeneration. The amount of tension that is acceptable is difficult to generally recommend, but if flexion of a joint is needed to approximate the nerve ends, the tension is doubtfully too high and reconstruction with nerve graft is recommended. The third step is *coaptation* of the proximal and distal nerve ends to their correct

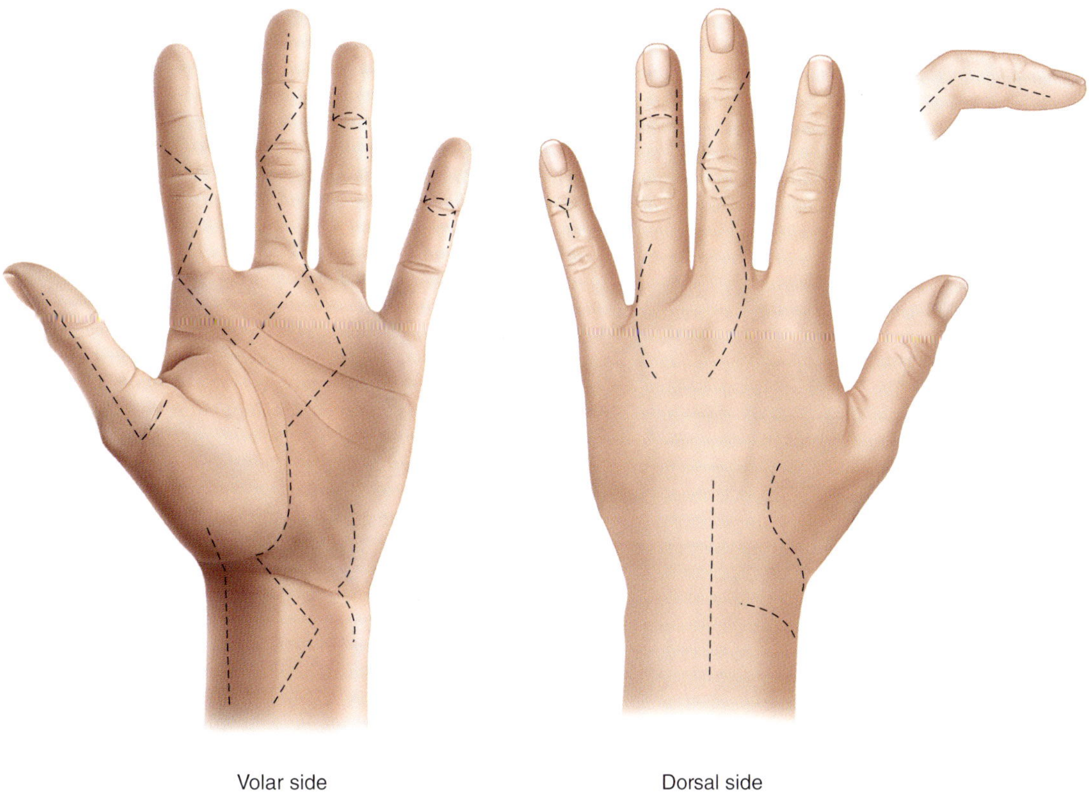

FIGURE 8-1 Preferred incisions in the hand and wrist used to explore different nerve injuries.

position without rotation of the nerve trunk. This can be done by identifying longitudinal epineurial blood vessels on the surface of the nerve trunk and aligning these when suturing the nerve. The final step in nerve repair is *maintenance*, where stitches or glue are applied. In a digital nerve repair, three or four 9-0 or 10-0 nylon sutures are suitable to maintain the coaptation (Fig. 8-2). The sutures should not be closed too tightly, since there is a risk for misalignment of the fascicles; thus, a minimal gap between the nerve ends may even be preferable. Fibrin glue can be used as an alternative, or in some circumstances as an adjunct. Our personal experience is that fibrin glue should be reserved for nerve reconstruction procedures. In repair of a median or ulnar nerve (Fig. 8-3) at wrist level the same principle is applied, but thicker sutures may be added, for example, 8-0 nylon sutures, with a few deeper sutures applied if the nerve trunk is thick. This epineurial nerve repair is the common technique applicable for most of the injured nerve trunks at wrist level and in the hand (Fig. 8-4). The ulnar nerve at wrist level contains 2 very specific nerve branches, that is, the superficial and deep ulnar branch, which actually can be dissected and repaired separately, that is, a group fascicular repair for the motor and sensory ulnar nerve branches.

NERVE RECONSTRUCTION

Some of the steps that were outlined for nerve repair are also relevant in nerve reconstruction, and include a proper approach, preparation of the nerve ends, calculation of the maximal gap that has to be bridged, calculation of the length of the graft, harvesting of a suitable nerve graft, and, finally, coaptation and maintenance of the nerve graft (Fig. 8-4). In the approach and preparation of the nerve grafts it may be advisable to use a longitudinal skin incision and raise a flap that can be utilized for closure of the wounds, thus enabling a proper coverage of the tissue and creating a well-vascularized surrounding for the nerve grafts. Again, the nerve ends

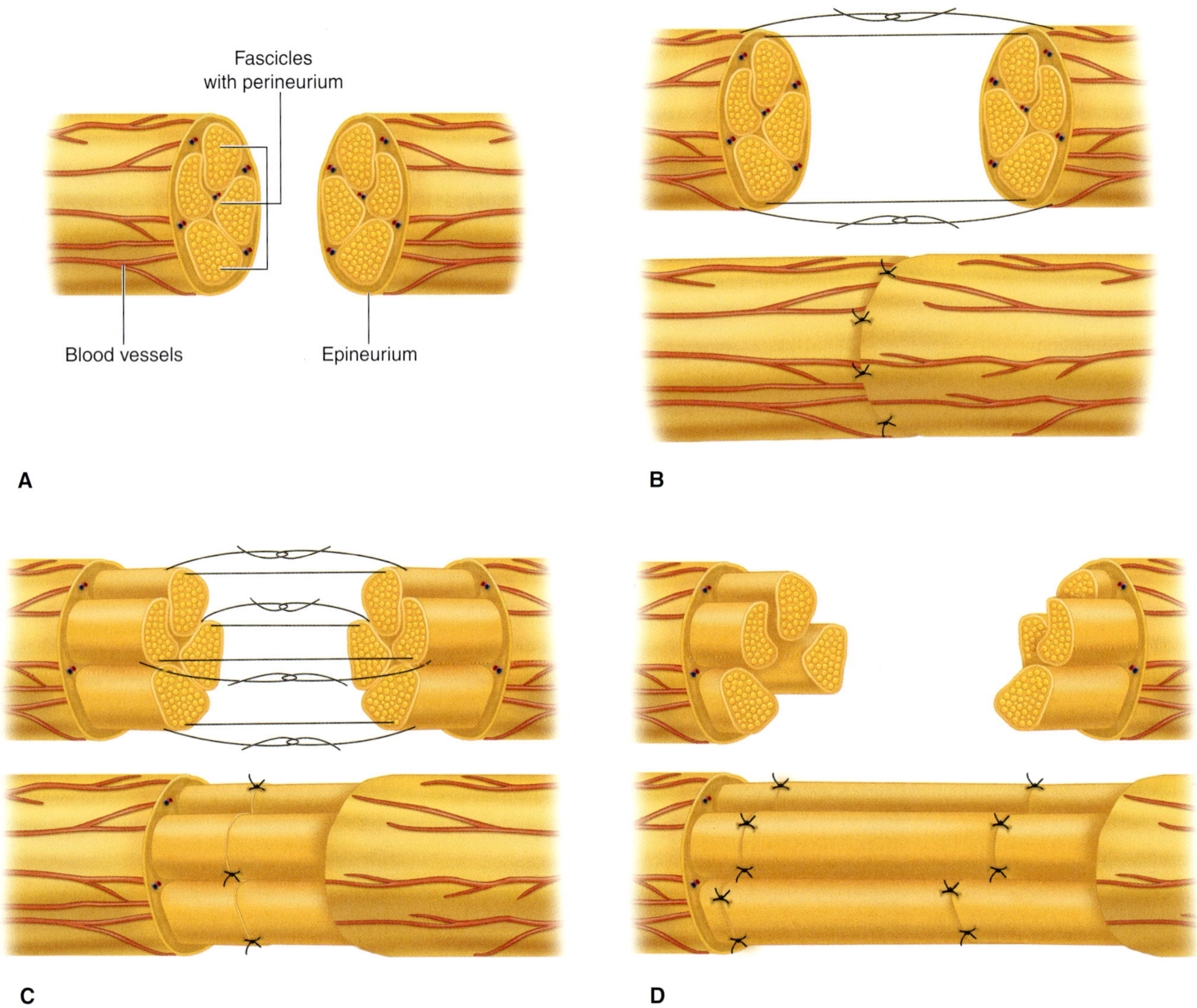

FIGURE 8-2 Different nerve repair and reconstruction techniques.

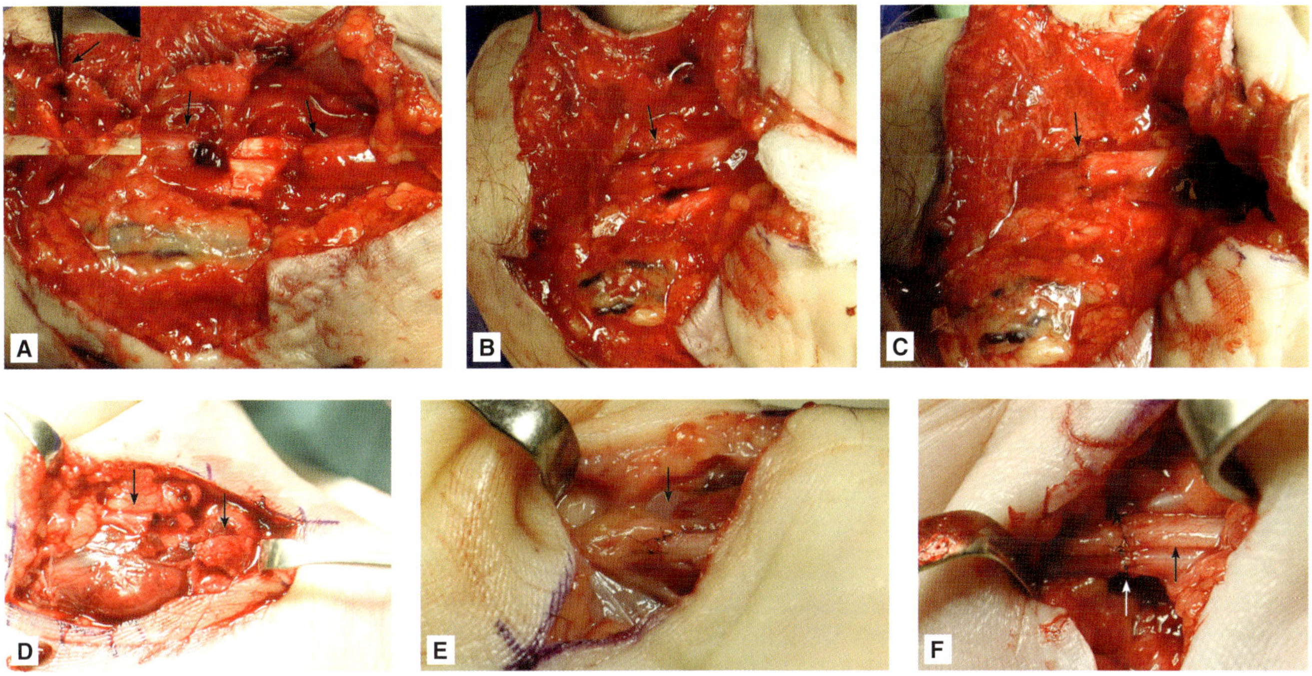

FIGURE 8-3 Photos of nerve repairs after injury. Transected median nerve at wrist level (**A-C**) with the proximal (with blood clot) and distal nerve ends marked with arrows (A) and the proximal nerve end with fascicles visible (inset in A; fascicle marked with arrowhead). The median nerve with three 9-0 sutures visible (B; arrows) and the final result after all the sutures (arrows) were applied (C). Transected proper (**D** and **E**) and common (**F**) digital nerves in hand before (D; proximal, with fascicles visible, and distal nerve ends marked with arrows) and after the nerve injury was repaired with several 9-0 sutures (E and F; black and white arrows, respectively, indicate the nerve repair). Note the superficial blood vessels in the nerve, which can be used to orient the nerve ends at apposition (F; marked with a black arrow). A Pacinian corpuscle is seen just above the nerve marked with an arrowhead in F.

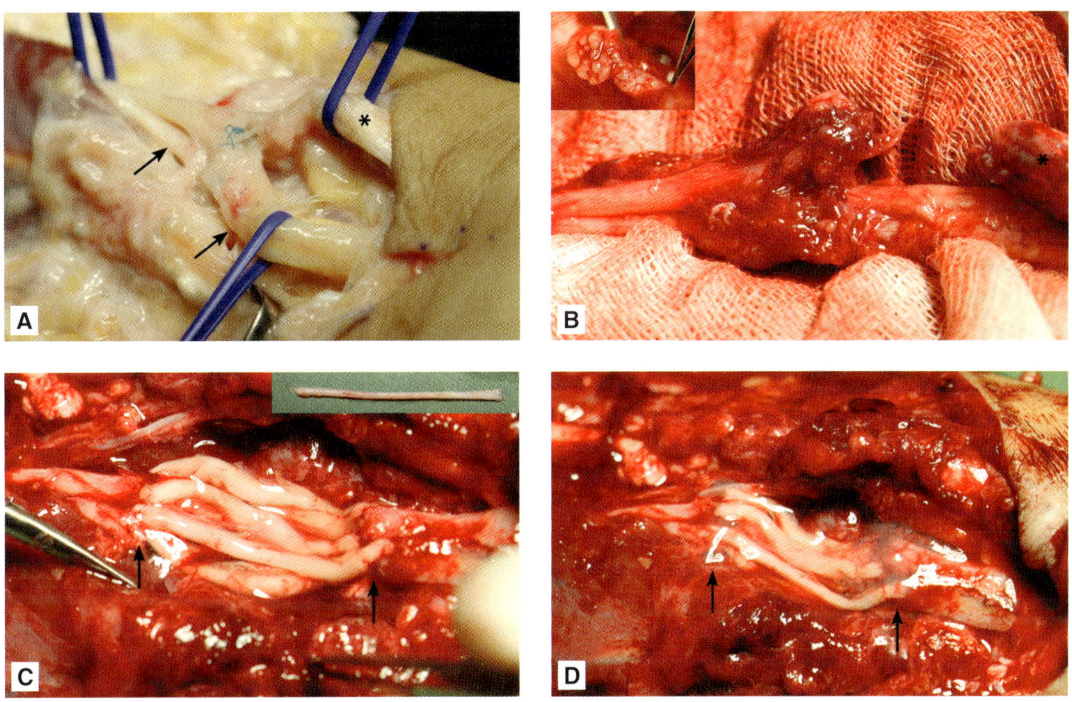

FIGURE 8-4 Reconstruction of a median nerve just proximal to the wrist (hand on the right) in a young patient 5 months after an open wound. Unfortunately, a nonqualified surgeon, who performed a repair partly with the tendon of the flexor carpi radialis muscle (marked by a star), treated the patient. **A.** The injured median nerve (arrows indicating proximal and distal nerve ends) with a blue suture on the top. **B.** The proximal and distal nerve ends were dissected and trimmed until a clear fascicular pattern was seen (inset). **C.** After resection several sural nerve grafts (a single one shown as inset) were attached to the proximal and distal nerve ends (arrows) and secured with single sutures (hardly visible at distal suture line). **D.** Maintenance is finally fulfilled by application of fibrin glue where it is possible to instantly glue the individual cable grafts to specific fascicles at the nerve ends.

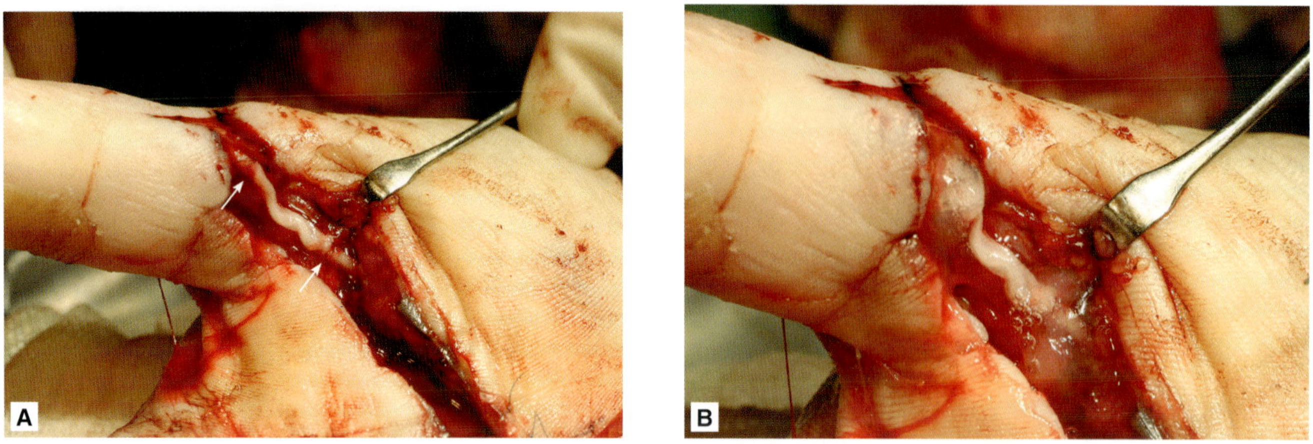

FIGURE 8-5 A digital nerve in a thumb reconstructed with a single nerve graft from the forearm (medial antebrachial nerve). **A.** Nerve graft attached and secured with a single 9-0 suture. **B.** Fibrin glue applied around the proximal and distal border between the radial nerve and the nerve graft.

have to exhibit a good appearance with mushrooming as a sign that necrotic and nonviable tissue has been removed. When the defect between the nerve ends is judged, one has to consider the possible change in length of the gap during rehabilitation and moving neighboring joints. The length of the nerve grafts should approximately be 15% longer than the maximum gap due to shrinkage of the graft as well as the nerve excursion. An important point is that the grafts should be applied when the defect is as long as possible, for example, with all adjacent joints fully extended.

Different grafts can be used to bridge nerve defects. For median or ulnar nerve at wrist level, a sural nerve graft is harvested through a longitudinal dorsal skin incision of the lower leg or through multiple transverse skin incisions. Up to a 30- to 40-cm sural nerve can be harvested, which is usually enough for an ulnar or median nerve injury. A soft dressing is applied on the lower leg and the patient is encouraged to directly mobilize the leg. Since the sural nerve is resected the postoperative complaints are similar to the patient's where the nerve is taken as a nerve biopsy, including loss of sensation, allodynia, neuroma problem, and cold intolerance. If a digital nerve or a common digital palmar nerve needs a nerve graft, there are 2 options: the medial antebrachial cutaneous nerve or the terminal branch of the posterior interosseous nerve (PIN). The first one can be harvested from the medial aspects of the forearm and the nerve, with its branches, usually matches the size of a digital nerve. The PIN is harvested just proximally to the wrist, where it is lying on the interosseous membrane. Through a dorsal incision a 4- to 5-cm long segment with a nerve containing 1 to 3 fascicles can easily be harvested without any complications or loss of function.[28]

In grafting a median or ulnar nerve defect (Fig. 8-4), single nerve cables are attached to appropriate groups of fascicles, matching the proximal and distal nerve ends, in the nerve. Single 9-0 or 10-0 nylon sutures are placed as maintenance just to facilitate determination of the length of the graft. A sufficient number of grafts are applied (for a median or ulnar nerve 3-4 sural nerve cables) and then the maintenance is fulfilled with fibrin glue as an adjunct, which allows instantly an optimal match between grafts and nerve ends. The same technique is used when a digital nerve is grafted, although only single cables are applied (Fig. 8-5). For a common palmar digital nerve it may be necessary to apply several small cables from the PIN or from the medial cutaneous antebrachial nerve.

POSTOPERATIVE CARE

A dorsal splint may be maintained for up to 3 weeks to protect a nerve repair in the hand. However, protected active mobilization over a 4-week period does not seem to impair the outcome after digital nerve repair.[29] A repair of the median or ulnar nerve at wrist level may be protected in a prolonged manner, that is, up to 6 weeks, to avoid extensive extension of the wrist. These general principles are applicable when nerve grafts are used in reconstruction.

SENSORY REEDUCATION

Outcome studies following nerve injury in adults usually show disappointing results as to the recovery of fine sensory function.[30] However, sensory outcome becomes substantially better if specific training programs, that is, sensory reeducation, are used following nerve repair.[31]

In the normal state, there is a distinct order, that is, a map, of the different body parts in the somatosensory cortex of the brain. Following a peripheral nerve injury profound cortical reorganization takes place. Immediately after a nerve injury and repair, no sensory signals from the injured area are sent to the somatosensory cortex resulting in a vacant area, which adjacent and contralateral cortical areas rapidly take over. When the new nerve fibers start to grow, there is a substantial misdirection of the outgrowing nerve fibers at the repair site resulting in a changed afferent nerve inflow resulting in a new and changed cortical hand map[6,7]; thus, "the hand speaks a new language to the brain"[30] (Fig. 8-6). The brain has to learn

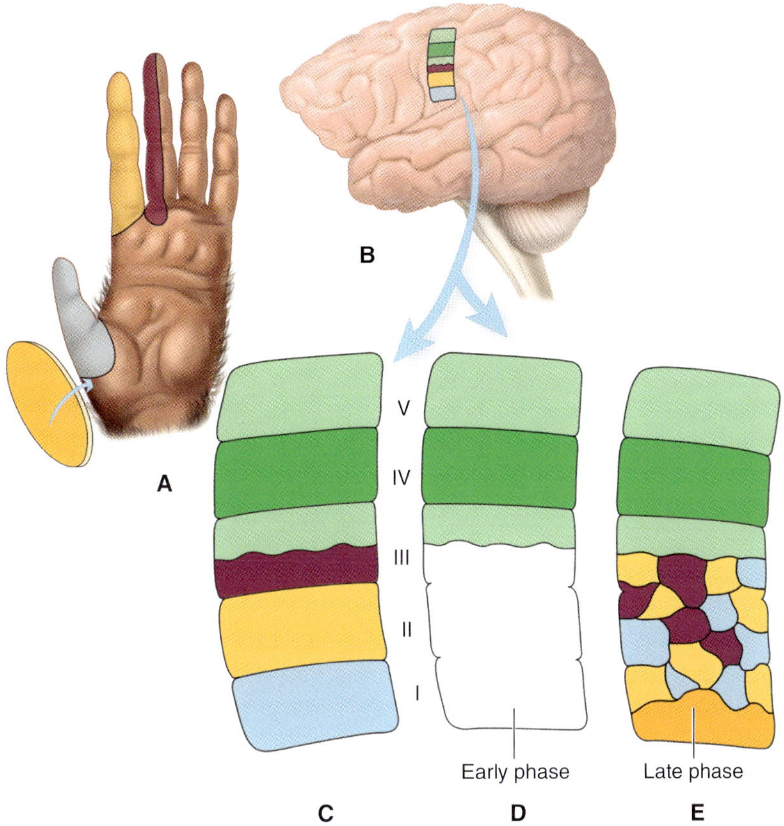

FIGURE 8-6 Cortical response of a peripheral nerve injury. Normally, each finger has a distinct cortical area in the primary somatosensory cortex responsible for processing sensory information from a specific finger, that is, finger somatotopy (**A-C**). Following a median nerve injury no nerve signals are sent to the primary somatosensory cortex resulting in an empty area (**D**; early phase), which is rapidly occupied by adjacent cortical areas. After nerve repair there is a substantial misdirection of outgrowing axons at the site of repair resulting in a changed signal pattern from the hand to the primary somatosensory cortex, thus a changed somatotopy in the cortical hand area (**E**; late phase). The illustration shows the brain and hand of a nonhuman primate, that is, the innervation of the fingers is different from that of humans, but the response is similar in nonhuman primates and humans. (Modified with permission from Lundborg.[30])

to interpret this new language, which is achieved by sensory relearning through sensory reeducational programs. Wynn-Parry published the first sensory reeducation program in 1966. The sensory reeducation programs designed in the 1960s and 1970s are still in use today despite the enormous advances during the last decade in neuroscience and neural plasticity.

Traditionally, sensory reeducation is first initiated when some perception of touch is demonstrated in the injured area[31] meaning that the training started months after the injury. New knowledge in basic neurobiology has shown that it is possible to differentiate between an early postoperative phase, before reinnervation has occurred, and a late postoperative phase, when some reinnervation of the hand has occurred. It has been suggested that different reeducational strategies should be used in the 2 phases.[30,31]

In the early phase, sensory bypass is one alternative using the brain's ability for cross-modal plasticity, the substitution of one sense with another. In this way the area in the primary somatosensory cortex, deprived of its sensory input, is activated and, theoretically, the organization within the primary somatosensory cortex is, to some extent, preserved. In the late phase, when the patient has regained some perception of touch and sensory information is sent from the periphery, sensory reeducation is classically based on vision-guided touch, but other sensory modalities can also be used to guide touch, thus improving the patients' ability to interpret afferent sensory nerve signals. Furthermore, bilateral tactile training can be used as sensory inputs are processed in both brain hemispheres[31] and since the two hemispheres are extensively interconnected. The aim of the training is to maintain cortical sensory input from the hand and thus to preserve the cortical organization during the time of nerve regeneration.

What about age? Should the sensory reeducation be different for different ages? Much speaks in favor of this. As pointed out earlier, it is well established that children gain excellent function after a nerve repair, whereas adults score lower.[3] The ability for plastic changes within the brain is not lost in aging, but it is changed. Most likely different mechanisms are important the sensory recovery after a nerve injury and thereby the sensory reeducation should be different depending on age of the patient.

The last decades' enormous advances in understanding how the brain can change and adopt, that is, brain plasticity,[31] have also made it possible to use plasticity mechanisms to treat patients with nerve injuries, that is, targeted plasticity. One such example is when the volar part of the forearm in patients with nerve injuries is deafferented by an anesthetic cream. This results in an area in the somatosensory cortex, where the neurons are devoted of input and these neurons rapidly start to respond to sensory information from the hand. Thus, more nerve cells are made available for the hand, resulting in a significantly improved sensory function in the hand. A prolonged improvement is seen when this deafferentation is repeated for several weeks. A better understanding of the effects of a peripheral nerve injury on the brain will likely result in more refined treatment programs in the future and a possibility to more precisely guide the sensory reeducation to achieve an optimal result.

ACKNOWLEDGMENTS

The papers referred in the chapter, which were based on the authors' research, were funded by the Swedish Research Council (Medicine), the Swedish Society for Medicine, and Skåne University Hospital in Region Skåne.

REFERENCES

1. Thorsen F, Rosberg HE, Steen Carlsson K, Dahlin LB. Digital nerve injuries: epidemiology, results, costs, and impact on daily life. *J Plast Surg Hand Surg*. 2012;46:184–190.
2. Lundborg G, Rosen B, Dahlin L, Holmberg J, Rosen I. Tubular repair of the median or ulnar nerve in the human forearm: a 5-year follow-up. *J Hand Surg Br*. 2004;29:100–107.
3. Chemnitz A, Bjorkman A, Dahlin LB, Rosen B. Functional outcome 30 years after median and ulnar nerve repair in childhood and adolescence. *J Bone Joint Surg Am*. 2013;95:329–337.
4. Fornander L, Nyman T, Hansson T, Ragnehed M, Brismar T. Age- and time-dependent effects on functional outcome and cortical activation pattern in patients with median nerve injury: a functional magnetic resonance imaging study. *J Neurosurg*. 2010;113:122–128.
5. Galanakos SP, Zoubos AB, Mourouzis I, Ignatiadis I, Bot AG, Soucacos PN. Prognostic scoring system for peripheral nerve repair in the upper extremity. *Microsurgery*. 2013;33:105–111.
6. Taylor KS, Anastakis DJ, Davis KD. Cutting your nerve changes your brain. *Brain*. 2009;132:3122–3133.
7. Chen R, Cohen LG, Hallett M. Nervous system reorganization following injury. *Neuroscience*. 2002;111:761–773.
8. Hart AM, Terenghi G, Wiberg M. Neuronal death after peripheral nerve injury and experimental strategies for neuroprotection. *Neurol Res*. 2008;30:999–1011.
9. Bjorkman A, Weibull A, Rosen B, Svensson J, Lundborg G. Rapid cortical reorganisation and improved sensitivity of the hand following cutaneous anaesthesia of the forearm. *Eur J Neurosci*. 2009;29:837–844.
10. de Ruiter GC, Malessy MJ, Alaid AO, et al. Misdirection of regenerating motor axons after nerve injury and repair in the rat sciatic nerve model. *Exp Neurol*. 2008;211:339–350.
11. Bjorkman A, Rosen B, Lundborg G. Acute improvement of hand sensibility after selective ipsilateral cutaneous forearm anaesthesia. *Eur J Neurosci*. 2004;20:2733–2736.
12. Rosen B, Lundborg G, Dahlin LB, Holmberg J, Karlson B. Nerve repair: correlation of restitution of functional sensibility with specific cognitive capacities. *J Hand Surg Br*. 1994;19:452–458.
13. Cederlund RI, Ramel E, Rosberg HE, Dahlin LB. Outcome and clinical changes in patients 3, 6, 12 months after a severe or major hand injury—can sense of coherence be an indicator for rehabilitation focus? *BMC Musculoskelet Disord*. 2010;11:286.
14. Ruijs AC, Jaquet JB, Kalmijn S, Giele H, Hovius SE. Median and ulnar nerve injuries: a meta-analysis of predictors of motor and sensory recovery after modern microsurgical nerve repair. *Plast Reconstr Surg*. 2005;116:484–494 [discussion 495–496].
15. Farnebo S, Thorfinn J, Dahlin LB. Peripheral nerve injuries of the upper extremity. In: Chang J, ed. *Neligan's 3rd edition of Plastic Surgery, Hand Surgery*. Vol. 6. Philadelphia: Saunders, Elsevier; 2012: 694–718.
16. Bloom OE, Morgan JR. Membrane trafficking events underlying axon repair, growth, and regeneration. *Mol Cell Neurosci*. 2011;48:339–348.
17. Twiss JL, van Minnen J. New insights into neuronal regeneration: the role of axonal protein synthesis in pathfinding and axonal extension. *J Neurotrauma*. 2006;23:295–308.
18. Liu K, Tedeschi A, Park KK, He Z. Neuronal intrinsic mechanisms of axon regeneration. *Annu Rev Neurosci*. 2011;34:131–152.
19. Saito H, Dahlin LB. Expression of ATF3 and axonal outgrowth are impaired after delayed nerve repair. *BMC Neurosci*. 2008;9:88.
20. Saito H, Kanje M, Dahlin LB. Delayed nerve repair increases number of caspase 3 stained Schwann cells. *Neurosci Lett*. 2009;456:30–33.
21. Tsuda Y, Kanje M, Dahlin LB. Axonal outgrowth is associated with increased ERK 1/2 activation but decreased caspase 3 linked cell death in Schwann cells after immediate nerve repair in rats. *BMC Neurosci*. 2011;12:12.
22. Saito H, Kanje M, Dahlin LB. Crossed over repair of the femoral sensory and motor branches influences N-CAM. *Neuroreport*. 2010;21: 841–845.
23. Zigmond RE. gp130 cytokines are positive signals triggering changes in gene expression and axon outgrowth in peripheral neurons following injury. *Front Mol Neurosci*. 2011;4:62.
24. Terenghi G, Hart A, Wiberg M. The nerve injury and the dying neurons: diagnosis and prevention. *J Hand Surg Eur*. 2011;36:730–734.
25. Efstathopoulos D, Gerostathopoulos N, Misitzis D, Bouchlis G, Anagnostou S, Daoutis NK. Clinical assessment of primary digital nerve repair. *Acta Orthop Scand Suppl*. 1995;264:45–47.
26. Vertruyen MF, Burgeon MA, Dachy BS, Ley RE. Sensory recovery after microsurgical repair of digital nerves. *Acta Chir Belg*. 1994;94: 325–328.
27. Yi C, Dahlin LB. Impaired nerve regeneration and Schwann cell activation after repair with tension. *Neuroreport*. 2010;21:958–962.
28. Thomsen NO, Mojaddidi M, Malik RA, Dahlin LB. Biopsy of the posterior interosseous nerve: a low morbidity method for assessment of peripheral nerve disorders. *Diabet Med*. 2009;26:100–104.
29. Henry FP, Farkhad RI, Butt FS, O'Shaughnessy M, O'Sullivan ST. A comparison between complete immobilisation and protected active mobilisation in sensory nerve recovery following isolated digital nerve injury. *J Hand Surg Eur*. 2012;37:422–426.
30. Lundborg G. *Nerve Injury and Repair. Regeneration, Reconstruction and Cortical Remodelling*. Philadelphia: Elsevier; 2004.
31. Skirven TM. *Rehabilitation of the Hand and Upper Extremity, Two-volume Set Expert Consult: Online and Print*. St. Louis: Elsevier; 2011.

9

Nerve Repair and Reconstruction: Elbow to Fingertips

David J. Slutsky, MD

BASIC CONSIDERATIONS

Nerve regeneration does not involve mitosis and multiplication of nerve cells. Instead, the cell body restores nerve continuity by growing a new axon. Axon sprouting has been demonstrated as early as 24 hours following nerve transection. One axon sends out multiple unmyelinated axon sprouts from the tip of the remaining axon or collateral sprouts from a nearby proximal node of Ranvier. The distal sprout contains the growth cone. This sends out filopodia that adhere to sticky glycoprotein molecules in the basil lamina of Schwann cells, such as laminin and fibronectin (neurite-promoting factors). The filopodia contain actin, which aids in pulling the growth cone distally. The basil lamina of 2 abutting Schwann cells forms a potential endoneurial tube into which the regenerating axon grows. These axons will deteriorate if a connection with a target organ is not reached. There are up to 50 advancing sprouts from 1 single axon. Initially there are many more nerve fibers crossing a nerve repair than in the parent nerve.[1] Although more than 1 axon may enter the same endoneurial tube, there is eventual resorption of the multiple sprouts leaving 1 dominant axon.

Axons grow between 1 and 2 mm per day. In general, axons grow approximately 1 to 2 mm per day. Motor end plates degrade at approximately 1% per week.[2] There is irreversible muscle fibrosis by 24 months. For practical purposes, the maximum length that a nerve can grow to restore motor function is approximately 35 cm. This in part accounts for the poor motor recovery when repairing nerve defects proximal to the elbow in adults. Sensory end organs remain viable since there is no end plate and they retain the potential for reinnervation. Reconstruction of a sensory nerve defect by comparison may provide protective sensation even after many years. Following nerve transection, the Schwann cell removes the axonal and myelin debris in both the severed nerve ends. Schwann cells produce an immediate source of nerve growth factor (NGF) that helps to support the proximal stump. The Schwann cell expresses NGF receptors that aid in directing the advancing growth cone. It also increases its production of other neurotrophic factors including ciliary neurotrophic factor, brain-derived neurotrophic factor, and fibroblast growth factor, which promote axonal growth. The laminin and fibronectin in the Schwann cell basil lamina act as a rail for the advancing axon sprouts to grow down. The Schwann cell produces a myelin sheath for the immature axon sprout.

A normal nerve has longitudinal excursion that subjects it to a certain amount of stress and strain in situ. A peripheral nerve is initially easily extensible, but this rapidly diminishes with further elongation due to the stretching of the connective tissue within the nerve. Chronically injured nerves become even stiffer. Elasticity decreases by as much as 50% in the delayed repair of nerves in which Wallerian degeneration has occurred. Experimentally, blood flow is reduced by 50% when the nerve is stretched 8% beyond its in vivo length. Complete ischemia occurs at 15%. Suture pullout does not occur until a 17% increase in length.[3] This suggests that ischemia and not disruption of the anastomosis is the limiting factor in acute nerve repairs.[3] This observation is also applicable to nerve grafting.

The nerve graft acts to provide a source of empty endoneurial tubes through which the regenerating axons can be directed. Any tissue that contains a basil lamina such as freeze-dried muscle or tendon can be substituted, but only the autogenous nerve graft also provides a source of viable Schwann cells. A normal nerve can compensate for the change in length with limb flexion and extension because it is surrounded by gliding tissue that permits longitudinal movement. A nerve graft becomes welded to its recipient bed by the adhesions through which it becomes vascularized. As a consequence, the nerve graft is exquisitely sensitive to tension because it has no longitudinal excursion. The harvested length of the graft must be long enough to span the nerve gap without tension while the adjacent joints are extended. This is also the position of temporary immobilization. If the limb or digit is immobilized with joint flexion, the graft will become fixed in this position. When the limb is then mobilized at 8 days, the proximal and distal stumps will be subject to tension even though the graft was initially long enough. Early attempts at lengthening the graft will lead to disruption of the anastomosis.

PRINCIPLES OF NERVE REPAIR

The location of fascicles varies somewhat within a nerve, and there are cross-connections between them as fibers migrate from 1 fascicle to another. This migration occurs because axons destined for a specific end-organ receptor may arise at more than 1 spinal cord level that results in a sorting and rearranging as it moves distally. There is a difference between a nerve gap and a nerve defect. A nerve gap refers to the distance between the nerve ends, whereas a nerve defect refers to the actual amount of nerve tissue that is lost. With simple nerve retraction following division, the fascicular arrangement is similar. As the nerve defect between the proximal and distal stumps increases, there is a greater fascicular mismatch between the stumps that leads to poorer outcomes, especially if the gap exceeds 5 cm. The use of intraoperative motor and sensory nerve differentiation can diminish the risk of fascicular mismatch when repairing or grafting a nerve. There is the anatomic method based on separate identification of groups of fascicles, and the electrophysiologic method and histochemical method that rely on staining for enzymes specific to motor or sensory nerves, which is time consuming and currently not in vogue.

Indications

The principal indication for surgery is a patient who presents with a laceration and a nerve deficit that does not recover within 1 week. A tension-free repair is the goal for any nerve anastomosis. When there is a clean transection of the nerve and the gap is caused by elastic retraction, an acute 1° repair is indicated. One should always discuss the possible need for a nerve graft or conduit with the patient however if a primary repair would lead to undue tension at the coaptation site.

Contraindications

Blast injuries that are heavily impregnated with debris or bacteria are better treated by staged reconstruction. Nerve repair cannot be performed in an infected wound. If the degree of the longitudinal injury cannot be determined, nerve repair should be delayed.

PRINCIPLES OF NERVE GRAFTING

Indications

When treatment of a nerve laceration is delayed, fibrosis of the nerve ends prevents approximation; hence, nerve grafting is required even though there is no loss of nerve tissue. Nerve grafting is indicated to bridge a defect when >10% elongation of the nerve would be necessary to bridge the gap. This is a better indication for grafting than the nerve gap per se, although 4 cm is often used as a critical defect.

Contraindications

Since the graft is vascularized from the tissue bed, nerve grafting cannot be performed in burned or irradiated tissue.

Donor Grafts

Small-diameter grafts spontaneously revascularize, but thick grafts undergo central necrosis with subsequent endoneurial fibrosis that ultimately impedes the advancement of any ingrowing axon sprouts. The donor-site defect must be acceptable for the patient and the harvested nerve must be long enough to ensure a tension-free anastomosis with the adjacent joints in full extension. For these reasons most of the available grafts are cutaneous nerves. Typical donor nerves include the medial and lateral antebrachial cutaneous nerves (LABCN) and the sural nerve (SN). The distal terminations of the anterior and posterior interosseous nerves (PIN) are suitable for digital nerve grafts at the distal interphalangeal (DIP) joint level.

MEDIAL ANTEBRACHIAL CUTANEOUS NERVE (MABCN)

The MABCN arises from either the medial cord or lower trunk of the brachial plexus. It travels down the arm medial to the brachial artery, and then pierces the deep fascia with the basilic vein about the middle of the arm. More than 90% of the time the MABCN will bifurcate into an anterior and a posterior branch proximal to the medial epicondyle that provide sensation to the medial forearm and posteromedial elbow, respectively. It is preferable to use the anterior branch to avoid a bothersome sensory loss over the elbow. The anterior branch crosses the elbow between the medial epicondyle and the biceps tendon usually in front of the cubital vein, and then travels superficial to the flexor carpi ulnaris muscle, ending 10 cm from the wrist. It is approached through an anteromedial incision on the proximal forearm. It provides a graft of up to 20 cm.

LATERAL ANTEBRACHIAL CUTANEOUS NERVE

The LABCN is the distal continuation of the musculocutaneous nerve. It exits from underneath the biceps tendon, and then divides into anterior and posterior branches at the elbow crease (Fig. 9-1). The donor-site defect corresponds to the anterolateral forearm, but it may also innervate the volar radial or dorsoradial thumb. For this reason, it is not harvested for grafting a sensory nerve deficit to the thumb. There is a partial or complete overlap of the sensory territory of the superficial radial nerve up to 75% of the time. The nerve is approached through an anterolateral incision on the proximal forearm, as it passes deep to the cephalic vein. The LABCN provides a nerve graft of 5 to 8 cm.

POSTERIOR INTEROSSEOUS NERVE

The terminal portion of the PIN provides proprioception to the joint capsule. Harvesting the nerve leaves no apparent

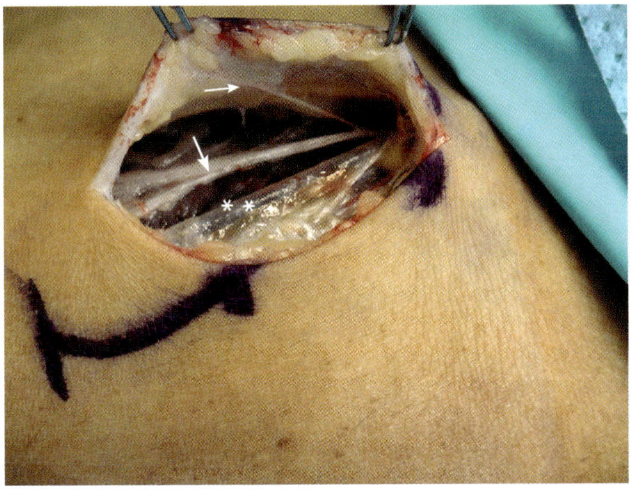

FIGURE 9-1 Lateral antebrachial cutaneous nerve branches (arrows) next to the cephalic vein (*) in the proximal forearm.

motor or sensory deficit. The PIN lies adjacent to the posterior interosseous artery on the dorsal surface of the interosseous membrane, deep to the fourth extensor compartment. It ranges from 1 to 5 mm and contains 1 to 5 fascicles. It is a good match for grafting digital nerve defects at the DIP. The nerve can be located through a dorsal wrist incision just proximal to Lister's tubercle, developing the plane between the third and fourth extensor compartments. The mean length of the PIN from its terminal expansion at the wrist to its most distal muscular branch (to the extensor pollicis longus) is 6 cm.

ANTERIOR INTEROSSEOUS NERVE (AIN)

The terminal portion of the AIN also provides proprioception to the joint capsule. Harvesting the nerve similarly leaves no apparent motor or sensory deficit. The nerve is located adjacent to the anterior interosseous artery on the anterior surface of the interosseous membrane, deep to the pronator quadratus (PQ). It can also be approached through a dorsal incision as for the PIN, after excising a window in the interosseous membrane (Fig. 9-2A and B). The primarily motor fibers of the AIN provide an expendable donor of adequate size and fascicle number suitable for grafting the recurrent motor branch of the median nerve or the deep motor branch of the ulnar nerve at the wrist.

SURAL NERVE

The SN is a common source of nerve graft material. It is formed from the medial cutaneous SN that originates from the tibial nerve. It descends between the 2 heads of the gastrocnemius piercing the deep fascia in the upper part of the leg, where it is joined by the lateral sural cutaneous branch off the peroneal nerve. It then passes downwards near the lateral margin of the tendo-Achilles to the interval between the lateral malleolus and the calcaneus. After giving off a medial calcaneal branch it runs forwards, below the lateral malleolus, and is continued along the lateral side of the foot. It supplies the skin of the lateral and posterior parts of the lower one third of the leg. In order to harvest the nerve, the patient is positioned supine on the operating table, with a sandbag placed at midcalf level. The leg is then flexed with the foot on the sandbag to maintain the flexed knee position. The nerve is located via a longitudinal incision that is 1 cm posterior and superior to the lateral malleolus, where it is often accompanied by the lesser saphenous vein. Traction is placed on the nerve until it can be palpated 3 cm proximally, and then a second transverse incision is made. In this manner, the nerve is followed as high as the popliteal fossa by dividing all of the sural communicating branches. The SN provides graft lengths of 30 to 40 cm (Fig. 9-3).

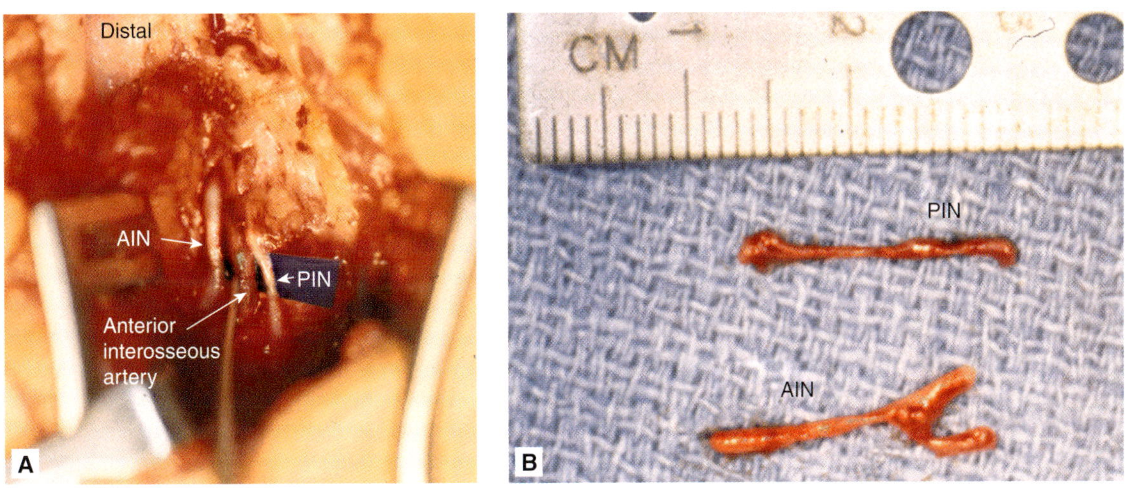

FIGURE 9-2 A. Intraoperative photo of PIN through a dorsal wrist incision. A window in the interosseous membrane allowed isolation of the AIN. B. Typical graft size.

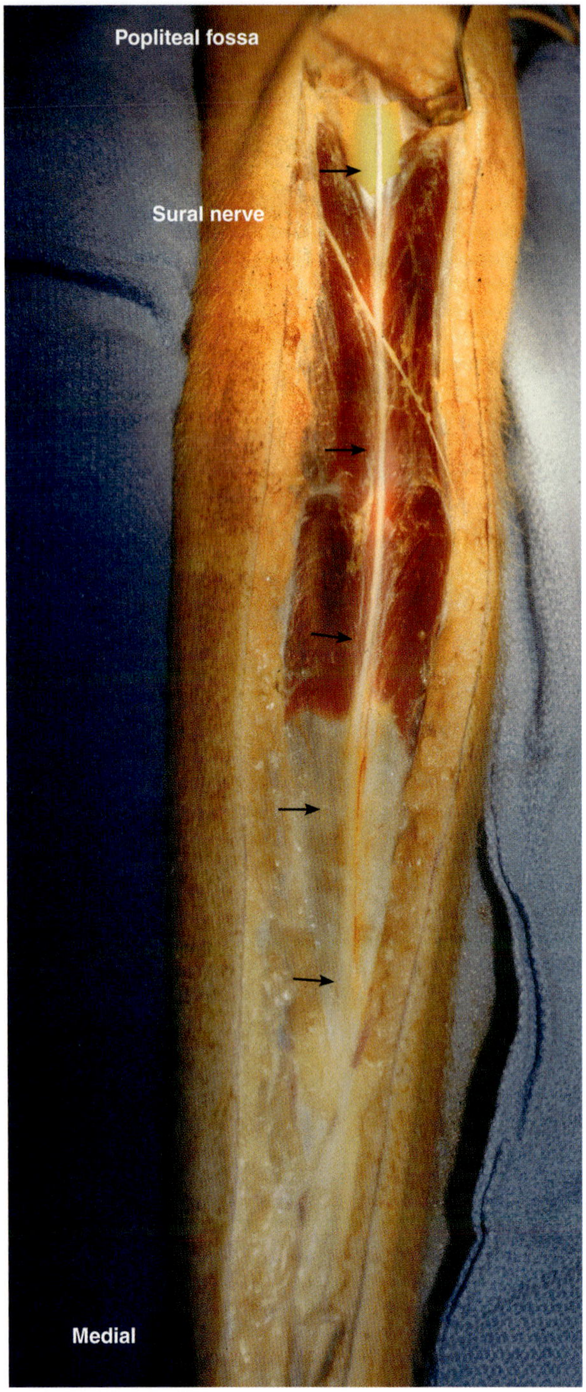

FIGURE 9-3 Demonstration of the sural nerve anatomy looking from the posterior aspect of a prone right leg (arrows).

Surgical Technique

Nerve repairs can be divided up into 3 types.

EXTERNAL EPINEURIAL SUTURE

This technique is appropriate for small nerves containing only 1 or 2 fascicles, such as digital nerves. Since they only contain sensory fibers, matching is not a problem. Usually 3 to 4 sutures with 9-0 nylon are sufficient. Alternatively, fibrin glue can be used that allows the placement of fewer sutures. Epineurial repairs are also indicated for mixed nerves where separate motor and sensory fascicle identification is not possible. Some authors only perform this type of repair regardless.

GROUP FASCICULAR SUTURE

The motor and sensory groups of fascicles are identified as described. In a major nerve such as the median or ulnar, 4 or 5 groups may be chosen for suture. These are then matched appropriately with the opposite end and approximated with sutures in both the internal and external epineurium. Alternatively, one can locate the motor fascicles proximally and distally, which are then repaired in a group fascicular manner. The sensory fascicles can then be coapted in an epineurial fashion.

EXTERNAL EPINEURIAL SPLINT

Jabaley has employed the external epineurium as a splinting device.[4] The external epineurium is incised longitudinally on its superficial surface and dissected away from the underlying fascicles. The epineurium is left attached on the deep surface, several millimeters from each nerve end. A few interrupted sutures with 8-0 nylon are used to join the ends of the external epineurial strips on the deep surface only, completing the construction of the splint. This maneuver provides for a coaptation of individual fascicles or groups of fascicles with little or no tension.

Millesi has written extensively on the technical aspects of nerve grafting.[5] If the recipient nerve is the approximate diameter of the graft, the 2 stumps are transected until normal-appearing tissue without fibrosis is seen and the graft is inserted by an epineurial repair. If the recipient nerve is larger than the graft, the fascicular pattern determines the type of preparation. If the nerve contains 1 to 4 fascicles, the stump is resected until healthy tissue is encountered. Multiple nerve grafts are used to completely cover the cross-sectional area of each fascicle in a 1:2 or 1:3 ratio. When there are 5 to 12 fascicles that are the size of the nerve graft, each fascicle is grafted individually. When there is a polyfascicular pattern with a group fascicular arrangement, interfascicular dissection is performed to isolate the fascicle groups, which are then grafted individually. If there is no group fascicular arrangement, interfascicular dissection is not performed. Graft insertion is then guided by the intraneural topography of the nerve for that specific level of injury.

GUIDELINES FOR DIGITAL NERVE GRAFT SELECTION

Higgins et al investigated the fascicular cross-sectional area and number of fascicles of 5 nerve graft sites to specific digital nerve segments.[6] In the fingertip distal to the DIP, the AIN, PIN, and MABCN were all appropriate choices for caliber-matched grafts. The LABCN however was the only similar donor nerve when the number of fascicles was assessed. It is also the best match in caliber and fascicle number for digital nerve deficits between the metacarpophalangeal (MP) joint and the DIP joint, and from the common digital nerve bifurcation to the MP joint. The SN was the most appropriate choice when grafting defects between the wrist and the common digital nerve bifurcation, even though there were considerably fewer fascicles and a smaller cross-sectional area than the common digital nerve.

Repair/Grafting Specific Nerves

MEDIAN NERVE

Anatomy. The median nerve arises from the medial and lateral cords of the brachial plexus. It contains the nerve root fibers from C6 to T1 and contains approximately 18,000 myelinated axons. It lies lateral to the axillary artery but then crosses medial to it at the level of the coracobrachialis. At the elbow it travels behind the bicipital aponeurosis but in front of the brachialis. The nerve and artery pass through the antecubital fossa underneath the lacertus fibrosis and give off branches to the palmaris longus (PL), flexor carpi radialis (FCR), flexor digitorum superficialis (FDS), and rarely the flexor digitorum profundus (FDP). The AIN arises from the median nerve on the dorsoradial surface about 5 to 8 cm distal to the medial epicondyle.

The median nerve then dives between the deep and superficial heads of the pronator teres (PT) to which it supplies 1 to 4 branches. The fibrous arch of the PT lies 3 to 7.5 cm below the humeral epicondylar line. The fibrous arch of the superficialis arch lies 6.5 cm below the humeral epicondylar line. The median nerve enters the forearm deep to the fibrous arch of the FDS and is adherent to the undersurface of the FDS muscle until it becomes superficial, 5 cm proximal to the wrist. It emerges beneath the radial side of the muscle belly of the middle finger superficialis where it is quite superficial and near the PL tendon. It then passes underneath the carpal transverse ligament giving off the recurrent motor branch and sensory branches to the thumb, index, middle, and radial side of the ring finger.

The AIN is the largest muscular branch that emerges from the median nerve. It innervates the FDP to the index and middle fingers, the flexor pollicis longus (FPL), and the PQ. The terminal portion also provides sensory innervation to the carpal joints. The AIN travels between the FDS and FDP, and then passes dorsally in the interval between the FPL and FDP, giving off 2 to 6 branches to each of these muscles. The nerve reaches the anterior surface of the interosseous membrane and travels with the anterior interosseous artery where it passes deep to the PQ that it also innervates. It ends by sending sensory afferent branches to the intercarpal, radiocarpal, and distal radioulnar joints.

Repair in the Arm. A straight medial approach is used. In the proximal third of the arm, the nerve lies in the sulcus between the coracobrachialis and the long head of the triceps. In the middle third, the nerve is located anterior to the medial intermuscular septum, in the groove between the biceps and the long head of the triceps, where it lies medial to the brachial artery and its venae comitantes. The medial brachial cutaneous nerve and MABCN lie posterior to the nerve. There are no branches in the arm, which allows easy mobilization of the nerve. A straight epineurial repair is performed for a primary repair. At this level, the motor and sensory fibers are intermingled, which precludes any fascicular grafting. If there is a nerve gap, a SN graft is used to cover the cross-sectional area of the nerve proximally and distally.

Repair at the Elbow. The median nerve is located through an S-shaped anteromedial incision at the cubital fossa. The lacertus fibrosis is divided taking care to preserve the LABCN. The median nerve and brachial vein lie medial to the artery. At this level the motor branches of the median nerve consistently collect into 3 fascicular groups. There is an anterior group (to the PT and FCR), middle group (to the FDS and hand intrinsics), and a posterior group (to the AIN branch). These branch groups can be traced proximally without harm, within the main trunk of the median nerve for 2.5 to 10 cm. This occasionally permits direct coaptation of the individual motor branches using 8-0 and 9-0 nylon. Any gap is treated with SN grafting similar to above (Fig. 9-4A-C).

Repair in the Forearm. The median nerve is approached through an S-shaped incision over the volar forearm. The nerve is identified on the undersurface of the sublimis muscle. In the upper third of the forearm the motor branches usually lie peripherally, typically on the radial and ulnar sides. The motor fascicles from the recurrent motor branch are in a slightly radial position at 100 mm proximal to the radial styloid. The motor branch can be separated from the main trunk without harm for up to 100 mm proximal to the thenar muscles. The central core of the proximal stump should be connected distally with the motor and sensory components of the hand, which typically lie centrally in the middle group. This can be done with a fascicular repair or graft (Fig. 9-5A and B). Any large identifiable motor branches to the PT or FCR should be attached about the periphery.

Repair at the Wrist. The median nerve at the wrist has approximately 30 fascicles. The motor recurrent branch often consists of 2 fascicles that are situated in a volar position, with the various sensory groups in the radial, ulnar, and dorsal positions (Fig. 9-6A and B). The motor fascicles in the recurrent motor branch are identified where they leave the median nerve trunk and then followed proximally to the distal nerve end. In order to maintain motor continuity when there is a median nerve gap at the wrist level, a fascicular repair or a SN graft should be sutured to the large bifascicular group of fascicles along the volar aspect of the distal stump, and connected to a matching radial group of fascicles in the proximal stump.

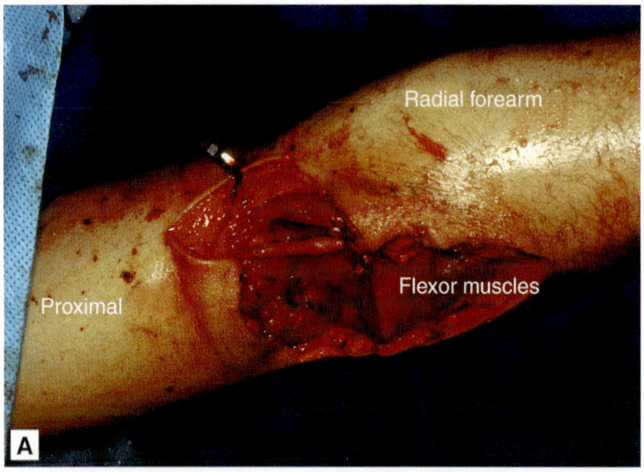

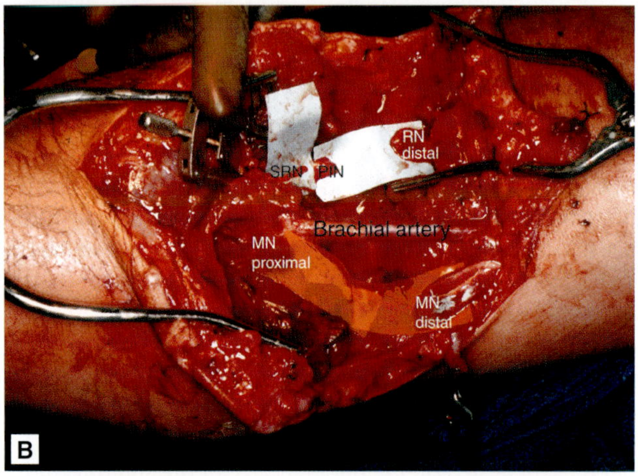

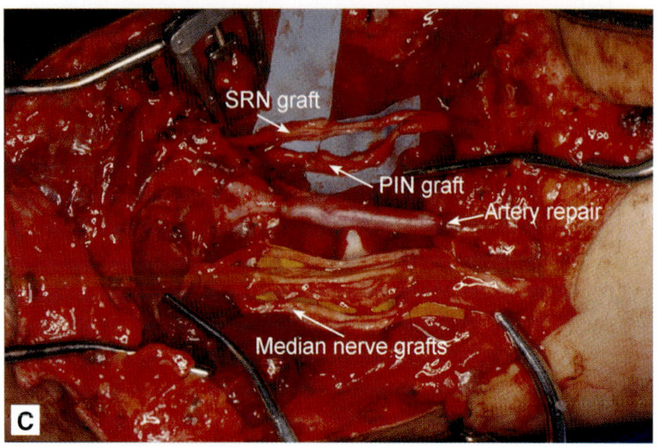

FIGURE 9-4 Proximal median and radial nerve grafts. **A.** Laceration through antecubital fossa. **B.** Note median nerve laceration (MN) and radial nerve (RN) laceration at bifurcation of superficial radial nerve branch (SRN) and posterior interosseous nerve (PIN). **C.** Multiple fascicular grafts to median nerve, superficial radial nerve, and PIN nerve.

Repair in the Hand. The median nerve is approached through an extensile carpal tunnel approach, with division of the transverse carpal ligament (TCL). The recurrent motor branch is most commonly found distal to the TCL as it enters the thenar muscles. Topographically, the motor

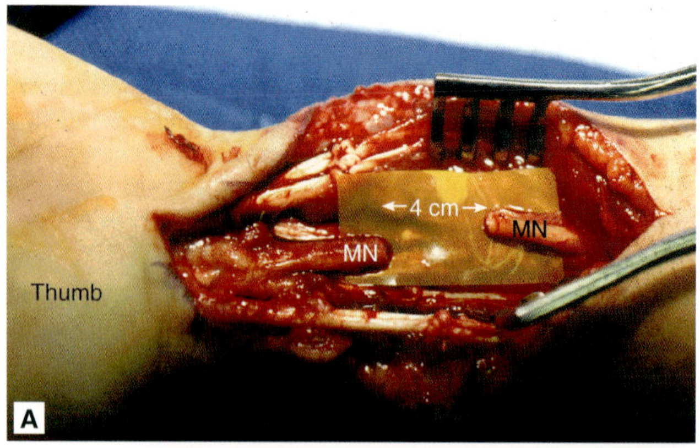

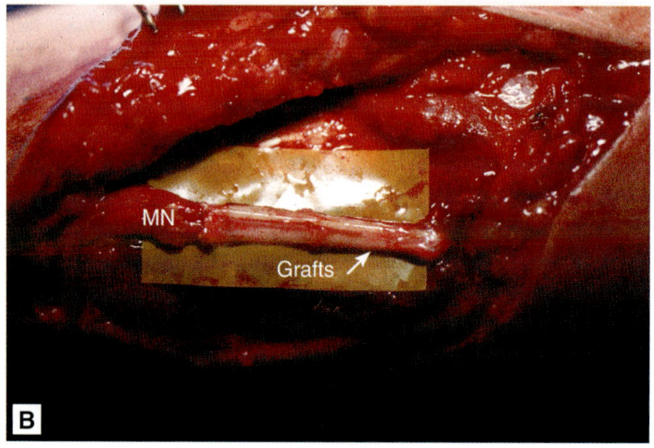

FIGURE 9-5 **A.** A 4-cm defect between median nerve (MN) ends. **B.** Sural nerve grafts with matching of volar radial fascicle groups.

branch is located on the radial-volar aspect 60% of the time, the central-volar aspect 22%, and between those 2 locations in 18%. In 56% the motor branch passes through a separate distinct fascial tunnel before entering the thenar muscles. A group fascicular repair of the motor branch and an epineurial repair of the remaining sensory fascicles are my preference, although some authors believe the outcomes are similar with a straight epineurial repair. The sensory fibers travel within the common digital nerves to the thumb, index, and middle, as well as the communicating branch to the third web space. The LACBN or MACBN is a suitable graft for nerve gaps at this level (Fig. 9-7A and B). When the median nerve defect is >5 cm and extends from the wrist to the common digital nerve bifurcation, sural grafts are more appropriate.

Digital Nerve Repair. There are often 2 fascicles in the typical digital nerve. An external epineurial repair gives the same results as a fascicular repair. Many authors recommend nerve grafting when the gap exceeds 1 cm, with the wrist and all 3 finger joints extended. The digital nerves are approached though a midlateral or a volar Brunner incision. The LACBN is a good caliber match at this level (Fig. 9-8A and B). The dorsal sensory branch that arises from the proper digital nerve can also be used as graft material. This branch most commonly arises proximal to the PIP flexion crease, and

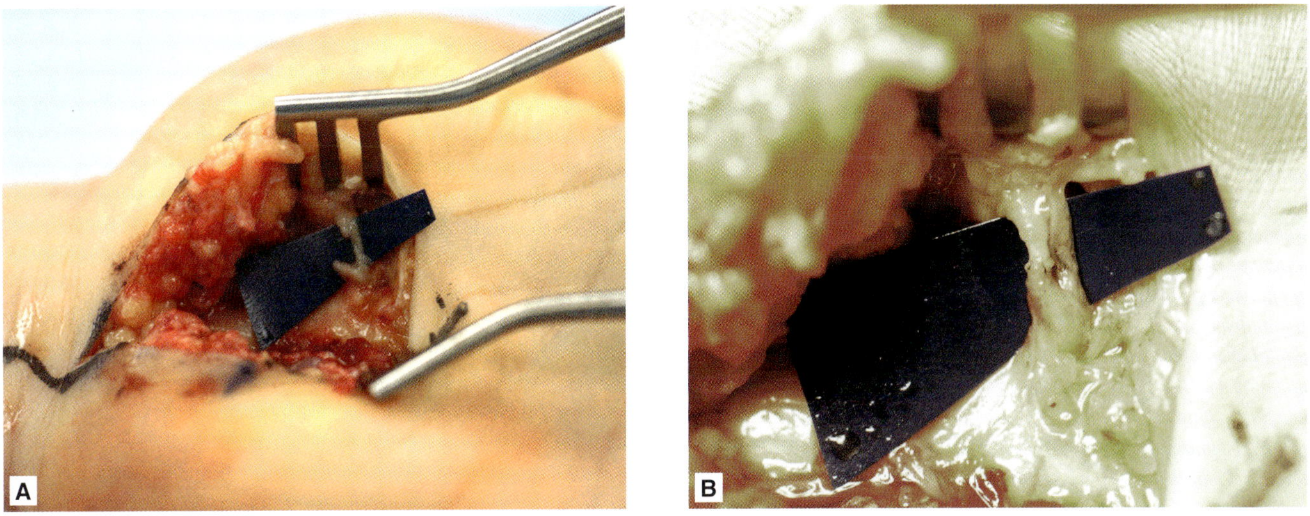

FIGURE 9-6 **A.** Laceration of 1 of 2 fascicles of recurrent branch. **B.** Fascicular repair of recurrent branch.

then crosses superficial or deep to the digital artery to lie just above the extensor mechanism, innervating the dorsum of the middle phalanx. This branch can provide a 1- to 2-cm nerve graft. Distal to the DIP joint the nerve trifurcates. The terminal PIN is a suitable graft at this level (Fig. 9-9A and B).

ULNAR NERVE

Anatomy. The ulnar nerve arises from the medial cord of the brachial plexus. It contains the nerve root fibers from C8 to T1. It provides the motor supply to the hypothenar

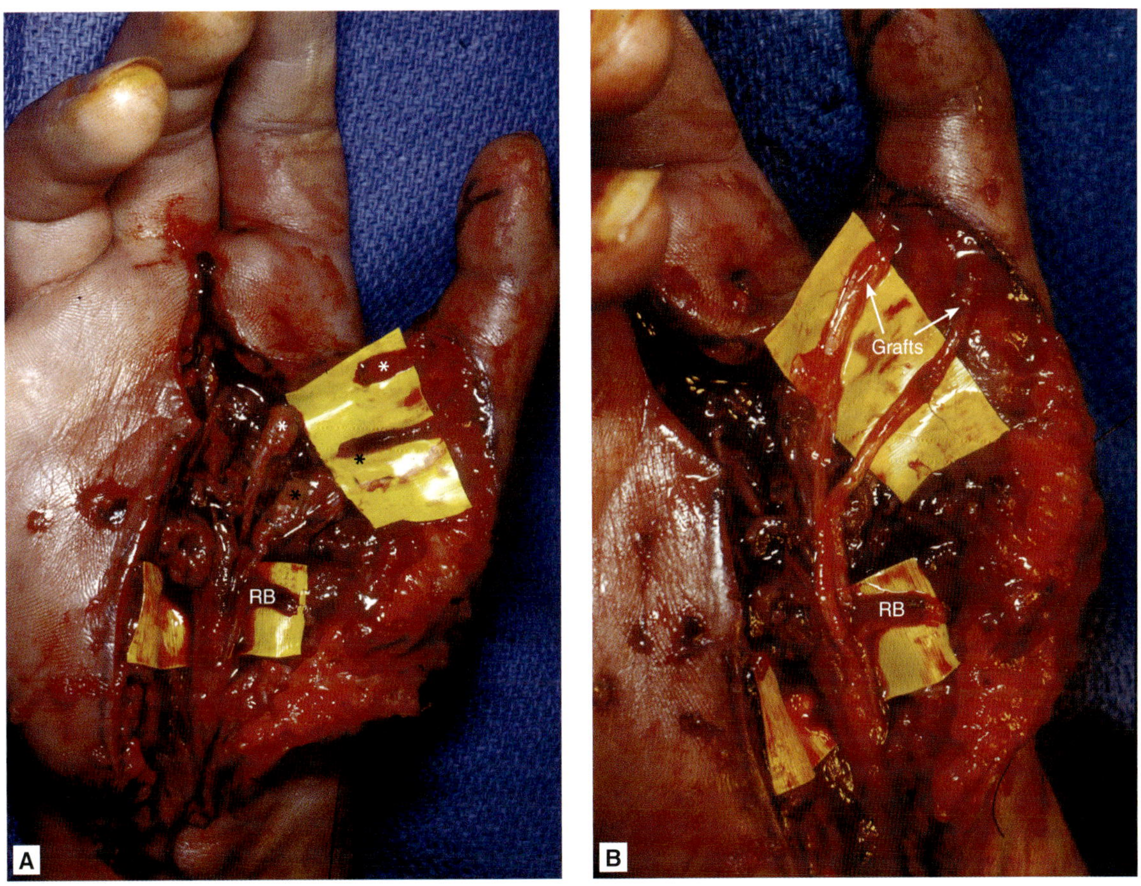

FIGURE 9-7 Median nerve laceration. **A.** Laceration of median nerve at junction of motor recurrent branch (RB) and digital sensory nerves to the thumb (*). **B.** Repair of recurrent branch, LABCN grafts to digital nerves.

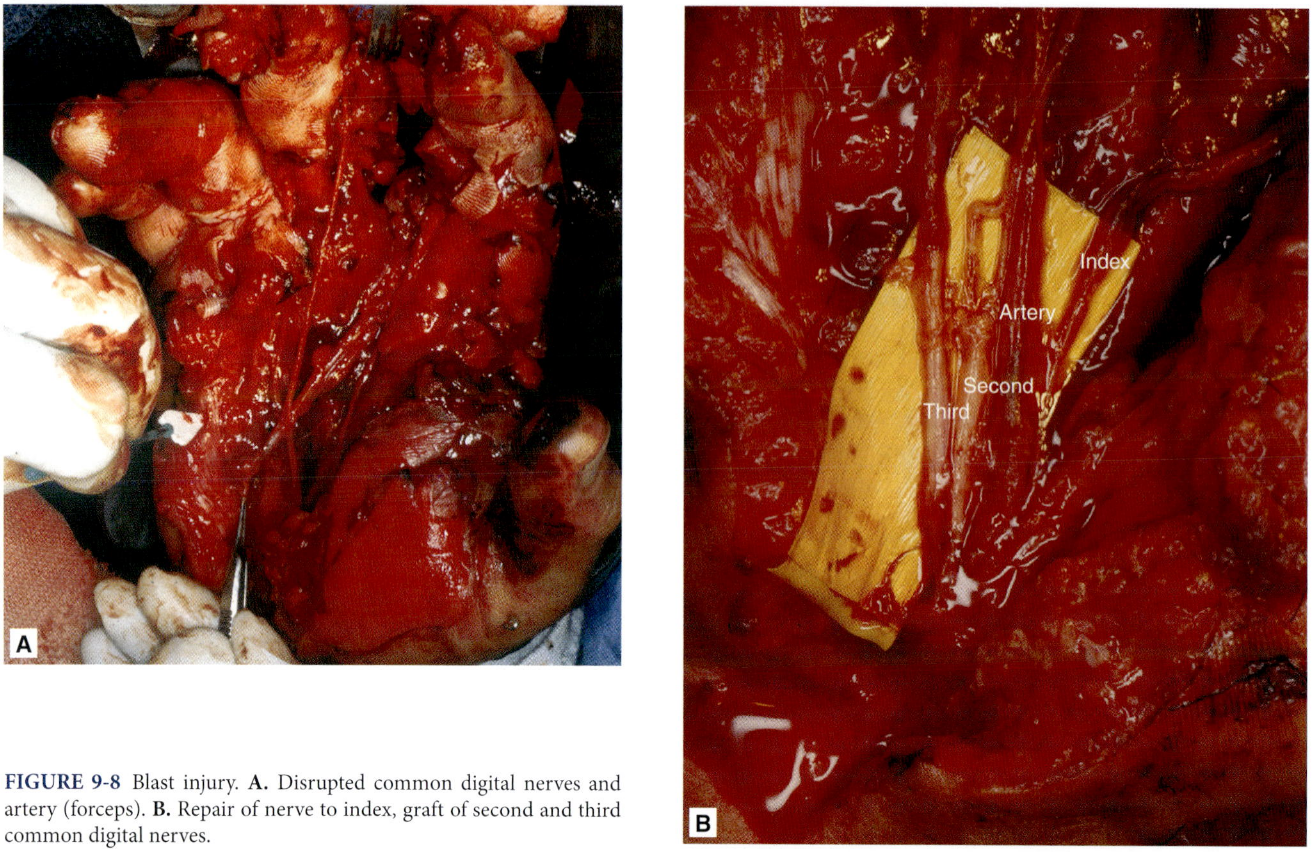

FIGURE 9-8 Blast injury. **A.** Disrupted common digital nerves and artery (forceps). **B.** Repair of nerve to index, graft of second and third common digital nerves.

muscles, the ulnar 2 lumbricals, the interosseous muscles, the adductor pollicis, FCU, and the profundus to the ring and small fingers. Its sensory distribution includes the palmar surface of the small and the ulnar half of the ring finger as well as the dorsoulnar carpus. It lies medial to the axillary artery and continues distally to the midarm where it pierces the medial intermuscular septum, approximately 8 cm proximal to the medial epicondyle. Historical investigations have concluded that Sir John Struthers did not actually describe an arcade in this area, and that an arcade of Struthers per se does not exist.[7] Rarely, fibrous bands may be seen crossing the ulnar nerve at this level. An internal brachial ligament (IBL) is present however in up to 73% of specimens.[8] The IBL consists of a fibrous band that originates from the medial intermuscular septum and travels laterally to lie on top of the epimysium of the triceps up to the medial condyle. When present, it forms a V-shaped opening with the medial intermuscular septum through which the ulnar nerve passes. The ulnar nerve lies on either the IBL or the triceps epimysium as it travels to the elbow. It then passes through the epicondylar

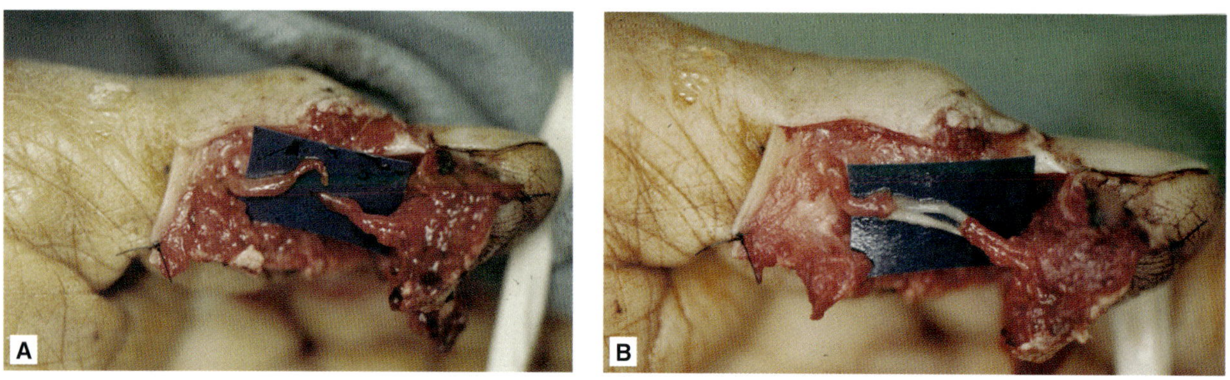

FIGURE 9-9 **A.** Saw injury to the radial digital nerve of the thumb at the IP joint. **B.** Terminal posterior interosseous nerve graft interposed between the 2 fascicles of the terminal digital nerve.

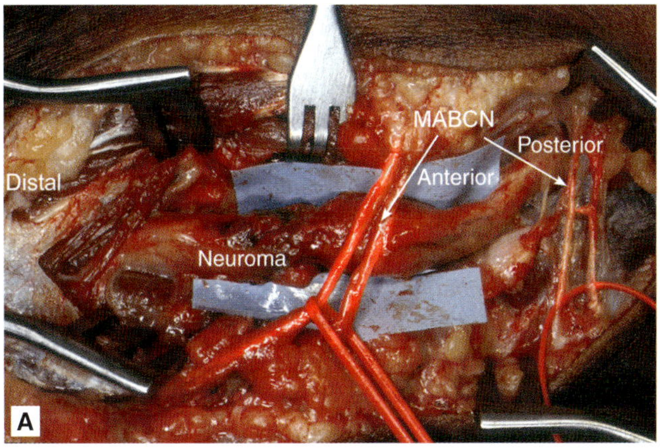

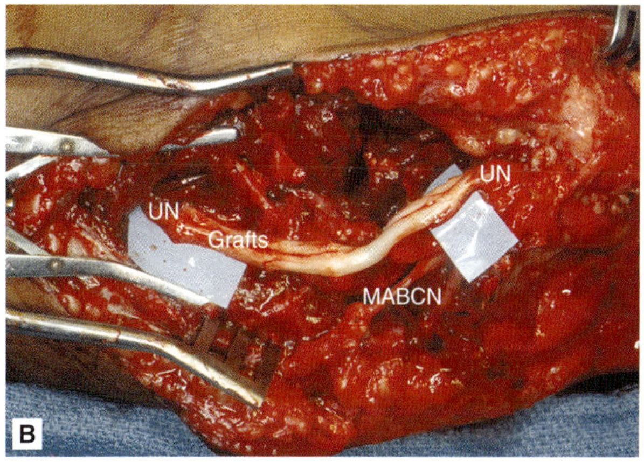

FIGURE 9-10 Neuroma of ulnar nerve at elbow. **A.** Medial aspect of the right elbow demonstrating an ulnar nerve neuroma. Note the anterior and posterior branches of the medial antebrachial cutaneous nerve (MABCN). **B.** Anterior transposition combined with sural nerve grafts to ulnar nerve (UN).

groove, which is a fibro-osseous tunnel bounded anteriorly by the medial epicondyle and laterally by the olecranon and ulnohumeral ligament and covered by a fibroaponeurotic band (ie, Osborne ligament, arcuate ligament, triangular ligament). The nerve then passes underneath the aponeurosis between the 2 heads of the flexor carpi ulnaris. The ulnar nerve is often accompanied by the superior ulnar collateral artery that forms an anastomosis with the inferior ulnar collateral artery around the medial epicondyle. It runs deep to the FCU until the distal forearm. At the wrist, it passes over the TCL, medial to the ulnar artery through Guyon canal. The deep motor branch is given off at the pisiform and passes underneath a fibrous arch to lie on the palmar surface of the interossei. It crosses the palm deep to the flexor tendons, to terminate in the adductor pollicis and ulnar head of the flexor pollicis brevis.

Repair at the Elbow. The ulnar nerve is located through a curved posteromedial incision behind the medial epicondyle. At the elbow the ulnar nerve contains about 20 fascicles including the motor branches to the forearm muscles. The motor fascicles to the FCU and the intrinsics are centrally located, whereas the sensory fibers are superficially located. The proximal motor branches to the FCU and FDP can often be traced for up to 6 cm prior to interfascicular connections. It is possible to distinguish between sensory and motor fascicles in the distal nerve end using low-intensity electrical stimulation, if performed within a few days of the injury. Occasionally fascicles innervating the flexor muscles can be separated from those supplying the intrinsic muscles in the hand. An external epineurial repair is the standard procedure. An anterior transposition of the nerve can be performed to gain 1 to 2 cm in length (Fig. 9-10A and B). If the ulnar nerve is transposed anteriorly, a 3-cm portion of the medial intermuscular septum should be resected to prevent secondary impingement. The SN is commonly used as graft material at this level. Care must be taken to avoid injury to accompanying veins of the inferior ulnar collateral artery that are just medial to the septum.

Repair in the Forearm. The motor fascicles lie dorsal and slightly ulnarly to the sensory fascicles at the wrist level, and usually maintain a dorsal relationship as one moves proximally. The motor component remains as a distinct entity up to 90 mm proximal to the styloid. At 50 to 85 mm proximal to the radial styloid the dorsal sensory branch joins the other groups. At the level of the midforearm, 50 mm from the ulnar styloid, the motor fascicles lie dorsal to the sensory fascicles (Fig. 9-11). A fascicular repair of the motor branch is desirable. If there is a gap, a nerve graft should be placed in the dorsal quadrant of the proximal nerve end and the dorsoulnar quadrant of the distal nerve end to restore motor continuity.

Repair at the Wrist. The ulnar nerve has 15 to 25 fascicles at the wrist. It can be clearly divided into a volar sensory component and a dorsal motor component (Fig. 9-12). The ulnar nerve is approached through an S-shaped incision over the volar ulnar forearm. The nerve is identified medial to the ulnar artery underneath the FCU muscle. If a muscle twitch

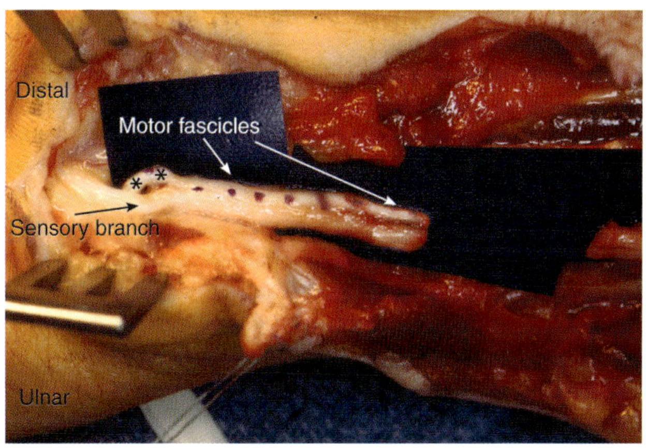

FIGURE 9-11 Ulnar nerve motor fascicles traced from the distal stump to the deep motor branch in the palm.

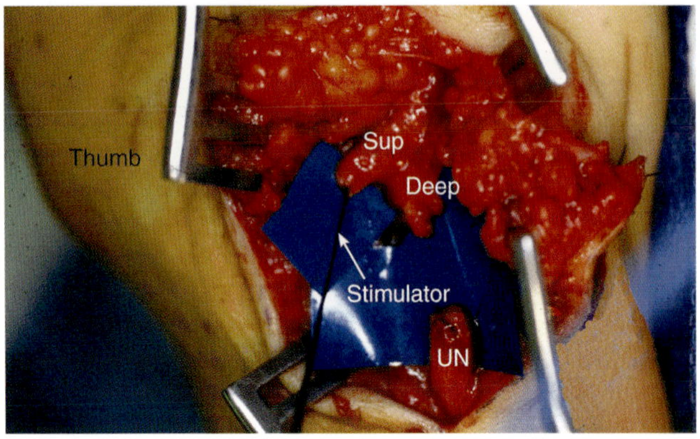

FIGURE 9-12 Laceration of the ulnar nerve in Guyon canal after it has separated into a deep motor and superficial sensory branch.

is no longer present, the motor branch can be traced from the takeoff of the deep motor branch to the distal nerve end and repaired primarily or grafted.

Repair in the Hand. The nerve is approached through a volar ulnar incision in line with the ring finger. The deep motor and more superficial sensory fascicles are easily separated at this level and allow separate grafting. The SN, LABCN, or MABCN provides suitable sized grafts (Fig. 9-13A and B). The DCBUN is not usually grafted since neuromas of this nerve are uncommon.

Digital Nerve Repair. Repair or grafting in the digits is similar to the median nerve.

RADIAL NERVE

Anatomy. The radial nerve arises from the posterior cord of the brachial plexus. It receives contributions from C5 to C8 spinal roots. The nerve contains approximately 16,000 myelinated fibers. It is the largest branch of the plexus and arises from the posterior cord. In the proximal third of the arm, the nerve descends behind the brachial artery until the junction of the proximal and middle thirds of the humerus, where it passes between the medial and long head of the triceps with the profundi brachii artery. The nerve reaches the lateral intermuscular septum lying on the medial head of the triceps that separates it from the spiral groove of the humerus and gives off branches to the triceps and the anconeus. At the midarm it pierces the lateral intermuscular septum to run between the brachialis and brachioradialis. In 10% of cases it may innervate the radial one third of the brachialis. It divides 2 cm distal to the elbow into a superficial radial sensory branch (SRN) and a deep motor branch, the PIN. It gives off branches to the extensor carpi radialis longus and brachioradialis before giving off the PIN branch. The extensor carpi radialis brevis is variably supplied by branches arising from the radial nerve, the PIN or the SRN. The PIN continues on between the superficial and deep head of the supinator muscle that it supplies, and then exits on the dorsal forearm. After it emerges from the distal border of the supinator, the PIN immediately sends short branches to the extensor digitorum communis, extensor carpi ulnaris, and extensor digiti quinti. It then sends off long fibers that split into a medial and a lateral branch. The medial branch supplies the extensor pollicis longus and the extensor indicis proprius, whereas the lateral branch supplies the extensor pollicis brevis and abductor pollicis longus in descending order, although there may be considerable variation.

Repair at the Elbow. The volar approach to the radial nerve is through an anterolateral incision, developing the intermuscular interval between the brachialis and brachioradialis (Fig. 9-14A and B). Recurrent branches from the radial artery must be divided to gain access to both nerve branches. Separate repair of the SRN and the PIN branch is relatively straightforward. In general, the SRN is not grafted in case some of the motor axons are misdirected.

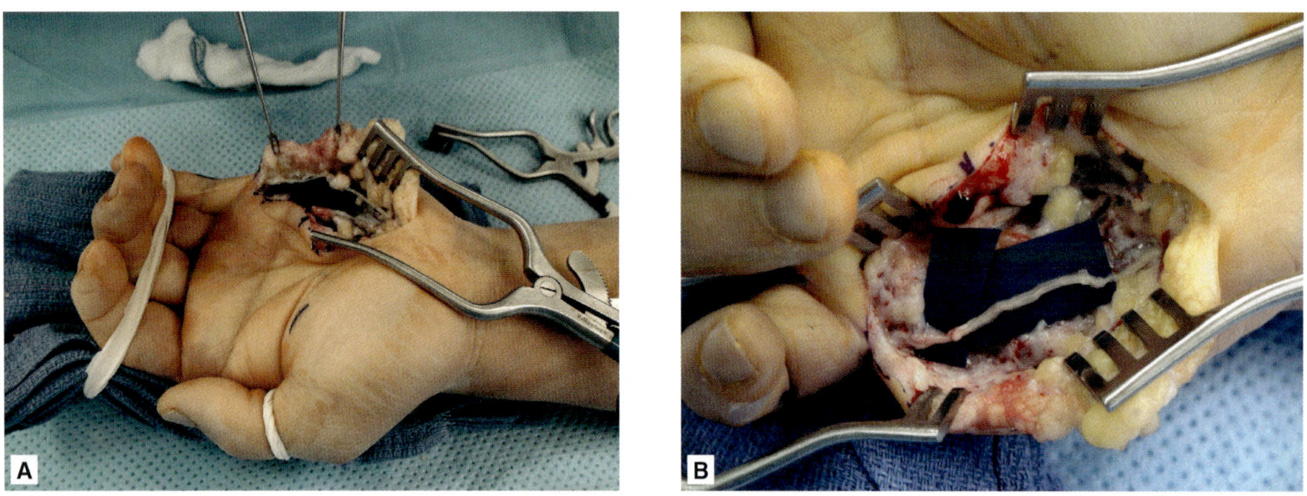

FIGURE 9-13 **A.** Neuroma-in-continuity of the ulnar nerve sensory branch to the small finger. **B.** LABCN graft after neuroma resection.

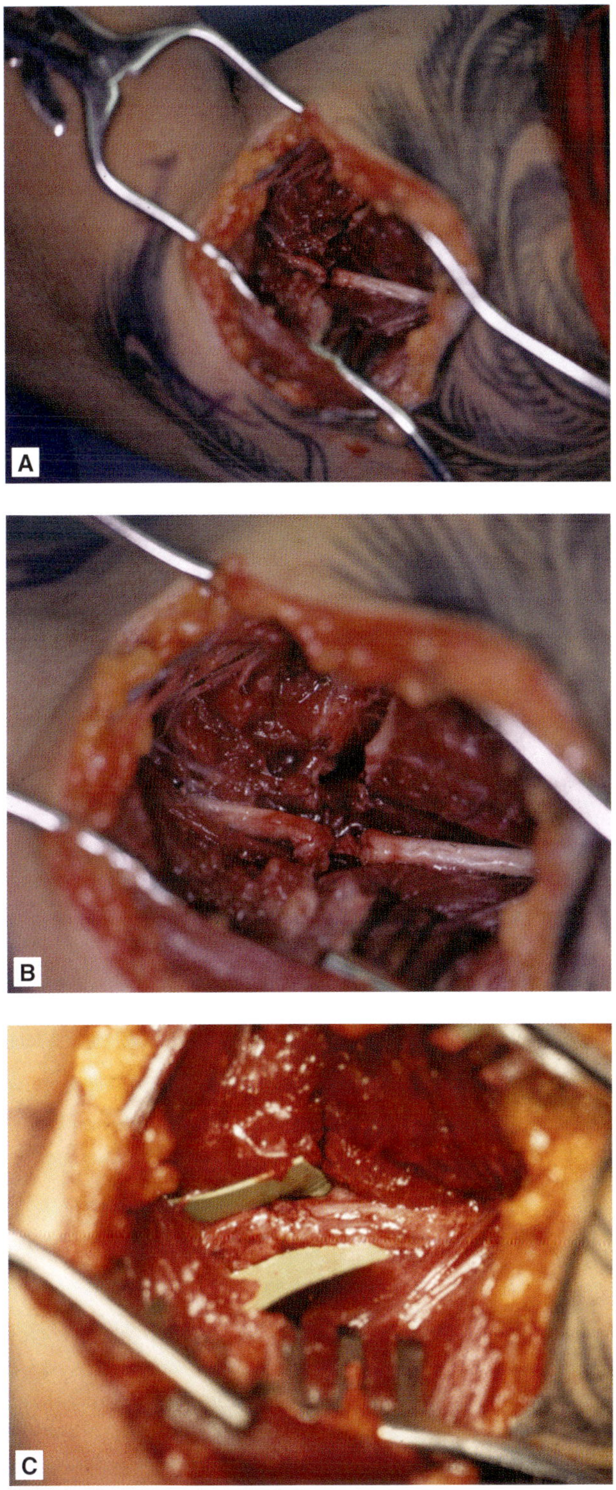

FIGURE 9-14 **A.** One-month-old proximal radial nerve laceration. **B.** Strip of posterior epineurium is sutured (arrow) to take the tension off the repair. **C.** Completed epineurial repair.

Repair in the Forearm and Wrist. The PIN nerve is approached through a dorsolateral approach, developing the plane between the extensor carpi radialis brevis and the extensor digitorum communis. At this level, the PIN contains motor fibers only; hence, separate fascicle identification is unnecessary. The PIN also has a short distance to travel to reinnervate the motor end plates, which accounts for the generally favorable results (Fig. 9-15A and B). Lacerations of the superficial branch in the forearm are not usually grafted, which allows harvest of the SRN for grafting adjacent nerve injuries. Some authors do advocate grafting the SRN at the wrist, mostly to prevent symptomatic neuroma formation.

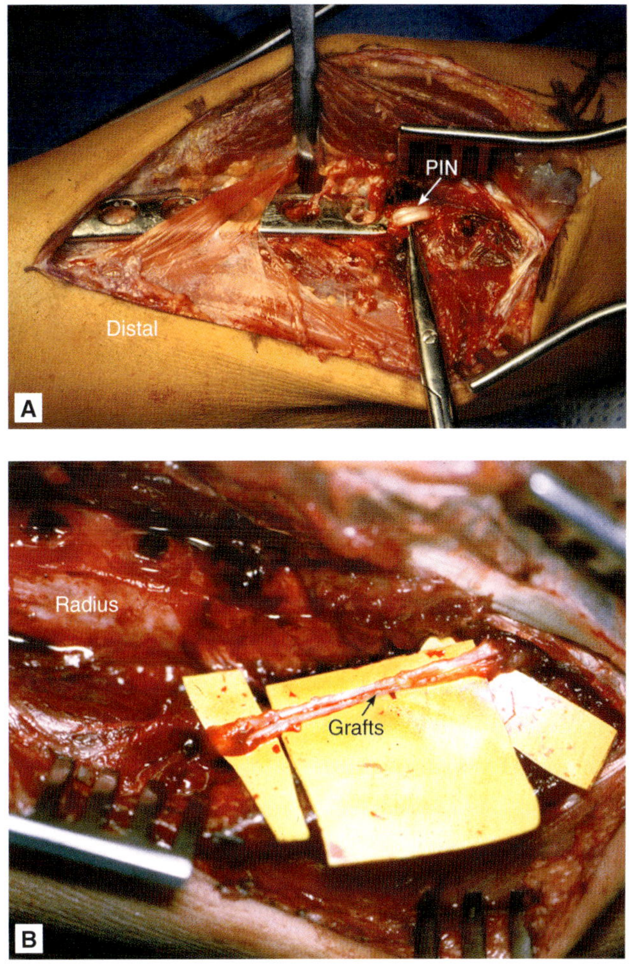

FIGURE 9-15 Posterior interosseous nerve injury. **A.** Dorsal approach to left forearm demonstrating a PIN injury after plating of a proximal radius fracture. **B.** Interposed nerve grafts.

POSTOPERATIVE REHABILITATION

After nerve repair the rehabilitation focuses on 3 areas: initial immobilization to protect the repair, joint mobilization to promote longitudinal excursion of the nerve, and sensory reeducation. Prior to wound closure, the adjacent joints are placed in various degrees of flexion and extension in order to determine the optimum limb position that unloads the repair site. This position is maintained with a blocking splint for 3 weeks, but a protected short arc of motion may be instituted to provide some nerve gliding.

Outcomes Following Repair/Graft

Most series report the results of nerve repair using the British Medical Research Council grading system that has been modified by Dellon.[9] In this classification, scores of S0 and M0 represent absent sensory and motor function, respectively, while scores of S1 or S2 and M1 or M2 represent detectable but less useful function. S3 equates to recovery of pain and touch sensibility, with 2-point discrimination (2-pd) of >15 mm, while S3+ equates to 2-pd of 7 to 15 mm, and S4 is normal sensation. A grade of M3 equates to a recovery of muscle strength that is sufficient to overcome gravity. M4 is strength with gravity and added resistance, while M5 is normal. As noted below, however, many other classifications are also in use, which can make comparison between studies difficult.

Ruijs et al performed a meta-analysis after microsurgical nerve repair of 623 median or ulnar nerve injuries.[10] Motor and sensory recovery were significantly associated. In ulnar nerve injuries, the chance of motor recovery was 71% lower than in median nerve injuries. Kallio and Vastamaki evaluated 132 patients (mean age 28 years) with injuries to the median nerve at an average 10.4 years after repair.[11] Most of the nerve lesions were sharp (76) or blunt (47) injuries. Division was total in 87 cases, and most were at the wrist level. Secondary repair was performed in 34 cases and fascicular grafting in 98 cases. The average gap was 5.8 cm. Excellent or good results were obtained in only 49.2%. The result of nerve repair was poor in patients aged over 54 years, when the level of the injury was more than 56 cm proximal to the fingertip, if the preoperative delay was more than 24 months, or if the graft length was more than 70 mm.

Secer et al reported the results of 407 ulnar nerve injuries caused by gunshot wounds. A good outcome was noted in 15% of patients who underwent high-level repair, 29% of patients who underwent intermediate-level repair, and 49% of patients after low-level repair.[12] The critical period for surgery was within 6 months of injury. Although the optimal graft length was found to be 5 cm, this finding was not statistically significant. Kim et al examined 45 patients following surgically treated PIN entrapments (21) or injuries (23).[13] Seven underwent suture repair, 7 were grafted, and the rest underwent neurolysis. Most muscles achieved LSUHSC Grade 3 or better. Kim et al reported M3/S3 in 72% of 50 patients.[13] Dauotis et al noted that M3 or better was achieved in 68% and S3 or better in 75% of 47 patients with median nerve grafts.[14] Millesi achieved M4 or better in 61% and S3 or better in 42%. For the ulnar nerve, he reported M4 or better in 49% and S3 or better in 27%, whereas he reported S3+ or better in only 22% for digital nerve repairs.[5] It is commonly accepted that the results are far better in children than in adults. Tomei et al evaluated 25 nerve repairs at the wrist in children under age 15 years with a minimum follow-up of 12 months.[15] The sensory results were often excellent (S4 or S3+ in 23/25 cases), whereas motor recovery ranged between M2 and M3.

Kallio studied 95 patients with 254 completely divided digital nerves at an average of 12.4 (5-20) years after repair.[16] Secondary epineurial suture was used in 53, fascicular grafting in 37, and fascicular suture in 5. Useful sensory function was recovered in 79% of the nerves operated on with epineurial or fascicular suture and in 56% with fascicular grafting.

ALTERNATE METHODS OF NERVE RECONSTRUCTION

Nerve Conduits

Neurotrophism is the ability of chemotactic hormonal or growth factors to enhance the rate of nerve regeneration. *Neurotrophic* factors produced by the target end organ undergo retrograde axonal transport and help support the cell body. *Neurotropism* describes the directional accuracy of that regeneration. The growth cone is attracted to *neurotropic* proteins that are derived from the distal degenerating nerve segment after nerve transection. These phenomena have been exploited through the use of synthetic or natural conduits to bridge the nerve gap. Histologically, fibrin clot develops inside the tube within hours. Within the first week longitudinally oriented fibrin matrix bridges span the nerve gap. In the second week, fibroblasts, Schwann cells, macrophages, and endothelial cells permeate the matrix. Axon sprouts from proximal nerve reach the distal stump and become myelinated by the fourth week. The axons elongate down intact the distal endoneurial tubes and reinnervate the target organs. Nondegradable tubes out of silicone were initially used. More recently, natural prosthetic tubes have included freeze/thawed muscle (which contains a basal lamina) and autogenous vein grafts. Biodegradable synthetic material includes polyglycolic acid (PGA), caprolactone, and collagen. The postoperative rehabilitation includes early mobilization of the part since tension on the repair site is not a consideration, followed by appropriate sensory and/or motor retraining.

INDICATIONS

Conduits are indicated for reconstruction of small-diameter, noncritical sensory nerves with a gap of less than 3 cm. They can be used with digital replantation with nerve gaps of less than 3 cm and in the mangled hand if a primary, tension-free nerve repair cannot be achieved in the acute setting and if the gap is less than 1 to 2 cm. They are indicated in association with flexor tendon repair in zone 2 to create a tension-free repair and allow early mobilization. Relative indications include nerve reconstruction after resection of a traumatic neuroma or a neoplasm. They can be used as a wrap around a partially injured nerve or after neurolysis of a scarred nerve. Large-diameter mixed sensorimotor nerves should be approached with caution. MacKinnon has noted the formula for volume ($V = \pi \times \text{radius} \times 2 \times \text{length}$); hence, doubling the radius would require using a conduit that is one fourth the length in order to maintain an equal volume and concentration of trophic factors.

CONTRAINDICATIONS

These include uncertainty about the viability of the nerve ends, especially with avulsion injuries, blast injuries, and gunshot wounds, local or systemic infection, and inadequate soft tissue coverage. When placed in superficial locations, the nerve conduit may be palpable for up to 1 year. PGA conduits are more likely to extrude due to their more rigid nature than collagen conduits and require thicker soft tissue coverage. Relative contraindications include nerve gaps greater than 3 cm and a pure motor nerve deficit.

SURGICAL TECHNIQUE

Synthetic Conduits. The procedure is done with the patient supine and the extremity on an arm board under tourniquet control. Microsurgical instruments are needed, but high-power loupe magnification is usually sufficient, although a fascicular dissection may be performed under the operating microscope. The proximal and distal nerve ends are identified and meticulous hemostasis is obtained. The tension-free gap is measured with the adjacent joints in full extension. The nerve stumps are trimmed under magnification until healthy fascicles are identified. The minimum distance between the ends is 5 mm with the maximum 3 cm. The diameter of the nerve is measured with a ruler to determine the appropriate size conduit. The inner diameter of the tube should be equal to or slightly larger than the diameter of the nerve to be implanted. Some synthetic conduits require saline immersion prior to implantation. Conduit size ranges from 2 to 10 mm and 4 cm in length. After the correct size is chosen, 1 nerve end is pulled into the conduit so that 2 to 5 mm of the nerve lies within the conduit or a distance equal to or greater than the nerve diameter. An 8-0 or 9-0 nylon is used to draw the nerve ends into the conduit using a horizontal mattress stitch (Fig. 9-16A and B). Either the proximal or distal end is sutured first. The stitch is passed from the outside to inside of the conduit wall at least 1 mm from its end. The suture is next passed transversely through the epineurium 2 to 3 mm from the stump and then back through the conduit from inside to out and tied after the stump is drawn into the conduit. The conduit lumen is filled with sterile saline for collagen tubes and heparinized saline for PGA tubes as per the manufacturer recommendation, to prevent air bubbles or blood clot formation that may impede axonal ingrowth.

Autogenous Vein Grafts. The use of autologous veins as a biologic tube to reconstruct a nerve gap has been well described over the past century. Chiu and Strauch have championed the use of autogenous venous nerve conduits (AVNC) for the reconstruction of digital sensory nerve defects of 3 cm or less.[17] They have demonstrated clinical results that compare favorably with autologous nerve grafts. Advantages of the AVNC include the avoidance of a cutaneous donor-site sensory defect and minimal cost as compared with the commercially manufactured synthetic conduits. The superficial veins on the dorsum of the hand are of an appropriate caliber for digital nerve reconstruction (Fig. 9-17A-C). Chiu has noted that there is a fairly constant dorsal vein that runs longitudinally in line with the fourth web space and is usually adjacent to the dorsal cutaneous branch of the ulnar nerve. The AVNC is reversed due to the possible presence of venous valves. The cut proximal end of the nerve is placed in the end of the vein that was distal (in situ) using a telescoping suture. The same is done to the other end of the nerve after the vein graft is cut to the appropriate length. Some authors prefer to use lower extremity veins only since they are thicker and have less of a tendency to collapse.

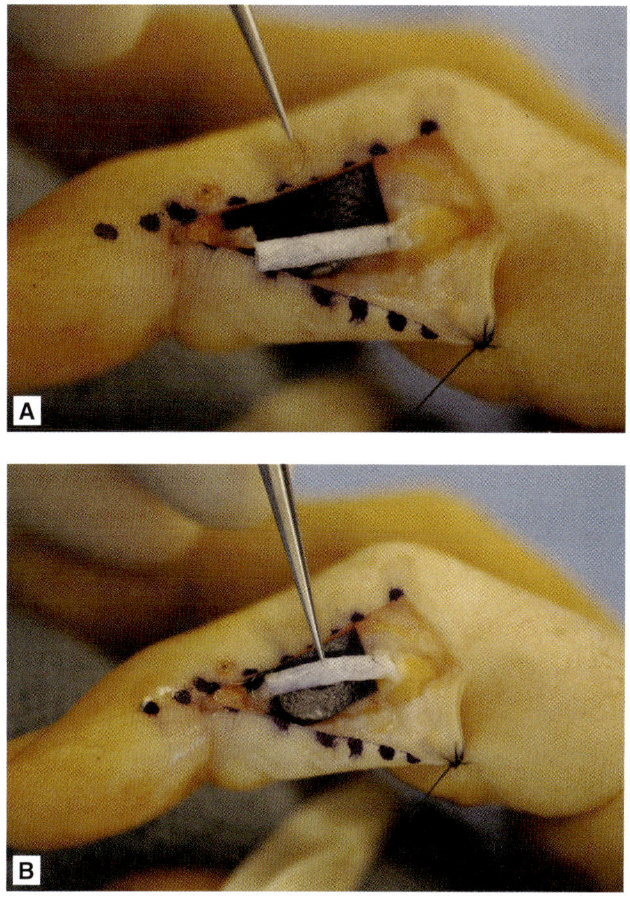

FIGURE 9-16 Collagen conduit for digital nerve reconstruction. **A.** Partially completed collagen conduit demonstrating the horizontal mattress suture. **B.** Conduit filled with saline.

POSTOPERATIVE REHABILITATION

Repair of other tendon or muscle injuries will influence the rehabilitation. With an isolated nerve reconstruction the affected part is immobilized with the adjacent joints in neutral. Composite extension or flexion in the opposite direction of the repair is avoided to prevent tension that could dislocate a nerve end from the conduit. Range of motion exercises

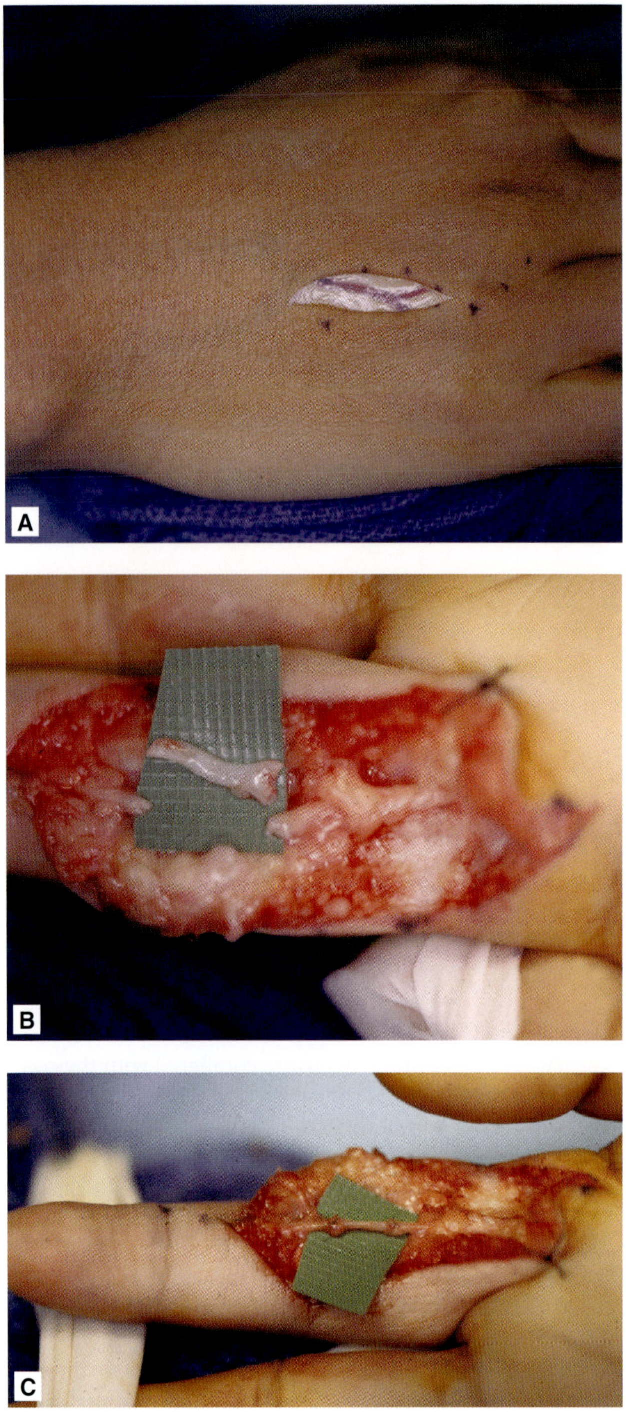

FIGURE 9-17 **A.** Harvest of dorsal vein conduit. **B.** Reversed vein graft prior to anastomosis. **C.** Completed repair.

are started at 10 days followed by strengthening exercises at 6 weeks and sensory reeducation for the next year.

OUTCOMES

Lundborg et al compared tubulation using a silicone conduit, after intentionally leaving a 3- to 4-mm nerve gap (11 cases) with a conventional microsurgical repair of transected median and ulnar nerve repairs (7 cases) in the forearm. The results showed no significant differences between the 2 techniques, although the silicone tubes had to be removed at a later date, due to compression of the reformed nerve.[18] Chiu and Strauch did a series of animal experiments bridging gaps of 1.0 to 6.0 cm using autogenous vein grafts.[17] The technique includes suturing a reversed vein graft in place distally so that the valves in the vein cannot collapse and block axonal migration. The proximal repair is performed after filling the vein with saline to present clot formation that will produce scarring that can obstruct the axons. In their clinical series, Chiu and Strauch reported comparable results to those obtained with nerve repair and grafting for sensory nerve defects of <3 cm.

Weber et al performed a randomized, prospective, multicenter evaluation on 98 subjects with 136 nerve transections in the hand comparing a polyglycolic conduit with either end-to-end or a nerve graft for nerve repair.[19] There were 56 nerves repaired in the control group and 46 nerves repaired with a conduit available for follow-up. The overall results showed no significant difference between the 2 groups as a whole. Nerves with gaps of 4 mm or less had better sensation when repaired with a conduit; the mean moving 2-point discrimination (MPD) was 3.7 ± 1.4 mm for PGA tube repair and 6.1 ± 3.3 mm for end-to-end repairs ($P = .03$). All injured nerves with deficits of 8 mm or greater were reconstructed with either a nerve graft or a conduit. This subgroup also demonstrated a significant difference in favor of the PGA tube. The mean MPD for the conduit was 6.8 ± 3.8 mm, with excellent results obtained in 7 of 17 nerves, whereas the mean MPD for the graft repair was 12.9 ± 2.4 mm, with excellent results obtained in none of the 8 nerves ($P < .001$ and $= .06$, respectively). Bertleff et al examined the results of using a caprolactone tube versus primary repair in 34 digital nerve lesions with gaps <2 cm.[20] The results with the conduits were equal to those of repair as evaluated by the pressure-specified sensory testing device and 2-pd.

Rinker and Liau performed a therapeutic level II study evaluating the sensory outcomes in 37 patients with 68 nerve injuries, with gaps of 3 cm or less, that precluded a direct repair.[21] The patients were randomized to a nerve repair with either a woven PGA conduit or autogenous vein graft. The median age was 35 years (range, 19-76). A power analysis determined 28 nerve repairs provided an 80% chance of detecting a statistical difference with a 95% confidence interval (CI). They repaired 36 nerves with the PGA conduit and 32 with vein. The nerve gaps ranged from 4 to 25 mm (mean, 10 mm). The mean static 2-point discrimination (SPD) and MPD at 12 months for the synthetic conduit group were 7.5 ± 1.9 and 5.6 ± 2.2 mm, compared with 7.6 ± 2.6 and 6.6 ± 2.9 mm for the vein group. When patients were divided up into a short gap <10 mm or long gap ≥10 mm, there were also no statistical differences between the PGA and vein conduit repairs. There were 2 extrusions in the synthetic conduit group requiring reoperation.

Marcoccio and Vigasio treated 17 patients with 21 digital nerve defects using a vein conduit filled with fresh skeletal muscle.[22] The donor vein and fresh muscle segments are obtained through a 5-cm skin incision in the proximal forearm. A suitable vein graft is harvested and a 22-gauge cannula is introduced into the lumen of the vein. A longitudinal segment of muscle fibers is harvested slightly longer than the vein graft. A 7-0 nylon suture is used to draw the muscle into the vein graft, and then removed. A tension-free repair is performed as described above. The average nerve gap was 2.2 cm (range, 1-3.5 cm). At a mean follow-up of 43 months (range, 18-96 months), 5 patients achieved S4 with complete recovery of SPD of 2 to 6 mm and MPD of 2 to 3 mm; 9 patients achieved S3+ with SPD of 7 to 15 mm and MPD of 4 to 7 mm but with good localization of stimulus; 3 patients achieved S3 with SPD of >15 mm, MPD >7 mm, and recovery of pain and touch sensibility; 1 had S2 with recovery of superficial pain and some touch sensibility; and 4 had S1 with recovery of superficial pain and some touch sensibility only.

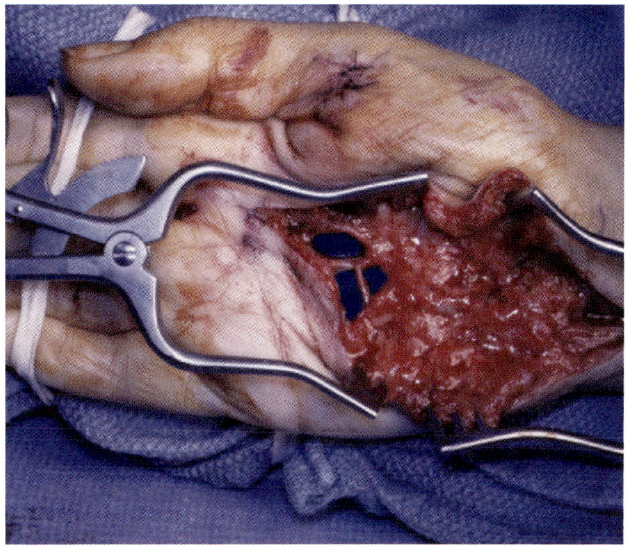

FIGURE 9-18 End-to-side repair to third common digital nerve.

End-to-side Repairs

Experimental data in both rabbit and primate models have shown that intact donor nerves have the ability to sprout lateral branches from their axons that can grow through endoneurium, perineurium, and epineurium and reinnervate target organs with functional sensory and motor results.[23] These results have also been duplicated in human studies that have included root avulsions of the brachial plexus, as well as patients with large gaps in peripheral nerves. A standard end-to-side anastomosis involves suturing the recipient nerve into an epineural window that is created in the donor nerve (Fig. 9-18). An advantage of this technique is that the donor nerve does not lose any function.

End-to-side repairs cannot replace a sound primary repair, but they have been used as an adjunctive procedure in the following situations: intact nerve to the musculocutaneous to neurotize the biceps muscle, distal stump of the ulnar nerve to the median nerve at the wrist in high ulnar nerve palsies or vice versa, and ulnar digital nerves to intact median sensory nerves. The limb is splinted for 3 weeks in a tension-free position, followed by motor and sensory reeducation. The procedure is best done early since the results deteriorate if delayed beyond 6 months. In Mennen's series of 56 patients that included 33 ulnar to median and 7 median to ulnar repairs, ≥M3/S3 was achieved in 56%.[24]

Neurotization

Brunelli et al pioneered the concept of direct neurotization of denervated muscles in situations where the motor nerve has been avulsed and direct nerve suture or grafting is not possible.[25] They demonstrated in rat and rabbit models that an axon that is in contact with a denervated muscular fiber can form a new neuromuscular junction. The motor end plate is, in fact, not an anatomic formation but rather a functional alteration of the axon endings and the muscular fibers that develop when they are in contact with each other. A prerequisite for this procedure is that there is some residual trophism of the muscle. This is manifested by the presence of fibrillation potentials on the EMG. The procedure is contraindicated if there is muscle atrophy without fibrillation potentials or if there is extensive scarring or joint stiffness. The donor nerve is retrieved and sectioned transversely until healthy fascicles are seen. The junction of the proximal one fourth and distal three fourths of the muscular belly is exposed. A SN graft of adequate length is harvested and sutured end to end to the donor nerve. The distal part of the nerve graft is freed from the epineurium and is divided into as many artificial fascicles as possible. The epineurium of the graft is sutured to the muscle epimysium in order to prevent graft retraction. A number of slits are made at different depths and as widely separated as the graft will permit. The artificial fascicles are then implanted into the muscle and held in place with fibrin glue and epineurial sutures and immobilized for 15 days, followed by mobilization. The limbs are immobilized for 15 days in order to prevent avulsion of the implanted nerve. Reeducation is started with joint mobilization and electrotherapy. In Brunelli's series of 80 patients, M4/M5 motor strength was achieved in 72 of the cases.

REFERENCES

1. Mackinnon SE, Dellon AL, O'Brien JP. Changes in nerve fiber numbers distal to a nerve repair in the rat sciatic nerve model. *Muscle Nerve.* 1991;14(11):1116–1122.
2. Wiertz-Hoessels EL, Krediet P. Degeneration of the motor end-plates after neurectomy, in the rat and the rabbit. *Acta Morphol Neerl Scand.* 1965;6:179–193.
3. Clark WL, Trumble TE, Swiontkowski MF, Tencer AF. Nerve tension and blood flow in a rat model of immediate and delayed repairs. *J Hand Surg Am.* 1992;17(4):677–687.
4. Jabaley ME. Technical aspects of peripheral nerve repair. *J Hand Surg Br.* 1984;9(1):14–19.

5. Millesi H. Techniques for nerve grafting. *Hand Clin.* 2000;16(1): 73–91, viii.
6. Higgins JP, Fisher S, Serletti JM, Orlando GS. Assessment of nerve graft donor sites used for reconstruction of traumatic digital nerve defects. *J Hand Surg Am.* 2002;27(2):286–292.
7. De Jesus R, Dellon AL. Historic origin of the "Arcade of Struthers". *J Hand Surg Am.* 2003;28(3):528–531.
8. Wehrli L, Oberlin C. The internal brachial ligament versus the arcade of Struthers: an anatomical study. *Plast Reconstr Surg.* 2005;115(2): 471–477.
9. Dellon AL. A numerical grading scale for peripheral nerve function. *J Hand Ther.* 1993;6(2):152–160.
10. Ruijs AC, Jaquet JB, Kalmijn S, Giele H, Hovius SE. Median and ulnar nerve injuries: a meta-analysis of predictors of motor and sensory recovery after modern microsurgical nerve repair. *Plast Reconstr Surg.* 2005;116(2):484–494 [discussion 495–496].
11. Kallio PK, Vastamaki M. An analysis of the results of late reconstruction of 132 median nerves. *J Hand Surg Br.* 1993;18(1):97–105.
12. Secer HI, Daneyemez M, Gonul E, Izci Y. Surgical repair of ulnar nerve lesions caused by gunshot and shrapnel: results in 407 lesions. *J Neurosurg.* 2007;107(4):776–783.
13. Kim DH, Murovic JA, Kim YY, Kline DG. Surgical treatment and outcomes in 45 cases of posterior interosseous nerve entrapments and injuries. *J Neurosurg.* 2006;104(5):766–777.
14. Daoutis NK, Gerostathopoulos NE, Efstathopoulos DG, Misitizis DP, Bouchlis GN, Anagnostou SK. Microsurgical reconstruction of large nerve defects using autologous nerve grafts. *Microsurgery.* 1994; 15(7):502–505.
15. Tomei F, Aubert JP, Benaim JL, Legre R, Magalon G. Results of nerve sutures in the wrist in children. *Chir Main.* 2000;19(1):23–30.
16. Kallio PK. The results of secondary repair of 254 digital nerves. *J Hand Surg Br.* 1993;18(3):327–330.
17. Chiu DT, Strauch B. A prospective clinical evaluation of autogenous vein grafts used as a nerve conduit for distal sensory nerve defects of 3 cm or less. *Plast Reconstr Surg.* 1990;86(5):928–934.
18. Lundborg G, Rosen B, Dahlin L, Danielsen N, Holmberg J. Tubular versus conventional repair of median and ulnar nerves in the human forearm: early results from a prospective, randomized, clinical study. *J Hand Surg Am.* 1997;22(1):99–106.
19. Weber RA, Breidenbach WC, Brown RE, Jabaley ME, Mass DP. A randomized prospective study of polyglycolic acid conduits for digital nerve reconstruction in humans. *Plast Reconstr Surg.* 2000; 106(5):1036–1045 [discussion 1046–1048].
20. Bertleff MJ, Meek MF, Nicolai JP. A prospective clinical evaluation of biodegradable neurolac nerve guides for sensory nerve repair in the hand. *J Hand Surg Am.* 2005;30(3):513–518.
21. Rinker B, Liau JY. A prospective randomized study comparing woven polyglycolic acid and autogenous vein conduits for reconstruction of digital nerve gaps. *J Hand Surg Am.* 2011;36(5):775–781.
22. Marcoccio I, Vigasio A. Muscle-in-vein nerve guide for secondary reconstruction in digital nerve lesions. *J Hand Surg Am.* 2010; 35(9):1418–1426.
23. Kelly EJ, Jacoby C, Terenghi G, Mennen U, Ljungberg C, Wiberg M. End-to-side nerve coaptation: a qualitative and quantitative assessment in the primate. *J Plast Reconstr Aesthet Surg.* 2007;60(1):1–12.
24. Mennen U. End-to-side nerve suture in clinical practice. *Hand Surg.* 2003; 8(1):33–42.
25. Brunelli G, Monini L, Brunelli F. Direct muscular neurotization. *Ann Chir Main Memb Super.* 1990;9(4):290–295.

Sensory Nerve Transfers

10

Ida K. Fox, MD
Andrew Yee, BS
Susan E. Mackinnon, MD

RATIONALE AND BASIC SCIENCE

Traditionally, the restoration of sensory nerve function has been through the use of direct end-to-end coaptation of the injured nerve ends. In the case of segmental nerve damage, sensory nerve grafts, conduits, or allogeneic materials have been used to bridge the gap. While these techniques are still popular, sensory nerve transfers are also useful in a variety of clinical scenarios.

Knowledge of the pathophysiology of the nerve injury is critical to determining whether a nerve transfer is an appropriate treatment option. Any sensory nerve that is likely to recover spontaneously should be left alone. These "favorable" nerve injury subtypes include a first-degree conduction block (neurapraxia) in the Seddon classification, which will recover fully within a few months, and second-degree (axonotmetic) and third-degree injuries where the connective tissue framework is still intact so that recovery is still possible, but incomplete. Third-degree nerve injuries may require repair if they are associated with severe neuropathic pain.[1]

Fourth-degree (neuroma-in-continuity) and fifth-degree (neurotmesis or transection) injuries will require repair and, in certain cases, a nerve transfer might be indicated. A nerve transfer might be especially indicated in the treatment of a sixth-degree or mixed injury because a nerve transfer may be done distal to the area of injury to restore critical sensation. This avoids the need for a potentially dangerous intrafascicular dissection within the zone, which may lead to downgrading any function that is preserved.

INDICATIONS

Sensory nerve transfers can be performed in cases where a proximal nerve stump is not available. One example of this is a brachial plexus injury. For example, in C5/6 nerve root avulsions, critical sensation to the thumb is absent. No proximal nerve is available for a direct repair; therefore, the only option for restoration of sensation in that territory is to reroute the sensory axons from an adjacent sensory territory such as from the intact neighboring nerve to the third web space.[2]

Technical factors may also influence the use of distal nerve transfers. Gunshot wounds or other trauma with multiple structures involved and incomplete distal return of sensory function are often better managed by a distal sensory nerve transfer. A previous vein grafted arterial repair or significant scarring might preclude direct exploration and grafting of the sensory nerve. With multiple nerve injuries, the autologous nerve grafts are preferentially used for the restoration of motor function; hence, sensory nerve transfers are a good option when donor grafts have been used up.[3]

While sensory nerve injuries are not as time sensitive as motor nerve injuries, they can be used to restore sensibility in months rather than years. In cases of brachial plexus injury or high median or ulnar nerve injury, nerve transfers have become our primary modality for sensory reconstruction in parallel to the senior author's (S. E. M.) development and use of motor nerve transfers in the forearm.

In contrast to the urgency necessitated by time constraints in nerve transfers for motor function, there is little, if any, time-related urgency in sensory reconstruction. According to contemporary data following delayed median nerve grafting, excellent results can be obtained despite long intervals to sensory reconstruction. Clinical judgment and electrodiagnostic examination are used to determine potential for sensory recovery following a closed nerve injury. In the setting of mixed motor and sensory loss, lack of recovery in proximal muscles leading to nerve transfers for motor function at 3 to 6 months post injury would suggest a similar need for sensory transfers for the digits. For proximal nerve injuries with progressing Tinel sign, distal motor nerve transfers (eg, AIN to deep motor branch of ulnar nerve) may be required due to long regeneration distances that obviate timely motor reinnervation. In these cases, however, sensory reinnervation may eventually occur as a result of ongoing regeneration from the original site of injury. Whether to perform nerve transfers for digital sensation is then at the discretion of the patient and the surgeon. If the decision is made to proceed with nerve transfers, the proximal end of the recipient nerve must be properly transposed since an eventual painful neuroma from regenerating nerve fibers is likely. When nerve discontinuity is known to exist, such as in traumatic disruption or surgical ablation, sensory reconstruction may essentially be performed at any time.

Nerve transfers can be performed in patients of any age; however, the results (as for any peripheral nerve procedure) are often superior in younger patients.

CONTRAINDICATIONS

The primary relative contraindication for nerve transfer is when a direct end-to-end nerve repair is possible.

If no donor nerves are readily available, a sensory nerve transfer cannot be performed such as in pan-plexus injuries where there are no readily available nearby donors. However, even in these relatively extreme cases, some investigators have tried using the sensory component of intercostal nerves to restore rudimentary sensation to the critical areas of the hand.[4,5]

Another contraindication to nerve transfer is in the case of a nerve injury that has some potential for recovery. If a nerve transfer is done, the recipient nerve is transected that may lead to neuroma formation of the proximal stump if there is any eventual axonal ingrowth. To prevent this it is good practice to bury the proximal stump in muscle, remote from the coaptation site.

SURGICAL TECHNIQUE

The patient position will depend on the nerve transfer being done. The radial to axillary sensory end-to-side transfer is typically done at the same time as the corresponding motor nerve transfers and is done with the patient in the prone position with the arm completely prepped from the posterior shoulder to the tips of the fingers. A curvilinear incision is made at the posterior border of the deltoid muscle and extending in a longitudinal fashion along the midaxis of the posterior arm for exposure of the donor and recipient nerves. For other sensory nerve transfers, the patient is positioned supine with the arm abducted on a hand table.

A tourniquet may be used; however, for cases where intraoperative stimulation of the motor components of the nerves is required, the tourniquet time should be limited to 20 minutes or stimulation should be done early in the case. Another option is to forgo use of the tourniquet and to infiltrate the incision with 1:100,000 epinephrine solution along with providing meticulous hemostasis.

General anesthesia is typically used as a Bier or other regional block precludes intraoperative stimulation. Limited use of short-acting paralytics is acceptable, but clear communication between anesthesiologist and surgeon is critical. Patients with preexisting complex regional pain syndrome might benefit from perioperative stellate ganglion blocks or (if intraoperative nerve stimulation is not required) use of a Bier block supplemented with dexmedetomidine.[6]

In all nerve transfers, the donor nerve should be cut as far distally as possible; it can then be transposed over toward the recipient nerve in a tension-free manner. Intraneural dissection of the recipient nerve is done at that point and more proximally to allow a loose, tension-free closure.

Intraoperative nerve stimulation can be helpful in identifying and mapping intact motor fascicles in the donor nerve and in the recipient nerve if present. A disposable handheld nerve stimulator set to 2 mA is used.

Once the donor and recipient nerves are properly identified and isolated, adequate length must be obtained to achieve tensionless coaptation at all extremes of joint position. The fascicles to be transferred are dissected with meticulous microneurosurgical technique as far proximally and distally as necessary or possible. We repeat the mantra, "Donor distal, recipient proximal," to recall that a favorable coaptation is achieved with distal length of the donor nerve, and proximal length of the recipient nerve. A fresh 15 blade and the use of a tongue depressor as a cutting board ensure a relatively clean nerve transection and microscissors can be used to trim back bulging fascicles. Coaptation is performed with the operating microscope using microsurgical instruments and 9-0 nylon suture for an epineurial repair. The nerve ends are gently apposed so that the fascicles are just touching. Too tight of an epineurial repair or a repair done under tension will impair subsequent regeneration.

Table 10-1 outlines the nerve transfer options for typical patterns of sensory loss. Some injury patterns have more than one option for donor nerve material. More detailed information is provided in the following text and attached figures.

Nerve Transfer for Upper Plexus Injury

For patients with upper brachial plexus nerve root avulsions, loss of sensation in the thumb (C6 dermatome) and index finger (C7 dermatome) will significantly affect normal prehension. Noncritical intact sensory nerves from the functioning fourth web space (C8 dermatome—spared in a C5-7 upper plexus injury) is used as donor material to restore more critical first web space sensation on the "pinch" surfaces of the thumb and index finger. (Occasionally, the sensation in the third web space will be functional on the ulnar side of the long [C7] and the radial side of the ring [C8] and this can also be used as a donor.) A similar transfer can be done in very proximal median nerve injury or in cases where direct repair of the median nerve is contraindicated or technically impossible.[7] In that case, again, the fourth web space common digital nerve is functioning because the ulnar nerve is uninjured. See Figure 10-1. The dorsal cutaneous branch of the ulnar nerve (DCU) can also be used for transfer material.[2,8]

Nerve Transfer for Axillary Nerve Injury

Also, in patients with upper brachial plexus or direct axillary nerve injury, there is loss of sensation at the lateral aspect of the shoulder. This numbness, while less critical for function, is annoying for patients and sensation can be restored

TABLE 10-1: Examples of Basic Sensory Nerve Transfer Techniques that can be Used with Location of Surgery (Incision, Dissection, and Coaptation Site)

Injury Pattern/Deficit	Nerve Transfer (Donor to Recipient *Nerve Branch*)	Location of Surgery
Upper plexus injury (C5/6/7)—loss of thumb sensation	For C5/6 injury—third web space *to* thumb For C5/6/7 injury—fourth web space *to* thumb	Distal forearm (extended CTR incision provides additional topographic landmarks)
Axillary nerve injury	Radial nerve *to* axillary sensory component (this should be done in an ETS fashion with axillary nerve end into side of radial nerve)	Posterior arm incision (follow border of posterior deltoid to midaxial posterior arm)
Median nerve injury	Fourth web space (or dorsal cutaneous branch of ulnar nerve) *to* first web space	Distal forearm (extended palmar incision with CTR can provide topographic landmarks)
Ulnar nerve injury	Third web space (median innervated) *to* ulnar nerve sensory component (ulnar ring and entire small finger)	Distal forearm (extended palmar incision with CTR can provide topographic landmarks)

CTR, carpal tunnel release; ETS, end to side. Additional end-to-side coaptations may provide restoration of rudimentary sensation to the donor nerve territory (please see figures for details).

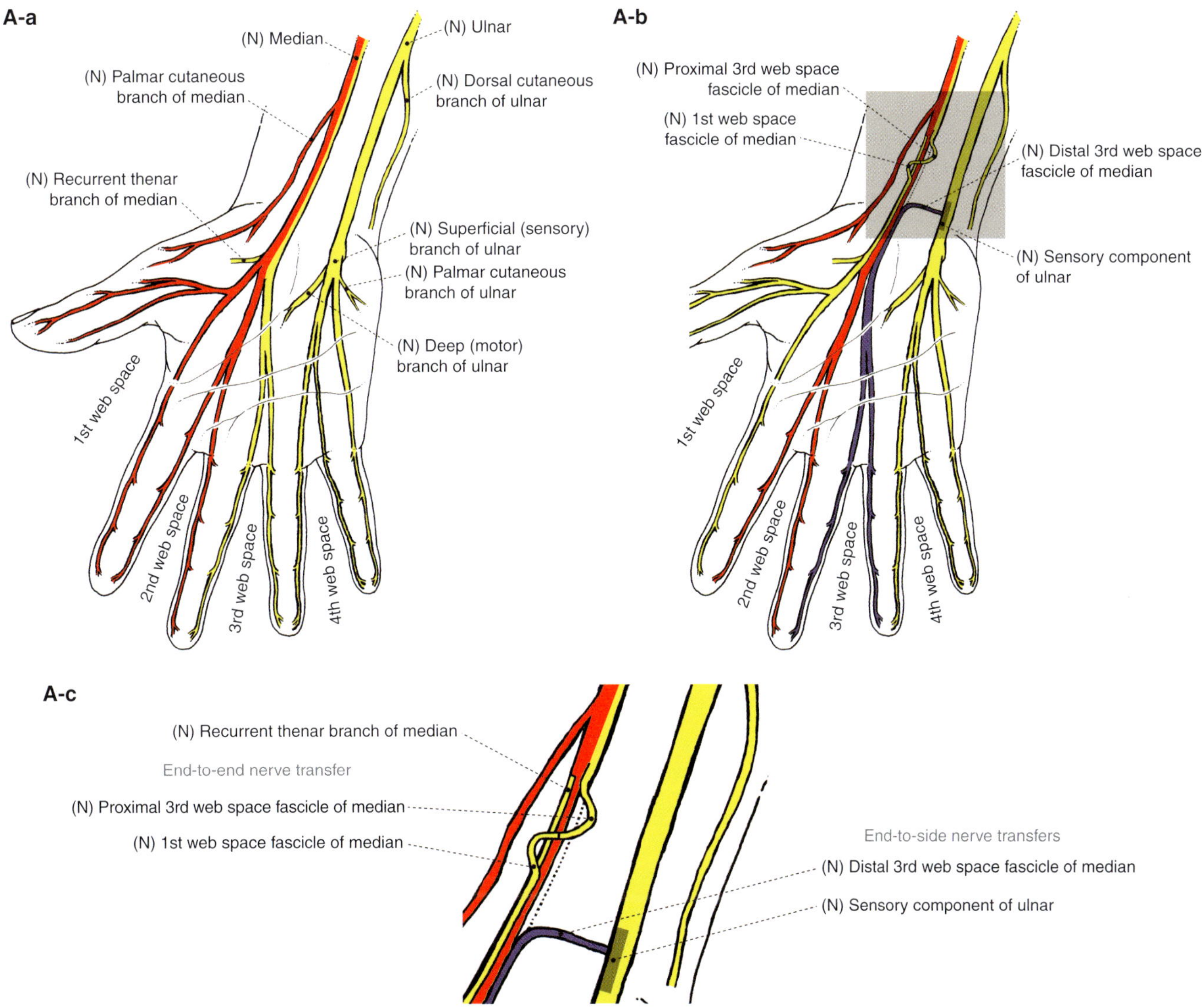

FIGURE 10-1 **A.** Nerve transfer to restore upper brachial plexus (C6/7) innervated critical sensory territory—anatomy and intraneural topography. **a.** With C5, C6 brachial plexus injury, sensation is lost in a dermatomal distribution. **b.** The goal is to restore sensation to the critical area of loss—the thumb. **c.** An end-to-end nerve transfer from the *donor* third web space fascicle of median nerve (C7 and C8 innervated) to *recipient* thumb and first web space fascicles of median nerve is performed. An end-to-side transfer from the ulnar nerve main sensory component is used to restore rudimentary sensation back to the third web space distal donor fascicle.

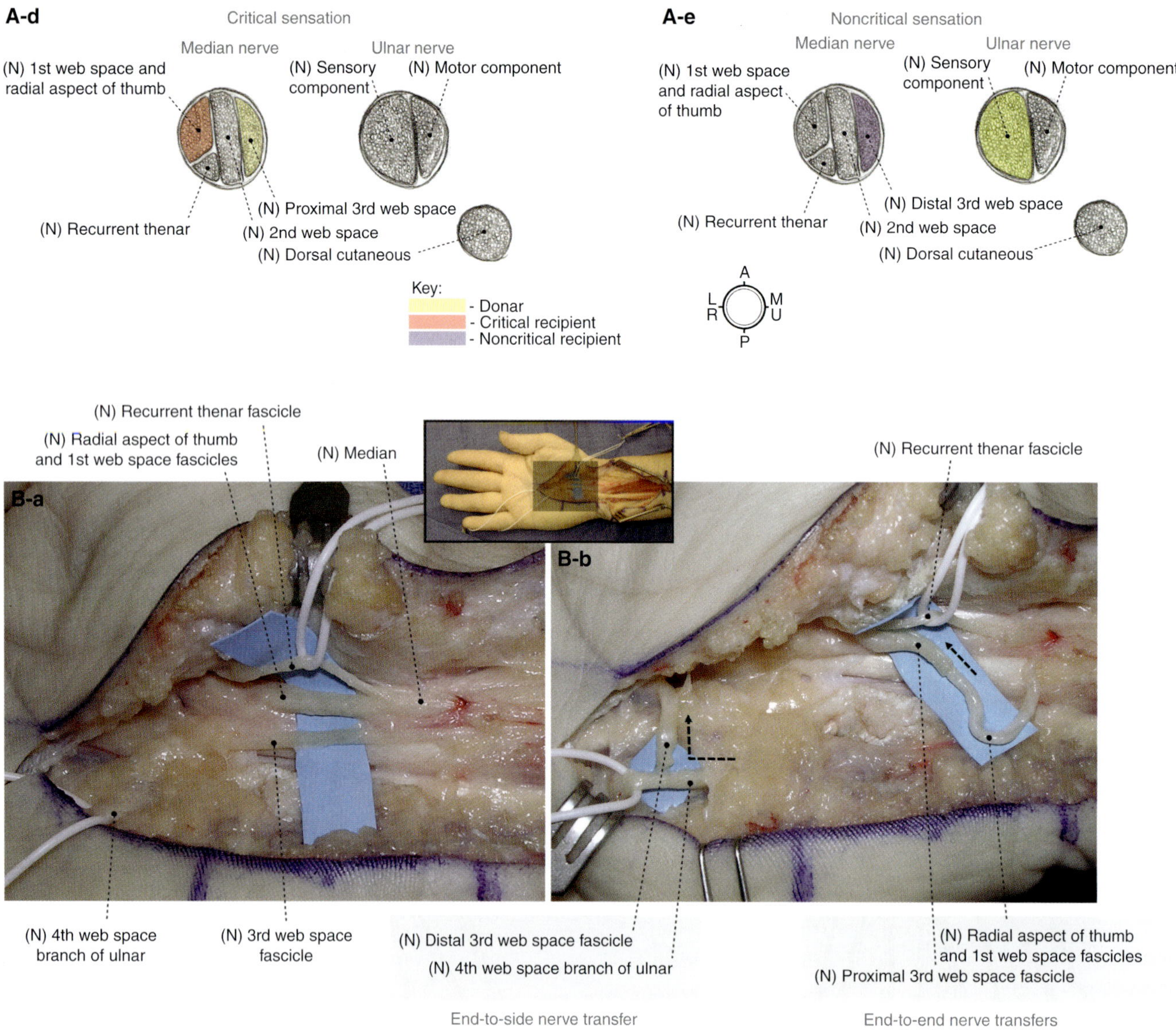

FIGURE 10-1 (*Continued*) **d.** Fascicular donor and recipient anatomy for restoration of critical sensation using end-to-end nerve transfer. **e.** Fascicular donor and recipient anatomy for restoration of rudimentary sensation using end-to-side nerve transfer. (Reproduced with permission, © 2011, nervesurgery.wustl.edu.) **B.** Nerve transfer to restore upper brachial plexus (C6/7) innervated critical sensory territory—surgical technique. **a.** The median nerve donor (third web space—C7/8 innervated) and recipient (thumb—C6 innervated) fascicles are identified. For restoration of critical sensation to the thumb, the donor third web space fascicle is identified on the medial aspect of the median nerve while the recipient fascicles are identified on the lateral aspect of the median nerve. The ulnar nerve sensory component may also be used as a donor in an end-to-side fashion to the distal third web space of median fascicle to restore rudimentary sensation. **b.** The *donor* third web space fascicle is coapted to the *recipient* fascicles of the median nerve to the thumb in an end-to-end fashion for restoring critical sensation. The *recipient* distal third web space fascicle of median nerve is coapted to the *donor* fourth web space branch of ulnar nerve in an end-to-side fashion for restoration of rudimentary sensation. Arrows portray direction of nerve regeneration. (Reproduced with permission, © 2011, nervesurgery.wustl.edu.)

by use of an end-to-side nerve transfer using the lateral side of the radial nerve (sensory component) as donor and the axillary nerve sensory component as the recipient. An end-to-end transfer should not be performed in this case because that would cause a donor-site deficit for this area of relatively noncritical loss of sensation. This is usually done as part of the motor nerve transfers to restore shoulder abduction and does not require any additional dissection.

Nerve Transfer for Median Nerve Injury

Ulnar to median sensory nerve transfer can be done in patients with very proximal median nerve injury or in cases where direct repair of the median nerve is contraindicated or technically impossible. In this case, the critical area of sensation to restore is the first web space. Transfer of the fourth web space functioning but noncritical ulnar innervated nerve fascicle into the sensory component (to thumb and index finger radial aspect) of the median nerve can be done. This restores sensation to the critical surfaces of the thumb and index finger to allow for prehension.

Digital nerve transfers were traditionally performed with distal dissection of proper digital nerves into the digits to obtain adequate length for transposition across the width of the hand. Later modification by our group limited dissection to the distal palm and, more recently (see Fig. 10-2), further limited dissection to the distal forearm. This minimizes incisions on the contact surface of the hand but does require intimate knowledge of the internal topography of the nerves.

If the transfers are done at the level of the palm, the proper digital nerves to be transferred are divided distally at the level of the web spaces with proximal neurolysis of the associated donor and recipient digital nerves from the main nerve trunks to allow adequate length for transposition.

A carpal tunnel incision with Bruner-type zigzag extensions is used to expose the distal median nerve and the nerves to the first and fourth web spaces. The transverse carpal ligament is divided along its ulnar border. Dissection of proper and common digital nerves is routine. Care is taken to maintain integrity of the digital arteries and superficial palmar arch, which lie superficial to the plane of the nerves in the palm. The nerves to the fourth web space are transected distally at the metacarpal heads, and then dissected proximally to the ulnar sensory group with neurolysis from the motor branch as needed to obtain adequate length for transposition. The nerves to the first web space are isolated from the median nerve trunk by internal neurolysis. The transfer is

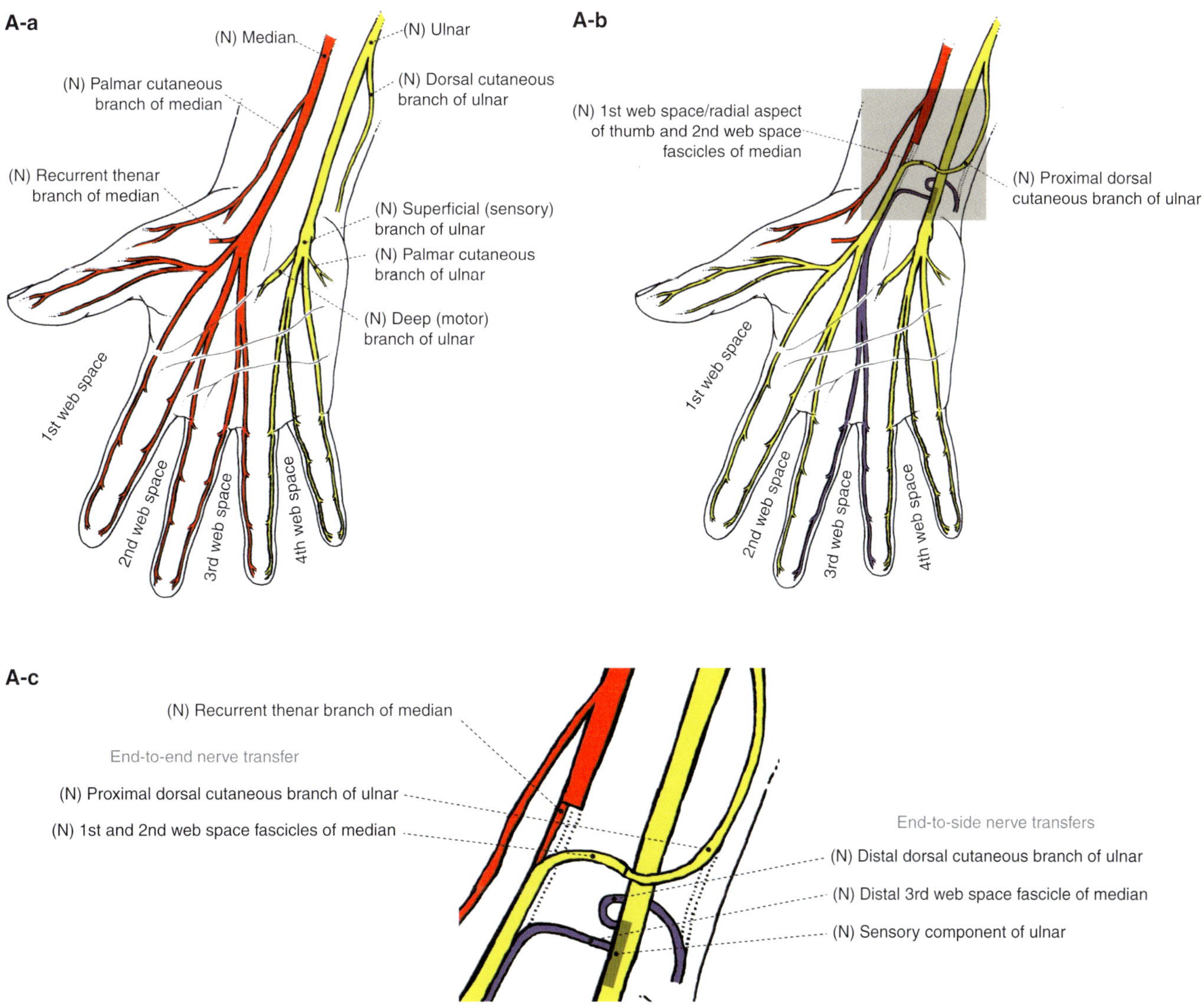

FIGURE 10-2 **A.** Nerve transfer to restore median innervated critical sensory territory—anatomy and intraneural topography. **a.** With loss of median nerve function, sensation is lost to the lateral and volar aspect of the hand including the thumb, index, long, and radial half of ring finger. **b.** The most critical area of sensory deficit is at the pinch surfaces of the thumb and index finger. To restore sensation, the dorsal cutaneous branch of the ulnar nerve (DCU) may be used as a relatively expendable sensory nerve donor. **c.** An end-to-end transfer of the *donor* DCU to the critical fascicles of the *recipient* median nerve is performed. This includes the median innervated radial aspect of thumb and first and second web space fascicles.

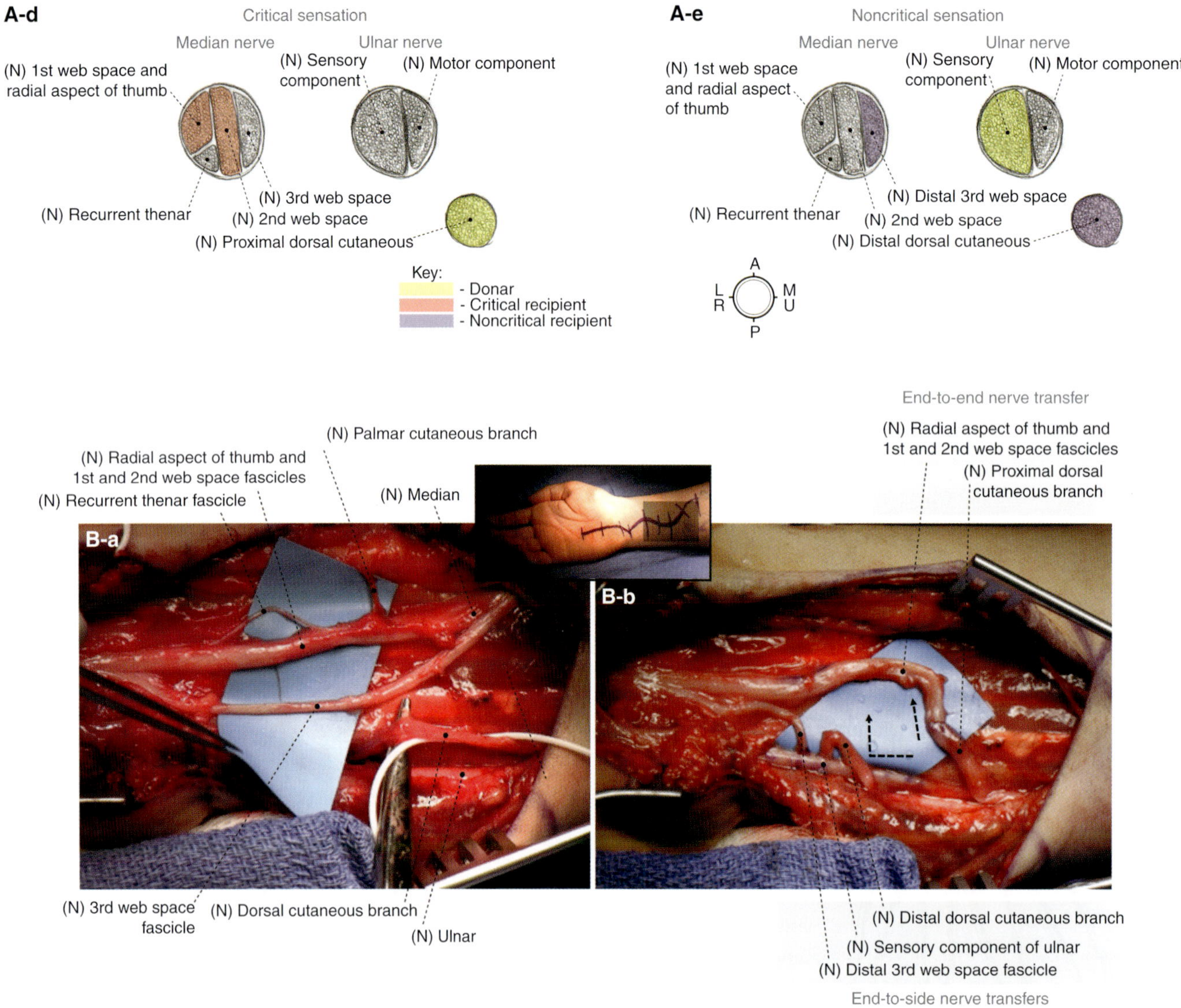

FIGURE 10-2 (*Continued*) End-to-side transfers may be performed to restore less critical sensory territories and include the following: (1) *donor* sensory component of the main ulnar nerve sensory fascicles *to recipient* DCU nerve (to restore rudimentary sensation back to the donor nerve territory) and (2) *donor* sensory component of the main ulnar nerve sensory fascicles to *recipient* distal third web space fascicle of median nerve (to restore rudimentary sensation back to a less critical area of lost median nerve sensation). **d.** Fascicular donor and recipient anatomy for restoration of critical median innervated sensation using end-to-end nerve transfer. **e.** Fascicular donor and recipient anatomy for restoration of noncritical sensation using end-to-side nerve transfers. (Reproduced with permission, © 2011, nervesurgery.wustl.edu.) **B.** Nerve transfer to restore median innervated critical sensory territory—surgical technique. **a.** The donor ulnar and recipient median nerve fascicular components are identified in the forearm. To identify the sensory components of the median nerve, the fascicle to the thenar muscles was separated away to avoid transferring sensory nerve fibers into this motor nerve. Additionally, the third web space fascicle was separated from the remaining median nerve sensory component to the radial aspect of the thumb, first web space, and second web space. **b.** The *donor* DCU nerve branch is coapted to the *recipient* main sensory component of the median nerve in an end-to-end fashion for restoration of the areas of critical sensation. The *recipient* distal DCU nerve branch and *recipient* distal third web space fascicle of the median nerve are coapted to the *donor* sensory component of the ulnar nerve in an end-to-side fashion for restoration of rudimentary sensation. Arrows indicate the direction of eventual nerve regeneration. (Reproduced with permission, © 2011, nervesurgery.wustl.edu.)

completed when sufficient length is obtained of the donor nerves distally and of the recipient nerves proximally. A caveat to this rule, owing to the more proximal location of the thumb, is that proximal dissection of the fourth web space donor nerves can also provide additional length for transfer. A tension-free end-to-end coaptation is performed.

Nerve Transfer for Ulnar Nerve Injury

Median to ulnar sensory nerve transfer can be done in patients with very proximal ulnar nerve injury, or in cases where direct repair of the ulnar nerve is contraindicated or technically impossible. In this case, the critical area of sensation to restore is the ulnar border of the hand. Transfer of the third web space functioning but noncritical median innervated nerve fascicle into the sensory component of the ulnar nerve can be done. This restores sensation to the volar and ulnar border of the hand as well as to the fourth web space. Restoration of sensation to the fourth web space is not critical for hand function, but the third web space nerve is a reasonably good size match to the entire sensory component of the ulnar nerve to the volar hand (the DCU is typically not included).[2,9] Sensation to the DCU territory can be achieved by either end-to-side or end-to-end transfer. The DCU can be coapted in an end-to-side fashion using the third web space nerve or median nerve proper as the donor nerve. Alternatively, the DCU can be coapted in an end-to-end fashion using the palmar cutaneous branch of the median nerve as donor material. We typically perform these nerve transfers in the distal forearm (see Fig. 10-3), but this does require detailed knowledge of the internal topography.

These transfers can also be done in the palm. For this approach an extended carpal tunnel incision, positioned just ulnar to the ring finger axis, is used to expose the median nerve at the wrist. The transverse carpal ligament is divided along its ulnar border, and the terminal median nerve branches are identified as they exit the carpal tunnel. Each

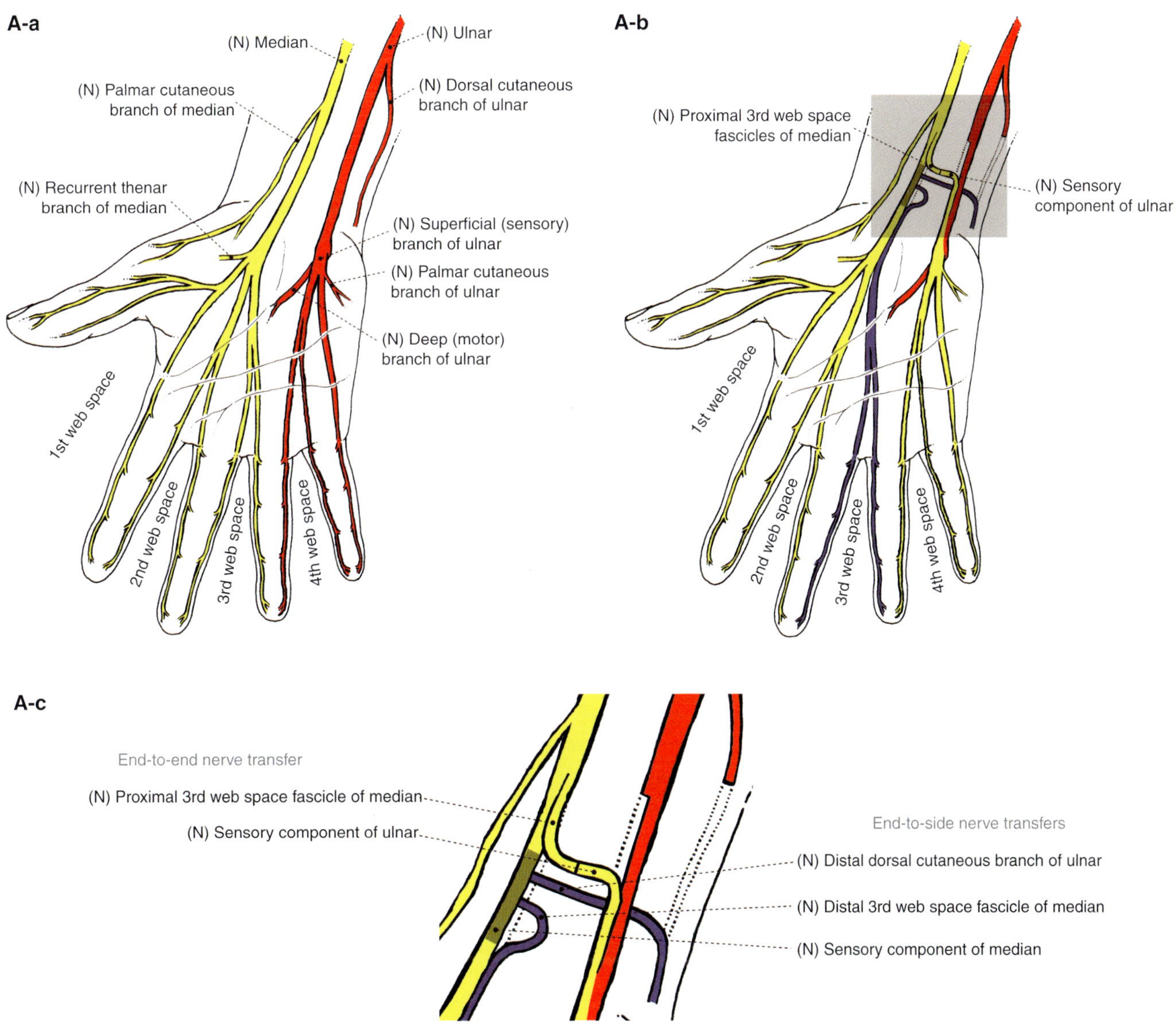

FIGURE 10-3 **A.** Nerve transfer to restore ulnar innervated critical sensory territory—anatomy and intraneural topography. **a.** With loss of ulnar nerve function, sensation is lost at the medial aspect of the hand. To restore sensation, the third web space fascicle of the median nerve may be used as a relatively expendable sensory nerve donor. **b.** The most critical area of sensory deficit is at the ulnar border or resting surface of the hand. The dorsal cutaneous branch of the ulnar nerve (DCU) and donor third web space fascicle of the median nerve can also be reinnervated by use of end-to-side transfers. **c.** An end-to-end transfer of the *donor* third web space fascicle (median nerve) to the *recipient* ulnar nerve sensory component is performed. End-to-side transfers from the (i) *donor* third web space fascicle of median nerve to *recipient* DCU and (ii) *donor* second web space fascicle of median nerve to *recipient* distal fascicle of third web space may also be performed to restore rudimentary sensation in noncritical areas.

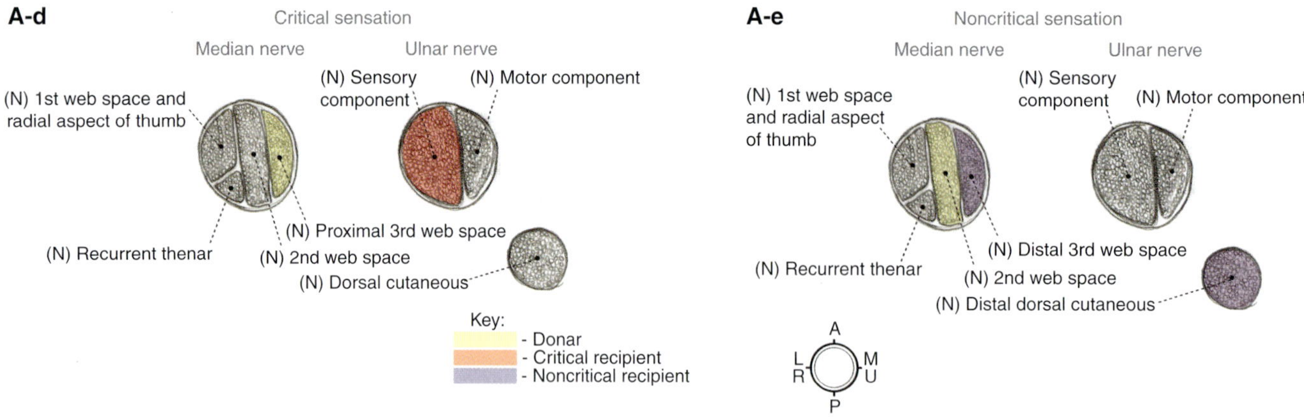

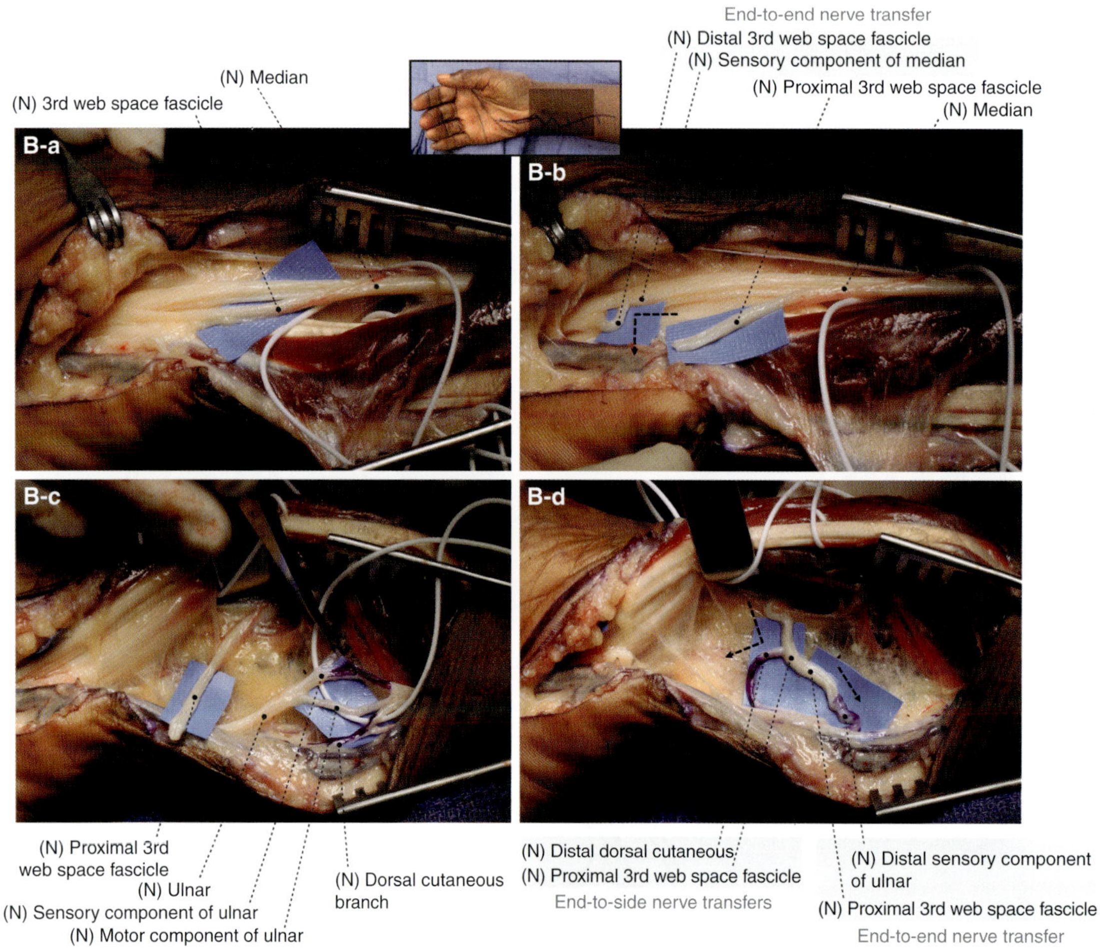

FIGURE 10-3 (*Continued*) **d.** Fascicular donor and recipient anatomy for restoration of critical ulnar innervated sensation using end-to-end nerve transfer. **e.** Fascicular donor and recipient anatomy for restoration of noncritical sensation using end-to-side nerve transfers. (Reproduced with permission, © 2011, nervesurgery.wustl.edu.) **B.** Nerve transfer to restore ulnar innervated critical sensory territory—surgical technique. **a.** The donor median and recipient ulnar fascicular components are identified in the forearm. The third web space fascicle is identified on the medial aspect of the median nerve and is separated from the remainder of the median nerve. **b.** The donor third web space fascicle of the median nerve is transected. The distal end is coapted in an end-to-side fashion to the remaining intact median nerve sensory component to restore rudimentary sensation back to the donor territory. **c.** The recipient sensory component of the ulnar nerve is identified on the lateral aspect of the ulnar nerve and is separated from the DCU and deep motor branches of the ulnar nerve. **d.** For critical sensation, the *donor* third web space fascicle is coapted to the *recipient* main sensory component of the ulnar nerve in an end-to-end fashion. For noncritical sensation, the *recipient* distal dorsal cutaneous branch of ulnar nerve is coapted in an end-to-side transfer to the *donor* proximal third web space fascicle of median nerve. Arrows portray direction of nerve regeneration. (Reproduced with permission, © 2011, nervesurgery.wustl.edu.)

branch can be tracked proximally within the ribbon-like median nerve visually, without necessarily physically separating one from the others. Specifically, the fascicles to the radial border of the thumb, the first web, the second web, and the third web are distinct in the distal-most median nerve beginning 13 mm proximal to the radial styloid line. This represents a conservative estimate based on Sunderland's histological data, with longer distances available if minor plexi are divided using meticulous technique and much discretion. The individual fascicular groups to be isolated, namely, the first or third web space nerves, are dissected as distinct bundles at the level of the wrist and tagged with vessel loops. To reiterate, Ross et al described the unique topography of the third web space nerves within the median nerve, and its relevance to use of the third web space fascicle as a donor nerve.[10] This article should be reviewed prior to performing this procedure for the first time. Of practical note, the fascicle to the radial border of the thumb should be left together with the fascicle to the first web space, without separating the two, due to the small size of the former and its relative importance to thumb sensation. The recurrent motor branch may be separated and excluded to prevent misdirection of transferred sensory axons. A special tip for distinguishing the border of the third web space group from the remainder of the median nerve is to gently "dunk" the fine point of a closed jeweler's forceps into the interval. Formal physical internal neurolysis from distal to proximal is performed as necessary.

The ulnar nerve is dissected through the same incision. Guyon canal is opened, and the terminal sensory fascicles of the ulnar nerve are observed. The ulnar sensory group is visually traced proximally as described above. At 20 mm distal to the radial styloid line, the deep motor branch joins the ulnar nerve on its dorsal and medial border. The deep motor branch usually requires release at the fibromuscular arch of the flexor digitorum quinti muscle origin. Proximal to this level, the motor group occupies the medial 40% of the nerve, and the sensory group occupies the lateral 60% of the nerve. The sensory and motor groups can be separated at the level of the wrist by using the techniques described above, up to a distance 75 mm proximal to the radial styloid line. At the wrist, the dorsal sensory branch may be encountered medial to the ulnar nerve proper. The dorsal sensory branch separates from the ulnar nerve 5 to 10 cm proximal to the wrist crease, and travels from volar to dorsal between the tendon of flexor carpi ulnaris and the head of the ulna to supply cutaneous innervation to the dorsal hand. The donor median nerve branch is cut distally and the recipient ulnar sensory component is cut proximally. The 2 ends are coapted in a tension-free fashion. The DCU and ulnar motor branches are deliberately excluded from this sensory transfer.

Unique Sensory Nerve Transfer

Additional sensory nerve transfers can be done to restore critical sensation and avoid long nerve grafts in a variety of unique clinical situations. For example, in the case of a blast injury to the hand and disruption of the sensory portion of the ulnar nerve, the goal was to prevent painful neuroma and restore critical sensation. Poor soft tissue coverage (skin graft to palm) and loss of the small finger created a situation where nerve grafting was not a viable option. Nerve grafts from the proximal nerve stump through a skin grafted bed to the single remaining distal ulnar sensory nerve fascicle would set the patient up for a forearm or palm level neuroma of the sensory component of the ulnar nerve. Therefore, distal nerve transfer was used to restore sensation to the new ulnar border of the hand (the ulnar aspect of the ring finger) and the proximal stump of the ulnar nerve was buried more proximally deep within the forearm muscles to prevent painful neuroma. In this case of blast injury to the medial border of the hand, there was concern for some neurapraxia of the medial portion of the median nerve, so the index ulnar digital nerve was used as donor material (Saheb-Al-Zamani M, Yee A, Fox IK. Interdigital sensory nerve transfer following digital amputation: case report and review. Unpublished data, 2012). See Figure 10-4.

For many of these sensory nerve transfers, the distal end(s) of the donor nerve may be dissected and coapted end-to-side to adjacent intact sensory nerves, without need for epineurotomy. The free proximal end of the recipient nerve should also be properly considered, since it must be appropriately transposed if there is any possibility that nerve regeneration from a more proximal source could eventually result in a painful neuroma.

The skin is closed following careful hemostasis to avoid excess scarring in the surgical field. Dressings are removed at the first postoperative visit, and the patient is allowed to shower. The wrist is immobilized with a volar splint for 7 to 10 days to protect the repair, and the fingers are left free to allow early range of motion. As nerve regeneration progresses and the patient regains sensation, a program of sensory reeducation is routinely initiated and critical to

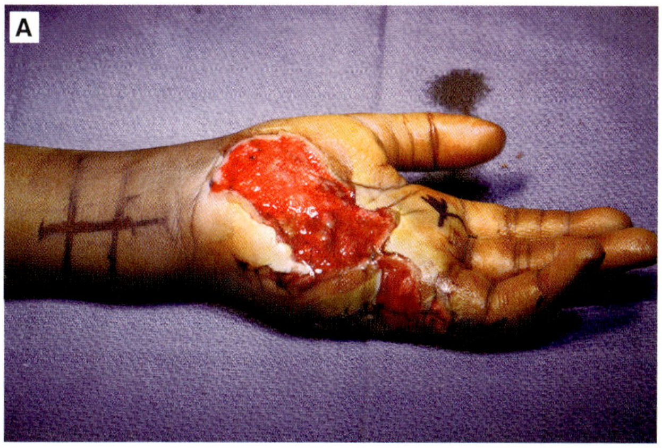

FIGURE 10-4 **A.** Case presentation of a gunshot wound to the hand. A 5-year-old female presented to our institution with a gunshot wound to the ulnar aspect of the hand. Initial exploration and small finger amputation were completed. The sensory component of the ulnar nerve was injured with segmental loss and need for soft tissue coverage. (Reproduced with permission, © 2011, nervesurgery.wustl.edu.)

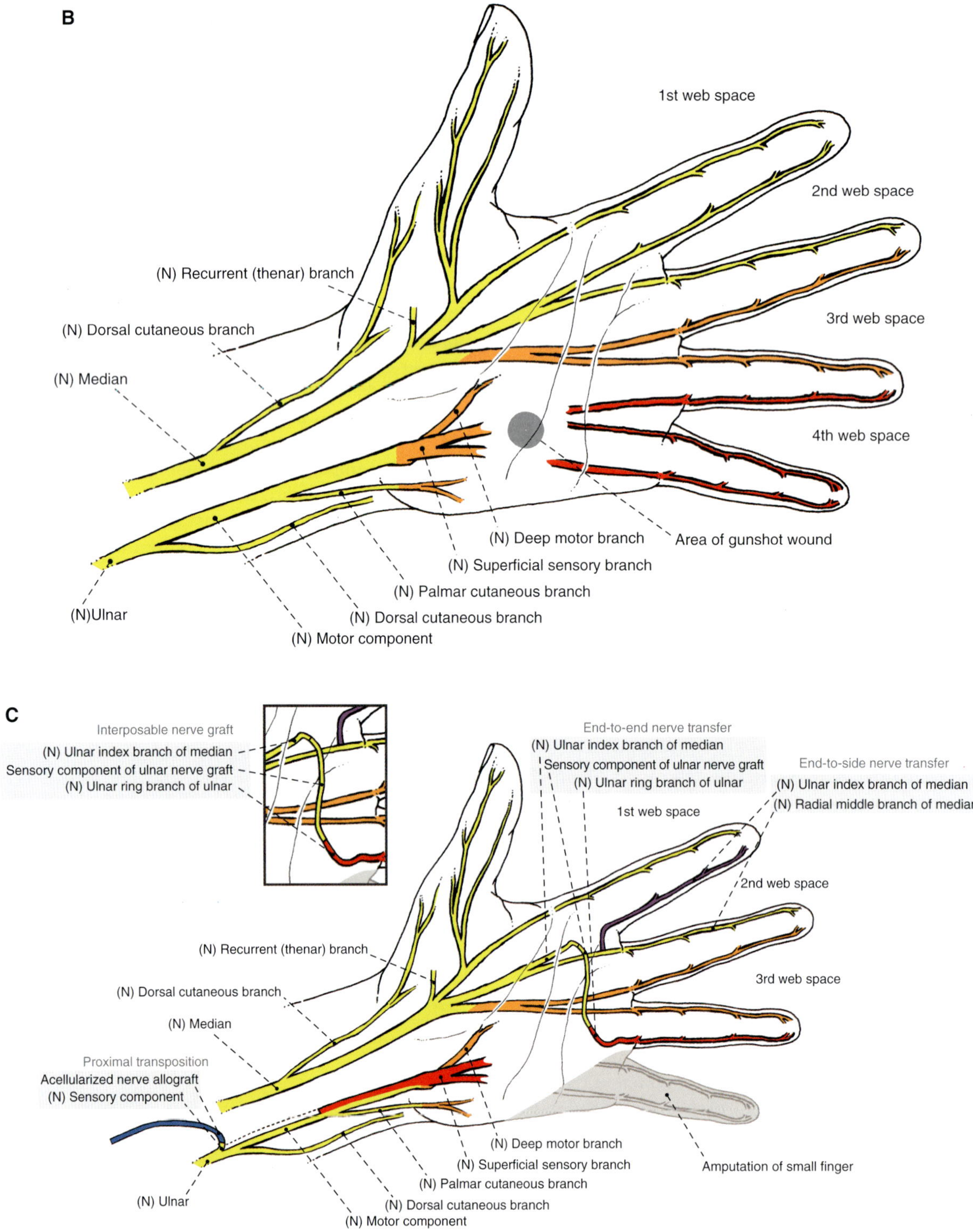

FIGURE 10-4 (*Continued*) **B.** Illustration of gunshot wound and nerve injury within the hand. The gunshot wound occurred at the ulnar palmar aspect of the hand that transected the ulnar sensory nerve branches distal to its branch point from the deep motor branch of the ulnar nerve. (Reproduced with permission, © 2011, nervesurgery.wustl.edu.) **C.** Surgical management and reconstruction of ulnar nerve sensation. The small finger required amputation. Due to the blast injury, there was poor soft tissue coverage at the palm preventing long nerve grafts. (1) Due to the distal injury, the median sensory nerve branch to the ulnar aspect of the index finger was selected as the donor nerve to transfer into the ulnar sensory nerve branch to the ulnar aspect of the ring finger for restoration of critical sensation. (2) Due to the required length needed, the ulnar nerve sensory component in the forearm was harvested proximally to bridge the gap as an autologous expendable nerve graft. (3) An acellularized nerve allograft was used as an extender to allow proximal transposition of the ulnar nerve sensory component intramuscularly at the forearm to prevent painful neuroma formation. (4) To restore rudimentary sensation back to the donor nerve sensory territory, an end-to-side nerve transfer to the median sensory branch to the radial aspect of the long finger was also performed. (Reproduced with permission, © 2011, nervesurgery.wustl.edu.)

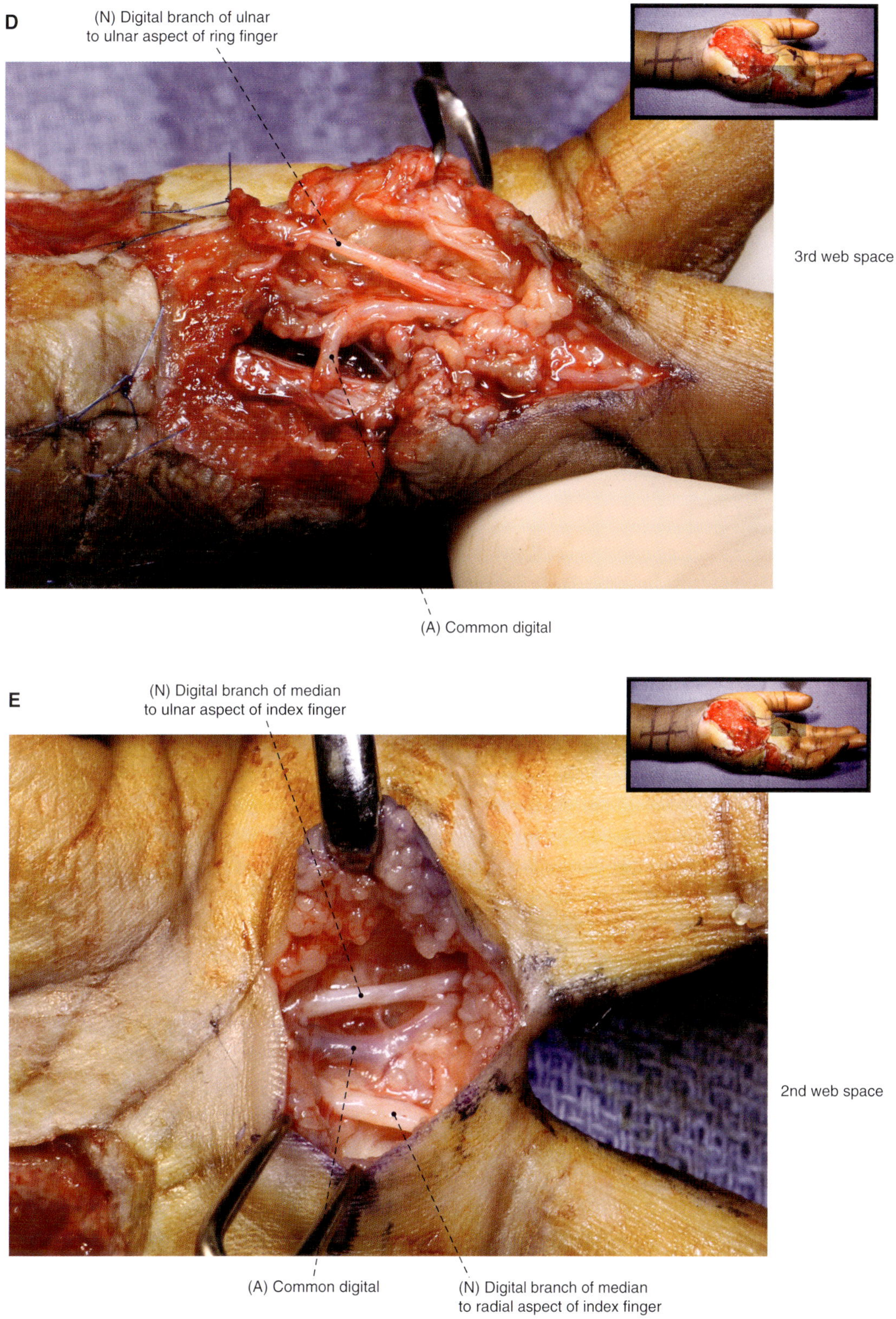

FIGURE 10-4 (*Continued*) **D.** Identification of the recipient digital nerve branch for nerve transfer. On the initial debridement, the transected digital nerve to the ulnar nerve to the ulnar aspect of the ring finger was identified and tagged with a suture. The adjacent common palmar digital artery was noted. (Reproduced with permission, © 2011, nervesurgery.wustl.edu.) **E.** Identification of the donor digital nerve branch for nerve transfer. An incision was made on the palmar aspect of the hand between the index and long finger. The digital nerve to the ulnar aspect of the index finger was identified as the donor nerve. This digital nerve was chosen as the donor for two reasons. The first is that the sensation to the ulnar aspect of the index finger is relatively expendable. The second is that the index finger was the furthest from the site of blast injury and was grossly intact. The adjacent digital nerve to the radial aspect of the long finger was also noted. (Reproduced with permission, © 2011, nervesurgery.wustl.edu.)

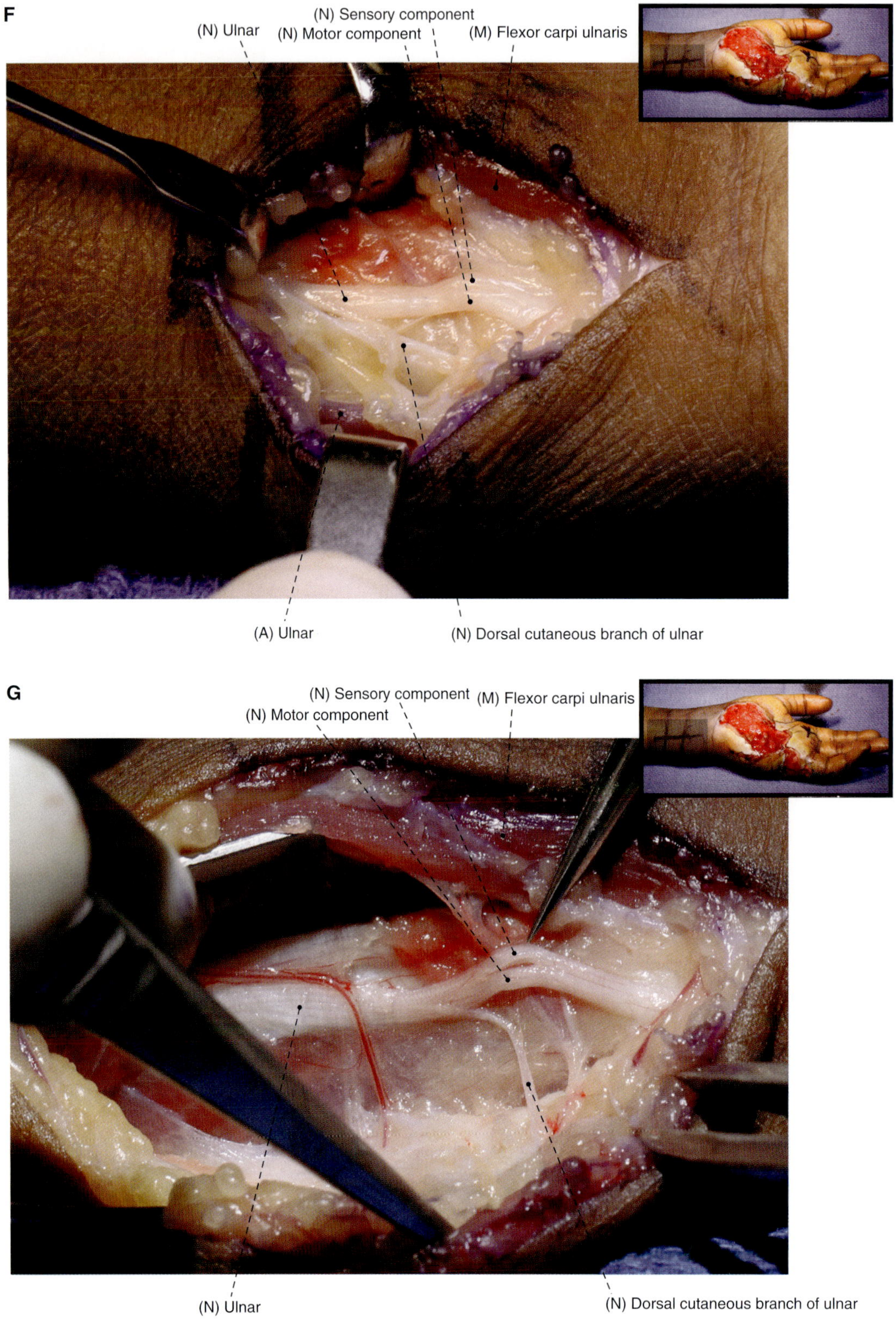

FIGURE 10-4 (*Continued*) **F.** Exposure of the ulnar nerve proximally in the forearm to harvest the nerve graft and to prevent neuroma formation. An incision was made proximally in the forearm to expose the ulnar nerve in order to harvest the sensory component of the ulnar nerve as a nerve graft. The dorsal cutaneous branch of the ulnar nerve was noted as well as the motor and sensory components of the ulnar nerve following initial intrafascicular neurolysis. (Reproduced with permission, © 2011, nervesurgery.wustl.edu.) **G.** Identification of the sensory component of the ulnar nerve as the nerve graft and prevention of neuroma formation. On further exposure and intrafascicular neurolysis, the sensory component of the ulnar nerve was identified on the radial aspect of the ulnar nerve. A microvessel is seen to separate the sensory from the motor component of the ulnar nerve. (Reproduced with permission, © 2011, nervesurgery.wustl.edu.)

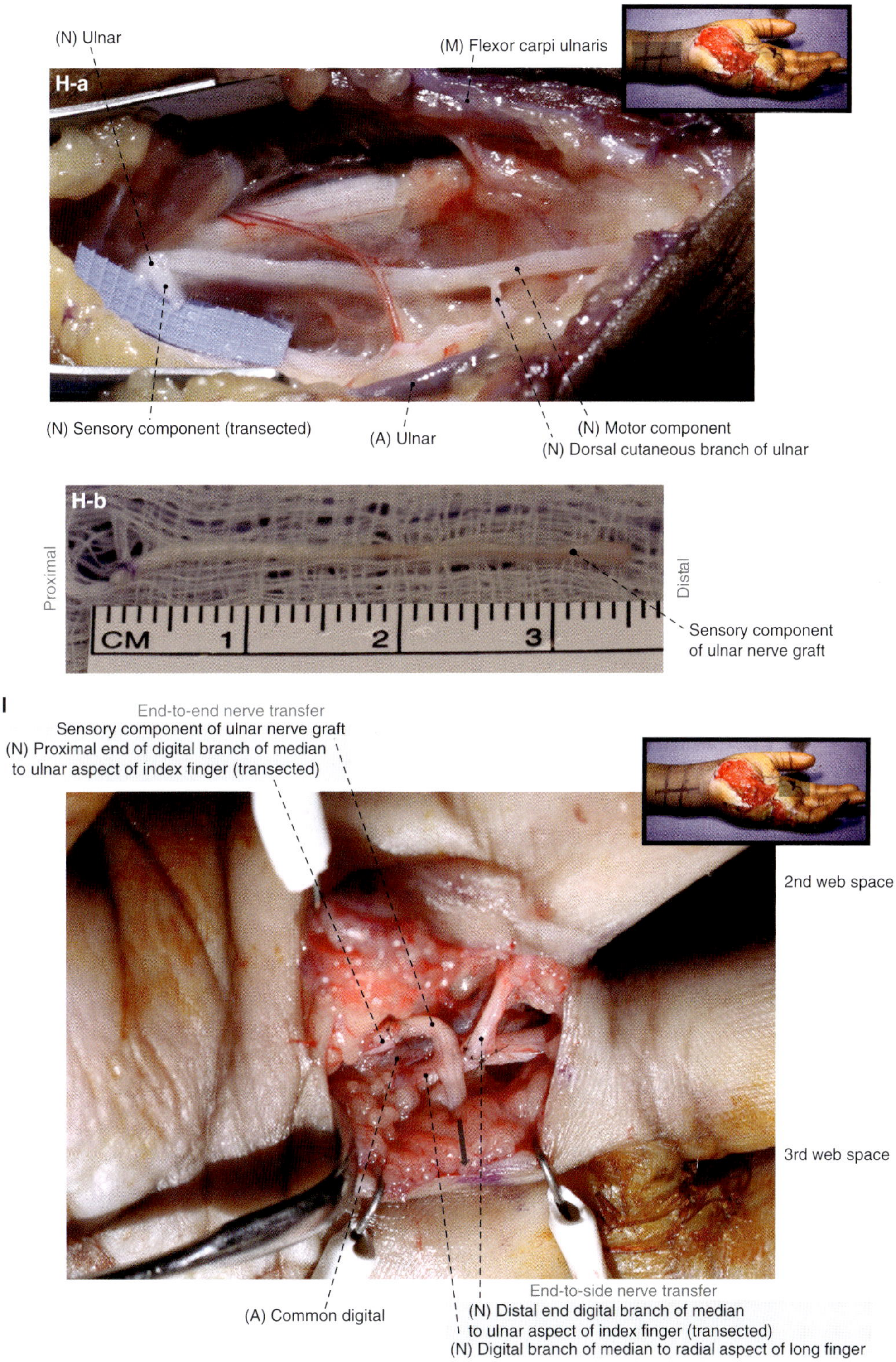

FIGURE 10-4 (*Continued*) **H.** Harvesting the sensory component of the ulnar nerve as the nerve graft. **a.** The sensory component of the ulnar nerve was harvested as the nerve graft. **b.** A 3.5-cm nerve graft was harvested from the ulnar nerve. The motor component of the ulnar nerve was protected and kept intact. (Reproduced with permission, © 2011, nervesurgery.wustl.edu.) **I.** Donor nerve and interposition nerve graft for nerve transfer and end-to-side nerve transfer to restore rudimentary sensation to the donor nerve territory. An interposition nerve graft from the "spare part" sensory component of the ulnar nerve was coapted to the proximal end of the donor digital palmar branch of the median nerve to the ulnar aspect of the index finger. To restore rudimentary sensation to the donor nerve territory, the distal end of the ulnar index finger branch of median was end-to-side transferred and coapted to the side of the radial middle branch of median. Please note that this is a very unique case where the ulnar nerve sensory component is being used as expendable graft material. This is due to the small finger being amputated as part of the initial injury. The objective was to reinnervate the ulnar aspect of the ring finger by distal nerve transfers. (Reproduced with permission, © 2011, nervesurgery.wustl.edu.)

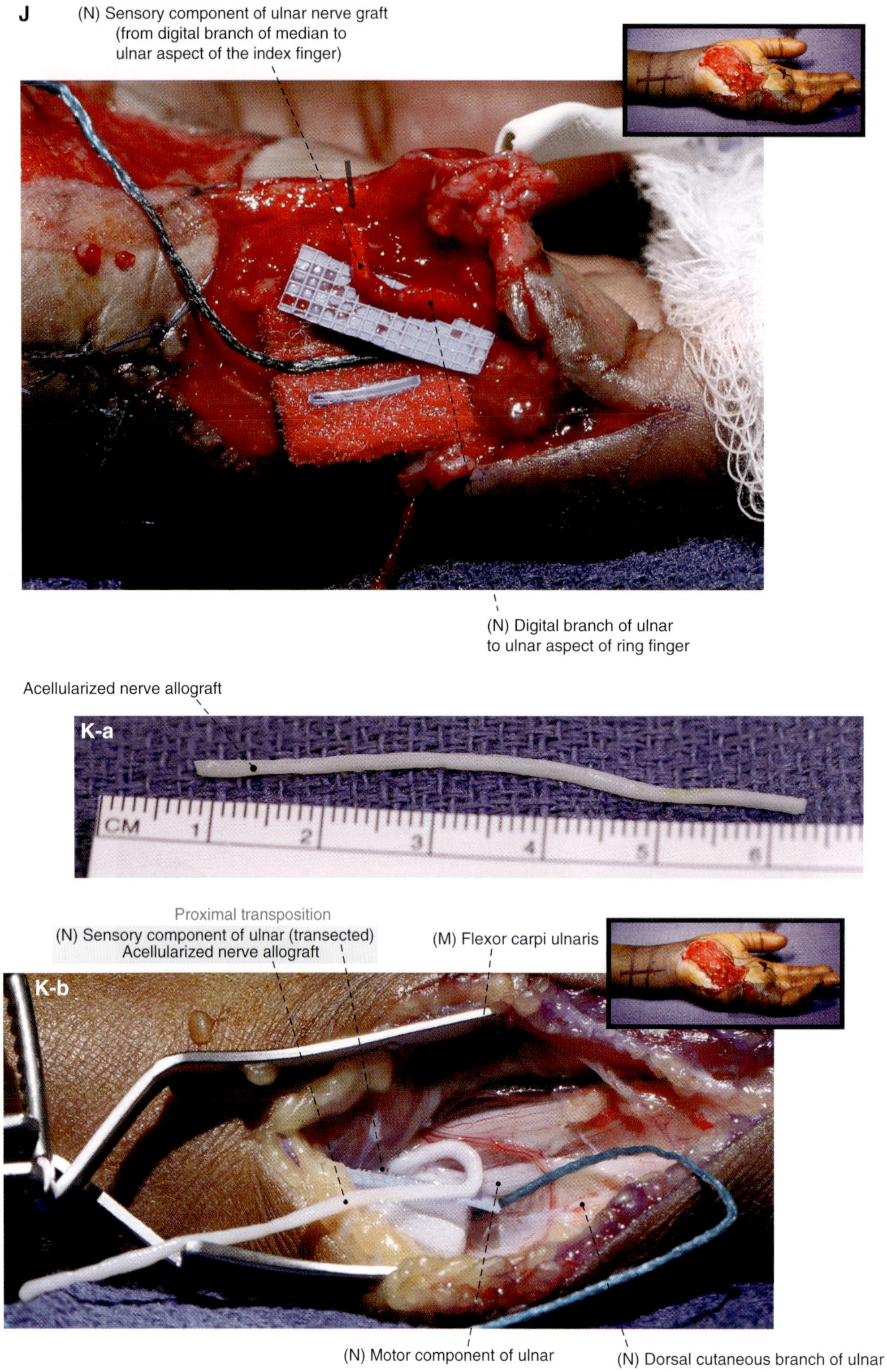

FIGURE 10-4 (*Continued*) **J.** Recipient nerve and interposition nerve graft for nerve transfer. The interposition nerve graft from the sensory component of the ulnar nerve was coapted to the distal end of the digital palmar branch of the ulnar nerve to the ulnar aspect of the ring finger. The nerve graft allows bridging the gap and reinnervating critical ulnar nerve sensation via nerve transfer. An autologous nerve graft was used to maximize reinnervation to this area of critical sensation. (Reproduced with permission, © 2011, nervesurgery.wustl.edu.) **K.** Acellularized nerve allograft as an extender from the sensory component of the ulnar nerve for intermuscular transposition. **a.** A 5.5-cm acellularized nerve allograft (Avance Nerve Graft, AxoGen, Inc) was used. **b.** The acellularized nerve allograft was coapted to the proximal end of the sensory component of the ulnar nerve, transposed proximally, and buried deep within the forearm musculature to prevent painful neuroma formation. (Reproduced with permission, © 2011, nervesurgery.wustl.edu.)

L

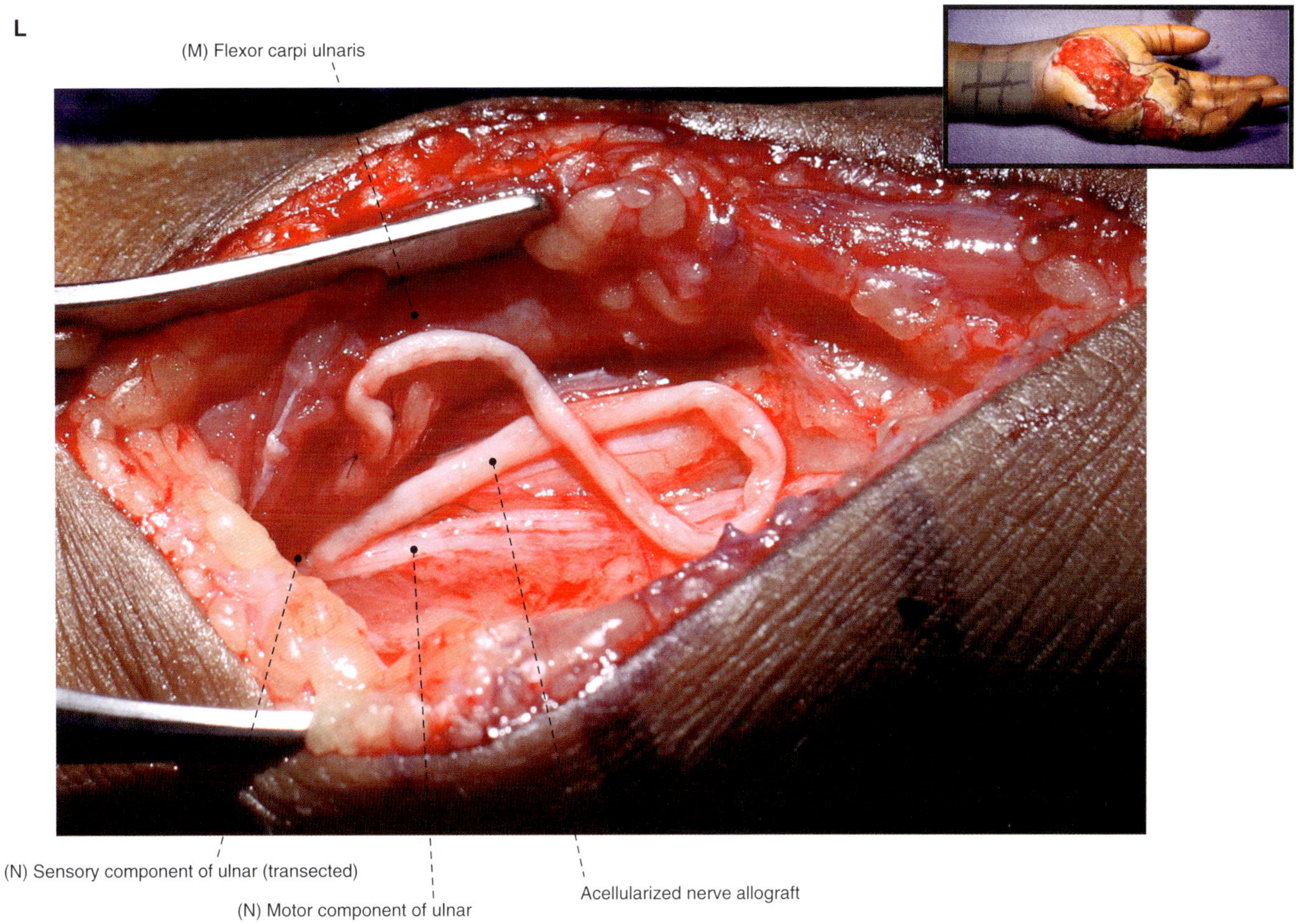

FIGURE 10-4 *(Continued)* **L.** Intermuscular proximal transposition of the sensory component of the ulnar nerve using an acellularized nerve allograft extender. The sensory component of the ulnar nerve was extended using an acellularized nerve allograft (Avance Nerve Graft, AxoGen) in order to more proximally transpose deeply within the flexor carpi ulnaris muscle—use of this allowed a segment of the ulnar nerve to be used as "spare part" autologous sensory nerve graft material. (Reproduced with permission, © 2011, nervesurgery.wustl.edu.)

maximizing the outcome. Specific training is provided for sensory localization from the donor digits to the newly reinnervated distal surfaces.

Controversies

End-to-side transfer has been controversial, especially in cases of motor nerve transfer.[11,12] There is, however, no significant disadvantage to transfer of the distal donor nerve stump in an end-to-side fashion to an intact sensory nerve. More recent experimental[13,14] and clinical work[2,15–17] does support the usefulness of this technique. In most cases, we do perform this transfer to restore rudimentary sensation back to the donor nerve territory. For example, where the third web space branch of the median nerve is used to restore sensation by end-to-end transfer to the sensory component of the ulnar nerve, the distal third web space nerve can be coapted back to the second web space nerve in an end-to-side fashion to restore some sensation to the donor nerve territory. See Figure 10-3.

COMPLICATIONS

Complications with nerve transfer are those of any upper extremity procedure and include scarring, stiffness, and wound healing problems. Complications specific to the nerve transfer include donor-site deficit, failure of reinnervation, and neuropathic pain. Loss of sensation in the donor nerve distribution may be mitigated by use of end-to-side transfer of the distal transected donor nerve stump to a proximal intact functional sensory nerve.

OUTCOMES

Our experience indicates that, at a minimum, recovery of protective sensation can be expected following primary nerve transfers for digital sensation, that is, with end-to-end coaptations.[18] Using the "10 test" for evaluation, sensory recovery even in the absence of sensory reeducation will be approximately 6/10 following end-to-end repair and 3/10 following end-to-side repair. Sensory testing following similar transfers in the series of Stocks et al showed a recovery of S3+ or S4 in 85% of patients.[19] This is consistent with values for microsurgical primary digital nerve repair, to which properly performed digital nerve transfer is theoretically equivalent. End-to-end microsurgical digital nerve repair has a reported outcome of >S3 in all patients, and >S3+ in 90%.[20] Despite less than optimal recovery of 2-point discrimination after digital nerve transfers, functional improvement beyond the existing anesthetic digits is subjectively[19] and objectively[21] favorable. These results have been confirmed by Brunelli.[22] Some tip sensibility returns within 3 to 4 months, with gradual maturation continuing past 2 years after nerve transfer. Localization of sensory stimuli to the donor digits persists for 2 to 3 years, with localization to the recipient digit improving with time, use, and sensory reeducation.[23]

ACKNOWLEDGMENTS

Research funding from AxoGen, Inc (manufacturer for Avance Nerve Graft; Ida K. Fox and Andrew Yee) and NIH (Susan E. Mackinnon) is gratefully acknowledged.

REFERENCES

1. Mackinnon SE, Dellon AL. *Surgery of the Peripheral Nerve.* New York: Thieme Medical Publishers Inc; 1988.
2. Boyd KU, Nimigan AS, Mackinnon SE. Nerve reconstruction in the hand and upper extremity. *Clin Plast Surg.* 2011;38(4):643–660.
3. Fox IK, Mackinnon SE. Adult peripheral nerve disorders: nerve entrapment, repair, transfer, and brachial plexus disorders. *Plast Reconstr Surg.* 2011;127(5):105e–118e.
4. Ihara K, Doi K, Sakai K, Kuwata N, Kawai S. Restoration of sensibility in the hand after complete brachial plexus injury. *J Hand Surg Am.* 1996;21(3):381–386.
5. Hattori Y, Doi K, Sakamoto S, Yukata K. Sensory recovery of the hand with intercostal nerve transfer following complete avulsion of the brachial plexus. *Plast Reconstr Surg.* 2009;123(1):276–283.
6. Memis D, Turan A, Karamanlioglu B, Pamukcu Z, Kurt I. Adding dexmedetomidine to lidocaine for intravenous regional anesthesia. *Anesth Analg.* 2004;98(3):835–840 [table of contents].
7. Brown JM, Yee A, Mackinnon SE. Distal median to ulnar nerve transfers to restore ulnar motor and sensory function within the hand: technical nuances. *Neurosurgery.* 2009;65(5):966–977 [discussion 977–978].
8. Tung TH, Mackinnon SE. Nerve transfers: indications, techniques, and outcomes. *J Hand Surg Am.* 2010;35(2):332–341.
9. Brown JM, Mackinnon SE. Nerve transfers in the forearm and hand. *Hand Clin.* 2008;24(4):319–340, v.
10. Ross D, Mackinnon SE, Chang YL. Intraneural anatomy of the median nerve provides "third web space" donor nerve graft. *J Reconstr Microsurg.* 1992;8(3):225–232.
11. Ray WZ, Kasukurthi R, Yee A, Mackinnon SE. Functional recovery following an end to side neurorrhaphy of the accessory nerve to the suprascapular nerve: case report. *Hand (N Y).* 2009;5(3):313–317.
12. Fernandez E, Lauretti L, Tufo T, D'Ercole M, Ciampini A, Doglietto F. End-to-side nerve neurorrhaphy: critical appraisal of experimental and clinical data. *Acta Neurochir Suppl.* 2007;100:77–84.
13. Brenner MJ, Dvali L, Hunter DA, Myckatyn TM, Mackinnon SE. Motor neuron regeneration through end-to-side repairs is a function of donor nerve axotomy. *Plast Reconstr Surg.* 2007;120(1):215–223.
14. Battiston B, Tos P, Conforti LG, Geuna S. Alternative techniques for peripheral nerve repair: conduits and end-to-side neurorrhaphy. *Acta Neurochir Suppl.* 2007;100:43–50.
15. Battiston B, Artiaco S, Conforti LG, Vasario G, Tos P. End-to-side nerve suture in traumatic injuries of brachial plexus: review of the literature and personal case series. *J Hand Surg Eur Vol.* 2009;34(5):656–659.
16. Dvali LT, Myckatyn TM. End-to-side nerve repair: review of the literature and clinical indications. *Hand Clin.* 2008;24(4):455–460, vii.
17. Artiaco S, Tos P, Conforti LG, Geuna S, Battiston B. Termino-lateral nerve suture in lesions of the digital nerves: clinical experience and literature review. *J Hand Surg Eur Vol.* 2009;35(2):109–114.
18. Rath RK, Mackinnon SE, Shenaq SM. New nerve transfers following peripheral nerve injuries. *Oper Tech Plast Reconstr Surg.* 1997;4:2–118.
19. Stocks GW, Cobb T, Lewis RC Jr. Transfer of sensibility in the hand: a new method to restore sensibility in ulnar nerve palsy with use of microsurgical digital nerve translocation. *J Hand Surg Am.* 1991;16(2):219–226.
20. Wray RC Jr. Repair of sensory nerves distal to the wrist. *Hand Clin.* 1986;2(4):767–772.
21. Novak CB, Kelly L, Mackinnon SE. Sensory recovery after median nerve grafting. *J Hand Surg Am.* 1992;17(1):59–68.
22. Brunelli GA. Sensory nerves transfers. *J Hand Surg Br.* 2004; 29(6):557–562.
23. Mackinnon SE, Novak CB. Nerve transfers. New options for reconstruction following nerve injury. *Hand Clin.* 1999;15(4):643–666, ix.

11

Flexor Tendon Repair and Reconstruction

Bradon J. Wilhelmi, MD, FACS
Saeed A. Chowdhry, MD

INTRODUCTION

The most challenging, controversial, and studied hand injuries over the years have been those to the flexor tendons. Historically, the poor results following flexor tendon repairs in the fingers led 1 expert hand surgeon, Boyes, to state, "Here in a small area we have two flexor tendons, one passing through the other in a close fitting sheath and snugly held to the proximal phalanx by a pulley which is unyielding so that either trauma or infection squeezes out the blood supply and the tendon dies of ischemia. Suturing of a divided tendon usually results in some thickening and this enlarged area cannot pass the constricting pulley and motion is prevented."[1] Also, Bunnell coined the term "No Man's Land" to emphasize the difficulties associated with flexor injuries in the area of the digital sheath.[2] However, if we exclude flexor tendon injuries within the digital sheath, the remaining flexor tendon injuries are less problematic. For those flexor injuries in the digital sheath, adherence to certain surgical techniques and postoperative therapy programs can optimize results and finger motion. In fact, Kleinert et al revolutionized the primary repair of acute flexor tendon injuries in the digital sheath after others treated these in a staged fashion with grafts for years.[3]

ANATOMY

Verdan classified flexor tendons by their location of transection relative to the extremity and their prognosis[4] (see Fig. 11-1). For simplicity of discussion, when the flexor is injured at certain levels, it is classified by 1 of 5 zones: distal to the flexor superficialis insertion (zone 1), within the digital sheath of the flexor superficialis and profundus (zone 2), palm (zone 3), within the carpal tunnel (zone 4), and in the forearm proximal to the carpal tunnel (zone 5). In general, flexor tendons repaired in zones 1, 3, 4, and 5 have a better prognosis than those in zone 2, known as "No Man's Land."

The flexor tendons originate in the forearm with muscles arranged in 3 different layers: superficial, intermediate, and deep. The superficial layer consists of the pronator teres, flexor carpi radialis, palmaris longus, and flexor carpi ulnaris proceeding in a radial to ulnar direction. The pronator teres, palmaris longus, and flexor carpi radialis are innervated by the median nerve, while the flexor carpi ulnaris is innervated by the ulnar nerve. The intermediate layer includes only the flexor digitorum superficialis, which is innervated by the median nerve. The deep layer consists of the flexor digitorum profundus, the flexor pollicis longus, and pronator quadratus. The median nerve innervates the flexor pollicis longus, pronator quadratus, and index/middle finger flexor digitorum profundus. The small and ring finger flexor digitorum profundus muscles are innervated by the ulnar nerve.

There are 9 flexor tendons. The flexor pollicis longus is the most radial structure and courses to insert onto the thumb distal phalanx to flex the interphalangeal joint of the thumb. The flexor digitorum profundus tendons are along the base of the carpal tunnel, aligned in order, traveling to insert into the base of the distal phalanx of the index through small fingers to flex the distal interphalangeal joint of each finger. The flexor superficialis tendons course under the carpal tunnel in a stacked array with the middle and ring tendon volar to the index and small tendons coursing to insert into the middle of the middle phalanx of each respective finger. In the palm, the flexor superficialis tendon decussates at the level of Camper chiasm, to allow the flexor digitorum profundus to become more volar in the finger. The flexor digitorum superficialis and flexor digitorum profundus tendons course in the finger in a fibro-osseous canal that is lined by synovium and reinforced by a pulley system.

The fibro-osseous canal is composed of different pulleys with varying arrangements lending to their function. There are annular (A1-A5) and cruciate pulleys (C0-C4). The A1, A3, and A5 pulleys prevent bowstringing of the flexor tendon across the metacarpal phalangeal joint, proximal interphalangeal (PIP) joint, and distal interphalangeal joint, respectively. The A2 and A4 pulleys prevent bowstringing of the flexor tendon across the proximal phalanx and middle phalanx, respectively. The A2 and A4 pulleys are thicker, longer, and in a more critical area to prevent bowstringing.

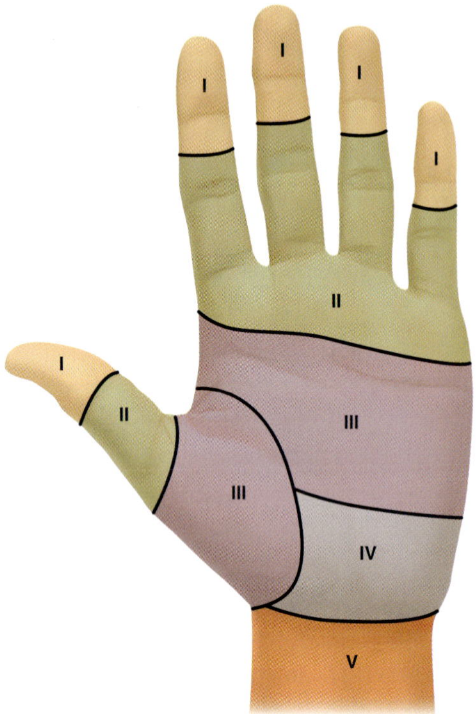

FIGURE 11-1 This is a diagram of the zones of injury to flexor tendons. When the flexor is injured at these levels, it is classified into the following zones: distal to the flexor superficialis insertion (zone 1), within the digital sheath of the flexor superficialis and profundus (zone 2), palm (zone 3), within carpal tunnel (zone 4), and in the forearm proximal to the carpal tunnel (zone 5). In general, flexor tendons repaired in zones 1, 3, 4, and 5 have a better prognosis than those in zone 2, known as "No Man's Land." (Figure modified from Hagberg L. Flexor tendon injuries. In: Blair WF, ed. *Techniques in Hand Surgery*. Baltimore, MD: Williams and Wilkins, 1996:138. With permission.)

The A2 and A4 pulleys are, therefore, termed the critical pulleys. A deficiency of 25% of either of these pulleys is known to potentially result in the condition of bowstringing and requires reconstruction to minimize moment and maximize finger motion with a certain tendon excursion (Fig. 11-2). Found between the annular pulleys, the cruciate pulleys (C0-C4) are of less biochemical and functional significance.

Digital flexor tendons receive nutrition by an intrinsic and an extrinsic source. The synovial fluid provides extrinsic nutrition to the digital flexor tendons by a pumping action facilitated by flexion and extension of the fingers. Flexor tendons receive intrinsic nutrition by 3 sources including longitudinal vessels entering the palm in the endotendinous channels, vessels that enter at the osseous insertion, and vincula (short and long). Most of the intrinsic nutrition is delivered on the dorsal side of the tendon.

Flexor tendon function depends on many factors including tendon excursion, an intact pulley system, joint motion, and the presence of lubricating synovial fluid. If bowstringing is present, a greater amplitude of muscle contraction and greater amount of tendon excursion are required to close the fingertip to palm (Fig. 11-3).

DIAGNOSIS

The most accurate means of detecting flexor tendon injuries is by clinical exam, wherein the patient is unable to actively flex the PIP joint with the adjacent finger hyperextended, with a sublimis tendon laceration and an inability to actively flex the DIP joint with a profundus laceration. There is a loss of the normal finger cascade and a loss of the tenodesis

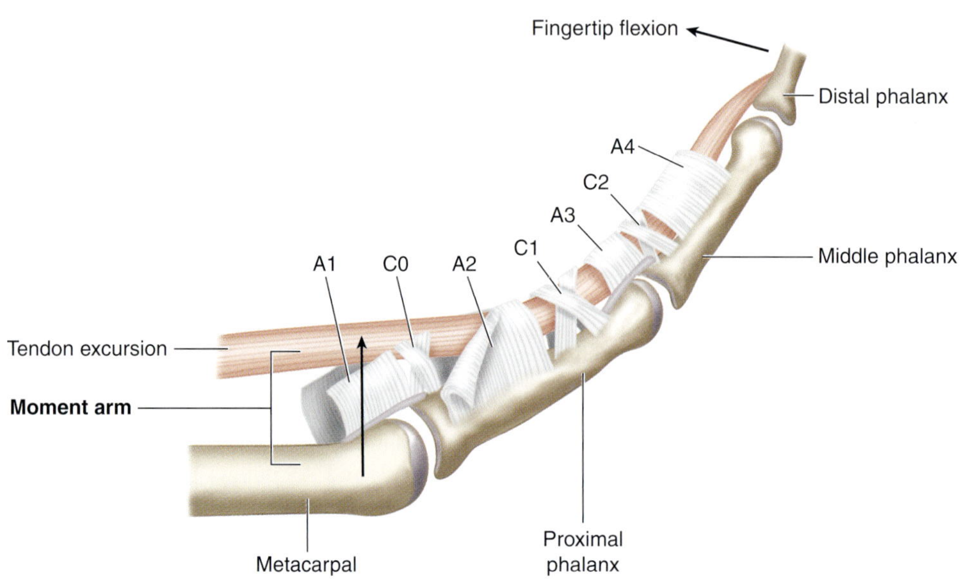

FIGURE 11-2 The A2 and A4 pulleys are the critical pulleys. When a certain amount of either of these pulleys is missing, the flexor is not held down to the bone that increases the moment of the system. Widening of the moment arm causes less motion of the fingertip with a given tendon excursion, resulting in bowstringing of the finger and loss of fingertip flexion. (Figure from Wilhelmi BJ, Snyder N, Verbesey JE, Ganchi PA, Lee WPA. Trigger finger release with hand surface landmark ratios: an anatomic and clinical study. *Plast Reconstr Surg*. 2001;108(4):902–907. With permission.)

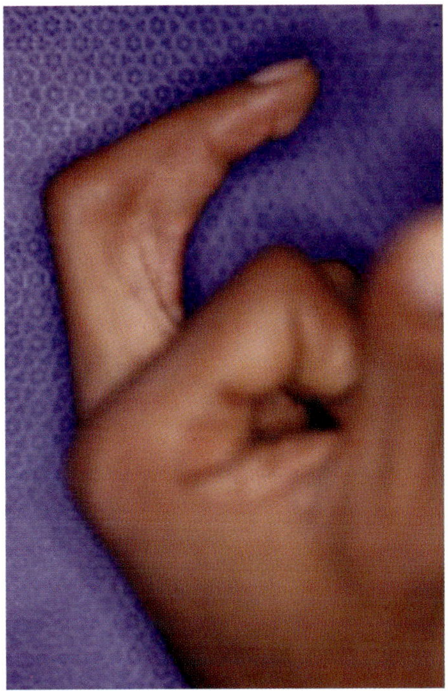

FIGURE 11-3 This figure demonstrates bowstringing as a result of loss of greater than 25% of either the critical A2 or A4 pulleys. (Photo copyrighted by Bradon J. Wilhelmi, MD.)

effect of passive finger flexion with passive wrist extension. Another useful technique is squeezing the flexors just proximal to the wrist that causes passive finger flexion.

Diagnostic studies are not as useful in detecting acute flexor tendon injuries. Plain radiographs, MRI, or ultrasound may help detect the location of the proximal tendon after zone 1 closed injuries (jersey finger injury).

INDICATIONS

Profundus avulsion classification of Leddy and Packer (reference) is as follows: type I, FDP tendon is avulsed from its insertion and retracts into the palm; type II, the profundus tendon is avulsed from its insertion, but the stump remains within the digital sheath, implying that the vinculum longum profundus is still intact; type III, a bony fragment is attached to the tendon stump, which remains within the flexor sheath. Further proximal retraction is prevented at the distal end of the A4 pulley.

When the FDP retracts into the palm (Leddy type 1), the tendon must be repaired within 4 weeks since the avulsion of the small and long vincula devascularizes the tendon. When the tendon retracts only to the PIP joint, the long vinculum remains intact; hence, the tendon remains viable longer and can be repaired up to 6 weeks (Leddy type 2). If the tendon only retracts to the A4 pulley (Leddy type 3), it remains viable indefinitely and can be repaired at a later date.[5]

Partial tendon injuries are suggested in patients with pain on resisted flexion. If the injury is more than 60% of the tendon's diameter, it should be repaired. If less than 60% of the tendon is injured, the free edges should be debrided to prevent catching on the pulleys.[6]

SURGICAL TECHNIQUE

The ideal flexor repair should be strong enough to allow for early active motion. The repair should be strong enough to resist gap formation, which can be a site for adhesion formation or rupture. The repair site should be smooth and nonbulky to facilitate tendon gliding. Usually full exposure of the proximal distal tendon requires extending the laceration in a zigzag (Brunner) or midaxial fashion. The distal end of the tendon can be found more distally when the injury occurs with the finger in flexion. When the finger is extended at the time of injury, the proximal and distal tendon ends are found at the laceration level. Excessive manipulation of the flexor tendons should be avoided to minimize adhesion formation. The flexor tendons should be grasped in the core of the severed end to avoid epitenon injury, which could be a nidus for adhesion formation. In general, the technique of flexor tendon repair is selected based on the zone of flexor injury.

Flexor repairs are generally performed in the operating room under a variety of anesthesia options to allow for use of a tourniquet. Alternatively, flexors can be explored and repaired with local anesthesia using epinephrine to avoid the use of a tourniquet.[6] According to a double-blinded randomized controlled study by Wilhelmi et al epinephrine can be safely used in digital, hand, and upper extremity procedures to prolong the duration of local anesthesia, reduce bleeding, and obviate the need for a tourniquet.[7] Furthermore, epinephrine has been safely used in upper extremity surgery in thousands of patients.[8,9] Performing a flexor tendon repair under straight local with epinephrine can allow for tendon repair site strength assessment and tendon balancing during the procedure.[10]

Our preferred repair method is the modified Becker (MGH) technique that has gained popularity for its strength and resistance to gap formation with early active range of motion.[11-17] The MGH technique is similar to the Becker repair as it involves placement of 4 strands through the core in a crisscross configuration[18] (Fig. 11-4A and B). However, the MGH technique is different in that the core sutures are 3-0 instead of 6-0, it includes augmentation with an epitenon suture, and it avoids a step-cut bevel.

The modified Becker technique first involves approximation of the epitenon with 6-0 nylon suture in a continuous fashion. Then 2 double-armed 3-0 sutures (Prolene) are used to place 4 crisscross sutures through the core. The crisscrosses of 2 of the 4 core sutures are placed on each side of the tendon, radially and ulnarly. The first 2 cores are started by placing the first needle purchase with the 3-0 suture (Prolene) transversely through the lateral aspect of the

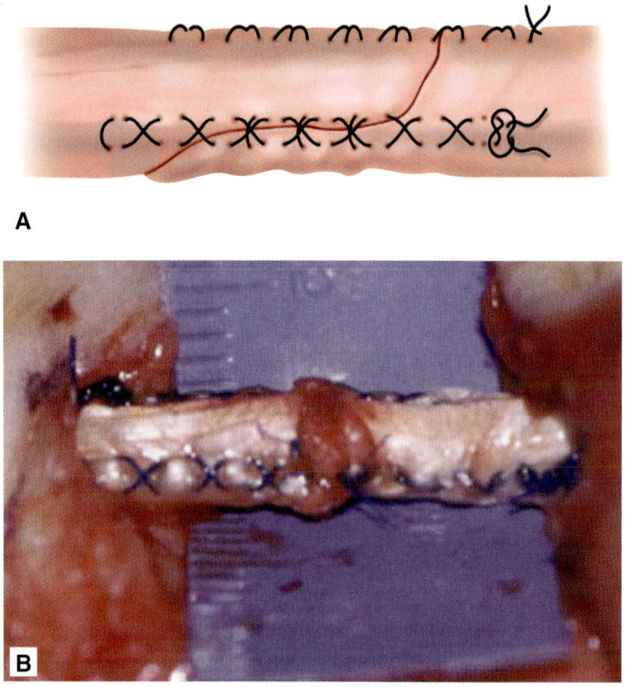

FIGURE 11-4 The modified Becker (MGH) technique is like the Becker repair (**A**) as it involves placement of 4 strands through the core in a crisscross configuration. **B.** However, the MGH technique is different in that the core sutures are 3-0 instead of 6-0, it includes augmentation with epitenon repair, and it avoids the step-cut bevel. (Photo copyrighted by Bradon J. Wilhelmi, MD.)

tendon at least 1.5 cm from the tendon end (Fig. 11-5A). Then 1 of the needles is driven in the oblique direction through the tendon (Fig. 11-5B). This is repeated 2 more times in a spiral fashion and brought out the core, creating oblique suture lines parallel to each other on the external surface of the tendon (Fig. 11-5B). Then the other needle of the first 3-0 suture (Prolene) is used to place sutures perpendicular to the previous spiral of sutures (Fig. 11-5C). These crisscrosses are created by passing the second needle in the oblique direction through the tendon between the parallel lines of the suture on the external surface in the proximal to distal direction to exit the core. This technique is repeated on the distal end of the tendon to complete the crisscross on both ends of the tendon (Fig. 11-5D). Then, the other double-arm 3-0 suture (Prolene) is used to complete the crisscross cores on the contralateral side of the tendon. In performing this technique 3 crisscrosses are placed on either end of the tendon. The sutures should be pulled taut at each suture purchase to facilitate tendon compression and preload the repair to prevent gapping. Furthermore, before tying the knot the suture is carefully seesawed to take the slack out and compress the tendon ends, preloading the repair to prevent gap formation.

A modification of the MGH technique involves laying this stack of knots longitudinally along the tendon with another purchase as far from the stack as the height of the stack (Fig. 11-5E). Then, 3 more ties can be performed to lay the stack of knots along the tendon (Fig. 11-5F). Also, a tapered needle is preferred to minimize the risk for suture attenuation with multiple needle passes through the tendon.

ZONE 1 INJURIES

Zone 1 flexor tendon injuries occur at the level distal to the flexor digitorum superficialis insertion and by definition can only involve the flexor digitorum profundus. An attempt should be made to repair the profundus tendon when it is disrupted by laceration or avulsion. If the patient presents too late for FDP repair, a distal interphalangeal joint arthrodesis can be considered only if the flexor superficialis is intact to avoid instability of the joint; however, with resultant loss in power grip. The tendon is exposed through a volar Brunner incision. If the proximal end has retracted, wrist and finger flexion with forearm compression can help milk the tendon distally to the opening in the sheath where it can be carefully grasped with a small Jacobson mosquito forceps and repaired to the distal stump. Usually, the long vincula prevent retraction of the profundus past the A2 pulley. As much of the A2 pulley as possible should be preserved in exposing the proximal tendon end. A hypodermic needle can be used through the proximal tendon and proximal pulley to hold it during the repair. If there is less than 1 cm of distal flexor digitorum profundus stump, the proximal tendon can be advanced to the decorticated distal phalanx with Keith needles and repaired dorsally over the sterile matrix of the nail with a button. Repair over the sterile matrix minimizes risk of nail deformity. For avulsion injuries of the flexor digitorum profundus, the Leddy classification can direct time constraints in management as discussed above (Fig. 11-6).

ZONE 2 INJURIES

Zone 2 injuries occur within the digital sheath from the distal palmar crease to the middle of the middle phalanx where the flexor digitorum superficialis inserts. Flexor repairs are more challenging in this area because of the pulley system and coursing of the flexor digitorum profundus through the chiasm of the flexor digitorum superficialis. A zigzag Brunner-type incision or midaxial incision is used. In exposing the tendon ends, it is important to preserve the critical A2 and A4 pulleys. The proximal profundus tendon should be pulled through the chiasms (Fig. 11-7).

ZONE 3, 4, 5 INJURIES

Wide exposure by dividing the carpal transverse ligament is generally required. In general, composite grip is usually recovered quite well for these patients with the flexor tendons moving en mass, even if adherent. However, recovery of the independent tendon glide for injuries at this level can be variable and optimized by use of the MGH technique, which allows for early active motion protocols to promote

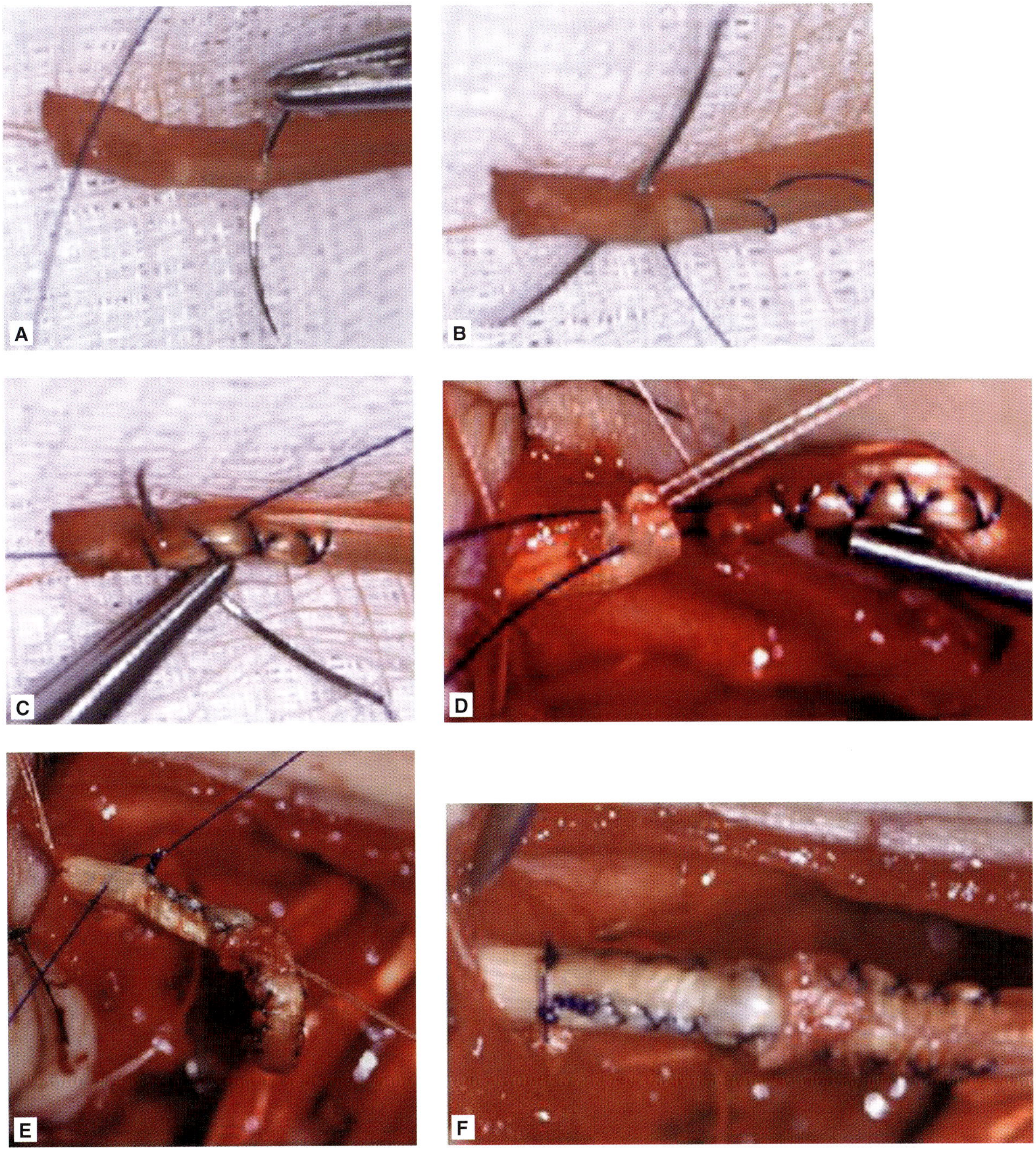

FIGURE 11-5 The first 2 core sutures are started by placing the first purchase 3-0 suture (Prolene) transversely through the lateral aspect of the tendon at least 1.5 cm from the tendon end (**A**). Then 1 of the needles is driven in the oblique direction through the tendon (**B**). This is repeated 2 more times in a spiral fashion and brought out the core, creating oblique suture lines parallel to each other on the external surface of the tendon (**B**). Then, the other needle of the first 3-0 suture (Prolene) is used to place sutures perpendicular to the previous spiral sutures (**C**). These crisscrosses are created by taking the second needle in the oblique direction through the tendon between the parallel lines of the suture on the external surface in the proximal to distal direction to exit the core. This technique is repeated on the distal end of the tendon to complete the crisscross on both ends of the tendon (**D**). Then, the other double-arm 3-0 suture (Prolene) is used to complete the crisscross cores on the contralateral side. In performing this technique 3 crisscrosses are placed on either end of the tendon. The sutures should be pulled taut at each suture purchase to facilitate tendon compression and preload the repair to prevent gapping. Furthermore, before tying the knot the suture is carefully seesawed to take the slack out and compress the tendon ends, preloading the repair to prevent gap formation. A monofilament suture (such as Prolene) slides through the tendon substance better and is preferred for preloading and minimizing gapping. However, the disadvantage of monofilament is the need for multiple knots, which can increase resistance to glide. A modification of the MGH technique involves laying this stack of knots longitudinally along the tendon with another purchase as far from the stack as the height of the stack (**E**). Then, 3 more ties can be performed to lay the stack of knots along the tendon (**F**). (Photo copyrighted by Bradon J. Wilhelmi, MD.)

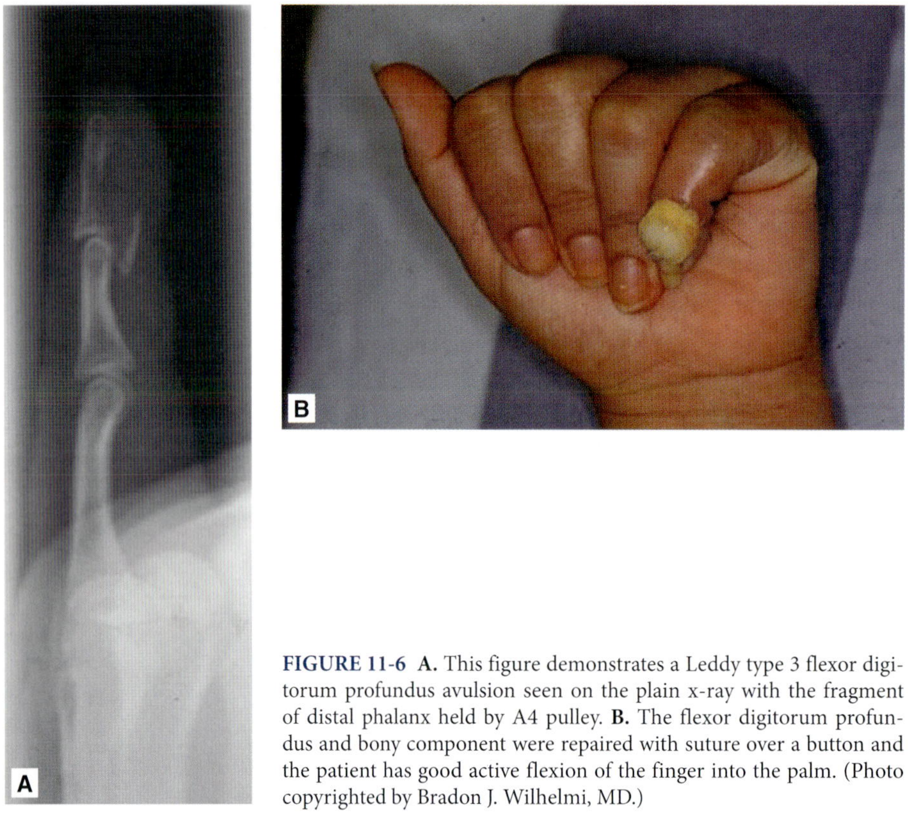

FIGURE 11-6 **A.** This figure demonstrates a Leddy type 3 flexor digitorum profundus avulsion seen on the plain x-ray with the fragment of distal phalanx held by A4 pulley. **B.** The flexor digitorum profundus and bony component were repaired with suture over a button and the patient has good active flexion of the finger into the palm. (Photo copyrighted by Bradon J. Wilhelmi, MD.)

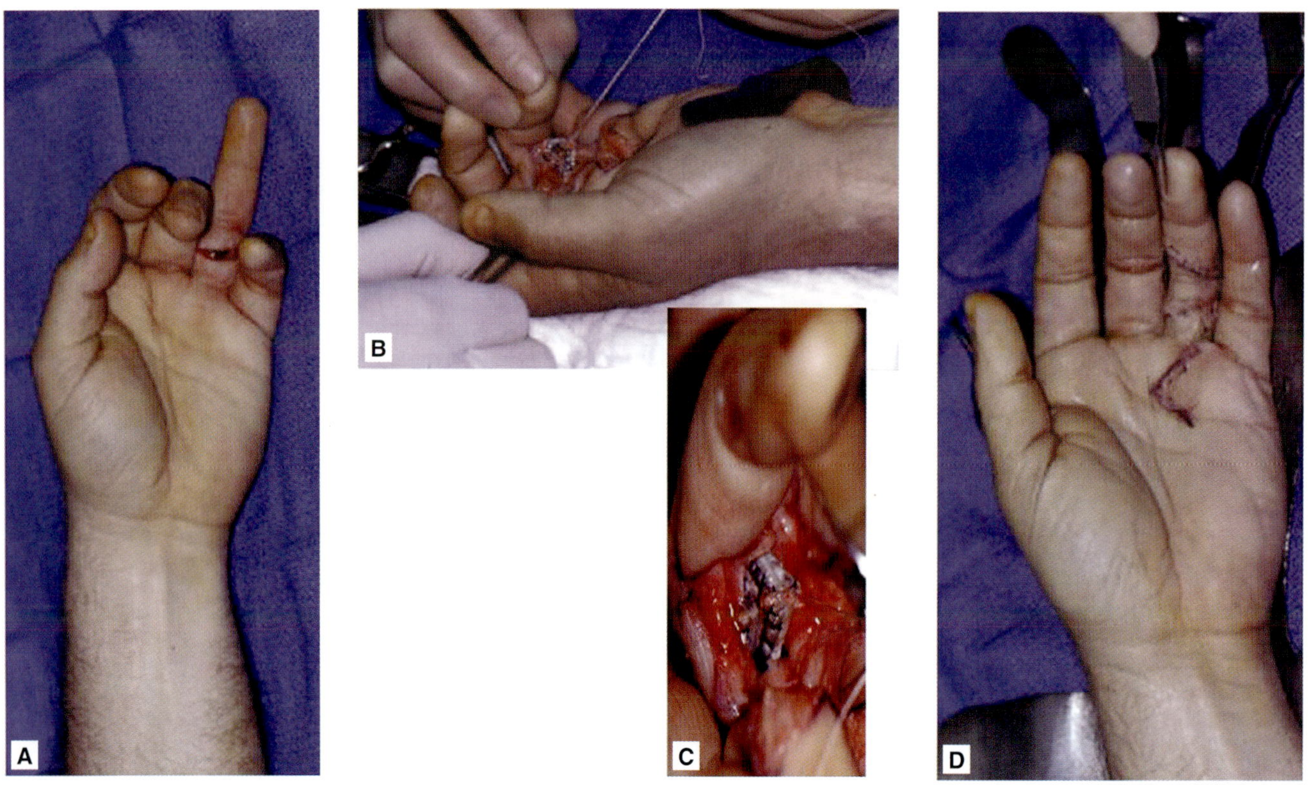

FIGURE 11-7 This series of photos demonstrates a zone 2 repair of both the flexor digitorum superficialis and profundus. **A.** The ring finger has lost cascade from flexor superficialis and profundus transection. **B** and **C.** This demonstrates repair of both the profundus and superficialis with the modified Becker MGH tenorrhaphy. **D.** This demonstrates restoration of cascade with flexor repairs.

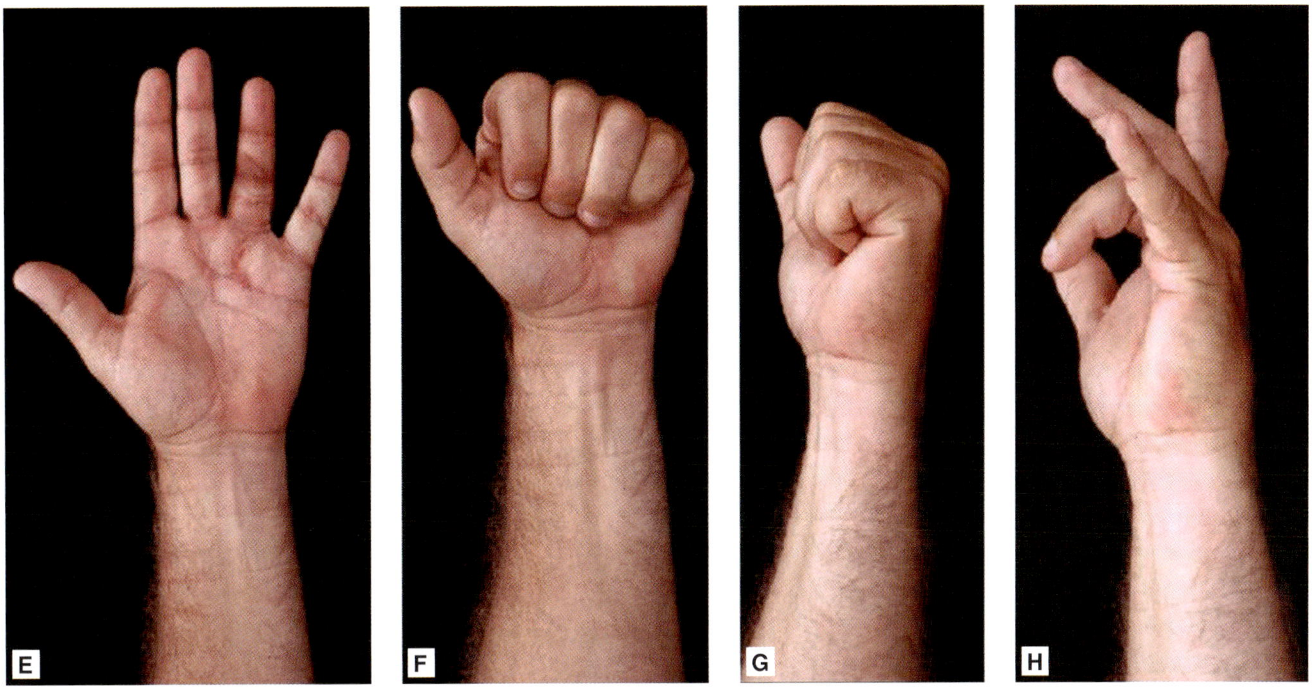

FIGURE 11-7 (*Continued*) **E** to **H.** These depict the postoperative photos of the patient to have recovering normal flexion with composite grip and differential gliding and near-normal extension. (Photo copyrighted by Bradon J. Wilhelmi, MD.)

individual tendon gliding during the healing process.[18] Reduced active and passive motion can occur due to adhesions in zone 5 injuries with adherence of all the tendons (Fig. 11-8).

THERAPY

Several flexor therapy regimens have been described. Passive range of motion programs include the Duran and Kleinert protocols. The Kleinert protocol involves the use of nail plate hooks with elastic bands attached proximally to the palm and wrist to passively draw the fingers into flexion. In both cases, patients actively extend their fingers into the dorsal blocking splint. Both protocols include the use of dorsal blocking splints with the wrist in 20° to 30° of flexion, metacarpophalangeal joints at 70° to 80° of flexion, and the interphalangeal joints straight. All the fingers are placed in the splint and permitted to actively extend to splint. Passive proximal and distal interphalangeal joint motion within the restrains of the dorsal blocking splint is encouraged 4 times a day. At 4 weeks, active composite flexion and extension is performed outside the splint, while dorsal blocking splint is continued between exercises. At the fifth week, the dorsal blocking splint is discontinued. Blocking exercises may be initiated at 6 weeks. Gentle passive extension is initiated and a static extension splint may be used if extrinsic flexor tightness is encountered. At 8 weeks, light strengthening is started and resisted exercises are begun at 10 weeks. By 12 weeks normal activities are performed.

An example of an active range of motion program, the MGH protocol, involves the use of a splint similar to the passive regimens (Table 11-1). However, in addition to passive flexion and active extension within the splint, this protocol also involves passive flex with active hold exercises. At 3 weeks gentle tenodesis exercises are begun out of the splint. Active composite flexion exercises without the splint are initiated at 4 weeks as well as differential tendon gliding exercises. The splint is discontinued at 6 weeks with initiation of passive extension exercises. At 7 weeks composite passive extension is started. Light strengthening is allowed at 8 weeks and normal activities at 12 weeks (Fig. 11-9).

Cast immobilization is necessary in children younger than 10 years of age due to lack of compliance with motion protocols.

OUTCOMES

In the Strickland Modified outcome assessment scale poor is 0% to 24% (<44°), fair 25% to 49% (44°-87°), good as 50% to 74% motion (88°-131°), and excellent as 75% to 100% motion (>132°).[19]

Osada et al[20] performed a 6-strand repair on 22 consecutive patients with 28 injured fingers. Postoperative motion was started combining active extension and passive or active flexion in a protective splint for the first 3 weeks after surgery. At an average follow-up of 13 months the results were excellent in 17 fingers, good in 9, and fair in 1. The average

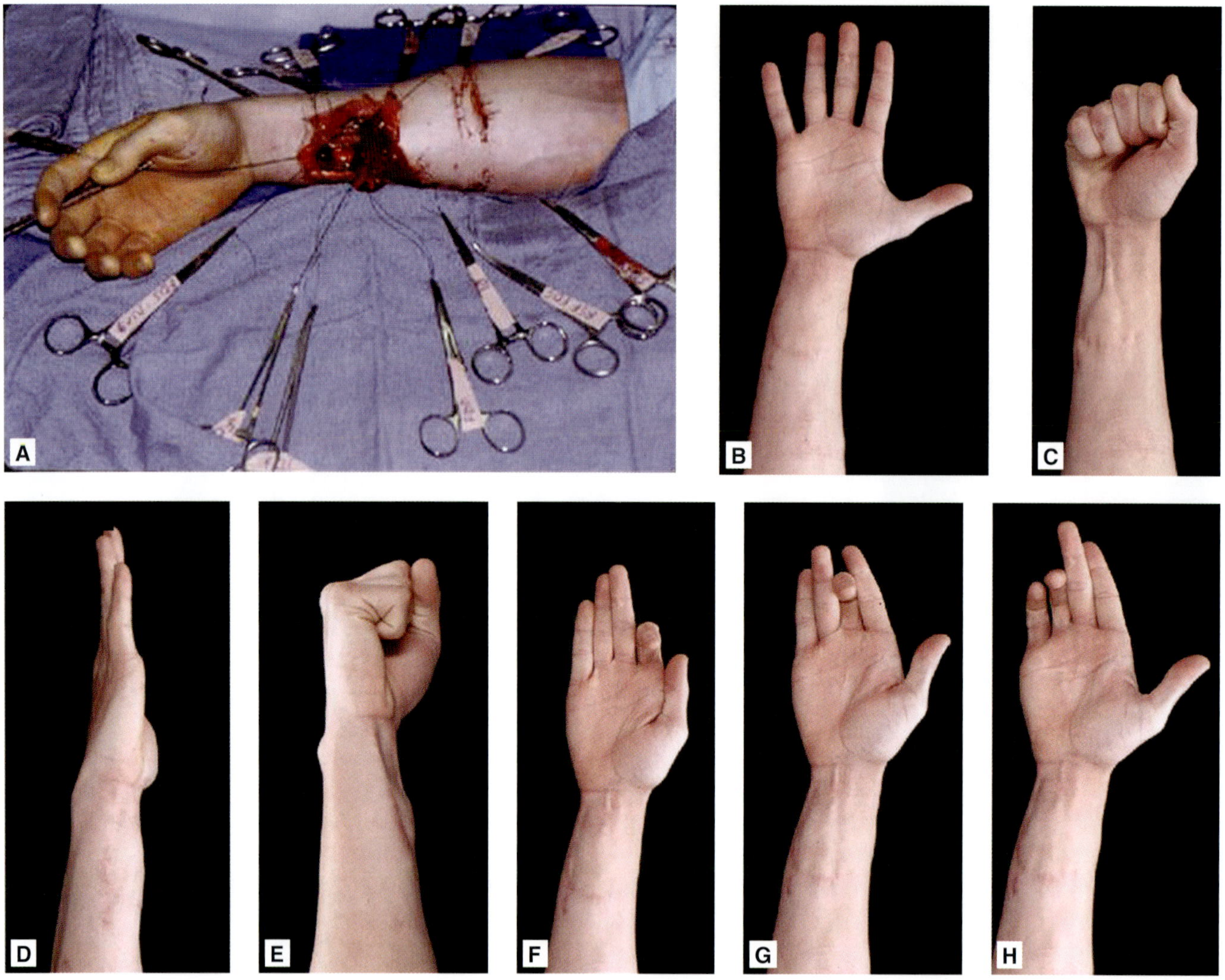

FIGURE 11-8 This series of photos demonstrates a zone 5 multiple flexor tendon repair (**A**) with recovery of normal composite grip and extension (**B-D**), as well as differential flexor gliding of the superficialis to the index, middle, ring and small fingers (**E-H**). (Photo copyrighted by Bradon J. Wilhelmi, MD.)

flexion was 62° for distal interphalangeal joints and 91° for PIP joints. None of the repaired tendons ruptured.

The type of injury influences the outcomes. Starnes et al[21] recently reviewed 2 groups of patients. The saw group injuries were from saws or from tearing mechanisms; the sharp group had clean transection injuries from knives or glass. The saw group had 13 patients with 17 fingers studied. The sharp group had 21 patients with 24 fingers studied. All patients had primary flexor digitorum profundus repairs in zone II. At an average follow-up of 4 years (range, 1-9 years), the TAM for the saw group was significantly worse than that for the sharp group ($86° \pm 14°$ vs $114° \pm 7°$; $P < .05$). The saw group fingers also had a worse average total passive motion TPM at the PIP and DIP joints than patients in the sharp group. In addition, there were larger flexion contractures for the combined PIP and DIP joints in the saw group compared with those in the sharp group. Secondary surgery was necessary in 9 of 17 digits in the saw group as compared with 3 of 24 digits in the sharp group.

Wilhelmi et al[18] performed a retrospective review of zone V finger flexor tendon repairs for 29 patients with an average age of 28 years, at a median follow-up of 24 weeks. These injuries involved 103 FDS and 65 FDP lacerations to 103 fingers. The total active motion for these zone V repairs was $236° \pm 5°$. Overall 97 of 103 digits attained good to excellent function and 88 of 103 developed some differential glide. One of these patients required a tenolysis. Three repairs ruptured in 1 patient owing to suture breakage that was associated with noncompliance with the dorsal extension block splint.

Trumble et al[22] compared active place-and-hold therapy with passive motion therapy. Ninety-three patients (106 injured digits) with zone II flexor tendon repairs were randomized to either early active motion with place-and-hold or a passive motion protocol. Range of motion was measured at 6, 12, 26, and 52 weeks following repair. At all time

TABLE 11-1: Early Active Motion Protocol

Day 1:	Dorsal blocking splint with wrist neutral, metacarpophalangeal joint 70°, and interphalangeal joints straight
	Digits strapped to splint
	Passive place (into flexion) and active hold (flexed into palm) and active extension to splint, composite and differential
3 weeks	
	Gentle tenodesis exercises out of splint
	No active composite flexion
	Continue passive place and active hold exercises
4 weeks	
	Active composite flexion exercises out of splint
	Differential tendon gliding exercises
	No passive extension, no blocking
	Continue dorsal blocking splint between exercises
5 weeks	
	Initiate blocking exercise
	Splint at night and for protection only during the day
6 weeks	
	Discontinue splint
	Initiate passive extension
7 weeks	
	Start composite passive extension
8 weeks	
	May start light strengthening (putty)
12 weeks	
	Normal activities

points, the patients treated with the active motion program had greater interphalangeal joint motion. At the time of the final follow-up, the interphalangeal joint motion in the active place-and-hold group was a mean of 156° ± 25° compared with 128° ± 22° ($P < .05$) in the passive motion group. The active motion group had both significantly smaller flexion contractures and greater satisfaction scores ($P < .05$). We could identify no difference between the groups in terms of the DASH scores or dexterity tests. When the groups were stratified, those who were smokers or had a concomitant nerve injury or multiple digit injuries had less range of motion, larger flexion contractures, and decreased satisfaction scores compared with patients without these comorbidities. Two digits in each group had tendon ruptures following repair.

COMPLICATIONS

The most common complications are related to tendon adhesions, especially in zone II. Flexor tendon rupture may also occur. Dy et al[23] did a meta-analysis of 29 studies on flexor tendon repairs. This included 1753 flexor tendon repairs; 58% were in zone II. In 12 studies a modified Kessler technique was used; 14 included an epitendinous suture. They found that the type of core suture technique or use of an epitendinous suture did not influence the rupture rate. However, the presence of an epitendinous suture decreased

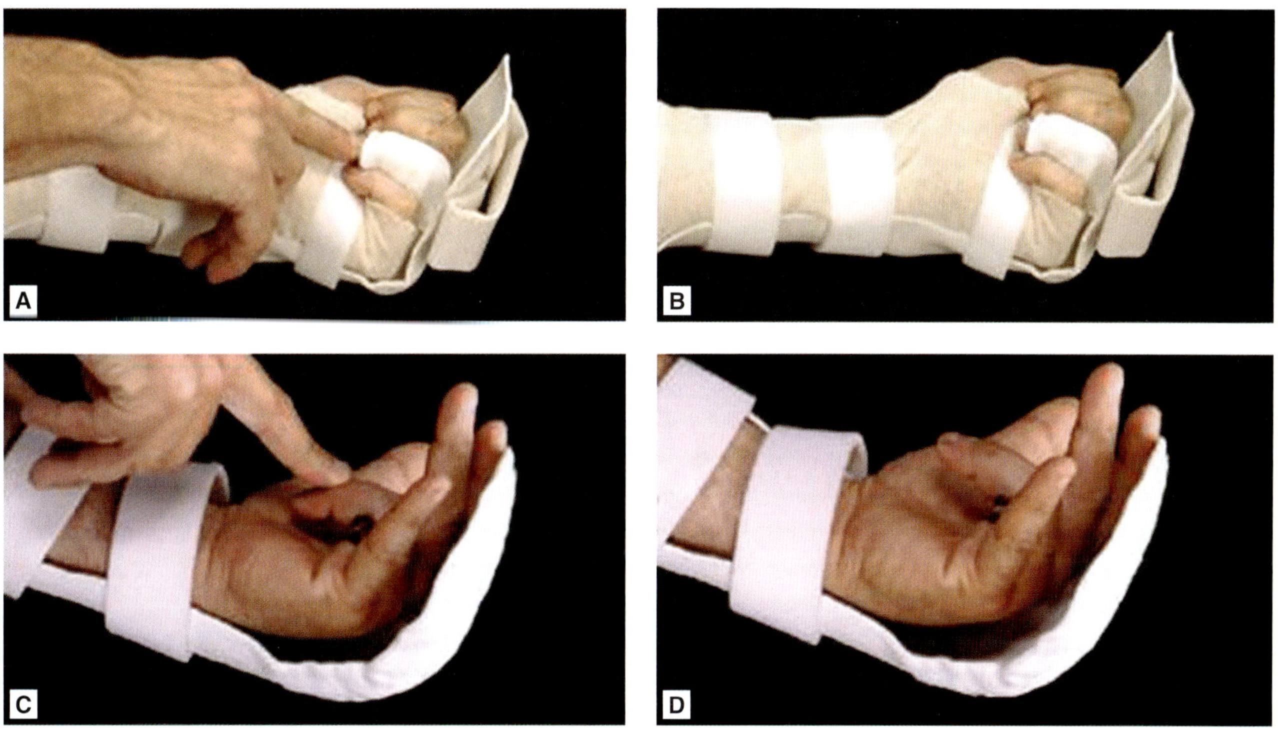

FIGURE 11-9 This photo demonstrates a patient performing the MGH active range of motion protocol with passive place and active hold exercises for composite grip (**A** and **B**) and differential flexor digitorum superficialis passive place and active hold exercises (**C** and **D**) within a protective splint. (Photo copyrighted by Bradon J. Wilhelmi, MD.)

the reoperation by 84%. Adhesion development was 57% lower when the modified Kessler technique was used.

TREATMENT OF LATER FLEXOR TENDON INJURIES

Flexor tendon grafting may be required in the late treatment of flexor tendon injuries including after later rupture of the flexor tendon repair, rupture of gap at the tenolysis site, and delay in treatment after flexor tendon injury. Flexor tendon grafting can be performed in a single stage or as 2 stages in which the first stage involves placement of a silicone rod, pulley reconstruction, and joint contracture release. Single-stage tendon grafting can be considered for tendon deficits in zones 3, 4, and 5. For coaptation of the tendon graft to the proximal distal ends of the tendon, the interweave technique is preferred because it has been shown to be the strongest in biomechanical studies.

Two-stage tendon grafting is recommended when patients require tendon grafting in conjunction with pulley reconstruction or joint contracture release. Two-stage grafting is also recommended if collapse of the sheath or excessive scarring is encountered at the time of tendon grafting or if soft tissue reconstruction is required over the graft.[24]

Several donor tendon site options are available: the palmaris, plantaris, extensor digitorum longus, extensor indicis proprius, and extensor digiti minimi. Selection of a tendon graft is based on the length requirement and the number of tendons requiring graft reconstruction. The palmaris longus provides 16 cm, or sufficient length to graft from the palm to the fingertip. If more graft is needed, lower extremity donors can provide longer tendons. The palmaris is generally the preferred graft because it is in the same operative field and provides sufficient length. The technique of harvesting a tendon involves dividing the tendon distally and pulling the tendon through a tendon stripper (Brand), which releases the tendon at the myotendinous junction. The palmaris longus is absent in 15% to 25% of patients. The presence of the palmaris longus can be determined by asking the patient to oppose the thumb to the small finger and flex the wrist against resistance. Another potential upper extremity donor is the injured flexor digitorum superficialis. When multiple tendon grafts or 1 long tendon graft from the wrist to the fingertip is required, the longer lower extremity donors are used. The plantaris provides 35 cm of tendon but is absent in 7% to 20% of patients. The plantaris can be located anterior and medial to the Achilles tendon. If the plantaris and palmaris are absent, the extensor digitorum longus from the second, third, and fourth toes can provide multiple segments of the tendon 30 cm in length. The extensor digitorum longus is harvested through an incision over the metatarsophalangeal joint. These tendons, however, can be fused at the ankle level, thus necessitating a second incision.

At the first stage of 2-stage tendon grafting for zone 2 reconstruction, the sheath is exposed with midaxial incisions. The flexor digitorum profundus can be used as the motor unit and is generally identified just proximal to the A1 pulley because it is held there by the origin of the lumbrical. The distal part of the flexor digitorum profundus is preserved to suture to the silicone rod and the tendon graft in the first and second stages, respectively. Alternatively, the flexor digitorum superficialis can be used as the motor unit to avoid the potential risk of tendon imbalance with quadrigia or a lumbrical plus posture. The distal end of the flexor digitorum superficialis is preserved to adhere to the flexor canal to prevent PIP joint hyperextension. If the PIP joint already hyperextends, the flexor superficialis tail can be tenodesed to the flexor canal to treat the hyperextension. Joint contractures should be released at the first stage. The distal portion of the silicon rod should be secured distally and left free proximally to prevent the rod from being pulled or migrating from the appropriate position. Pulley reconstruction should be performed at the first stage over the silicone rod. Of the various techniques described, the encircling repair technique with a tendon graft has been shown to be the strongest. In this technique, the tendon graft is passed circumferentially around the silicone rod and proximal phalanx volar to the extensor for the A2 pulley and dorsal to the extensor for the A4 pulley. For reconstruction of the pulley system of the thumb, the oblique pulley has been shown to be the most critical.

The second stage should be performed at 3 months to allow time for development of a pseudosheath. Radiographs can be obtained to confirm appropriate position of the rod. After limited proximal and distal incisions, the tendon graft is sutured to the rod proximally and pulled distally, delivering the graft into the pseudosheath. Of the various distal juncture techniques, repairing the tendon to tendon has been shown to heal most reliably. The distal juncture can also be repaired with a pull-through suture through the sterile matrix of the nail bed and nail plate over a button. The proximal end of the tendon graft is repaired to the motor unit with the interweave technique, which allows for size discrepancy and tendon balancing 1 cm tighter than cascade to allow for tendon stretching. This technique also allows for setting the appropriate length of the tendon graft. If the tendon graft is too short, quadrigia and weakened grip can result. If the tendon graft is too long, a lumbrical plus posture results with paradoxical hyperextension of the PIP joint on attempted finger flexion. These potential complications can be avoided by using the proximal flexor digitorum superficialis as the motor unit to avoid quadrigia and lumbrical plus posture. Immediately after the second-stage operation, early active motion can be initiated with passive flexion and active hold exercises. Patients can begin active flexion exercises at 4 weeks postoperatively. At 6 weeks, the dorsal blocking splint can be discontinued. The patient is allowed to participate in regular activities at 12 weeks (Fig. 11-10).

Some of the possible complications following tendon grafting include adhesions, infection, rod exposure, synovitis, rupture, and tendon imbalance.

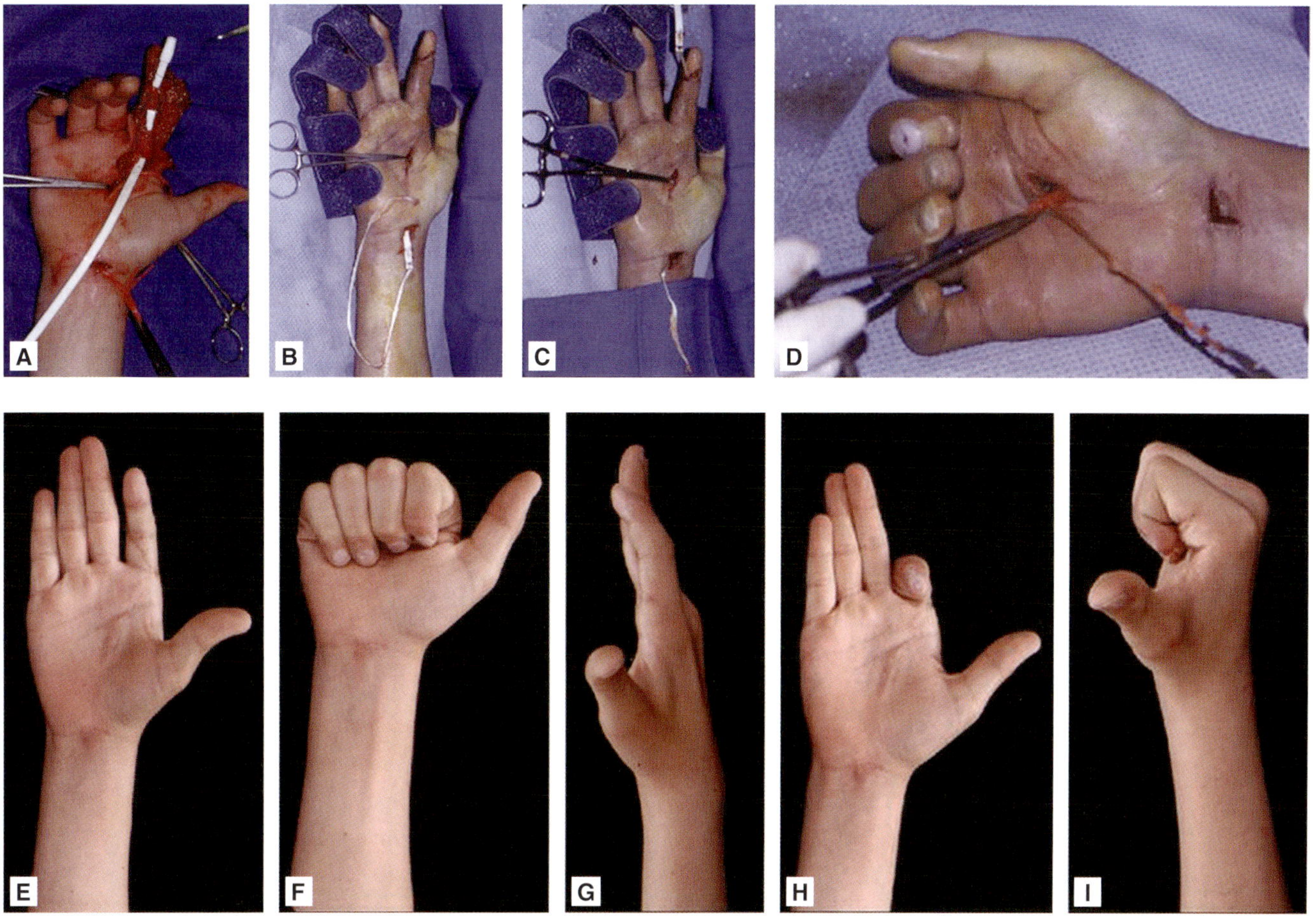

FIGURE 11-10 This series of photos demonstrates a patient who has undergone a 2-stage tendon graft procedure with initial pulley reconstruction over a silicone rod (**A**). At the second stage the silicone rod is replaced with a tendon graft (**B** and **C**). After completion of the distal juncture repair over a button the proximal tendon is repaired with interweave technique to set the proper tension across the graft (**D**). Postoperative photos demonstrate the recovery of full composite grip, differential flexion, and full extension (**E-I**). (Photo copyrighted by Bradon J. Wilhelmi, MD.)

Outcomes

In general, the outcomes after flexor tendon grafting are inferior to the results of primary flexor tendon repair. Leversedge et al[25] using an intrasynovial graft from the second toe in 9 patients reported 2 excellent, 4 good, 2 fair, and 1 poor. Two required a tenolysis and 1 graft ruptured. Coyle et al[26] performed a fingertip to palm reconstruction method in 35 patients using a 2-stage reconstruction method and reported 13 excellent, 11 good, 7 fair, and 4 poor. There were 3 tendon graft ruptures, 2 tenolysis, 1 lumbrical plus deformity, 1 PIP joint arthrodesis, and 2 silicone rod complications. Finsen[27] reported on a cohort of 43 patients treated with a 2-stage tendon grafting method. There were 0 excellent, 11 good, 16 fair, and 15 poor. The time away from work was 44 days after the first procedure and 104 days after the second procedure. Reoperation was necessary in 16 of 43 including 5 tenolysis, 2 PIP joint release, 1 PIP/distal interphalangeal joint fusion, 3 amputations, 5 infections, and 4 silicone rod complications.

REFERENCES

1. Boyes JH. Immediate versus delayed repair of the digital flexor tendons. *Ann West Med Surg*. 1947;1:145–152.
2. Bunnell S. *Surgery of the Hand*. Philadelphia: Lippincott; 1944:434.
3. Kleinert HE, Kutz JE, Ashbell TS, et al. Primary repair of lacerated flexor tendons in No Man's Land. *J Bone Joint Surg Am*. 1967;49:577.
4. Verdan C. Primary repair of flexor tendons. *J Bone Joint Surg Am*. 1960;42:617–657.
5. Leddy JP. Avulsions of the flexor digitorum profundus. *Hand Clin*. 1985;1:77–83.
6. Wilhelmi BJ, Blackwell SJ, Miller J, Mancoll JS, Phillips LG. Epinephrine in digital blocks: revisited. *Ann Plast Surg*. 1998;41(4):410.
7. Wilhelmi BJ, Blackwell SJ, Miller JH, et al. Don't use epinephrine in digital blocks: myth or truth with prospective, randomized, double-blinded study of epinephrine in digital block anesthesia. *Plast Reconstr Surg*. 2001;107(2):393.
8. Chowdhry S, Seidenstricker L, Cooney DS, Wilhelmi BJ. Do not use epinephrine in digit blocks; myth or truth? Part II. A retrospective review of 1111 cases. *Plast Reconstr Surg*. 2010;126(6):2031.
9. Lalonde D, Bell M, Benoit P, et al. A multicenter prospective study of 3110 consecutive cases of elective epinephrine in the fingers. *Plast Reconstr Surg*. 2005;30(5):1061.
10. Lalonde DH. Wide awake flexor tendon repairs. *Plast Reconstr Surg*. 2009;132(2):623.

11. Neumeister MW, Wilhelmi BJ. Flexor tendon repair. In: McCarthy JG, Galiano RD, Boutros S, eds. *Current Therapy in Plastic Surgery*. Philadelphia, PA: Elsevier Science; 2005:535–540.
12. Greenwald DP, Hong HZ, May JW Jr. Mechanical analysis of tendon suture techniques. *J Hand Surg Am*. 1994;19A:641.
13. Greenwald DP, Randolph MA, Hong HZ, May JW Jr. Augmented Becker versus modified Kessler tenorrhaphy in monkeys: dynamic mechanical analysis. *J Hand Surg Am*. 1995;20A:267.
14. Wasserman RJ, Howard R, Markee B, et al. Optimization of the MGH repair using an algorithm for tenorrhaphy evaluation. *Plast Reconstr Surg*. 1997;99:1688.
15. Yang C, Zhao C, Amadio PC, Tanaka T, Zhao KD, An KN. Total and intrasynovial work of flexion of human cadaver flexor digitorum profundus tendons after modified Kessler and MGH repair techniques. *J Hand Surg Am*. 2005;30(3):466.
16. Moriya T, Zhao C, Yamashita T, An KN, Amadio PC. Effect of core suture technique and type on the gliding resistance during cyclic motion following flexor tendon repair: a cadaveric study. *J Orthop Res*. 2010;28(11):1475.
17. Becker H, Orak F, Duponselle E. Early active motion following a beveled technique of flexor tendon repair: report on fifty cases. *J Hand Surg Am*. 1979;4(5):454–460.
18. Wilhelmi BJ, Kang RH, Wages DJ, Lee WP, May JW Jr. Optimizing independent finger flexion with zone V flexor repairs using the Massachusetts General Hospital flexor tenorrhaphy and early protected active motion. *J Hand Surg Am*. 2005;30(2): 230–236.
19. Strickland JW, Glogovac J. Digital function following flexor tendon repair in zone II; a comparison of immobilization and controlled passive motion techniques. *J Hand Surg Am*. 1980;5:537–543.
20. Osada D, Fujita S, Tamai K, Yamaguchi T, Iwamoto A, Saotome K. Flexor tendon repair in zone II with 6-strand techniques and early active mobilization. *J Hand Surg Am*. 2006;31(6):987–992.
21. Starnes T, Saunders RJ, Means KR Jr. Clinical outcomes of zone II flexor tendon repair depending on mechanism of injury. *J Hand Surg Am*. 2012;37(12):2532–2540.
22. Trumble TE, Vedder NB, Seiler JG 3rd, Hanel DP, Diao E, Pettrone S. Zone-II flexor tendon repair: a randomized prospective trial of active place-and-hold therapy compared with passive motion therapy. *J Bone Joint Surg Am*. 2010;92(6):1381–1389.
23. Dy CJ, Hernandez-Soria A, Ma Y, Roberts TR, Daluiski A. Complications after flexor tendon repair: a systematic review and meta-analysis. *J Hand Surg Am*. 2012;37(3):543–551.e1.
24. Derby BM, Wilhelmi BJ, Zook EG, Neumeister MW. Flexor tendon reconstruction. *Clin Plast*. 2011;38:607–619.
25. Leversedge FJ, Zelouf D, Williams C, Gelberman RH, Seiler JG III. Flexor tendon grafting to the hand: an assessment of the intrasynovial donor tendon—a preliminary single-cohort study. *J Hand Surg Am*. 2000;25:721–730.
26. Coyle MP Jr, Leddy TP, Leddy JP. Staged flexor tendon reconstruction fingertip to palm. *J Hand Surg Am*. 2002;27:581–585.
27. Finsen V. Two-stage grafting of digital flexor tendons: a review of 43 patients after 3 to 15 years. *Scand J Plast Reconstr Surg Hand Surg*. 2003;37:159–162.

Extensor Tendon Injuries in the Hand: Acute and Chronic

12

Christopher J. Dy, MD, MPH
Lauren Rosenblatt, BS
Steve K. Lee, MD

RATIONALE AND BASIC SCIENCE

Epidemiology

Injuries to the intricate extensor mechanism of the hand and fingers are common. An epidemiologic survey revealed that mallet finger injuries and extensor tendon injuries of the forearm and hand were 2 of the most frequently diagnosed soft tissue injuries encountered in the emergency department, with a combined annual incidence of 27.76 injuries per 100,000 persons.[1] Men are more likely than women to suffer from these injuries, with male:female ratios of 79:21 for extensor tendon injuries in hand and forearm and 60:40 for mallet fingers.[1] These injuries tend to occur in the fourth and fifth decades of life, which is a younger age than those who suffer fractures.[2]

Despite their common occurrence, extensor tendon injuries have not received a proportional amount of attention in the peer-reviewed literature. There are knowledge gaps in the current literature with regards to optimal surgical treatments and rehabilitation protocols; specifically, there is a marked deficiency in level I evidence.[3] Although one may be tempted to apply principles from the copious body of flexor tendon research, there are unique anatomic, biomechanical, and functional differences that need to be considered when treating extensor tendon injuries.

Anatomy

An in-depth understanding of the anatomy of the extensor tendons is critical to inform treatment strategies. During their muscular course in the forearm, the extensors of the wrist, hand, and fingers are divided into superficial and deep groups. The superficial group is composed of the extensor carpi radialis longus (ECRL), extensor carpi radialis brevis (ECRB), extensor digitorum communis (EDC), extensor digiti minimi (EDM), and extensor carpi ulnaris (ECU), while the abductor pollicis longus (APL), extensor pollicis brevis (EPB), extensor pollicis longus (EPL), and extensor indicis proprius (EIP) are the deep group. The ECRL and ECRB are innervated by the radial nerve, and the remaining extensor muscles are innervated by the posterior interosseous nerve.

There are numerous anatomic variations of the extensor tendons, including the presence of additional structures such as the extensor carpi radialis intermedius, extensor medii proprius, extensor indicis et medii, and extensor digitorum brevis manus.[4] The hand surgeon should be aware of the potential existence of these structures so as to aid in the diagnosis of extensor tendon–related pathology and for their potential use as tendon grafts.

The musculotendinous junctions of the extensors are 4 cm proximal to the wrist joint, except for the EIP, which has muscle fibers up to the level of the wrist joint. When crossing the wrist joint to reach the hand, the extensor tendons pass through the 6 extensor compartments, which are individual synovial-lined fibro-osseous sheaths. The extensor retinaculum transversely spans the wrist to prevent bowstringing of the extensor tendons. After passing through the extensor compartments, the extensor tendons flatten and become more superficial.

On the dorsum of the hand, there are stout fibrous bands (juncturae tendinae) that connect the ring EDC to the EDC tendons of the middle and small fingers. There is also a less substantial band that connects the middle and index EDC tendons. By linking the EDC tendons of adjacent digits, the juncturae tendinae restrict independent extension of the fingers. The juncturae tendinae can also allow a digit's extensor mechanism to function after an extensor tendon laceration, provided that the injury is proximal to the level of the juncturae and the adjacent extensor tendon is intact.

As the extensor tendons cross the metacarpal-phalangeal (MP) joint, they are secured to the dorsal axial midline by the sagittal bands. These fibrous thickenings originate on the volar plate of the MP joint and the intermetacarpal ligaments and traverse circumferentially to insert along the extensor hood. There is no actual tendinous attachment of the EDC to the proximal phalanx, with extension of the MP joint provided by the sagittal bands. Injuries to the sagittal bands, from either acute open injuries or chronic attenuation, can lead to subluxation of the EDC tendon off the dorsal axial midline, which can compromise extension of the MP joint.

The complexity of the extensor mechanism increases distal to the MP joint. The intrinsic tendons of the interossei and lumbricals join to form the lateral bands, which rise to the dorsal portion of the finger at the level of the proximal phalanx. The EDC trifurcates proximal to the proximal interphalangeal (PIP) joint, with the central portion becoming the central slip and attaching to the middle phalanx, where it helps to initiate PIP extension. The 2 lateral portions of the trifurcated EDC join with the lateral bands to form the conjoined lateral bands.

The conjoined lateral bands continue distally along the dorsal aspect of the finger, where they cross the distal interphalangeal (DIP) joint, converge to form the terminal tendon, and attach onto the distal phalanx 1.2 mm proximal to the germinal nail matrix.[4] The position of the conjoined lateral bands along the dorsal/volar axis of the finger is critical to ensuring appropriate function of the extensor mechanism. The conjoined lateral bands are stabilized to their dorsal position by the triangular ligament, which prevents palmar subluxation of the conjoined lateral bands during PIP flexion, and the transverse retinacular ligament, which prevents dorsal subluxation of the conjoined lateral bands during PIP extension. Incompetence of the triangular ligament leads to the boutonniere deformity, with PIP flexion and DIP hyperextension, while incompetence of the transverse retinacular ligament leads to the swan neck deformity, with PIP extension and DIP flexion.

Anatomy—Zones of Injury

Extensor tendon injuries can be described according to their anatomic location using the classification described by Kleinert and Verdan that was later modified by Doyle.[4] The zones can be easily remembered by recalling that the zones over the joints are assigned to odd numbers (starting with zone I at the DIP and ending with zone VII at the wrist). Because there is only 1 interphalangeal joint of the thumb, the numbering of the zones is slightly different than that of the digits, with the thumb IP joint labeled as T1 and the thumb MP joint labeled as T3. The different anatomic and biomechanical features of the tendons in each of the individual zones should be considered when planning treatment strategies, particularly the type of suture configuration used during operative management.

Biomechanics

The amplitude of tendon excursion for the finger extensors is 5 cm, but the majority of this excursion occurs proximal to the digits in the musculotendinous portions. Because there is minimal tendon excursion in the digits, the extensor mechanism is very sensitive to minor changes in tendon length and tension. Even slight lengthening of the tendon, as either a direct consequence of tendon injury or relative sequelae from a fracture, can lead to extensor lag.[4] This is particularly apparent in the fingers, as opposed to the hand, because the MP joints can hyperextend at baseline, which helps in accommodating for any extensor lag created by extensor mechanism injury.[4] Conversely, slight shortening of the tendon can restrict flexion in the digit. The sensitivity of the extensor mechanism to slight changes in length and tension provides insight into the challenges inherent to treating extensor mechanism injuries of the hand.

Suture Configurations

Selection of the appropriate suture configuration for repair of acute extensor tendon lacerations depends on the morphology of the tendon at the location of laceration. Unlike flexor tendons, there is no paratenon (except in zone VII) and the collagen of extensor tendons is longitudinally oriented with minimal or no cross-linking. The extensor tendons flatten as they reach the hand, tapering to thicknesses of 1.75 mm in zone II and 0.65 mm in zone I.[4] The thicker proximal tendon can hold core sutures, while the thinner distal tendons are broad and cannot generally accommodate core sutures.

Compared with flexor tendon injuries, there are relatively few biomechanical studies of suture configuration. Previous work by Newport and colleagues has demonstrated the biomechanical superiority of the Kleinert modification of the Bunnell repair in zones IV and VI.[5,6] More recent work has shown superior strength of the MGH repair in zone VI and the modified Becker technique in zone IV.[7,8]

The senior author recently performed a biomechanical comparison of the modified Becker, modified Bunnell, and a running interlocked horizontal mattress (R-IHM) suture (Fig. 12-1A and B).[9] The R-IHM suture, which does not require core sutures, was stiffer than the other techniques, in addition to having less tendon shortening. Additionally, the R-IHM suture can be rapidly performed, addressing 1 of the challenges of the modified Becker technique noted by Woo et al.[8] It is our experience that the R-IHM suture configuration is ideal for a broad tendon that cannot accommodate core sutures, and we continue to use this suture configuration in our practice because it provides strong fixation that can permit early mobilization (Fig. 12-2A and B).

INDICATIONS

Operative management is indicated in patients with complete or ≥25% transection of the extensor tendon, those with partial lacerations who cannot actively extend the digit, those with associated injuries that require formal irrigation and debridement (such as a "fight bite"), those with an unstable joint, and those who have failed a complete trial of nonoperative management. Patients who are initially evaluated

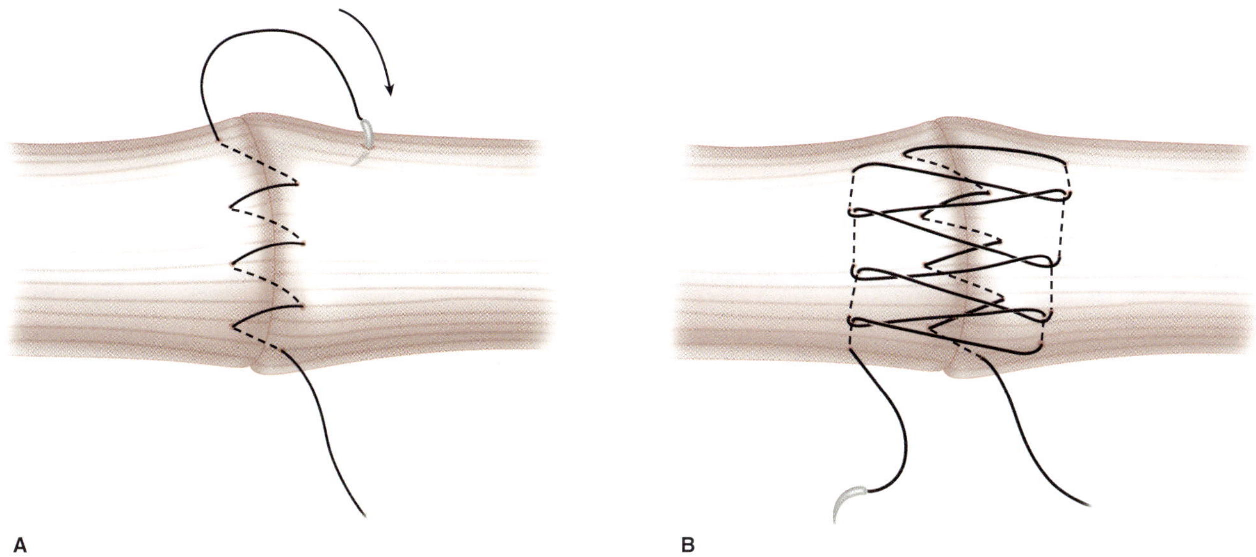

FIGURE 12-1 **A.** How to perform the new extensor tendon running interlocking horizontal mattress repair technique: begin the simple running suture at the near end. (Reprinted with permission from Lee et al.[9] Copyright Elsevier.) **B.** How to perform the new extensor tendon running interlocking horizontal mattress repair technique: run the interlocking horizontal mattress suture by starting at the far end. The suture needle passes underneath the prior crossing suture to lock each throw. Finish the suture and tie at the near end. (Reprinted with permission from Lee et al.[9] Copyright Elsevier.)

and treated in the emergency department or by a primary care physician should be referred for early evaluation (ideally, within 1 week) by a hand surgeon.

Chronic injuries involving the sagittal bands, central slip, triangular ligament, and transverse retinacular ligament may present with more subtle physical exam findings and/or visible deformities of the digits. While acute open injury to the sagittal bands will present with visible subluxation of the EDC, closed chronic injuries to the sagittal band may present with a subtle snapping sensation, pain, swelling, and decreased MP joint motion without any detectable instability. Elson's test is helpful in diagnosing both acute and chronic central slip injuries. In this test, the PIP joint is passively flexed to 90° and the subject attempts to actively extend the PIP joint against examiner resistance.[10] With central slip injuries, there is no detectable active extension of the PIP joint, but instead rigid extension or hyperextension of the DIP joint. In patients with finger deformities, such as boutonniere and swan neck, careful assessments of passive and active range of motion of both the PIP and DIP joints are critical. Serial casting or splinting is initially recommended for patients with early deformities, with serial reassessment of extensor deficiency and joint motion used to guide surgical management.

The ideal candidate for surgical repair is a patient who has a medical profile favorable to tendon healing (nondiabetic,

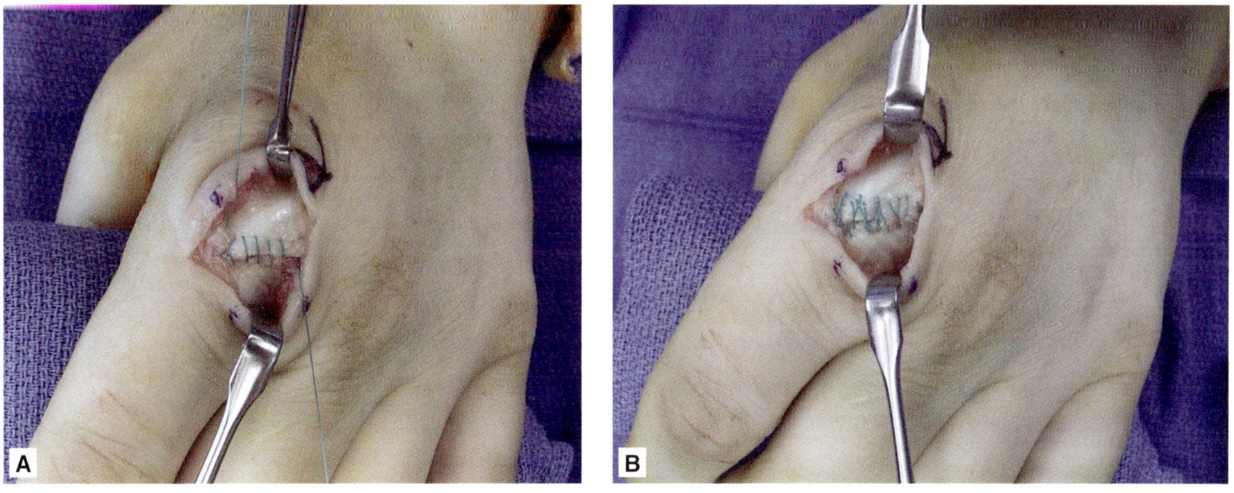

FIGURE 12-2 **A.** Running interlocking horizontal mattress (R-IHM) suture, running portion. **B.** Completed R-IHM.

nonsmoker, adequate nutritional status) who can be compliant with postoperative splinting and rehabilitation. While generally not emergent, repair of an acute laceration that meets operative criteria should be performed as soon as reasonably possible, generally within a few days.

CONTRAINDICATIONS

Nonoperative management is attempted for patients with incomplete extensor tendon lacerations, provided that active finger extension distal to the level of injury is intact. Patients with intact active extension of the wrist, hand, and fingers without any detectable deficit in strength should be treated nonoperatively. Noncompliance with attempted nonoperative treatment using splints is a relative contraindication for progression to surgical treatment.

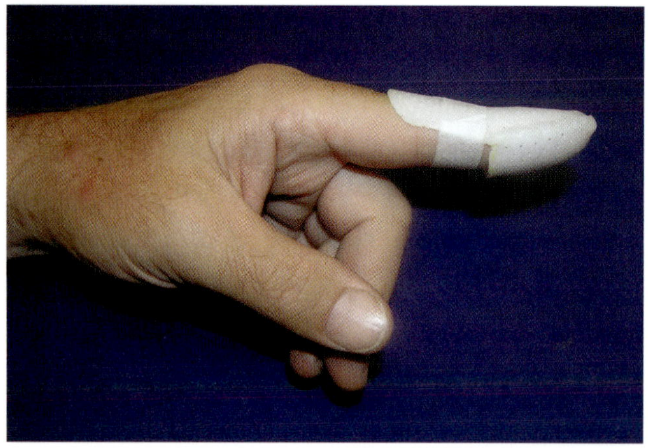

FIGURE 12-3 Mallet finger splint, custom made with thermoplastic material by a certified hand therapist. It immobilizes the distal interphalangeal joint yet allows for motion at the proximal interphalangeal joint. (Image reproduced with permission from Hand Therapy at Hospital for Special Surgery, New York, New York.)

SURGICAL TECHNIQUE

In general, we prefer to perform these procedures in the operating room under sterile conditions. We prefer regional anesthesia, such as an infraclavicular block. The patient is positioned supine with a hand table and pneumatic tourniquet is generally used. We prefer 4-0 FiberWire (Arthrex, Naples, Florida) for suture material because of its favorable biomechanical properties, although any braided nonabsorbable suture preferred by the surgeon is suitable.[11] Larger suture sizes (such as 3-0) can be used in rounder portions of the tendon, such as zones VI to IX.

Zone I

Acute injuries: Most closed acute zone I (mallet finger) injuries are amenable to nonoperative management with full-time splinting for 8 weeks, followed by night splinting for 4 weeks. While we prefer a therapist-created custom mallet splint (Fig. 12-3), other similar splints (either made of other materials or purchased "off the shelf") are acceptable, given that the patient follows instructions for constant wearing and appropriate splint changing techniques. The splint should keep the DIP joint extended to 0° and allow for active motion of the PIP joint. Patients should be instructed that the finger should not be allowed to flex past 0° for 24/7 for 8 weeks. They should also be instructed to evaluate the skin for breakdown or other issues. For bony mallet injuries with more than 40% articular involvement or subluxation/instability of the DIP joint, extension block pinning is preferred.[12-14] A 0.035- or 0.045-in K-wire is inserted in a distally directed orientation at approximately 45° into the distal aspect of the dorsal middle phalanx just dorsal to the fractured bony fragment of the distal phalanx with the DIP joint flexed (Fig. 12-4A). The DIP joint is then extended to 0° that will reduce the bony fragment by the bony block technique. The DIP joint is then fixed using a K-wire inserted longitudinally in a retrograde fashion across the joint (centered on AP and lateral fluoroscopic images) (Fig. 12-4B). The wires are removed at 6 weeks provided that the fracture heals radiographically and clinically (Fig. 12-5A-E).

A number 11 blade is used to make a small longitudinal skin incision where the dorsal-block pin will rest to avoid skin necrosis.

Regardless of the treatment technique used, it is important to instruct patients to continue motion of their PIP joint to avoid the unintended consequence of adjacent joint stiffness.

Chronic injuries: For chronic mallet injuries, decisions for treatment are made based on the patient's symptoms. For patients who are asymptomatic, nonoperative treatment with careful counseling is chosen. If the patient has pain, the DIP joint is evaluated clinically and radiographically for degenerative arthritis and DIP arthrodesis is considered.

If the patient has functional deficits resulting from persistent extensor lag, we prefer a terminal tendon imbrication procedure that takes up the "slack" present in the elongated terminal tendon. Using an H-type dorsal incision, the terminal tendon is exposed to gain access to the radial and ulnar aspects of the tendon. A tenolysis is performed to assure the palmar portion of the tendon is free of adhesions. The DIP joint is pinned in extension using a longitudinal, retrograde K-wire centered on AP and lateral fluoroscopic images. The terminal tendon is then transversely cut in the region of the DIP joint. The proximal portion of the tendon is advanced distally until the "slack" in the extensor mechanism is no longer present and imbricated to the distal terminal tendon with a horizontal mattress suture using a nonabsorbable braided suture (Fig. 12-6A and B). While success after tenodermodesis and skin imbrication techniques has previously been described, we prefer to not remove tendon or skin in an attempt to preserve the soft tissue envelope.

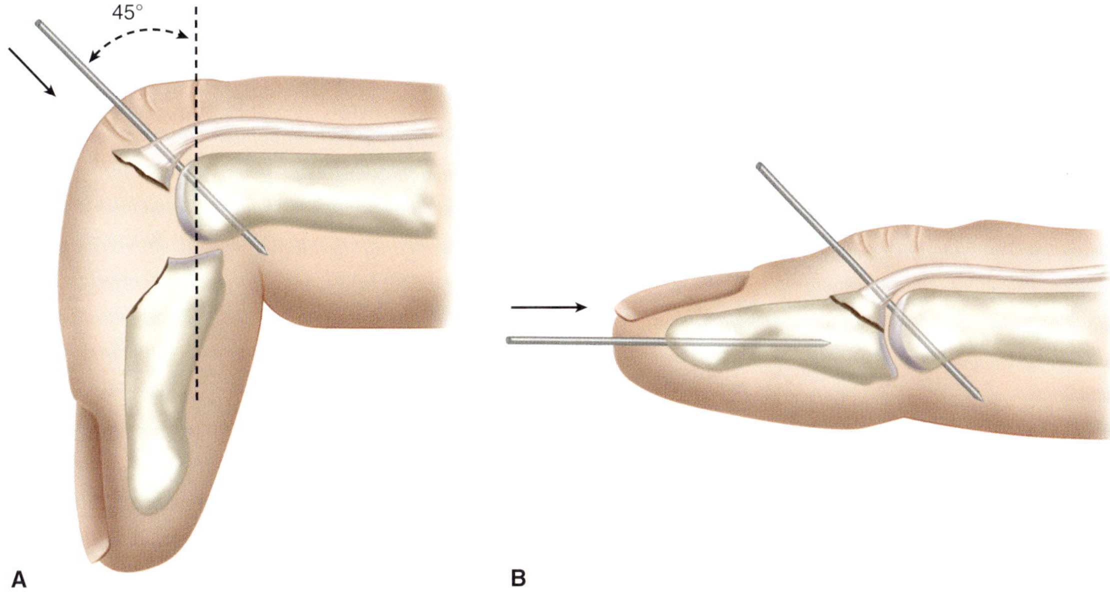

FIGURE 12-4 **A.** A 1.4-mm (0.045-in) K-wire is introduced under fluoroscopic guidance through the extensor tendon at a 45° angle into the distal portion of the middle phalanx with the distal interphalangeal joint flexed. The distal phalanx is then extended and translated, compressing the fragment and acting as an extension block. Occasionally, manipulation of the distal phalanx against the extension block K-wire is required to obtain an anatomic reduction. (Reprinted with permission from Hofmeister et al.[14] Copyright Elsevier.) **B.** A second K-wire is inserted longitudinally from distal to proximal across the DIP joint with the DIP joint extended. (Reprinted with permission from Hofmeister et al.[14] Copyright Elsevier.)

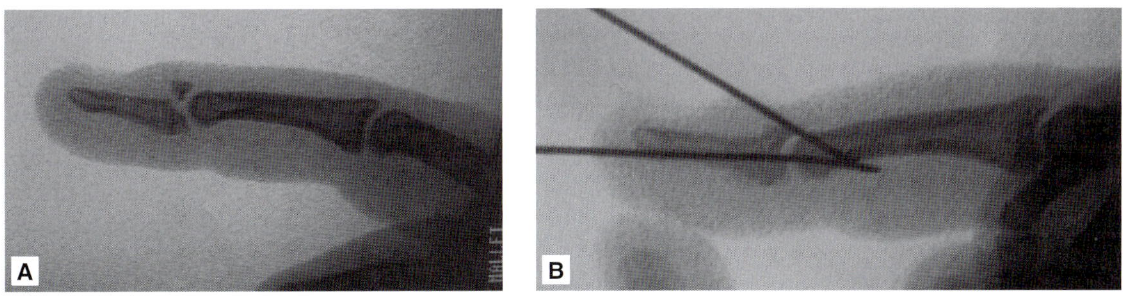

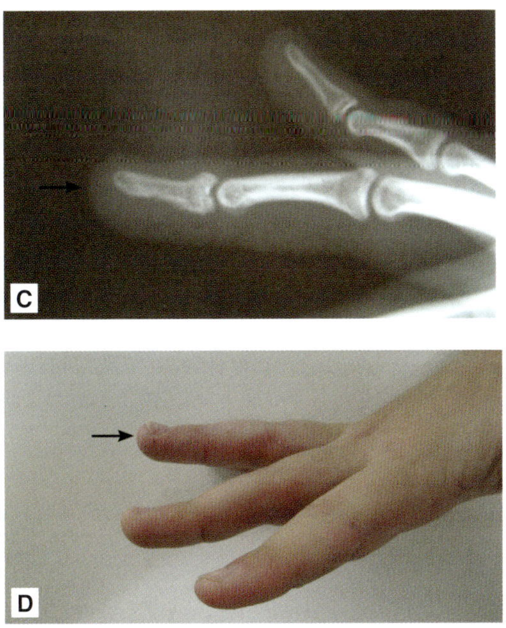

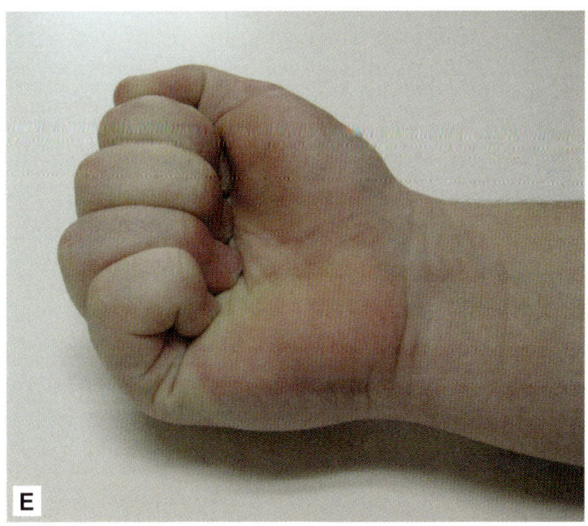

FIGURE 12-5 **A.** Lateral radiograph of bony mallet finger. **B.** Extension block pinning. **C.** Three months postoperative, healed fracture. **D.** Postoperative range of motion, extension. **E.** Postoperative range of motion, flexion.

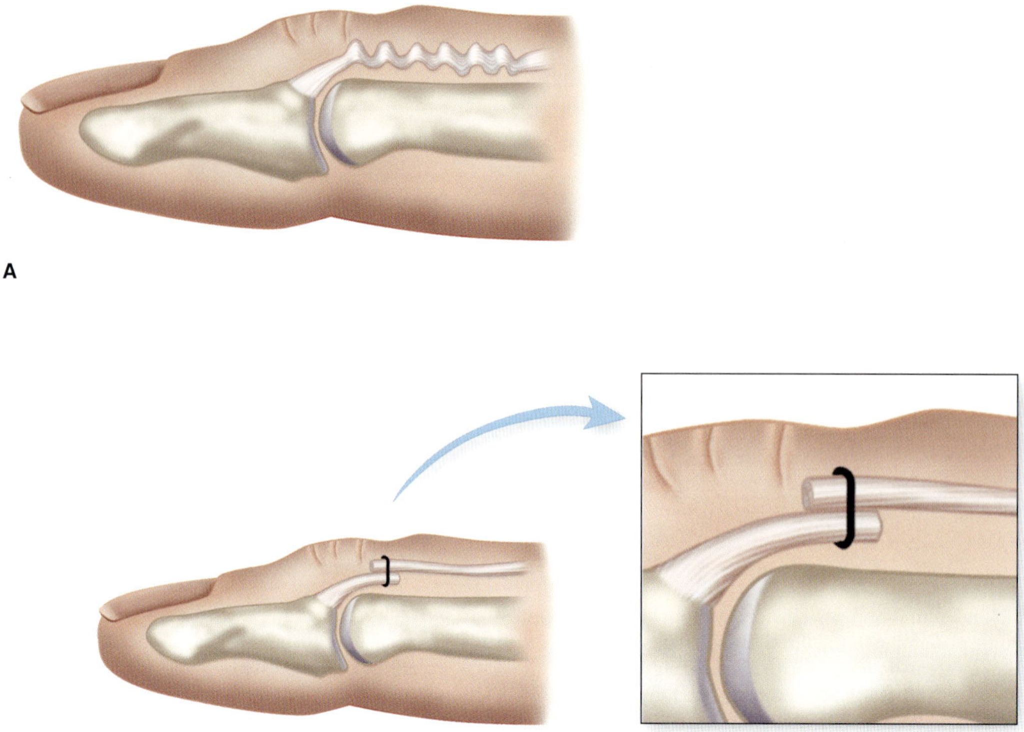

A

B

FIGURE 12-6 **A.** In a chronic mallet finger from a closed injury, the terminal tendon is present but lacks appropriate tension. **B.** The DIP joint is extended and pinned using a 0.045- or 0.035-in Kirschner wire. The terminal tendon is transected and imbricated with 1 or 2 horizontal mattress sutures.

Zones II and IV

Acute injuries: For these injuries, early surgical repair is recommended if more than 25% of the tendon is transected or the extensor mechanism is nonfunctional. For the flatter tendons in zones II and IV, we prefer the R-IHM suture using 4-0 FiberWire.[9] The technique begins with a simple running suture, starting along the "near" portion of the tendon and advancing away from the surgeon. After reaching the "far" portion of the tendon, the suture is brought back to the surgeon with a R-IHM (Figs. 12-1A and 12-2A). The suture needle is passed beneath the prior crossing suture, which locks each step of the mattress configuration. After finishing the last horizontal mattress throw, the suture is tied at the near end (Figs. 12-1B and 12-2B).

While we prefer to immobilize patients for 4 weeks before beginning extensor tendon motion protocols, the R-IHM suture is strong enough to allow early motion if required for other injuries (such as a concomitant flexor tendon injury that has been repaired).

Zone III—Central Slip

Acute injuries: For acute closed injuries, initial management consists of splinting the finger with the PIP in extension and the DIP free for 4 weeks. For open injuries, the central slip is repaired under direct visualization using a running suture or figure-of-8 suture configuration. If there is inadequate distal tendon, a bone suture anchor on the middle phalanx base may be used.

Chronic injuries: For chronic boutonniere deformities with flexible PIP motion, splinting is attempted to stretch the tight transverse retinacular ligaments. If splinting fails, there are many described surgical techniques to treat chronic deformities, such as the Curtis staged reconstruction.[4,15] In our experience, a customized "a la carte" approach can be taken, depending on the joint flexibility and degree of deformity present. Release of the tight transverse retinacular ligaments may be sufficient to rebalance the extensor/flexor mechanism at the PIP joint. Additionally, the triangular ligament can be effectively reconstructed by suturing the lateral bands together distal to the PIP joint (Fig. 12-7). The finger is then splinted with the PIP extended for 4 weeks with the DIP free.

If the lateral bands are sutured together proximal to the PIP joint, PIP flexion will be impeded.

Zone V—Sagittal Band

Acute injuries: For acute closed injuries, initial management consists of splinting the finger with the MP in extension

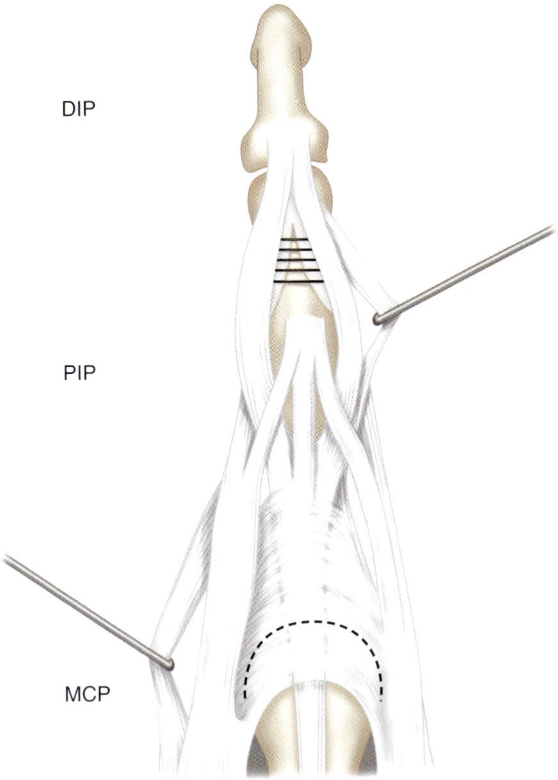

FIGURE 12-7 Reconstruction for chronic boutonniere finger. After the transverse retinacular ligaments are released and the lateral bands mobilized so they may be moved dorsally, the lateral bands are sutured together distal to the PIP joint. The suturing is started distally and after each suture, the finger is ranged to assure continued adequate ability to flex the PIP joint. The proper number of sutures is achieved when the lateral bands are dorsal to the axis of rotation at the PIP joint when the finger is extended, yet still allow for full PIP flexion.

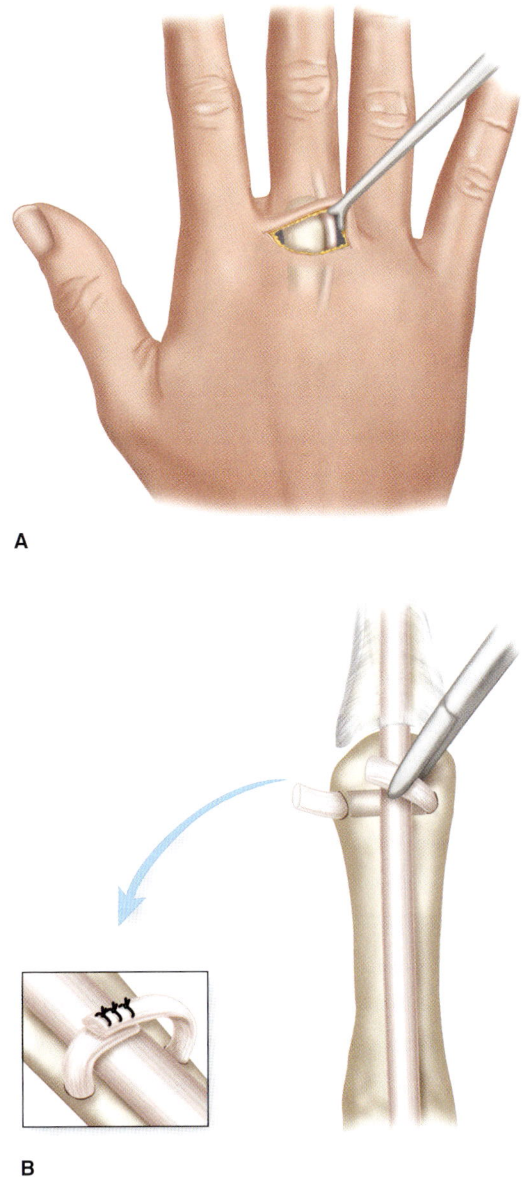

FIGURE 12-8 **A.** Skin incision and exposed subluxated extensor digitorum communis tendon. (Reprinted with permission from Kang and Carlson.[16] Copyright Elsevier.) **B.** Tendon graft in position within the bone tunnel. (Reprinted with permission from Kang and Carlson.[16] Copyright Elsevier.)

and the IP joints free for 4 weeks. For open injuries or those that fail attempted splint management, the sagittal bands are repaired under direct visualization using a running suture or figure-of-8 suture configuration.

Chronic injuries: For chronic injuries, a primary repair technique is preferred. However, if the local tissue is not amenable to repair or imbrication, we prefer the extensor tendon centralization technique described by Kang and Carlson.[16] Following a dorsal midline exposure to reveal the subluxated extensor tendon, a palmaris longus tendon graft (or other graft such as EIP or half flexor carpi radialis if palmaris longus is not present) is harvested if primary repair of the sagittal band cannot be performed. A transverse bone tunnel is created with a 1.6-mm drill bit at the level metacarpal head–neck junction (Fig. 12-8A). The palmaris longus graft is woven through the bone tunnel while the extensor tendon is held in a centralized position without ulnar or radial subluxation (Figs. 12-8B and 12-9A). Graft tension is checked by bringing the MP joint through a passive range of motion and ensuring that there is no ulnar or radial deviation of the extensor tendon. The newly created graft pulley is sutured using 3-0 braided nonabsorbable suture with a horizontal mattress configuration (Fig. 12-9B). Passive range of motion of the MP joint is checked to ensure that there is no tendon subluxation. Following hemostasis and skin closure, the MP joint is splinted in extension until the first postoperative visit.

The orientation of the drill bit for the bony tunnel should be customized based on the location of extensor tendon instability. Further sutures in the sagittal band may be necessary to "fine-tune" the tendon balancing.

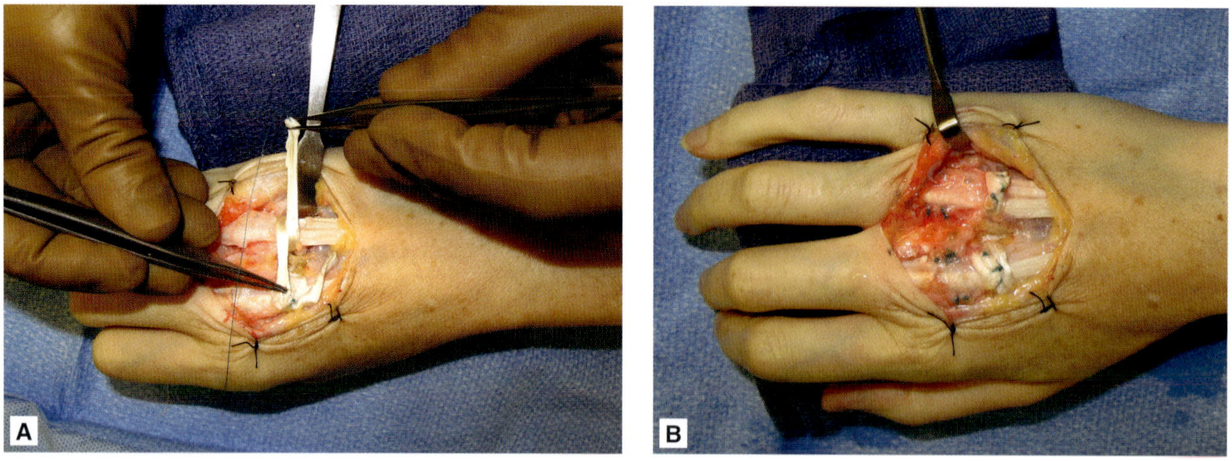

FIGURE 12-9 **A.** Extension pulley reconstruction, tendon through bone tunnel. **B.** Extension pulley reconstruction, status post reconstruction.

Zones VI, VII, VII, IX

Acute injuries: For the larger and more rounded tendons in zone VI, we prefer a modified Kessler technique to allow core suture placement. We prefer using a larger suture (such as a 3-0) for these tendons.

Chronic injuries: For chronic injuries in the more proximal zones, we use strategies similar to those employed for rheumatoid arthritis–related tendinopathy. If possible, we prefer tendon transfers to adjacent extensor tendons.

COMPLICATIONS

As reported in work of Newport et al from 1990, static immobilization intended to protect extensor tendon repair can have the unplanned effect of joint stiffness.[17] In their series of 62 patients who underwent 101 extensor tendon repairs and static splinting, more patients suffered from loss of flexion than from extensor lag, and those with distal injuries (zones III and IV) were more likely to experience joint stiffness.[3,17] The loss of flexion affects functionality more than loss of extension, as grip strength and the ability to grasp objects can be quite limited. Dynamic motion protocols have decreased the frequency of this complication.

The complications classically associated with tendon repairs are less common. Repair rupture is infrequent, with rates ranging from 0% to 8%.[17-21] While tenolysis rates reported in the literature range from 0% to 17%, all of the complications generally associated with extensor tendon repair have decreased since the implementation of early motion protocols and modern suturing techniques.[5,17,19,20]

OUTCOMES

The seminal work of Newport et al provides a strong base for a description of outcomes following extensor tendon repair.[17] Better outcomes were seen in more proximal zones (V-VIII) compared with distal injuries (I-IV). Less than 50% of patients who had distal injuries had good/excellent outcomes according to Miller's scoring system,[24] while 63% to 83% of those with proximal injuries had good/excellent results. The implementation of early controlled motion has improved outcomes, particularly for proximal injuries, with good to excellent outcomes exceeding 90%.[22-24] While the outcomes for zones III and IV remain less favorable, the results have improved with early motion protocols.[19,25-28]

REFERENCES

1. Clayton RA, Court-Brown CM. The epidemiology of musculoskeletal tendinous and ligamentous injuries. *Injury*. 2008;39:1338–1344.
2. Court-Brown CM, Caesar B. Epidemiology of adult fractures: a review. *Injury*. 2006;37:691–697.
3. Matzon JL, Bozentka DJ. Extensor tendon injuries. *J Hand Surg Am*. 2010;35:854–861.
4. Doyle JR. Extensor tendons—acute injuries. In: Green D, ed. *Operative Hand Surgery*. 4th ed. New York: Churchill Livingstone; 1999:195–198.
5. Newport ML, Pollack GR, Williams CD. Biomechanical characteristics of suture techniques in extensor zone IV. *J Hand Surg Am*. 1995;20:650–656.
6. Newport ML, Williams CD. Biomechanical characteristics of extensor tendon suture techniques. *J Hand Surg Am*. 1992;17:1117–1123.
7. Howard RF, Ondrovic L, Greenwald DP. Biomechanical analysis of four-strand extensor tendon repair techniques. *J Hand Surg Am*. 1997;22:838–842.
8. Woo SH, Tsai TM, Kleinert HE, Chew WY, Voor MJ. A biomechanical comparison of four extensor tendon repair techniques in zone IV. *Plast Reconstr Surg*. 2005;115:1674–1681 [discussion 1682–1683].
9. Lee SK, Dubey A, Kim BH, Zingman A, Landa J, Paksima N. A biomechanical study of extensor tendon repair methods: introduction to the running-interlocking horizontal mattress extensor tendon repair technique. *J Hand Surg Am*. 2010;35:19–23.
10. Elson RA. Rupture of the central slip of the extensor hood of the finger. A test for early diagnosis. *J Bone Joint Surg Br*. 1986;68:229–231.
11. Miller B, Dodds SD, deMars A, Zagoreas N, Waitayawinyu T, Trumble TE. Flexor tendon repairs: the impact of fiberwire on grasping and locking core sutures. *J Hand Surg Am*. 2007;32:591–596.
12. Ishiguro T, Itoh Y, Yabe Y, Hashizume N. Extension block with Kirschner wire for fracture dislocation of the distal interphalangeal joint. *Tech Hand Up Extrem Surg*. 1997;1:95–102.

13. Tetik C, Gudemez E. Modification of the extension block Kirschner wire technique for mallet fractures. *Clin Orthop Relat Res.* 2002;(404):284–290.
14. Hofmeister EP, Mazurek MT, Shin AY, Bishop AT. Extension block pinning for large mallet fractures. *J Hand Surg Am.* 2003;28:453–459.
15. Stark HH, Boyes JH, Wilson JN. Mallet finger. *J Bone Joint Surg Am.* 1962;44A:1061.
16. Kang L, Carlson MG. Extensor tendon centralization at the metacarpophalangeal joint: surgical technique. *J Hand Surg Am.* 2010;35:1194–1197.
17. Newport ML, Blair WF, Steyers CM Jr. Long-term results of extensor tendon repair. *J Hand Surg Am.* 1990;15:961–966.
18. Browne EZ Jr, Ribik CA. Early dynamic splinting for extensor tendon injuries. *J Hand Surg Am.* 1989;14:72–76.
19. Chow JA, Dovelle S, Thomes LJ, Ho PK, Saldana J. A comparison of results of extensor tendon repair followed by early controlled mobilisation versus static immobilisation. *J Hand Surg Br.* 1989;14:18–20.
20. Crosby CA, Wehbé MA. Early protected motion after extensor tendon repair. *J Hand Surg Am.* 1999;24:1061–1070.
21. Howell JW, Merritt WH, Robinson SJ. Immediate controlled active motion following zone 4–7 extensor tendon repair. *J Hand Ther.* 2005;18:182–190.
22. Sameem M, Wood T, Ignacy T, Thoma A, Strumas N. A systematic review of rehabilitation protocols after surgical repair of the extensor tendons in zones V-VIII of the hand. *J Hand Ther.* 2011;24:365–372 [quiz 373].
23. Newport ML, Tucker RL. New perspectives on extensor tendon repair and implications for rehabilitation. *J Hand Ther.* 2005;18:175–181.
24. Miller H. Repair of severed tendons of the hand and wrist. *Surg Gynecol Obstet.* 1942;74:693–698.
25. Hung LK, Chan A, Chang J, Tsang A, Leung PC. Early controlled active mobilization with dynamic splintage for treatment of extensor tendon injuries. *J Hand Surg Am.* 1990;15:251–257.
26. Saldana MJ, Choban S, Westerbeck P, Schacherer TG. Results of acute zone III extensor tendon injuries treated with dynamic extension splinting. *J Hand Surg Am.* 1991;16:1145–1150.
27. Walsh MT, Rinehimer W, Muntzer E, Patel J, Sitler MR. Early controlled motion with dynamic splinting versus static splinting for zones III and IV extensor tendon lacerations: a preliminary report. *J Hand Ther.* 1994;7:232–236.
28. Evans RB. Early active short arc motion for the repaired central slip. *J Hand Surg Am.* 1994;19:991–997.

13

Soft Tissue Coverage of the Hand

David J. Slutsky, MD

Protective sensibility is desirable when providing soft tissue coverage of the dorsum of the hand and palm, but critical sensibility of the digits is important for functional hand use. Moberg stated that precision sensory grip or tactile gnosis requires 2-point discrimination (2pd) of <6 mm, whereas gross sensory grip would be possible at 6 and 15 mm.[1] As a result, neurosensory flaps are commonly used. A neurosensory flap can therefore be considered to be an innervated flap that provides sensory feedback, either immediately or following a neurorrhaphy. Incorporating a cutaneous nerve in a skin flap provides a means for sensory innervation, and may also aid the flap circulation since the skin vascularity partly depends on the vessels around these nerves.[2] Noninnervated flaps may also acquire some degree of sensibility through peripheral innervation, but often to a lesser degree. Pedicled flaps have a number of advantages in comparison to free tissue transfers. The arterial supply is often more reliable, which simplifies postoperative monitoring and lends itself to outpatient procedures. Most of these flaps can be dissected under loupe magnification and permit early active motion, which is desirable in acute injuries. Microvascular technique may be of use, but it is not an absolute prerequisite. Finger flaps may be harvested from the same finger (homodigital) or an adjacent finger (heterodigital). Pedicled flaps may be antegrade or retrograde (reverse flow).

It is a good practice to add 10% to 15% more to both the length and size of the flap. Incorporating a small skin island along the vascular pedicle simplifies insetting and aids in avoiding skin bridges. Methods of salvaging a failing flap may include suture removal, leech therapy, or even conversion to a free flap. Some general contraindications to pedicled flaps include any cause of massive hand swelling such as crush-avulsion and wringer injuries, high-energy trauma, or prior arterial injury. Some pitfalls common to pedicled flaps include an inadequate arc of rotation, a short pedicle, vascular insufficiency due to tunneling, or inadequate flap size.

There are myriad pedicled flaps described for fingertip and thumb coverage. Flap selection will ultimately be based on the size of the defect, the requirements for sensibility, the surgeon's comfort level, and the patient profile such as gender, age, or systemic disease. A knowledge of the skin topography and flap anatomy is integral to the success of any flap.

HUESTON FLAP

This is a local transposition flap for fingertip skin loss that is pedicled on 1 neurovascular bundle. It was described by Hueston in 1966[3] and subsequently modified by Souquet and Souquet in 1986 to include both neurovascular bundles.[4]

Anatomy

The flap is an asymmetric arterial advancement flap based on either the radial or ulnar neurovascular bundle. It relies on cutaneous perforators from the digital artery. The flap is drained by the venae comitantes as well as the intact subdermal venous plexus. It receives its innervation from the proper digital nerve. The advancing free edge of the flap is initially insensate but regains sensibility with time. It has a range of advancement of 12 to 18 mm.

Indications

The flap is used to cover a loss of the pulp tissue of the fingers and thumb. It is indicated in situations where it is important to preserve bone length to diminish the risks of a hook nail deformity and where there is no possibility of distal replantation. The flap is homodigital and provides satisfactory texture for resurfacing fingertips. It is simple, reliable, and allows immediate finger motion.

Contraindications

The flap cannot be used with injury to a neurovascular bundle. It is not indicated when more than 18 mm of transposition is required.

Surgical Technique

The skin is advanced on the side of relatively less functional importance, such as the radial pulp of the thumb and small finger or the ulnar border of the middle digits. An L-shaped incision is made proximal to the fingertip defect. The longitudinal limb extends along the midlateral line while the transverse limb is placed in the metacarpophalangeal (MP) or proximal interphalangeal (PIP) flexion crease. The plane of dissection passes superficial to the neurovascular bundle that is closest to the midlateral incision. The contralateral neurovascular bundle is incorporated into the base of the flap, which is then advanced obliquely to cover the amputation stump. A proximally based triangle of skin raised along the longitudinal border of the flap can be rotated transversely to cover the donor site.

The flap can be modified by including both neurovascular bundles (Fig. 13-1A-C). This was thought to preserve the sensibility of the flap, at the expense of restricting some distal advancement. The longitudinal incision is made in the same manner as above, while the transverse incision is extended to the opposite midlateral line, ending with a back cut. The plane of dissection proceeds deep to both neurovascular bundles, which are incorporated into the skin flap. The flap is then advanced and inset as above.

Outcomes

In the series of Foucher et al of 43 flaps, 2pd averaged 7 mm in the standard Hueston flap (31 cases) and 6 mm with the modified flap (12).[5]

Complications

The palmar tension pulls on the nail matrix that causes a tendency toward a parrot beak nail deformity. This can be minimized by skewering the tip of the flap with a transfixing needle. The free edge of the flap can lead to a dog-ear deformity, which can be corrected by excising a segment of dorsal skin. Cold intolerance is common during the first year, and correlates with poorer return of sensation. Persistent fingertip sensitivity may occur due to neuroma formation. A contracture of the distal or PIP joint may result if there is excessive joint flexion during flap insetting.

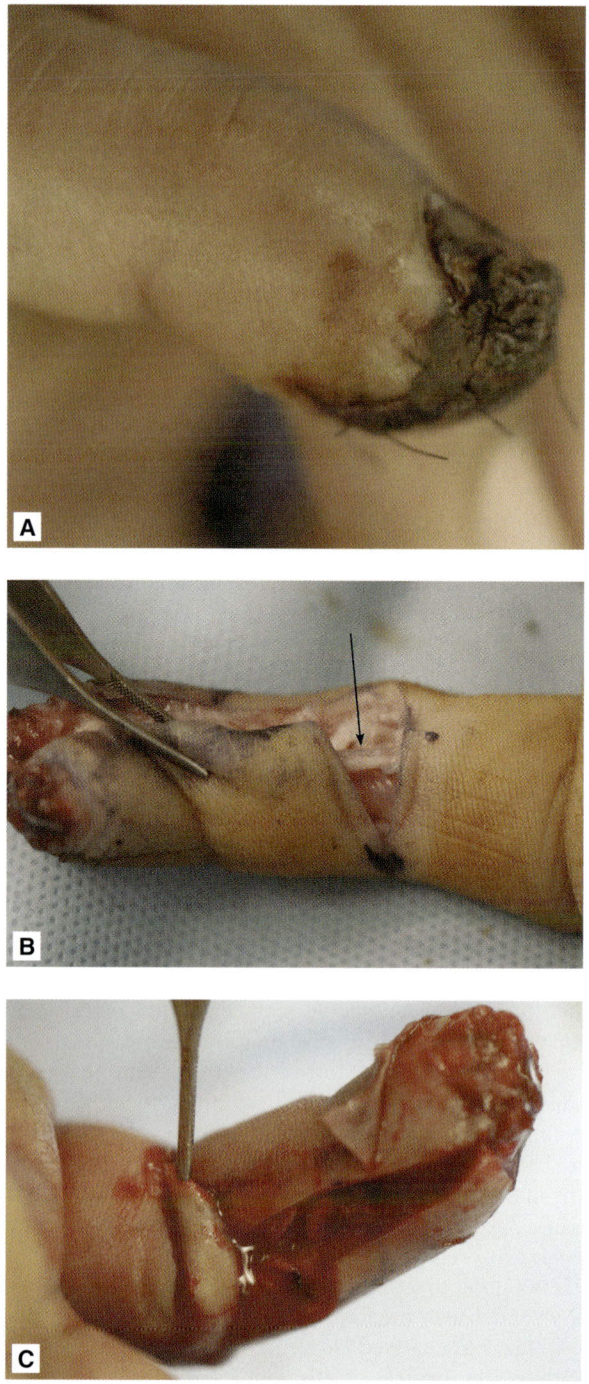

FIGURE 13-1 Modified Hueston flap. **A.** Necrosis of distal fingertip following a laceration. **B.** Note amount of advancement based on radial neurovascular bundle (arrow). **C.** A proximally based triangle of skin raised along the longitudinal border of the flap is rotated transversely to cover the exposed pedicles.

CROSS-FINGER FLAP

More than 60 years after its description, the cross-finger flap is still widely in use.[6] In cases where the dorsal digital networks cannot be used or when elaborate microsurgical procedures are not available, cross-finger flaps are still useful for finger coverage distal to the PIP joint. Sensory return, however, is unpredictable and can mar the ultimate functional result. The innervated cross-finger flap was developed to improve upon this by transferring the dorsal skin over the middle phalanx along with its sensory nerve. A neurorrhaphy is performed between this nerve and 1 of the severed digital nerve ends of the injured finger.

Anatomy

The initial blood supply of this random pattern flap comes from 1 of the paired dorsal branches arising from the palmer digital artery at the proximal one-third of the middle phalanx.[7] The venous drainage is initially from the venae comitantes and subdermal veins. The major dorsal branch of the superficial radial nerve (SRN) and the dorsal cutaneous branch of the ulnar nerve innervate the dorsum of the hand up to the level of the PIP joints. Distal to this, the dorsal skin is innervated by a dorsal sensory branch that arises from the proper digital nerve. This branch most commonly arises proximal to the PIP flexion crease. It then crosses superficial or deep to the digital artery to lie just above the extensor mechanism, innervating the dorsum of the middle phalanx. The arc of rotation of the cross-finger flap is short, since the skin is pedicled on the midlateral line of the finger. The flap is left attached to the donor finger until sufficient peripheral arterial and venous anastomoses have occurred, and then divided.

Indications

The cross-finger flap is indicated in cases of full-thickness loss of the entire pulp of an adjacent finger, especially with exposed bone or tendon. The long finger is used for coverage of the thumb pulp. It can be used for larger defects that may not be suitable for homodigital flaps. With the innervated flap, no additional donor finger denervation occurs because the dorsal sensory branch is ordinarily transected when elevating the standard cross-finger flap. Suturing this branch to the transected digital nerve in the recipient finger allows reinnervation without any need for cortical reorientation.

Contraindications

The cross-finger flap cannot be used when there is concomitant injury to adjacent digits. Flap innervation is not possible if there has been damage to either the dorsal sensory branch or the proximal digital nerve. Patient age greater than 40 years is a relative contraindication, due to the finger stiffness that results from 2 weeks of immobilization to an another digit.

Surgical Technique

The dissection is performed under tourniquet control. A pattern of the defect is outlined over the dorsum of the middle phalanx of an adjacent finger. Two transverse incisions delineate the proximal and distal extent of the flap. A longitudinal incision is then made on the side opposite the injured finger. The incision should not extend volar to the midlateral line to prevent a scar contracture. The dorsal sensory branch is isolated through a separate proximal incision that extends to the edge of the flap. The nerve is sectioned proximally, leaving a 1.5- to 2-cm tail. The flap is then elevated along with the nerve branch. The plane of dissection proceeds superficial to the paratenon of the extensor mechanism. The flap is dissected laterally to the opposite midlateral line, until it can be transposed without acute angulation.

The tourniquet is released ensuring flap viability. A full-thickness skin graft is placed over the donor site and secured with a tie-over bolster. The flap is transposed and inset so that the deep surface of the flap lies against the finger defect (Fig. 13-2A-D). For an innervated flap, the digital nerve end is isolated along the opposite border of the injured digit. An epineurial repair between the dorsal sensory nerve branch and the digital nerve stump is performed with 9-0 nylon. A finger spica splint or bulky dressing is applied to prevent tension on the suture sites. At the time of flap division 2 weeks later, no special care for the nerve repair is necessary since the nerve junction is on the side opposite the flap base.

Lassner et al have used a bilaterally innervated sensory cross-finger flap.[8] First, the contralateral dorsal sensory branch is elevated with the flap at the PIP joint level, and sutured to the digital nerve end on the far side of the injured finger. After 3 weeks, when the pedicle is dissected, the remaining dorsal sensory branch is dissected and sutured to the remaining digital nerve of the injured finger. Because the regenerative distance is only 1.5 to 2 cm, there is excellent sensory reinnervation, with 2pd ranging from 2 to 6 mm. Gaul described an innervated cross-finger flap from the index that provides immediate sensation for resurfacing volar defects of the thumb.[9] The flap is transferred along with the dorsoradial digital nerve to the index, which is a continuation of the major dorsal branch of the SRN. This sensory branch is mobilized at the same time the cross-finger flap is transposed, and transferred subcutaneously to lie under the volar skin envelope of the thumb. In an effort to improve the ultimate sensibility, Hastings modified this index finger flap by turning it into a dual innervated flap (Fig. 13-3A-D).[10] The superficial radial sensory nerve is mobilized and transposed as above. The dorsal sensory branch of the proper radial digital nerve of the index is then sutured to the severed end of the radial digital nerve of thumb. Sensory reinnervation is reported to be rapid and does not require cortical reorientation.

A reversed cross-finger flap can be used to cover a dorsal digital defect. This is done by de-epithelializing the dorsal aspect of the cross-finger flap, which can then be transposed to cover the dorsum of an adjacent digit. The donor site is then skin grafted (Fig. 13-5A-C).

Outcomes

In 1 series of innervated cross-finger flaps, 7/8 patients achieved an average 2pd of 4.8 mm as compared with non-innervated cross-finger flaps in whom patients achieved a mean value of 9 mm.[11]

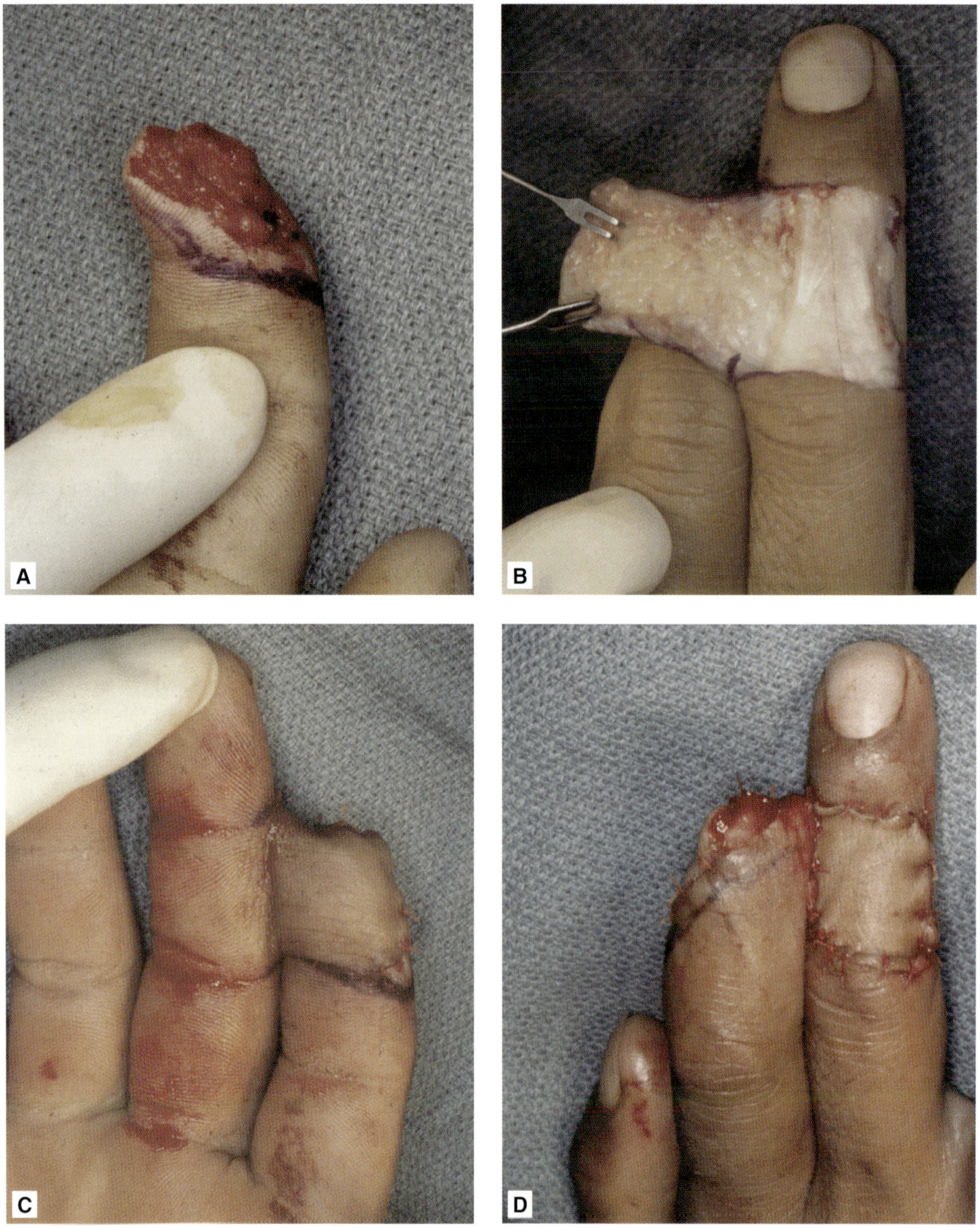

FIGURE 13-2 Cross-finger flap. **A.** Fingertip saw injury. **B.** Pedicled cross-finger flap. **C.** Insetting of flap. **D.** Skin graft of donor-site defect.

Complications

Joint stiffness is common. The flap may be hair bearing. Donor finger morbidity includes poor skin graft color match and a visible contour deformity. If only 1 digital nerve anastomosis is performed, a painful neuroma may develop from the unrepaired digital nerve stump. The functional outcome of the radial sensory innervated cross-finger flap is compromised in some patients by double sensitivity. In this case, sensation from the ulnar side of the flap is interpreted as arising from the dorsum of the index finger, whereas sensation on the radial side of the flap is interpreted as coming from the thumb. Sensory testing shows that after transfer to the thumb, the ulnar side of the flap still receives its innervation from the superficial sensory branch of the radial nerve.

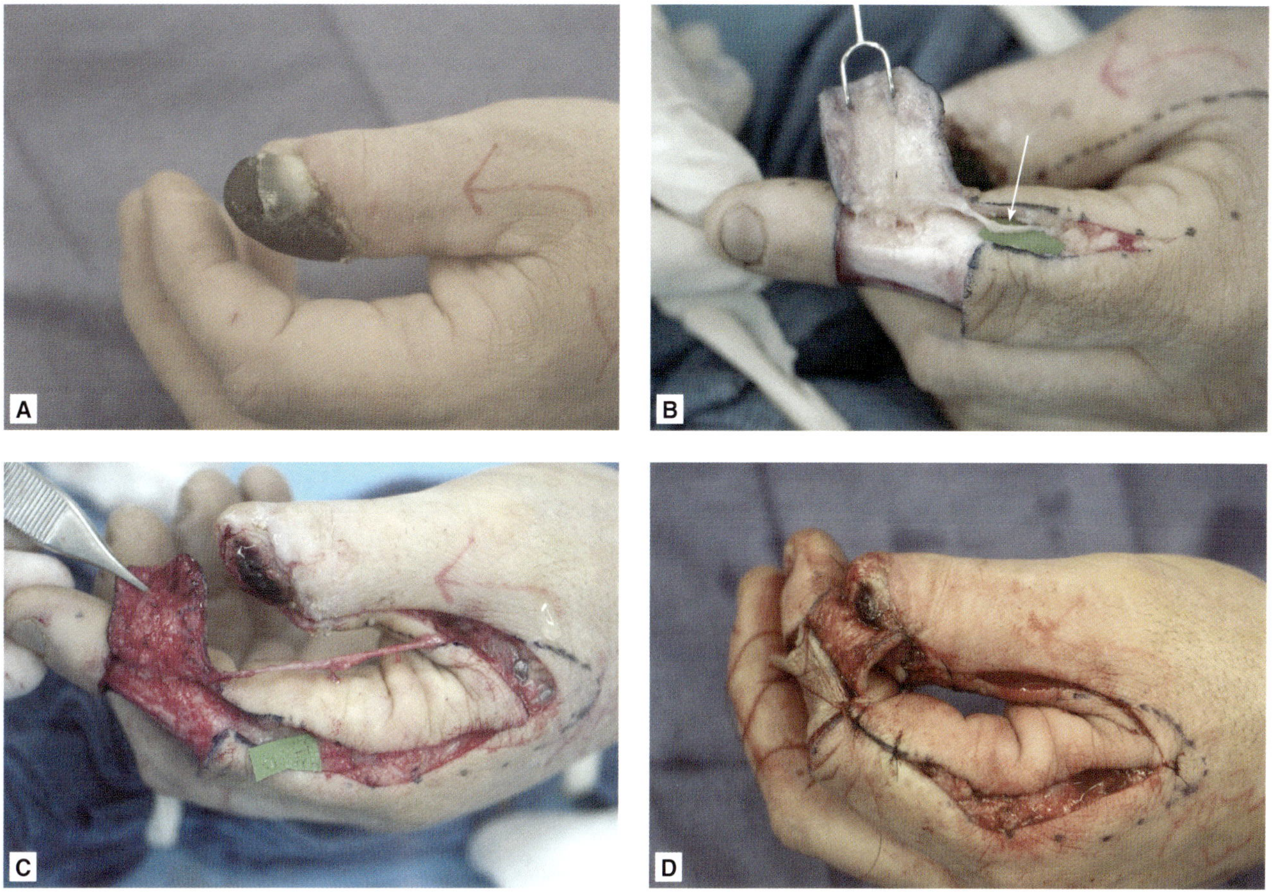

FIGURE 13-3 Dual innervated cross-finger flap. **A.** Full-thickness skin necrosis of distal thumb. **B.** Elevation of cross-finger flap incorporating the radial sensory branch (arrow). **C.** Mobilization of superficial radial nerve (SRN). **D.** After transposition of the SRN.

REVERSED DIGITAL ARTERY FLAP

The reversed digital artery (RDA) flap described in 1986 by Kojima et al is used for 1-stage reconstruction of finger pulp defects.[12] The flap can be innervated by including the dorsal sensory nerve branch.

Anatomy

The RDA flap is harvested from the dorsolateral skin of the proximal phalanx, which derives its blood supply from the opposite digital artery through abundant communicating branches. There are 3 transverse palmar arches connecting the radial and ulnar digital arteries. The proximal and middle arches are always in association with the limbs of the C1 and C3 pulleys (Fig. 13-4). The distal arch lies just beyond the insertion of the profundus tendon.[13]

When the proximal digital artery is ligated, the blood crosses over from the opposite digital artery through the middle and distal transverse palmar arches. The blood then flows down the ligated artery in a retrograde fashion. The RDA flap is designed over the dorsolateral area of the proximal phalanx, which is nourished by a proximal dorsal cutaneous branch. This small branch, 0.3 to 0.6 mm in size, arises from the palmar digital artery at the midpoint of the proximal phalanx. It passes through Cleland's ligament, running close to the bone, and emerges on the dorsal aspect of the finger. Histological studies have revealed the presence of venules and capillaries in the perivascular fat tissue that appear to represent adequate channels for venous drainage.

The dorsal sensory nerve branch can be harvested with the skin flap. In the border digits the terminal branches of the SRN or dorsal cutaneous branch of the ulnar nerve can also be transferred. The arc of rotation is around the midpoint of the middle phalanx, which allows the flap to easily reach the fingertip. The digital artery cannot be elevated beyond the middle phalanx for fear of disrupting the distal transverse arch.

Indications

This flap is indicated for coverage of acute and chronic fingertip defects (Fig. 13-5A-C). It can be used for fingertip reconstruction to correct a hook nail deformity. Some authors recommend the RDA flap for coverage of large

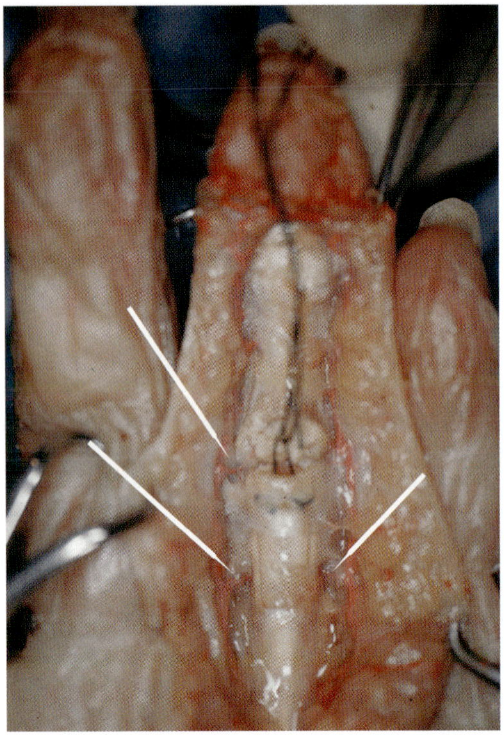

FIGURE 13-4 Cadaver dissection demonstrating the transverse palmar arches connecting the radial and ulnar digital arteries (arrows).

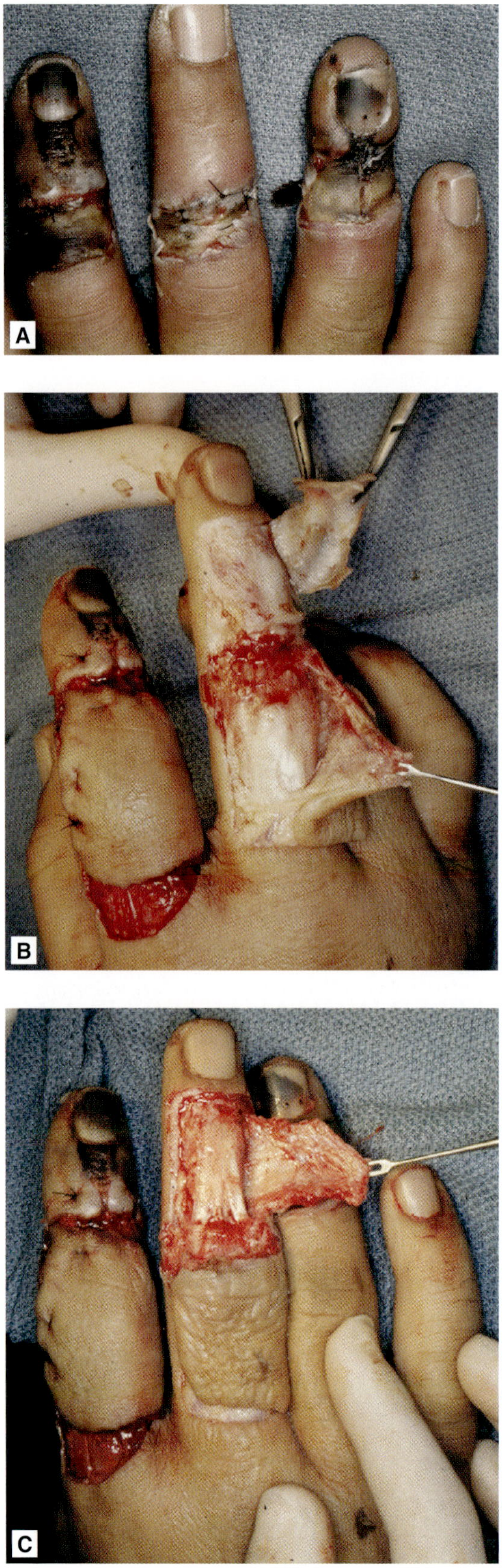

FIGURE 13-5 Reversed cross-finger flap. **A.** Full-thickness burn to dorsum of ring finger. **B.** De-epithelialization of middle phalanx. **C.** De-epithelialized skin is rotated 90° to cover dorsum of ring finger.

defects of the dorsal aspects of the middle and distal phalanx, which cannot be covered with other local digital sensory flaps. It may also be useful following release of volar scar contractures of the fingers. Neurorrhaphy between the dorsal sensory branch and the terminal digital nerve allows for flap innervation through the normal anatomic pathway, so that cortical misinterpretation can be avoided.

Contraindications

A disadvantage of this procedure is that it sacrifices a digital artery, and a nerve repair is required. The RDA flap cannot be used if there is only 1 patent digital artery, or if there has been an injury to the distal transverse palmar arch.

Surgical Technique

A digital Allen test with or without Doppler is used to ascertain that both digital arteries are intact. Under tourniquet control, the injured tip is debrided and a pattern of the defect is outlined over the proximal phalanx. The flap margins are incised and elevated, including the subcutaneous tissue and the digital artery. The dorsal sensory branch is identified and divided 10 mm proximal to the flap margin. A midlateral incision is then made from the distal flap margin, as far as the midpoint of the middle phalanx. The artery is separated from the digital nerve, leaving as much surrounding fat as possible for venous drainage.

A microvascular clamp is applied to the digital artery proximal to the skin flap while the tourniquet is released to check the circulation of both the finger and the flap. The proximal artery is then divided and elevated to the midportion of the middle phalanx. The skin island is rotated 180° into the fingertip defect, taking care to avoid kinking the pedicle. Leaving a tail on the flap or skin grafting the pedicle can avoid arterial compression. The dorsal sensory nerve branch is sutured to the recipient nerve prior to insetting. Donor-site defects up to 2 × 3 cm can be closed primarily. Flaps up to 5 × 2 cm can be harvested.

Lai et al described an extended RDA flap in which the dorsal skin over the MP joint may be included. This skin extension is a fasciocutaneous flap that survives on the rich anastomosis between the first dorsal metacarpal artery (FDMA) and the digital artery near the metacarpal head. Lai et al noted that the sensory recovery of this skin extension was relatively poor.[14] In an effort to overcome this, both the dorsal sensory branch from the proper digital nerve and the superficial sensory branch from the corresponding radial or ulnar nerve are sectioned at their proximal ends and included with the RDA flap. For bilaterally innervated flaps, these branches are sutured to both digital nerve ends. Static 2pd of 5 mm was obtained in the series of Lai et al of 3 patients.

In cases where 1 of the digital arteries has been injured, an innervated RDA cross-finger flap harvested from the proximal phalanx of the adjacent finger can be used to cover defects of the middle and distal phalanges. A piece of skin graft is placed over the pedicle, which is divided at 2 weeks. In situations in which the fingertip pulp is lost completely some authors have included the proper digital nerve in the pedicle that is then sutured to the stump of the opposite proper digital nerve.

Outcomes

In a study of 120 fingers, the mean values for 2pd range between 6 and 10 mm.[15] Noninnervated flaps have also been reported to regain <10 mm of 2pd sensation.[16]

Complications

Flap edema secondary to impaired venous drainage from kinking of the pedicle, or due to an inadequate amount of perivascular fat for venous drainage, is common. The flap tends to be bulky if applied over subcutaneous tissue rather than bone. Skin grafting the pedicle at the distal interphalangeal joint may be necessary. Inadequate finger perfusion occurring when the digital artery proximal to the island flap is clamped may preclude use of this flap. Numbness over the dorsum of the middle phalanx due to transection of the dorsal sensory branch may be bothersome. If the margin of the flap extends volar to the midaxial line, a PIP flexion contracture can develop. Cold intolerance is a risk, especially for outdoor workers in cold climates.

DORSAL THUMB FLAPS

The arterial supply of the thumb is quite different from that of the fingers. The direct- or reverse-flow volar island flaps centered on only 1 arterial pedicle that have been described for the fingers are not possible for the thumb. Through their anatomic studies, Brunelli et al discovered a consistent artery along the dorsoulnar aspect of the thumb that they used as the basis for a reverse pedicled skin flap.[17] They simultaneously described a pedicled flap based on a dorsoradial artery. The flaps can be innervated by incorporating the terminal branches of the SRN and can be used for coverage of distal thumb defects. The flaps provide satisfactory texture for resurfacing the prehensile surfaces and they are homodigital, which allows immediate thumb motion. Because of the distal nature of their pedicle, the flaps can easily reach the tip of the thumb. Primary closure of the donor site is possible for smaller flaps.

Anatomy

The princeps pollicis artery divides into 2 palmer digital arteries at the level of the MP flexion crease. As a consequence, any pedicled flap of the thumb that is based on the palmar arteries has a short pedicle. This would require marked IP joint flexion in order to prevent undue tension on the princeps pollicis. The dorsal arteries of the fingers are extremely segmental, inconstant, and dependent on palmar anastomoses. In the thumb there is a constant dorsoulnar artery that originates from the palmar arteries at the neck of the thumb metacarpal and runs along the dorsoulnar side of the thumb. It may be as large as 0.1 mm and travels superficially within the subcutaneous tissue, above the aponeurosis. The dorsoulnar artery is reinforced by an anastomosis with the palmer digital artery at the neck of the proximal phalanx, approximately 2.3 cm from the nail fold. The artery terminates in a dorsal arcade within 0.7 mm of the nail. Venae comitantes can be present when the artery is of a large size (about 50% of cases). In the remaining cases, venous drainage is mostly based on tiny venules in the perivascular fatty tissue. The terminal sensory branch of the SRN is located 1 to 2 cm from the median axis of the thumb.

Moschella et al also identified a similar, but less constant and smaller artery that may be found 72% of the time along the dorsoradial aspect of the thumb.[18] The dorsoradial artery arises from the radial artery at the level of the anatomic snuffbox and passes palmar to the extensor pollicis brevis tendon. It then travels subcutaneously along the radial side of the thumb adjacent to a SRN branch and remains at an average distance of approximately 1 cm from the medial axis. This artery consistently communicates with the palmar vessels near the middle third of the proximal phalanx. In their study, the dorsoradial artery communicated with the nail matrix arcade of vessels in only 4/25 cadaver dissections; hence, a reverse-flow flap cannot be pedicled past the middle portion of the proximal phalanx (Fig. 13-6A-C).

Indications

Dorsal thumb flaps are indicated for reconstruction of extensive loss of the thumb pulp. They can be used for coverage of amputation stumps at the IP joint level or for coverage of dorsal skin loss over the proximal and distal phalanx. The flap provides satisfactory texture for resurfacing fingertips and is homodigital that allows immediate thumb motion. Because of the distal nature of its pedicle, the flap can easily reach the tip of the thumb. Innervated flaps can be used to resurface posttraumatic painful neuromas at the thumb tip. Primary closure of the donor site is possible for smaller flaps.

Contraindications

The flaps cannot be used with injury to the princeps pollicis or digital arteries. It is also contraindicated when there is a significant soft tissue injury at the base of the thumb.

Surgical Technique

THE DORSOULNAR THUMB FLAP

According to Brunelli et al, the flap can be pedicled distally at 2 levels, which determines the arc of rotation. It can be pedicled at the dorsal nail fold arcade for cases of distal amputation, or for loss of palmar or dorsal tissue. Dissection of the pedicle must be limited to 1 cm from the nail base.

When used for more proximal amputation stumps, it is pedicled on the palmar anastomosis at the neck of the proximal phalanx. In this case, the dissection should be limited to 2.5 cm from the nail base.

The following points are first marked on the skin: (1) the dorsal arcade of the proximal nail fold, 0.9 cm proximal to the nail base; (2) the palmar anastomosis at the level of the neck of the proximal phalanx, 2.5 cm proximally; (3) the course of the dorsoulnar artery, 1 cm from the median axis of the thumb at the level of the neck of the proximal phalanx (Fig. 13-7A-D). The flap dimensions are then marked out on the dorsoulnar aspect of the MP joint, centered over the dorsoulnar artery. The flap is raised in a proximal to distal direction. The terminal sensory branch of the radial nerve is located and divided 2 cm from the proximal flap edge. A midlateral incision is then extended along the ulnar side of the thumb connecting to the distal area of soft tissue loss. This incision is very superficial in order to avoid damaging the arterial pedicle. Two dermoepidermis skin flaps are raised in a dorsal and palmar direction starting from the ulnar incision, taking care not to harm the subcutaneous tissue. A 1-cm-wide, full-thickness strip of subcutaneous tissue is harvested en bloc, centered around the arterial axis of the flap, leaving the extensor aponeurosis in situ. The flap artery may be quite small and is not directly isolated during harvesting to avoid damage. Care should be taken to avoid any tension or compression where the subcutaneous pedicle is reflected on itself.

An adipofascial extension of the proximal flap allows primary closure of the donor site and avoids tightness of the

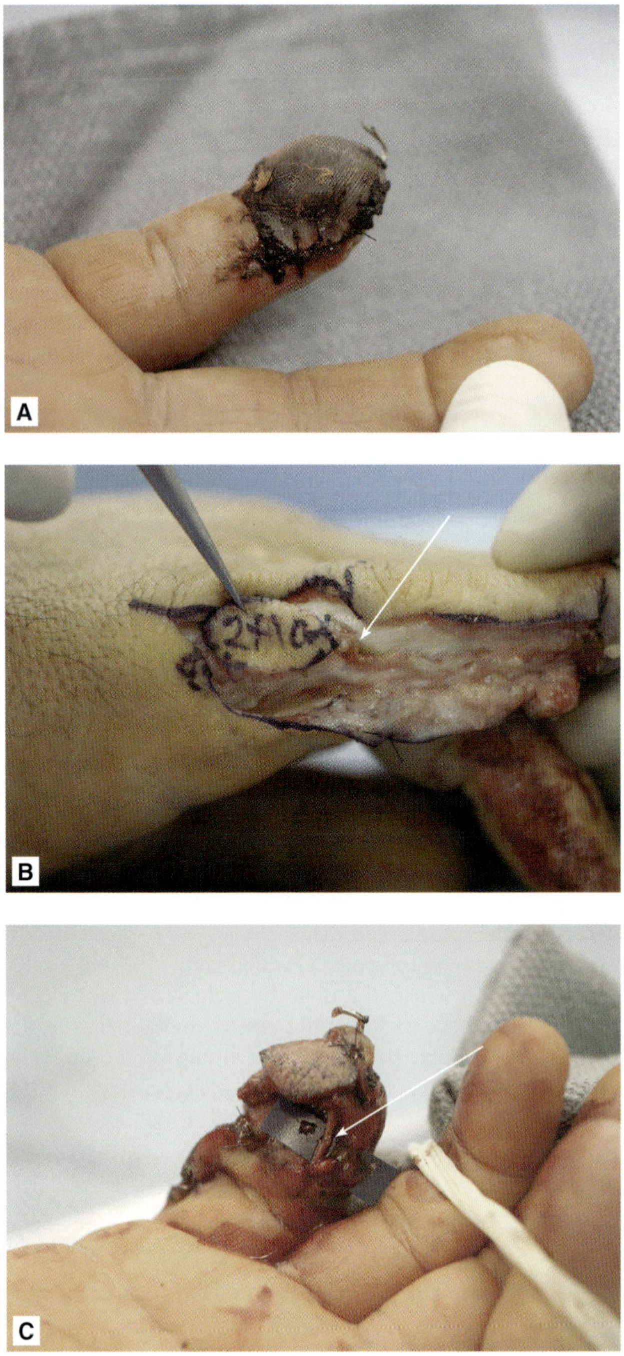

FIGURE 13-6 **A.** Full-thickness necrosis of distal small finger following a crush injury. **B.** Elevation of a 2 × 1 cm skin flap pedicled on the ulnar digital artery (arrow). The ulnar digital nerve is left undisturbed. **C.** Transposition of the flap to cover the distal pulp. A neurorrhaphy is performed between the dorsal sensory branch incorporated in the skin flap and the terminal cut end of the radial digital nerve (white arrow).

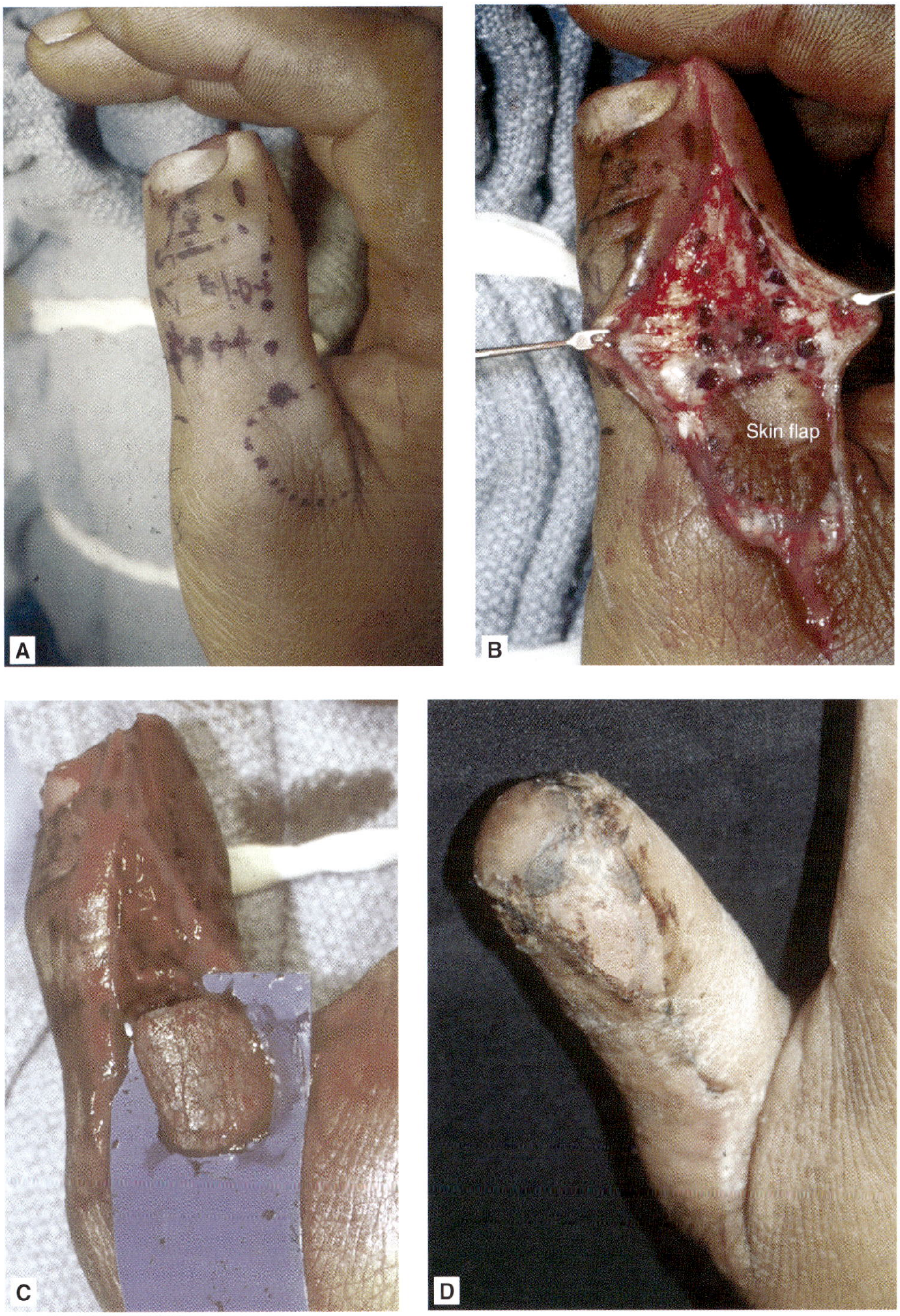

FIGURE 13-7 **A.** Skin markings for dorsoulnar thumb flap. **B.** Fascial pedicle outlined over dorsoulnar artery. **C.** Skin flap elevated. **D.** Good color match and contour of distal thumb at 3 weeks.

first web and reduced MCP joint motion. This extension and the pedicle are covered by a split-thickness graft to avoid vascular compromise.

The flap can be used as a cross-finger variant for coverage of skin loss of the fingers. Any part of the hand is accessible to this flap based on the distal end of a mobile thumb. The temporary pedicle, composed of a 1-cm-wide band of skin and subcutaneous tissue, is divided at 15 days after a clamping test confirms that the flap has become autonomous.

The dorsoulnar artery sends several periosteal and osseous branches to the neck of the first metacarpal. Vascularized bone from the metacarpal neck can be harvested with a reversed pedicled dorsoulnar skin flap for reconstruction of combined skin and bone defects of the distal phalanx.[19]

THE DORSORADIAL THUMB FLAP

The course of the dorsoradial artery of the thumb is identified by Doppler ultrasound the course of the dorsal radial digital artery from the snuffbox to the middle point of the proximal phalanx. The expected pivot point of the flap on the middle third of the radial aspect of the proximal phalanx is marked. The arc of rotation of the flap allows soft tissue coverage of palmar or dorsal aspects of distal thumb as well as soft tissue defects along the radial side of the proximal and distal phalanx. The dissection is performed under loupe magnification using tourniquet control. The skin island is drawn approximately 10% greater than the defect and centered over the course of the dorsoradial artery over the thumb metacarpal. Flaps as large as 5 × 4 cm can be harvested. A 1-cm strip of subcutaneous tissue is included to provide venous outflow and to avoid kinking of the pedicle. No attempt is made to visualize the artery. A cutaneous tail is included in the proximal margin of the flap in order to avoid tunneling, and to facilitate skin closure after rotation of the flap. The dissection halts at the level of the pivot point at the midportion of the proximal phalanx, and then the flap is rotated 180° and inserted into the defect. Raising the flap with a wide base near the pivot point protects the anastomosis with the palmar vessels and avoids kinking of the pedicle. The skin island is incised down to the level of the paratenon and the flap is raised in the plane immediately dorsal to the paratenon in a proximal to distal direction. The tourniquet is released at this point to assess the flap perfusion.

In order to innervate the flap a branch of the SRN can be elevated with the skin flap and coapted with the distal termination of the palmer radial digital nerve.

If the donor site cannot be closed primarily, a full-thickness skin graft is applied. Because of the risk of flap edema, any remaining skin bridge between the defect and the pivot point is incised to prevent pressure on the flap pedicle. The skin above the pedicle must not be under any tension. To avoid compression of the pedicle, the wound is left partially open or the pedicle is skin grafted. The donor site can be closed primarily with flaps up to 4 × 3 cm. Unlike the dorsoulnar flap, hair growth is rare on the radial side of the thumb. There is no risk of a first web contracture from harvesting the skin flap. Postoperatively, the thumb is immobilized in a finger spica splint for 2 weeks, followed by thumb motion.

Outcomes

Brunelli et al reported their experience with 32 dorsoulnar thumb flaps.[17] In 25 cases this flap was used for distal skin loss coverage (palmar or dorsal) of the thumb as an island flap. In 7 cases it was used for reconstruction of the finger pulp (5 index and 2 middle fingers) in the form of a cross-finger flap. There was no significant difference in sensibility between innervated and noninnervated flaps that ranged from 10 mm of 2pd to protective sensibility.

The same group separately reported their experience with the use of the homodigital dorsoradial flap in 16 patients to repair distal thumb defects.[18] The flap size ranged from 2 × 2 to 5 × 4 cm. In 3 cases, there was venous congestion that resolved by removing the sutures over the pedicle. Partial necrosis of the distal 4 mm in 1 patient healed spontaneously. All the other flaps survived completely. The donor site was closed primarily in 14/16 patients. The final results were good for reliability, coverage, and from an aesthetic point of view for both the reconstructed area and the donor site. Full thumb flexion and extension was maintained. In pulp reconstruction (9 patients), there was a good recovery of sensibility with 2pd ranging from 7 to 11 mm (mean 9.7 mm). Only 1 flap was innervated, without any apparent improvement in the ultimate 2pd.

Li et al used this flap in 12 cases with a soft tissue defect along with exposed bone at the distal thumb.[20] Ten flaps were pedicled distally at the proximal rotation point, 2.5 cm proximal to the cuticle. Two flaps were pedicled distally at the distal rotation point, 1.0 cm proximal to the cuticle. The flaps harvested in this study were 1.1 × 1.3 to 1.8 × 2.5 cm. All the flaps survived. At a follow-up of 2 to 14 months the appearance of the thumbs was satisfactory, save for 2 bulky distally based flaps. In 6 cases a finger pulp defect was repaired, with 2pd ranging from 8 to 10 mm. Thumb IP motion was equal to the opposite side in all cases.

Complications

Raising the flap proximal to the MP joint may exclude the nutrient artery, resulting in flap failure. Harvesting the terminal radial sensory nerve branch of the thumb leads to sensory loss over the dorsum of the thumb, and could result in neuroma formation. Harvesting the skin from the dorsoulnar aspect of the thumb MP can result in a restriction of MP motion along with a decrease in the first web space span. The donor area is hair bearing and debulking of the flap may be necessary due to overlap of the pedicle.

FIRST DORSAL METACARPAL ARTERY FLAP

This is a fasciocutaneous flap first described by Holevich in 1963.[21] It was modified and used as a neurosensory island flap by Foucher and Braun in 1979.[22] It is based on the FDMA or its dorsal digital branches. It is innervated by terminal sensory branches of the SRN.

Anatomy

The FDMA arises from the radial artery just distal to the extensor pollicis longus tendon, before the artery dives between the 2 heads of the first dorsal interosseous (FDI) muscle (Fig. 13-8A). The FDMA typically measures 1.2 to 1.5 mm in diameter. There is usually more than 1 accompanying vein. The artery runs superficial to the FDI fascia and divides into 3 terminal branches: a radial (FDMAr), ulnar

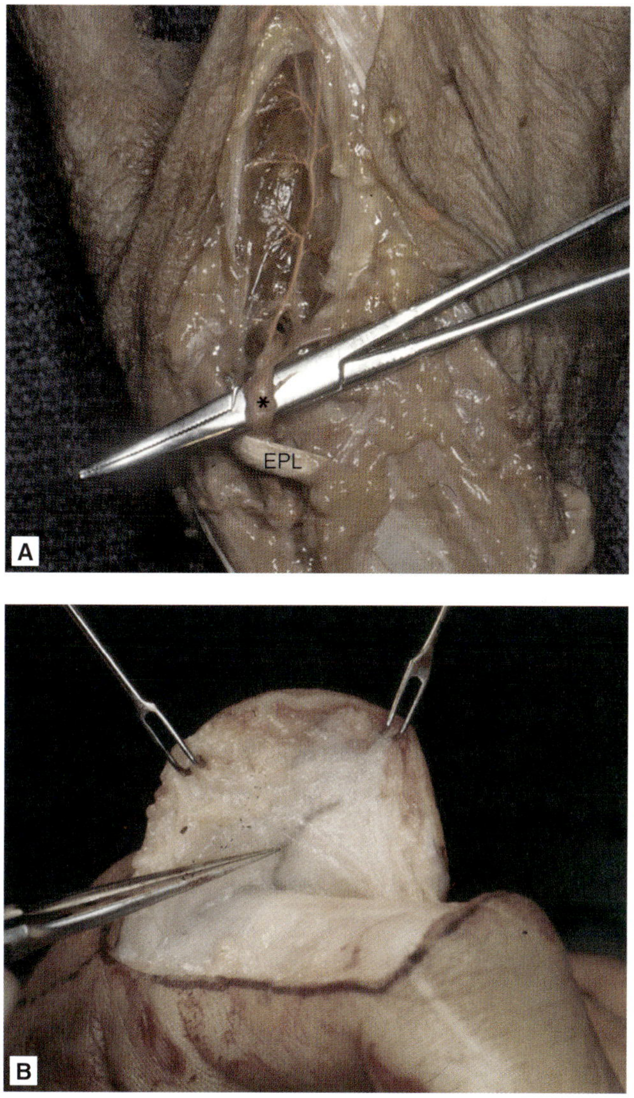

FIGURE 13-8 **A.** Cadaver injection studies demonstrating the origin of the first dorsal metacarpal artery (FDMA) from the radial artery (*). **B.** Demonstration of the FDMAu that terminates in a plexus over the dorsal fascia of the index.

(FDMAu), and intermediate branch. The radial branch runs along the thumb metacarpal and becomes or anastomoses with the dorsoulnar artery. The ulnar branch runs along the index metacarpal up to the MP joint, giving branches to the periosteum and adjacent extensor tendons. It terminates in a plexus over the dorsal fascia of the index (Fig. 13-8B). The intermediate branch runs toward the first web space and anastomoses with branches from the other 2. The flap is based on either the radial or ulnar branch of the FDMA. A proximally based flap is rotated around the point of origin of the artery at the base of the FDI space. The arc of rotation can include the palmar or dorsal thumb, wrist, and palm to the third metacarpal.

The venous drainage is that of the accompanying superficial veins. The superficial branch of the radial nerve becomes subcutaneous after it leaves the brachioradialis, and then bifurcates into 2 major branches 4 cm proximal to the styloid. Both branches pass radial to Lister's tubercle. The major palmar branch passes over the first dorsal wrist compartment, and then continues distally to become the dorsoradial digital nerve of the thumb. The major dorsal branch also bifurcates into the dorsoulnar digital nerve to the thumb and the dorsoradial digital nerve to the index, which supplies the adjacent sides of the second web space.

Indications

The FDMA is indicated for resurfacing either volar or dorsal defects of the distal thumb as far distal as the IP joint. It can be used to cover the ulnar surface of the dorsum of the hand and the wrist, or the palm up to the third metacarpal. The FDMA flap is useful for first web space reconstruction following contracture and it can provide soft tissue coverage of the index finger up to the level of the proximal phalanx. Some of the advantages of this flap are its variable size, stability, and pliability. It provides innervated skin with no major donor-site morbidity. Its elevation does not sacrifice a major artery. It can be transferred as a pedicled flap or an island flap. The innervated FDMA flap allows immediate postoperative mobilization and the avoidance of a nerve repair. It restores sensibility, particularly in the older patient.

Contraindications

The flap cannot be used with radial artery injury in the snuffbox. If the skin overlying the first web space is included in the flap, skin grafting the donor-site defect may lead to a secondary contracture. The arterial pedicle is difficult to dissect. The flap is at risk of partial necrosis if pedicled on a nondominant branch.

Surgical Technique

PEDICLED FLAP

A Doppler probe may be used to check the pulse of the FDMAr and FDMAu against the first and second metacarpals. The flap is drawn over the dorsum of the index, thumb, or back of the hand according to the skin defect. Under tourniquet the flap is raised from distal to proximal, in the areolar plane over the extensor paratenon. The skin incision is continued along the radial aspect of the index metacarpal to include a large subcutaneous vein in the pedicle. At the second metacarpal neck a large perforator is consistently present and should be ligated. The entire interosseous fascia over the FDI is included to avoid a meticulous dissection of the pedicle, and to avoid raising the flap on a nondominant branch. A small cuff of muscle of the FDI may be included to ensure the artery is included in the pedicle. Either the major palmar or dorsal branch of the SRN is incorporated into the flap. The fascia is released from the metacarpal until the flap can reach the defect. If the flap is used for first web reconstruction, the interosseous fascia is released from both the thumb and index metacarpals. The flap is enlarged ulnarly toward the third metacarpal so that the skin extension lies on the first web space, avoiding a first web contracture.

ISLAND FLAPS

The flap is pedicled on the FDMAu when used to cover defects over the volar surface of the distal thumb (Fig. 13-9A-C). Alternatively, the dorsal skin over the proximal phalanx of the thumb, which is supplied by the FDMAr, can resurface the radial side of the index. The flap is outlined over the dorsum of the index proximal phalanx. A proximal longitudinal incision is made over the FDI muscle. The flap is elevated starting distally, developing the plane between the subcutaneous tissue and the extensor tendon paratenon up to the level of the MP joint. The dorsoradial branch of the SRN is harvested with the skin island. The subdermal fascia can be quite thin; hence, care is taken to preserve its continuity with the FDI fascia. Inclusion of a small strip of extensor hood along the radial aspect of the extensor hood is recommended to protect the vascular connection from the pedicle to the skin island. Flap dimensions extend from the base of the proximal phalanx to the PIP extension crease, and can be up to 4 × 2 cm. The pedicle can be up to 9 cm in length.

The proximally based flap is rotated around the origin of the FDMA at the base of the first web space. It can be rotated and passed through a subcutaneous tunnel, taking care not to compress the pedicle at the thumb IP joint. Harvesting a proximal tail with the island flap simplifies insetting and avoids the need for tunneling. The donor site is skin grafted.

Harvesting the dorsal skin over the middle phalanx of the index as a random extension allows coverage of larger defects than a standard FDMA flap, in a normal length thumb. Composite flaps can include the extensor indicis proprius or communis tendon that can be transferred as a vascularized tendon graft. An insensate fascial flap may also be used for soft tissue coverage only, but it requires skin grafting.

Reverse-flow fascial flaps can be used for coverage of the dorsum of the digits proximal to the PIP joints. Unfortunately, this flap variant cannot be innervated. The reverse-flow flap can reach as far ulnarly as the fifth metacarpal head. In this variation, the FDMA is ligated at its origin from the radial artery. The interosseous fascia is then elevated up to the level of the metacarpal neck. The donor site is skin grafted if primary closure is not possible.

Outcomes

In 1 large series, the average 2pd was 10.8 mm (range 4-15 mm).[23] There was no difference in patients younger or older than 50 years of age. The average loss of 2pd over the flap area compared with the donor area was 2.7 mm.

Complications

Postoperative complications may include flap edema from kinking of the pedicle. Flap necrosis can occur with injury to the thin fascial extension between the index island flaps and the FDI. Numbness over the dorsum of the middle phalanx of the index or hair growth over the volar aspect of the thumb may be an irritation. Loss of index finger motion and/or poor take of the skin graft over the index extensor tendon are possible. Cold intolerance and dysesthesia can occur.

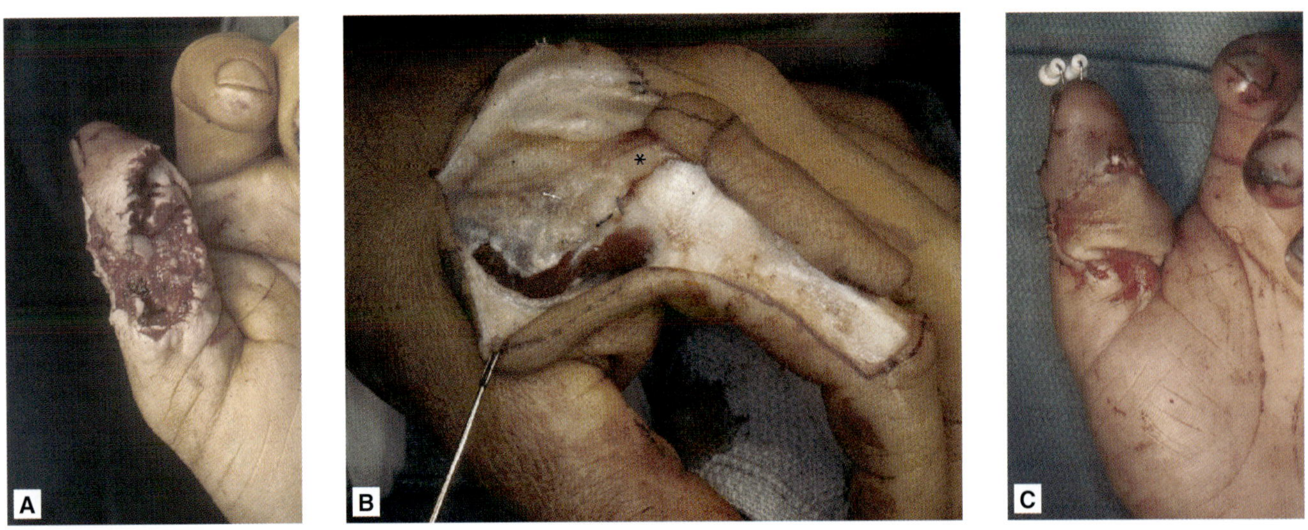

FIGURE 13-9 **A.** Saw injury to right thumb with destruction of the IP joint. **B.** FDMA flap raised from dorsum of index with a proximal skin tail. Note preservation of the continuity of the fascia (*) between the skin island and the interosseous muscle. **C.** Insetting of flap following IP joint fusion.

THE PEDICLED RADIAL FOREARM FLAP

The radial forearm flap is a useful and versatile fasciocutaneous flap designed on the radial artery. It was initially developed as a free flap in 1978 by Yang et al.[24] It was subsequently described as a pedicled flap using either antegrade or retrograde blood flow.[25] The flap includes the volar forearm skin, the underlying antebrachial fascia, and the intermuscular fascia that contains the radial artery and its cutaneous branches. It can be innervated by the medial and lateral antebrachial cutaneous nerves. With retrograde flaps, neurorrhaphy to the local nerves is required.

Anatomy

The skin of the forearm flexor surface does not have any truly axial artery. An axial pattern flap is in effect created by raising a flap including the fascial and subcutaneous vessels with their longitudinal orientation and interconnections. The entire radial artery from its brachial artery origin to the wrist can be transferred. For most of its course, the radial artery lies under the brachioradialis. The pronator teres, flexor pollicis longus, and pronator quadratus lie deep to the artery. The SRN is lateral to the artery under the brachioradialis. After giving off the radial recurrent artery near its origin, the radial artery has no named branches until it reaches the wrist. Here it gives off a superficial palmar branch and a palmar carpal branch. Cadaver studies have demonstrated between 9 and 17 branches from the radial artery to the fascia along the flexor surface of the forearm. The branches supplying the skin are contained in an intermuscular septum between the brachioradialis and the flexor carpi radialis (FCR). These branches are arranged into a proximal and distal group with corresponding zones of perfusion.[26] In the distal half of the forearm, there are branches every 1 to 2 cm. As elsewhere, 1 vascular zone can be extended into another. The distal zone vessels can perfuse a fasciocutaneous flap as far proximal as the elbow. In a reverse pedicled flap, the skin blood supply is dependent on retrograde flow from the ulnar artery through the deep palmar arch.

Venous drainage of the radial forearm flap is by means of both the superficial and deep veins. There are 3 subcutaneous veins including the cephalic, basilic, and the median forearm vein as well as the paired deep venae comitantes of the radial artery. A reverse pedicled flap is drained by means of retrograde flow through the venae comitantes. Normally the venous valves prevent backflow. When a distally based flap is raised, the veins are denervated. The veins are kept filled by blood from the wrist and hand that leads to an increased venous pressure after ligation of their proximal ends. Timmons believes that the combination of these factors allows reverse flow through the venous valves.[26]

The SRN, the brachioradialis, FCR, and palmaris longus tendons are each supplied by direct branches and branches off cutaneous vessels. The medial and lateral antebrachial cutaneous nerves enter the proximal margin of the flap and supply sensibility to the volar forearm.

The radial artery gives off at least 2 periosteal branches of 0.2 to 0.5 mm in size along the lateral aspect of the radius, immediately distal to the pronator teres insertion. These branches are accompanied by 2 small venae comitantes and pass along the fascial layer deep to the extensor carpi radialis longus and brevis. Musculoperiosteal vessels form a constant source of blood supply over the anterior aspect of the distal shaft. They are in turn fed by branches of the radial artery supplying the flexor pollicis longus and pronator quadratus.

Over the distal volar forearm the flap is thin with little fat, but it leaves a poor bed for skin grafting, consisting of tendons covered only by paratenon. A proximal flap is hair bearing and thicker since it has more subcutaneous fat. The donor site contains muscle bellies, which is more favorable for skin grafting. The skin can be innervated by including the medial or lateral antebrachial cutaneous nerve. The flap can include the entire volar forearm skin from the subcutaneous border of the ulna around to the radial dorsum of the forearm, extending as far proximal as the antecubital fossa. Forearm flaps as large as 35 × 15 cm have been reported.

Indications

The flap is useful for thumb reconstruction (Fig. 13-10A-G). It can be used for coverage of the palm or extensor surface of the carpus, with or without vascularized tendon. It can be used to cover dorsal finger defects in selected cases (Fig. 13-11A and B).

Distally based radial forearm flaps designed on the proximal forearm can easily reach the dorsal and palmar surfaces of the hand. They can include vascularized tendon and bone. Pedicle lengths up to 15 cm are possible. If the flap is less than 6 cm in width, the donor site can be closed primarily.

The flap arc of rotation can be increased by freeing the radial artery in the snuffbox and passing the flap underneath the thumb extensors. This allows the flap to reach as far as the thumb tip. The forearm flap permits postoperative elevation and early mobilization of the injured limb. Proximally based flaps can be used to resurface defects well above the elbow joint. These flaps are directly innervated by including the medial or lateral cutaneous nerve of the forearm.

Contraindications

Underdevelopment of the radial artery or injury to the superficial and deep palmar arches would preclude the use of this flap, as would the absence of a connection between the radial and ulnar arteries. In Coleman and Anson's dissection of 650 cadaver arms only 3.2% had no communication between the radial and ulnar arteries, and 3% had an incomplete deep arch.[27] If both of these variations are present, the thumb will be dependent on the radial artery (approximately

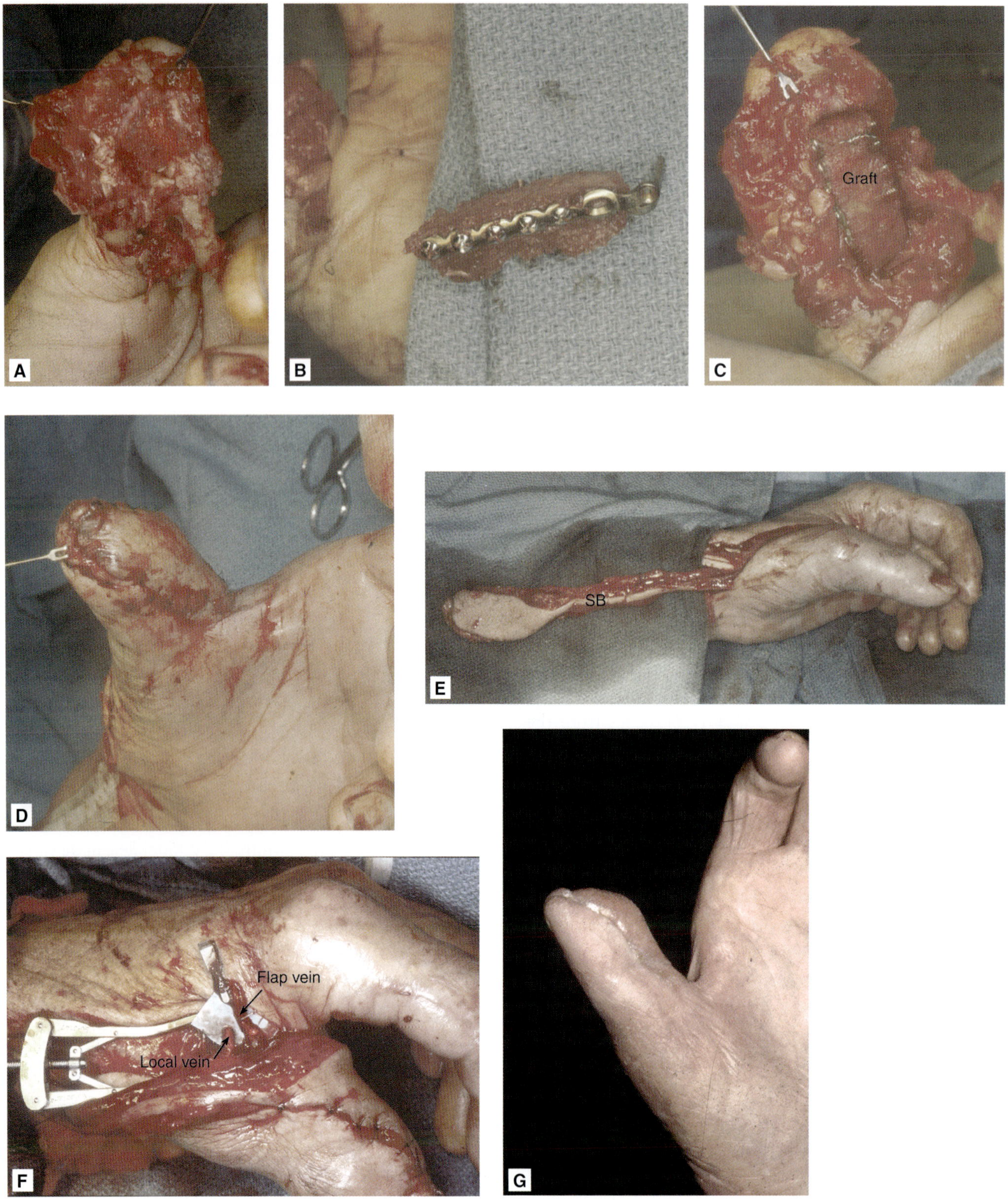

FIGURE 13-10 **A.** Saw injury with skin and bone loss of distal thumb. **B.** Bone reconstruction using iliac crest graft and minicondylar plate. **C.** Reconstruction of thumb ray with graft. **D.** Pedicle reverse-flow radial forearm flap. Note skin bridge (SB) over the pedicle. **E.** Supplemental venous anastomosis. **F.** Insetting of flap. **G.** Long-term result.

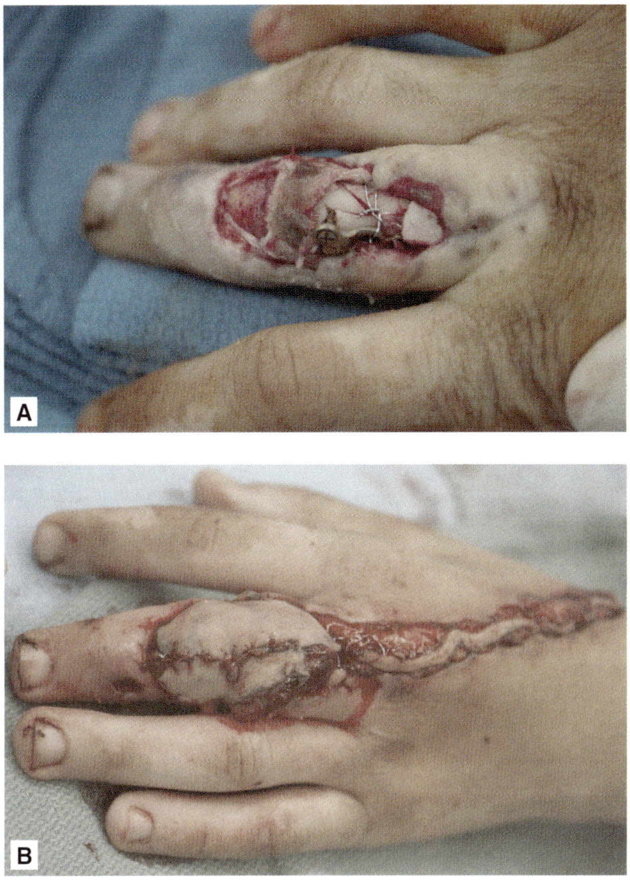

FIGURE 13-11 A. Skin breakdown following bony reconstruction of a gunshot wound to the proximal phalanx. B. Pedicled retrograde flap based.

1 in 1100). This can be identified by a preoperative Allen test. Vein graft reconstruction of the radial artery would be necessary in these cases. Care should be exercised in acute trauma when hematoma extends to the snuffbox.

Surgical Technique

The course of the radial artery is marked. Using a pattern from the recipient site, outline the size of the defect on the proximal forearm. If the flap is outlined over the proximal ulnar forearm, it will be thinner and less hair bearing. A thin skin island can be left over the course of the radial artery to prevent the need for skin grafting the pedicle later on and to avoid an overlying skin bridge. Incise the flap down to the deep fascia. Harvest veins along the proximal medial border of the flap. This allows an easier anastomosis with local veins once the flap has been rotated 180°. Identify the medial or lateral antebrachial cutaneous nerve, and then make a proximal extensile incision for a longer nerve pedicle. The SRN should be protected to preserve sensation to the radial aspect of the hand.

Develop a plane deep to the radial artery at the wrist and find the intermuscular septum between the FCR and the brachioradialis. Incise the deep fascia over the FCR muscle belly, well medial to the intermuscular septum. Dissect the interval between the deep fascia and the muscle. Suture the deep fascia to the skin flap to minimize shear on the septocutaneous perforators. Continue the dissection deep to the radial artery on both sides of the septum. The fascia superficial to the radial artery is left undisturbed since it contains the septocutaneous perforators that supply the skin flap. After the flap dissection is complete, apply a microvascular clamp to the proximal radial artery prior to releasing the tourniquet. If there is adequate perfusion to the flap and the thumb, then the artery is divided. Raise the flap, ligating all the perforators deep to the artery. Transpose the flap to the dorsum of the hand. If desired, perform a venous anastomosis prior to insetting the flap.

The radial forearm flap can be raised as a composite skin flap including vascularized bone and tendon for thumb reconstruction. A purely fascial radial forearm flap can be used to cover exposed tendons on the dorsum of the hand, but it has to be skin grafted and innervation is not possible. A reverse radial fascial-fat flap preserves the radial artery and has been used to cover a scarred median nerve.

Outcomes

In 1 series the moving 2pd averaged 13.2 mm. This was more sensitive than the donor forearm; hence, it was postulated that the sensory return was more dependent on the recipient nerve than on the donor nerve.[28]

Complications

Postoperative complications include flap edema, unstable skin graft over tendons, hand swelling, and SRN injury. Flap edema is common due to associated forearm injury or impaired venous drainage. Additional venous anastomoses will help minimize this. Skin graft failure is most likely to occur over tendons, especially the FCR. Even when they have successfully taken on tendons, skin grafts may suffer recurrent breakdown. Avoidance of the distal forearm as a donor site and covering the tendons with adjacent muscle fibers from portions of the brachioradialis, flexor digitorum superficialis, and flexor carpi ulnaris provide a better skin graft bed. Unmeshed skin grafts can be used to maximize the bridging phenomenon. Preoperative tissue expansion can also be used.

The donor-site defect is quite noticeable. The flap is hair bearing and often bulky. A radial shaft fracture can occur following harvest of vascularized one; hence, above-elbow casting or splinting for up to 8 weeks is recommended. Although digital temperature comparisons show an average 2.5% decrease following the use of the radial forearm flap, cold intolerance is often transient.[29]

SUMMARY

It is apparent that any particular soft tissue defect of the hand can be managed in a variety of ways. Oftentimes the simplest procedure with the fewest potential complications will suffice. Soft tissue coverage is merely 1 component in the management of complex hand injuries, which may also require bony stabilization, neurovascular repair, and tendon reconstruction. Although not specifically addressed, the role of aggressive hand therapy with edema control, early active motion, and functional retraining cannot be overemphasized. Providing stable soft tissue coverage with the potential for sensibility, however, expands the subsequent reconstructive options and enhances the ultimate functional result.

REFERENCES

1. Moberg E. Aspects of sensation in reconstructive surgery of the upper extremity. *J Bone Joint Surg Am.* 1964;46:817.
2. Bertelli JA, Catarina S. Neurocutaneous island flaps in upper limb coverage: experience with 44 clinical cases. *J Hand Surg Am.* 1997;22:515.
3. Hueston J. Local flap repair of fingertip injuries. *Plast Reconstr Surg.* 1966;37:349.
4. Souquet R, Souquet JR. The actual indications of cross finger flaps in finger injuries. *Ann Chir Main.* 1986;5:43.
5. Foucher G, Dallaserra M, Tilquin B, et al. The Hueston flap in reconstruction of fingertip skin loss: results in a series of 41 patients. *J Hand Surg Am.* 1994;19:508.
6. Cronin TD. The cross finger flap: a new method of repair. *Am Surg.* 1951;17:419.
7. Endo T, Kojima T, Hirase Y. Vascular anatomy of the finger dorsum and a new idea for coverage of the finger pulp defect that restores sensation. *J Hand Surg Am.* 1992;17:927.
8. Lassner F, Becker M, Berger A, et al. Sensory reconstruction of the fingertip using the bilaterally innervated sensory cross-finger flap. *Plast Reconstr Surg.* 2002;109:988.
9. Gaul JS Jr. Radial-innervated cross-finger flap from index to provide sensory pulp to injured thumb. *J Bone Joint Surg Am.* 1969;51:1257.
10. Hastings H 2nd. Dual innervated index to thumb cross finger or island flap reconstruction. *Microsurgery.* 1987;8:168.
11. Cohen BE, Cronin ED. An innervated cross-finger flap for fingertip reconstruction. *Plast Reconstr Surg.* 1983;72:688.
12. Kojima T, Hayashi Y, Sakurai N, et al. Eleven cases of vascular pedicle island flap for difficult skin defects on the hand. *J Jpn Soc Surg Hand.* 1986;3:350.
13. Strauch B, de Moura W. Arterial system of the fingers. *J Hand Surg Am.* 1990;15:148.
14. Lai CS, Lin SD, Chou CK, et al. Innervated reverse digital artery flap through bilateral neurorrhaphy for pulp defects. *Br J Plast Surg.* 1993;46:483.
15. Han SK, Lee BI, Kim WK. The reverse digital artery island flap: clinical experience in 120 fingers. *Plast Reconstr Surg.* 1998;101:1006.
16. Sapp JW, Allen RJ, Dupin C. A reversed digital artery island flap for the treatment of fingertip injuries. *J Hand Surg Am.* 1993;18:528.
17. Brunelli F, Vigasio A, Valenti P, et al. Arterial anatomy and clinical application of the dorsoulnar flap of the thumb. *J Hand Surg Am.* 1999;24:803.
18. Moschella F, Cordova A, Pirrello R, Brunelli F. Anatomic basis for the dorsal radial flap of the thumb: clinical applications. *Surg Radiol Anat.* 1996;18:179–181.
19. Cavadas PC. Reverse osteocutaneous dorsoulnar thumb flap. *Plast Reconstr Surg.* 2003;111:326.
20. Li J, Wang J, Yang W, Tong Z. Application of the dorsoulnar arterial retrograde flap of the thumb to repair of soft tissue defect at the distal thumb. *Zhongguo Xiu Fu Chong Jian Wai Ke Za Zhi.* 2004;18:420–422.
21. Holevich J. A new method of restoring sensibility to the thumb. *J Bone Joint Surg Br.* 1963;45:496.
22. Foucher G, Braun JB. A new island flap transfer from the dorsum of the index to the thumb. *Plast Reconstr Surg.* 1979;63:344.
23. Trankle M, Sauerbier M, Heitmann C, et al. Restoration of thumb sensibility with the innervated first dorsal metacarpal artery island flap. *J Hand Surg Am.* 2003;28:758.
24. Yang G, Chen B, Gao Y, et al. Forearm free skin flap transplantation. *Natl Med J China.* 1981;61:139.
25. Song R, Gao Y, Song Y, et al. The forearm flap. *Clin Plast Surg.* 1982;9:21.
26. Timmons MJ. The vascular basis of the radial forearm flap. *Plast Reconstr Surg.* 1986;77:80.
27. Coleman SS, Anson BJ. Arterial patterns in the hand based upon a study of 650 specimens. *Suvr Med (Sofiia).* 1961;113:409.
28. Yamauchi T, Yajima H, Kizaki K, et al. Sensory reconstruction in sensate radial forearm flap transfer. *J Reconstr Microsurg.* 2000;16:593.
29. Kleinman WB, O'Connell SJ. Effects of the fasciocutaneous radial forearm flap on vascularity of the hand. *J Hand Surg Am.* 1993;18:953.

14

Hand and Finger Replantation

Clara WY Wong, MBChB, MRCS, FRCSEd(Orth), FHKAM(Orthopedic Surgery), FHKCOS
WL Tse, MBChB, MRCS, FRCSEd(Orth), FHKAM(Orthopedic Surgery), FHKCOS
PC Ho, MBBS, FRCS(Edinburgh), FHKAM(Orthopedic Surgery), FHKCOS

INTRODUCTION

Through decades of researches on microvascular surgeries, successful limb replantation in humans became a reality in May 1962, when Malt and McKahn successfully replanted an arm amputation in a boy at Massachusetts General Hospital in Boston.[1] The first report of replantation was by Chen et al, who successfully replanted a distal forearm complete amputation in January 1963 in Shanghai Sixth People's Hospital in China.[2] The first successful replantation of a thumb was achieved by Komatsu and Tamai in July 1965 with the use of an operating microscope.[3] Replantation surgery is now well established worldwide, and the results obtained with replantation are superior to the results achieved following an amputation.[4–8]

INDICATIONS

The indications for replantation are not absolute. These can be evaluated through a full understanding of the patient and the injury, which includes the patient's age, gender, occupation, hand dominance, smoking history, mechanism, severity, and the complexity of the injury, level of amputation, ischemic time, and concomitant injuries, as well as patient comorbidities including diabetes mellitus, peripheral vascular disease, chronic obstructive airway disease, peptic ulcer disease, and psychopathology. The decision should be discussed with the patient and the family, with pros and cons balanced. It depends on:

1. The expected chance of survival of the replanted parts
2. The expected outcome of the replanted parts
3. The ability of the patient to endure the perioperative morbidities physically and psychologically, and the possible subsequent reconstructive surgeries
4. The demand and desire of the patient

Good candidates for replantation include any amputation level in children or young women; sharp-cut amputations; amputation distal to the flexor digitorum superficialis (FDS), or the distal interphalangeal joint (DIPJ); and thumb amputation, multiple digit amputations, and hand and wrist amputations with a short warm ischemia time.

Replantation of almost any amputated part generally is recommended for healthy children. They are able to adapt to replantation better than adults. Epiphyseal growth continues and sensibility is usually restored.[9,10] On the other hand, advanced age increases the potential morbidity of the procedure as chronic medical conditions are more prevalent in older patients.

The zone of tissue damage in sharp-cut or guillotine amputation is limited, which requires minimal debridement and gives the most favorable results. Crushing amputations may be associated with more extensive injury than indicated by the external appearance. Adequate debridement is required, but the distinction between vital and nonvital tissues is often difficult to make. Avulsion amputations have the most extensive zone of tissue damage because of the tearing mechanism.

Replantation distal to the FDS generally functions well and is cosmetically superior to an amputation stump or prosthesis.[11] Distal replantation, replantation at or distal to the DIPJ, is the ideal and the only technique to restore the original tissue, with a high survival rate, and good cosmetic and functional qualities.[12–14]

The function of a replanted thumb is definitely superior to that of prosthesis.[15–19] Hand function is severely affected if thumb or multiple fingers are not present to oppose each other. For multiple digit amputation, the priority should be given to the less damaged parts, those parts that can be transferred from their original position to a more functional and important position or to a more suitable stump to increase the chances of survival.[20] Replantation priority should be given to the thumb, middle finger (MF), ring finger (RF), then little finger (LF), and lastly to the index finger (IF). Wrist and palm replantation generally gives better functional results than a prosthesis.[21,22] Although intrinsic muscle recovery is sometimes poor or may result in contracture that requires a subsequent release, a restoration of protective sensation can usually be achieved and enough useful grasp can be obtained from undamaged extrinsic muscle function.

CONTRAINDICATIONS

There are some conditions in which replantation is not recommended:

1. Minimal viable structures in the distal and proximal parts of the amputation, as a result of severe or multiple avulsion/crush injury or severe contamination
2. Patients with multiple injuries or medical diseases, for whom prolonged replantation surgery would be life-threatening
3. Patients with peripheral vascular disease, such as vasculitis, Raynaud disease, or chronic renal failure
4. A mentally unstable patient who is not able to comply with the perioperative care
5. Prolonged warm ischemic time

These contraindications, however, may not be absolute.

Successful outcomes have been observed in avulsion and crush-type injuries (Fig. 14-1). Successful replantation of badly contaminated and damaged digits has also been reported. One case involved a girl with a 4-finger amputation secondary to a guillotine that were then eaten by a chicken. Her fingers were retrieved from the chicken's esophagus and 1 finger was successfully replanted. There was another case of successful finger replantation following retrieval of the amputated part from a dog's stomach.[23] Whether a digit is replantable or not can sometimes only be determined following an inspection under the operating microscope.

Preexisting diseases may preclude the patient's ability to withstand the perioperative blood volume changes, the anticoagulation, and long anesthetic and operative times. Finger and hand replantation, however, can be performed under brachial plexus anesthesia (PA). Finger replantation can be done under local anesthesia (LA). Perioperative anticoagulation is not mandatory, especially in a clean-cut amputation with healthy vessels (Fig. 14-2) and in children. Bleeding can be minimized with tourniquet use, vein-first-anastomosis technique, and good hemostasis.

Replantation survival rates drop with longer ischemic times.[24] Ideally replantation of a digit at room temperate should not exceed 6 hours, at which time irreversible tissue damage occurs. Prolonged cold ischemic time should not be an absolute contraindication for replantation, although the success rate drops. Leung reported the successful transfer of a toe to hand after 36 hours of cold ischemia.[25] Wei et al reported the successful replantation of 3 fingers in a patient after 84, 86, and 94 hours of cold ischemic time.[26] Muscle is the tissue that is most vulnerable to anoxia. Fortunately, there is no muscle in the digits, and the muscles in hand are not as abundant as in the forearm or arm. Revascularization of the fingers and hands after a prolonged period of ischemia rarely carries the same systemic risk as a proximal replantation.

The patient's desire and special needs should be respected. Restoration of full length and preservation of the nail may be necessary in certain professions such as musicians. In Chinese and some Oriental countries, the concern of body integrity is very strong. Some would define health as body integrity. Some regard it as a religious belief. And some emphasize the importance of body integrity at one's death. Moreover, physical appearance can be more important than

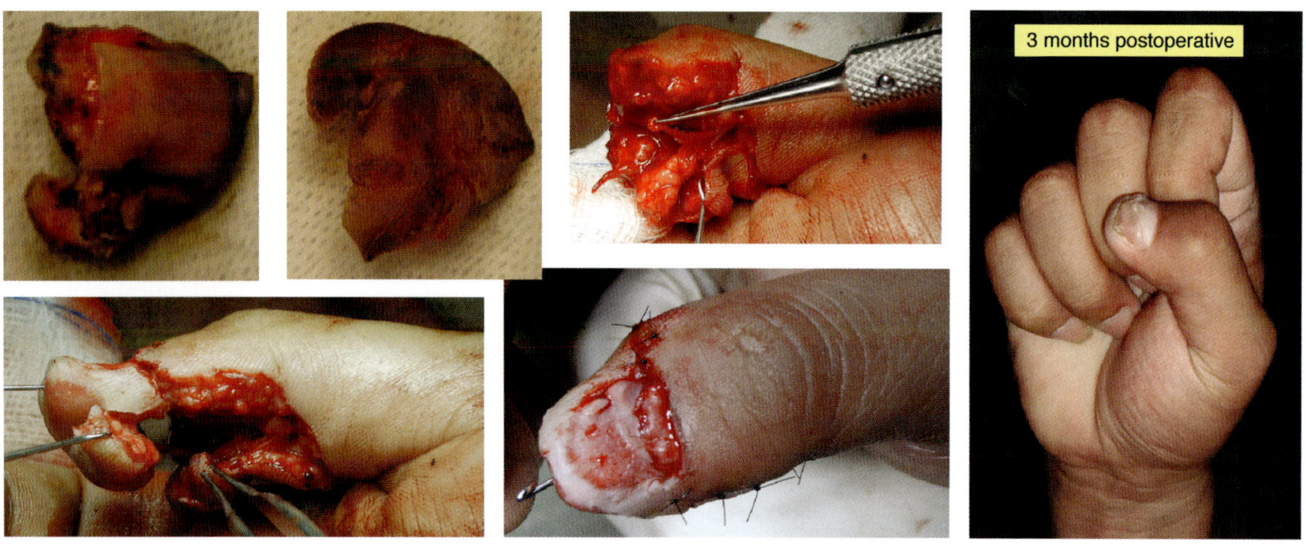

FIGURE 14-1 Badly crushed right thumb tip. After debridement and inspection under the microscope, a viable artery and volar vein were identified and anastomosed. Results at postoperative 3 months were good.

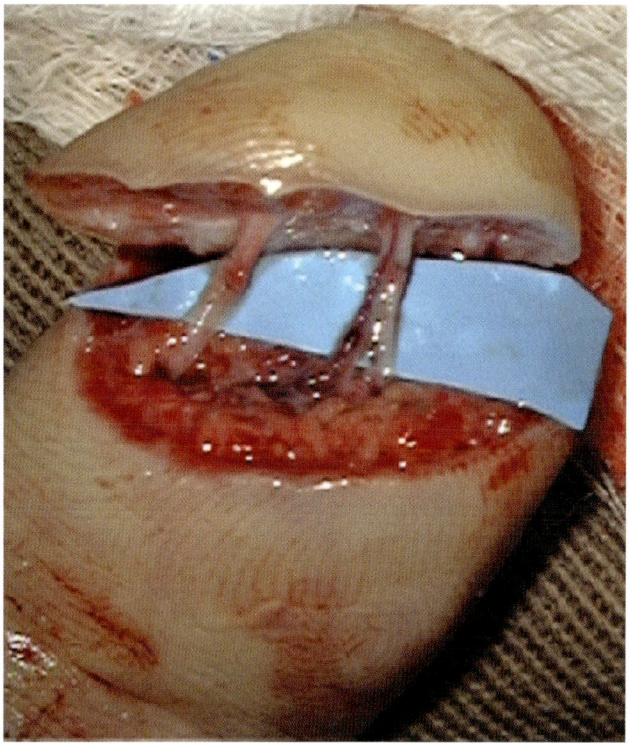

FIGURE 14-2 Sharp-cut amputation. No anticoagulation was necessary.

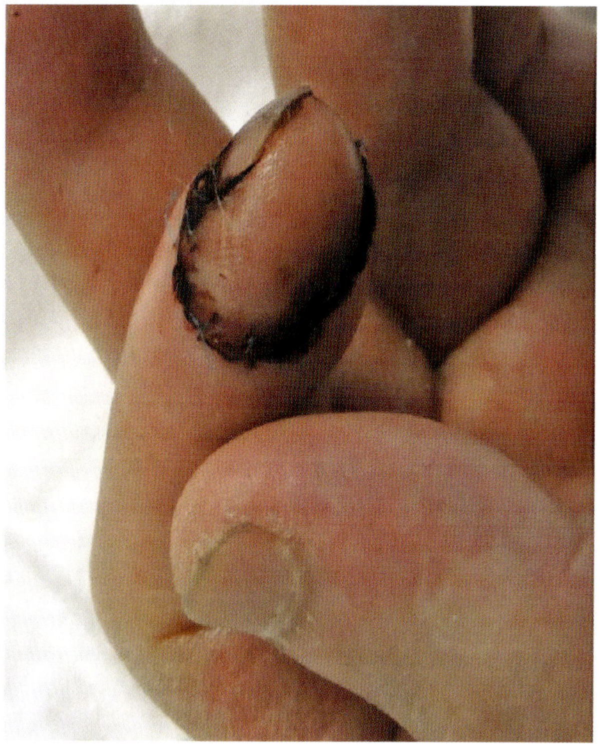

function in some individuals. Patients often request replantation even after a detailed discussion and the understanding that the procedure would not improve the overall hand function.

Therefore, the decision should be individualized.

SURGICAL TECHNIQUES

Once the suitability of replantation has been determined, every minute of delay counts. It is an emergency surgery. Collaboration with all of the involved parties, including nurses, anesthetists, the operating room, and the surgeons of the replantation team, is important. The initial management determines the final outcome, not only the limb survival but also later reconstructive options.

Preoperative Measures

The immediate management of a patient with an amputation injury follows the Advanced Trauma Life Support guidelines. The amputated part and stump are inspected and photographed for preoperative planning. X-rays of both the amputated and proximal parts should be available. The amputated part is then immediately wrapped with gauze soaked in physiological saline, sealed in a waterproof plastic bag and placed in ice with water, or refrigerated at 4°C. One surgeon starts the preparation of the distal part, while the other prepares the patient for surgery.

General Aspects

The operation is performed under general anesthesia (GA), or PA, which aids vessel dilatation and is the most common mode of anesthesia for replantation in China. Children need GA. Finger or distal replantation can be performed under LA. The patient is kept warm. A Foley catheter is inserted. A tourniquet is applied but not inflated unless there is profuse bleeding from the proximal part. Excessive arm abduction is avoided; otherwise it is difficult to hypersupinate or hyperpronate the forearm and hand during surgery, which will create difficulties especially when replanting a thumb. The lower limb is draped for the possible harvesting of vein grafts and skin graft for hand replantation.

DEBRIDEMENT, LABELING, AND BONE SHORTENING

A meticulous debridement of the distal and proximal parts of the amputation is a basic requirement to the success of replantation and is part of the process to identify and label the vital structures.

To save time, it is better to have 2 teams, 1 working on the distal part and the other on the proximal part. For the proximal part, the inflation of tourniquet is not routine, unless the bleeding obscures the field or affects the vascular dissection. The tourniquet time should be minimized to prevent the subsequent refractory vasospasm. Vascular clamps are applied to the vessels to decrease the tourniquet time.

The debridement is done under the operating microscope. All devitalized and contaminated tissues are removed. The neurovascular structures are identified and marked. Avoid immersing the distal part into normal saline for cleansing or squeezing the parts; otherwise, the blood clots and the vessel lumen are diluted or removed, and the tissue at the amputation end becomes swollen making the identification of the neurovascular structures difficult. Stabilize and mount the distal part on a towel with a needle, over the nail plate (Fig. 14-3). It can be placed on a wet gauze on top of a small ice pack to reduce the warm ischemic time.

The digital nerves lie medial and volar to the digital arteries. The diameter of the radial and ulnar digital arteries is similar in the MF. But in the other fingers, the dominant artery is the one facing the MF. At the distal phalanx, about 5 mm distal to the distal finger crease, the digital artery turns toward the midline, crossing dorsal to the digital nerve, anastomoses with the contralateral digital artery, and forms an arcade in the pulp, just distal to the insertion of the flexor digitorum profundus (FDP) tendon, about half way along the distal phalanx. In distal replantation, in the proximal half of the distal phalanx, the artery can be traced along the sides of the pulp; in the distal half, the artery is identified in the central portion. Usually the most central artery is the longest and has the largest diameter.

It is easier to anastomose the dorsal veins as compared with the volar veins, which are fixed tightly to the dermis, and have a smaller diameter and thinner wall. The dorsal venous system also has a characteristic pattern for easy identification. It tends to lie at the sides of the distal phalanx at the DIPJ level and form a cross-network at the phalangeal level. Since the veins form a network, when 1 vein is identified, the second can be found when followed distally in the distal part and proximally in the proximal part. Three to 4 veins are enough. If the dorsal veins are insufficient, the volar veins are traced. Elevation of triangular skin flaps as advocated by Tsai et al gives a good exposure of the volar veins.[27] Both the arteries and veins can be identified in the region of dots of blood clot. Milking the finger refills the vessel lumen with blood that makes it more visible. If a vein cannot be identified, especially in a distal replantation, it can be left until after the arterial anastomosis has been completed when the blood outflow refills the vein that makes it easier to visualize.

The damaged vessel wall is excised. The zone of vascular damage depends on the mechanism of injury. In a crush injury, the vascular injury can be segmental and multiple, and not confined to the level of amputation. In an avulsion injury, the zone of injury is more extensive and there may be a ribbon sign and red-line sign, which is indicative of more extensive vessel damage, where a red line can be seen along the course of the artery. The damaged segment of the vessel that should be excised includes vessel wall with a loss of the normal elasticity, a swollen vessel wall with unidentifiable layers, adventitial injury, muscle layer injury, intimal damage with exfoliation, irregular vessel wall, and vessel wall with an adherent fibrinous material. Pulsatile flow from the proximal artery is a sign of good blood flow, which should be steady and sustained. One should not hesitate to excise the unhealthy vessel; otherwise it will be much longer to revise the anastomosis. In a crush and avulsion amputation, the digits can be salvaged with multiple vein grafts.[28] In a distal replantation, however, an arterial defect is unusual. Since the artery in the pulp is tortuous, dissection of a short segment and straightening the artery is sufficient to overcome any length defect and allow opposition to the proximal artery.

Vessel irrigation is useful in order to assess the condition of the vascular bed and to flush out the metabolic products and thrombi of the distal part. It is not necessary in a sharp-cut distal amputation where the distal vascular bed is healthy. Heparinized saline is injected slowly and gently into the arterial opening. If the vascular bed is patent, saline will flow out from the cut ends of the communicating branches of the artery, bone medullary cavity, and veins. If there is resistance to the injection, there may be a distal occlusion secondary to vasospasm or clot, or a vessel tear or rupture, in which saline will escape into the subcutaneous tissue. Dissection distally to identify and deal with the rupture or occlusion is necessary. If the resistance is mild and the irrigating saline slowly outflows from the vein, this may be secondary to tissue edema from a prolonged ischemia time. In extensive rupture of capillary bed, which commonly occurs in a compression or crush injury, punctate hemorrhage is found in the skin, and the distal part is swollen with no saline outflow when irrigated. If no arterial rupture or occlusion can be identified after an extensive dissection, the replantation may need to be abandoned.

Next, identify and label the nerves. Excise the flimsy torn nerve ends in avulsion amputation. In a distal replantation, good sensory recovery can still be observed even if no nerve is repaired, probably because of good distal neurotization.[29]

Bone shortening is necessary for a primary tension-free neurovascular anastomosis and soft tissue coverage, without compromising length and function. Shorten the bone for about 4 to 5 mm in adults, 3 to 4 mm in children, and 2 to 3 mm in a distal replantation where tension in the neurovascular anastomosis is seldom a problem. If the amputation is close to a joint, shorten the side with the longer bony length in order to preserve the joint. If the joint is disrupted, excise the subchondral bone for an arthrodesis. Use a sterile glove as a tissue protector during the bone excision (Fig. 14-4).

APPROXIMATION OF THE 2 PARTS

The order of repair for various structures varies according to the surgeon's preference and the clinical scenario. Our preferred sequence is: osteosynthesis, flexor tendon repair, extensor tendon repair, dorsal vein anastomosis, digital nerve coaptation, digital artery repair, volar vein anastomosis if necessary, and skin closure/coverage. If the distal tendon stump is short, the tendon sutures are placed prior to osteosynthesis. If a vein graft is needed to bridge the vascular

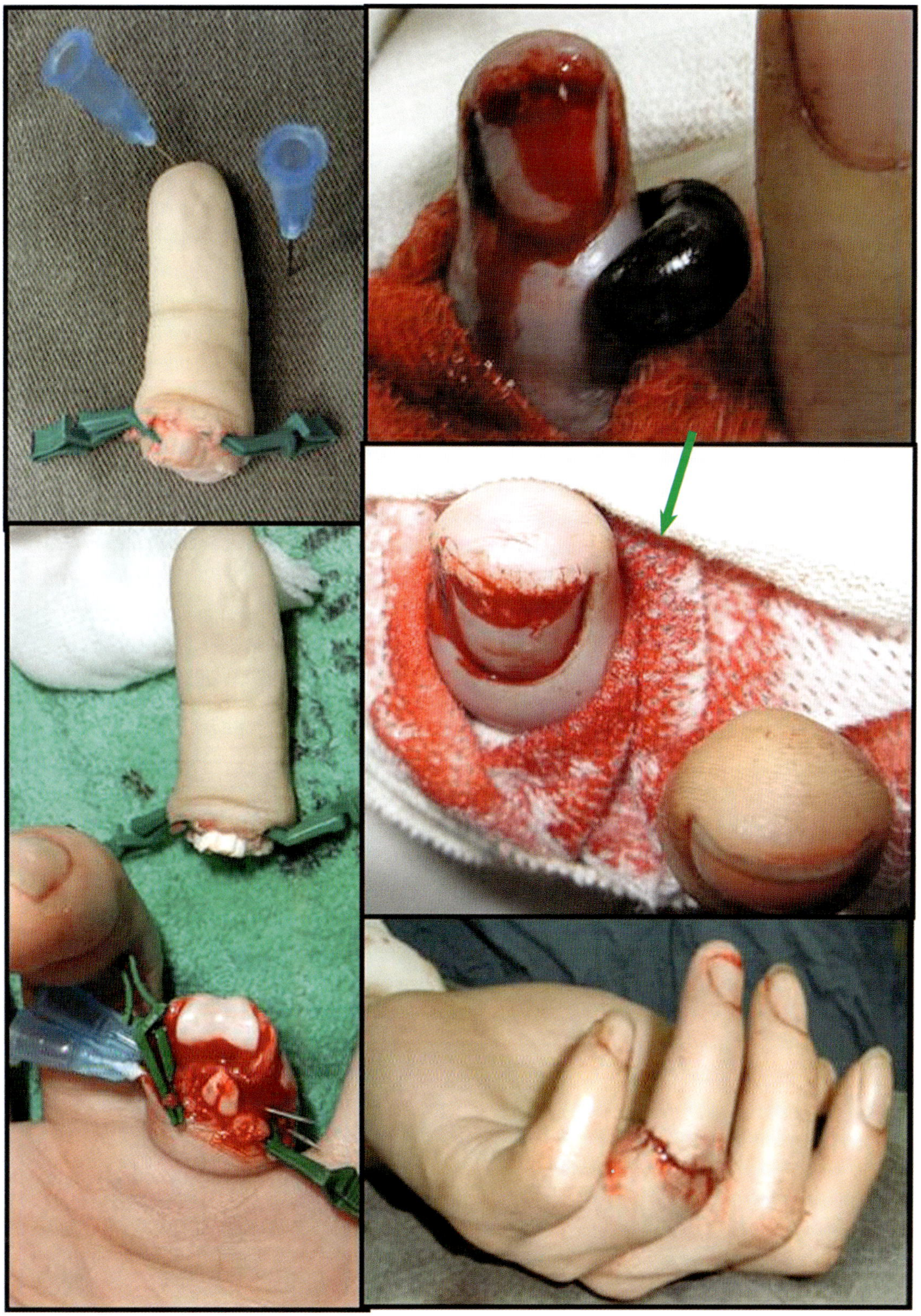

FIGURE 14-3 Left RF was amputated at the PIPJ level. It was replanted with 1 artery and 3 dorsal veins. The joint was successfully preserved without bone shortening. Postoperative venous congestion was salvaged with leech therapy.

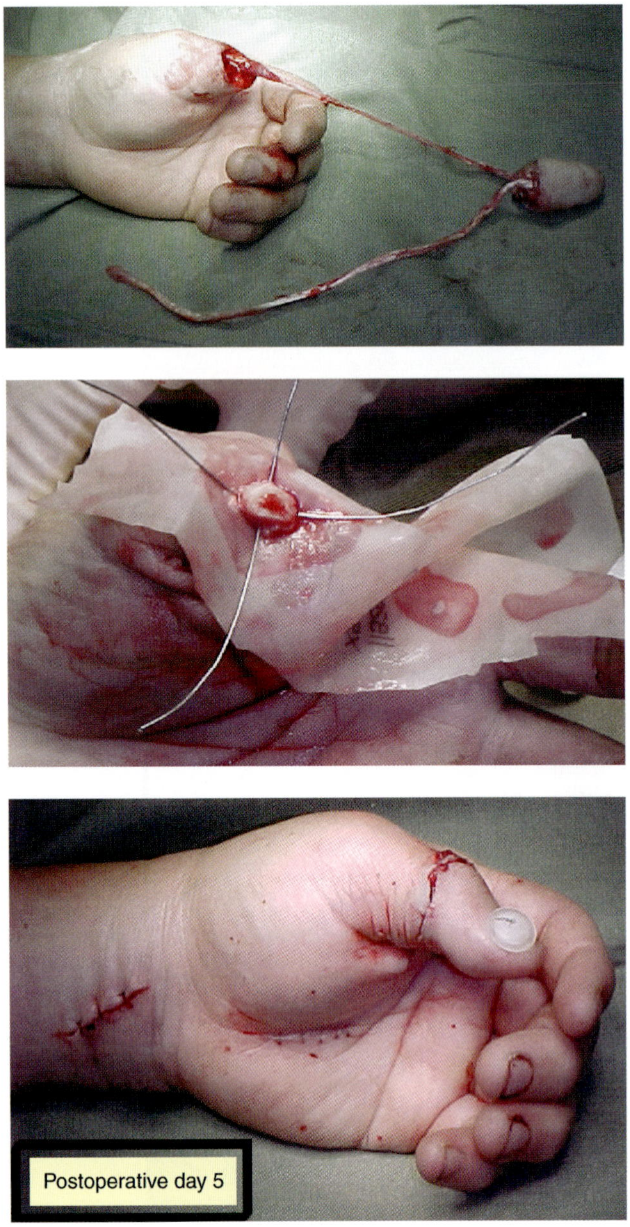

FIGURE 14-4 Thumb avulsion amputation. A sterile glove was used as tissue protector during bone shortening and skeletal fixation with 90-90° wiring loops. FDS of the ring finger was transferred to the FPL. The EIP was transferred to the EPL and reinforced with pullout wiring. The digital arteries were anastomosed at the proximal phalangeal base with interposition vein grafts. Two dorsal veins and digital nerves were directly repaired.

defect, it can be anastomosed to the distal part before osteosynthesis in order to shorten the warm ischemia time. If the ischemic time is short, the trauma is not severe, and the vascular status is satisfactory, a vein-first-anastomosis can establish the venous return after arterial anastomosis, reduce the bleeding, provide a cleaner operative field, avoid venous stasis and tissue edema, and eliminate the possibility of vasospasm or blood clotting when inflating the tourniquet after arterial anastomosis. Repairing digital nerve early ensures a meticulous repair in a bloodless field.

Osteosynthesis. Bony stabilization is the first step in the approximation of the 2 parts. This provides a stable construct to protect against excessive tension on multiple microanastomoses. Without a stable bony framework, the nerves or vessels that have already been anastomosed may become twisted or lacerated, and the soft tissue will not be restored, making tensioning of the tendons difficult. Rigid bony fixation also allows early rehabilitation to prevent tendon adhesion or joint stiffness. However, if the exposure and completion of the microvascular anastomosis are difficult after osteosynthesis, such as in a volar oblique distal amputation, the K-wire that is used to fix the fracture can be initially inserted to the distal part and then advanced into the proximal part after the vascular anastomosis has been completed.

Techniques for bone fixation are numerous. They should be simple, quick, effective, and secure. They include the use of K-wires, intramedullary screw, interosseous wires, and plate fixation. Crossed K-wires are commonly used. They are quickly applied and produce acceptable results.[30] But they do not support vigorous mobilization. Stiffness, nonunion, or malunion may result. Interosseous wiring in concert with a screw or K-wire as described by Lister[31] and 90-90° wiring are our preferred techniques (Fig. 14-5). Other configurations include Cassel's tetrahedral cerclage,[32] and tension band wiring.[33] Interosseous wiring techniques are relatively easy, speedy, require little additional dissection, provide compression at the fracture site, give reliable healing, and permit early and intensive postoperative mobilization.[30,34,35] Dorsal and lateral plating provides a very stable construct, but needs more extensive dissection and takes longer. Lag screws are used to secure oblique fractures that are not commonly seen in amputation injuries. Intramedullary screws are commonly used in DIPJ fusion or phalangeal fractures. The stability is reliable and the soft tissue dissection is minimal. The bone ends must be perpendicular to the longitudinal axis of the phalanx so that the distal part can be completely screwed into the proximal one without impinging on the opposite bone end. Care must be taken to avoid trapping the tagged vessels or nerves in the fracture site. If the joint is disrupted, fuse the joint at functional position.

Flexor Tendon and Extensor Tendon Repair. The standard flexor tendon repair includes 4 strands of core sutures and an epitendinous running stitch. Sturdy tendon repair facilitates early mobilization and minimizes tendon adhesion. In a zone II flexor tendon injury, the FDS can be excised without repair unless it is a sharp-cut amputation. In a proximal interphalangeal joint (PIPJ) arthrodesis and multiple digit amputations, no FDS repair is necessary. Some advocate performing the arterial anastomosis before the flexor tendon repair in zone II in order to allow finger extension and better exposure for the neurovascular repair. The proximal and distal core sutures are placed beforehand and tied after the arterial anastomosis and nerve repair. The forearm is then pronated for the extensor tendon repair.

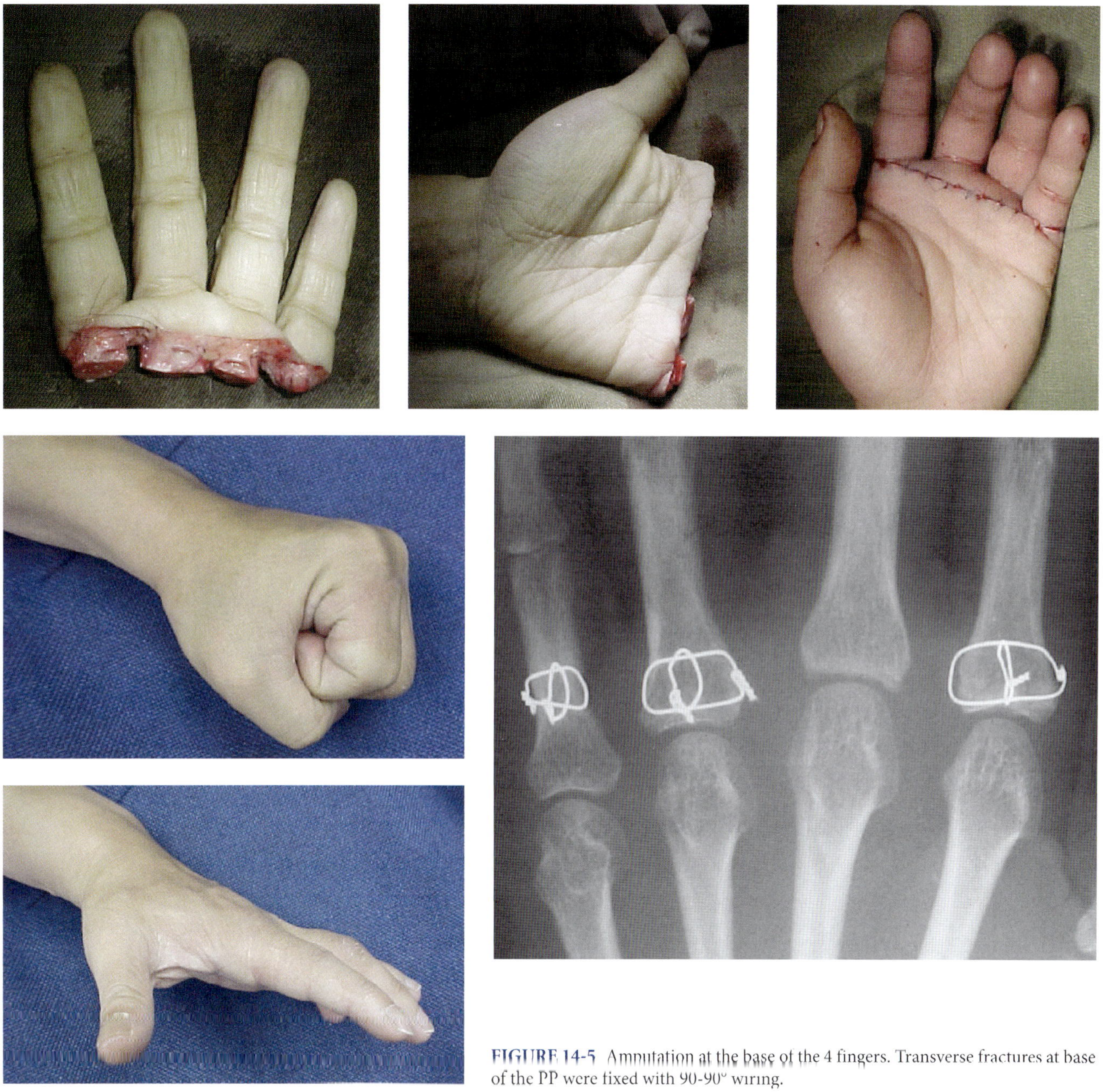

FIGURE 14-5 Amputation at the base of the 4 fingers. Transverse fractures at base of the PP were fixed with 90-90° wiring.

Dorsal Vein Anastomosis. Choose the biggest and best-quality vein for anastomosis first. Excise the segment with a valve if it is close to the anastomosis site. Use 10-0 nylon sutures. Release the vascular clamp to allow filling of the collapsed vein. If the tourniquet is inflated, squeeze the forearm to force some blood flowing across the anastomosis and refill the lumen. In a more distal amputation, the vein is smaller, adhered to the skin, and fragile with a thinner wall, which does not allow for a long dissection or use of a vascular clamp. The posterior wall is sutured first, with intermittent heparinized saline irrigation to clear the view. Venous blood refluxing into the repairing lumen fills up the distal vein and avoids suturing the opposite wall when repairing the anterior wall. Anastomose at least 2 to 3 veins in a finger replantation and more in a hand replantation. For a distal replantation, although an arterial-only anastomosis also gives successful results using a bloodletting technique for venous drainage postoperatively,[36] a venous anastomosis decreases a postoperative venous congestion, improves the chances of survival of the replantation, decreases the bleeding risk, and simplifies the postoperative care. A venous anastomosis should still be attempted at least once, and is mandatory if more than 1 artery is anastomosed in a distal replantation. If no distal vein is available, anastomosing the distal artery to a proximal vein is also a viable option for venous drainage.

As soon as the anastomosis is completed, a bolus of heparin 3000 to 5000 IU is administrated intravenously if there is no contraindication.

Digital Nerve Repair. Contused and flimsy nerve ends are excised. Use 9-0 nylon sutures. Use about 4 epineurial stitches for each nerve.

Arterial Anastomosis. Confirm there is good pulsatile proximal arterial flow before anastomosis. A weak arterial flow signifies arterial spasm due to a proximal arterial injury, a cold environment, low patient blood pressure and dehydration, vasospasm secondary to pain when brachial PA is wearing off, or external pressure from retracted skin or swollen adjacent damaged tissue. All these factors should be reversed. Dissect the artery proximally and release the adjacent tissues and adventitia. Local injection of lignocaine and papaverine is usually helpful.

Anastomose both digital arteries if possible. If the smaller-sized digital artery is not repairable, ensure that there is flow through the larger vessel. If a primary repair of the larger vessel is not possible, it needs to be reconstructed, in addition to anastomosing the smaller one. Reconstructive options include:

- An interpositional vein graft, which can be harvested from the volar wrist, anterior forearm, or dorsum of the foot. Ensuring an appropriate length of the vein graft is important. The diameter of a vein graft of insufficient length undergoes narrowing on tension. A graft that is too long kinks, thus decreasing flow and increasing the risk of thrombosis. Reverse the graft for arterial interposition.
- Interpositional artery graft. This can be harvested from the nonreplantable digits in multiple digit amputations.
- Arterial transposition from an adjacent finger (Fig. 14-6). This is a good option especially for a long vascular defect and is commonly used in a thumb avulsion amputation. Apply a vascular clamp on the donor artery before transfer to test for the adequacy of arterial supply to the normal finger. An adequate arterial length and straight course of the transferred artery are also important.

If there are arterial defects of both digital arteries, an arterial cross-transfer in the same digit is helpful to restore vascularity. It is done by anastomosing the longer artery of each side (Fig. 14-6).

Release the tourniquet or vascular clamp after the arterial anastomosis. Assess the patency of the arterial and venous anastomosis by assessing the color, capillary refill, and turgor of the distal part. Anastomose additional veins if necessary.

Skin Coverage/Closure. Achieve meticulous hemostasis before closure. Take care not to injure the anastomosed veins during closure. If there is a dorsal skin defect with loss of venous tissue, the surgical options include:

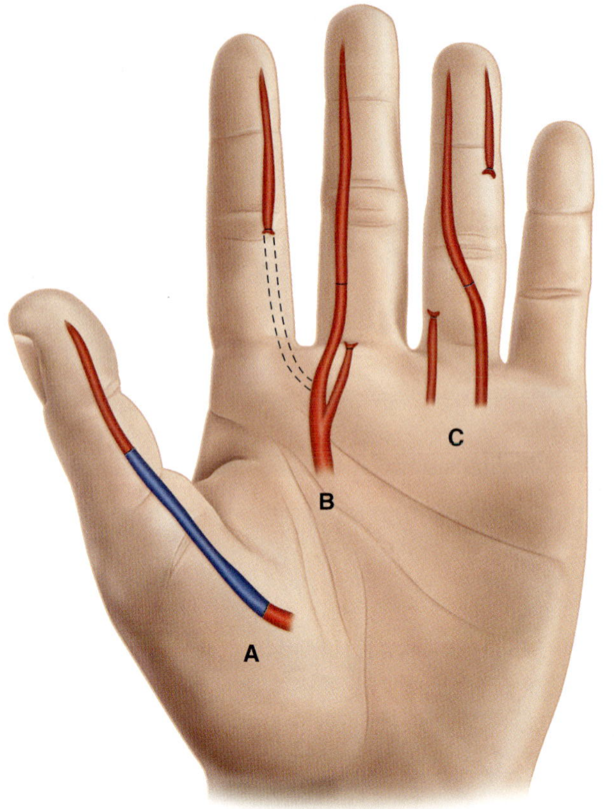

FIGURE 14-6 Arterial reconstructions for arterial defects. **A.** Interposition vein graft. **B.** Arterial transposition from an adjacent finger, length of the transposed artery must be longer than the arterial defect. **C.** Arterial cross-transfer in the same finger.

- Vein grafting and then covering the defect with a skin graft.
- A Foucher venous flow-through flap. Raise a flap from an adjacent finger, including the underlying cutaneous veins that are divided at the PIPJ level. The flap is used to cover the skin defect after the flap veins are anastomosed to the veins of the finger being replanted. This is particularly well suited for a thumb avulsion amputation.

Remove the distal one third of nail plate for possible later bloodletting techniques.

POSTOPERATIVE MONITORING AND CARE

In general, keep the patient in a warm room that is 80°F if available. Maintain good hydration and oxygenation. We usually give dextran 40 at 40 mg daily and intravenous fluid for 5 days if not contraindicated. Monitor the hemoglobin level and administer a blood transfusion when necessary. Give anticoagulants for about 10 days if not contraindicated, in concert with an H_2 receptor antagonist or proton pump inhibitor. Give aspirin for a month if not contraindicated. Continue antibiotics and monitor the circulation hourly. The height of hand elevation is according to the circulatory status. Bloodletting is performed if there is venous congestion. It can be achieved by pricking the exposed nail bed with needle. Gently massage the finger. Apply a small piece of heparin-soaked gauze over the nail bed. Remove any blood clot on the nail bed when formed. Alternatively, one can use medical leeches along with prophylactic antibiotic for *Aeromonas hydrophila* infection (Fig. 14-3).

Change the dressing to avoid constriction by dried blood 2 days after the operation. Blood-soaked dressings also offer a bacterial culture medium and can augment the conditions for local infection. Trim any necrotic skin edges when necessary to avoid infection.

Reexploration is performed in the event of a vascular crisis. In a distal replantation, reexploration for vascular crisis is usually futile and only 1 attempt is performed. Educate the patient to avoid tobacco, and caffeine-based food.

SPECIFIC CIRCUMSTANCES

Ring Avulsion Amputation. Urbaniak classified this injury into 3 types: type I, soft tissue injuries with preserved circulation; type II, circulation compromised; type III, complete degloving or amputation. Avulsion injuries are usually associated with a poor functional outcome especially for a complete amputation (type III) at the PP or PIPJ level. Urbaniak advocated revision amputation for type III injuries, but a recent systemic review reported a mean survival of 66%, total action motion of 174°, and a mean 2-point discrimination of 10 mm.[37] The success relies on the techniques of:

- Adequate bone shortening to allow a primary soft tissue envelope and neurovascular repair
- Aggressive debridement of avulsed vessels with use of interpositional grafts
- Arterial or venous transposition from adjacent fingers or hand dorsum (Fig. 14-7)
- Use of skin graft and venous flow-through flaps to provide wound coverage[38]

Multiple Digits, Multiple Level Amputation. This is a great challenge that requires surgical expertise, experience, creativity, and a dedicated team approach to meet the surgical complexity and prolonged operative time. There are some tricks:

- When each part is still connected by a skin bridge, the part can be placed on a wet gauze on an ice bag to cool the digits and reduce the warm ischemic time during the operation.
- If the parts are separated, we prefer a sequential approach in which they are replanted individually, with the others kept on ice until replantation.
- A priority is given to the less damaged parts, with the best chance of survival, the best expected recovery, and a most significant contribution to the overall hand function. Those parts can be transferred from their original position to a more functional and important position, for example, moving a digit to the thumb position, or to a more suitable stump to increase the chance of survival.[20]

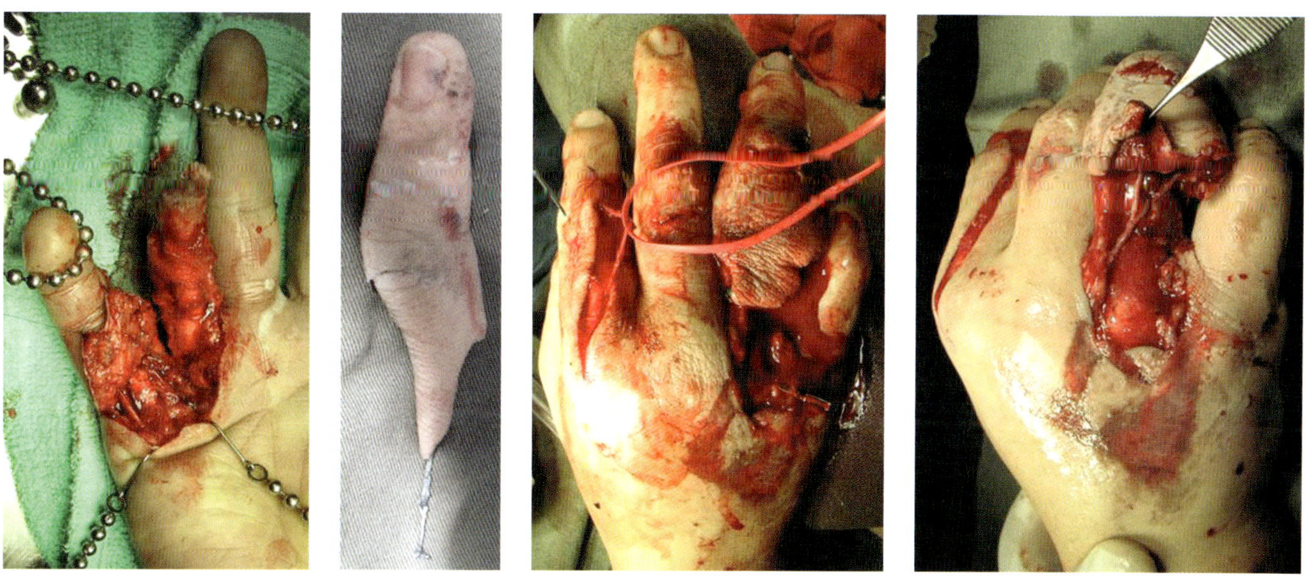

FIGURE 14-7 Urbaniak type III ring avulsion amputation of right RF. The radial digital artery was reconstructed with a vein graft. A dorsal vein was transposed from the index with the distal ends of the Y-bifurcation anastomosed to the RF. The digital nerves were repaired with a nerve graft.

- If all parts are similarly damaged, the priority is based on patient's functional demands. Replantation of the MF and IF is a priority if pinching function is more desirable; replantation of the RF and LF is a priority if better gripping and grasping are needed. Controversies exist with regards to replantation of the IF and LF. The patient will bypass a stiff and insensate replanted IF and use the MF. The IF also limits the first web space span and impedes the function and opposition of the other fingers to the thumb. On the other hand, the function of the other fingers is not uncommonly interfered with by a stiff LF. In multiple digit replantation, however, the function of the other fingers is similar, and LF replantation helps to restore hand span. Therefore, in general, we recommend the priority of replantation should be the thumb, MF, RF, LF, and lastly the IF.
- Replant as many fingers as possible in case any of the replants fail.
- Part salvage is important. Make use of the spare parts, such as artery, veins, tendon, nerve, and even skin as donor tissue, from the unreplantable amputated parts, to reconstruct the injured replantable parts.
- Two to 3 teams participate, in order to reduce the ischemia time when operating on different parts concurrently, and to change off after every digit, to minimize the surgeon's fatigue during a prolonged operation.
- To shorten the ischemic time, the sequence of repair can be: osteosynthesis, extensor tendon repair, 1 dorsal vein anastomosis, core sutures placed at the flexor tendons (not yet tied), and 1 digital artery anastomosis. Once the circulation is established in 1 finger, proceed to another. Then complete all by anastomosis of another dorsal vein, another digital artery, digital nerves, and finally the flexor tendons.
- Arterial-first anastomosis if the injury condition is not favorable, that is, in crush and avulsion injuries, and long ischemic time.

Thumb Amputation. The thumb constitutes 40% to 50% of the total hand function. Successful replantation provides a significant restoration of the hand function. The ulnar digital artery is twice the size of the radial digital artery, which has a more variable anatomy.[39] Anastomosing the ulnar digital artery gives a more reliable circulation to the thumb. Sensory recovery of the ulnar pulp is also more important than the radial side in the thumb. However, exposure and repair of the ulnar digital artery and nerve are difficult even with the hand in hyperpronation. The digital arteries are branched from princeps pollicis or directly from the palmar arches. The branches are so short that once ruptured, they retract between the first dorsal interosseous and adductor pollicis muscles, and make their identification and exposure for anastomosis difficult. There are some techniques that help to make thumb replantation easier and more successful:

- Avoid too much abduction of the shoulder during positioning after the administration of anesthesia so that forearm hyperpronation can be easier.
- Radical debridement is important to make sure that healthy tissues are left for repair and the risk of infection and inflammation causing tissue edema is minimal. Do not hesitate to use an arterial interposition vein graft, which was shown to improve the survival rate significantly.[40,41]
- Anastomose the ulnar digital artery and repair the ulnar digital nerve before osteosynthesis. This solves the positioning problem, gives a better exposure, keeps the plane of anastomosis in plane with the hand, and widens the field of focus of the operating microscope. The sequence of repair is: insertion of K-wire into the distal bone, insertion of the core sutures in the proximal and distal stumps of the flexor pollicis longus (FPL), ulnar digital artery repair (proximal vascular clamp in place), ulnar digital nerve repair, osteosynthesis by advancing the K-wires proximally after reduction, radial digital nerve repair, radial digital artery repair if available, extensor tendon repair, dorsal vein anastomosis, and release of the vascular clamp and tying of the FPL sutures. If the ischemic time is long, release the proximal vascular clamp on the ulnar digital artery and reapply if necessary.
- If the amputation level is at the metacarpophalangeal joint, use an arterial interposition vein graft from the radial artery in the anatomic snuffbox (end-to-side anastomosis) to the ulnar digital artery of the distal part.[40,42] Prepare a subcutaneous tunnel at the ulnar aspect of the thumb base to the snuffbox, and dissect the radial artery for end-to-side anastomosis. The sequence of repair is: insertion of the K-wire in the distal bone, insertion of the FPL core sutures, vein graft anastomosis to the distal ulnar digital artery, passage of the vein graft to the snuffbox, ulnar digital nerve coaptation, osteosynthesis, radial digital nerve coaptation, radial digital artery repair if available, extensor tendon repair, dorsal vein anastomosis, end-to-side anastomosis of the vein graft to the radial artery, and tying of the FPL sutures.

Thumb Avulsion Amputation. Replantation of an avulsed thumb is more complicated. The vessels are avulsed into a ribbon shape, the digital nerves into a "rat-tail" appearance, the tendons are torn at the musculotendinous level, and the skin is degloved. The decision as to whether to perform a 1-stage replantation and reconstruction or a 2-stage reconstruction depends on the status of the residual vascular bed that is determined after debridement. One-stage surgery is advocated for thumbs with a reasonable expectation of survival. The surgical techniques required for success are:

- A team approach. One team prepares the distal and the other prepares the proximal. When the preparation of the proximal part is not completed, preserve the distal part cold.
- Radical debridement is important.
- The proximal veins are usually badly torn. A vein transfer from the IF is a viable option. An adequate length of subcutaneous vein from the IF is harvested, with distal

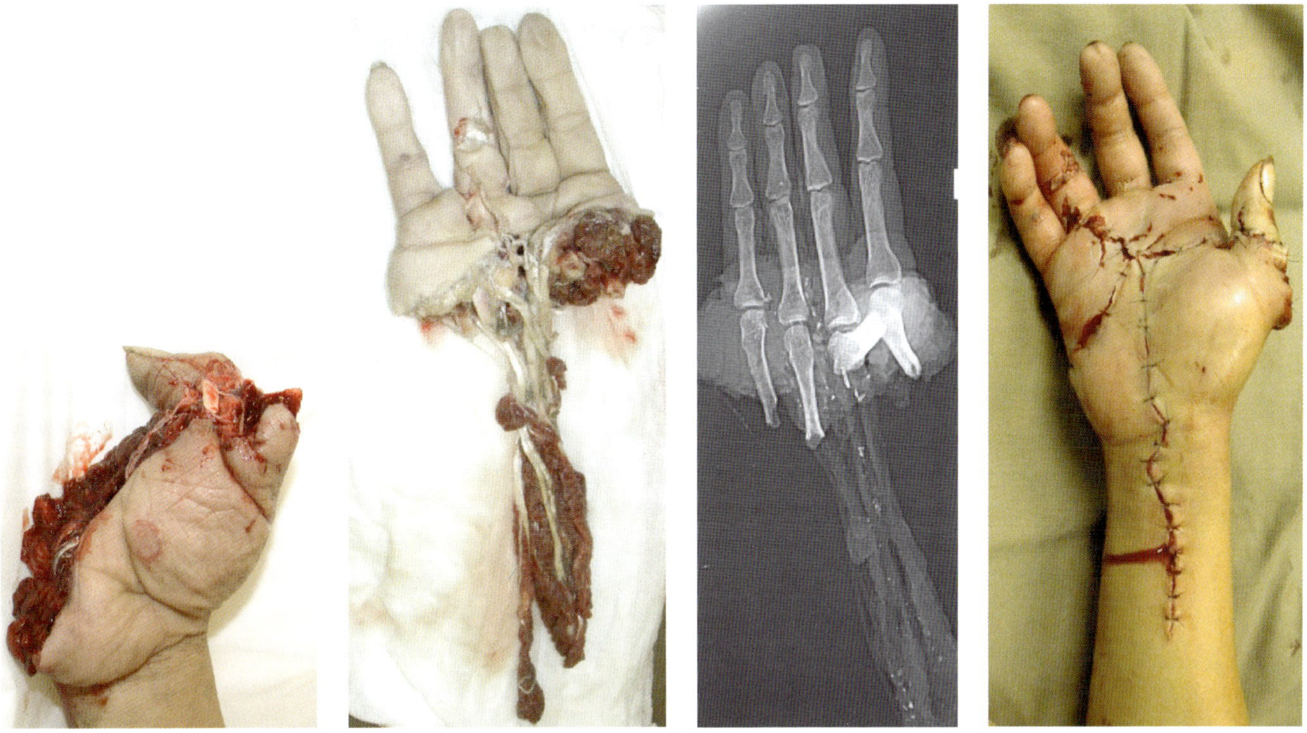

FIGURE 14-8 Honda type B hand avulsion amputation. This was an avulsion type. The devitalized muscles were excised; metacarpals were shortened and fixed with plates.

end of Y-shaped bifurcation for anastomosis to 2 dorsal veins of the thumb. If there is dorsal skin defect, a venous flow-through flap from the IF can be prepared for transfer.

- If it is decided to proceed with a 1-stage procedure, an adequate preparation of the proximal part before osteosynthesis is crucial to reduce the warm ischemia time. This includes harvesting and transferring the extensor indicis proprius (EIP) to the extensor pollicis longus (EPL) and the FDS of the RF to the FPL (Fig. 14-4). Prepare for a digital nerve transfer from the IF, by transferring either the ulnar digital nerve of the IF or radial slip of the radial digital nerve of the IF. Interposition nerve graft is another option. Use interposed vein graft for digital artery anastomosis. If it is decided to transfer the radial digital artery of the IF to the ulnar digital artery of the thumb, prepare an adequate length and make sure the circulation of the IF is not compromised.
- Liberal use of interposition vein graft and skin grafts is helpful.

Hand Amputation. Honda et al classified hand amputation into 5 types: type A, amputation through the carpus; type B, amputation through all 5 metacarpals (Fig. 14-8); type C, amputation through the second to fourth metacarpals and thumb PP; type D, amputation through the second to fourth metacarpals; type E, amputation through the first to fourth metacarpals.[43] However, hand replantation is generally regarded as the replantation of the proximal palm, wrist, and distal forearm level. Surgical techniques are similar to any replantation, but soft tissue tensioning is very important to the final functional outcomes. All flexor tendons should be repaired so that the FDS can be later transferred if intrinsic muscle function of the hand does not return after reinnervation. A volar incision and carpal tunnel release help expose the tendon and nerves for proper identification and repair. The knowledge of the arrangement of flexor tendons in the wrist must be clear, where the FDS of the MF and RF are volar to the IF and LF. The recurrent motor branch should be traced and repaired. If the articular cartilage is mostly preserved in a type A amputation, a proximal row carpectomy (PRC) helps both to achieve bone shortening and to preserve joint motion.[44,45] A secure and strong repair of the joint capsule and extrinsic ligaments of the wrist prevents later ulnar translocation of capitate from the lunate fossa of the radius[46,47] (Fig. 14-9). If the wrist joint is fused, it is held in 20° of extension (Fig. 14-10A and B). The tendon repair is very time-consuming. The warm ischemic time can be reduced by placing core sutures at the flexor tendons before osteosynthesis. In general, the sequence of repair is: PRC/bone shortening; osteosynthesis; dorsal extrinsic ligament repair; extensor tendon repair; 2 dorsal vein anastomosis; radial artery/ulnar artery anastomosis; once circulation is established, volar extrinsic ligament repair, otherwise, anastomose the other artery; flexor tendon repair; median nerve and ulnar nerve repair under microscope; more dorsal vein

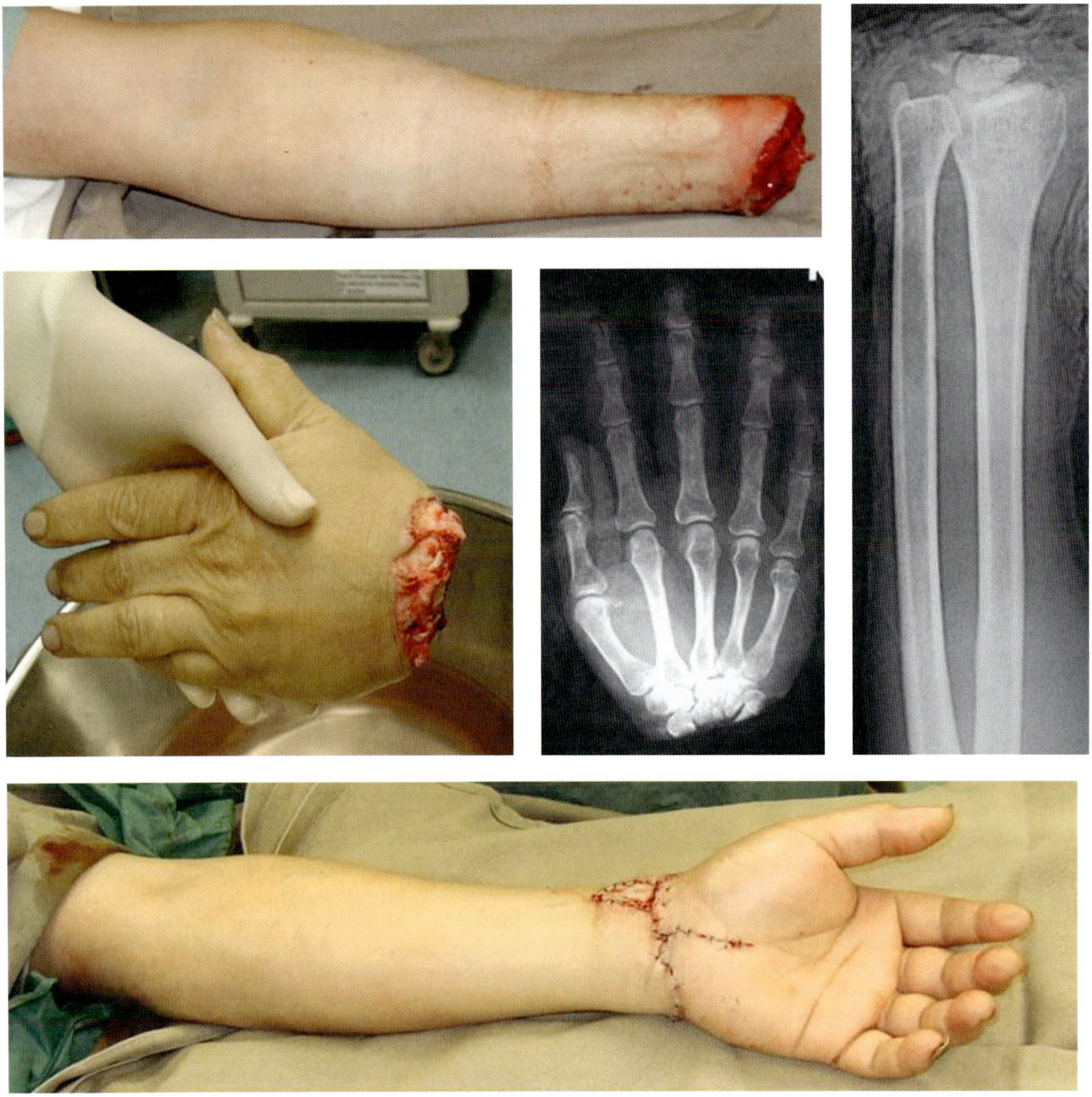

A

FIGURE 14-9 **A.** Honda type A hand amputation. A 47-year-old man, left wrist saw cut injury. The capitate fracture was fixed. A proximal row carpectomy was done and the wrist was fixed with K-wires. Three dorsal veins, the radial artery, and ulnar artery were anastomosed.

and artery anastomosis to achieve a circulatory equilibrium. A prophylactic fasciotomy is usually not necessary. If ischemic time is long, artery is anastomosed after osteosynthesis. Tourniquet is periodically inflated and deflated to stay within safe time limits. This is particularly true in wrist avulsion amputation, which demands a much longer operative time. The tricks for success are to minimize ischemic time by team approaches and arterial-first anastomosis and sometimes arterial shunting, radical debridement and excision of devitalized muscles, preservation of tendons, and primary tendon transfer (Fig. 14-10A and B).

OUTCOMES AND COMPLICATIONS

It is more common to encounter failures and complications if the meticulous steps are not followed. In general, the overall survival rates of finger and hand replantation

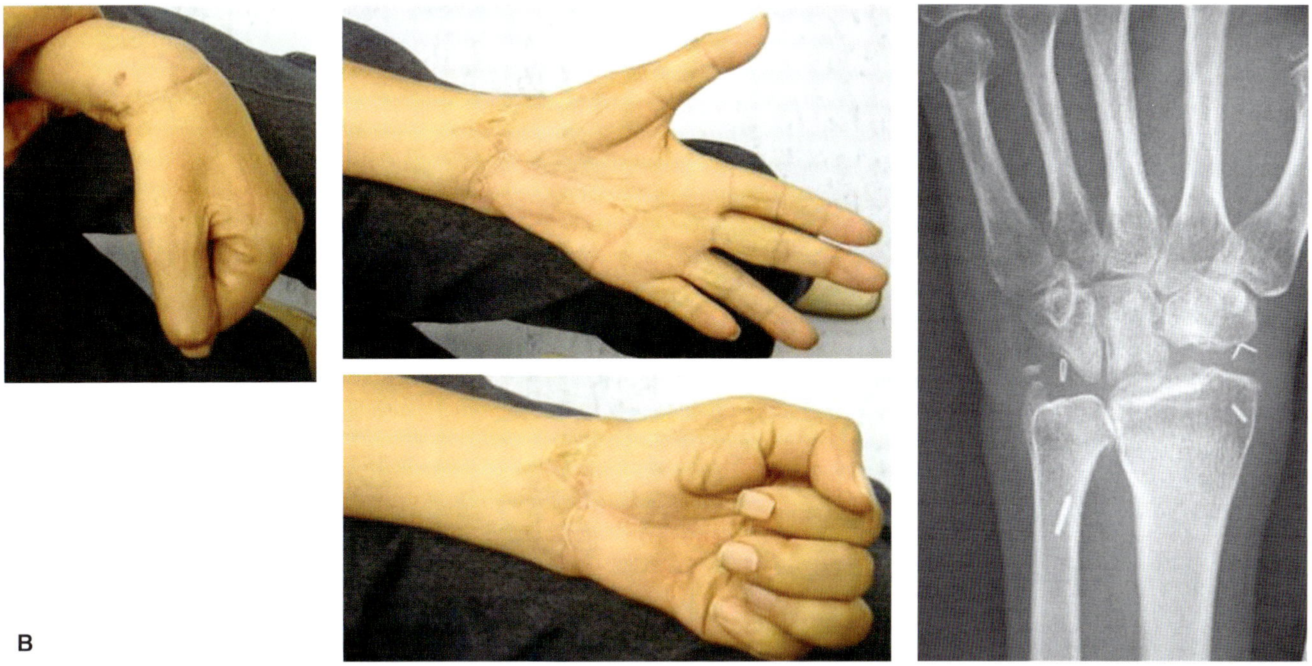

FIGURE 14-9 (*Continued*) **B.** Results at 3.5 years after replantation. X-rays showed maintenance of the joint space between the lunate fossa of radius and capitate without evidence of an ulnar translocation.

are high. In Mainland China, for a 10 years' time, from 1992 to 2003, of the reported 25,221 replanted fingers, the survival rate ranged from 75.5% to 98.3%.[47] It is much higher in hand replantation but lower in crush and avulsion amputations, and with long ischemic time. Complications should be looked for and corrected promptly. Early complications include vascular crisis, bleeding, and infection. Arterial insufficiency occurs at a time when edema was at its peak on the second to fourth day when the wounds should be checked routinely for tissue tension, tight stitching, or hematoma collection. When arterial insufficiency is detected early, exploration and thrombectomy often save the replantation. Venous congestion can be earliest detected by a throbbing sign when an obvious throb is felt on the pulp.[48] In distal replantation, gentle massage usually can save the finger. However, if it is allowed to persist in a more proximal replantation, frank venous congestion will develop and circulatory shutdown will be resulted. Loose bulky dressing, hand elevation, and sometimes medical leeches are helpful (Fig. 14-4). If these are not effective, exploration, venous reanastomosis, vein grafting, loosely placed stitches, and skin grafting to prevent tissue tension should be done promptly. Despite careful hemostasis, bleeding commonly occurs after anticoagulation and bloodletting, which may require blood transfusion. Oozing usually stops spontaneously in a few days and bedside coagulation to the bleeders of the proximal part is sometimes necessary. Infection can be prevented by extensive debridement with bone shortening and skin grafting or local flaps. Finger stiffness is expectedly a common late complication for amputation proximal to the FDS insertion. Tenolysis and joint contracture release are performed 6 months after replantation to achieve maximum function. Rigid fracture fixation helps to minimize fracture nonunion and hasten early mobilization to reduce joint stiffness and tendon adhesion. In primary nerve repair, the recovery of sensibility is nearly as good as the results of an isolated peripheral nerve.

Functional recovery represents the true success in replantation. The more distal the replantation, the more complete the functional recovery. Young patients have a particular good prognosis. Although the survival rate of hand replantation is high, recovery of motor and sensory function is variable.[22,49,50] Nevertheless, high probability of returning to work and having useful hand function made the patients satisfied with the replantation surgery.[22,49,50] In the series of Honda et al, the worst results were observed in type A, which was associated with reflex sympathetic dystrophy; the best results were achieved in type C to D, whereas type B and E results depended on the resultant thumb function.[43] For finger replantation, the total active motion (TAM) of more than 50% of the contralateral finger, total grip strength approaching two-thirds of the healthy hand, the pinch power of at least half of the contralateral finger, satisfactory sensory recovery, and patient satisfaction were commonly reported. We performed a detailed review of 37 distal finger replantation cases over 5 years, with 77% resulting from avulsion and crush injuries, gave 85.7% survival rate, with pinch power 78.4%, grip power 90%, and TAM 92% of the contralateral side, and 2-point discrimination averaged 5.7 mm.[29]

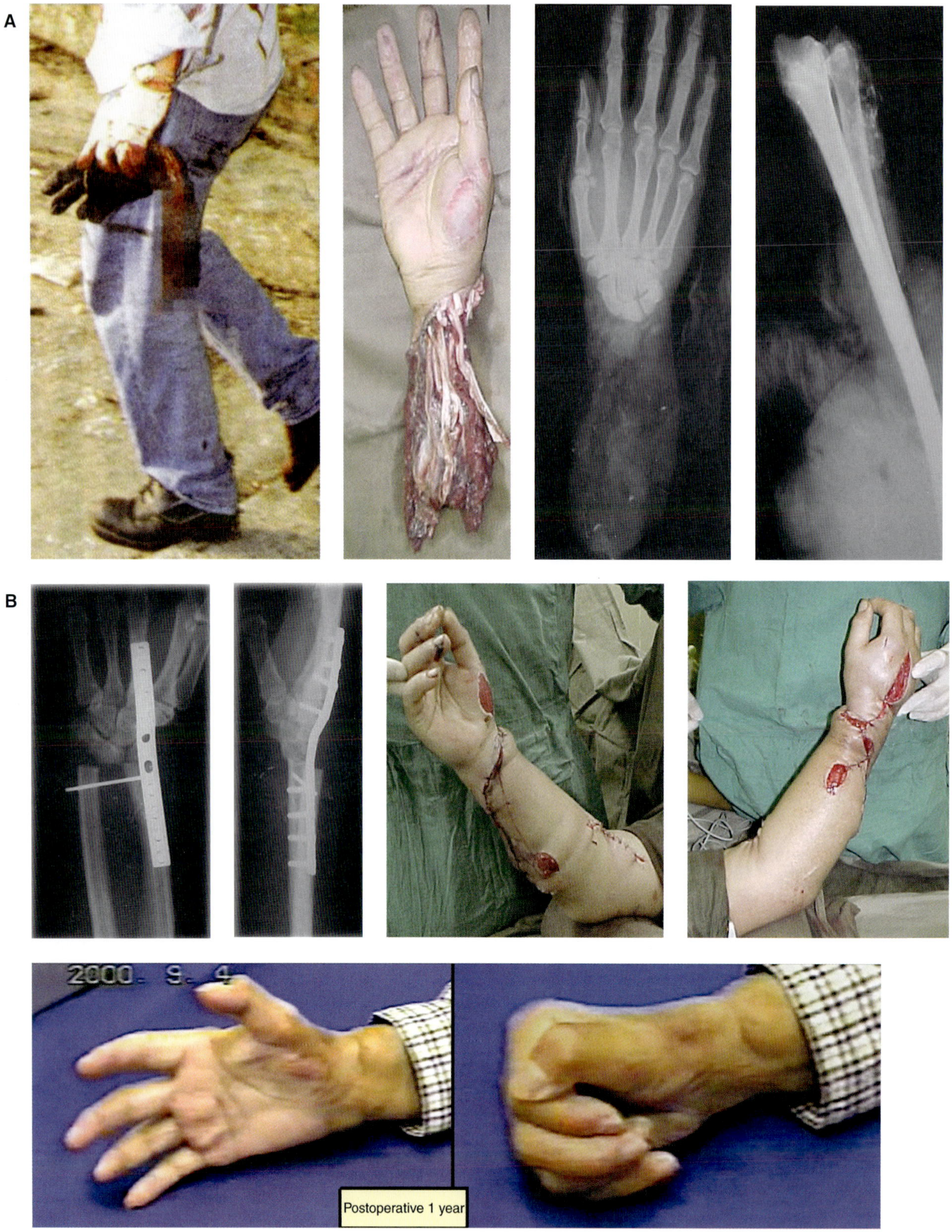

FIGURE 14-10 **A.** A 50-year-old man sustained a traumatic amputation at a construction site. He picked up his amputated hand and walked to the hospital. The finger tendons were avulsed at the musculoskeletal junction, whereas the wrist flexors and extensors were avulsed at the wrist level. Both the median and ulnar nerves were avulsed at the midforearm level. **B.** The distal radius and ulna were shortened 3 cm and a primary wrist fusion was done. The radioulnar joint was stabilized with a K-wire. The flexor carpi radialis was transferred to the FPL, the FDP tendons were repaired to the FDP muscle, the extensor carpi radialis brevis was transferred to the EPL, the extensor carpi radialis longus was transferred to the abductor pollicis longus, and the extensor digitorum communis (EDC) tendons were repaired to the EDC muscles.

REFERENCES

1. Malt RS. Replantation of severed arms. *JAMA*. 1964;189(10):114.
2. Chen CW, Chien YC, Pao YS. Salvage of the forearm following complete traumatic amputation: report of a case. *Chin Med J (Engl)*. 1963;82:633–638.
3. Komatsu S, Tamai S. Successful replantation of a completely cut off thumb. *J Plast Reconstr Surg*. 1968;42:374–377.
4. Nylander G, Vilkki S, Ostrup L. The need for replantation surgery after traumatic amputations of the upper extremity—an estimate based upon the epidemiology of Sweden. *J Hand Surg Br*. 1984;9(3):257–260.
5. Atroshi I, Rosberg HE. Epidemiology of amputations and severe injuries of the hand. *Hand Clin*. 2001;17(3):343–350.
6. Friedrich JB, Poppler LH, Mack CD, Rivara FP, Levin LS, Klein MB. Epidemiology of upper extremity replantation surgery in the United States. *J Hand Surg Am*. 2011;36(11):1835–1840.
7. Vilkki SK, Goransson H. Traumatic amputations and the need for a replantation service in Finland. *Ann Chir Gynecol*. 1982;71(1):2–7.
8. Richards WT, Barber MK, Richards WA, Mozingo DW. Hand injuries in the state of Florida, are centers of excellence needed? *J Trauma*. 2010;68(6):1480–1490.
9. Demiri E, Bakhach J, Tsakoniatis N, Martin D, Baudet J. Bone growth after replantation in children. *J Reconstr Microsurg*. 1995;11(2):113–122.
10. Saies AD, Urbaniak JR, Nunley JA, Taras JS, Goldner RD, Fitch RD. Results after replantation and revascularization in the upper extremity in children. *J Bone Joint Surg Am*. 1994;76(12):1766–1776.
11. May JW Jr, Toth BA, Gardner M. Digital replantation distal to the proximal interphalangeal joint. *J Hand Surg Am*. 1982;7(2):161–166.
12. Chen CT, Wei FC, Chen HC, Chuang CC, Chen HT, Hsu WM. Distal phalanx replantation. *Microsurgery*. 1994;15:77–82.
13. Foucher G, Norris RW. Distal and very distal digital replantations. *Br J Plast Surg*. 1992;45:199–203.
14. Yamano Y. Replantation of fingertips. *J Hand Surg Br*. 1993;18:157–162.
15. Schlenker JD, Kleinert HE, Tsai TM. Methods and results of replantation following traumatic amputation of the thumb in sixty-four patients. *J Hand Surg Am*. 1980;5:63–69.
16. Morrison WA, O'Brien BM, MacLeod AM. The surgical repair of amputations of the thumb. *Aust N Z J Surg*. 1980;50:237–243.
17. Earley MJ, Watson JS. Twenty-four thumb replantations. *J Hand Surg Br*. 1984;9:98–102.
18. Goldner RD, Howson MP, Nunley JA, Fitch RD, Belding NR, Urbaniak JR. One hundred eleven thumb amputations: replantation vs revision. *Microsurgery*. 1990;11(3):243–250.
19. Ward WA, Tsai TM, Breidenbach W. Per primam thumb replantation for all patients with traumatic amputations. *Clin Orthop*. 1991;266:90–95.
20. Soucacos PN, Beris AE, Malizos KN, Vlastou C, Soucacos PK, Georgoulis AD. Transpositional microsurgery in multiple digital amputations. *Microsurgery*. 1994;15(7):469–473.
21. Meyer VE. Hand amputations proximal but close to the wrist joint: prime candidates for reattachment (long term functional results). *J Hand Surg Am*. 1985;10(6 Pt 2):989–991.
22. Vanstraelen P, Papini RP, Sykes PJ, Milling MA. The functional results of hand replantation. The Chepstow experience. *J Hand Surg Br*. 1993;18(5):556–564.
23. Cheng GL. Replantation of amputated finger. In: Cheng GL, ed. *Replantation and Reconstruction of Fingers*. China: People's Medical Publishing House;. 2008:145–146 [chapter 5].
24. Arakaki A, Tsai TM. Thumb replantation: survival factors and re-exploration in 122 cases. *J Hand Surg Br*. 1993;18:152–156.
25. Leung PC. Prolonged refrigeration in toe-to-hand transfer—case report. *J Hand Surg Am*. 1981;6(2):152.
26. Wei FC, Chang YL, Chen HC, Chuang CC. Three successful digital replantations in a patient after 84, 86, and 94 hours of cold ischemia time. *Plast Reconstr Surg*. 1988;82(2):346–350.
27. Tsai TM, McCabe SJ, Maki Y. A technique for replantation of the fingertip. *Microsurgery*. 1989;10:1–4.
28. Alpert BS, Buncke HJ, Brownstein M. Replacement of damaged arteries and veins with vein grafts when replanting crushed, amputated fingers. *Plast Reconstr Surg*. 1978;61:17.
29. Wong C, Ho PC, Tse WL, Cheng S, Chan DK, Hung LK. Do we need to repair the nerves when replanting distal finger amputations? *J Reconstr Microsurg*. 2010;26(5):347–354.
30. Whitney TM, Lineaweaver WC, Buncke HJ, Nugent K. Clinical results of bony fixation methods in digital replantation. *J Hand Surg Am*. 1990;15:328–334.
31. Lister G. Intraosseous wiring of the digital skeleton. *J Hand Surg Am*. 1978;3(5):427–435.
32. Gordon L, Monsanto EH. Skeletal stabilization for digital replantation surgery. *Clin Orthop*. 1987;214:72–77.
33. Brown ML, Wood MB. Techniques of bone fixation in replantation surgery. *Microsurgery*. 1990;11:255–260.
34. Gingrass RP, Fehring B, Matloub H. Intraosseous wiring of complex hand fractures. *Plast Reconstr Surg*. 1980;66:383–394.
35. Hoffmann R, Buck-Gramco D. Osteosynthesis in digital replantation surgery. *Ann Chir Gynecol*. 1982;71:14–18.
36. Lee BH, Park CI, Lee JM. Intermittent bleeding method after replantation of the distal phalanx. *J Korean Soc Microsurg*. 2011;20(1):38–42.
37. Sears ED, Chung KC. Replantation of finger avulsion injuries: a systemic review of survival and functional outcomes. *J Hand Surg Am*. 2011;36:686–694.
38. Brooks D, Buntic RF, Kind GM, Schott K, Buncke GM, Buncke HJ. Ring avulsion: injury pattern, treatment, and outcome. *Clin Plast Surg*. 2006;34(2):187–195.
39. Earley MJ. The arterial supply of the thumb, first web and index finger and its surgical application. *J Hand Surg Br*. 1986;11:163–174.
40. Hamilton RB, O'Brien BM, Morrison WA, MacLeod AM. Survival factors in replantation and revascularization of the amputated thumb—10 years experience. *Scand J Plast Reconstr Surg*. 1984;18(2):163–173.
41. Biemer E. Experience in replantation surgery in the upper extremity. *Ann Acad Med Singapore*. 1979;8:393.
42. Shafiroff BB, Palmer AK. Simplified technique for replantation of the thumb. *J Hand Surg Am*. 1981;6(6):623–624.
43. Honda T, Nomura S, Yamanouchi S, et al. Clinical survey of the replanted hands at the level of the palm. *Orthop Surg*. 1983;34:1758–1760.
44. Woo SH, Lee YK, Lee HH, Park JK, Kim JY, Dhawan V. Hand replantation with proximal row carpectomy. *Hand*. 2009;4:55–61.
45. Cannon DL, Urbaniak JR. Transcarpal and radiocarpal wrist amputation and replantation. In: Watson HK, Weinzweig J, eds. *The Wrist*. 1st ed. New York: Lippincott Williams & Wilkins; 2001:269–276.
46. Jebson PJ, Hayes EP, Engber WD. Proximal row carpectomy: a minimum 10-year follow-up study. *J Hand Surg Am*. 2004;9:257–261.
47. Cheng GL. Overview and advancement in replantation of amputated finger and reconstruction of thumb or finger. In: Cheng GL, ed. *Replantation and Reconstruction of Fingers*. China: People's Medical Publishing House; 2008:3–5 [chapter 1]
48. Leung PC. The "throbbing sign"—an indication of early venous congestion in replantation surgery. *J Hand Surg Br*. 1979;4:409–411.
49. Hoang NT. Hand replantations following complete amputations at the wrist joint: first experiences in Hanoi, Vietnam. *J Hand Surg Br*. 2005;31(1):9–17.
50. Syrko M, Jablecki J. Quality of life-oriented evaluation of late functional results of hand replantation. *Ortop Traumatol Rehabil*. 2010;12(1):19–27.

II

CARPUS

15

Kienböck Disease

David M. Lichtman, MD
Kathryn A. Heim, MD
Timothy R. Niacaris, MD, PhD

INTRODUCTION

In 1910, Dr Robert Kienböck, a Viennese radiologist, described collapse of the lunate and attributed it to traumatic disruption of the bone's blood supply.[1] Over 100 years later, Kienböck disease is still best characterized as avascular necrosis of the lunate.

In 1947, Stahl classified Kienböck disease based on x-ray morphology combined with pathologic changes in the bone.[2] In 1977, Lichtman et al refined the staging system to make it more clinically relevant (Table 15-1).[3] Today, to enhance its clinical applicability, investigators are looking at MRI and arthroscopic findings in order to understand the implications of vascular and cartilage changes on the individual stages of Kienböck disease.

Controversy and uncertainty still exist regarding the best treatment options. Several factors can account for this. First, Kienböck disease is a relatively uncommon disorder, making it difficult to assemble large enough series to generate effective studies. Next, in most cases, the precise etiology of the disorder is unknown; consequently, preemptive treatment is problematic. This is aggravated by the fact that most patients are diagnosed relatively late in the course of the disease, making it difficult to identify proximate inciting causes. Finally, the natural history is largely unknown since there are few well-designed studies that follow the longitudinal course of the disease or that prospectively compare the outcomes of treated versus untreated patients.

Despite the lack of significant progress over the past century, there are indications that newer technology will soon enable surgeons to more accurately assess the appropriate treatment options for specific cases of Kienböck disease. This chapter will explore these possibilities from the perspective of creating a more clinically relevant treatment algorithm for patients with this very challenging diagnosis.

ETIOLOGY

Negative ulnar variance may be a risk factor for the development of Kienböck disease. To determine the ulnar variance, a posteroanterior radiograph of the wrist should be obtained with the forearm in neutral rotation. In 1928, Hülten speculated that negative ulnar variance may increase shear forces across the lunate and predispose patients to developing lunate AVN.[4] He observed that 78% of his patients with Kienböck disease had ulnar negative variance, compared with only 23% in the unaffected population. In contrast, D'Hoore et al found no significant difference between the mean ulnar variance of 125 patients without Kienböck disease and 52 patients with the disorder.[5] Nakamura et al studied Japanese patients with normal wrists and those with Kienböck disease and found no significant difference in ulnar variance between the 2 groups when corrected for gender and age.[6]

A cadaveric study published in 1980 by Gelberman et al identified 3 distinct patterns of the lunate's intraosseous blood supply.[7] These anatomic variations led the authors to conclude that Kienböck disease may be the result of compression fractures due to repeated trauma to poorly vascularized lunates. One criticism of this conclusion, however, is that none of the lunates showed signs of avascular necrosis; therefore, lunates with Kienböck disease could possibly have a fourth as yet unspecified vascular pattern.

In another study, Schiltenwolf et al measured the intraosseous pressure in 12 normal lunates and 12 lunates with Kienböck disease and found increased pressures in the necrotic lunates.[8] Based on these results, they hypothesized that impaired venous congestion with subsequent restriction of arterial flow is a risk factor for the development of osteonecrosis. However, it is impossible to know if these increased pressures were the cause of Kienböck disease or were merely a result of the inherent changes in the lunate subsequent to its onset.

Scattered case reports also exist of Kienböck disease in association with other systemic conditions such as septic emboli, sickle cell disease, hepatitis C, and gout.[9] There are also reports of familial occurrence that may indicate a genetic predisposition or heritable component of the disorder. The variety of theories on the etiology of Kienböck disease demonstrates that its pathogenesis is not yet fully understood. In fact, the etiology is likely multifactorial with several anatomic, environmental, and/or genetic predispositions that make certain lunates susceptible to injury, which

TABLE 15-1: Stages of Kienböck Disease

	Radiographic Findings
Stage I	Normal radiographs Decreased MRI signal on T1; increased/decreased on T2
Stage II	Increased lunate density Normal wrist architecture
Stage III	Lunate collapse
IIIA	Carpal alignment maintained; radioscaphoid angle <60°
IIIB	Fixed scaphoid rotation ("ring sign"); radioscaphoid angle >60°
Stage IV	Lunate collapse Degenerative change in radiocarpal, midcarpal, and/or STT joints

may act as the catalyst for development of AVN. The progression of Kienböck disease may then occur gradually due to minor, repeated trauma or may develop rapidly following a single major traumatic event. The role of osteoclastic regulation of bone resorption is also being studied as a factor in the rate and severity of lunate collapse.[10]

CLASSIFICATION

The classification system described by Lichtman et al in 1977 was originally designed for the purposes of research.[3] Without a standardized system to categorize the severity of disease, comparing the results of treatment modalities was challenging. Today, the system is also used as a treatment algorithm for patients with Kienböck disease.

Current Staging of Kienböck Disease

Plain radiographs are normal in Stage I, and there is no evidence of sclerosis or lunate collapse. The remainder of the carpus is also unaffected. On MRI the lunate shows low signal on T1-weighted images, and on the T2-weighted images the signal may be decreased or increased depending on whether bone edema is present or revascularization is occurring (Fig. 15-1). Clinically, patients in Stage I present with symptoms similar to wrist sprains. Typically there is intermittent dorsal wrist pain, exacerbated by wrist extension and axial loading.

In Stage II, radiographs of the wrist reveal increased lunate density, but carpal architecture is maintained (Fig. 15-2). The lunate may have 1 or more fracture lines present at this stage. Patients with Stage II Kienböck disease typically have a clinical presentation of synovitis with persistent pain during the day and even at night. The T1 MRI findings are similar to those in Stage I; however, T2 sequences may now show larger areas of decreased signal, indicating sclerosis.

Stage III Kienböck disease was originally described as lunate collapse with disruption of the carpal alignment on plain radiographs. It was modified in 1990 to include

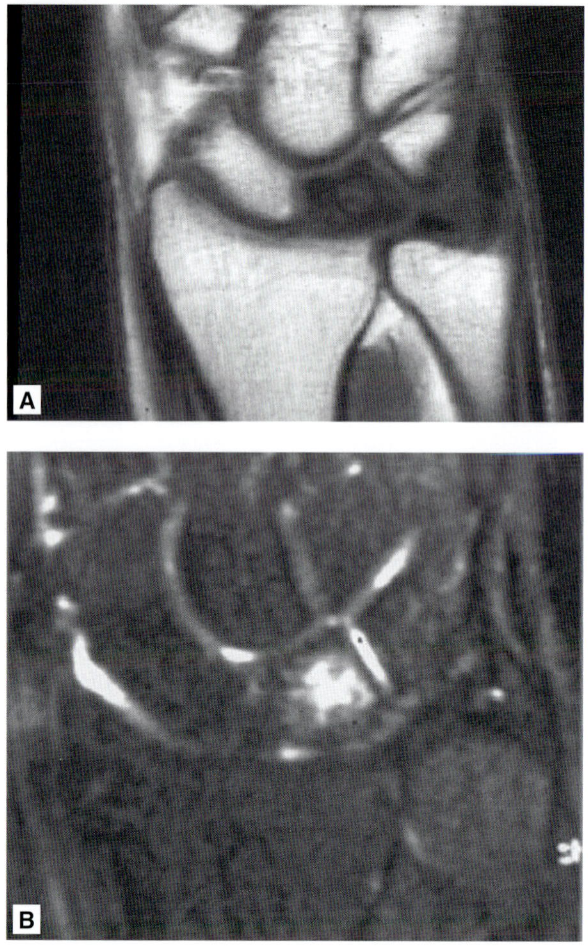

FIGURE 15-1 MRI of a patient with Stage I disease showing (**A**) decreased signal on the T1 image and (**B**) increased uptake on the T2 image.

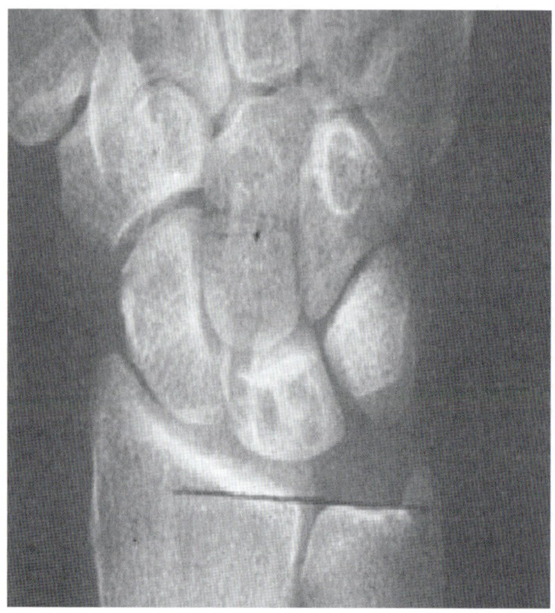

FIGURE 15-2 In Stage II disease, the lunate shows increased density on radiographs.

Stages IIIA and IIIB.[11] Both subdivisions of Stage III involve lunate collapse. In Stage IIIA there is maintenance of carpal alignment, but in Stage IIIB the scaphoid is fixed in a hyperflexed position, demonstrated by a "ring sign" on radiographs. In addition, the capitate migrates proximally. The radioscaphoid angle can be measured to distinguish between Stages IIIA and IIIB; an angle of less than 60° is consistent with Stage IIIA and one greater than 60° defines Stage IIIB. Goldfarb et al showed that the use of the radioscaphoid angle to distinguish between Stages IIIA and IIIB increases the interobserver reliability of the system.[12] Clinically, patients in Stage IIIA demonstrate progressive wrist pain and stiffness, whereas patients in Stage IIIB often develop signs of mechanical wrist instability. This instability is a result of the overall inflammatory wrist synovitis with subsequent loss of ligamentous support to the necrotic lunate.

Stage IV Kienböck disease is defined by lunate collapse and secondary degenerative changes in the radiocarpal, scaphotrapeziotrapezoid (STT), and/or midcarpal joints (Fig. 15-3). We believe the pathogenesis of these radiographic findings is chronic mechanical instability and synovitis, similar to scaphoid nonunion advanced collapse (SNAC) or scapholunate advanced collapse (SLAC) wrists, prompting us to refer to this condition as Kienböck disease advanced collapse (KDAC). The clinical picture in Stage IV is that of degenerative arthritis of the wrist with intermittent swelling, pain, and limited range of motion.

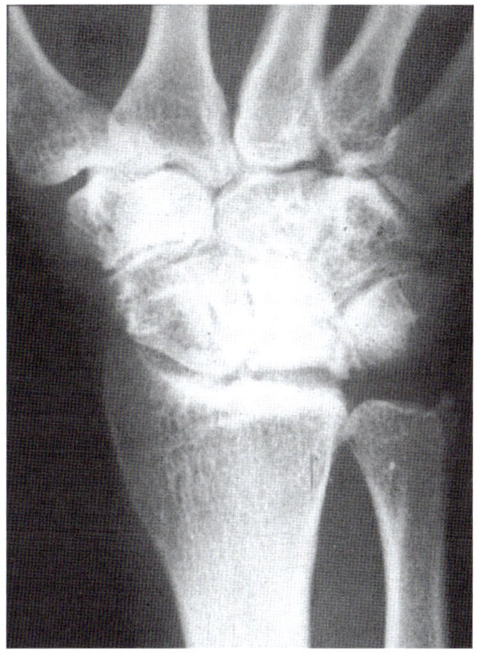

FIGURE 15-3 Stage IV disease.

Further categorizing the stages using newer diagnostic modalities may help to more precisely select the best treatment for individual patients. In addition to changes in bone morphology, as characterized by the current classification system, there is clearly a need to account for changes in the cartilage surfaces of the wrist bones as well as the vascular status of the lunate. In 2006, Bain and Begg described a classification system and treatment algorithm for Kienböck disease based on arthroscopic findings of the affected joint surfaces (Fig. 15-4).[13] The classification system is based on the number of degenerative articular surfaces seen during wrist arthroscopy. Combined with the radiographic evidence,

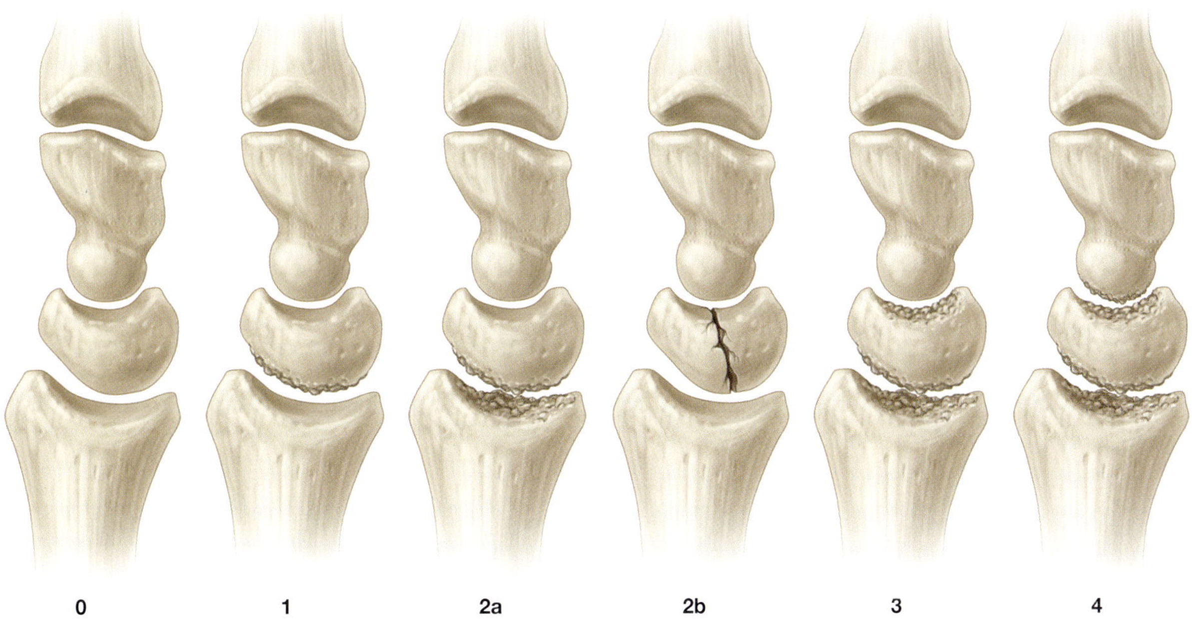

FIGURE 15-4 The arthroscopic classification system of Kienböck disease. (From Bain and Begg.[13])

TABLE 15-2: MRI-Based Classification of Kienböck Disease

Stage	Contrast-enhanced T1 Images	Interpretation
A	Homogenous enhancement in proximal lunate	Edema; perfusion intact
B	Inhomogenous enhancement in proximal lunate	Partial osteonecrosis
C	No contrast enhancement in the proximal lunate	Complete osteonecrosis; poor prognosis

this information may assist the surgeon in selecting the most appropriate treatment option. Although potentially useful, it is important to recognize that arthroscopic images tend to magnify small anatomic changes and that the clinical significance of cartilage changes in Kienböck disease has yet to be determined. Based on this classification the authors have proposed an algorithm for treatment. In Grade 0, all articular surfaces are normal; hence, an extra-articular unloading procedure may be indicated. In Grade 1, where there is 1 nonfunctional proximal lunate surface, a proximal row carpectomy (PRC), radioscapholunate fusion or lunate excision, and scaphocapitate (SC) fusion can be performed. In Grade 2, the proximal and distal lunate surfaces are nonfunctional, which requires a PRC or SC fusion (with lunate excision). Grades 3 and 4 require total wrist fusion or arthroplasty.

In 2007, Schmitt and Lanz described a classification system of Kienböck disease based on changes seen on gadolinium-enhanced MRI images (Table 15-2).[14] These images provide information on the vascularity of the lunate and, by inference, its healing potential. By combining this information with the degree of osseous collapse, carpal instability, and cartilage surface changes, a more nuanced classification could be created to assist in the development of a comprehensive treatment guide or algorithm.

There is also some rationale for the inclusion of a stage that precedes Stage I of Kienböck disease. A proposed "Stage 0" would include patients with intermittent wrist pain, normal radiographs, and a normal MRI. The concept of a Stage 0 Kienböck disease is analogous to the preclinical Stage 0 of the Ficat classification of AVN of the hip. One way to identify these patients would be to perform a contrast-enhanced MRI immediately after repetitive axial loading of the wrist, similar in concept to performing an EKG while running on a treadmill during a cardiac stress test. In a Stage 0 patient, we would expect to see increased signal in the lunate on this "wrist stress test." As we learn more about the etiology and natural history of Kienböck disease, this stage may be an ideal point to intervene and arrest the progression of the disorder.

TREATMENT

Over the years, a variety of procedures have been performed for Kienböck disease. These procedures, some of which are no longer performed, can be broadly categorized as immobilization, direct lunate revascularization, indirect revascularization/lunate unloading, lunate excision with or without replacement, and salvage procedures (Table 15-3). Despite the large volume of work that has been done, the appropriate treatment choices for patients with Kienböck disease remain a matter of debate. Innes and Strauch performed a retrospective systematic review of 37 uncontrolled studies with a minimum 1-year follow-up on the treatment of Kienböck disease from 1998 to 2008.[25] They concluded that there was no active treatment that was superior in the treatment of Kienböck disease and that there were insufficient data to determine whether the outcomes of any intervention were superior to placebo or the natural history of the disease.

Our Recommended Treatment Protocol

For the past 30 years we have linked the treatment of Kienböck disease with the staging system described above (Table 15-4). For patients with Stage I disease, we usually suggest a trial of immobilization for 3 months. This is accomplished by cast immobilization or, rarely, by external fixation. MRI is used to assess the results of treatment, with increased signal on T2-weighted images indicating attempts at revascularization and a positive prognosis. Immobilization is often successful in young adults and children. Due to a better prognosis,[26] we sometimes refer to this group as having "Teenbock disease."

In Stage II and IIIA Kienböck disease, the treatment is aimed at direct or indirect revascularization of the lunate.

TABLE 15-3: Treatment Categories for Kienböck Disease

Immobilization	Cast immobilization External fixation[15] Temporary STT pinning[16]
Direct revascularization	Vascularized pisiform[17] Fourth and fifth extensor compartment artery distal radius transfer[18] Vascularized segment of distal radius and pronator quadratus[19] Second dorsal metacarpal artery transfer[20]
Indirect revascularization (lunate unloading)	Radial shortening osteotomy Ulnar lengthening osteotomy Radial wedge osteotomy[21] Capitate shortening osteotomy[22] STT fusion Scaphocapitate fusion
Lunate excision (± replacement)	Excision without replacement Silicone replacement[3] Titanium replacement Tendon interposition[23] Pisiform transfer
Salvage	Proximal row carpectomy[24] Total joint arthroplasty Partial wrist fusion Total wrist fusion

TABLE 15-4: Recommended Treatment of Kienböck Disease

Stage I	Immobilization; cast or external fixation
Stages II and IIIA	
Ulnar negative	Joint unloading; radial shortening
Ulnar positive/neutral	Capitate shortening with or without direct revascularization
Stage IIIB	Limited intercarpal arthrodesis or proximal row carpectomy
Stage IV	Proximal row carpectomy or wrist arthrodesis

Direct revascularization options include a vascularized pisiform transfer, vascularized transfer of a segment of the distal radius, or a transfer of branches of 1 of the dorsal metacarpal arteries. Indirect revascularization involves relieving the pressure on the lunate with procedures such as radial shortening, ulnar lengthening, or capitate shortening osteotomies. The goal of indirect revascularization is elimination of the source of repetitive trauma so that the lunate can regenerate its own blood supply. If the patient has an ulnar negative wrist, we usually recommend a joint leveling procedure such as radial shortening to unload the lunate. In ulnar neutral or ulnar positive patients, however, we perform a capitate shortening with or without a direct lunate revascularization procedure. In general, we prefer indirect revascularization procedures for Stages II and IIIA. Another option for Stages II and IIIA is core decompression of the distal radial metaphysis in an attempt to stimulate revascularization of the lunate.[27]

Once the patient has progressed to Stage IIIB, ulnar variance becomes less of a factor as the treatment now must address the carpal instability. At this stage, we recommend either limited intercarpal arthrodesis or a PRC. The purpose of these treatments is to address the symptoms of mechanical instability and/or slow the progression of arthritis in the radiocarpal and midcarpal joints (KDAC). Intercarpal fusions, either STT or SC, can be performed with or without excision of the lunate. The goal is to restore the scaphoid to a neutral position of 45° of flexion relative to the long axis of the radius. In addition, if it is determined that the necrotic lunate is contributing to overall synovitis, it should be excised as part of the procedure.

In Stage IV Kienböck disease, we consider salvage procedures for pain relief in patients with significant degenerative changes of the wrist. Salvage treatment options include PRC or wrist arthrodesis when the degenerative changes are extensive.

TYPES OF PROCEDURES

Vascularized Bone Graft

In the older literature, a vascular bundle implantation was the preferred method of lunate revascularization. Hori et al implanted the dorsal metacarpal vascular pedicle directly into the lunate of 9 patients and found evidence for revascularization of the lunate.[28] Tamai et al reported improvement in pain and grip strength in 50 of 51 patients after implantation of a vascular bundle into the lunate.[29]

The pedicled graft most commonly used for Kienböck disease is based on the 4 + 5 extensor compartment artery (ECA). The origins of the fourth and fifth ECAs are identified at the posterior division of the anterior interosseous artery, which is ligated proximal to the origins of these vessels, and a bone graft based on the fourth ECA is harvested from the distal radius approximately 1 cm proximal to the radiocarpal joint. This graft provides a large pedicle diameter and long pedicle length.

INDICATIONS

A vascularized bone graft (VBG) is indicated in Stage I and II Kienböck disease. It can also be used in Stage IIIA if the collapse is minimal.

CONTRAINDICATIONS

A fracture of the lunate precludes this procedure. Smoking is a general contraindication to VBG, and it is not indicated in patients over 40 years old.

SURGICAL TECHNIQUE OF THE 4 + 5 ECA VASCULARIZED GRAFT

A straight skin incision is made over the dorsal wrist from the third metacarpal base to the distal forearm. The fifth dorsal extensor compartment is exposed and incised and the extensor tendons are retracted radially. The fifth ECA, which originates from the dorsal branch of the anterior interosseous artery, is identified. The fourth ECA originates from the fifth ECA or anterior interosseous artery and supplies nutrient branches to the dorsal aspect of the radius within the fourth extensor compartment. A bone graft proximal to the radiocarpal joint and overlying the fourth ECA including the nutrient vessels is outlined. The lunate is then exposed, and the necrotic part is removed through a dorsal cortical window. The anterior interosseous artery is ligated proximal to the fourth and fifth ECAs. The graft is then inset into the lunate. Postoperatively, the extremity is immobilized in a below-elbow cast for 6 weeks.

OUTCOMES

De Smet and colleagues reviewed 8 patients at a mean follow-up of 29 months (range 13-42).[5] The mean range of movement was 65% of the unaffected side (range 43%-76%). Using the modified Mayo wrist score, there were 3 excellent, 3 good, and 1 fair result. The mean postoperative DASH score was 29.8 versus 40.0 preoperatively.

Moran et al retrospectively reviewed 26 patients who underwent the 4 + 5 ECA VBG along with supplemental external fixation or SC pinning for 6 to 8 weeks, at an average follow-up of 31 months.[18] Twenty-six 4 + 5 ECA VBGs were performed as treatment for Kienböck disease. The average patient age was 32 years (range, 13-59). At the time of surgery, 12 patients were graded as Stage II, 10 as IIIA, and 4 as IIIB. The mean follow-up time was 31 months. Twenty patients showed no radiographic progression of disease or collapse after surgery. Two patients progressed from Stage II to IIIA, 1 progressed from Stage II to IV, 1 progressed from Stage IIIA to IIIB, 1 progressed from Stage IIIA to IV, and 1 progressed from Stage IIIB to IV. The average Mayo wrist score was 77 (range, 35-100). According to the Mayo wrist scores 6 patients had an excellent result, 6 had a good result, 9 had a fair result, and 3 had a poor result. Satisfactory results were seen in 22 patients, based on the Lichtman scoring system.

Vascularized Pisiform Graft

INDICATIONS

This technique is indicated in Stage IIIA and IIIB Kienböck disease.

CONTRAINDICATIONS

This procedure should not be performed in Stage I when the lunate may be salvaged by direct or indirect revascularization. It is contraindicated in Stage IV, when there is complete lunate collapse associated with radiocarpal and midcarpal osteoarthritis.

SURGICAL TECHNIQUE

The procedure follows Saffar's original description.[30] A longitudinal incision is made parallel to the FCU tendon at the anteromedial aspect of the forearm, beginning 4 cm proximal to the distal wrist crease. At the level of distal wrist crease, it is curved radially and continued distally for 2 cm into the palm. The FCU tendon is retracted. A vessel loop is placed around the ulnar nerve that is protected throughout the procedure. The cubitodorsal artery and venae comitante are dissected distally up to the pisiform, ligating any horizontal branches. The pisiform is then detached from the triquetrum by dividing the capsule, taking care to preserve the periosseous arterial circle coming from the cubitodorsal artery. The pisiunciform ligament underneath the ulnar nerve is preserved and harvested with the pisiform. The FCU tendon is detached from the pisiform along with the tissue covering this bone and sutured to the capsule of the triquetrum or abductor digiti minimi tendon. Alternatively, it may be transferred attached to the pisiform. The flexor tendons are retracted radially to expose the palmar wrist capsule and the palmar aspect of the lunate is exposed. The articular surface of the proximal lunate is usually depressed or fragmented. The cartilage is elevated from the lunate and sutured to the scapholunate ligament that is sectioned near its attachment to the lunate. The lunotriquetral ligament is divided and the lunate is then removed in a piecemeal fashion, preserving the posterior wall to prevent dorsal dislocation of the transferred pisiform. The pedicled pisiform is passed under the FCU tendon and the ulnar nerve, taking care not to twist the pedicle and transferred to the lunate fossa. The pedicled pisiform is rotated 90° so that the triquetral facet faces the proximal surface of the capitate. Two K-wires are prepositioned to stabilize the pisiform. The first is placed through the triquetrum until it is just visible in the lunate cavity; the second one penetrates the radial aspect of the distal radius at the apex of the anatomic snuffbox, 2 cm proximal to the tip of the radial styloid, avoiding the tendons and the superficial nerves. It is angled in the direction of the lunate fossa until it is seen penetrating the lunate fossa. The K-wires are then advanced to stabilize the pisiform after the transposition. Two sutures are passed through the remaining scapholunate ligament and the pisiunciform ligament. A limited closure of the capsule is performed without compressing the pedicle. A plaster splint is applied for 3 days followed by a forearm cast for 3 weeks. A soft splint is then substituted, followed by protected wrist motion. The K-wires are removed at 6 weeks.

Daecke et al modified this procedure by leaving the lunate in situ and inserting the vascularized pisiform into a hollowed-out defect in the lunate.[17] The pisiform is freed from the muscular attachment and the flexor carpi ulnaris. The short blood vessels from the ulnar artery, passing dorsally and volarly across the ulnar nerve to the radial side of the pisiform, are preserved. The dorsal branch to the ulnar side of the pisiform is identified and preserved after incising the pisotriquetral capsule. With the proximal attachment still preserved, the articular cartilage and the cortical bone of the pisiform are abraded, preserving the vascular bundle on the ulnar side. Finally, the proximal pisotriquetral ligaments are cut and the vascular pedicle is dissected from distal to proximal including the surrounding soft-tissue bundle without separating the blood vessel from it.

COMBINED PROCEDURES

If there is a significant discrepancy of the distal radius and ulna, a radial shortening osteotomy can be performed along with the direct revascularization. In Stage IIIB, when the radioscaphoid angle is greater than 60°, an STT fusion or SC fusion can be added to unload the joint.

OUTCOMES

Saffar described his experience with 51 cases in Stages IIIA and IIIB with a maximum follow-up of 15 years. There was an improvement in the pain level by 3 grades. The average flexion–extension improved by 35°, radial and ulnar deviation improved by 14°, and strength improved by 10%.[31]

Daecke et al reviewed 23 patients at an average of 12 years who underwent a vascularized pisiform transposition to a cored-out lunate for Stages II and III.[17] The pain improved in 20 patients. Patients with negative ulnar variance underwent an additional radial shortening. The wrist motion increased significantly, and the grip strength averaged 84% of the contralateral hand. The mean DASH score was 15.3 ± 17.9. Out of 20 patients with preoperative x-rays the radiographic stage was unchanged in 11, improved in 3, and progressed in 6 patients. Osteoarthritis was found in 7 of 22 patients.

In another study, 18 patients with Kienböck disease Stage II were treated with transposition of a pedicled pisiform. In 8 cases of negative ulnar variance, a radius shortening osteotomy was performed. There was an average follow-up of 30 months. Seventeen patients had less pain. Fourteen patients showed an improved range of motion of 30°. Magnetic resonance imaging showed perfusion of the pisiform in 16 cases.[32]

Leveling Procedures of the DRUJ: Radial Shortening Osteotomy

INDICATIONS

Radial shortening osteotomy is more commonly performed than ulnar lengthening. This procedure is indicated in Stage II and IIIA wrists with a significant negative ulnar variance. Caution should be exercised if there is a protruding lip of the radius into the proximal DRUJ.

CONTRAINDICATIONS

Ulnar positive wrist or potential DRUJ impingement is a contraindication to radial shortening (Fig. 15-5A-D). Stage IIIB is a relative contraindication, whereas Stage IV should not be treated with this technique. Smoking is a relative contraindication to all osteotomies.

SURGICAL APPROACH

The distal third of the radius is exposed through a standard volar approach. A 6-hole dynamic compression plate or a volar locking plate is applied on the volar surface. The bone is marked to determine the level of the osteotomy and the correct rotation of the radius. The osteotomy is performed removing 2- to 3-mm section of bone and the plate is attached with screws (Fig. 15-6A-D). The patients are started on early wrist motion postoperatively.

OUTCOMES

Weiss et al performed a radial osteotomy in 29 patients (30 wrists).[33] They noted that most of the patients did not progress from Stage III to IV. The wrist motion averaged 32% of extension and 27% of flexion compared with the uninjured side, and grip strength averaged 49% of the uninvolved side. Quenzer and coworkers reviewed 68 patients at a mean follow-up of 52 months. The pain improved in 93% and grip strength improved in 76%, but motion was limited to 60% to 65% of the uninvolved side.[34] Similarly, Wada et al found that there was radiographic progression in 8/13 patients at the 10-year follow-up after a closing wedge osteotomy.[35]

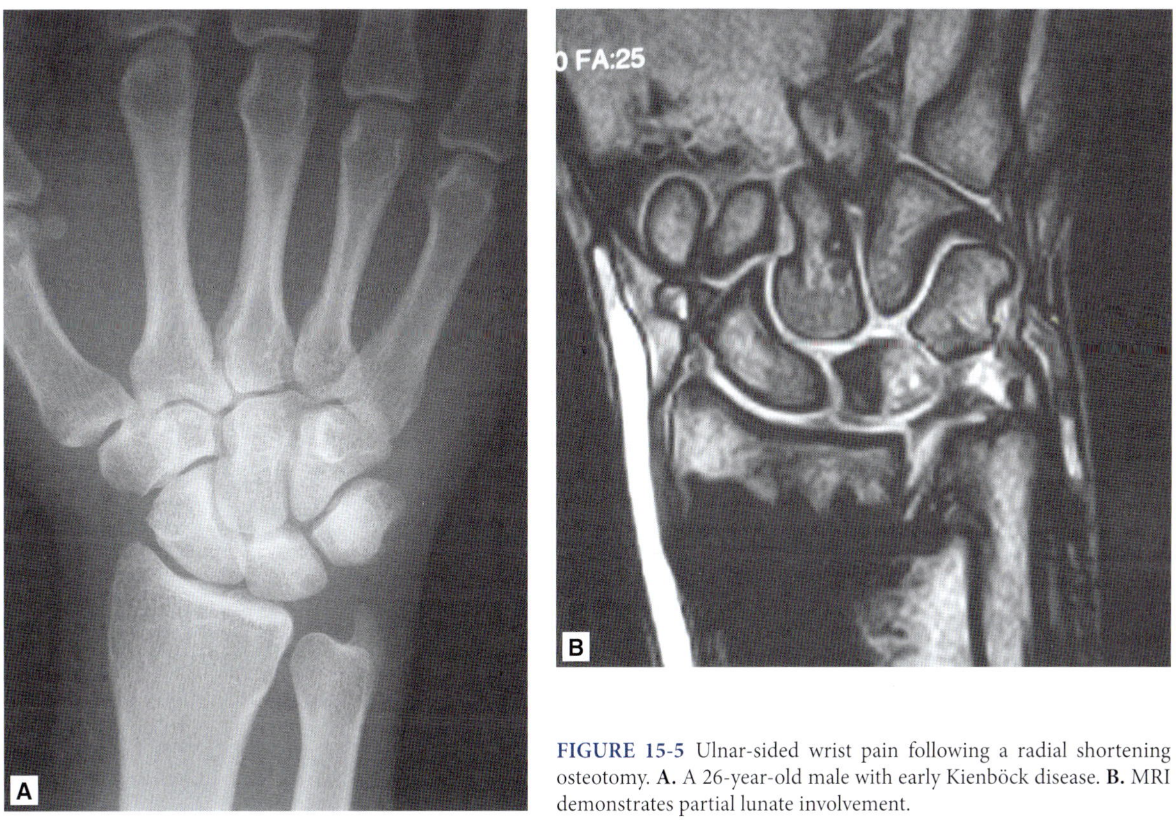

FIGURE 15-5 Ulnar-sided wrist pain following a radial shortening osteotomy. **A.** A 26-year-old male with early Kienböck disease. **B.** MRI demonstrates partial lunate involvement.

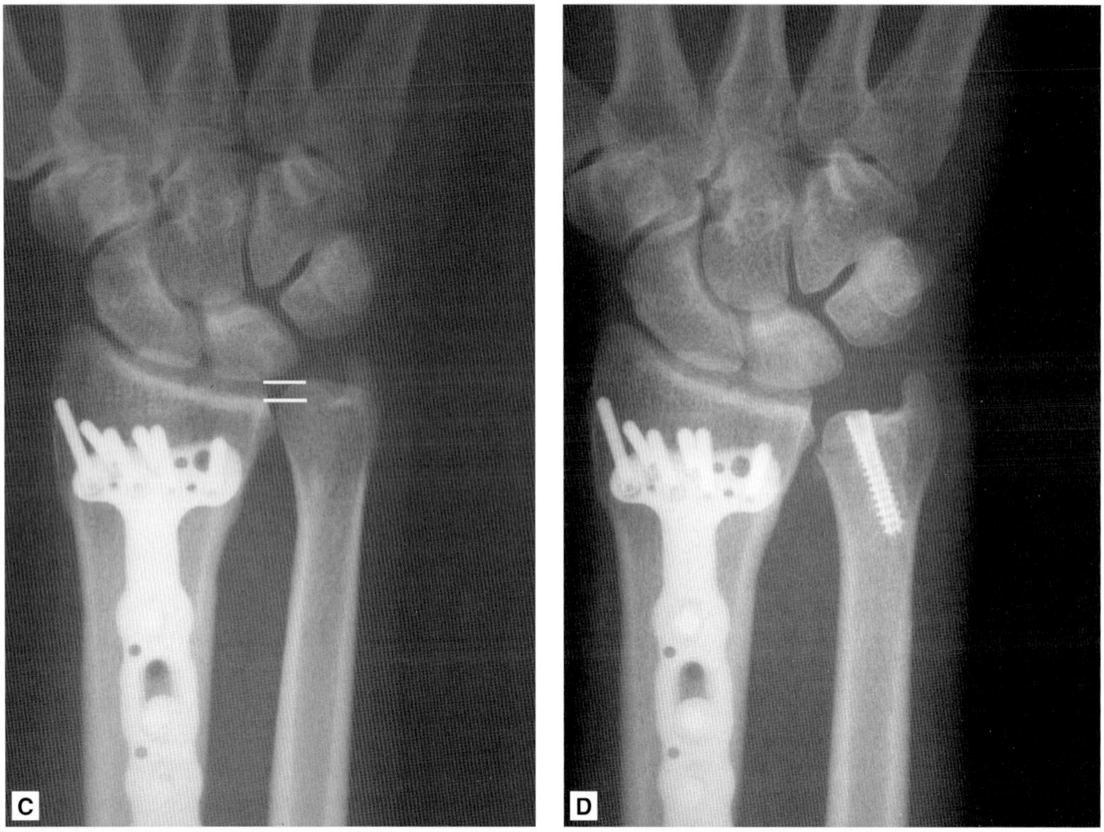

FIGURE 15-5 (*Continued*) **C.** Radial shortening procedure done by referring physician. Note the ulnar positive variance. **D.** Closing wedge osteotomy of ulnar head restores ulnar neutral variance. (Copyright David J. Slutsky, MD.)

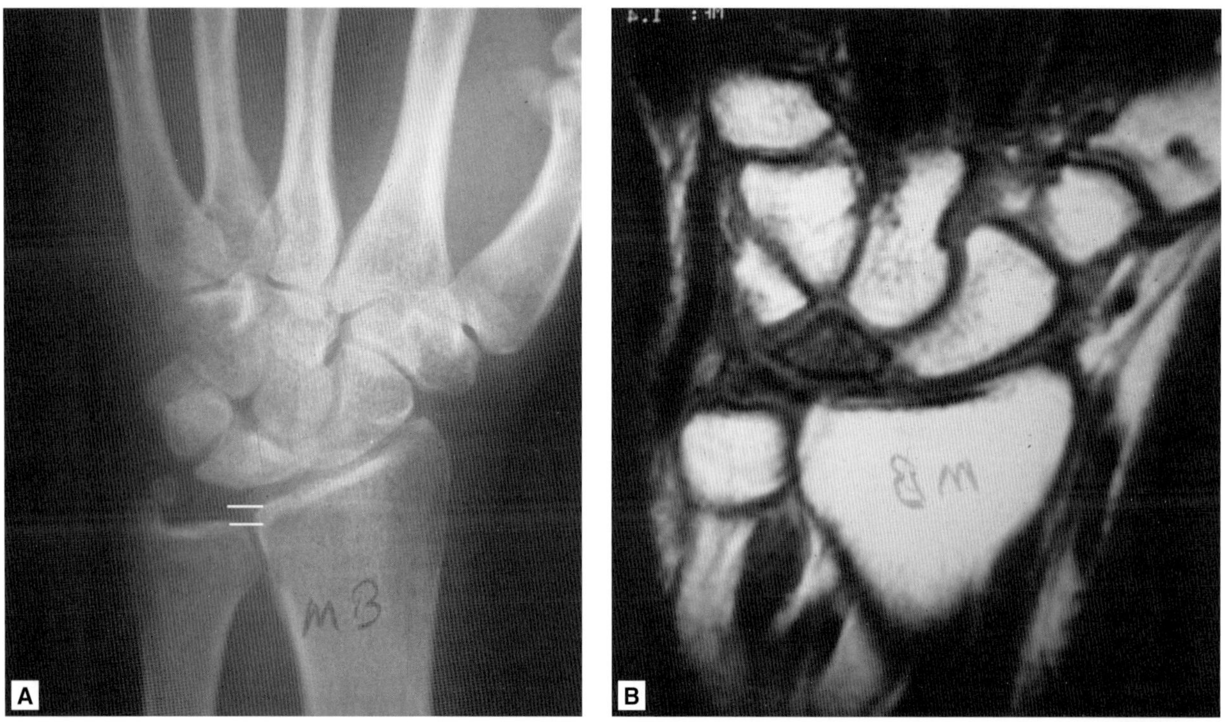

FIGURE 15-6 Radial shortening. **A.** A 30-year-old male with Stage II Kienböck disease. Note the ulna minus 2 mm variance. **B.** MRI confirms hypoperfusion of entire lunate on T1-weighted image.

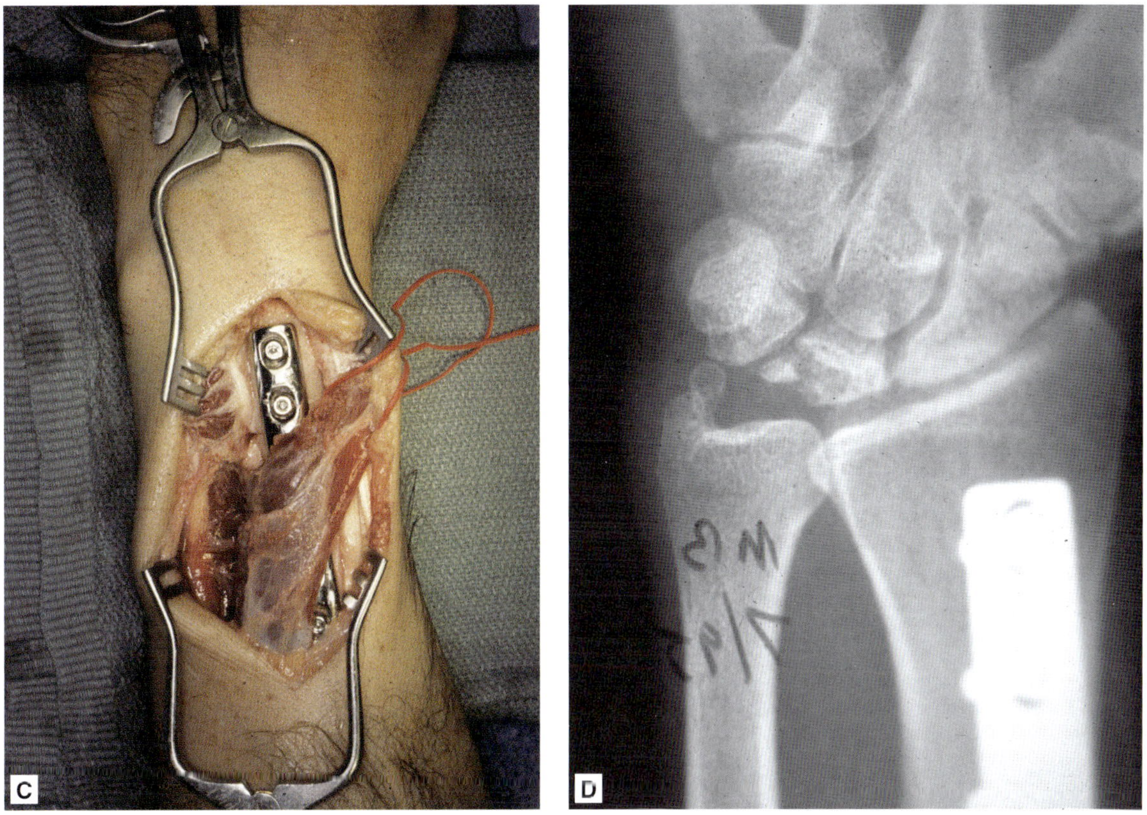

FIGURE 15-6 (*Continued*) **C.** Radial shortening and dorsal dynamic compression plate. **D.** Two-year follow-up demonstrates further collapse of lunate. (Copyright David J. Slutsky, MD.)

Some authors believe it is the change in blood supply that results in the clinical improvement rather than the shortening per se. Blanco and Blanco followed 11 patients aged 18 to 42 years, with Kienböck disease with a distal radius osteotomy and plate fixation without modifying the radial length or inclination.[36] According to the radiographic classification, 3 patients were Stage II, 5 were Stage IIIA, and 3 were Stage IIIB. One patient was ulnar positive; otherwise, there was an average negative ulnar variance of 1.8 mm (range, 1.5-3 mm). At a minimum 10-year follow-up, 6 patients reported no pain, 3 reported mild pain, and 2 reported moderate pain. Active wrist motion increased approximately 30%. Grip strength improved 65% to 80% compared with the nondominant side. Radiographically, the lunate showed some sclerosis in 3 cases and fragmentation in 2. No patient developed evidence of osteoarthritis at the radiocarpal joint at the final follow-up. The radiographic stage deteriorated in 1 patient. The average carpal height ratio did not change. The ulnar variance and the radioulnar joint showed no change.

Salvage Procedures

Both limited wrist arthrodesis with scaphotrapezial trapezoid fusion and SC fusion are options for Stage IIIB. PRC is another option for advanced stages of Kienböck disease.[37]

SURGICAL TECHNIQUE: SCAPHOCAPITATE FUSION

The branches of the radial sensory nerve are identified and protected. The distal termination of the posterior interosseous nerve can be excised at the surgeon's discretion. The radiocarpal and intercarpal articular cartilage surfaces are carefully inspected for significant arthrosis. The status of the lunate is evaluated in Kienböck disease and is left in place if the cartilage shell is intact (Fig. 15-7); otherwise it is excised. The adjacent articular surfaces of the scaphoid and capitate are removed. The ideal radioscaphoid angle is between 30° and 57° based on a cadaver study and the SC joint is stabilized with 2 guidewires. Cancellous bone graft is then packed into the SC interval. There are several options for final fixation including Kirschner wires, screws, staples, or even small plates (Fig. 15-8A-C). Occasionally a radial styloidectomy may be performed in situations of radial styloid impingement. Prior to wound closure, final radiographs are obtained to evaluate hardware placement, the radioscaphoid angle, and alignment of the fusion. The wrist is immobilized in a splint with slight wrist extension for about 6 weeks after operation.

OUTCOMES

Sennwald and Ufenast performed a SC arthrodesis in 11 patients with Kienböck disease with a median age of

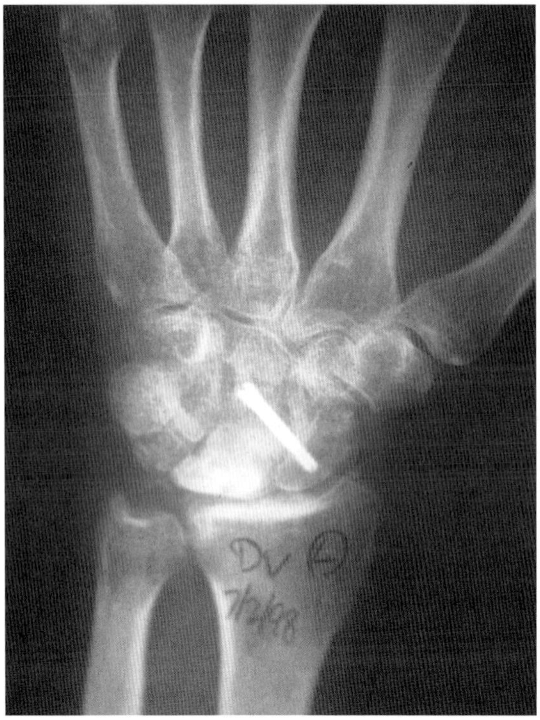

FIGURE 15-7 Scaphocapitate fusion with retention of the lunate. (Copyright David J. Slutsky, MD.)

26 years.[38] Ten patients had Grade III and 1 had Grade II disease by the Lichtman classification. The lunate was left in situ and a SC arthrodesis was performed with 2 lag screws and corticocancellous bone graft. At an average follow-up of 36 months 10 patients had complete pain relief and 1 had persistent pain. The average loss of the flexion/extension arc was 52%.

INDICATIONS FOR PROXIMAL ROW CARPECTOMY

A PRC is indicated for patients with Stage IIIB and IV disease with reasonable preservation of the cartilage on the capitate head and lunate fossa of the radius.

CONTRAINDICATIONS

These include severe damage to the cartilage in the lunate fossa, ulnar translocation of the wrist, a damaged capitate head, or a previous intercarpal arthrodesis. Caution should be exercised when the radial styloid has been excised along with attachment of the stabilizing volar radiocarpal ligaments.

SURGICAL TECHNIQUE

A transverse or longitudinal dorsal incision is made. The dorsal retinaculum is opened over the third compartment, and a Mayo ligament-sparing capsulotomy or longitudinal

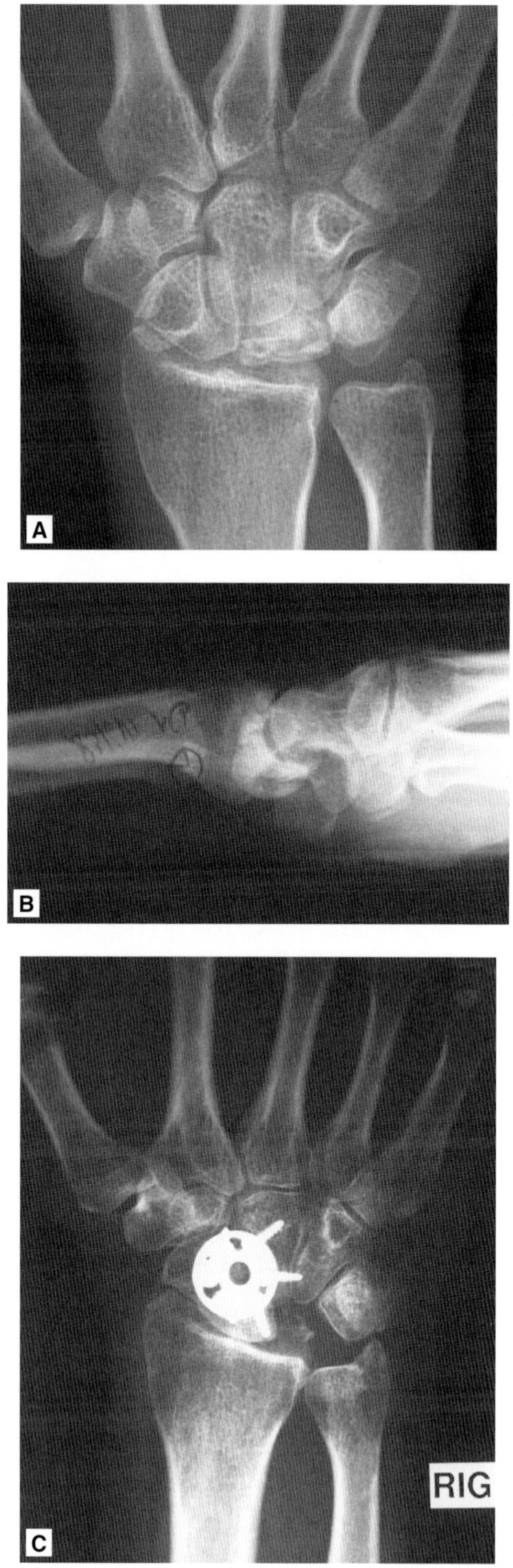

FIGURE 15-8 Scaphocapitate fusion with lunate excision. **A.** Stage IIIB Kienböck disease. **B.** Note the DISI deformity. **C.** Successful scaphocapitate fusion with a circular plate combined with lunate excision, but note the scapholunate narrowing. (Copyright David J. Slutsky, MD.)

capsulotomy is performed to expose the carpus. A K-wire can be used to manipulate the carpal bones, which can be removed intact starting with the lunate, or each bone can be osteotomized and morselized, and then removed piecemeal. The capitate is seated in the lunate fossa and the wrist stability is assessed. The capsule and retinaculum are anatomically repaired. If the capitate is unstable, it can be held with temporary K-wire fixation, but there is a risk of pin-tract infection. If there is styloid carpal impingement with radial deviation, then 1 cm or less of radial styloid can be excised through the same incision. The wrist is immobilized in a cast for 4 weeks followed by wrist motion exercises.

OUTCOMES

Jebson et al reported results in 18 patients who were evaluated at an average follow-up of 13.1 years after PRC (range, 10.0-17.2 years).[39] The average wrist range of motion was 63% and the average maximal grip strength was 83% of the opposite extremity. Seventeen patients were satisfied with their outcome. One patient complained of persistent pain and was not satisfied but did not want further surgery. Follow-up radiographs showed flattening of the proximal capitate in 6 patients. Radiocapitate arthrosis was absent or minimal in 13 patients and moderate to severe in 4 patients. The presence of radiographic changes did not correlate with patient satisfaction or degree of wrist pain. DiDonna et al reviewed 22 patients at a mean of 14 years.[40] The mean range of motion values were 36° flexion, 36° extension, 9° radial deviation, and 31° ulnar deviation. The average grip strength was 91% of the contralateral hand. Half of the patients reported mild-to-moderate pain with activity, but all of these patients were satisfied with the procedure. Eighty-seven percent of patients had radiographic evidence of arthritis between the head of the capitate and the radius, but neither the presence nor the degree of arthritis correlated with clinical outcome. Four patients were dissatisfied with the procedure and elected to proceed with wrist arthrodesis. Lumsden et al recently reviewed 17 patients with Stage IIIA and IIIB with a minimum 15-year follow-up.[41] Using the Glickel and Milender scale there were 5 excellent, 7 good, 1 fair, and no poor results. Total arc of motion averaged 73% of the uninvolved side. Grip strength averaged 92% of the uninvolved side. Compared with preoperative values, range of motion improved an average of 16% and grip strength improved an average of 129%. Radiographically 2 patients demonstrated no degenerative changes, 5 showed minimal changes, 3 had moderate changes, and 1 patient demonstrated severe degeneration. However, these radiographic findings did not correlate with clinical outcome or time since surgery.

Other Procedures

Afshar treated 9 patients with Stages II and IIIA with ulnar neutral or ulnar positive wrists with capitate shortening and reported MRI evidence of partial revascularization at a mean of 4.7 months postoperatively (Fig. 15-9A-C).[42] Illarramendi

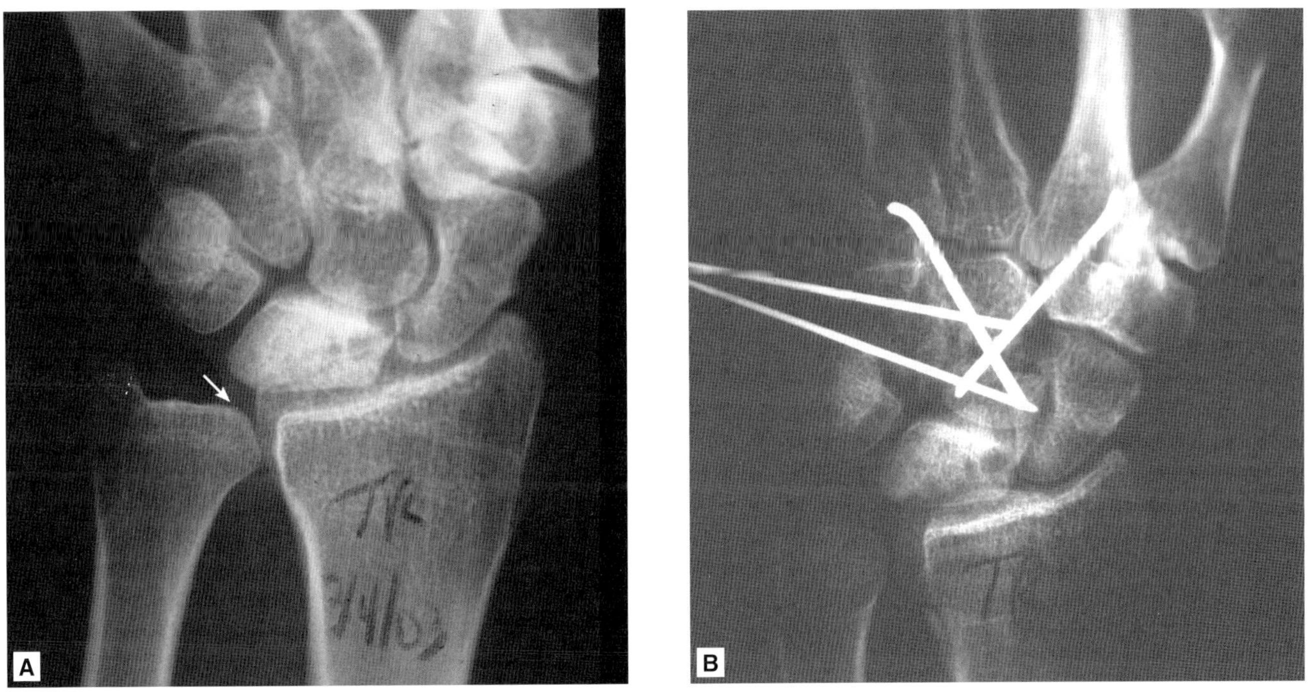

FIGURE 15-9 Capitate shortening. **A.** Kienböck disease Stage II, the ulnar positive variance (arrow) precludes a radial shortening. **B.** Capitate shortening osteotomy and capitohamate fusion.

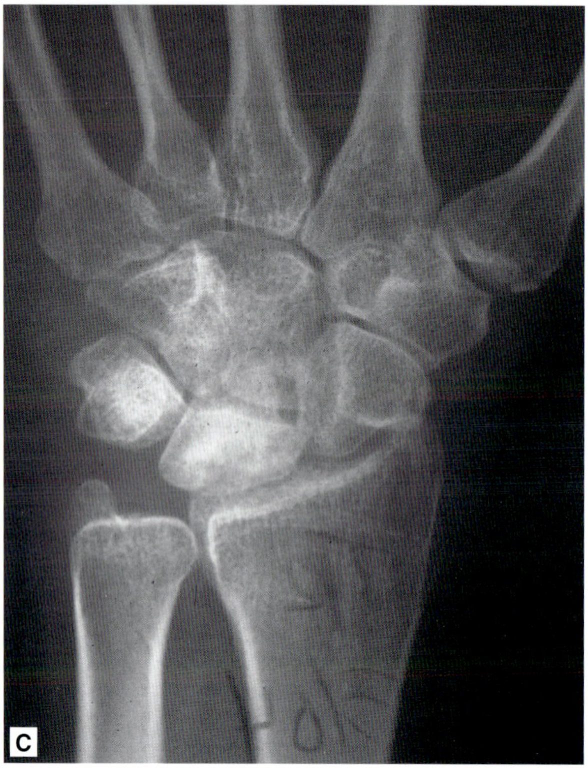

FIGURE 15-9 (*Continued*) **C.** One-year follow-up with a healed C-H fusion and no further lunate collapse. (Copyright David J. Slutsky, MD.)

et al reported their results using a core decompression of the distal radius and ulna in 22 patients aged 18 to 64 years with Stage I to IIIA disease (Fig. 15-10A and B).[27] A small cortical window was created in the distal radius and ulna, and the metaphysis was decompressed using small curettes. At a mean follow-up of 10 years, 16 patients were pain free, 4 had occasional pain, and 1 had moderate pain. Radiographically 17/22 had the same radiographic stage, whereas 5 progressed. The average wrist extension was 59° (range, 32°-80°) and the average wrist flexion was 57° (range, 30°-80°). The average grip strength was 75% (range, 37%-112%) compared with the contralateral side. Wrist denervation and the Graner operation have also been used, but there are no large reported series.

CONCLUSION

In summary, many procedures have been utilized for the treatment of Kienböck disease, and the success of the various procedures can be difficult to distinguish. In the future, we need to be more precise in selecting the proper procedure for each patient. As our knowledge of the various factors that affect the natural history and treatment outcomes of Kienböck disease increases, it is logical that a more comprehensive classification system incorporating the radiographic, cartilaginous, and vascular changes ("the triple threat") will be developed to guide treatment selection. This comprehensive guide could, in certain cases, change the recommended treatment when compared with that based solely on the radiographic classification. For example, if a patient with radiographic Stage II Kienböck disease has Stage 0 changes in the cartilage and Stage B changes in the vascularity, a radial shortening procedure might be an appropriate treatment. In contrast, if the same Stage II patient had Stage 4 cartilage and Stage C vascularity, then a radiocarpal arthrodesis might be a better option. All of the available information could then be used to guide treatment (Table 15-5). We have recently passed the centennial anniversary of Kienböck disease. Unfortunately, our clinical knowledge has not kept pace

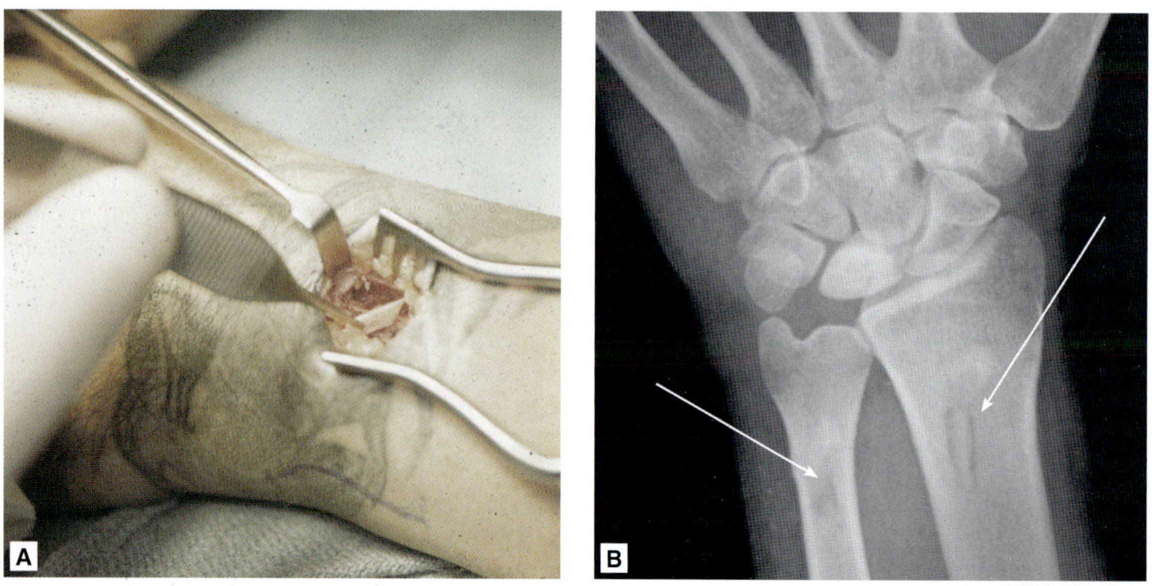

FIGURE 15-10 A. Removal of dorsal cortex from distal radius. **B.** Core decompression of radius and ulna (arrows). (Copyright David J. Slutsky, MD.)

TABLE 15-5: Integrated Kienböck Disease Classification System

Radiographic	Cartilaginous	Vascular
0	0	A
I	0, 1	A, B, or C
II	0, 1, 2	A, B, or C
IIIA or IIIB	3, 4	A, B, or C
IV	4	C

with the passage of time. There is reason to believe, however, that further research and new technology may assist our understanding of this disease in the future. The key to better patient care will be to apply this research to translational studies that test the long-term outcomes of treatment and the natural history of the disorder. This task will only be accomplished with multicenter trials facilitated by international communication and cooperation.

REFERENCES

1. Peltier LF. The classic. Concerning traumatic malacia of the lunate and its consequences: degeneration and compression fractures. Privatdozent Dr. Robert Kienböck. *Clin Orthop Relat Res.* 1980;149:4–8.
2. Stahl F. On lunatomalacia (Kienbock's disease), a clinical and roentgenological study, especially on its pathogenesis and the late results of immobilization treatment. *Acta Chir Scand.* 1947;126:1–133.
3. Lichtman DM, Mack GR, MacDonald RI, Gunther SF, Wilson JN. Kienböck's disease: the role of silicone replacement arthroplasty. *J Bone Joint Surg.* 1977;59:899–908.
4. Hülten O. Überanatomischevariationen der handgelenkknochen. *Acta Radiol Scand.* 1928;9:155–168.
5. D'Hoore K, De Smet L, Verellen K, Vral J, Fabry G. Negative ulnar variance is not a risk factor for Kienböck's disease. *J Hand Surg Am.* 1994;19:229–231.
6. Nakamura R, Tanaka Y, Imaeda T, Miura T. The influence of age and sex on ulnar variance. *J Hand Surg Br.* 1991;16(1):84–88.
7. Gelberman RH, Bauman TD, Menon J, Akeson WH. The vascularity of the lunate bone and Kienböck's disease. *J Hand Surg Am.* 1980;5:272–278.
8. Schiltenwolf M, Martini AK, Mau HC, Eversheim S, Brocai DR, Jensen CH. Further investigations of the intraosseous pressure characteristics in necrotic lunates (Kienböck's disease). *J Hand Surg Am.* 1996;21:754–758.
9. Castagnoli M, Giacomello A, Argentina RS, Zoppini A. Kienböck's disease in gout. *Arthritis Rheum.* 1981;24:974–975.
10. Irisarri C. Aetiology of Kienböck's disease. *Handchir Mikrochir Plast Chir.* 2010;42:157–161.
11. Alexander AH, Turner MA, Alexander CE, Lichtman DM. Lunate silicone replacement arthroplasty in Kienböck's disease: a long-term follow-up. *J Hand Surg Am.* 1990;15:401–407.
12. Goldfarb CA, Hsu J, Gelberman RH, Boyer MI. The Lichtman classification for Kienböck's disease: an assessment of reliability. *J Hand Surg Am.* 2003;28:74–80.
13. Bain GI, Begg M. Arthroscopic assessment and classification of Kienbock's disease. *Tech Hand Up Extrem Surg.* 2006;10:8–13.
14. Schmitt R, Krimmer H. Osteonecrosis of the hand skeleton. In: Schmitt R, Lanz U, eds. *Diagnostic Imaging of the Hand.* 1st ed. Stuttgart, NY: Georg Thieme Verlag; 2007:351–364.
15. Lichtman DM, Roure AR. External fixation for the treatment of Kienböck's disease. *Hand Clin.* 1993;9:691–697.
16. Ando Y, Yasuda M, Kazuki K, Hidaka N, Yoshinaka Y. Temporary scaphotrapezoidal joint fixation for adolescent Kienböck's disease. *J Hand Surg Am.* 2009;34:14–19.
17. Daecke W, Lorenz S, Wieloch P, Jung M, Martini AK. Vascularized os pisiform for reinforcement of the lunate in Kienböck's disease: an average of 12 years of follow-up study. *J Hand Surg Am.* 2005;30:915–922.
18. Moran SL, Cooney WP, Berger RA, Bishop AT, Shin AY. The use of the 4 + 5 extensor compartmental vascularized bone graft for the treatment of Kienböck's disease. *J Hand Surg Am.* 2005;30:50–58.
19. Lee JC, Lim J, Chacha PB. The anatomical basis of the vascularized pronator quadratus pedicled bone graft. *J Hand Surg Br.* 1997;22:644–646.
20. Simmons SP, Tobias B, Lichtman DM. Lunate revascularization with artery implantation and bone grafting. *J Hand Surg Am.* 2009;34:155–160.
21. Nakamura R, Tsuge S, Watanabe K, Tsunoda K. Radial wedge osteotomy for Kienböck disease. *J Bone Joint Surg.* 1991;73:1391–1396.
22. Almquist EE. Capitate shortening in the treatment of Kienböck's disease. *Hand Clin.* 1993;9:505–512.
23. Küçük L, Ozdemir O, Coşkunol E, Süğün TS, Ozaksar K. The effect of excisional arthroplasty with palmaris longus tendon on carpal height ratio in Stage 3 Kienböck's disease. *Acta Orthop Traumatol Turc.* 2011;45:393–398.
24. Begley BW, Engber WD. Proximal row carpectomy in advanced Kienböck's disease. *J Hand Surg Am.* 1994;19:1016–1018.
25. Innes L, Strauch RJ. Systematic review of the treatment of Kienbock's disease in its early and late stages. *J Hand Surg Am.* 2010;35:713–717, 717.e1–717.e4.
26. Kalb K, Pillukat T, Schmitt R, Prommersberger KJ. Kienböck's disease in paediatric and juvenile patients. *Handchir Mikrochir Plast Chir.* 2010;42:187–197.
27. Illarramendi AA, Schulz C, De Carli P. The surgical treatment of Kienböck's disease by radius and ulna metaphyseal core decompression. *J Hand Surg Am.* 2001;26:252–260.
28. Hori Y, Tamai S, Okuda H, Sakamoto H, Takita T, Masuhara K. Blood vessel transplantation to bone. *J Hand Surg Am.* 1979;4A:23–33.
29. Tamai S, Yajima H, Ono H. Revascularization procedures in the treatment of Kienbock's disease. *Hand Clin.* 1993;9(3):455–466.
30. Saffar P. Replacement of the semilunar bone by the pisiform. Description of a new technique for the treatment of Kienbock's disease. *Ann Chir Main.* 1982;1:276–279.
31. Saffar P. Vascularized pisiform transfer in place of lunatum for Kienböck's disease. *Chir Main.* 2010;29(suppl 1):S112–S118.
32. Wustner-Hofmann MC, Hofmann AK. Vascular pedicled transposition of the pisiform bone for treatment of lunate malacia. *Handchir Mikrochir Plast Chir.* 1997;29(4):171–177.
33. Weiss APC, Weiland AJ, Moore JR, Wilgis EFS. Radial shortening for Kienbock disease. *J Bone Joint Surg.* 1991;73A:384–391.
34. Trail IA, Linscheid RL, Quenzer DE, Scherer PA. Ulnar lengthening and radial recession procedures for Kienbock's disease. Long-term clinical and radiographic follow-up. *J Hand Surg Am.* 1996;21(B):169–176.
35. Wada A, Miura H, Kubota H, Iwamoto Y, Uchida Y, Kojima T. Radial closing wedge osteotomy for Kienbock's disease: an over 10 year clinical and radiographic follow-up. *J Hand Surg Br.* 2002;27:175–179.
36. Blanco RH, Blanco FR. Osteotomy of the radius without shortening for Kienbock disease: a 10-year follow-up. *J Hand Surg Am.* 2012;37:2221–2225.
37. Croog AS, Stern PJ. Proximal row carpectomy for advanced Kienböck's disease: average 10-year follow-up. *J Hand Surg Am.* 2008;33:1122–1130.
38. Sennwald GR, Ufenast H. Scaphocapitate arthrodesis for the treatment of Kienbock's disease. *J Hand Surg Am.* 1995;20A:506–510.
39. Jebson PJ, Hayes EP, Engber WD. Proximal row carpectomy: a minimum 10 year follow-up study. *J Hand Surg Am.* 2003;28(4):561–569.
40. DiDonna ML, Kiefhaber TR, Stern PJ. Proximal row carpectomy: study with a minimum of ten years follow-up. *J Bone Joint Surg Am.* 2004;86-A(11):2359–2365.
41. Lumsden BC, Stone A, Engber WD. Treatment of advanced-stage Kienböck's disease with proximal row carpectomy: an average 15-year follow-up. *J Hand Surg Am.* 2008;33:493–502.
42. Afshar A. Lunate revascularization after capitate shortening osteotomy in Kienbock's disease. *J Hand Surg Am.* 2010;35:1943–1946.

16

Preiser Disease

David B. Jones, Jr., MD
Steven L. Moran, MD
Marco Rizzo, MD

RATIONALE AND BASIC SCIENCE PERTINENT TO THE PROCEDURE

Avascular necrosis (AVN) of the scaphoid is a rare, potentially debilitating condition. First described by Preiser in 1910 in patients with a history of wrist trauma, *idiopathic* AVN of the scaphoid is now commonly referred to as Preiser disease.[1] It is differentiated from the more common posttraumatic AVN of the proximal pole that results from disruption of the blood supply by a fracture or nonunion.

Patients generally present with radial-sided or dorsal wrist pain, loss of motion, and weakness secondary to pain. There may or may not be a history of trauma or repetitive strain, but the onset tends to be insidious. Tenderness to palpation is often localized to the anatomic snuffbox, although more generalized synovitis, swelling, and wrist irritability are possible.

The etiology of Preiser disease remains uncertain. Several risk factors have been implicated in the development of idiopathic osteonecrosis including high-dose systemic corticosteroid therapy,[2-4] chemotherapy,[5,6] systemic lupus,[4,7,8] progressive systemic sclerosis,[9] excessive alcohol intake,[10,11] congenital scaphoid hypoplasia,[12,13] and repetitive trauma.[11] Multiple factors seem to likely ultimately contribute to the development of the disease.[11] While the exact etiology and risk factors may not be clear, the end result is ischemic osteonecrosis of the scaphoid.

Several anatomic and biomechanical features of the scaphoid make it susceptible to vascular disruption and AVN. The majority of the scaphoid is covered with articular cartilage. The primary vascular supply is from the radial artery with up to 80% of the intraosseous vascularity arising from branches entering the scaphoid through the dorsal ridge.[14] The distal 20% to 30% of the scaphoid is supplied by vessels entering the tubercle volarly, but there is no significant intraosseous anastomosis between the volar and dorsal vessels. The entire proximal pole is supplied in a retrograde manner by branches entering dorsally.[14,15] These branches pass through a thin intra-articular membrane between the capsule and dorsal ridge.[15]

Biomechanical studies have demonstrated increased pressure across the dorsal ridge from the extensor carpi radialis brevis tendon during wrist flexion.[15] These increased pressures may exceed the intraluminal pressure of the nutrient arterioles, thereby compromising blood flow to the scaphoid particularly with prolonged or repetitive wrist flexion activities and loading. Flow through these dorsal vessels may be further compromised by increased intra-articular pressure within the wrist caused by effusion, synovitis, or capsular thickening.

Regardless of the specific cause of vascular disruption, lack of adequate blood flow to the bone ultimately leads to scaphoid osteonecrosis. Histopathologic evaluation of the bone demonstrates empty lacunae and necrotic bone marrow.[16] Loss of viable bone ultimately leads to structural collapse and progressive degenerative arthritis at the radioscaphoid and midcarpal joints.

This progression has been classified by Herbert and Lanzetta into 4 stages based on the radiographic appearance of the bone (Table 16-1).[17] Stage 1 follows the initial vascular insult and is characterized by negative x-rays and a positive bone scan demonstrating the inflammatory response at the scaphoid. MRI is currently used more frequently than bone scans and demonstrates diminished marrow signal in the scaphoid on T1- and T2-weighted images (Fig. 16-1). Stage 2 demonstrates increased density of the proximal pole and generalized osteopenia resulting from increased osteoblast and osteoclast activity. Failure of this reparative phase to restore viable, vascularized bone leads to progression of the disease. Stage 3 is characterized by fragmentation of the proximal pole with or without a pathologic fracture resulting from the progressive necrosis and loss of architectural strength of the bone. Stage 4 represents the end stage of the disease and is characterized by carpal collapse and osteoarthritis.

While traditionally Preiser disease has been described to involve the entire scaphoid, Kalainov et al recently evaluated the MRI findings of patients with Preiser disease.[16] Two patterns of the disease were identified (Table 16-2). Type 1 is characterized by diffuse involvement of the scaphoid with MRI signal change throughout the entire scaphoid. Type 2

TABLE 16-1: Herbert and Lanzetta Classification[17]

Stage 1	Normal x-rays with abnormal bone scan (or decreased marrow signal on MRI)
Stage 2	Increased density in the proximal pole with osteopenia
Stage 3	Fragmentation of the proximal pole with or without pathologic fracture
Stage 4	Carpal collapse with osteoarthritis

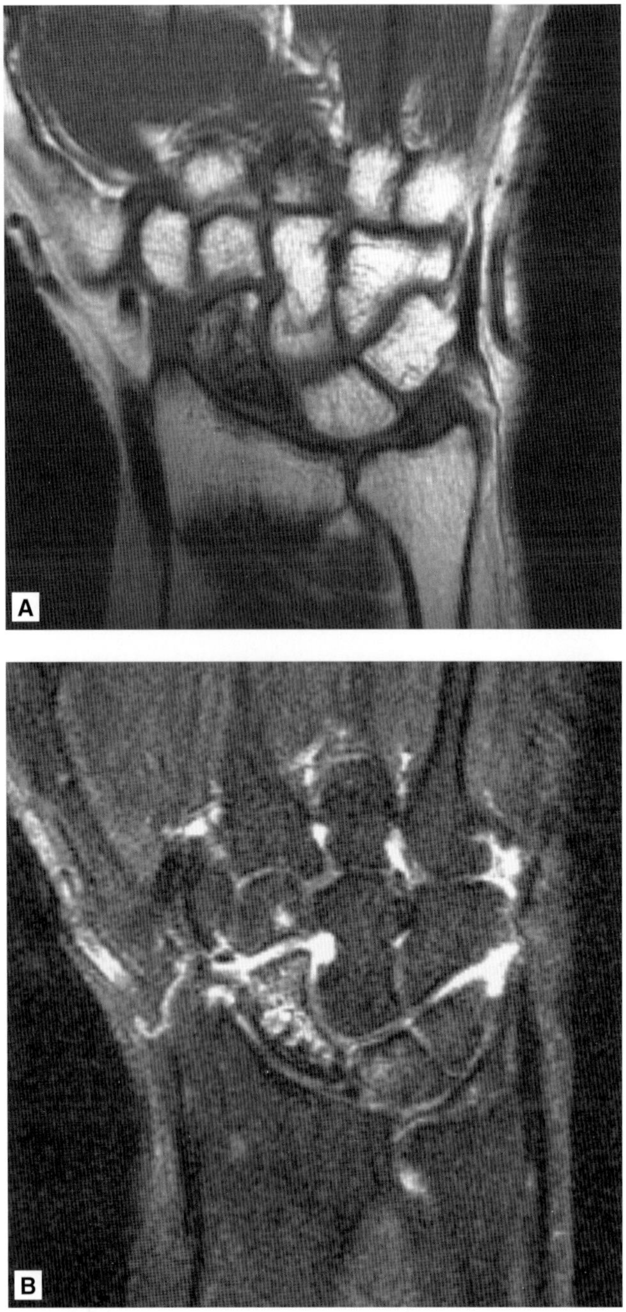

FIGURE 16-1 T1- and T2-weighted magnetic resonance imaging demonstrates diminished marrow signal in the scaphoid.

TABLE 16-2: Kalainov Classification[16]

Type 1	Diffuse avascular necrosis of the scaphoid
Type 2	Localized avascular necrosis of the scaphoid

is characterized by partial scaphoid involvement averaging 42% (range 33%-66%) of the scaphoid. Patients in the type 1 group were more likely to have a systemic risk factor such as corticosteroid use, while patients in the type 2 group were more likely to have a history of trauma. Patients in the type 1 group with avascularity of the entire scaphoid had worse clinical outcomes following treatment than the patients in the type 2 group.

Treatment strategies, therefore, must take into account the stage of the disease and degree of involvement of the scaphoid. Given the rare nature of Preiser disease, all treatment recommendations are based on relatively small, retrospective studies. Nonoperative management includes activity modification, immobilization, electrical stimulation, anti-inflammatory medications, physiotherapy, and corticosteroid injections.[16,18] Results of nonoperative modalities are variable with several patients' symptoms reportedly stabilizing or improving.[13,16,18] However, frequently the disease continues to progress despite conservative management to fragmentation and collapse.[16]

While there may be debate about the best treatment of stage 1 or 2 disease, there is general consensus that for patients with stage 3 or 4 disease attempts at revascularization of the scaphoid are not warranted. Once the scaphoid has fragmented and collapsed and certainly once degenerative changes are present, treatment options are limited to palliative and salvage procedures.

In patients with stage 3 or 4 disease with symptoms refractory to nonoperative management, several surgical procedures can be considered. Historically some patients were treated with partial or complete scaphoid excision and silicone replacement,[17,19] but because of concerns for silicone synovitis, implant fracture, progressive arthrosis, and carpal collapse, this has fallen out of favor.[20] Simple arthroscopic debridement and removal of loose bodies has been reported to be successful in improving symptoms and function in a case report of a patient with stage 3 Preiser disease.[21] Partial wrist denervation with selective anterior interosseous nerve (AIN) and posterior interosseous nerve (PIN) neurectomy has been shown to provide some relief of wrist pain in cases of radiocarpal arthritis.[22] Neurotomy of the articular branches from the superficial branch of the radial nerve (SBRN) and lateral antebrachial cutaneous (LABC) nerve in addition to AIN/PIN neurectomies has also been described and may improve pain relief with radial-sided pathology such as Preiser disease.[23] Results of partial wrist denervation for Preiser disease are limited and have been variable.[10] Nonetheless, it is an option for patients in whom a larger surgery is medically contraindicated or who are reluctant to consider partial or total wrist arthrodesis.

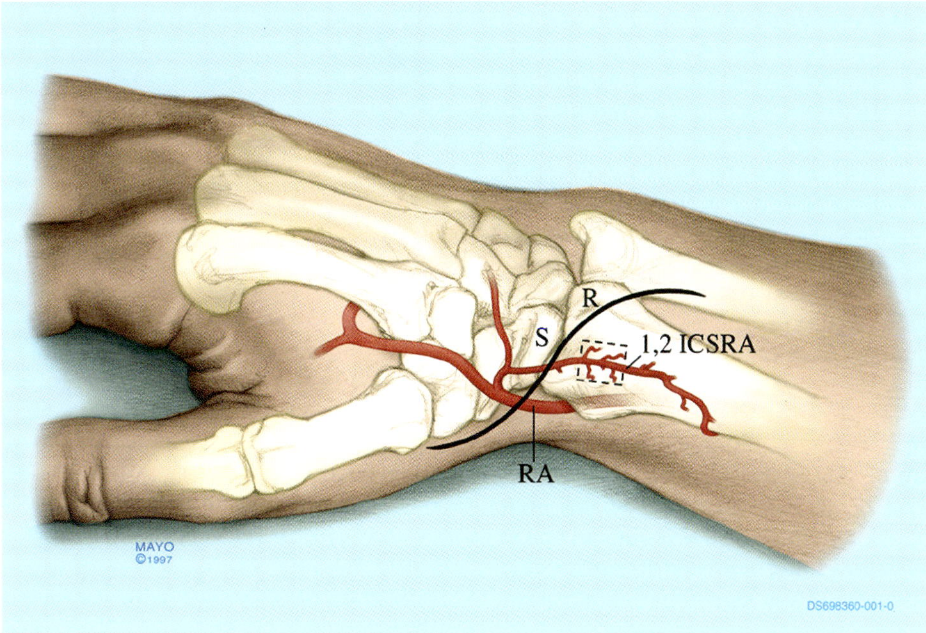

FIGURE 16-2 The reverse-flow 1,2 ICSRA vascularized bone graft from the dorsal distal radius. (With permission of Mayo Foundation for Medical Education and Research. All rights reserved.)

Definitive treatment of patients with stage 3 or 4 Preiser disease is limited to salvage procedures. Proximal row carpectomy (PRC) has been reported with largely satisfactory results.[10,24] The advantage of this procedure is that it is not dependent on achieving bony union and therefore may be advantageous in smokers and others with risk factors for nonunion. However, it requires an intact lunate fossa of the distal radius and capitate head and thus is not a good option in patients with more extensive radiocarpal or midcarpal arthritis. Furthermore, there are limited long-term studies of PRC and given the difference in radius of curvature of the capitate head and lunate fossa, the new articulation is less congruent and may be prone to increased wear.[25]

Scaphoid excision and 4-corner fusion has also been used in the treatment of advanced Preiser disease.[26] Although the wrist must be immobilized until bony union is achieved, this procedure maintains carpal height and preserves the radiolunate articulation. Long-term outcomes are similarly limited but demonstrate largely satisfactory results with preservation of approximately 50% of motion and 75% grip strength.[27] If patients continue to have pain despite PRC or limited arthrodesis, total wrist arthrodesis is the final resort.

In stage 1 or 2 Preiser disease, the cartilage shell of the scaphoid is intact. Therefore, treatment aims to unload the scaphoid or restore vascular supply to the bone to reverse the process of osteonecrosis. Closing wedge radial osteotomy[28] and arthroscopic drilling[29] have been reported successful in single case reports. Simple curettage with or without nonvascularized bone grafting has been also described for Preiser disease.[13,17,30]

However, vascularized bone grafting offers several potential advantages over the above procedures. Vascularized bone grafts restore blood supply to the devascularized bone, preserve viable osteocytes that accelerates consolidation without the need for creeping substitution, have biological and mechanical properties superior to nonvascularized grafts, and have been shown to be superior to nonvascularized grafts in treating scaphoid AVN of the proximal pole associated with nonunion.[31–35] Several pedicled vascularized bone grafts from the distal radius have been described for treating Preiser disease.[36–38] Our preference is the 1,2 intercompartmental supraretinacular (1,2 ICSRA) graft from the distal dorsal distal radius[38,39] (Fig. 16-2).

INDICATIONS

Use of vascularized bone grafts in the treatment of Preiser disease is limited to Herbert stage 1 or 2 disease in which the cartilage shell of the scaphoid is intact and in which the radioscaphoid and midcarpal joints are without arthritic change. If arthritic change is limited to the radial styloid, a radial styloidectomy could be performed at the time of vascularized bone grafting. More extensive degenerative change or collapse of the scaphoid warrants 1 of the palliative or salvage procedures described above.

Surgical treatment is warranted when patients' symptoms do not resolve with conservative measures. A prolonged trial of nonoperative management without improvement in pain may lead to progression of the disease resulting in fragmentation of the scaphoid or degenerative change that may preclude scaphoid preserving options.

CONTRAINDICATIONS

Fragmentation of the scaphoid and arthritic change beyond just the radial styloid (Herbert stage 3 or 4 Preiser disease) constitute contraindications to vascularized bone grafting procedures. The degree of arthritis may not be fully appreciable until intraoperative assessment of the articular cartilage. As such, the surgeon should be prepared to convert to 1 of the palliative or salvage procedures outlined above.

Additionally, previous dorsal wrist surgery is a relative contraindication as the vascular pedicle may have been compromised by the prior operation. In that case alternative vascularized grafts such as the pedicled distal radius graft based on the 4 + 5 extracompartmental artery or the free vascularized medial femoral condyle graft should be considered.[40] Finally, patients with peripheral vascular disease, smokers, and females have had higher rates of failure of this graft when used for scaphoid nonunions and may similarly be at higher risk of failure in the setting of Preiser disease.

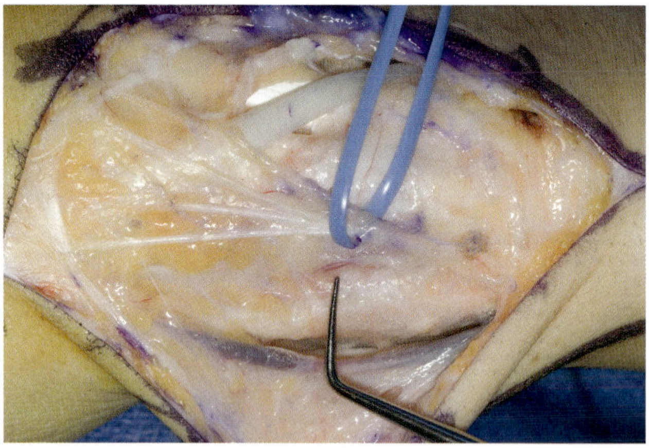

FIGURE 16-4 The 1,2 ICSRA vessels identified on the superficial surface of the extensor retinaculum between the first and second extensor compartments just deep to the branches of the superficial radial nerve.

SURGICAL TECHNIQUE

The procedure is performed with the patient supine with the operative extremity on a hand table under regional or general anesthesia. The arm is exsanguinated by elevation alone prior to tourniquet inflation to facilitate pedicle identification. A gentle curvilinear incision centered over the radioscaphoid joint along the extensor pollicis longus provides adequate exposure of the scaphoid and distal radius (Fig. 16-3). The branches of the superficial radial nerve are identified and protected during superficial dissection. The 1,2 ICSRA vessel is then identified on the superficial surface of the extensor retinaculum between the first and second extensor compartments (Fig. 16-4). This can be dissected distally to its anastomosis with the radial artery in the anatomic snuffbox. The retinaculum is incised on either side of the vessel creating a cuff of retinaculum with the pedicle. The pedicle is protected during the exposure and preparation of the scaphoid.

A transverse dorsoradial capsulotomy facilitates exposure, examination, and preparation of the scaphoid. The integrity of the scaphoid cartilage as well as midcarpal and radiocarpal joints is confirmed. A dorsal trough is made in the scaphoid with a high-speed burr or osteotomes (Fig. 16-5) and the necrotic bone thoroughly debrided with curettes taking care not to violate the scaphoid shell of subchondral bone and cartilage (Fig. 16-6).

Once the scaphoid is prepared, the pedicled graft is harvested. A rectangle centered 15 mm proximal to the joint line centered over the perforating nutrient vessels is marked out on the distal radius. The 1,2 ICSRA vessels are ligated proximal to the graft harvest site but remain in continuity with the radial artery distally creating a reverse-flow pedicled graft (Fig. 16-7). The vessels are mobilized from the underlying radius and capsule to allow protection during graft harvest and rotation toward the scaphoid. The graft is then harvested

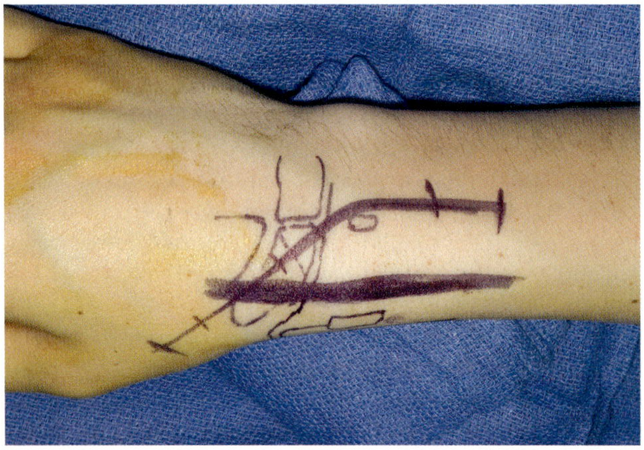

FIGURE 16-3 The dorsal curvilinear incision along the extensor pollicis longus tendon centered over the radioscaphoid joint.

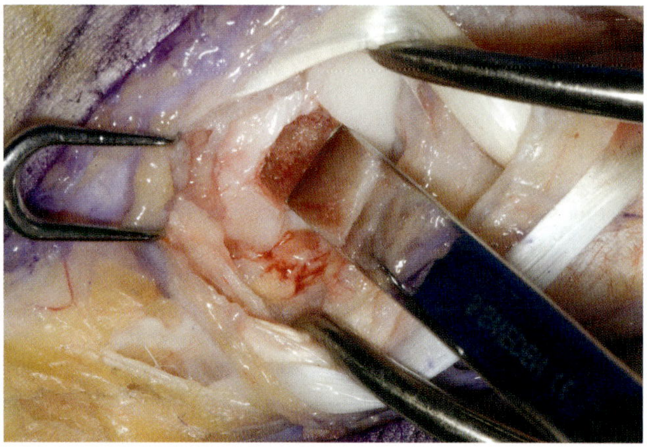

FIGURE 16-5 A trough is made along the dorsal surface of the scaphoid to receive the vascularized graft.

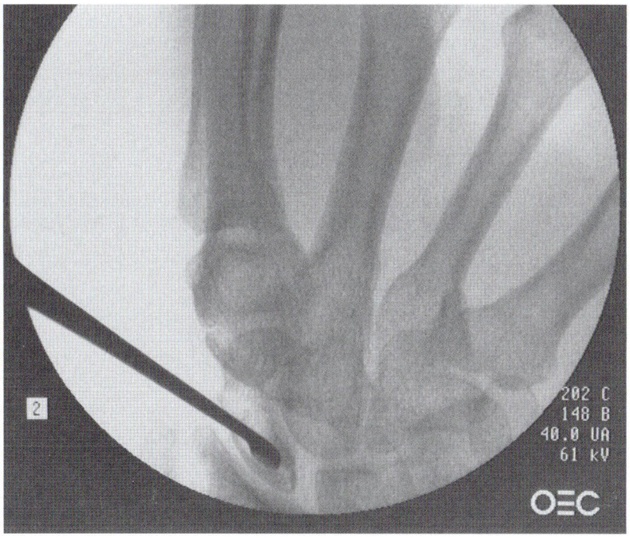

FIGURE 16-6 The necrotic bone is debrided with a curette through the dorsal trough taking care to avoid penetrating the cartilage shell of the scaphoid.

with sharp osteotomes or sagittal saw taking care to protect the pedicle and avoid shearing the periosteum and cortex from the underlying cancellous bone. An additional cut can be made proximal to the graft and angled toward the base of the graft to facilitate harvest of the intact graft. Once the graft is elevated, additional cancellous graft can be harvested from

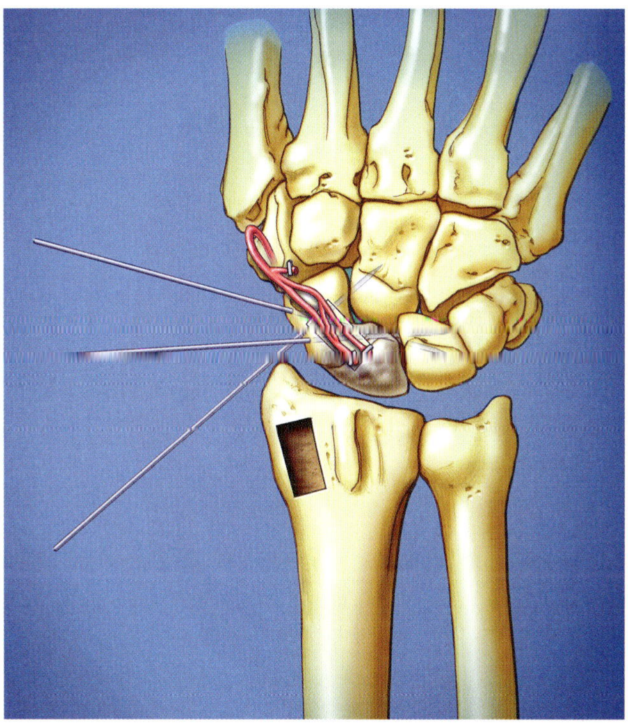

FIGURE 16-7 The 1,2 ICSRA vessels are ligated proximally but remain in continuity with the radial artery distally creating a reverse-flow pedicled graft that can be rotated to the scaphoid. (With permission of Mayo Foundation for Medical Education and Research. All rights reserved.)

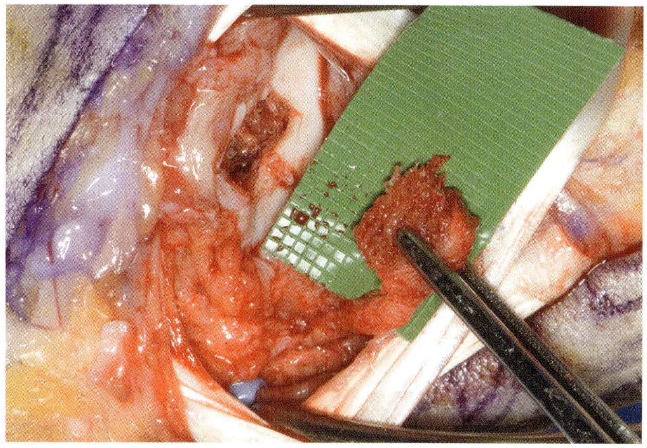

FIGURE 16-8 The graft is elevated, trimmed to size, and rotated on its pedicle toward the dorsal aspect of the scaphoid.

the distal radius and used to fill the remainder of the scaphoid after the graft is inset. The graft is then trimmed to size as necessary, rotated, and passed beneath the wrist extensors (Fig. 16-8), and press-fit into the dorsal trough in the scaphoid, taking care not to impact or compress the pedicle itself while insetting the graft (Fig. 16-9). Temporary K-wires are used to prevent graft extrusion. Additionally, scaphocapitate pins can be used to protect the midcarpal joint during the healing process (Fig. 16-10). The capsule is then partially closed taking care to avoid any compression or kinking of the vascular pedicle.

After the skin is closed, the wrist is immobilized with either an external fixator or sugar-tong thumb spica splint. The external fixator offers the theoretical benefit of unloading the scaphoid that may protect it during the healing phase, although this benefit has not been demonstrated clinically.[38] We more commonly use a sugar-tong splint and then cast to immobilize the wrist for 6 to 8 weeks at which time gentle range of motion exercises are initiated using a removable splint for an additional 4 to 6 weeks.

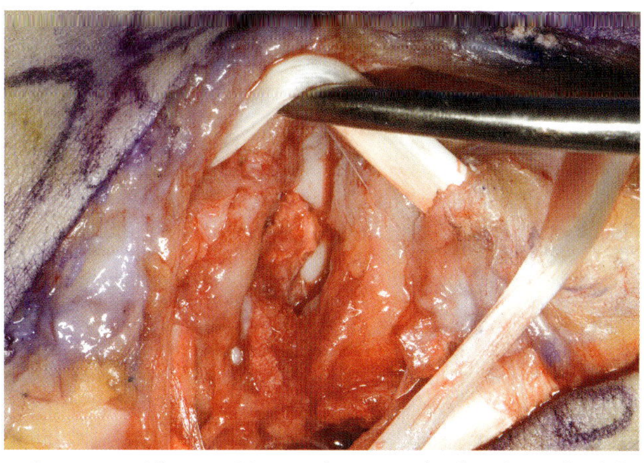

FIGURE 16-9 The 1,2 ICSRA graft inset in the dorsal trough of the scaphoid.

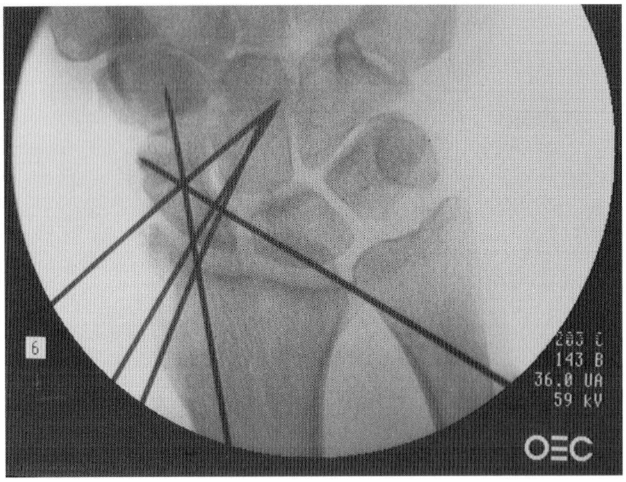

FIGURE 16-10 Temporary K-wires are used to prevent graft extrusion and prevent midcarpal motion for approximately 6 weeks postoperatively.

COMPLICATIONS

In addition to potential complications inherent in any surgical procedure, several are related specifically to the use of the 1,2 ICSRA pedicled bone graft for Preiser disease. As mentioned above, the subchondral bone and cartilage shell of the scaphoid can become quite thin in the process of debridement and perforation with damage to the articular cartilage is possible. Additionally, the vascular pedicle can be compromised at any step from the initial dissection to the elevation of the bone graft, to the insetting, to the closure of the capsule. If the pedicle is compromised from prior procedures or intraoperatively, the 2,3 ICSRA or the 4 + 5 extracompartmental artery grafts can be used.

Complications may also be related to the graft itself. The periosteum may shear off the cortex or the cortex may shear off the cancellous bone during harvest or insetting. Additionally, the graft may extrude dorsally if inadequately captured with K-wires or after K-wire removal. Finally, complications or suboptimal clinical outcomes with progressive scaphoid collapse, degenerative radiocarpal and midcarpal arthritis, limited range of motion, and persistent or progressive pain requiring additional salvage procedures are also possible.

OUTCOMES

The results of patients with Preiser disease treated at our institution over a 10-year period with pedicled vascularized bone grafts were described by Moran et al.[38] Eight patients were followed for a mean of 36 months (range 8-72) postoperatively. All patients had preoperative MRI findings consistent with Kalainov type 1 Preiser disease. Postoperatively all patients had MRI evidence of revascularization; however, all had only partial revascularization of the proximal pole. All patients reported improved pain postoperatively. Wrist motion averaged 55% and grip strength averaged 67% of the contralateral side. The average Mayo wrist score was 68 (range 45-90). Radiographic radial styloid arthritis was present in 2 patients, dorsal intercalated segment instability (DISI) deformity in 1, and 2 had continued collapse as evidenced by narrowing of the scaphoid waist and proximal pole. One patient had persistent pain requiring salvage with PRC 8 months postoperatively.

These results are comparable to other reported series. Kalainov et al[16] described 9 patients with Preiser disease (4 type 1, 5 type 2) who underwent vascularized bone grafting. Mayo wrist scores averaged 50 at an average of 33 months postoperatively. They noted improved outcomes in patients with type 2 Preiser disease compared with those who had global ischemic changes. Three of the 4 with type 2 progressed to stage 3 or 4 disease. One went on to wrist arthrodesis. In de Smet's report of 22 patients with Preiser disease, 12 were treated with PRC with satisfactory results in 10. Range of motion averaged 74.8° (range 60-90). Given the rarity of the disorder, there are no prospective studies comparing revascularization with PRC or limited arthrodesis. But the potential to preserve normal wrist anatomy and biomechanics makes revascularization procedures such as the 1,2 ICSRA graft appealing. Further study is necessary on the long-term outcomes of these various treatment options in alleviating pain and optimizing function for patients with Preiser disease.

REFERENCES

1. Preiser G. Eine typische posttraumatische und zur spontanfraktur fuhrende ostitis des naviculare carpi. *Fortschr Geb Roentgenstr.* 1910;15:189–197.
2. Yamamoto T, Irisa T, Sugioka Y, Sueishi K. Effects of pulse methylprednisolone on bone and marrow tissues: corticosteroid-induced osteonecrosis in rabbits. *Arthritis Rheum.* 1997;40(11):2055–2064.
3. Chernetsky SG, Mont MA, LaPorte DM, Jones LC, Hungerford DS, McCarthy EF. Pathologic features in steroid and nonsteroid associated osteonecrosis. *Clin Orthop Relat Res.* 1999;(368):149–161.
4. Zizic TM, Marcoux C, Hungerford DS, Dansereau JV, Stevens MB. Corticosteroid therapy associated with ischemic necrosis of bone in systemic lupus erythematosus. *Am J Med.* 1985;79(5):596–604.
5. Harper PG, Trask C, Souhami RL. Avascular necrosis of bone caused by combination chemotherapy without corticosteroids. *Br J Med.* 1984;288:267–268.
6. Beckmann J, Gotz J, Grifka J, Borisch N. Necrosis of the carpal scaphoid after chemotherapy. Case report. *Orthopade.* 2005;34(9):938–940.
7. Dubois EL, Cozen L. Avascular (aseptic) bone necrosis associated with systemic lupus erythematosus. *JAMA.* 1960;174:966–971.
8. Urman JD, Abeles M, Houghton AN, Rothfield NF. Aseptic necrosis presenting as wrist pain in SLE. *Arthritis Rheum.* 1977;20:825–828.
9. Kawai H, Tsuyuguchi Y, Yonenobu K, Inoue A, Tada K. Avascular necrosis of the carpal scaphoid associated with progressive systemic sclerosis. *Hand.* 1983;15:270–273.
10. De Smet L. Avascular nontraumatic necrosis of the scaphoid. Preiser's disease? *Chir Main.* 2000;19:82–85.
11. Assouline-Dayan Y, Chang C, Greenspan A, Shoenfeld Y, Gershwin ME. Pathogenesis and natural history of osteonecrosis. *Semin Arthritis Rheum.* 2002;32(2):94–124.
12. Parkinson RW, Noble J, Bale RS, Freemont AJ. Rare abnormalities of the scaphoid in association with congenital radial ray defects of the hand: a report of two cases. *J Hand Surg Br.* 1991;16(2):208–211.
13. Vidal MA, Linscheild RL, Amadio PC, Dobyns JH. Preiser's disease. *Ann Chir Main Memb Super.* 1991;10:227–235.

14. Gelberman RH, Menon J. The vascularity of the scaphoid bone. *J Hand Surg Am*. 1980;5:508–513.
15. Buttermann GR, Putnam MD, Shine JD. Wrist position affects loading of the dorsal scaphoid: possible effect on extrinsic scaphoid blood flow. *J Hand Surg Br*. 2001;26B:34–40.
16. Kalainov DM, Cohen MS, Hendrix RW, Sweet S, Culp RW, Osterman AL. Preiser's disease: identification of two patterns. *J Hand Surg Am*. 2003;28A:767–778.
17. Herbert TJ, Lanzetta M. Idiopathic avascular necrosis of the scaphoid. *J Hand Surg Br*. 1994;19:174–182.
18. Imam S, Aldridge C, Lyall H. Bilateral idiopathic avascular necrosis of the scaphoid: a rare case of Preiser's disease. *J Bone Joint Surg Br*. 2009;91(10):1400–1402.
19. Ferlic DC, Morin P. Idiopathic avascular necrosis of the scaphoid: Preiser's disease? *J Hand Surg Am*. 1989;14:13–16.
20. Haussman P. Long-term results after silicone prosthesis replacement of the proximal pole of the scaphoid bone in advanced scaphoid nonunion. *J Hand Surg Br*. 2002;27(5):417–423.
21. Menth-Chiari W, Poehling GC. Preiser's disease: arthroscopic treatment of avascular necrosis of the scaphoid. *Arthroscopy*. 2000;16:208–213.
22. Weinstein LP, Berger RA. Analgesic benefit, functional outcome, and patient satisfaction after partial wrist denervation. *J Hand Surg Am*. 2002;27(5):833–839.
23. Wilhelm A. Denervation of the wrist. *Tech Hand Up Extrem Surg*. 2001;5(1):14–30.
24. De Smet L, Aerts P, Walraevens M, Fabry G. Avascular necrosis of the carpal scaphoid: Preiser's disease. Report of 6 cases and review of the literature. *Acta Orthop Belg*. 1993;59:139–142.
25. Richou J, Chuinard C, Moineau G, Hanouz N, Hu W, Le Nen D. Proximal row carpectomy: long-term results. *Chir Main*. 2010;29(1):10–15.
26. Ashmead D 4th, Watson HK, Damon C, Herber S, Paly W. Scapholunate advanced collapse wrist salvage. *J Hand Surg Am*. 1994;19(5). 741–750.
27. Dacho A, Grundel J, Holle G, Germann G, Sauerbier M. Long-term results of midcarpal arthrodesis in the treatment of scaphoid nonunion advanced collapse (SNAC-Wrist) and scapholunate advanced collapse (SLAC-Wrist). *Ann Plast Surg*. 2006;56(2):139–144.
28. Hayashi O, Sawaizumi T, Nambu A, Ito H. Closing radial wedge osteotomy for Preiser's disease: a case report. *J Hand Surg Am*. 2006;31(7):1154–1156.
29. Viegas SF. Arthroscopic treatment of osteochondritis dissecans of the scaphoid. *Arthroscopy*. 1988;4(4):278–281.
30. Ekerot L, Eiken O. Idiopathic avascular necrosis of the scaphoid. *Scand J Plast Reconstr Surg*. 1981;15:69–72.
31. Arata MA, Wood MB, Cooney WP 3rd. Revascularized segmental diaphyseal bone transfers in the canine. An analysis of viability. *J Reconstr Microsurg*. 1984;1(1):11–19.
32. Han CS, Wood MB, Bishop AT, Cooney WP III. Vascularized bone transfer. *J Bone Joint Surg*. 1992;74A(10):1441–1449.
33. Goldberg VM, Shaffer JW, Field GA, Davy DT. Biology of vascularized bone grafts. *Orthop Clin North Am*. 1987;18(2):197–205.
34. Shaffer JW, Field GA, Goldberg VM, Davy DT. Fate of vascularized and nonvascularized autografts. *Clin Orthop*. 1985;197:32–43.
35. Merrell GA, Wolfe SW, Slade JF 3rd. Treatment of scaphoid nonunions: quantitative meta-analysis of the literature. *J Hand Surg Am*. 2002;27(4):685–691.
36. Braun JJ, Birkenhager-Frenkel DH, Rietveld AH, Juttmann JR, Visser TJ, Birkenhager JC. Influence of 1 alpha-(OH)D3 administration on bone and bone mineral metabolism in patients on chronic glucocorticoid treatment; a double blind controlled study. *Clin Endocrinol (Oxf)*. 1983;19(2):265–273.
37. Shin AY, Bishop AT. Pedicled vascularized bone grafts for disorders of the carpus: scaphoid nonunion and Kienbock's disease. *J Am Acad Orthop Surg*. 2002;10:210–216.
38. Moran SL, Cooney WP, Shin AY. The use of vascularized grafts from the distal radius for the treatment of Preiser's disease. *J Hand Surg Am*. 2006;31(5):705–710.
39. Sheetz KK, Bishop AT, Berger RA. The arterial blood supply of the distal radius and its potential use in vascularized pedicled bone grafts. *J Hand Surg*. 1995;20A:902–914.
40. Moran SL, Shin AY. Vascularized bone grafting for the treatment of carpal pathology. *Orthop Clin North Am*. 2007;38(1):73–85, vi.

Carpal Instability—Scapholunate, Lunotriquetral, and Midcarpal

17

Alex Lluch Bergadà, MD
Marc Garcia-Elias, MD, PhD

A normal wrist supports considerable compressive forces and shear stresses; yet, it remains stable throughout its entire range. To achieve this, a perfect balance between bone architecture, capsular-ligamentous constraints, and muscle forces around the joint is necessary.[1,2] When that balance is disrupted, by fracture, ligament injury, or tendon rupture, instability may appear.

For a wrist to be considered clinically unstable, it needs to have a kinetic and/or kinematic dysfunction causing pain and weakness.[3] From a kinetic viewpoint, the wrist is unstable when it is not able to sustain its alignment under physiological loads. From a kinematic viewpoint, a wrist is unstable when it exhibits sudden, unexpected changes in the alignment of the carpal bones. In a stable wrist, the carpal bone motion is smooth and congruous, with no abrupt shifts in alignment. And finally, from a clinical point of view, a wrist is said to be unstable when it has a kinetic and/or kinematic instability, plus symptoms, most often in the form of pain and loss of function.[1]

CLASSIFICATION OF CARPAL INSTABILITIES

There are 2 main types of instability: dissociative and nondissociative.[4] Dissociative carpal instabilities, known by the acronym CID ("carpal instability dissociative"), are secondary to a disruption (ligament rupture or bone fracture) between bones of the same row. Depending on which row is affected, the CID may be proximal or distal. A nondissociative "carpal instability" (CIND) applies to radiocarpal or midcarpal instability without a disruption of either the proximal or distal carpal rows. When a carpal instability has features of both CID and CIND, the case is classified as a "carpal instability complex" (CIC). And finally, when an abnormal carpal alignment is secondary to pathology located outside of the carpus, such as dorsal midcarpal instability that occurs secondary to a distal radius malunion that has healed with an abnormal dorsal tilt, the condition is referred to as a "carpal instability adaptive" (CIA).

From a radiological point of view, when a carpal instability pattern is identified with a standard AP and lateral view, the instability is said to be "static."[4] Conversely, if the carpal instability can only be seen under certain loading conditions or in specific wrist positions (stress radiographs), this is referred to as a "dynamic" instability. A "predynamic" instability is an older term coined by Watson et al to apply to instability demonstrable on physical examination but not by radiographic studies.[5]

Dissociative Instabilities (CID)

The most common causes of CID are scaphoid nonunion, scapholunate (SL) dissociations, and lunotriquetral (LTQ) dissociations.

SCAPHOID NONUNION

Scaphoid nonunions may be stable or unstable. A nonunion is stable when there is no visible interfragmentary mobility under thumb traction, when the 2 ends of the fractured bone are strongly connected by fibrous tissue. On the contrary, a nonunion is unstable when the 2 fragments are disconnected and move independently of each other. If the fracture is at the waist of the bone, the distal scaphoid fragment tends to rotate into flexion and pronation, while the proximal fragment is pulled by the lunate and triquetrum to an abnormal extension. This leads to the typical dorsal apex angulation of the scaphoid with loss of carpal height ("humpback deformity"). By contrast, if the unstable nonunion is located proximal to the waist, the distal fragment tends to slide dorsally over an extended proximal fragment, thus impinging the dorsal rim of the radius.

Treatment of the unstable nonunion consists of: (1) reduction of the 2 fragments in order to recover the external dimensions of the bone, (2) insertion of an intercalary bone graft to replace the portion of bone that is missing, and (3) bone fixation with wires or headless screws. A more detailed description of this technique is discussed elsewhere in this book.

SCAPHOLUNATE DISSOCIATION

Complete rupture of the SL-supporting ligaments produces a carpal malalignment similar to the one caused by an unstable scaphoid nonunion, except that in this case the entire scaphoid is abnormally flexed and pronated, its proximal pole subluxing over the top of the dorsoradial rim of the radius. The lunate, once devoid of its lateral constraints, follows the triquetrum into an abnormal extension, supination, and ulnar translation. This pattern of displacement is known by the acronym DISI ("dorsal intercalated segment instability"), and it is characterized by a SL diastasis and radioscaphoid and midcarpal joint incongruity[1,6–8] (Fig. 17-1).

When in front of a symptomatic SL dissociation, aside from the age, etiology, profession, and vocational activities of the patient, it is important to collect detailed information about the extent and nature of the injury.[9] In this regard, it is useful trying to answer the following 5 questions: (1) Is dorsal SL ligament still intact? (2) Does the ligament have good healing potential? (3) Are secondary stabilizers (scaphocapitate and scaphotrapeziotrapezoid ligaments) still competent? (4) Is the malalignment still easily reducible? (5) Is the cartilage still normal? By answering these questions in a "yes" or "no" format, each case can be allocated into 1 of 6 groups or stages indicated in Table 17-1. In theory, each grade has a specific treatment. In practice, each patient deserves individualized treatment, taking into consideration all aspects of the problem. What follows is a swift review of the most commonly used surgical techniques for each stage of SL instability.

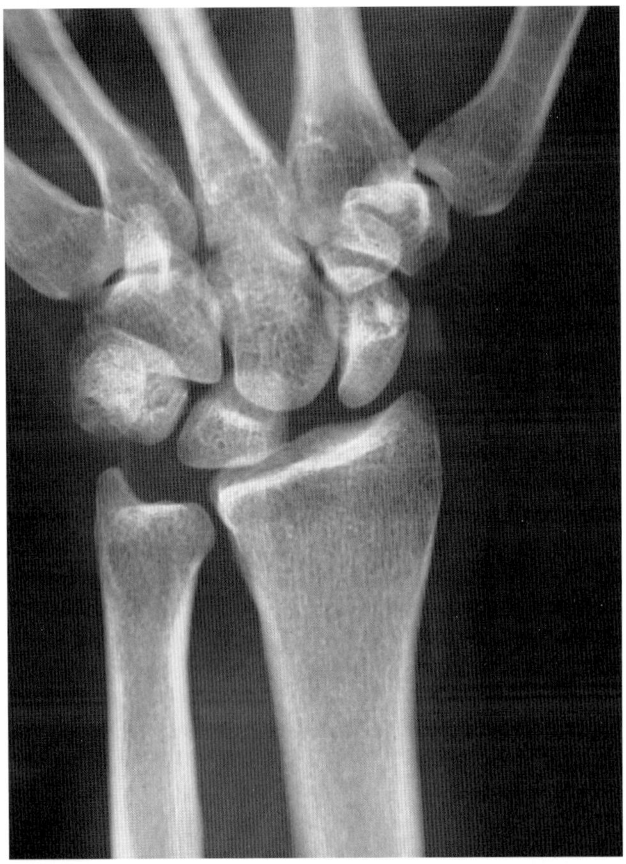

FIGURE 17-1 Posterioanterior view of a wrist with a scapholunate dissociation. Note the flexed and pronated scaphoid and the increased SL joint space. The scaphoid follows the distal row, whereas the lunate keeps attached to the triquetrum.

TABLE 17-1: Clinical Staging of Patients with SL Dissociation[a]

Stage 1:	Partial SL ligament tear
Stage 2:	Complete, repairable, SL ligament disruption
Stage 3:	Complete, unrepairable, SL ligament rupture
Stage 4:	Complete SL disruption with carpal collapse, easily reducible
Stage 5:	Irreducible carpal collapse, without cartilage degeneration
Stage 6:	Chronic SL dissociation with osteoarthritis (SLAC wrist)

[a]Data from Garcia-Elias et al.[9]

Stage 1: Several surgical options have been described for the symptomatic partial SL ligament tear; the least morbid, most effective method to relieve pain is an arthroscopy guided joint synovectomy and debridement.[10] Indeed, in most cases, patient's discomfort is secondary to excessive SL motion and interposition of ligament remnants that cause synovial irritation. If the scaphoid tends to sublux dorsoradially, aside from removing the synovium arthroscopically, percutaneous fixation of the SL joint with Kirschner (K) wires for 6 to 8 weeks is recommended.[1,6–8] In all instances, surgery needs to be followed by a controlled program of reeducation of the SL muscle stabilizers (abductor pollicis longus, flexor carpi radialis, and flexor carpi ulnaris).[11]

Stage 2: When there is optimal healing potential, direct repair of a complete SL ligament rupture is ideal. Ligaments can be repaired by direct sutures, transosseous sutures, or metal anchors.[1,7,8,12] Obviously, the best scenario would be the uncommon situation in which the ligament is attached to an avulsed bony fragment (Figs. 17-2 to 17-4). In all instances, it is recommended to neutralize the repair with K-wires across the joint for a period of at least 6 weeks. Undoubtedly, the results published after an acute repair of the injured ligaments are better than joint immobilization without ensuring that the 2 ends of the ligament are closed enough as to heal spontaneously.[12]

Stage 3: When the dorsal SL ligament has poor healing potential, different options are possible. One is to replace that ligament with a "bone–ligament–bone" graft (B-L-B) obtained from the distal row.[1] Another is to reconstruct the missing ligament with a tendon graft, and will be detailed later. The first alternative is technically demanding, with a relatively high index of complications, including nonunion of the graft, stiffness, or recurrence of the instability. Adding a dorsal capsulodesis may improve the clinical results obtained with B-L-B reconstruction.[13]

Stage 4: Different types of ligament reconstruction using tendon grafts have been described for the easily reducible SL dissociation with good cartilage. Most techniques

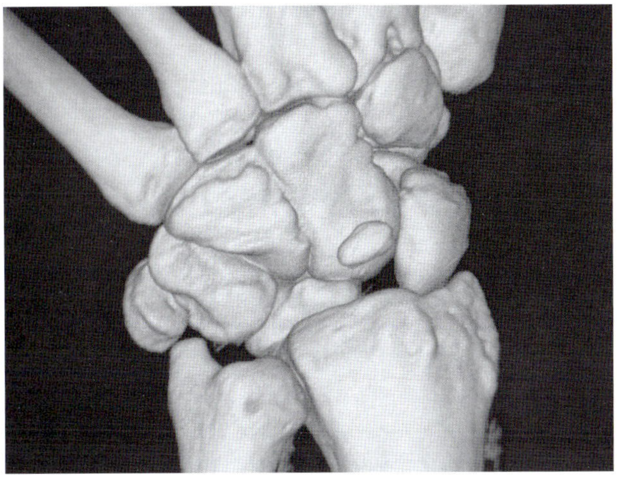

FIGURE 17-2 CT scan of a complete lesion of the SL ligamentous complex. In this case the dorsal SL ligament is avulsed from the lunate with a bony fragment.

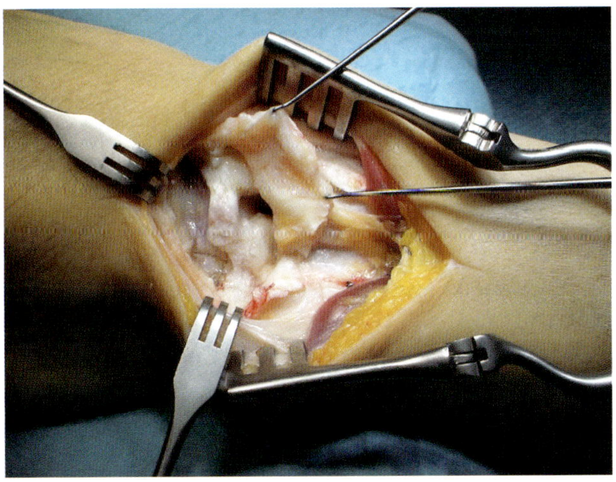

FIGURE 17-3 Intraoperative view. The optimal healing potential and possibility of reattachment of the bony fragment are confirmed.

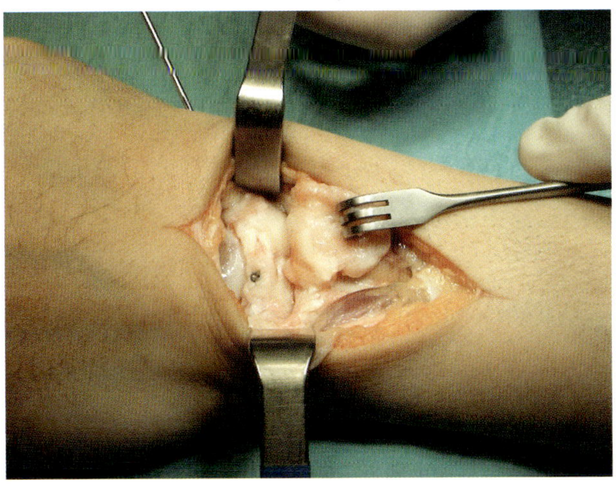

FIGURE 17-4 Fragment fixation with a 2.0-mm cancellous screw. By this, complete SL lesion is transformed into a partial lesion. Additional K-wire stabilization is needed.

consist of passing strips of tendon through tunnels to recreate the missing ligaments. In our hands, the so-called 3-ligament tenodesis (3LT) has been consistently successful.[9] In this technique, a slip obtained from flexor carpi radialis (FCR) tendon is passed obliquely through the scaphoid from palmar to dorsal, emerging at the point of insertion of the dorsal SL ligament. The slip is then fitted in a trough created in the dorsum of the lunate, passed through a slit made in the dorsal radiotriquetral ligament, looped around, and sutured onto itself in the adequate tension (see detailed description in the section "Treatment of Reducible Scapholunate Dissociation With Preserved Cartilage").

In general, the more anatomic the reconstruction, the more acceptable the results. Yet, it is important to note that a tendon graft cannot normalize proprioception; only the original ligaments contain mechanoreceptors to ensure proper neuromuscular control of the unstable wrist.[11]

Another alternative to prevent carpal collapse consists of increasing tightness of the capsular segment opposite to the direction of collapse: to prevent the scaphoid to collapse into flexion, a dorsal capsular tether between the radius and the scaphoid has been described by Blatt.[1] To prevent the scaphoid from rotating into pronation, a dorsal intercarpal capsuloplasty has been suggested by Szabo.[1] Although effective in the short term, most capsulodesis tend to deteriorate over time, often allowing the carpus to return to its initial malalignment.

Stage 5: It is important emphasizing that soft tissue–stabilizing procedures are not indicated if the carpal malalignment cannot be easily reduced. If substantial force is needed to bring the collapsed bones back into its original alignment, not even the best capsulotenodesis will be strong enough to maintain that reduction: loads across the carpus are too high.

The treatment of choice, when carpal collapse is not easily reducible, is a partial fusion.[14] When carefully planned and executed, partial arthrodesis may return stability to the carpus without completely losing its global mobility. The main requirement for such an intervention is that the articular surfaces surrounding the arthrodesis are to be perfectly healthy. It is also important to align the joints as anatomically as possible, so that the shape and dimensions of the bone block are as similar as possible to the initial state.

One of the most frequently attempted partial arthrodesis in SL dissociations has been the SL fusion. Theoretically, it should be most effective in SL instability. In practice, a SL fusion is very difficult to obtain, given the small articular surface between the 2 bones and the magnitude of the forces acting on that joint. The complication rate of this technique is high. Interestingly enough, the functional results of the cases that failed consolidating are consistently better than those that succeeded. Based on this, there are authors suggesting temporary transfixion of the SL joint with 1 or 2 screws in order to create a beneficial arthrofibrosis. Along this concept, the so-called reduction association of the SL joint (RASL procedure) has shown early promising results.[1] Whether they will maintain good function down the line is not known.

Arthrodesis of the scaphoid-trapezium-trapezoid (STT) joints is another frequently used solution, popularized by Watson et al.[14] It is particularly indicated when there is an irreducible rotary subluxation of the scaphoid. It stabilizes the scaphoid by fusing the STT joint, thereby preventing the progression of carpal collapse. Most common complication is the emergence of short-term overload of the radioscaphoid joint space. To avoid this complication it is important to follow Watson's technique very precisely.

In our experience, the most effective way to recover good function in stage 5 SL dissociation is to perform a radioscapholunate fusion plus a distal scaphoidectomy.[15] The rationale for this operation is based on 3 facts: first, from a functional point of view, the midcarpal joint is more important than the radiocarpal joint because it is there where the so-called dart-throwing motion occurs; second, if the scaphoid is fused to the radius, the midcarpal joint cannot flex or radially deviate; and third, if the distal portion of a stiff scaphoid is excised, the midcarpal joint is allowed to recover both its normal flexion and radial deviation. Promising midterm results have been published with this strategy that, again, is indicated in irreducible SL dissociations, but also in radiocarpal osteoarthritis.

Stage 6: When a chronic SL dissociation has evolved into an osteoarthritic joint, the so-called scapholunate advanced collapse (SLAC) wrist, only salvage procedures such as a proximal row carpectomy or a scaphoidectomy plus a midcarpal fusion are indicated. The published results using these techniques are encouraging in terms of pain relief. Obviously, the long-term function of these operations is a matter of concern.

Treatment of Reducible Scapholunate Dissociation with Preserved Cartilage

Indications and Contraindications. Tendon reconstruction of the SL linkage is recommended only in SL dissociation stage 3 or 4. For this to be successful, however, it is very important that the malalignment is easily reducible, and the periscaphoid cartilages are completely normal.

Although this condition is usually seen in young males, there is no theoretical limit of age for the procedure provided that the 2 previously mentioned requirements are present. Heavy manual workers are not good candidates for this treatment modality; they may require a more solid form of stabilization, such as a partial fusion.

Preoperative Planning. A complete set of plain radiographic views and stress views are mandatory.

- CT scan is useful to see bone positioning, and 4D CT scan (if available) provides information about scaphoid movement and may differentiate partial from complete SL lesions.
- Arthroscans (tomograms taken after 3-compartment injection of dye) are very useful to assess cartilage status.
- Best-quality magnetic resonance imaging may provide useful accessory information regarding bone vascularity, synovitis effects, and soft tissue status.
- Arthroscopy is by far the best tool for preoperative planning.

Surgical Technique. An axillary block is preferable. The patient is in the supine position. Tourniquet is placed in the arm and inflated up to 250 mm Hg after the extremity is exsanguinated.

Approach

- An 8-cm dorsal zigzag, lazy S, or longitudinal incision of the skin and subcutaneous tissue is centered on the tubercle of Lister. Dorsal sensory branches of the radial and ulnar nerves are identified and protected.
- The extensor retinaculum is divided along the third compartment and the extensor pollicis longus (EPL) tendon is retracted radially. This allows easy repositioning of EPL in its compartment after reconstruction is performed.
- The retinacular septa between compartments II and V are sectioned and the 2 retinacular flaps so created are retracted. Most septa contain intraseptal vertical vessels that need to be carefully coagulated.

Dorsal Capsulotomy

Dorsal Fiber-splitting Capsulotomy. Described by Berger et al,[16] dorsal fiber-splitting capsulotomy avoids transverse cutting of the dorsal capsular ligaments and provides excellent view (Fig. 17-5):

- The first incision is made along the dorsal rim of the radius to the center of the lunate fossa.
- The second incision is made from the end of the first incision following the fibers of the dorsal radiotriquetral ligament to its distal insertion onto the dorsal ridge of the triquetrum.
- The third incision is made from the STT joint progressing medially along the dorsal intercarpal ligament to its insertion onto the dorsum of the triquetrum.
- By connecting the last 2 incisions, a radially based capsular flap is created. This flap is carefully elevated by sectioning its connections to the dorsal edge of the 3 bones of the proximal row.
- It is important to leave enough dorsal RTq ligament attached to the triquetrum in order to facilitate later tensioning of the tendon reconstruction.

Nerve-sparing Dorsal Approach. This capsulotomy can be used in those cases in which the posterior interosseous nerve, placed in the radial side of the floor of the fourth extensor compartment, has a normal aspect and the proprioception transmitted by the nerve wants to be preserved.[17]

Capsular flap is proximal, thus protecting the entrance of nerve fibers inside the capsule, and, as in Berger's capsulotomy, no transverse section of the dorsal capsular ligaments is performed.

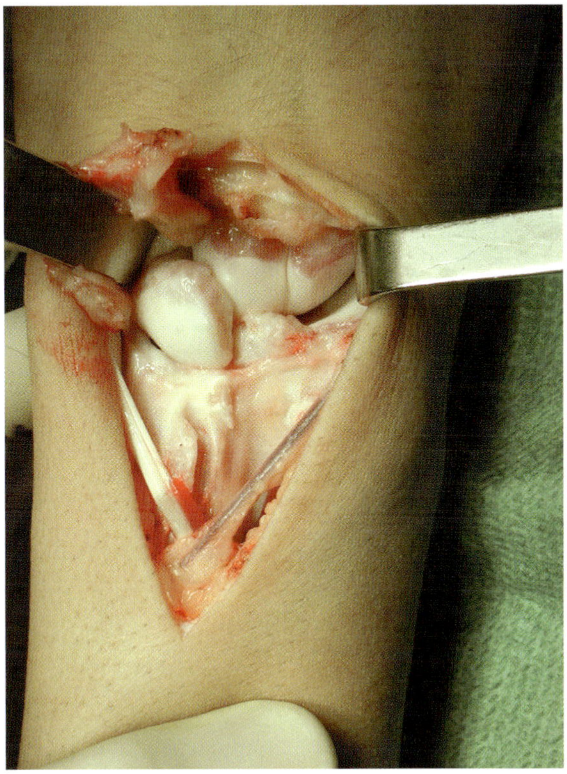

FIGURE 17-5 Stage 4 SL dissociation treated by a 3LT technique. Easy reduction and good cartilage are mandatory conditions for ligament reconstruction.

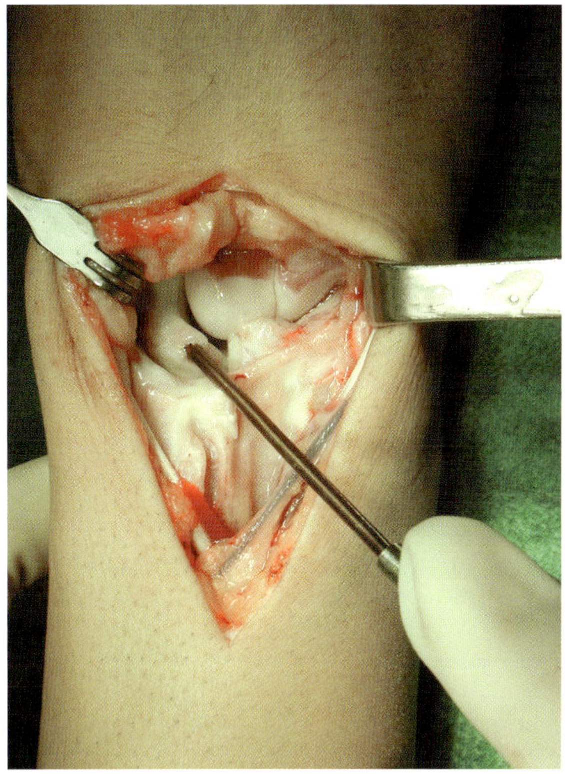

FIGURE 17-6 An oblique tunnel is created following the axis of the scaphoid.

Three-ligament Tenodesis

- The wrist joint is explored from the dorsum.[9] Normal cartilage surface of the carpal bones is confirmed. Easy reduction by traction of the SL dissociation should be achieved. Remaining tissue in the SL space is excised in order to facilitate the correct reduction of the bones.
- An oblique tunnel along the longitudinal axis of the scaphoid is created, from dorsal to palmar, entering at the level of the original insertion site of the dorsal SL ligament, and aiming at the palmar tuberosity. So as not to damage the medial or lateral articular surfaces of the scaphoid, we recommend using a 2.7- to 3.2-mm cannulated drill over a K-wire preset under fluoroscopic control (Fig. 17-6).
- A strip of the FCR tendon is then obtained. At the level of the distal pole of the scaphoid, a small transverse palmar incision is made and the distal part of FCR is identified. The skin is incised at the musculotendinous junction; a strip is incised and left attached distally. The strip is passed under the skin through multiple transverse incisions or using a wire loop. The size of graft harvested depends on the size of the scaphoid and bone tunnel created.
- The FCR tendon strip is passed through the oblique scaphoid tunnel using a wire loop or a tendon passer (Fig. 17-7).
- A transverse trough or channel is then made over the dorsum of the lunate with a rongeur. This trough needs to uncover cancellous bone, the only tissue able to generate

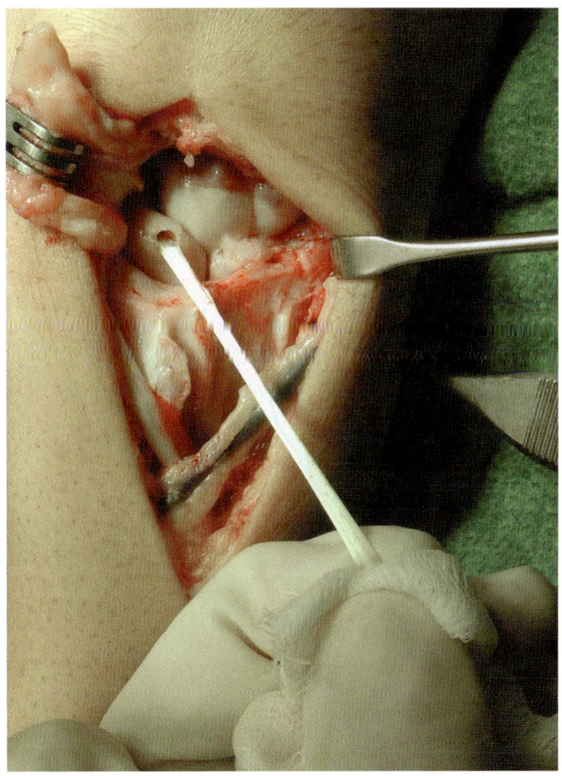

FIGURE 17-7 A strip of the FCR is obtained and passed through the scaphoid tunnel.

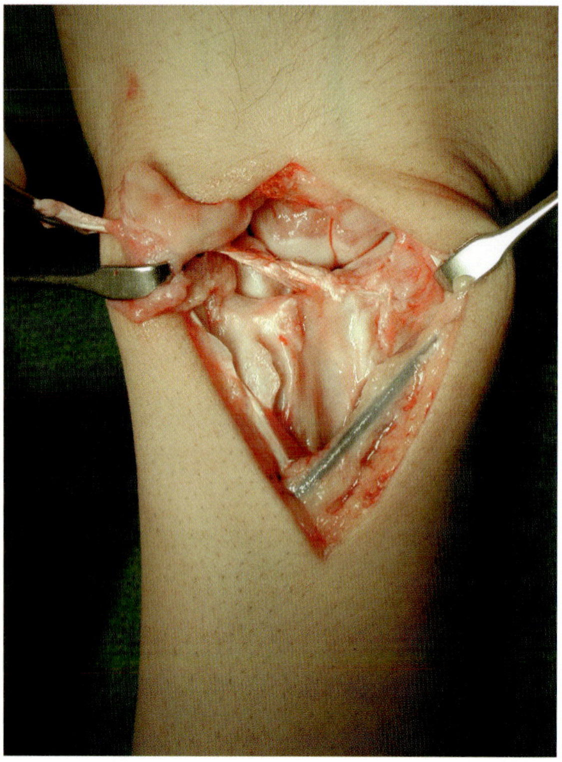

FIGURE 17-8 The slip is the fitted in a though created in the dorsum of the lunate, passed through a slit made in the dorsal radiotriquetral ligament, looped around and sutured onto itself (see text).

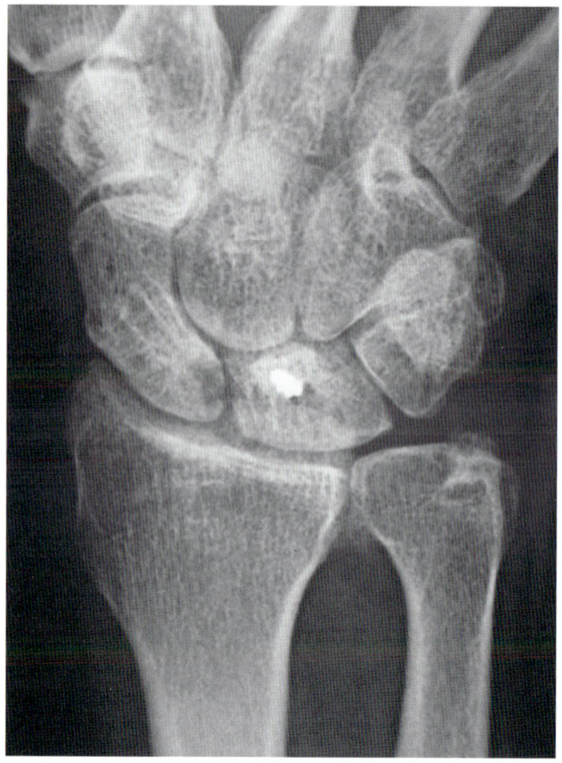

FIGURE 17-9 Radiographic long-term follow-up. Note the oblique tunnel in the scaphoid and the bony anchor that has been used to keep the tendon in the dorsum of the lunate.

proper healing of the tendon into bone. To obtain intimate contact between the tendon strip and the lunate cancellous bone, a small anchor suture is placed into the floor of the trough.

- The distal end of the dorsal radiotriquetral ligament is then localized. By its insertion on the bone, a slit is created through which the tendon strip is passed volar to dorsal. The ligament is used as a pulley to tension the strip (Fig. 17-8).
- The scaphoid, lunate, and capitate are reduced and stabilized with two 1.5-mm K-wires prior to tensioning the tendon graft. One wire is placed across the SL joint and 1 across the scaphocapitate joint. It is critical to ensure reduction of the scaphoid and the lunate, elimination of any DISI deformity, and proper placement of the wires using fluoroscopy.
- Radially directed tension is applied to the tendon graft already placed around and through the dorsal radiotriquetral ligament. After that, the tendon graft is secured tightly into the cancellous bone channel created in the lunate using the suture anchor.
- The end of the tendon strip is sutured onto itself with 3-0 sutures (Fig. 17-9).
- The capsular flap is brought back, over the tendon reconstruction, to its original position by suturing side-by-side the split fibers of the 2 ligaments involved in the capsulotomy. Some sutures are also placed connecting the capsule and the tendon loop to reestablish the normal capsular attachment to the dorsum of the SL joint.
- The extensor retinaculum is finally reconstructed, drains are placed, and the skin is closed.

Pearls and Pitfalls

Indications: Never perform the 3LT if malalignment is not easily reducible or if there is cartilage wear. Inform the patient about the need to change the indication depending on intraoperative findings.

Scaphoid tunnel: Drill the tunnel from proximal to distal following scaphoid axis. Entry should be at the original insertion of dorsal SL ligament. Use first a K wire; check the position with fluoroscopy and then use a cannulated drill. Fit the tunnel size to scaphoid size. It is best to have a tighter fit rather than a looser fit in the tunnel so that there is less "slop" in the system and potentially less likelihood of loss of reduction. It is easier to adapt the size of the strip to the width of the tunnel, and not the opposite way. Pass the strip with a wire loop or tendon passer and avoid hemostatic forceps or similar instruments.

Pin stabilization: One KW enters from the dorsoradial corner of the scaphoid and crosses the bone, aiming at the level of the hook of the hamate. A second KW enters from the palmar–radial corner of the scaphoid tuberosity, aiming at the lunate. Avoid K-wires across the anatomic snuffbox (radial artery at risk).

Fixation to the lunate: The anchor suture in the lunate is not to be used as anchor point for tendon tensioning, but only as a means to maintain the split tendon in full contact to cancellous bone. Tension of the tenodesis relies on the dorsal radiotriquetral ligament.

Tensioning of the tenodesis: Avoid excessive reduction of the DISI by applying too much tension to the graft. A "volar intercalated segment instability" (VISI) may be created, aside from affecting motion, or may even lead to necrosis.

Postoperative Care

- The wrist is immobilized in a well-padded splint including the metacarpophalangeal joint of the thumb for 10 days. After stitch removal, the wrist is maintained in a short arm thumb spica cast for 5 more weeks.
- A protective removable splint is then fabricated. This will allow resting the joint between sessions of supervised physiotherapy. The splint is used for an additional 4 weeks.
- Before wire removal, at 8 weeks, therapy consists of only gentle radiocarpal mobilization. After pin removal, global active mobilization is emphasized. Aggressive passive mobilization is never recommended.
- Muscle strengthening exercises are not initiated until 10 weeks after surgery. Contact sports are to be avoided for 6 months after surgery.

Outcomes. A review of 38 patients with symptomatic SL dissociation who had a 3LT procedure, with a mean follow-up of 46 months, showed an average range of motion of about 75% of the contralateral side.[9] Average grip strength was 65%. Pain relief at rest was obtained in 28 patients, with 8 complaining of mild discomfort during strenuous activity, and 2 having pain in most activities of daily life. Twenty-nine resumed their normal occupational–vocational activities. There were no signs of scaphoid necrosis. Recurrence of carpal collapse occurred in only 2 wrists. Nine patients showed mild signs of degenerative osteoarthritis at the tip of the radial styloid, but none had substantial symptoms.

Complications. Recurrence of the malalignment and subsequent development of degenerative arthritis is common when the technique is used inappropriately, in cases with a poorly reducible SLD (stage 5), or when cartilage deterioration is already present (SLAC).

When reducibility is in doubt, a more aggressive treatment (partial fusion or proximal row carpectomy) is recommended.

LUNOTRIQUETRAL DISSOCIATION

Rupture or insufficiency of the interosseus ligaments binding the LTQ joint produces a carpal instability different from the SL instability.[18,19] The resultant malfunction is further enhanced if the extrinsic radiotriquetral ligaments are also attenuated. In this case the lunate is devoid of any control by the triquetrum and it is dragged by the scaphoid into flexion and pronation, the so-called VISI. The triquetrum, by contrast, becomes completely unstable and, not having a rigid support to lean on, it migrates proximally. This generates midcarpal joint incongruity, and consequently substantial dysfunction characterized by a typical crepitation in ulnar deviation (Figs. 17-10 and 17-11).

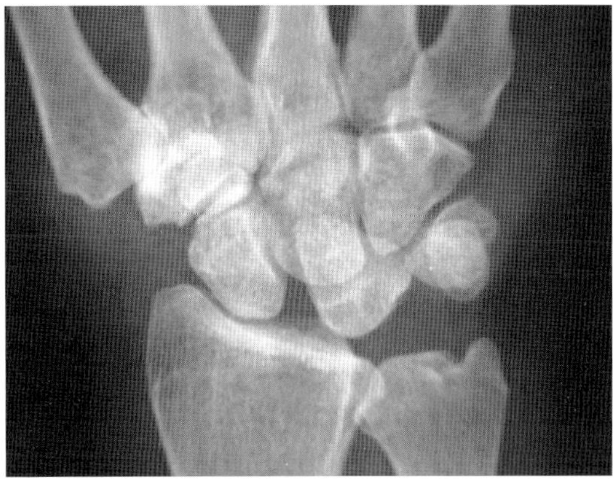

FIGURE 17-10 Plain x-ray of a patient with a static lunotriquetral dissociation. Note the flexed and pronated position of the lunate following the scaphoid, and the incongruency at LTQ joint space. In PA view the lunate is flexed when it shows a triangular shape, meaning that the narrow dorsal pole is located distally than the volar and broader part of the bone.

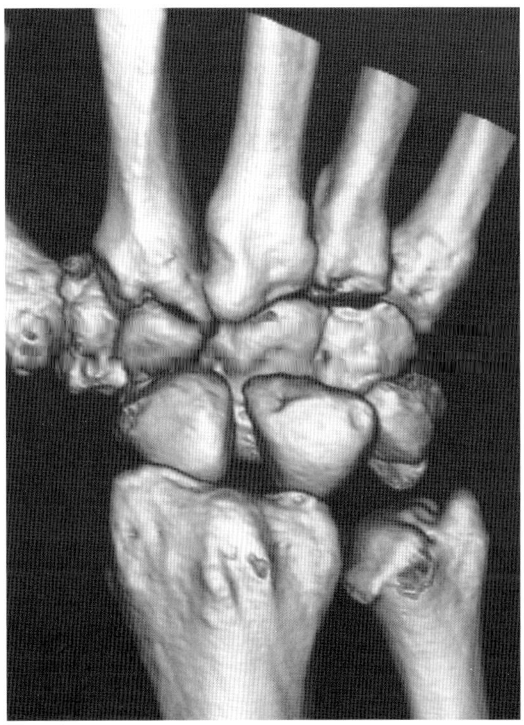

FIGURE 17-11 CT scan-3D reconstruction of the same patient. From a dorsal view, the flexed position of the lunate is obvious (VISI). Although sometimes the SL joint space seems to be widened in plain x-rays, in this 3D image a normal dorsal SL relationship is confirmed.

As highlighted when discussing the treatment of SL dissociations, a number of factors may influence the management of LTQ dissociations: extent of the injury, chronicity, reducibility, status of cartilage, presence of other local injuries, etc. Based on these factors, one may decide between percutaneous LT joint fixation with K-wires (indicated in the acute injury), LTQ fusion (indicated in the chronic instability without carpal collapse), tendon reconstruction of the LTQ ligaments (indicated in chronic instability with partial LTQ tears), or more radical procedures (proximal row carpectomy, radiocarpal or midcarpal fusion) for the chronic carpal collapse into VISI.[19]

Treatment of Lunotriquetral Dissociation Without Carpal Collapse. Chronic dynamic lunate triquetrum dissociation means that the 2 ends of LTQ ligaments have degenerated, making the chances for a successful direct repair very low, but no radiographic evidence of static instability is seen (VISI or step-off in the lunate in the lunate triquetrum interval).

Indications

- Dynamic LTQ instability secondary to complete intrinsic ligament rupture without ulnocarpal abutment syndrome (normal TFCC) and normal midcarpal joint. In the case of a relatively long ulna, lunate triquetrum fusions or even ligament reconstructions may remain symptomatic. In such instances, a wafer procedure or ulnar shortening may be performed in addition.
- No radiographic evidence of VISI should be present.

Preoperative Evaluation

- Positive lunate triquetrum ballottement test.
- Fluoroscopic evaluation of abnormal proximal–distal shift of the triquetrum during radioulnar movement.
- CT, 4D CT, and MRI can help in the diagnosis, mainly confirming the dynamic condition and the joint surface and soft tissue status.
- Arthroscopy is by far the best tool for preoperative planning. It will confirm a complete or partial LT ligament lesion, and will rule out TFCC degeneration secondary to ulnocarpal abutment or triquetrum–hamate impingement.

Surgical Technique. An axillary block is preferable. The patient is in the supine position. Tourniquet is placed in the arm and inflated up to 250 mm Hg after the extremity is exsanguinated.

Approach and Capsulotomy

- Perform a dorsal (zigzag, lazy "S," or longitudinal) incision centered at IV-V septum. As a reference, remember that extensor indicis proprius tendon (contained in V compartment) is at the level of DRUJ.
- The dorsal branch of the ulnar nerve can be identified dorsally just distal to the ulnar head.

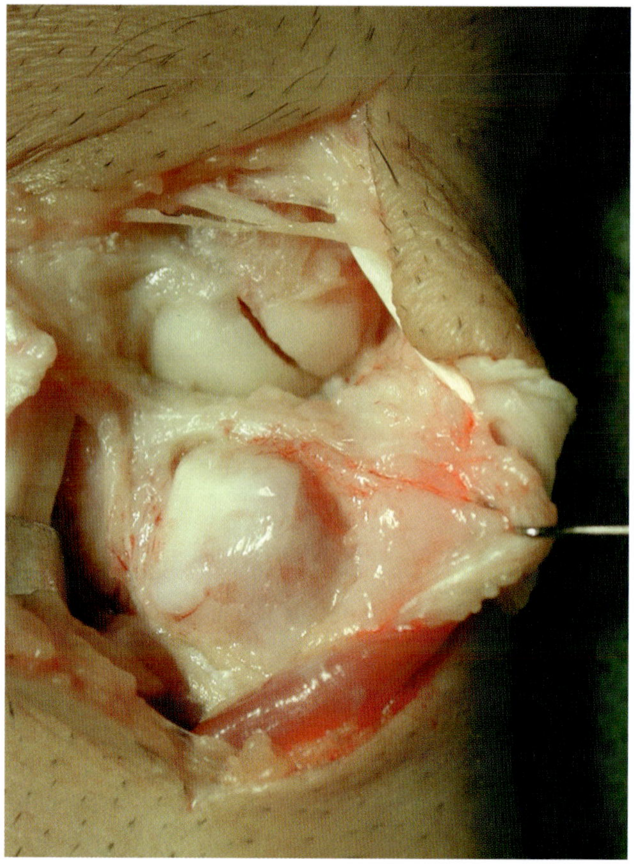

FIGURE 17-12 Intraoperative view of a LTQ fusion for a dynamic instability. A dorsal approach through the IV to V compartments, creating an ulnarly based capsular flap, provides excellent view of both the lunate-triquetrum space and DRUJ.

- Open the septum between IV and V; coagulate intraseptal artery.
- Perform a "Z" capsulotomy creating 2 flaps following the "fiber-splitting" concept.[20]

Lunate Triquetrum Arthrodesis

- Complete section of the remnants of lunate triquetrum ligaments (Fig. 17-12).
- Open the LTQ joint space as a book, and remove the joint surfaces with a rongeur to expose cancellous bone. Create a biconcave cavity, but do not excise the rim of the opposing cortical edges to preserve the normal interosseous separation.
- Cancellous bone is harvested from the radius. It can easily be done through a window created at the floor of the opened IV extensor compartment.
- Place K-wires in the ulnar aspect of the triquetrum (Fig. 17-13). If the fusion has to be done with a cannulated screw, have in mind that 1 of the wires will be used to place the screw. If it is going to be done with KW, place multiple wires in a nonparallel configuration.

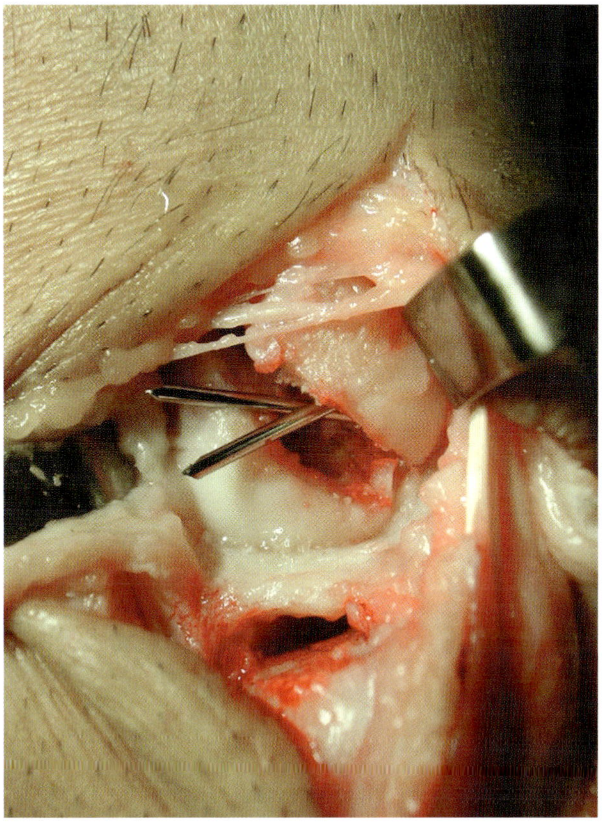

FIGURE 17-13 A concave cavity is created, filled with cancellous bone, and stabilized in this case with KW (see text for explanation).

- Bone graft is densely packed in the cavity. The joint is reduced, KW driven into the lunate, and fixation completed with a headless compression cannulated screw or KW. In the case that screw is used, leaving an extra KW is recommended. All the wires are cut below the skin surface (Figs. 17-14 and 17-15).
- Standard capsular and retinacular closure.

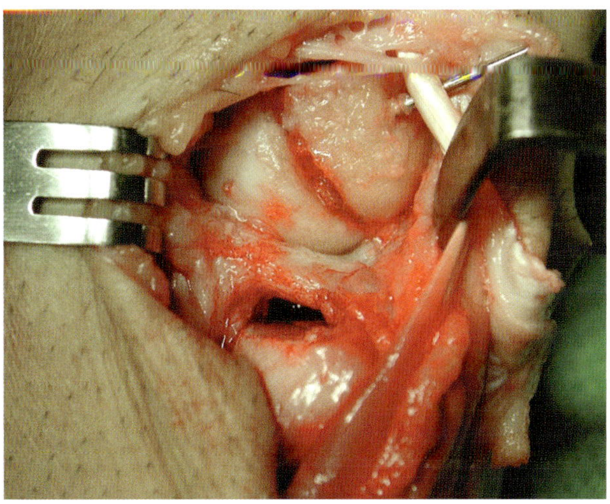

FIGURE 17-14 Final intraoperative view of the procedure. Note that a "wafer" procedure was also performed in this case.

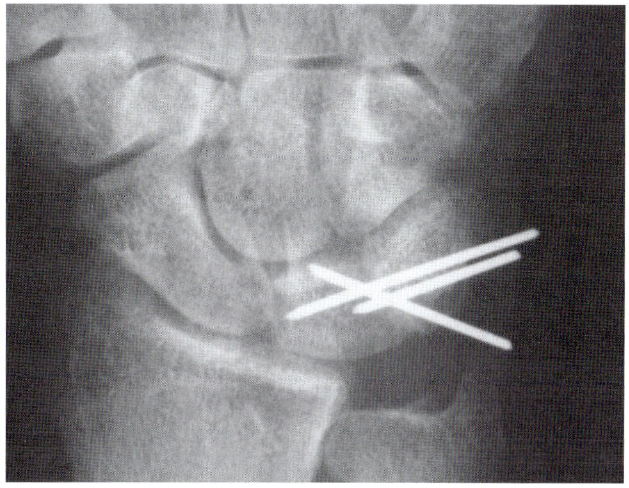

FIGURE 17-15 X-ray at 8 weeks. Several KW were used in this case. Removal of the KW is not performed until fusion is obvious.

Postoperative Care

- Short arm thumb spica cast for 6 weeks, changed at 10 days for stitch removal and x-rays.
- At 6 weeks x-rays. Perform out-of-cast x-rays, but maintain immobilization until healing is obvious. At that time, removal of KW under local anesthesia.
- Rehabilitation after cast removal to regain motion and grip strength. Contact sport not allowed until 6 months postoperatively.

Outcomes and Complications. Although a nonunion rate of 26% and complication rate of 43% have been reported, most of the complications with this procedure appear when it is incorrectly planned or secondary to technical problems. One should expect that 75% of patients have a painless wrist, with 80% of global motion and 75% grip strength.[21]

Nondissociative Instabilities (CIND)

As stated above, CIND instability implies integrity of the transverse intercarpal ligaments binding bones of the same row. In contrast to CID, a dysfunction of the entire proximal carpal row happens, and may predominate in the radiocarpal joint (radiocarpal CIND), in the midcarpal joint (midcarpal CIND), or, more frequently, in both.

RADIOCARPAL CIND

This instability is characterized by the inability to maintain the carpal condyle in its normal position in relation to the radius. The most common causes are an abnormal tilt of the distal radial surface and/or a failure of the ligaments that prevent radiocarpal subluxation.[22,23] When the distal surface of the radius is abnormally inclined (most often toward the ulna), high tangential forces acting on the carpal condyle may develop; if they are high enough, abnormal ligament tensions may elongate the radiocarpal ligaments and induce a serious global subluxation of the entire carpal condyle. Madelung distal radial deformity may lead to this situation, as well as rheumatoid arthritis. In the first case, the nonphysiological ulnarly inclined distal radius is the one to be blamed; in the second, it is the rupture of the ligaments in charge of maintaining the carpal condyle in normal position. In both circumstances the carpus may appear subluxed both ulnarly and palmarly, with the subsequent alteration of the kinematics. A radiocarpal corrective osteotomy, or more often a radiocarpal fusion, is the usual treatment for this condition.[23]

MIDCARPAL CIND

This group includes palmar and dorsal midcarpal nondissociative instabilities. Palmar CIND is by far the most common, and is a particular type of instability in which the primary defect is in the palmar midcarpal crossing ligaments, namely, the palmar triquetrum–hamate–capitate ligaments, the scaphocapitate, and the STT ligaments.[24] Ligament failure may be idiopathic, due to chronic laxity, or secondary to carpal malalignment after fracture of the distal radial epiphysis. Patients with symptomatic palmar CIND typically complain of a painful "clunk" (so-called "catch-up clunk") when moving the wrist from radial to ulnar deviation. This occurs when the flexed proximal row pops suddenly into an extended position close to the end of ulnar deviation (Fig. 17-16). Most authors advocate fusing the triquetrum–hamate joint. In our experience a radiolunate arthrodesis is as effective a proximal row stabilizer as a midcarpal fusion, with the added benefit of not eliminating the midcarpal joint. Indeed, if we preserve midcarpal rotation, the patient will be allowed good dart-throwing rotation, the one used in most activities of daily living (Figs. 17-17 and 17-18).

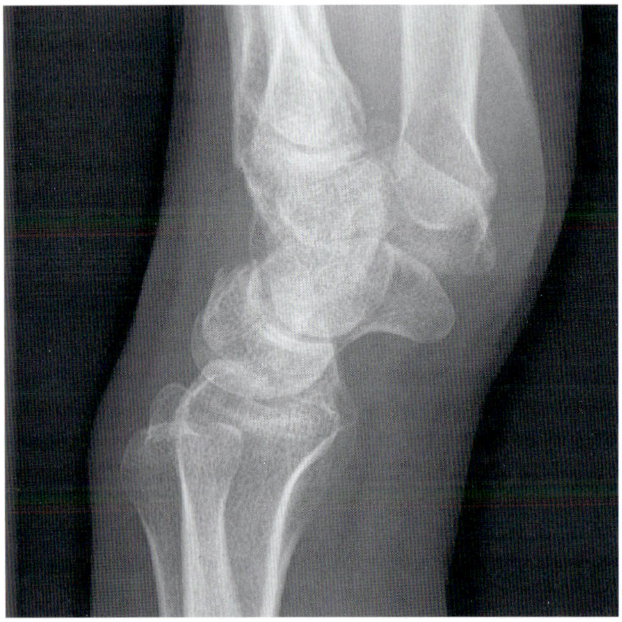

FIGURE 17-16 Typical lateral view of a patient with a palmar midcarpal nondissociative instability. The entire proximal row is in a flexed position until the wrist is in complete ulnar deviation. Note the visible volar depression at the midcarpal level that is usually seen in these cases just by visual inspection of the wrist.

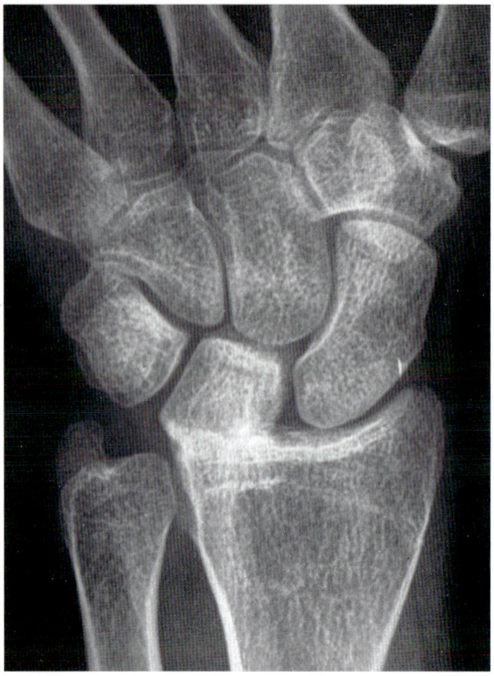

FIGURE 17-17 Long-term x-ray of a radiolunate fusion in the case of a palmar midcarpal instability in a lax individual. The KW used in this case for fixation had been previously removed.

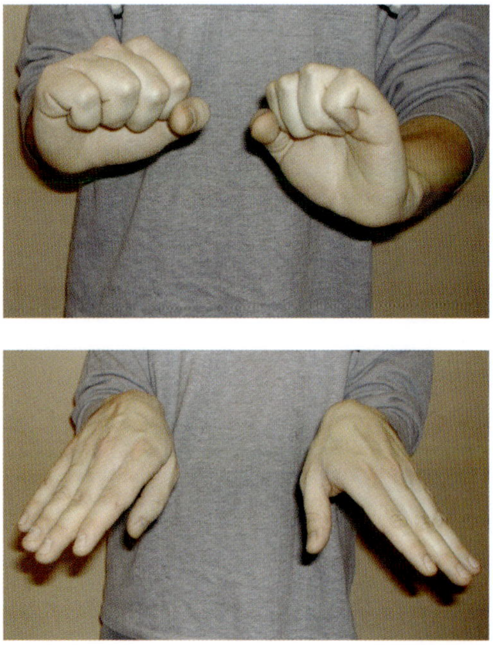

FIGURE 17-18 Range of motion after RL fusion. Note that extension is in radial deviation and flexion in ulnar deviation in the so-called "dart-throwing motion."

REFERENCES

1. Garcia-Elias M. Carpal instability. In: Wolfe S, Hotchkiss R, Pederson W, Kozin S, eds. *Green's Operative Hand Surgery*. 6th ed. Philadelphia: Churchill Livingstone Elsevier; 2011:465–521.
2. Berger RA. The ligaments of the wrist: a current overview of anatomy with considerations of their potential functions. *Hand Clin*. 1997;13:63–82.
3. The Anatomy and Biomechanics Committee of the IFSSH. Position statement: definition of carpal instability. *J Hand Surg Am*. 1999;24:866–867.
4. IWIW Terminology Committee. Wrist: terminology and definitions. *J Bone Joint Surg Am*. 2002;84(suppl 1):1–69.
5. Watson H, Ottoni L, Pitts EC, Handal AG. Rotary subluxation of the scaphoid: a spectrum of instability. *J Hand Surg Br*. 1993;18(1):62.
6. Linscheid RL, Dobyns JH, Beabout JM, Bryan RS. Traumatic instability of the wrist: diagnosis, classification and pathomechanics. *J Bone Joint Surg Am*. 1972;54:1612–1630.
7. Kuo CE, Wolfe SW. Scapholunate instability: current concepts in diagnosis and management. *J Hand Surg Am*. 2008;33:998–1013.
8. Manuel J, Moran SL. The diagnosis and treatment of scapholunate instability. *Orthop Clin North Am*. 2007;38:261–277.
9. Garcia-Elias M, Lluch A, Stanley KJ. Three-ligament tenodesis for the treatment of scapholunate dissociation: indications and surgical technique. *J Hand Surg Am*. 2006;31:125–134.
10. Chloros GD, Wiesler ER, Poehling GG. Current concepts in wrist arthroscopy. *Arthroscopy*. 2008;24:343–354.
11. Salva-Coll G, Garcia-Elias M, Leon-Lopez MT, Llusa-Perez M, Rodríguez-Baeza A. Effects of forearm muscles on carpal stability. *J Hand Surg Eur*. 2011;36:553–559.
12. Lavernia CJ, Cohen MS, Taleisnik J. Treatment of scapholunate dissociation by ligamentous repair and capsulodesis. *J Hand Surg Am*. 1992;17:354–359.
13. Cuénod P, Gray A, Papalöizos M. Bone–ligament–bone and dorsal capsulodesis reconstruction for chronic scapholunate instability. A mid-term review. *J Hand Surg Eur*. 2012;37(suppl 1):S82.
14. Watson HK, Weinzweig J, Guidera PM, Zeppieri J, Ashmead D. One thousand intercarpal arthrodeses. *J Hand Surg Br*. 1999;24:307–315.
15. Garcia-Elias M, Lluch AL, Ferreres A, Papini-Zorli I, Rahimtoola ZO. Treatment of radiocarpal degenerative osteoarthritis by radioscapholunate arthrodesis and distal scaphoidectomy. *J Hand Surg Am*. 2005;30:8–15.
16. Berger RA, Bishop AT, Bettinger PC. New dorsal capsulotomy for the surgical exposure of the wrist. *Ann Plast Surg*. 1995;35:54–59.
17. Hagert E, Ferreres A, Garcia-Elias M. Nerve-sparing dorsal and volar approaches to the radiocarpal joint. *J Hand Surg Am*. 2010;35(7):1070–1074.
18. Reagan DS, Linscheid RL, Dobyns JH. Lunotriquetral sprains. *J Hand Surg Am*. 1984;9:502–514.
19. Shin AY, Battaglia MJ, Bishop AT. Lunotriquetral instability: diagnosis and treatment. *J Am Acad Orthop Surg*. 2000;8:170–179.
20. Berger RA. A method of defining palpable landmarks for the ligament-splitting dorsal wrist capsulotomy. *J Hand Surg Am*. 2007;32:1291–1295.
21. Guidera PM, Watson HK, Dwyer TA, et al. Lunotriquetral arthrodesis using cancellous bone graft. *J Hand Surg Am*. 2001;26:422–427.
22. Rayhack JM, Linscheid RL, Dobyns JH, Smith JH. Posttraumatic ulnar translation of the carpus. *J Hand Surg Am*. 1987;12:180–189.
23. Zebala LP, Manske PR, Goldfarb CA. Madelung's deformity: a spectrum of presentation. *J Hand Surg Am*. 2007;32:1393–1401.
24. Garcia-Elias M. The non-dissociative clunking wrist: a personal view. *J Hand Surg Eur*. 2008;33:698–711.

18

Wrist Arthroscopy

David J. Slutsky, MD

INTRODUCTION

Wrist arthroscopy has steadily grown from a mostly diagnostic tool to a valuable adjunctive procedure in the treatment of myriad wrist disorders. A thorough wrist examination is integral to any arthroscopic assessment. Although wrist arthroscopy can identify an anatomic abnormality, it cannot be used to differentiate between an asymptomatic degenerative condition and a pathologic lesion that is the cause of wrist pain.

ANATOMY

The standard portals for wrist arthroscopy are mostly dorsal (Fig. 18-1A and B). This is in part due to the relative lack of neurovascular structures on the dorsum of the wrist as well as the initial emphasis on assessing the volar wrist ligaments. The dorsal portals are named in relation to the extensor compartments. One anatomic study determined that branches of the superficial radial nerve (SRN) pass within 3 mm (range, 1-6 mm) of the 1-/,2 portal.[1] The radial artery was found at an average of 3 mm radial to the portal (range, 1-5 mm). Either partial or complete overlap of the lateral antebrachial cutaneous nerve (LABCN) with the SRN occurs up to 75% of the time.[2] Steinberg et al recommended placing this portal no more than 4.5 mm dorsal to the first extensor compartment and within 4.5 mm of the radial styloid.[3] Branches of the SRN that were radial to the 3-/,4 portal were located at a mean distance of 16 mm and were generally remote from the 4-/,5 portal. Branches of the SRN were found radial to the midcarpal radial (MCR) portal at a mean of 7.2 mm. The dorsal cutaneous branch of the ulnar nerve (DCBUN) passes within 2.5 mm of the 6R portal and 17.5 mm from the dorsal distal radioulnar portal.[4]

In an anatomic study of the volar radial (VR) portal performed by the author, there was a safe zone comprising the width of the flexor carpi radialis (FCR) tendon plus at least 3 mm or more in all directions at the level of the proximal wrist crease, which was free of any neurovascular structures.[96] There was no true safe zone for the volar ulnar (VU) portal; hence, careful dissection and wound spread technique should be observed.[5]

METHODOLOGY

The patient is positioned supine under general anesthesia with the arm abducted under tourniquet control. A 2.7-mm 30° angled scope along with a camera attachment is used along with some method of overhead traction. The structures that should be visualized as a part of a standard examination include the radius articular surface, the proximal scaphoid and lunate, the volar carpal ligaments, the scapholunate interosseous ligament (SLIL) and lunotriquetral interosseous ligament (LTIL), and the triangular fibrocartilaginous complex (TFCC). It is the author's practice to establish the dorsal portals first but then to start the arthroscopic examination with the VR portal in order to visualize the palmar SLIL and the dorsal radiocarpal ligament (DRCL) to minimize artifact 2° to iatrogenic trauma to the dorsal capsular structures. If the patient has ulnar-sided wrist pain, the VU portal is utilized to assess the palmar LTIL and dorsal radioulnar ligament (DRUL), extensor carpi ulnaris (ECU) subsheath (ECUS), and radial TFCC attachment. The scope is then inserted in the 3-/,4 portal followed by various combinations of the 4-/,5 portal and 6R portal. The 6U portal is mostly used for outflow, but it may be used for instrumentation when debriding palmar LTIL tears. Midcarpal arthroscopy is performed next to assess the integrity of the intercarpal ligaments and to inspect for chondral lesions or loose bodies in the midcarpal joint. The special use portals such as the dorsal and volar distal radioulnar joint (DRUJ) portals and the 1-/,2 portal are used as needed.

3-/,4 Portal

The surgeon is initially seated facing the dorsal surface of the wrist. The concavity overlying the lunate between the extensor pollicis longus (EPL) and the extensor digitorum

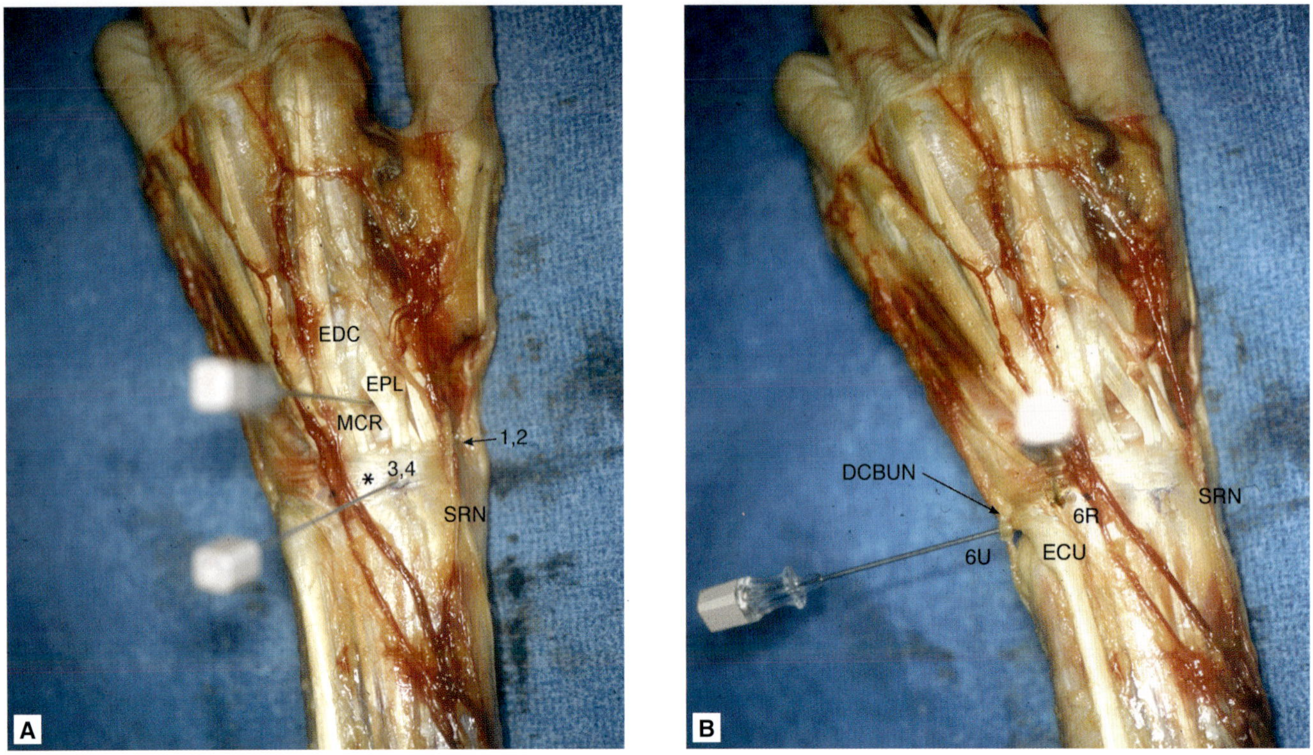

FIGURE 18-1 Dorsal portal anatomy. **A.** Cadaver dissection of the dorsal aspect of a left wrist demonstrating the relative positions of the dorsoradial portals. EDC, extensor digitorum communis; EPL, extensor pollicis longus; SRN, superficial radial nerve. (*) Lister's tubercle. **B.** Relative positions of the dorsoulnar portals. DCBUN, dorsal cutaneous branch of the ulnar nerve.

communis (EDC) is located just distal to Lister's tubercle, in line with the second web space. The radiocarpal joint is identified with a 22-gauge needle that is sloped 10° palmar to account for the volar inclination of the radius. The joint is injected with 5 cm^3 of saline. A shallow skin incision is made to avoid injuring small branches of the SRN or superficial veins. Tenotomy scissors or blunt forceps are then used to spread the soft tissue and pierce the dorsal capsule. This technique is repeated for each portal. The vascular tuft of the radioscapholunate ligament (RSL) is directly in line with this portal. Superior to the RSL is the membranous portion of the SLIL. The insertion of the dorsal capsular attachment can often be visualized by rotating the scope dorsally while looking ulnarwards. The RSL and long radiolunate ligament (LRL) are radial to the portal and can be probed with a hook in the 4-/,5 portal. The LTIL, TFCC, ulnolunate ligament (ULL), and ulnotriquetral ligament (ULT) are ulnar to the portal.

4-/,5 Portal

The interval for the 4-/,5 portal is identified with a 22-gauge needle inserted between the EDC tendons and the extensor digiti minimi (EDM), in line with the ring metacarpal. Due to the normal radial inclination of the distal radius, this portal lies slightly proximal and about 1 cm ulnar to the 3-/,4 portal. Views of the ulnar one half of the lunate are obtained by moving the scope radially, whereas the triquetrum is seen by angling the scope in a superior and ulnar direction. The LTIL is often difficult to differentiate from the carpal bones without probing. The ULL and ULT can be seen on the far end of the joint. Proximally, the radial insertion of the TFCC blends imperceptibly with the sigmoid notch of the radius, but it can be palpated with a hook probe in either the 3-/,4 or 6R portal. The peripheral insertion of the TFCC slopes upwards into the ulnar capsule. The volar and DRULs can be probed for laxity/tears, but they are not seen as distinct structures since they blend with the TFCC. The pisotriquetral orifice (PTO) is just distal and anterior to the prestyloid recess and is found within the substance of the ULT just anterior to the proximal articular surface of the triquetrum.

6R, 6U Portals

The 6R portal is identified on the radial side of the ECU tendon, just distal to the ulnar head. The scope should be angled 10° proximally to avoid hitting the triquetrum. The TFCC is immediately below the entry site. The LTIL is located radially and superiorly, whereas the ulnar capsule is immediately adjacent to the scope. The 6U portal is located ulnar to the ECU tendon. This portal can be used to view the dorsal rim of the TFCC or for instrumentation when debriding the palmar LTIL.

Midcarpal Portals

The MCR portal is found 1 cm distal to the 3-/,4 portal. The scaphotrapezial trapezoidal (STT) joint lies radially and can be seen by rotating the scope dorsally. The scapholunate (SL) articulation that is proximal to this portal can be probed for instability or step-off. By moving the scope in an ulnar direction, the lunotriquetral (LT) articulation comes into view. Superiorly, the proximal surface of the capitate, the interosseous ligament, and the hamate are seen. The midcarpal ulnar (MCU) portal is located 1 cm distal to the 4-/,5 portal or 1.5 cm ulnar and slightly proximal to the MCR portal, in line with the ring metacarpal axis. Normally there is very little step-off between the distal articular surfaces. When there is any doubt, the traction should be released and the SL joint should be viewed with the scope in the MCU, whereas the LT joint should be viewed with the scope in the MCR.

Volar Portals

To establish the VR radial portal, the surgeon is seated facing the volar aspect of the wrist. A 2-cm transverse or longitudinal incision is made in the proximal wrist crease overlying the FCR tendon (Fig. 18-2). It is not necessary to specifically identify the adjacent neurovascular structures, provided that the anatomic landmarks are adhered to. The tendon sheath is divided and the FCR tendon is retracted ulnarly. The radiocarpal joint space is identified with a 22-gauge needle and distended with 5 cm^3 of saline. Tenotomy scissors or forceps are used to pierce the volar capsule. A blunt obturator and trocar are then introduced followed by the arthroscope.

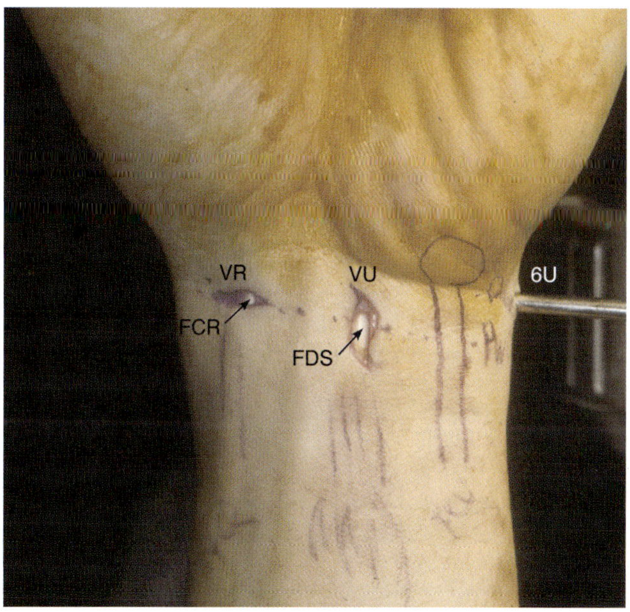

FIGURE 18-2 Relative positions of the volar radial (VR) portal and the volar ulnar (VU) portal. FCR, flexor carpi radialis; FDS, flexor digitorum sublimus.

The midcarpal joint can be accessed through the same skin incision by angling the trocar 1 cm distally and approximately 5° ulnarwards. A hook probe is inserted through the 3/-,4 portal and it is used to assess the palmar aspect of the SLIL and the DRCL. A useful landmark when viewing from the VR portal is the intersulcal ridge between the scaphoid and lunate fossae. The origin of the DRCL is seen immediately ulnar to this ridge, just proximal to the lunate. The VU portal is established via a 2-cm longitudinal incision centered over the proximal wrist crease along the ulnar edge of the finger flexor tendons. The tendons are retracted to the radial side and the radiocarpal joint space is identified with a 22-gauge needle. Blunt tenotomy scissors or forceps are used to pierce the volar capsule, followed by insertion of a cannula and blunt trocar, and then the arthroscope. The ulnar nerve is protected by use of the cannula and a more radial entry site. The median nerve is protected by the adjacent flexor tendons. The palmar region of the LTIL can usually be seen slightly distal and radial to the portal. A hook probe is inserted through the 6R or 6U portal.

DRUJ Portals

The dorsal aspect of the DRUJ joint can be accessed through a proximal and a distal portal. The proximal portal is mostly for outflow and can be identified by inserting a 22-gauge needle horizontally at the neck of the distal ulna. The distal portal (DDRUJ) is identified just proximal to the 6R portal, underneath the DRUL. This portal can be used for outflow drainage or for instrumentation. It lies on top of the ulnar head but underneath the TFCC.

The topographical landmarks and establishment of the volar distal radioulnar (VDRU) portal are identical to those of the VU portal. The capsular entry point lies 5 to 10 mm proximally.[6] There is more room on the VU aspect of the DRUJ for insertion of an arthroscope with relatively unimpeded views of the proximal articular disc and the foveal attachments. The VDRU portal is accessed through the VU skin incision. A 1.9 mm small joint arthroscope can be used since gaining access to the DRUJ can be difficult, especially in a small wrist, but a standard 2.7-mm scope provides a better field of view. It is useful to leave a needle or cannula in the ulnocarpal joint for reference. The DRUJ is located by angling a 22-gauge needle 45° proximally, and then injecting the DRUJ with saline. Once the correct plane is identified, the volar DRUJ capsule is pierced with tenotomy scissors followed by a cannula with a blunt trocar and then the arthroscope. Alternatively, a probe can be placed in the DDRUJ portal and advanced through the palmar incision to help locate the joint space. It can then be used as a switching stick over which the cannula is introduced. Initially, the DRUJ space appears quite confined, but over the course of 3 to 5 minutes the fluid irrigation expands the joint space, which improves visibility. A burr or thermal probe can be substituted for the 3-mm hook probe through the DDRUJ as necessary (Fig. 18-3A-D).

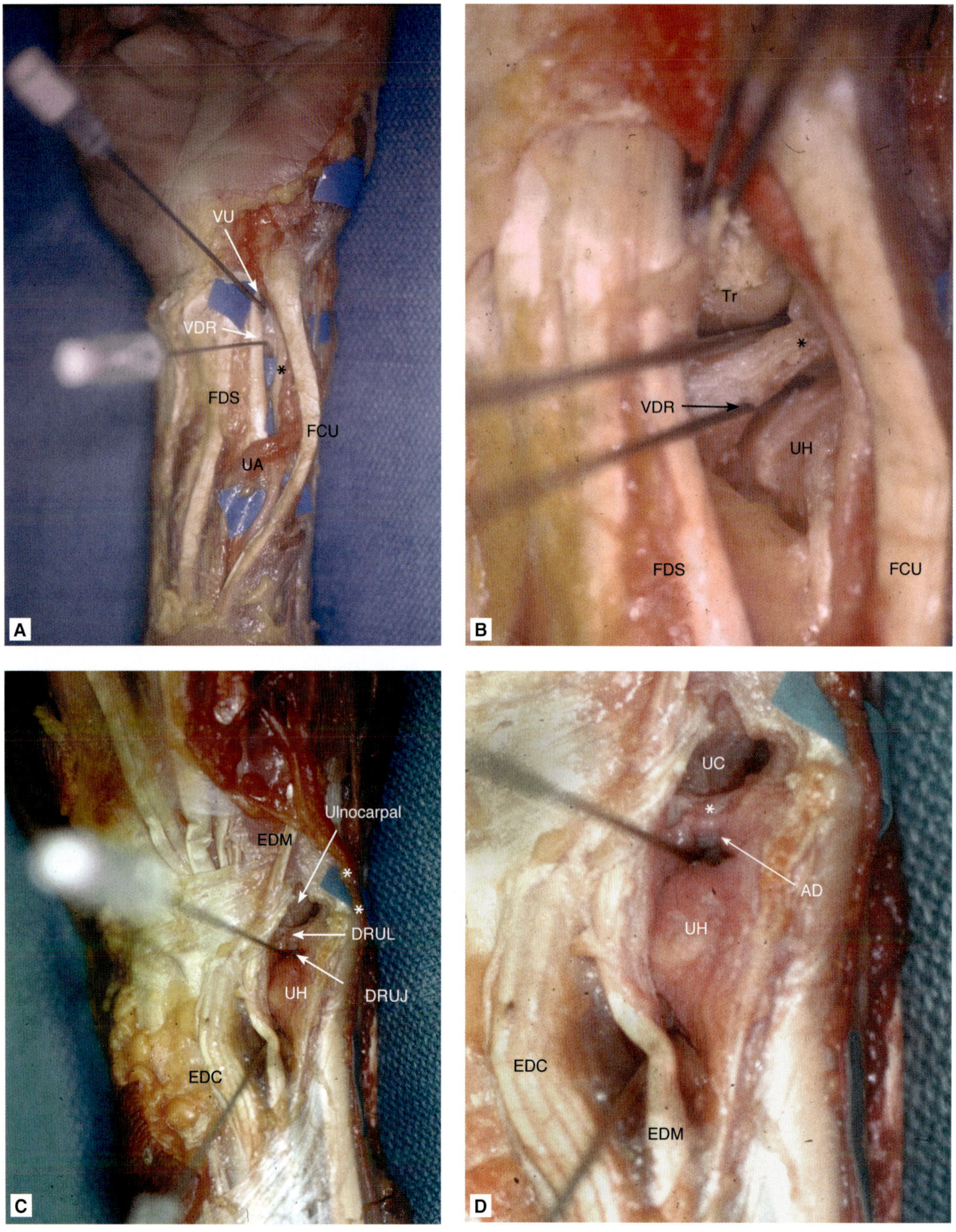

FIGURE 18-3 **A.** Volar aspect of a left wrist demonstrating the relative positions of the VU and volar DRUJ (VDR) portals in relation to the ulnar nerve (*) and ulnar artery (UA). FCU, flexor carpi ulnaris; FDS, flexor digitorum sublimus. **B.** Close-up view after the volar capsule is removed showing position of needles in relation to the volar radioulnar ligament (*). Tr, triquetrum; UH, ulnar head. **C.** Relative position of the proximal (PDRUJ) and distal (DRUJ) portals. **D.** Close-up view with the dorsal capsule removed demonstrating the position of the needles in relation to the dorsal radioulnar ligament (*). AD, articular disk; UC, ulnocarpal joint; UH, ulnar head.

SYNOVIAL BIOPSY

Indications

A synovial biopsy is mostly indicated in inflammatory conditions where a tissue sample is required to aid in the diagnosis. These would include inflammatory arthritis, gout, sarcoidosis, and granulomatous infections. Synovial biopsy is also of use when quantitative analysis of the inflammatory response in a rheumatoid patient is indicated for prognostic reasons.

Contraindications

This should be done with caution in any patient who is on anticoagulation medication or with a bleeding disorder.

Outcomes

Kraan et al demonstrated that the inflammation in 1 inflamed joint is generally representative of that in other inflamed joints and that it is possible to use serial samples from the same joint, selecting either large or small joints, for the evaluation of antirheumatic therapies.[7] They examined 9 patients with rheumatoid arthritis and performed an arthroscopic synovial biopsy of both an inflamed knee joint and an inflamed wrist or metacarpophalangeal joint. Multiple biopsy specimens were collected and stained for macrophages, T cells, plasma cells, fibroblast-like synoviocytes, and interleukin-6 (IL-6) by immunohistochemistry. They found no significant differences in mean cell numbers for all markers investigated in samples from the knee joint compared with samples from the small joints, but they did find a statistically significant correlation for the numbers of sublining macrophages, T cells, and plasma cells, as well as for IL-6 expression, between the knee joint and the small joints. It is most efficient to take a sample directly using arthroscopic forceps, although a full radius resector and arthroscopic scalpel may also be used.

A radiographic association between calcium pyrophosphate dihydrate crystal deposition disease (CPPD) and chronic SL dissociation[8] and scaphotrapezial (ST) osteoarthritis[9] has been noted, but the question of cause and effect has not been completely settled. A recent report has linked gout and SL and LT ligament pathology as well. Wilczynski et al recently reported the arthroscopic findings in 7 patients with the diagnosis of gout and nontraumatic wrist pathology.[10] All 7 wrists had diffuse synovitis, with crystalline deposits throughout the radiocarpal joint (positive histology for urate crystals available in 4 patients) as well as focal crystalline precipitates on the SL and LT ligaments but not on the triangular fibrocartilage complex. SL (6 cases) or LT ligament (5 cases) disruption was noted in addition to an early scapholunate advanced collapse (SLAC) pattern of arthritis in 6 of the 7 patients.

SYNOVECTOMY

Indications

An arthroscopic synovectomy is mostly indicated in rheumatoid patients who have not responded to 6 months of appropriate medical management with a stable wrist joint and well-preserved articular surfaces. It is also beneficial in patients who have juvenile rheumatoid arthritis, systemic lupus, and postinfectious arthritis. Preoperatively, MR imaging of the wrists in patients with early RA can help to predict the future course.

Contraindications

Similar to a biopsy, a synovectomy should be done with caution in any patient who is on anticoagulation medication or with a bleeding disorder. It is not recommended in psoriatic arthropathy.[11]

Surgical Technique

The synovectomy is performed systematically using a 3.5-mm resector and a thermal probe, starting on the radial side of the wrist. Synovitis is especially localized around the radial styloid the radioscaphocapitate (RSC) ligament, the prestyloid recess, and the ECUS (Fig. 18-4A and B). The surgeon may interchange instruments and the scope between the 3-/4, 4-/5, and VR portals for access. The ulnocarpal joint is then addressed through the 4-/5, 6R, and VU portals. The midcarpal joint is explored through the MCR, MCU, and STT portals. A DRUJ synovectomy can be performed with the scope in the VDR portal and the instruments in the DDRUJ portal. Occasionally the DRUJ can be accessed through a central TFCC tear. Early motion is instituted postoperatively to limit adhesions.

Outcomes

Adolfsson and Frisen warn against using it for psoriatic arthropathy based on the poor results in a small number of patients who had been treated with an arthroscopic synovectomy.[11] They noted that the synovitis was less pronounced and there was a tendency for ankylosis with this disease. Adolfsson interviewed 18 patients 12 to 15 years after they had undergone an arthroscopic synovectomy and noted they generally experienced a long period of comfort following the synovectomy with only 1 patient requiring additional surgery.[12]

CHONDROPLASTY AND LOOSE BODIES

Indications

Articular cartilage damage is a common cause of wrist pain and may result from osteochondral fractures, chronic

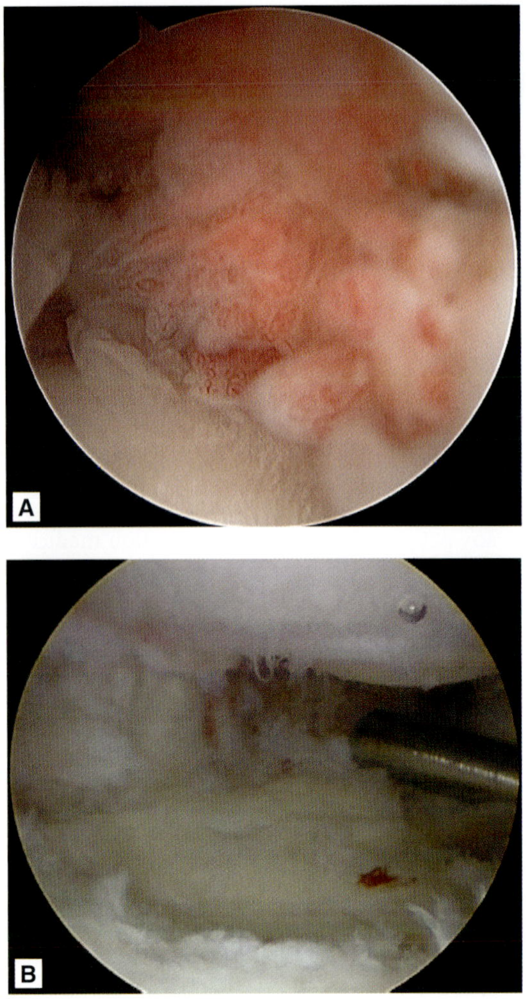

FIGURE 18-4 **A.** Rheumatoid synovitis in the ulnar capsule. **B.** View of the ulnar capsule from the 3,4 portal following a synovectomy.

carpal instability, sloughing of a cartilage defect in avascular necrosis, or idiopathically. Intermittent locking from loose bodies constitutes an ideal indication for wrist arthroscopy (Fig. 18-5A). Articular defects often go undetected by preoperative imaging studies and they are best seen at the time of arthroscopy. Culp et al have provided a modified Outerbridge classification for chondral lesions in the wrist where grade 1 represents softening of the hyaline surface, grade II consists of fibrillation and fissuring, grade III represents a fibrillated lesion of varying depth in the articular surface, and grade IV has a full-thickness defect down to bone (Fig. 18-5B).[13] Grade I to III lesions are treated with debridement and localized synovectomy. Localized grade IV lesions can be treated with abrasion chondroplasty and subchondral drilling.

Contraindications

Chondroplasty is not indicated if there is widespread cartilage loss.

Surgical Technique

Once a focal area of chondral damage is identified, an arthroscopic burr or 0.62-mm K-wire is used to make multiple perforations into the subchondral bone plate. These perforations are made 1 to 2 mm apart while maintaining an adequate bony bridge (Fig. 18-5C).

Outcomes

Bain and Roth noted improvement in 83% of patients with 1° chondral defects that were treated with debridement.[14] Whipple stated that patients often have relief after abrasion arthroplasty if the defect is <5 mm.[15]

ARTHROSCOPY AND AVASCULAR NECROSIS

Bain and Begg described an arthroscopic classification for Kienböck disease based on the number of articular surfaces.[16] Grade 0 is where all articular surfaces are normal; hence, an extra-articular unloading procedure may be indicated. Grade I consists of 1 nonfunctional proximal lunate surface that can be treated with a proximal row carpectomy (PRC), radioscapholunate fusion or lunate excision, and scaphocapitate (SC) fusion (Fig. 18-6). Grade II is when the proximal and distal lunate surfaces are nonfunctional that requires a PRC or SC fusion. Grades III and IV require total wrist fusion or arthroplasty. Menth-Chiari et al utilized arthroscopic debridement alone of the necrotic lunate in 7 patients with Lichtman stages IIIA and IIIB.[17] All patients reported significant improvement in pain relief and complete relief of mechanical symptoms at an average of 19-month follow-up. There are scant reports on arthroscopic treatment of Preiser disease, but the same investigators reported good pain relief and improved wrist motion in a patient following debridement of a necrotic scaphoid at a 31-month follow-up.[18]

ARTHROSCOPIC WRIST GANGLIONECTOMY

Osterman and Raphael pioneered the arthroscopic resection of dorsal wrist ganglia and reported on 150 procedures with only 1 recurrence.[19] Volar wrist ganglia that originate from the radiocarpal joint are amenable to arthroscopic resection. Arthroscopic resection of ganglia from the STT joint has not been reported.

Indications

The indication for arthroscopic removal of a dorsal ganglion is similar to those for an open method. An ideal indication is when patients have concomitant wrist pain and a positive

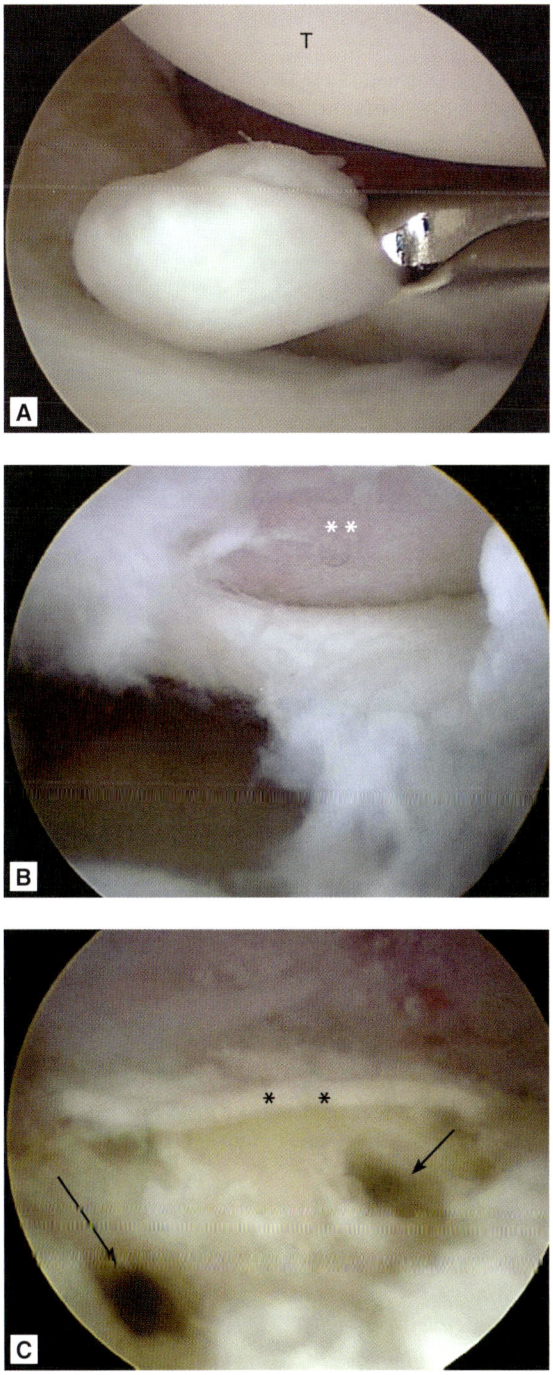

FIGURE 18-5 **A.** Arthroscopic forceps in the 4-/,5 portal are used to remove a loose body in the ulnocarpal joint. T, triquetrum. **B.** Full-thickness chondral defect (*) of the lunate. **C.** A chondral defect is viewed from the MCR. Note the rim of remaining cartilage (*) and the 2 drill holes (arrows) separated by a bone bridge.

scaphoid shift test where evaluation of any associated SLIL instability is desirable. The occult ganglion that is entirely intracapsular and cannot be visualized during open surgery is another good indication. Preoperative x-rays should be performed to rule out intraosseous communication or other carpal pathology. It is important to ensure the lesion is in fact a ganglion with transillumination, an MRI, or needle aspiration. An Allen test should be performed with volar ganglia to ensure adequate hand perfusion from the ulnar artery in the event of radial artery perforation, and to rule out an aneurysm masquerading as a cyst.

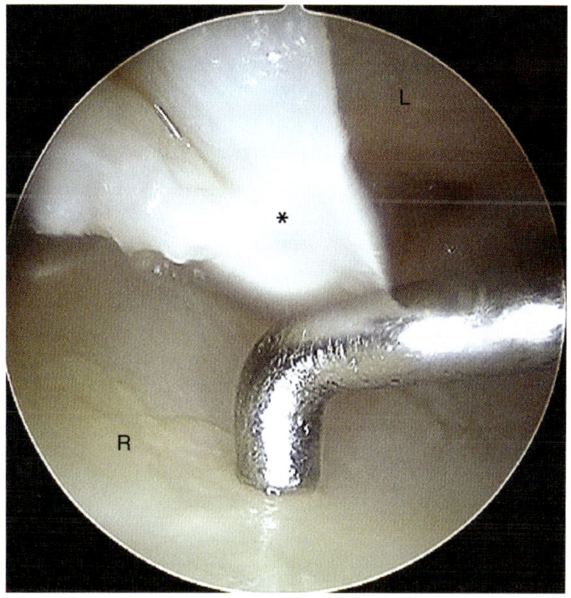

FIGURE 18-6 Staging of Kienböck disease. A flap of nonviable cartilage (*) is hanging into the joint exposing the subchondral bone of the lunate (L). The cartilage on the lunate fossa of the radius (R) is still viable.

Contraindications

Scarring in the area due to previous injury or surgery for recurrence may distort the anatomy and make it difficult to establish the portals.

Surgical Technique: Dorsal Ganglionectomy

Since the ganglion overlies the 3-/,4 portal, it is my preference to view the ganglion through the VR portal, which provides a direct line of sight and allows one to rule out a tear of the DRCL. Alternatively, the 1-/,2 or 6R portal can be used. A shaver is then introduced into the ganglion through the 3-/,4 portal to perforate the ganglion and resect the stalk. The intra-articular ganglion is completely debrided along with a 1-cm area of surrounding dorsal capsule. The extensor tendons may be visible through the defect. Midcarpal arthroscopy should be performed to debride any midcarpal extension of the ganglion and to assess the status of the SL and LT joints (Fig. 18-7A and B).

Surgical Technique: Volar Ganglionectomy

The ganglion is amenable to arthroscopic resection only if it arises from the radiocarpal joint that can be determined

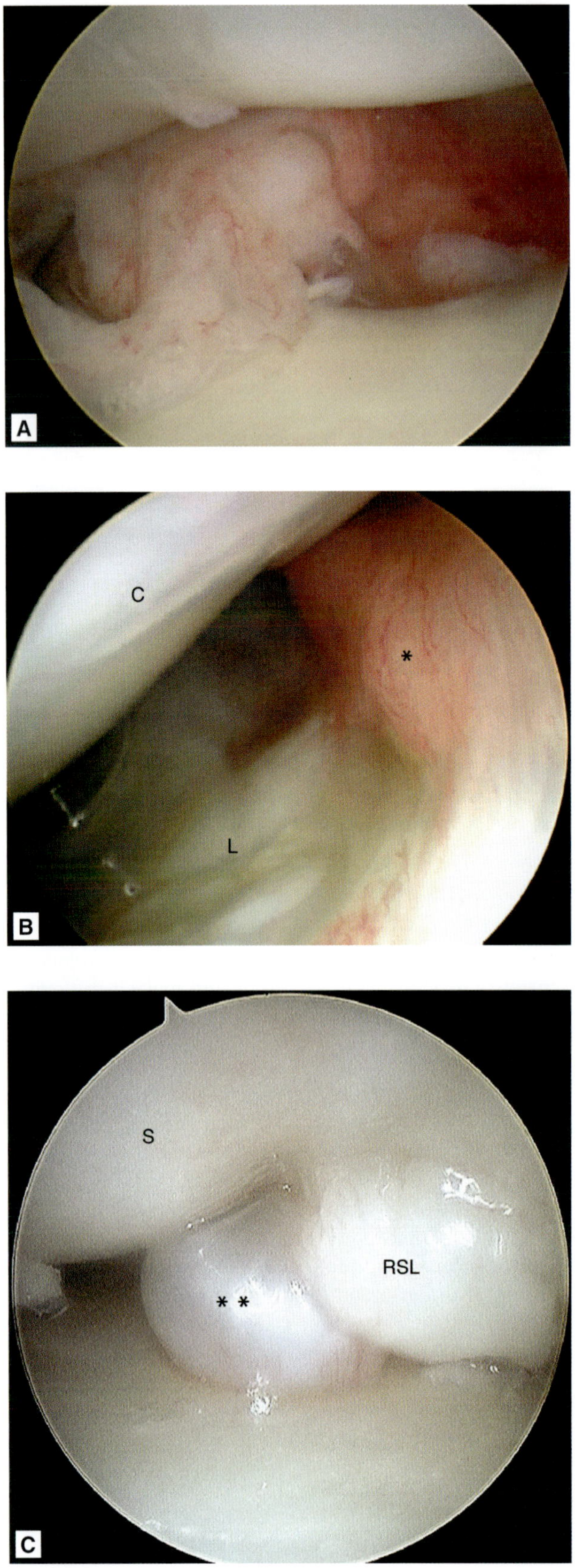

FIGURE 18-7 **A.** Dorsal wrist ganglion seen from the VR portal. **B.** Midcarpal extension of a dorsal wrist ganglion (*) as seen from the MCR. C, capitate; L, lunate. **C.** Volar wrist ganglion (*) viewed from the 3-/4 portal. RSL, radioscapholunate ligament; S, scaphoid.

by injecting the cyst with dye intraoperatively under fluoroscopy.[20] The joint is surveyed in the standard fashion starting with the 3-/,4 portal. When a volar ganglion is present, there may be an outpouching in the sulcus between the RSC and LRL (Fig. 18-7C). Volar pressure on the cyst can deliver it into the joint space. A resector is placed through the VR, 1-/2, or 4-/,5 portal to resect the ganglion and 1 cm of surrounding capsule until the FCR tendon is seen. Postoperatively, the wrist is splinted for 1 week for comfort followed by protected range of motion. Loss of wrist flexion following dorsal ganglia excision or loss of wrist extension with volar ganglia can be treated with dynamic splinting at 6 to 8 weeks.

Outcomes

Rizzo et al performed an arthroscopic resection of 41 dorsal ganglia. At 2 years, patients demonstrated improved wrist motion and grip strength, excellent pain relief, and only 2 recurrences.[21] Mathoulin et al performed an arthroscopic resection on 32 patients with a volar cyst with no recurrences at an average follow-up of 26 months and an arthroscopic resection of 96 dorsal ganglia with 4 recurrences at a mean follow-up of 34 months.[22] At the 1-year follow-up, Kang et al reported a recurrence rate of 3/28 in patients undergoing an arthroscopic resection and 2/23 in patients treated with an open ganglion resection.[23] Edwards and Johansen had no recurrences at a minimum 2-year follow-up in 55 patients following an arthroscopic dorsal ganglion resection.[24] They noted a high incidence of interosseous ligament laxity. Using the Geissler classification, the SL joint demonstrated laxity types I (2 of 45 cases), II (22 of 45 cases), III (20 of 45 cases), and IV (1 of 45 cases). The LT joint demonstrated laxity types II (6 of 45 cases) and III (39 of 45 cases). Good results are not invariable in patients with associated intracarpal pathology however. Povlsen and Tavakkolizadeh reviewed 16 patients with painful dorsal wrist ganglia and arthroscopically confirmed ligament abnormalities. They documented the presence of an abnormal SL joint in 10/16 patients and an abnormal LT joint in 2/16 patients. At a 5-year follow-up there were no recurrences of the ganglia, but only 1 patient remained pain free.[25] Langner et al reported a high incidence of TFCC lesions in association with painful volar or dorsal wrist ganglia.[26] They noted an incidence of 22 TFCC lesions in 46 patients who underwent an arthroscopic ganglion resection. The TFCC lesions were treated with debridement or repair depending on the locations and type of tear. At 1 year, the DASH scores had improved in all patients, but there was a 17% recurrence rate.

ARTHROSCOPIC RELEASE OF WRIST CONTRACTURE

Indications

Patients lacking a functional arc of wrist motion who have failed a trial of dynamic/static progressive splinting are candidates for this procedure. Lee et al devised a classification

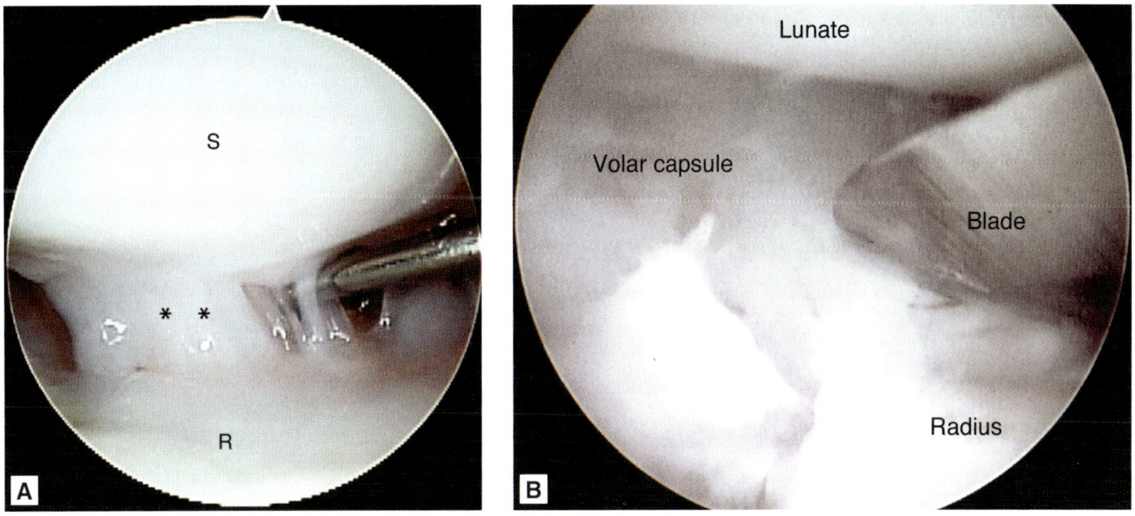

FIGURE 18-8 **A.** Arthrofibrosis between the radius (R) and scaphoid (S) viewed from the 3-/4 portal. **B.** Volar capsulotomy. The arthroscope is in the 3-/4 portal and the blade is inserted in the 4-/5 portal.

system based on pathologic anatomic location.[27] Type I represents intrinsic adhesions that are subdivided into radiocarpal (A), midcarpal (B), DRUJ (C), and combined (D). Type II represents extrinsic contracture that can be dorsal (A), volar (B), DRUJ (C), and combined (D). The operative approach should be wrist arthroscopy for types IA (radiocarpal adhesions) and IB (midcarpal adhesions) where intra-articular adhesions are present. Types IC (DRUJ adhesions) and IIC (DRUJ capsular contracture) are best approached in an open manner where dorsal and palmar capsulectomies of the DRUJ are performed. For types IIA, B, and D (dorsal, palmar, and combination extrinsic contracture, respectively), both open and arthroscopic methods are utilized.

Contraindications

A frank carpal instability pattern is a contraindication since release of the volar and/or dorsal extrinsic ligaments would likely exacerbate this condition. Similarly, significant posttraumatic OA will limit any ultimate gains. Division of the RSC, LRL, and short radiolunate ligament (SRL) should be performed with caution in patients who are at risk for ulnar translocation such as those patients with rheumatoid arthritis and those who have undergone previous radial styloidectomies. Patients who cannot comply with postoperative dynamic/static progressive splinting due to low pain threshold or psychological disorder are not appropriate candidates.

Surgical Technique: Volar Capsulotomy

A blunt trocar and a cannula are initially inserted in the 3-/,4 portal and used in a sweeping fashion to clear a path. A full radius resector is used to clear adhesions. The radial artery passes within 5.2 mm, the median nerve 6.9 mm, and the ulnar nerve passes within 6.7 mm of the volar capsule, which should be kept in mind.[28] An arthroscopic knife is introduced through a cannula in the 4-/,5 portal (Fig. 18-8A and B). The RSC ligament is gently divided until the volar capsular fat and/or the FCR tendon is seen. The ULL and ULT should not be released in the presence of an LT joint instability since in sectioning studies this combination results in a volar intercalated segmental instability (VISI) pattern, especially when the DRCL is also released.

Surgical Technique: Dorsal Capsulotomy

It is my preference to view through the VR portal, although the 1-/,2 portal may be substituted. In patients with a partial or complete SLIL tear, sectioning the DRCL should be done with caution since it may exacerbate any preexisting SL instability. An arthroscopic knife is introduced through a cannula placed in the 3-/,4 portal. The dorsal capsule and the DRCL are gently sectioned until the dorsal capsular fat and/or the extensor tendons can be seen. Verhellen and Bain use an umbilical tape to retract and protect the extensor tendons.[28] If it is desirable to release the dorsoulnar capsule, it is necessary to establish a VU portal, or to view through the 6U portal. The adhesions are cleared through utilizing the 4-/,5 and 6R portals and then a capsulotomy is performed in a similar fashion. Postoperatively, the patient is placed in a bulky splint for 2 to 3 days to reduce hematoma formation, followed by aggressive wrist mobilization.

Outcomes

Osterman described his experience with 23 patients with an average preoperative wrist flexion of 5° and extension of 15° (A. L. Osterman, personal communication, 2000). At a 2-year follow-up flexion improved to 48° and extension to 58°. Hattori et al noted an average increase of 22° in their series of 11 patients.[29] Luchetti et al reported on 28 patients. Radiocarpal, midcarpal, and distal radioulnar portals were used. At a mean of 28 months, wrist flexion/extension increased from an average of 84° to 99° and mean pronation/supination increased from 144° to 159°.[30]

INTEROSSEOUS LIGAMENT INJURIES

Arthroscopy has perhaps influenced the diagnosis and treatment of interosseous ligament injuries more than any other type of carpal disorder. Geissler et al proposed an arthroscopic grading scale of interosseous ligament instability that can be applied to both the SL and LT ligaments.[31] This classification quantifies the resultant instability and not the actual size of the tear. When examining the SL joint with a Geissler I instability, a 1-mm hook probe placed through the MCU portal can be inserted between the scaphoid and lunate. In a grade II lesion the probe can be rotated 90° due to none to minimal instability from ligament attenuation but no tearing. This magnitude of instability was previously undetected since despite clinical symptoms, the imaging studies including MRI, plain x-rays, and dynamic motion studies are normal. In a grade III lesion abnormal scaphoid flexion and lunate extension produces a midcarpal step-off at the SL joint when viewed arthroscopically. Ulnar deviation and grip view x-rays may show an increased SL gap. In a grade IV lesion there is a complete SLIL tear that allows one to pass the arthroscope from the midcarpal joint to the radiocarpal joint through the diastasis.

Scapholunate Ligament Injuries

It has become clear that the stability of the SL joint is not dependent wholly on the SLIL but rather on both primary and secondary stabilizers that form a scapholunate ligament complex (SLLC).[32] Each case of SL instability is unique and therefore should be treated with tissue-specific repairs, which may partly explain why 1 procedure cannot successfully restore joint stability in every case. Wrist arthroscopy has a pivotal role in both the assessment and treatment of the SLLC derangements. Elsaidi et al sequentially divided the RSC, LRL and SRL, the SLIL, and finally the dorsal capsule insertion on the scaphoid.[33] There was no appreciable change in the radiographic appearance of the wrist. When the DRCL was then divided, a dorsal intercalated segmental instability (DISI) deformity occurred. Short et al determined that the SLIL is the primary stabilizer of the SL articulation and that the DRCL, the dorsal intercarpal (DIC) ligament, the ST ligaments, and the RSC ligaments are secondary stabilizers.[34] Dividing the DRCL alone only caused increased radial deviation of the lunate with the wrist in maximum flexion, whereas dividing the SLIL after any of the ligaments tested produced increased flexion and ulnar deviation of the scaphoid and lunate extension. The SL joint stability is therefore dependent on a complex of ligaments, each having a separate role but working in concert. Any given reconstructive procedure should be designed for 1 specific function rather than multiple functions, which may be a reason for failure in some cases. Rather than grouping procedures into those that

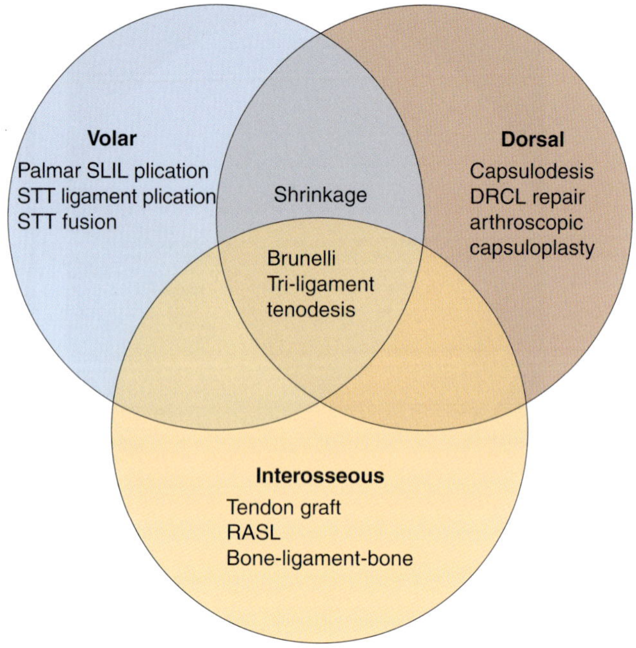

DIAGRAM 1

provide sagittal plane stability versus those that provide coronal plane stability, it is preferable to consider the individual subcomponent(s) of the SLLC. The reconstructive procedures can be therefore grouped into those that stabilize the volar components of the SLLC (the palmar SLIL, RSC, ST ligaments), the dorsal components (dorsal capsule, dorsal SLIL, DRCL, DIC), and the interosseous component (SLIL) that is illustrated in the Venn diagram (Diagram 1).

INDICATIONS

Arthroscopic assessment of the SLLC is indicated in any patient with radial-sided wrist pain and with a positive scaphoid shift test who has not responded to conservative measures. It is also indicated when there is a SL gap without a DISI deformity. It then guides the subsequent treatment by allowing the staging of the degree of injury and the severity of instability.

CONTRAINDICATIONS

Complete and repairable SLIL tears as well as static carpal instabilities are best managed with open techniques. Rosenwasser et al have treated complete but irreparable ligament tears with the reduction and association of the scaphoid and lunate (RASL) procedure, which uses a cannulated Herbert screw to create a stable pseudarthrosis.[35] Hausman has reported favorable results with an arthroscopic version of the RASL.[36]

SURGICAL TECHNIQUE: ARTHROSCOPIC DEBRIDEMENT

Arthroscopic debridement alone is indicated for acute or chronic Geissler I and II lesions. Palmar tears are best seen through the VR portal (Fig. 18-9).[37] The tear is debrided to

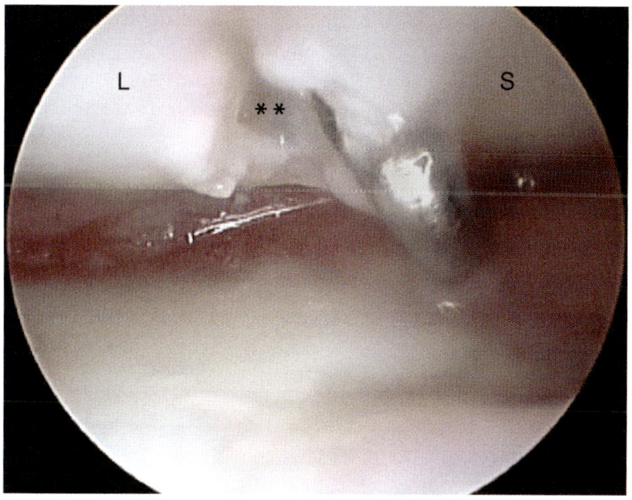

FIGURE 18-9 Palmar tear of the scapholunate ligament (*) as seen from the VR portal. L, lunate; S, scaphoid.

stable margins while preserving any intact fibers by switching the arthroscope and resector between the VR, 3-/,4, and 4-/,5 portals. Early wrist motion is instituted postoperatively. Dynamic wrist arthroscopy can be performed in a similar manner to motion studies under live fluoroscopy. With the scope in the 3-/,4 portal the wrist is taken out of traction and passively moved into flexion and extension and radial and ulnar deviation while observing the relative motion of the scaphoid and lunate. This same step is repeated with the scope in the MCU portal. The SL joint is then observed while performing a scaphoid shift test. Without traction one gets a better sense of the normal and pathologic wrist kinematics.

SURGICAL TECHNIQUE: THERMAL SHRINKAGE

The indications for thermal shrinkage are the same as for debridement, but it may have some use if there is an associated dynamic instability. The dorsal SLIL is treated using a thermal probe in the 4-/,5 portal. The palmar SLIL can be treated with the probe in the 3-/,4 portal while viewing through the VR portal. It is important to use rapid irrigation to limit possible thermal damage to the cartilage. The probe is applied using multiple strokes like a paintbrush for only a few seconds at a time. In the midcarpal joint, the radial limb of the arcuate ligament is seen at the palmar junction of the scaphoid and lunate. Danoff et al have shown this tissue actually represents a continuation of the palmar SLIL.[38] Short bursts of thermal energy to this tissue tighten the SL and scapholunocapitate articulations.[39] When midcarpal examination reveals SL joint congruency without gapping, the thermal shrinkage is complete. K-wire fixation is often used following shrinkage for 8 weeks, followed by wrist motion.

SURGICAL TECHNIQUE: ARTHROSCOPIC-ASSISTED PERCUTANEOUS K-WIRE FIXATION

In patients with partial tears without carpal malrotation (Geissler II), temporary K-wire fixation may improve SL stability. If necessary, individual K-wires can be inserted dorsally into the lunate and the distal scaphoid and used as joysticks to derotate the scaphoid and lunate. The K-wires should be introduced in a safe zone that is no more than 4.5 mm dorsal to the first extensor compartment and within 4.5 mm of the radial styloid.[3] A second K-wire is inserted between the distal scaphoid and the capitate. The reduction is checked with both fluoroscopy and arthroscopy.

OUTCOMES

The current available literature consists mostly of level IV, retrospective case series, with a short follow-up and small numbers. Despite this, some useful information can be gleaned.

DORSAL SLLC

O'Meeghan et al demonstrated that milder grades of instability do not necessarily culminate in a static carpal instability.[40] At a 7-year follow-up, 11 patients with untreated Geissler I or II SLIL injuries still showed no radiologic signs of instability, but they continued to experience considerable pain, loss of motion, and functional limitation. In Whipple's series of 40 patients treated with arthroscopic reduction and pinning, 85% of patients with a <3-mm side-to-side SL gap and symptoms of <3 months' duration maintained comfort and stability at 2 to 7 years.[13] Only 53% of the patients with a >3-mm side-to-side SL gap or symptoms >3 months were symptom free at 1 to 3 years. This supported the concept that both the chronicity of the lesion and the degree of instability impact the eventual outcomes.

Darlis et al treated 16 patients with a mean age of 34 years, who had a Geissler I/II SLIL injury.[41] The average duration of pain was 5.4 months (range, 3-14 months). Each patient underwent debridement and thermal shrinkage of the SLIL and dorsal capsule, followed by 2 weeks of immobilization. At an average follow-up of 19 months, there were 14 excellent/good results and 2 fair/poor results using the modified Mayo wrist score. Others have reported similar outcomes. Darlis et al found that arthroscopic debridement and pinning provides inconsistent results with more advanced degrees of ligamentous instability.[42] They treated 11 patients with a Geissler III/IV SLIL instability with aggressive debridement down to bleeding bone and percutaneous pinning for 4 to 8 weeks. Three patients failed within the first year and required a partial carpal fusion. At the 3-year follow-up, only 6/11 achieved a good result without further revision surgery.

Mathoulin et al reported the preliminary results of treatment of chronic Geissler II or reducible grade III lesions by an arthroscopic capsuloplasty between the SLIL and the dorsal capsule.[43] Thirty-six patients with a mean age of 38.5 years (range, 25-58 years) were treated with this technique, supplemented by percutaneous pinning in the 16 patients with a grade III lesion. At a mean follow-up of 11.4 months (range, 7-19 months) the mean DASH was 6.1 points (range, 0-100). Nineteen of the 22 patients reached 85% or more of the contralateral wrist range of movement. Using the visual analogue score (VAS) the mean preoperative pain was 3.4 (range, 0-10) and the postoperative VAS was 0.31. The average grip strength of the injured wrists was 96% of the contralateral side.

PALMAR SLLC

Danoff et al reported good short-term outcomes in 7/8 patients with Geissler grade II SL instability after arthroscopic debridement and radio-frequency shrinkage of the palmar SLIL.[38]

INTEROSSEOUS SLLC

Rosenwasser et al popularized the RASL procedure using a cannulated Herbert screw.[35] They recently reported excellent long-term results in 31 patients with a chronic static SL instability at an average follow-up of 6.4 years (range, 16 months to 18.0 years).[44] The mean DASH score was 17.0 (range, 0-50.8); the mean VAS was 1.65 (range, 0-7.3) with moderate activity. The results of an arthroscopic RASL (ARASL) were subsequently reported by Aviles et al in 7 patients aged 28 to 77 years with static SL instability.[45] At a mean follow-up of 19 months, good pain relief was achieved in 6/7 patients with 1 failure in a patient with advanced radiocarpal and midcarpal OA. The total arc of wrist motion was reduced 17.6%. The mean SL gap was reduced from 4.2 to 1.75 mm and the mean SL angle was reduced from 81.6° to 61.8°. The authors stressed that the key to a successful result was dependent on proper screw placement. Caloia et al reported the results of an ARASL in 8 patients/9 wrists with a chronic reducible SL ligament tear.[46] The mean age was 44.5 years (range, 38-56 years). At a follow-up of 34.6 months (range, 12-43 months) the VAS improved from 5.4 (range, 0-10) preoperatively to 1.5 (1-3). The postoperative grip strength was 78% of the contralateral side and the average postoperative wrist ROM was reduced by 20%. The SL angle decreased from 70.5° to 59.3°. Three patients required screw removal secondary to loosening or hardware irritation.

THERMAL SHRINKAGE

Hirsh et al treated 10 patients (mean age, 37 years) having Geissler II SLIL injuries with shrinkage and 4 to 6 weeks of immobilization. Symptom duration was >6 months in 8 patients. At 28 months, the pain had resolved in 9/10 patients.[47] Similarly, Shih and Lee studied 19 patients (mean age, 23 years) with symptomatic dynamic and predynamic SL instability present for 17 months. At 28 months following thermal shrinkage, 15/19 patients were fully satisfied with the results and returned to their preinjury activity. Four patients had recurrent laxity of the SL joint. The loss of wrist motion averaged 5°.[48] Battistella et al divided 120 patients into 4 groups. Group A consisted of 20 patients with a Geissler I SLIL instability.[49] They were treated with thermal shrinkage alone. Group B consisted of 20 patients with a grade I instability treated with debridement alone. Group C consisted of 40 patients with a grade II or III instability treated with thermal shrinkage and pinning for 6 weeks. Group D consisted of 40 patients with a grade II or III instability treated with debridement and pinning for 6 weeks. At an average of 24-month follow-up, patients treated with thermal shrinkage with and without pinning had superior Modified Mayo scores and less pain as compared with the debridement groups.

Lunotriquetral Ligament Injuries

INDICATIONS

LTIL ligament tears often coexist with a TFCC tear and an ulnar positive variance. An LTIL debridement may be combined as necessary with TFCC debridement and a wafer resection or an open ulnar shortening osteotomy.

CONTRAINDICATIONS

Patients with static carpal instability may be staged arthroscopically, but they will usually require an open procedure for definitive treatment.

SURGICAL TREATMENT

The 4-/,5 portal is the usual working portal, but superior views of the LTIL can be obtained through the 6R and 6U portals. Palmar tears of the LTIL are best seen through the VU portal (Fig. 18-10A and B).[5] They can also be seen obliquely through the 6U portal. Grade I tears are debrided. Grade II tears are treated with arthroscopic reduction, thermal shrinkage ± K-wire fixation for 8 weeks. Acute grade III tears are treated similar to grade II injuries, but consider open treatment for injuries >6 months old. Grade IV acute tears may be pinned in selected circumstances, but chronic injuries are usually beyond arthroscopic management.

OUTCOMES

If there is no instability, debridement alone can be successful. Ruch and Poehling reported the relief of mechanical symptoms in 13/14 treated for membranous flap tears of the LTIL with no progression of instability at 34 months.[50] In their study of 43 patients, Weiss et al noted symptom improvement at 27 months with no evidence of a carpal instability pattern in 100% of patients with a partial LTIL tear versus 78% with a complete tear.[51]

ARTHROSCOPIC DORSAL RADIOCARPAL LIGAMENT REPAIR

In most series, the DRCL is overlooked during the standard arthroscopic since it is difficult to visualize through the standard dorsal portals. The DRCL is best viewed through the VR portal due to the straight line of sight.[52]

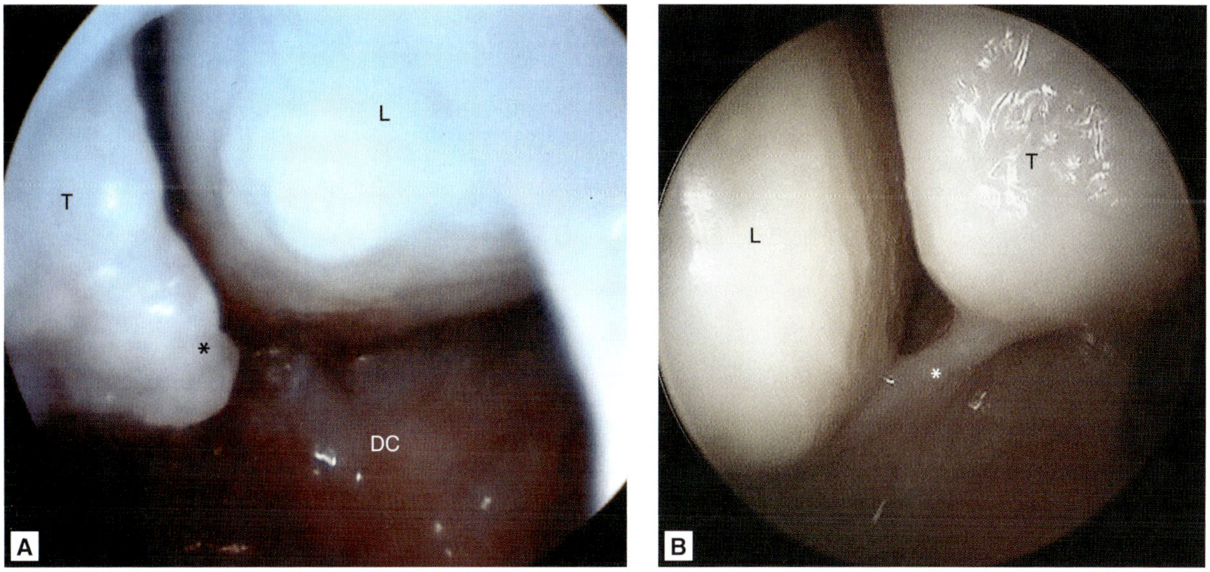

FIGURE 18-10 **A.** Palmar tear of the lunotriquetral ligament as seen from the VU portal using a dry technique. The ligament (*) is still attached to the triquetrum. DC, dorsal capsule; L, lunate. **B.** Dorsal tear of the lunotriquetral ligament as seen from the 6U portal using a dry technique. The membranous portion of the ligament (*) is still intact. L, lunate; T, triquetrum.

Indications

Isolated DRCL tears respond favorably to repair. Repairs may also be considered in cases where the associated interosseous ligament tear or TFCC tear can be treated arthroscopically.

Contraindications

If any associated interosseous ligament tear or carpal instability requires open repair, the dorsal capsulotomy renders any separate DRCL repair unfeasible.

Surgical Technique

A VR portal is established as described. The DRCL is visualized just ulnar to the 3-/4 portal, underneath the lunate. Fluid irrigation and use of the hook probe will reveal the torn edge of the ligament. It can also be seen obliquely from the 6R portal (Fig. 18-11A and B). The torn edge may appear rounded in long-standing cases, which should not be confused with a redundant dorsal capsule. A 2-0 absorbable suture is passed through a curved spinal needle that is introduced through the 4-/,5 portal. The end of the suture is retrieved with a grasper in the 3-/,4 portal. After both ends of the suture are

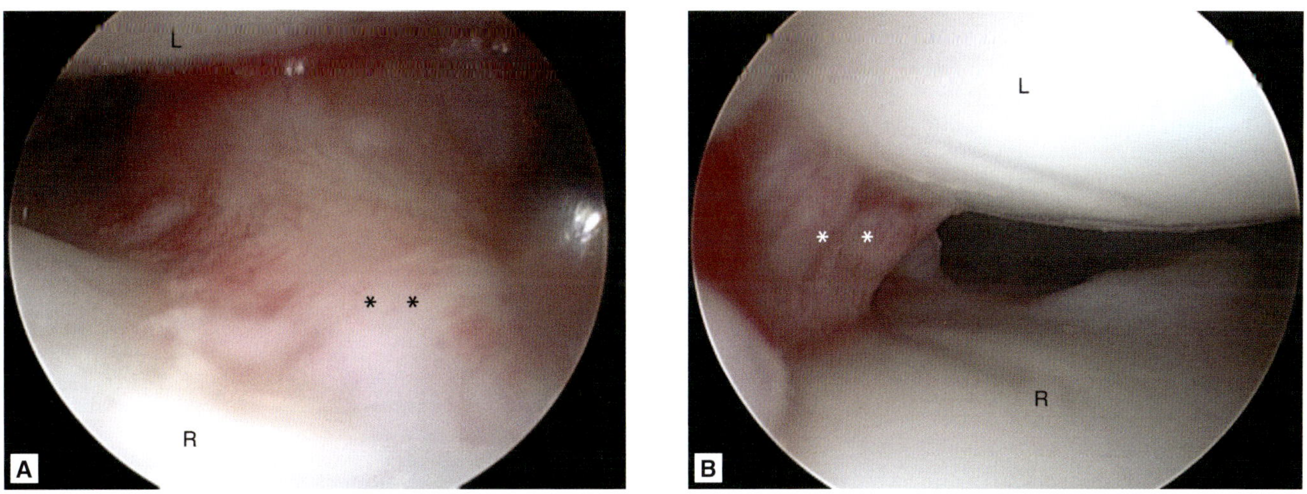

FIGURE 18-11 **A.** View from the VR portal using a dry technique demonstrating the torn edge of the DRCL (*) protruding into the joint space. L, lunate; R, radius. **B.** View from the 6R portal using a dry technique that provides oblique views of the torn DRCL (*). L, lunate; R, radius.

withdrawn, dorsal traction can be seen to pull the torn edge of the DRCL up against the dorsal. One suture is usually sufficient. A curved hemostat is used to pull either end of the suture underneath the extensor tendons, and the knot is tied either at the 3/-,4 or 4/-,5 portal after the wrist traction has been released (Fig. 18-12A-C). Following the repair, the patient is placed in a below-elbow cast with the forearm in neutral rotation for 4 weeks followed by wrist mobilization.

Outcomes

In my own series from 1998 to 2006, 64 patients underwent diagnostic wrist arthroscopy for chronic wrist pain or carpal instability.[53] DRCL tears were found at the time of arthroscopy in 35 patients or 55%. None of these tears could be identified preoperatively, by either examination or imaging studies. In 5 of the patients, the DRCL tear was the first manifestation of the carpal instability and was the sole cause of the wrist pain. Fourteen patients in this series had an SLIL instability and/or tear: 7/14 also had a DRCL tear. Seven patients had an LTIL instability and/or tear: 2/7 also had a DRCL tear. A DRCL tear was found in 1 of 2 patients with a capitohamate ligament tear. There were 9 patients with both a DRCL tear and a TFCC tear. Two or more lesions were present in 23 patients; DRCL tears were present in 12/23 patients. At an average follow-up of 15.8 months, all 5 patients with an isolated DRCL tear had an excellent result with no or mild pain following an arthroscopic repair. When there were other intercarpal derangements, the results were quite mixed and largely dependent on the treatment of the associated pathology.

MIDCARPAL INSTABILITY

There are no arthroscopic findings that are diagnostic of midcarpal instability (MCI). Laxity of the LTIL may be seen, although this is not invariable. Midcarpal arthroscopy may reveal laxity of the triquetrohamate-capitate ligament (THCL), but this is difficult to gauge. Nonsurgical treatment consists of activity modification, NSAIDs, and splinting. Various pisiform support splints have been described. Definitive treatment of this condition ultimately requires surgical treatment. Lichtman et al have performed an open dorsal capsular reefing in milder cases.[54] Many authors recommend a midcarpal arthrodesis as the definitive long-term solution for more severe cases.[55] Arthroscopic thermal shrinkage has enjoyed some success for milder cases.[56]

Indications

Arthroscopy is indicated in MCI to rule out associated intercarpal ligament pathology and to inspect the midcarpal joint to assess for chondral damage. Milder forms of MCI can be treated with a thermal capsulorraphy.

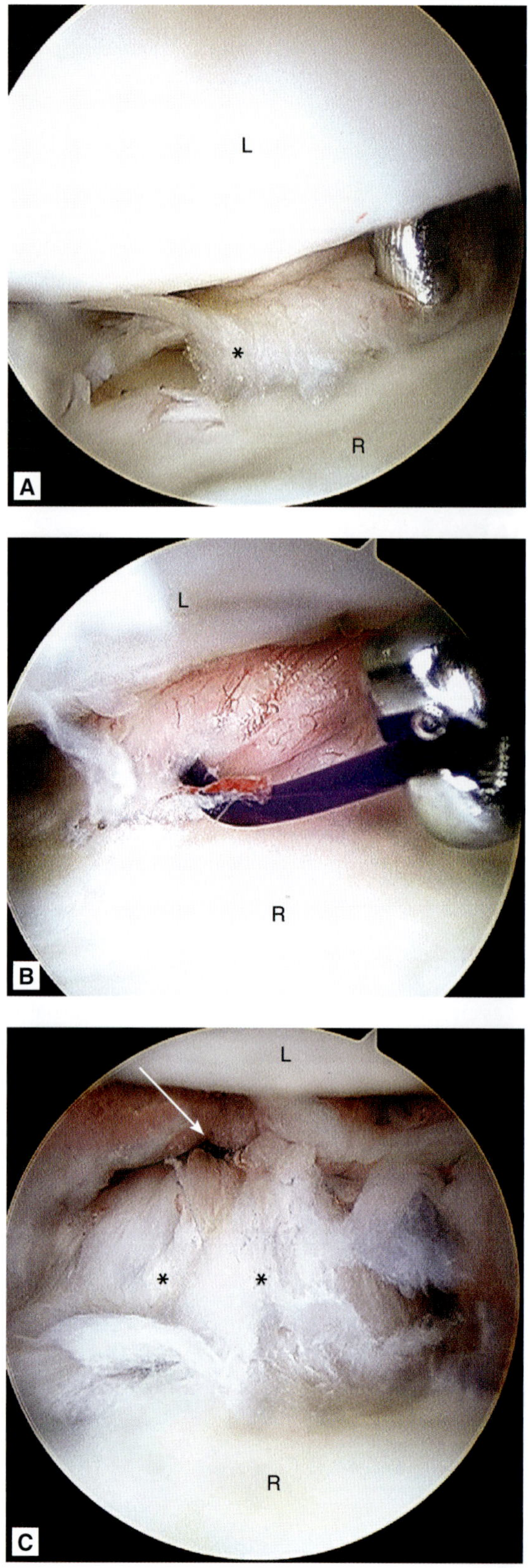

FIGURE 18-12 Dorsal radiocarpal ligament repair. **A.** View from the VR portal demonstrating the torn edge of the DRCL (*) protruding into the joint space. L, lunate; R, radius. **B.** The suture is entering from the 4-,/5 portal and being retrieved by a grasper in the 3-/,4 portal. **C.** Note how the suture (arrow) pulls the DRCL (*) up against the dorsal capsule.

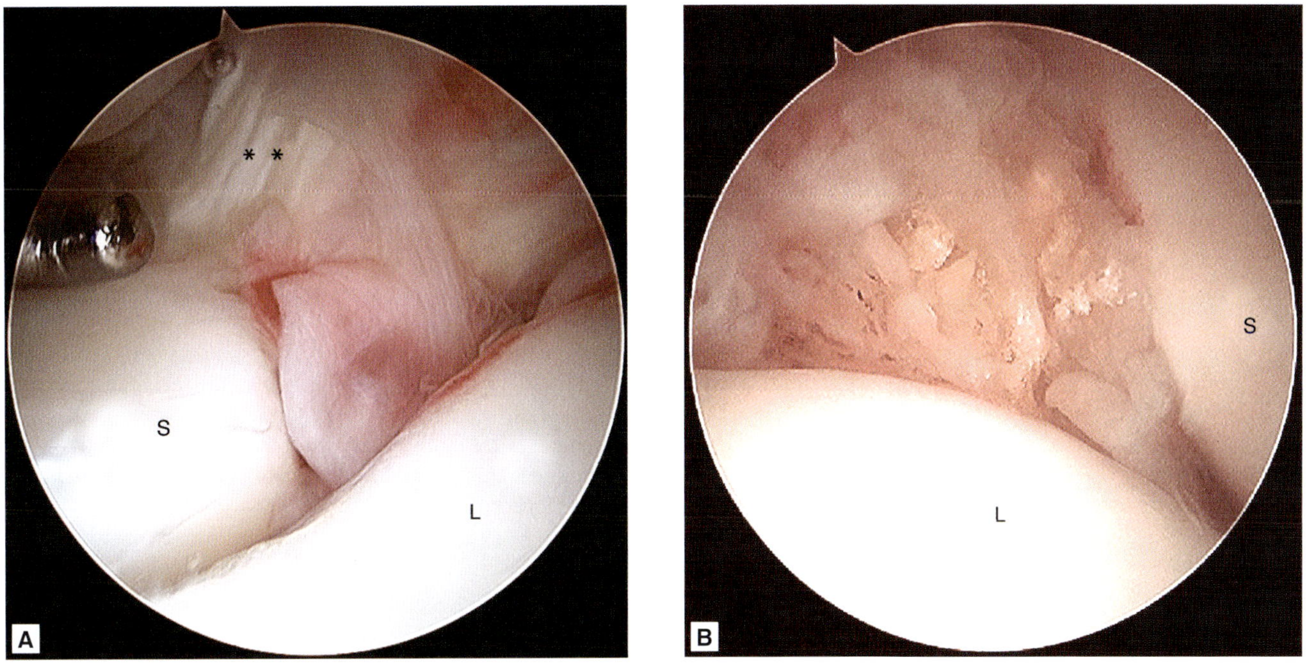

FIGURE 18-13 Arcuate limb shrinkage. **A.** View from the MCU portal demonstrating the radial limb (*) of the arcuate ligament. L, lunate; S, scaphoid. **B.** Following thermal shrinkage. L, lunate; S, scaphoid.

Contraindications

A static VISI, severe cases, and combined palmar and dorsal MCI are not amenable to arthroscopic treatment. Extrinsic MCI due to a dorsally malunited distal radius fracture is treated with a distal radius osteotomy.

Surgical Technique of Arthroscopic Capsular Shrinkage

The standard dorsal portals including 3-/,4 and 4-/,5, 6R, MCR, and MCU portals are used. A thermal probe is applied to the LRL and SRL and dorsal capsule using a stripe technique, leaving sections of untouched ligament in between. The thermal probe is introduced through the MCR and applied to the radial limb (RSC), and ulnar limb (ulnocapitate, ulnotriquetral, and triquetrocapitate) of the arcuate ligament (Fig. 18-13A and B). A VR portal is established and the thermal probe is applied to the DRCL. The wrist is immobilized for 6 weeks.

Outcomes

There is a paucity of literature on the use of arthroscopy for MCI. Culp and coworkers reported their experience of 5 patients who underwent an arthroscopic capsular shrinkage.[56] The average age was 33 (29-57) years. Follow-up averaged 9 months (3-18). The midcarpal clunk resolved in 6 of the 8 patients with pain resolution. Range of motion decreased 20% in the flexion/extension plane, while grip strengths increased by an average of 15%. Mason and Hargreaves recently reported the results of a prospective study of 13 patients (15 wrists) with painful wrist clunking due to palmar MCI who underwent arthroscopic thermal capsulorrhaphy after at least 6 months of failed conservative treatment.[57] The mean duration of symptoms was 5 years (8 months to 20 years). A thermal probe was applied to the arcuate ligament and the accessible parts of the dorsal capsule in both the radiocarpal and midcarpal joints. Postoperatively the patients' wrists were splinted for 6 weeks. At a mean follow-up of 42 months (14-67), complete resolution of the symptoms occurred in 4 patients and almost complete in the remaining 11 patients. The mean DASH score improved from 34 (13-67, SD 16) preoperatively to 12 (0-48, SD 14) at the final follow-up. The ulnar shift test was negative in 12/14 wrists that were available for examination. Wrist movement was reduced by a mean of 16° in flexion and 10° in extension in 9 wrists as compared with the opposite side, but there was no reduction in grip strengths.

TRIANGULAR FIBROCARTILAGE TEARS

Relevant Anatomy and Biomechanics

The TFCC consists of the articular disc, the meniscus homologue, the palmar radioulnar ligament (PRUL) and DRUL, the ECUS, the ulnar capsule, and the ULL and ULT.[58]

The PRUL and DRUL contain a superficial and a deep portion that are conjoined at the radius attachment. The superficial portion surrounds the articular disc but has no clear definable insertion into the ulnar styloid. The fibers of the deep portion of the DRUL and the PRUL interdigitate to form a conjoined tendon as they converge toward their insertion into the fovea at the base of the ulnar styloid along with the ulnocapitate ligament. Although Kauer noted that Henle and Fick originally designated the ligamentum subcruentum as a vascularized fissure between the ulnar styloid and the deep foveal fibers,[59] Kleinman has suggested that this term now refers to the deep fibers themselves.[60] The deep foveal fibers have a greater effect on rotational stability than the superficial fibers and may be a cause of DRUJ instability if detached.[61] With an intact foveal ligament attachment, patients still may suffer from a peripheral TFCC tear but they may not experience the same instability as those with a total avulsion of the ulnar ligament attachments, which can be seen with an avulsion fracture of the entire ulnar styloid.[62] When examined from a coronal perspective, the ulnar styloid lies relatively dorsal on the end of the ulnar head. The DRUL drapes over the dorsal aspect of the ulnar head as it converges toward the fovea. These factors limit the field of view and make it difficult to insert anything larger than a 1.9-mm scope through a dorsal DRUJ portal. There is more room on the VU aspect of the DRUJ for insertion of an arthroscope with relatively unimpeded views of the proximal articular disc and the foveal attachments. The dorsal DRUJ portals remain useful, however, for outflow and for instrumentation.

Mechanism and Classification

TFCC injuries may occur when the wrist is axially loaded in extension with carpal pronation, which occurs with a fall onto an outstretched hand or from a forceful rotational injury or a distraction force.[61] Lindau et al found that TFCC tears occurred in 39/51 displaced distal radius fractures and that DRUJ instability was common at the 1-year follow-up.[63] Palmer classified traumatic TFCC tears into 4 categories.[64] A type 1A lesion represents an isolated tear in the central portion of the articular disc. Type 2B lesions represent a peripheral TFCC tear, and it may be associated with DRUJ instability. Type 1C lesions represent a disruption of the TFCC from the volar ulnocarpal extrinsic ligaments and may result in a supination deformity of the carpus on the ulna. Type 1D lesions represent avulsions of the TFCC from its radial attachment on the sigmoid notch and they are often seen with distal radial fractures.

Diagnosis and Nonoperative Treatment

Patients typically present with ulnar-sided wrist pain and sometimes clicking, which is exacerbated by ulnar deviation and by forceful forearm rotation. Tay et al noted that tenderness over the fovea has a sensitivity of 95% and specificity of 86% in detecting foveal disruptions and/or split tears of the ULT.[65] Patients may have a positive TFCC compression test, which consists of pain with axial loading and ulnar deviation. DRUJ stability should be tested with the forearm in pronation and supination, and the ulnar head should be checked for a positive piano key sign.[66] An associated LTIL ligament tear may demonstrate localized tenderness and a positive LT shear test. ECU subluxation should be ruled out. Most acute tears heal or become asymptomatic with immobilization for 4 to 6 weeks. Cortisone injections may be of use in subacute cases.

All patients should have AP and lateral views, including a pronated grip view to determine the ulnar variance.[67] Double and triple row arthrography had been the standard for years, especially with digital subtraction, but it is no longer in vogue having been supplanted by 1.5T and 3.0T MRI. MR arthrography does not significantly improve the ability to evaluate the central disk of the TFCC with reported sensitivities of 74% and specificity of 80%. CT arthrography is highly sensitive for detecting central TFCC tears but is not accurate for peripheral tears.[68] Arthroscopy, however, remains the gold standard in both the diagnosis and treatment of TFCC tears.

Indications

Arthroscopy is indicated in patients who have failed 3 months of nonoperative treatment unless there is associated DRUJ instability, which should be addressed immediately.[13] Repairable peripheral tears of the TFCC are either type 1B lesions or type 1C lesions. Symptomatic radial TFCC tears with a stable DRUJ may be treated with arthroscopic debridement alone, whereas those that are associated with DRUJ instability are repaired. Type 1A lesions are debrided since they are in an avascular zone and are not amenable to suture repair.

Contraindications

Gross DRUJ instability, an arthritic radiocarpal joint, and ulnocarpal abutment preclude repair. TFCC tears that cannot be adequately reapproximated or reduced should undergo debridement to a smooth rim.

Surgical Treatment—Traumatic TFCC Lesions

TYPE 1B LESIONS

The arthroscope is placed in the 3-/,4 portal and either the 4-/,5 or 6R portal is used for instrumentation. I also use a VU portal to facilitate triangulation of the instruments and to allow better visualization of the dorsal ulnar corner of the TFCC. Any synovitis obscuring the view is debrided. The site of the lesion is then defined to differentiate between a radial-sided tear, central tear, and a peripheral tear. If the ulnar head

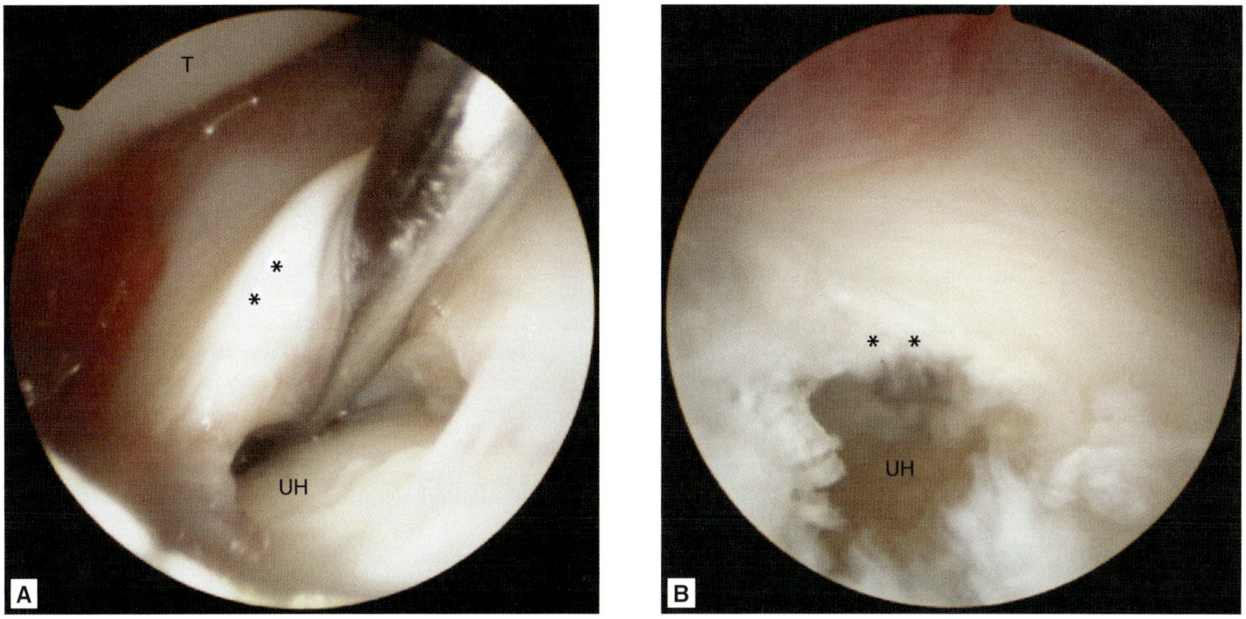

FIGURE 18-14 Central TFCC tear. **A.** A central TFCC tear is seen from the 4-/5 portal after debridement back to a stable rim (*) with exposure of the ulnar head (UH). **B.** A central TFCC tear is seen from the VU portal after debridement back to a stable rim (*) following a wafer resection of the ulnar head (UH).

is visible, then there is a central tear that is debrided back to a stable rim (Fig. 18-14A and B). The ulnar head is usually still covered with a peripheral tear. If no tear is seen but there is a loss of TFCC tension, a positive hook test and a foveal detachment may be present (see below). This diagnosis is made through either a small capsulotomy or an inspection of the deep insertion through the volar DRUJ portal. If present, a direct open or all arthroscopic foveal reattachment is necessary.

Once a peripheral lesion is identified, it is debrided to provide a stimulus for fibrin clot formation at the repair site. An outside-in technique described by Trumble et al uses either vertical or horizontal mattress sutures.[69] A 22-gauge needle is placed into the wrist joint at the level of the tear. A 1- to 2-cm longitudinal dorsoulnar incision is then made centered over the needle and carried down to the wrist capsule, avoiding injury to the DCBUN. An 18-gauge needle is passed just inferior (for horizontal tears) or radial (for vertical tears) to the torn edge of the TFCC. A 2-0 PDS suture (Ethicon, Somerville, New Jersey) is then threaded into the 18-gauge needle and retrieved with arthroscopic grasping forceps or a wire suture lasso through a separate puncture wound. The tissue bridge between the just inserted suture grasper and the 18-gauge needle is the area over which the repair will be tied down. Two or 3 sutures are passed and tied with the traction released (Fig. 18-15A-C). The patient is placed in an above-elbow splint with the wrist in neutral for 4 weeks, followed by a below-elbow splint for an additional 2 weeks. After 6 weeks, passive range of motion exercises and gentle strengthening are instituted with a return to full activities after approximately 10 to 12 weeks.

TYPE 1C LESIONS

The type 1C tear is a rare lesion and consists of a rupture along the volar attachment of the TFCC or tears from the ULL and ULT ligaments. More proximal split tears may be amenable to arthroscopic repair if the ligamentous injury is vertically oriented, but distal transverse tears or avulsion of the ULT ligament off the triquetrum require open treatment. If the lesion is repairable, Culp et al describe making a 1-cm incision volar to the ECU tendon in the area of the triquetral snuffbox.[13] Needles are passed through the capsule in the area of the defect in the ulnar extrinsic ligaments. The looped sutures of 2-0 PDS are then brought out and tied over the capsule. Attenuation of the ULL and ULT may require a tenodesis procedure as described by Moskal et al.[70] Tay et al described an arthroscopic repair of longitudinal split tears of the ULT, which were not recognized in the Palmar classification.[65]

TYPE 1D LESIONS

The scope is placed in the 4-/,5 portal or the VU portal. The radial-sided tear is debrided back to stable edges, and then a curette or burr is used to roughen the sigmoid notch. An arthroscopic cannula is inserted through the 6U portal. Under direct vision a 2.5-mm drill bit is advanced through the cannula and into the sigmoid notch, angling toward the radial metaphysis. Two separate drill holes are made. A double-armed meniscal repair needle with a 2-0 absorbable suture is then threaded through the cannula. The first needle is inserted through the radial edge of the TFCC approximately

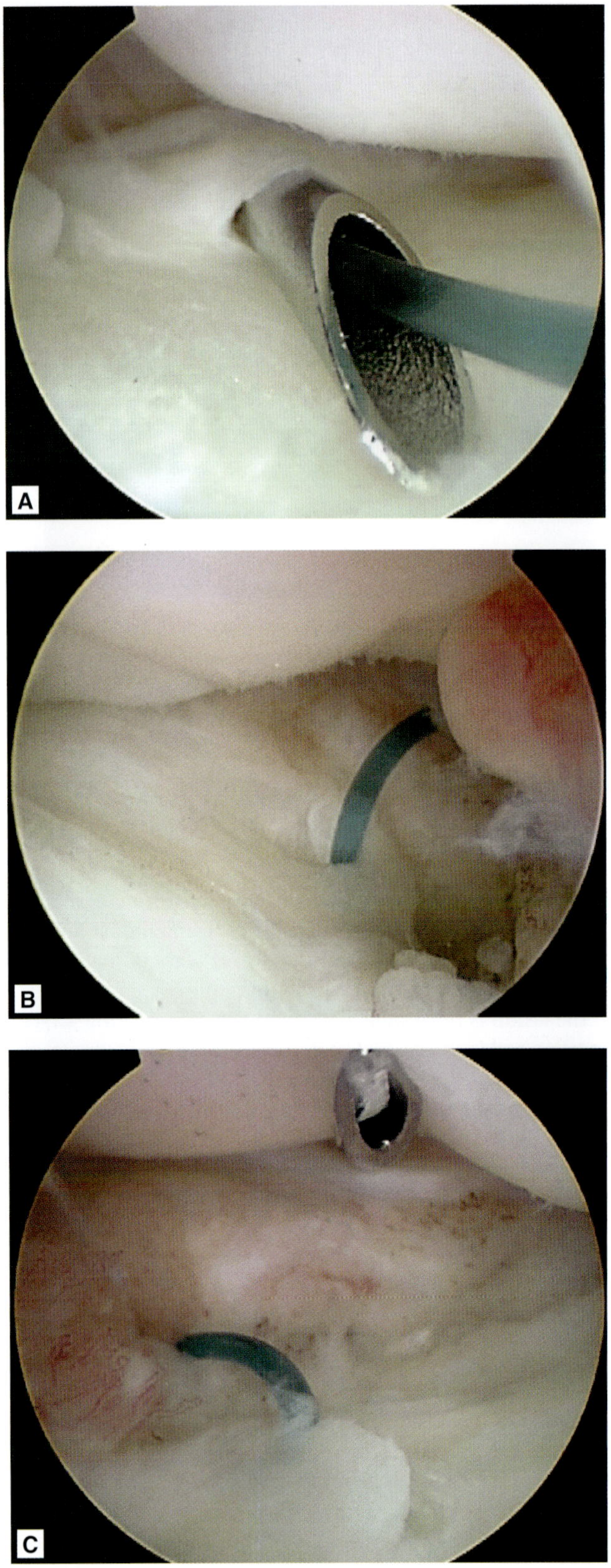

FIGURE 18-15 Dorsoulnar TFCC tear. **A.** View of a 22-gauge needle from the VU portal inserted through the dorsoulnar rim of a TFCC tear. **B.** View of the suture from the 3-/4 portal. **C.** View of the suture from the VU portal.

5 mm from the tear, then advanced through the drill hole, and brought out through the proximal and radial side of the wrist. The second needle is then advanced in a similar fashion through the TFCC edge and the second drill hole. A small skin incision is made between the first and second compartments while protecting the SRN, and the sutures are tied with the traction released. More recently I have used a cannulated drill bit and then inserted both of the sutures through the same drill hole, which are then tied over the lateral periosteum and fixed with a push-lock screw. The repair is inspected arthroscopically and additional sutures are placed as necessary (Fig. 18-16A-C). The patient is immobilized in a Munster splint allowing elbow flexion but restricting forearm rotation for 4 weeks, followed by wrist mobilization.

Debridement

The setup and portals are identical to that of a repair. A motorized shaver or a thermal probe is inserted through the 6R or 6U portal to debride any synovitis and to smooth the edges of the defect. Unstable flaps are resected using small joint suction punches. Once the arthroscopic procedure is complete, the wrist is reexamined to rule out any DRUJ instability. A wrist splint is worn for comfort for 4 weeks followed by gradual strengthening.

Outcomes

Reiter et al reviewed the results of an inside-out arthroscopic repair of Palmer B tears in 46 patients.[71] The average age was 34 years (range, 10-58 years). The average follow-up was 11 months (range, 6-23 months), and the delay to surgery was 9.7 months. Postoperative ROM averaged 128° ± 23° for the extension/flexion arc, 41° ± 11° for the radial/ulnar deviation arc, and 171° ± 19° for the pronation/supination arc of motion. However, no relation could be found between ulna length and clinical outcome. The modified Mayo wrist score was rated excellent in 22% of patients, good in 41%, fair in 27%, and poor in 10%. The average DASH score was 21.70 ± 17.17 (range, 0-58.33). A delay to surgery did not affect clinical outcome.

Estrella et al reviewed 35 patients who underwent an arthroscopic TFCC repair.[72] The average age was 33 years (range, 13-51 years). The average follow-up was 39 months (range, 4-82 months). TFCC tears were classified by the Palmer classification as follows: IB (11), IC (5), and ID (1). The remaining 18 were not classified according to the Palmer classification. Seventy-four percent of patients had reduction in pain after surgery, with improvement in grip strength and daily activities ($P < .05$). The modified Mayo wrist score was excellent in 54%, good in 20%, fair in 12%, and poor in 14%. Nineteen of 28 working patients returned to their original work. Ulnar nerve dorsal branch neuritis occurred in 17%. A "second-look" arthroscopy was performed on 9 patients with healing shown in 7. Additional procedures were performed

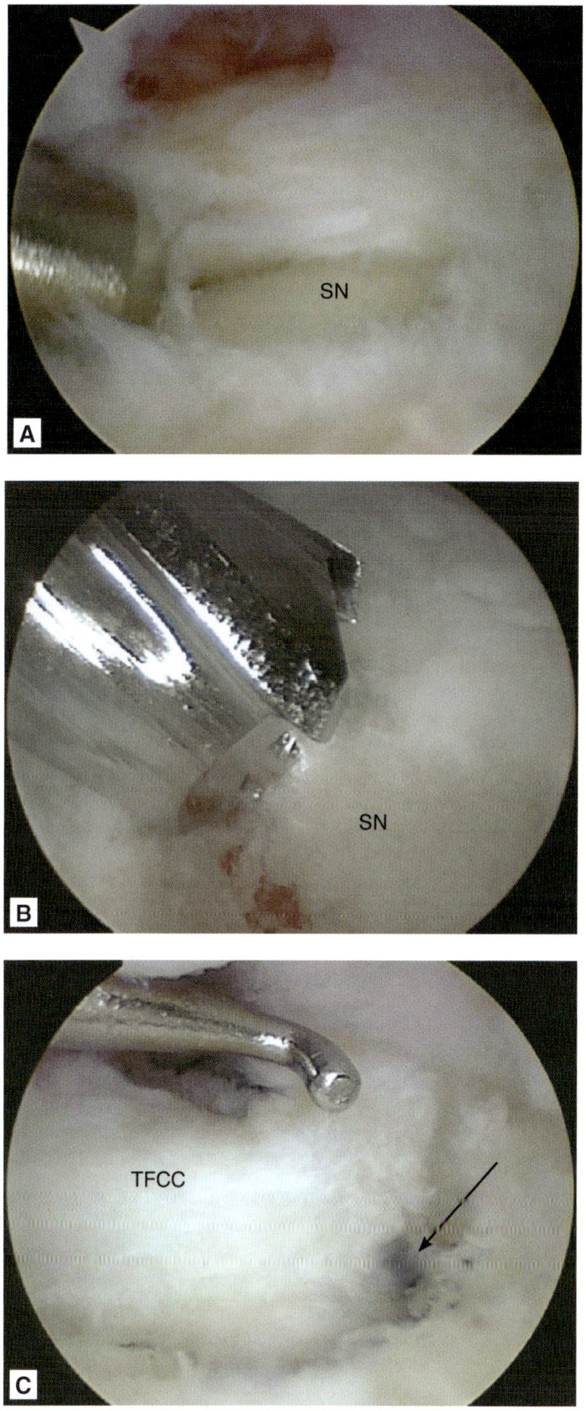

FIGURE 18-16 Radial TFCC tear. **A.** View of a radial TFCC tear from the 4-/5 portal. SN, sigmoid notch. **B.** Burring of the sigmoid notch (SN). **C.** View of the completed repair after tying the suture (arrow).

on 10 patients (29%) to improve the functional outcome. Tatebe et al performed second-look arthroscopies in 32 patients with central TFCC tears treated with an ulnar shortening osteotomy.[73]

All arthroscopic repairs have been previously reported, but clinical series are lacking. Yao and Lee, however, recently described the use of the FasT-Fix suture device (Smith and Nephew Endoscopy, Andover, Massachusetts), which uses 2 absorbable poly-l-lactate (PLLA) blocks that are deposited outside the capsule.[74] There were 12 patients with Palmer 1B tears with a mean age of 42 years (range, 19-69) who underwent repair followed by an above-elbow cast for 6 weeks. At a mean follow-up of 17.5 months (range, 11-27), 11/12 patients demonstrated excellent subjective outcomes with a mean QuickDASH score of 11 (range, 0-43) and a mean PRWE score of 19 (range, 2-53). The wrist motion was normal and the mean supination was 78° (range, 60°-90°), with a mean grip strength of 64% (range, 38%-86%) of the other side. One patient required an ulnar shortening at 1 year for persistent pain.

Osterman presented his results on a retrospective study of 19 patients with Palmer class ID TFCC lesions without DRUJ instability that compared the clinical outcomes after TFCC reattachment versus debridement.[75] He concluded that debridement was equally effective as repair in alleviating wrist pain, improving grip strength, and restoring range of motion.

Nakamura identified 4 different types of radial TFCC tears.[76] Those that involve the central disc only are stable and can be treated with debridement. Those that involve a tear of the volar and/or DRULs can cause DRUJ instability and require repair. If the DRUJ is unstable with noticeable clunking during forearm compression and passive rotation, then the ulnar styloid fracture should undergo internal fixation.

FOVEAL TEARS

The diagnosis of a foveal tear requires a high index of suspicion since it cannot be seen through the standard radiocarpal portals. Ruch et al first described the hook test as an indirect method to test the foveal insertion of the TFCC.[77] If the TFCC can be pulled dorsally and radially with a hook probe, this is indicative of a foveal detachment. This has been recently confirmed by Tay et al[65] and Atzei et al.[78] With these methods, however, one must ultimately perform a DRUJ capsulotomy to directly observe the foveal fibers in order to definitively make the diagnosis. MR imaging can detect these tears in some instances, but this requires not only a high-power magnet with a dedicated wrist coil and a high-resolution grid with a narrow field of view but also an experienced musculoskeletal radiologist who can interpret these findings. Amrami and Felmlee recently described an MRI technique to evaluate DRUJ instability that correlated well with a foveal tear.[79] They found that subluxation of the ulnar head relative to the sigmoid notch of the radius on the MRI, with the wrist in pronation, is a predictor of tears of the foveal attachment of the TFCC. Thirty-four patients with intraoperatively confirmed foveal tears had a mean dorsal ulnar subluxation measurement of 16% ± 4%, whereas the 11 controls had a mean subluxation measurement of 5% ± 4%.

I have been using a VDRU portal to assess the deep foveal fibers directly.[80] A 2-cm longitudinal incision is made centered over the proximal wrist crease along the ulnar edge of the finger flexor. The tendons are retracted to the radial side and the radiocarpal joint space is identified with a 22-gauge needle. The capsular entry point lies 5 to 10 mm proximal to the ulnocarpal joint. A 1.9-mm small joint arthroscope can be used since gaining access to the DRUJ can be difficult, especially in a small wrist, but I have found that a standard 2.7-mm scope provides a better field of view. Initially, the DRUJ space appears quite confined, but over the course of 3 to 5 minutes the fluid irrigation expands the joint space, which improves visibility. A burr or thermal probe can be substituted for the 3-mm hook probe through the dorsal DRUJ portal as necessary. Gross DRUJ instability or chronic foveal tears greater than 6 months in duration are not amenable to a foveal repair and require some type of open ligament reconstruction (Fig. 18-17A-C).

Atzei and Luchetti published a new classification for foveal TFCC repairs as well as an arthroscopically assisted (AA) open reattachment technique.[81] They reviewed 18 patients with a mean age of 34.2 years. All patients had a history of trauma and complained of pain in the ulnar fovea with clinical signs of slight (10 patients) to mild (8 patients) DRUJ instability. At arthroscopy, 14 patients had a combined Palmer type 1B peripheral tear and a foveal disruption (class 2), while 4 patients had an isolated foveal tear (class 3). At a mean follow-up of 18 months, 94% of the patients had an excellent or good result using the modified Mayo wrist score with increased range of motion (90.7%-96% of the contralateral side) and improved grip strength (73%-90% of the contralateral side). The VAS decreased from 8.3 to 1.2 and the average DASH score was 10.5.

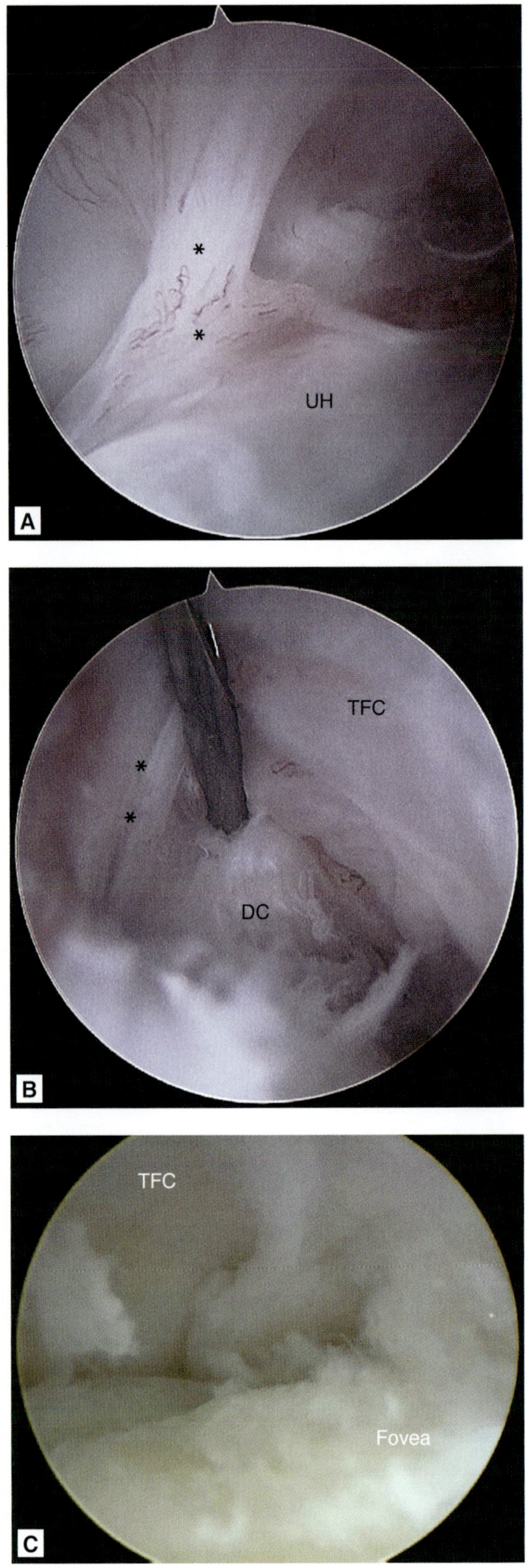

FIGURE 18-17 View from the VDRU portal. **A.** View of the intact deep fibers of the TFCC (*). UH, ulnar head. **B.** The needle is in the dorsal DRUJ and is used to tense the foveal attachment (*). DC, dorsal capsule. **C.** Chronic tear demonstrating an absence of the foveal fibers.

Type 2: Degenerative TFCC Lesions (Ulnocarpal Impaction Syndrome)

Degenerative central tears of the articular disk occur more frequently with advancing age. In a cadaver study of 180 wrist joints, Mikic noted an incidence of 53% over age 60 as compared with 7% in the third decade.[82] Clinical experience has shown, however, that not all of these tears are symptomatic. Most symptomatic degenerative tears of the TFCC are related to chronic overloading of the ulnocarpal joint. Primary ulnar impaction syndrome is related to an increased ulnar variance. Viegas and Ballantyne dissected 100 cadaver wrists and found a 73% incidence of TFCC tears in specimens with an ulnar positive variance versus 17% when there was a negative ulnar variance.[83] Acquired ulnar positive deformities can occur with distal radius fractures that heal with radial shortening, distal radial growth arrest, and Galeazzi fractures. Ulnar impaction may also be dynamic and occur with power grip in the pronated position.[84] This is because of the approximate 1.95 cm of radial shortening that occurs as the radius rotates across the ulna during pronation that leads to a dynamic impingement. Ulnocarpal impaction syndrome consists of the triad of a TFCC tear, a LT ligament tear, and an ulnar positive variance, which is treated by unloading the ulnocarpal joint. This can be accomplished with an arthroscopic wafer resection. In a biomechanical study, excision of 3 mm of subcondylar bone decreased the force transmitted across the ulnar head by 50%; further bone resection did little to decrease this force farther.[85] The goal is to resect sufficient ulna to produce a 2-mm negative ulnar variance.

In Palmer classification, degenerative TFCC tears are subdivided into 5 categories: type 2A, wearing of the TFCC without perforation or chondromalacia; type 2B, wearing of the TFCC with chondromalacia of the lunate or ulna; type 2C, true perforation of the TFCC with lunate chondromalacia; type 2D, TFCC perforation plus lunate and/or ulnar chondromalacia and LTIL tears without carpal instability; type 2E, TFCC perforation with an LTIL tear and ulnocarpal arthritis.

Surgical Treatment—Degenerative TFCC Lesions

TYPES 2A AND 2B

Symptomatic incomplete TFCC tears are treated with debridement. Osterman and Terrill recommend an open ulnar shortening osteotomy with these lesions.[86]

Tomaino and Elfar have reported good results with an arthroscopic TFCC disc excision and wafer resection for the treatment of ulnar abutment before a TFCC tear has occurred.[84]

TYPE 2C

After an initial arthroscopic radiocarpal and midcarpal survey, the scope is placed in the 4-/,5 portal. The 6R and 6U portals are used for instrumentation, although it is useful to assess the completeness of ulnar head resection with the scope in the 6U portal (Fig. 18-18A and B). The VU portal may also be used for viewing while the burr is placed in the 4-/,5 or 6R dorsal portal since this increases the space for triangulation of the instruments. Rapid irrigation is needed to clear the debris. The edges of the TFCC tear are debrided back to stable margins. A 2.9-mm burr is then used in a back-and-forth motion to resect 2 to 3 mm of the ulnar head. The diameter of the burr can be used as a gauge of the amount of bony resection, but this should also be checked fluoroscopically. The arm must be pronated and supinated in order to avoid leaving a shelf of bone. Care must be taken to avoid injury to the deep foveal insertion of the TFCC as well as the sigmoid notch. I have performed a wafer resection through the DRUJ portals.[87] This allows for a more conservative TFCC debridement since the ulnar head resection is performed underneath the TFCC tear and not through it. The DRUJ wafer resection also facilitates preservation of the volar and DRULs as well as the deep foveal attachment. Postoperatively the patient is placed in a below-elbow splint for 4 weeks and started on protected range of motion including pronation and supination.

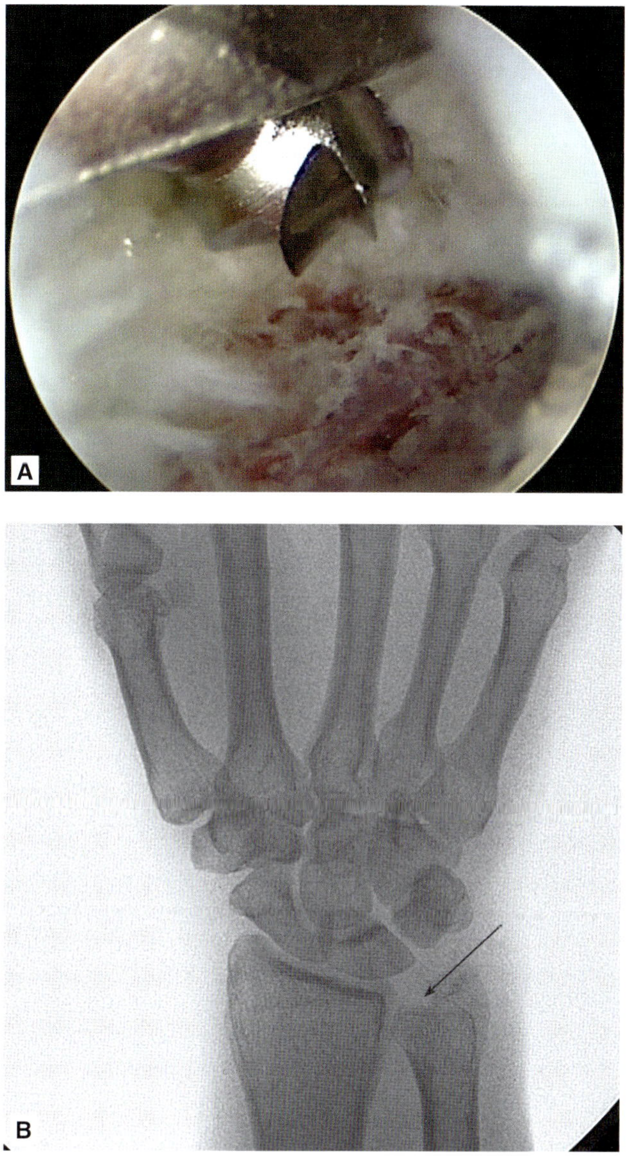

FIGURE 18-18 Arthroscopic wafer resection. **A.** The completeness of the wafer resection of the ulnar head is viewed from the 6U portal with the burr in the 4-/,5 portal. **B.** AP x-ray demonstrating the amount of bony resection (arrow).

TYPES 2D AND 2E

The status of the LT joint determines whether open or arthroscopic methods are indicated. With a Geissler III, LTIL instability, the LT joint can be pinned or it can be stabilized with an arthroscopic plication of the ulnocarpal ligaments.[65] The TFCC tear is debrided and the joint is unloaded with a wafer procedure or open ulnar shortening. A below-elbow cast is applied for 6 to 8 weeks followed by pin removal and mobilization. With a Geissler IV LTIL instability, an open ligament repair or reconstruction with the ECU tendon is often needed.[88]

Outcomes

In a study by Bernstein et al on ulnar impaction syndrome, 11 patients treated with arthroscopic TFCC debridement and arthroscopic wafer resections were compared with 16 patients who were treated with arthroscopic TFCC debridement and an open ulnar shortening.[89] At mean follow-up times of 21 and 15 months, respectively, 9/11 patients showed good to excellent results after arthroscopic treatment as compared with 11/16 following an open ulnar shortening. The authors concluded that a combined arthroscopic TFCC debridement and wafer procedure provides similar pain relief and restoration of function with fewer secondary procedures when compared with an open shortening. Tatebe et al performed 75 ulnar shortening osteotomies for ulnar wrist disorders.[73] There were 32 tears that involved the central, avascular zone of the TFCC disc. At the time of a second-look arthroscopy 16 of these tears were found to be healed, demonstrating that the avascular zone of the TFCC possesses some potential for healing, but factors promoting spontaneous repair of this tissue were not identified.

PROXIMAL POLE OF HAMATE RESECTION

Cartilage erosion of the proximal pole of the hamate is a common site of arthrosis within the wrist. Viegas et al described 2 types of lunate morphology: type I, in which there was no medial facet, was evident in 34.5% of the dissected specimens and type II, in which there was a medial (hamate) facet, was evident in 65.5% of the dissected specimens.[90] Significant cartilage erosion at the proximal pole of the hamate (Fig. 18-19), which was not identifiable by radiographs, was evident at dissection in 44.4% of the type II lunates but 0% of the type I lunates.[91] Harley et al noted a strong association between hamate arthrosis and LTIL tears and coined the acronym "HALT" or hamate arthrosis lunate ligament tear. In a biomechanical study they found that resection of 2.4 mm of the proximal hamate pole completely unloaded the hamatolunate articulation.[92]

Indications

Arthroscopy is indicated in patients with persistent ulnar-sided wrist pain who have failed an adequate trial of conservative treatment. The history and physical findings are not diagnostic of this condition. Occasionally one might find cystic change of the proximal hamate pole on x-ray or marrow edema on an MRI. Most often the condition is diagnosed at the time of arthroscopy and is found in association with other ulnar-sided wrist pathology.

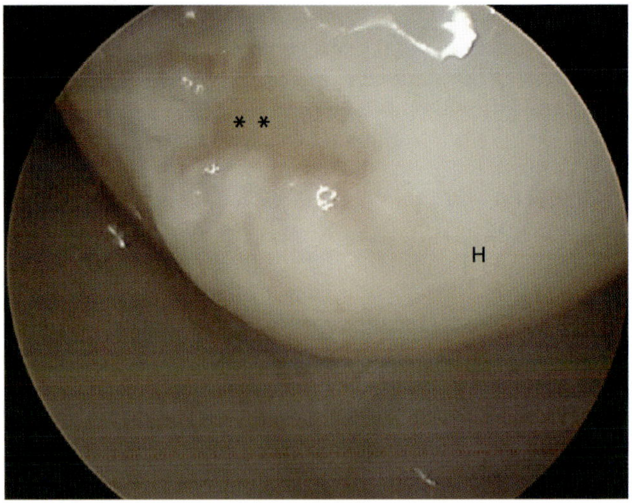

FIGURE 18-19 View of chondromalacia (*) on the proximal pole of the hamate (H).

Contraindications

Inflammatory arthritis or autoimmune disease that involves the wrist is a contraindication. Resection of the proximal hamate in a patient with minimal or focal chondromalacia is controversial. Patients with diffuse degenerative change and/or interosseous ligament tears will have compromised outcomes and may be more suitable for partial fusions or PRC.

Surgical Treatment

With the arthroscope in the MCR portal, a 2.7-mm full radius resector and a 2.9-mm burr are placed alternately into the MCU portal. After the subchondral bone of the proximal hamate has been exposed with the shaver, 2 to 4 mm of the proximal pole of the hamate can be excised using the burr. It is often necessary to view through the MCU portal in order to clearly visualize the full extent of resection, which is confirmed fluoroscopically. Any associated LTIL or TFCC tears are treated concomitantly as described above.

Outcomes

Harley et al examined 21 patients at an average of 4.7 years postoperative.[92] Eighteen patients had good or excellent results. There were 1 fair and 2 poor results using a modified Mayo wrist scale. All 14 patients with isolated HALT pathology had good or excellent results following a hamate resection. Four of 6 patients with TFCC perforations, LTIL tears, and midcarpal synovitis had good or excellent results, whereas only 1 of the 2 patients with LTIL, TFCC, and SLIL tears achieved these outcomes. No patients with preexistent radiocarpal arthritis (scaphoid or lunate facet of distal radius) had good or excellent outcomes.

RADIAL STYLOIDECTOMY

Indications

Radial styloidectomy is an early salvage procedure that may provide short-term relief of mechanical pain from radial styloid impingement. It is an acceptable alternative to more aggressive procedures in patients with low functional demands or those who wish to defer more definitive treatment by means of a PRC or limited wrist fusion. Radial styloid impingement due to a SLAC or scaphoid nonunion advanced collapse (SNAC) wrist is a common indication, although it has been used following an STT fusion.

Contraindications

The main risk following a radial styloidectomy is ulnar translocation of the carpus. Nakamura et al observed significantly increased radial translation with ulnar and palmar carpal displacement after 6- and 10-mm radial styloidectomies and therefore recommended a styloidectomy of no more than 3 to 4 mm.[93] Patients who do not have an intact RSC ligament are at risk for ulnar translocation and are not candidates for this procedure, especially if a PRC is contemplated. Ulnar translocation is a frequent sequela of long-standing rheumatoid disease; hence, any patient with chronic wrist involvement is a poor candidate for this procedure.

Surgical Treatment

This is 1 procedure where the 1-/,2 portal is particularly helpful for debridement (Fig. 18-20A-C). The author also uses the VR portal interchangeably with the 3-/,4 portal in order to gain complete access to the dorsoradial aspect of the styloid. The origins of the RSC and LRL on the distal radius mark the ulnar extent of the resection. The diameter of the burr will give a rough guide as to the amount of bony resection, but this needs to be confirmed fluoroscopically. Enough bone should be resected so that there is no residual impingement between the scaphoid and the radial styloid when the wrist is radially deviated with the traction released. Postoperatively the patient is splinted for the first week followed by progressive wrist motion and strengthening.

PROXIMAL ROW CARPECTOMY

Indications

PRC is another motion-preserving salvage procedure for wrist arthritis that may be performed arthroscopically. It is indicated for a wide range of conditions that culminate in radiocarpal arthrosis including long-standing SL instability, scaphoid nonunion, chronic unreduced lunate/perilunate dislocation, and early Kienböck disease. The potential

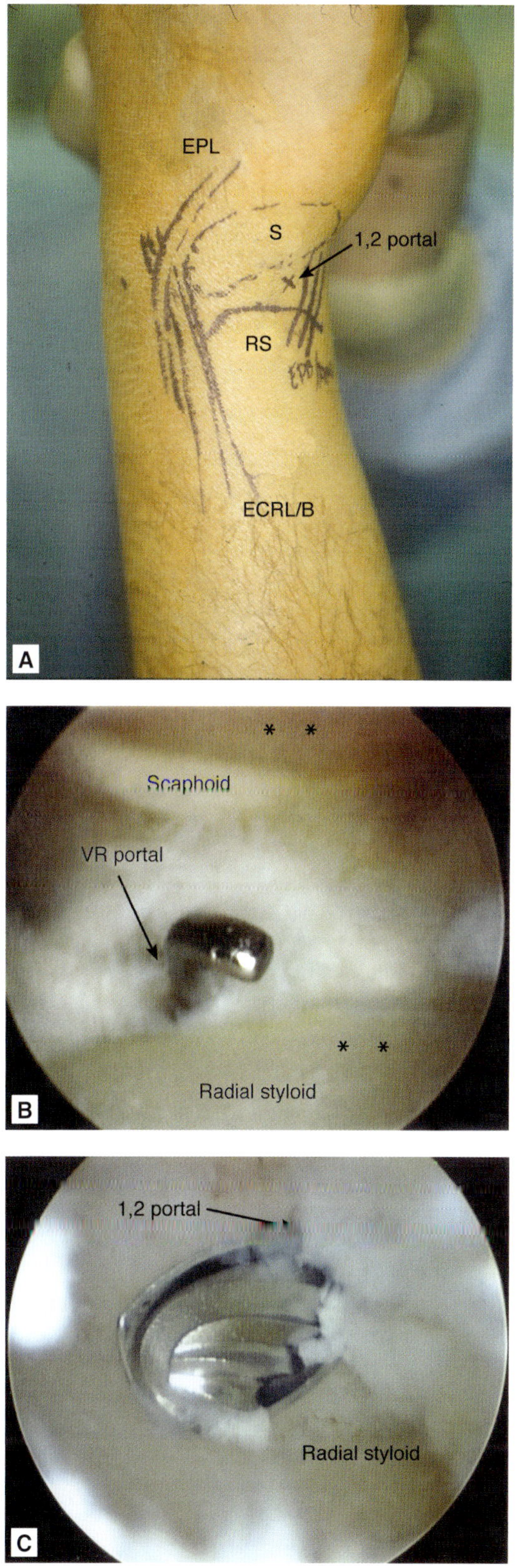

FIGURE 18-20 **A.** Surface landmarks for 1,2 portal. ECRL/B, extensor carpi radialis longus/brevis; RS, radial styloid; S, scaphoid. **B.** View from the 1-/,2 portal, probe is in the VR portal. Note the chondromalacia (*). **C.** Abrader introduced through 1-/,2 portal as seen from the VR portal.

advantages of an all arthroscopic PRC (APRC) include avoiding the need for a capsulotomy with reduced pain and scarring and relative sparing of the capsular ligaments.

Contraindications

A prerequisite for this procedure is a preserved lunate fossa. An unstable carpus that is common in rheumatoid patients or previous radial styloidectomy of more than 4 mm is a relative contraindication due to the risk of ulnar translocation.

Surgical Treatment

An initial arthroscopic survey is performed to assess the cartilage on the lunate fossa and proximal pole of the capitate. Then an arthroscopic ARPC is performed through the midcarpal portals, initially with a 3.0-mm arthroscopic burr introduced through the MCR portal, with the MCU portal used for viewing. The burr is used to decorticate the medial corner of the scaphoid at the midcarpal SL joint, with care being taken not to injure the articular cartilage of the head of the capitate. Once an adequate portion of the corner of the scaphoid is removed, a larger 4.0-mm burr is substituted. The scaphoid is then removed from ulnar to radial and distal to proximal. The STT portal is used to facilitate removal of the distal pole of the scaphoid while viewing in the MCR portal. After scaphoid excision, the arthroscope is placed in the STT or MCR portal. The burr is placed in an enlarged MCR or MCU portal, and then the lunate (distal to proximal) and triquetrum (distal to proximal) are sequentially removed. Confirmation of a complete APRC is made with fluoroscopy. Traction is then released, and arthroscopy and fluoroscopy are used to confirm seating of the head of the capitate in the lunate fossa. If there is residual radiocarpal impingement with radial deviation of the wrist, an arthroscopic radial styloidectomy can be performed, with the burr in the 1/2 portal and the arthroscope in the 3/4 portal. Postoperative motion is started immediately. The wrist is immobilized in a cast for approximately 4 to 5 weeks, followed by protected wrist motion, and then strengthening.

Outcomes

This is an uncommon procedure. Weiss et al reported their results in 16 patients who underwent an APRC.[94] At an average follow-up of 24 months (range, 12-48 months), the mean flexion–extension arc was 94° (range, 50°-130°), the average radial–ulnar deviation arc was 40° (range, 20°-55°), and the average maximum grip strength was 81% of the contralateral side. Five patients reported no pain, 5 had mild pain, and 6 had moderate pain. The authors noted however that the results were comparable but not superior to an open PRC.

DISTAL SCAPHOID RESECTION FOR SCAPHOID NONUNION

Indications

Distal scaphoid resection can be regarded as a temporizing procedure for a chronic scaphoid waist nonunion that is not amenable to internal fixation. It can relieve pain by alleviating the painful mechanical impingement between the hypertrophic distal pole and the radial styloid. It is especially indicated ideal when the cartilage degeneration and osteophyte formation and deformity are confined mainly to the radial styloid. It enables early wrist motion and does not burn any bridges with regards to more definitive salvage procedures.

Contraindications

Advanced degenerative change involving the entire scaphoid fossa or the capitolunate joint is a contraindication to this procedure. An intact SL ligament and RSC ligament are prerequisites to the procedure in order to minimize the risk of a DISI deformity.

Surgical Technique

The patient is positioned supine under general anesthesia with the arm abducted under tourniquet control. The thumb is suspended by finger traps with 10 lb of countertraction. Intraoperative fluoroscopy is employed to assess the adequacy of bone resection and for locating the portals as needed. The arthroscopic scaphoidectomy is performed through the midcarpal joint. With arthroscope introduced in the MCU portal, a 2.0-mm shaver is inserted into the MCR portal and used to debride the nonunion site. The STT-U portal is useful for distal 1/3 nonunions. A 2.9-mm and then a 3.5-mm arthroscopic burr are inserted into the MCR or STT-U portal and used to resect the distal scaphoid fragment starting at the nonunion site and moving toward the distal tubercle until the articular surfaces of the trapezoid and trapezium can be seen (Fig. 18-21A-D). Rapid fluid irrigation and intermittent suction is used to remove the debris. In order to protect the adjacent chondral surfaces, the cancellous bone of the fragment can be resected from the inside while preserving the outer cartilage shell, which can then be removed piecemeal with arthroscopic forceps or a small rongeur. Fluoroscopy is used to monitor the completeness of resection. An arthroscopic radial styloidectomy can be added if residual impingement is noted.

Outcomes

Most of the reports involve an open resection of the distal scaphoid fragment for a chronic scaphoid nonunion. Ruch et al reported good pain relief in 3 patients with a chronic scaphoid nonunion associated with avascular necrosis following an arthroscopic resection of the distal scaphoid

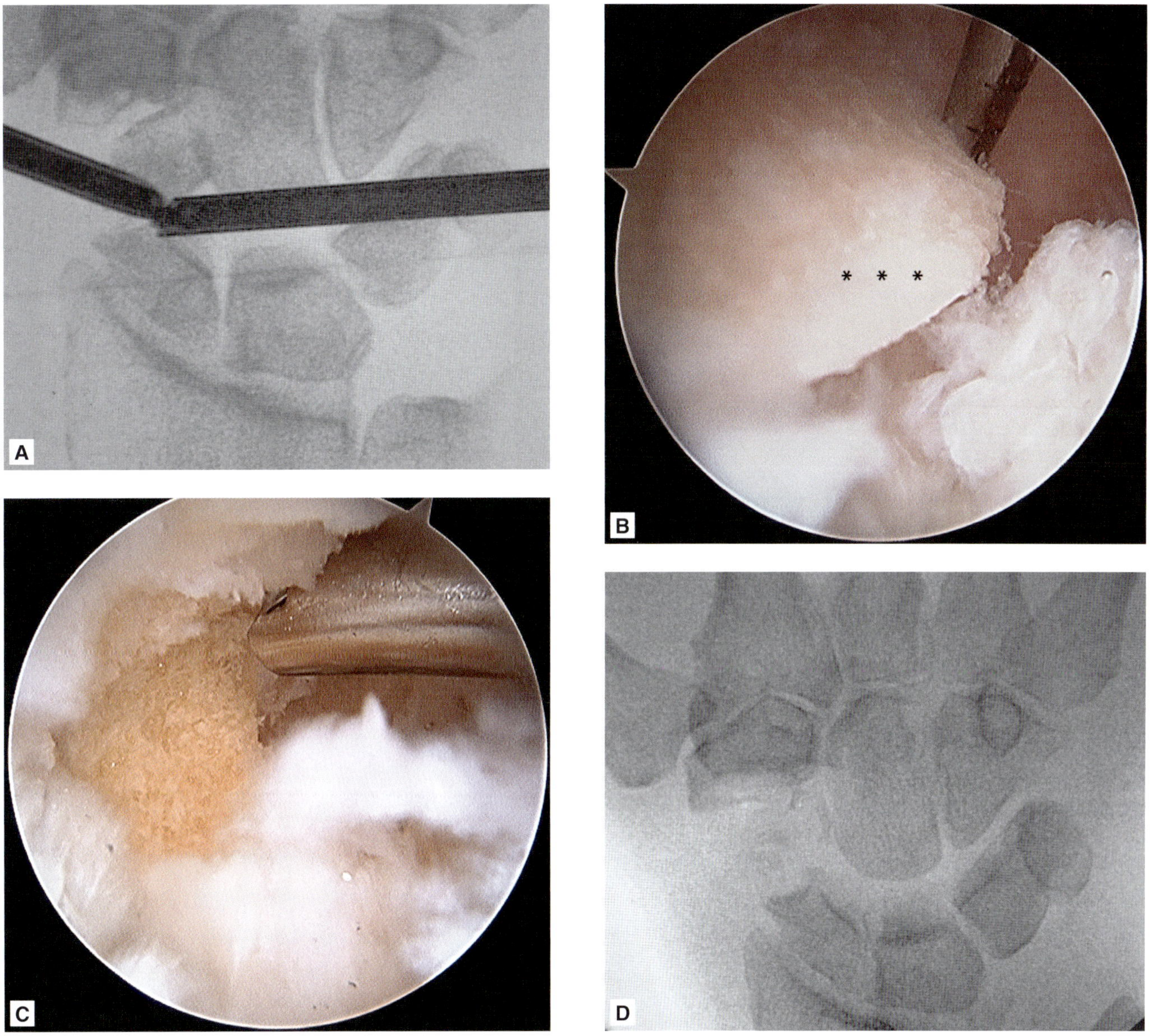

FIGURE 18-21 Arthroscopic distal scaphoid resection. **A.** AP x-ray view showing relative positions of the arthroscope and burr. **B.** View of the unstable distal scaphoid pole (*) from the MCU portal. **C.** View of a partial resection of the distal pole. **D.** AP x-ray view showing the completed resection.

combined with arthroscopic radial styloidectomy.[95] His group then reported the outcomes in 13 patients with persistent scaphoid nonunion after previous unsuccessful surgical treatment.[96] The authors performed an initial arthroscopic survey to assess the degree of cartilage loss and perform a limited debridement of any partial SLIL tears. They then performed an open resection of the distal pole. Eleven patients achieved complete pain relief while 2 patients had mild pain only during strenuous activity. The mean wrist flexion improved by 23° and extension increased by 29°. The postoperative DASH was 25 ± 19 points. There was a significant increase in the radiolunate angle, indicative of a dorsal intercalated segment instability deformity in 6 patients.

ARTHROSCOPIC-ASSISTED FIXATION: DISTAL RADIUS

Indications

More than 2 mm of articular displacement or gap is a typical indication for surgical treatment. Isolated radial styloid fractures and simple 3-part fractures are most suited to this technique. Displaced intra-articular fractures of the distal radius are often associated with unrecognized intra-articular soft tissue injuries; hence, a suspicion of a significant acute SLIL or LTIL tear or DRUJ instability due to a suspected TFCC tear is an additional indication. Traction views will help to sort out the fracture anatomy. It is the author's preference to perform a CT scan along with coronal views to rule out an unrecognized sagittal split as well as to assess the congruency of the sigmoid notch.

Contraindications

Large capsular tears that carry the risk of marked fluid extravasation, active infection, neurovascular compromise, and distorted anatomy are some typical contraindications. Marked metaphyseal comminution, shear fractures, and volar rim fractures require open treatment, although the arthroscope can be inserted to check the adequacy of the joint reduction. Due to the risk of late collapse, adjuvant internal fixation with locking plates is advised in elderly and osteopenic patients since fracture site settling may occur for up to 6 months.[97]

Surgical Treatment

Intraoperative fluoroscopy is used frequently throughout the case, with the C-arm positioned horizontal to the floor. I prefer to use much of the procedure without fluid irrigation using the dry technique of del Piñal et al,[98] which eliminates the worry of fluid extravasation. Intermittent fluid irrigation is used with a 10-cm^3 syringe while the field is kept dry with a suction on the shaver. The working portals include the VR and 6R portals for fracture visualization and the 3-/,4 portal for instrumentation, but all of the portals are used interchangeably.

RADIAL STYLOID FRACTURES

It is easiest to obtain the reduction through ligamentotaxis while the arm is suspended in the traction tower. A Freer elevator may also be placed in the fracture site to facilitate this step. A 1-cm incision is made over the styloid to prevent injury to the SRN, and two 0.62-mm K-wires are inserted for manipulation of the styloid fragment. The fracture site is best assessed by viewing across the wrist with the scope in the 6R portal, in order to gauge the rotation of the styloid. The K-wires are used as joysticks to manipulate the fragment, and then 1 K-wire is driven forward to capture the reduction. One or 2 cannulated screws are used to stabilize the fracture fragment (Fig. 18-22A-C).

THREE- AND 4-PART FRACTURES

Three-part fractures are composed of a radial styloid fragment and a medial or lunate fragment. The radial styloid fracture is reduced and pinned as above. It is then used as a landmark to which the depressed lunate fragment is reduced. An elevator, shoulder arthroscopic hook probe, or large pin is inserted percutaneously to elevate the lunate fragment. Tenaculum forceps with large jaws are used to hold the reduction and to prevent crushing the SRN. The reduction

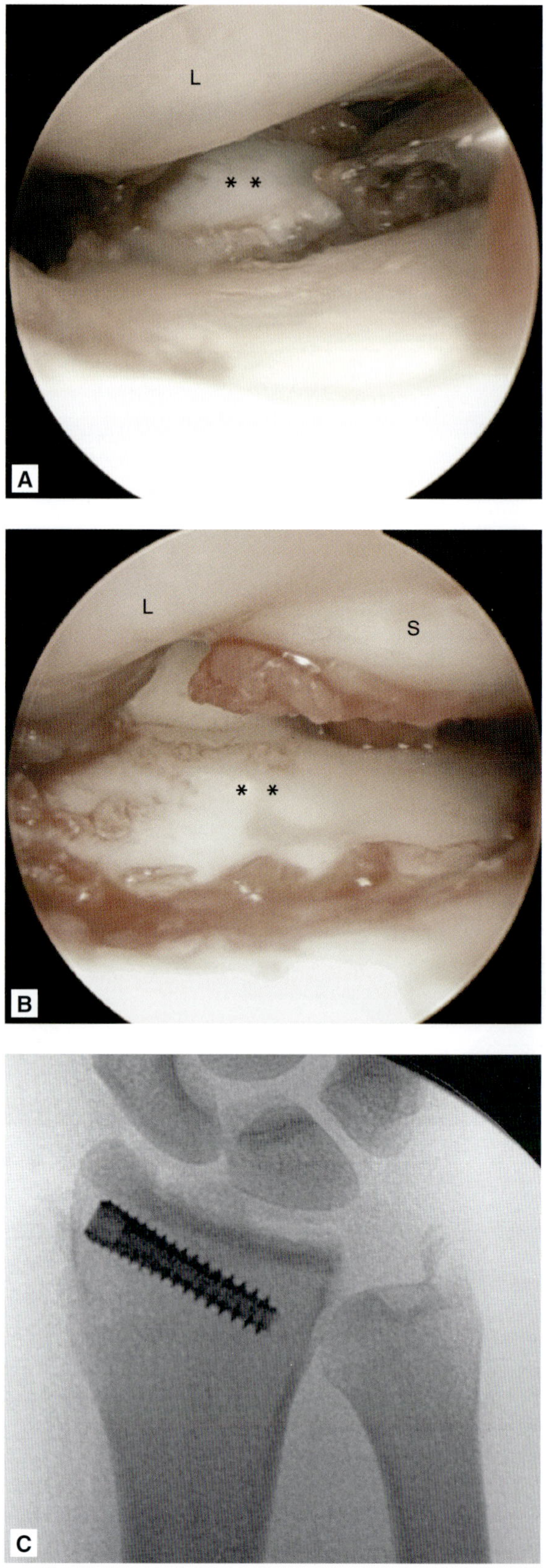

FIGURE 18-22 Arthroscopic-assisted fixation of radial styloid fracture. **A.** View of the radial styloid fracture (*) from the 6R portal, using a dry technique. L, lunate. **B.** Following reduction and screw fixation. L, lunate; S, scaphoid. **C.** AP x-ray view following screw fixation.

is captured with horizontal subchondral K-wires, stopping short of the DRUJ. Mehta et al described a 5-level algorithm for reducing the fracture fragments.[99] This included the "London technique" where the K-wires were advanced through the distal ulna into the subchondral distal radius and withdrawn from the radial aspect so that they do not encroach on the DRUJ. The VR portal aids in the reduction of any dorsal die-punch fragments.

In 4-part fractures, the lunate facet is split into volar and dorsal fragments. The radial styloid fragment is reduced with ligamentotaxis and temporarily held with K-wires. The volar medial fragment must usually be reduced through an open incision since wrist traction rotates this fragment and prevents reduction by closed means. An FCR volar approach or a limited VU incision can be made. The volar medial fragment is reduced under direct observation by pinning it back to the shaft and the radial styloid fragment. A standard locking volar plate or 2.4-mm volar locking plate is provisionally applied and held with K-wires. The reduction is checked through the 6R and VR portals and any fine-tuning of the reduction is performed before the distal locking screws are inserted. A small locking dorsal plate can be applied if necessary or alternatively the distal screws of the volar plate can be used to lag the volar medial and dorsomedial fragments. In this event, 1 or more of the distal screws should be placed in a nonlocking fashion to help compress the fragments.

Outcomes

Doi et al performed a prospective study comparing 34 intra-articular distal radius fractures treated with arthroscopic reduction, pinning (ARIF), and external fixation versus 48 fractures treated with open plate fixation (ORIF) or with pinning ± external fixation.[100] At an average follow-up of 31 months, the ARIF group had significantly better ranges of flexion–extension, radial–ulnar deviation, and grip strength ($P < .05$). Radiographically, the ARIF group had better reduction of volar tilt, ulnar variance, and articular gap reduction. Ruch et al compared the functional and radiologic outcomes of AA percutaneous pinning and external fixation versus fluoroscopically assisted (FA) pinning and external fixation of 30 patients with comminuted intra-articular distal radius fractures. Patients who underwent AA surgery had significantly improved supination compared with those who underwent FA surgery (88° vs 73°). AA reduction also resulted in improved wrist extension (77° vs 69°) and wrist flexion (78° vs 59°).[101] Varitimidis et al performed a randomized prospective study comparing 20 patients with intra-articular fractures of the distal radius who underwent AA and FA reduction and external fixation plus percutaneous pinning versus 20 patients with the same fracture characteristics who underwent FA reduction alone and external fixation plus percutaneous pinning.[102] At 24 months the patients who underwent AA and FA treatment had significantly better supination, extension, and flexion, although the mean DASH scores were similar for both groups.

INTRA-ARTICULAR MALUNIONS

An outside-in osteotomy for an intra-articular malunion is unpredictable since the cleavage plane may not always go through the original articular fracture site. del Piñal et al have described a technique for an arthroscopic inside-out osteotomy for the treatment of malunited intra-articular fractures.[103] This is indicated in any malunion with an intra-articular step-off of 2 mm or more. Posttraumatic radiocarpal osteoarthritis is a contraindication to this procedure, which should be managed with a salvage procedure. del Piñal recommends the use of 15° and 30° angle shoulder periosteal elevators (Arthrex, Naples, Florida), as well as straight and curved osteotomes due to the limited intra-articular working space.

The osteotomes are typically inserted through a dorsal portal to ostetotomize a volar fragment and vice versa. After exsanguination of the arm, a volar approach to the radius is performed with the arm extended on a hand table. In order to control the fracture cleavage plane, an incomplete external osteotomy is performed. Any external callus is removed with a rongeur and then an osteotomy is made starting in the metaphysis and moving distally, but stopping short of the articular surface. No attempt is made to lever the fragments at this point because of the risk of fragmentation. Provisional application of a volar locking plate with K-wires is then performed. The hand is then suspended in traction with 10 to 15 lb of distraction. A 2.7-mm scope is introduced through the 3/,-4 portal with a shaver through the 6R portal for debridement of intra-articular adhesions. A dry technique is used as described above with intermittent irrigation through the scope and suction through the shaver. The portals are enlarged by 0.5 cm, to facilitate passage of the osteotomes and shoulder elevators, which are introduced vertically to prevent injury to the extensor tendons. The VR portal can be established through the volar wrist incision as necessary. Provided there is no major loss of the articular surface, the healed fracture lines are identified, and then gently osteotomized. They are then carefully pried apart until they connect with the extra-articular osteotomy and mobilized. Disimpacted fragments can be elevated by hooking them with a strong shoulder probe and pulling upwards. Any granulation tissue impeding the reduction is resected with small curettes, shaver, or burrs. Retrograde K-wire insertion into the fragments can help with both reduction and provisional fixation. Once the reduction is acceptable, the fragments are stabilized with the locking plate or headless screws as needed (Fig. 18-23A-G).

Outcomes

del Piñal et al reviewed 11 patients following an arthroscopically guided osteotomy of an intra-articular malunion of the distal radius from 1 to 5 months after the injury.[104] The preoperative step-off ranged from 2 to 5 mm (average, 2.5 mm). The original fracture patterns included 1 radial styloid fracture, 1 radiocarpal fracture–dislocation, and 9 comminuted

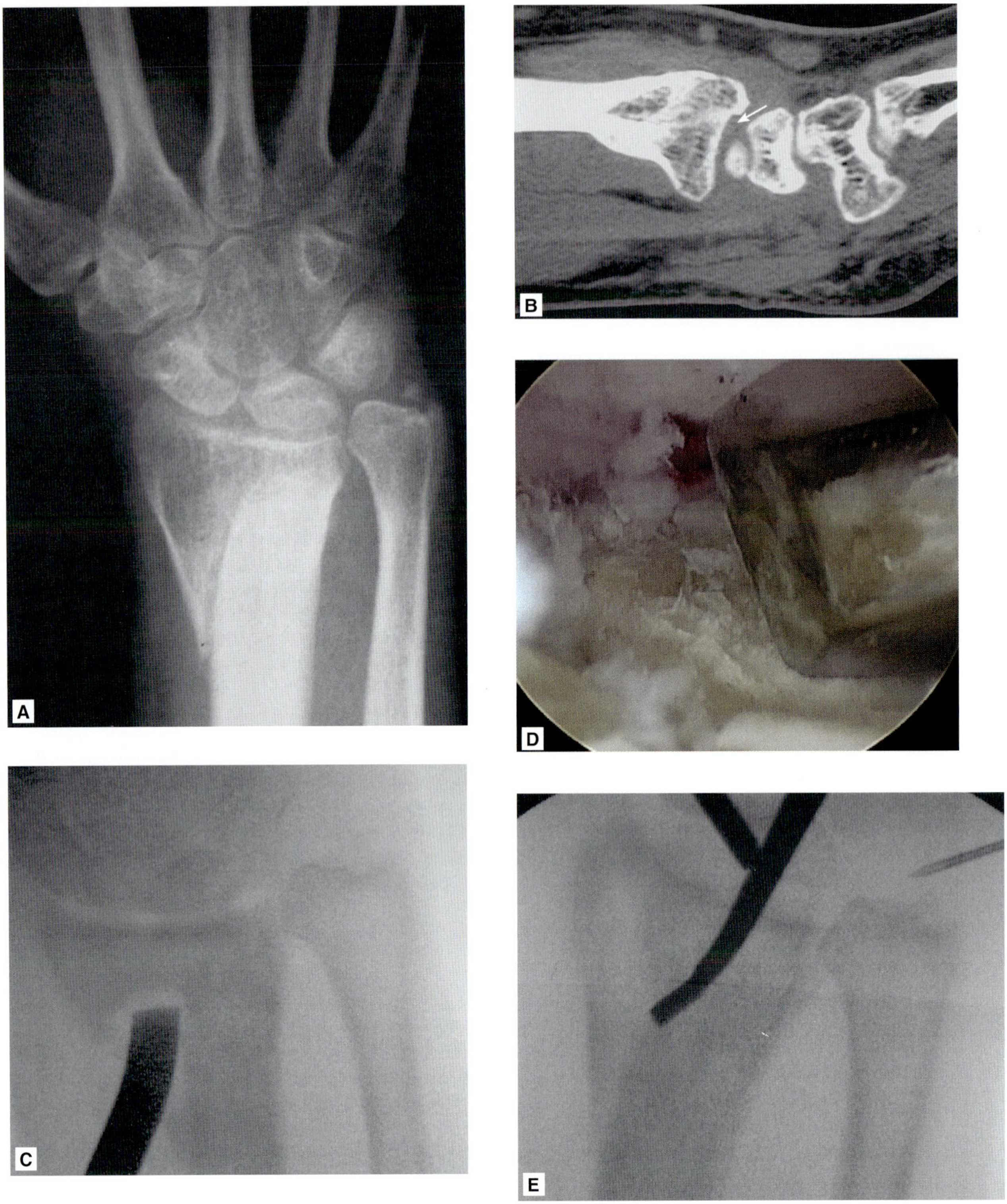

FIGURE 18-23 Arthroscopic-assisted osteotomy of distal radius malunion. **A.** AP x-ray view of a malunited intra-articular fracture. **B.** Lateral CT scan demonstrating a 6-month-old malunited volar Barton fracture with an intra-articular step-off (arrow). **C.** Fluoroscopic view of partially completed osteotomy. Note the ulnar positive variance. **D.** Intra-articular osteotomy viewed from the 6R portal. Osteotome is in the 3-/4 portal. **E.** AP x-ray of the intra-articular osteotomy.

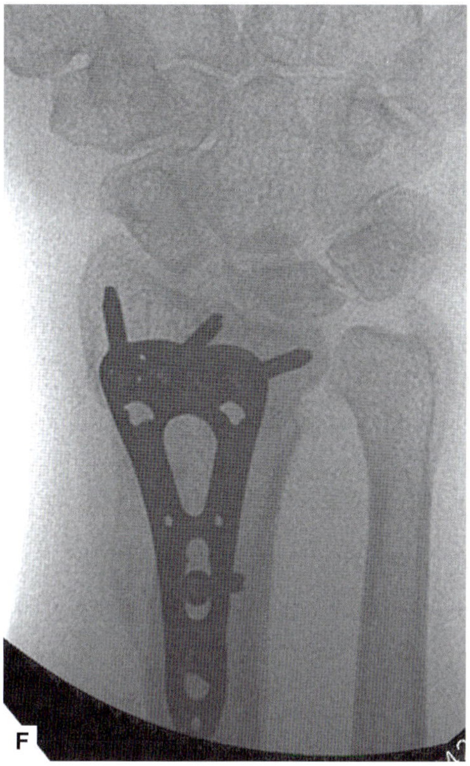

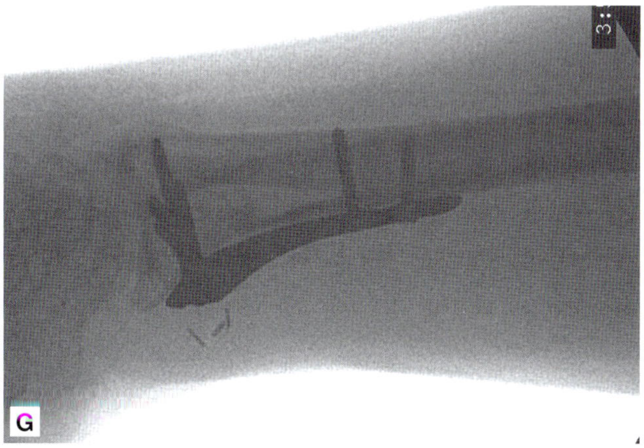

FIGURE 18-23 (*Continued*) **F.** Following plate fixation. Note the ulnar neutral position and restored radial height. **G.** Congruent articular surface (arrow).

intra-articular fractures. In 5 cases an anterior ulnar or radial styloid fragment was repositioned. In the others 2 to 3 fragments were osteotomized. In 1 patient, the articular osteotomy was combined with an ulnar shortening osteotomy. The step-offs were reduced in most cases to 0 mm; however, localized gaps (<2 mm) and cartilage defects were commonly seen intraoperatively because the fragments did not accurately fit. At a follow-up of 12 to 48 months, the average improvement in wrist motion was 44° of flexion/extension and 59° of pronosupination. The grip strength average was 85% of the contralateral side. There were 4 excellent and 7 good results (mean score of 2.8) using the Gartland and Werley score. The modified Green and O'Brien system achieved a mean score of 83, with 3 excellent, 5 good, and 3 fair results. One patient showed radiolunate narrowing on follow-up radiographs. In 1 patient the fragment redisplaced due to poor fixation and 1 patient required hardware removal.

ARTHROSCOPIC-ASSISTED INTERNAL FIXATIO N: SCAPHOID

Most scaphoid screws can be inserted percutaneously or through a mini-open approach. There are some instances, however, where an arthroscopic assist can be useful. It can guide the starting point for guidewire placement in the proximal pole with dorsal insertion. It is a valuable aid to assessing the quality of the reduction, to guard against screw cutout, and to evaluate the rigidity of fixation since seeming good screw purchase may not adequately stabilize a comminuted segment. The fracture position is assessed with an AP, lateral, and oblique x-rays, although a CT scan is helpful in difficult cases. I prefer to obtain an MRI in all scaphoid nonunions preoperatively to rule out AVN. Dorsal screw insertion is recommended for scaphoid fractures of the proximal pole, whereas distal pole fractures are best approached through a volar percutaneous approach. Waist fractures can be stabilized through either approach. Volar implantation often requires eccentric screw placement through the distal pole since one has to ream through the trapezium in order to gain access to the central scaphoid axis, but the screw can still be placed centrally through the waist and proximal pole.[105]

Indications

The indications are synonymous with percutaneous scaphoid screw insertion, which parallel those for an open reduction. This includes any acute displaced proximal pole or waist fracture of the scaphoid with >1 mm of displacement or translation, or any fractures with significant comminution or angulation. Nondisplaced fibrous scaphoid nonunions without evidence of avascular necrosis are also suitable candidates.

Contraindications

Partial or complete avascular necrosis of the scaphoid is a relative contraindication to percutaneous techniques. A small proximal pole fragment does not allow adequate screw purchase. Nonunions with a humpback deformity and secondary DISI require an open volar wedge graft. The presence of significant radiocarpal and/or midcarpal degenerative changes mandates an alternate approach.

Surgical Treatment

DORSAL APPROACH

The patient is positioned supine on the operating room table with the arm abducted on a hand table. Guidewire insertion is accomplished free handed and percutaneously using fluoroscopic control, initially without tourniquet. I prefer antegrade screw insertion for proximal pole and waist fractures. The fluoroscopy unit is positioned over the arm board, parallel to the floor. The ARC traction tower (ARC Medical, Beaverton, Oregon) is ideally suited for this procedure since it has no central pole to obstruct instrumentation and the wrist can be flexed to 45° in traction that allows one to alternate fluoroscopic and arthroscopic assessment without moving the C-arm or extending the wrist and hence avoid the "dance of the K-wires." Alternatively the wrist is flexed 45° over folded towels, which places the scaphoid axis at 90° to the beam and facilitates placing the screw down the central axis. I hand insert 2 K-wires into the midline of the STT joint to act as targeting aids for guidewire insertion. The first guidewire is placed through the ulnar (STT-U) arthroscopy portal that is located in line with the midshaft axis of the index metacarpal, just ulnar to the EPL tendon. A second guidewire is inserted through a radial portal (STT-R) that is radial to the abductor pollicis longus (APL) tendon at the level of the STT joint. The targeting wires should intersect at the midpoint of the STT joint. The ideal starting point for the guidewire is at the most proximal tip of the scaphoid pole immediately adjacent to the insertion of SLIL. I place a third K-wire into the dorsal aspect of the SL interval just ulnar to this point. Alternatively, with the scope in the 3/4 or 4/5 portal, the tip of the guidewire can be directed to the soft spot on the proximal pole bordering the SLIL insertion.

Using a power drill, the guidewire is driven from an ulnar dorsal to a radial volar direction while keeping the wrist flexed. Aiming toward the intersection point of the dorsal STT K-wire on an AP fluoroscopic view guides the medial/lateral alignment of the guidewire. Pointing toward the intersection point of the radial STT K-wire on the semipronated fluoroscopic view guides the dorsal/volar alignment. The guidewire is then advanced distally through the trapezium and out through the skin. The wrist can be extended if necessary once the trailing end clears the radiocarpal joint. If the fracture is displaced, the guidewire is withdrawn distally until it lies solely within the distal fragment. Percutaneous 0.62-mm K-wires can then be inserted into the proximal and distal fragments and used as joysticks to align the scaphoid as described by Slade. The alignment of the concave scaphoid surface on the AP x-ray view can be used as a reference for fracture reduction. Once it is satisfactory, the reduction is captured by driving the guidewire proximally. A second antirotation K-wire should be inserted prior to reaming. The targeting K-wires are removed and the reamer is then introduced over the guidewire. Reaming stops 2 mm short of the distal pole.

The arm is exsanguinated and the tourniquet is elevated at this point. When using some other type of traction tower, the arm is suspended with 10 to 15 lb of traction with the wrist in extension and the quality of the fracture site reduction is visualized by inserting the arthroscope into the MCU portal with the probe in the MCR portal. Adjustments to the fracture reduction can be performed by withdrawing the guidewire into the distal fragment and using a Freer elevator alternately inserted in the MCR and STT-U portals. Once the reduction is acceptable, the guidewire is positioned within 2 mm of the STT joint with the wrist maintained in flexion. Most of the screw measuring guides from different types of headless screws overestimate the screw length; hence, a second wire of equal length is placed percutaneously at the proximal scaphoid pole and parallel to the guidewire. The difference in length between the trailing end of each wire is the scaphoid length. The screw length selected should be 4 mm less than the scaphoid length. This permits 2 mm of clearance of the screw at each end of the scaphoid, thus ensuring complete implantation without screw exposure. If it is necessary to take the wrist out of traction for this part, the screw length can be gauged by driving the guidewire volarly and distally until the trailing end is in the subchondral bone of the distal scaphoid pole and the process is repeated. A recent anthropometric study determined that the average scaphoid length in adult males was 31.3 ± 2.1 mm while the average female scaphoid was 27.3 ± 1.7 mm; hence, the longest screw lengths may range from 23 to 27 mm.[106]

The guidewire is driven volarly once more so that it is left protruding both proximally and distally. This prevents guidewire migration during reaming and screw insertion. The wrist must remain flexed during this part; otherwise the guidewire will bend and block both reaming and screw insertion. The scaphoid is then power reamed to within 2 mm of the distal pole. Care is taken not to ream through the subchondral bone since this reduces compression along the fracture site. A headless screw is advanced under fluoroscopic guidance to within 1 to 2 mm of the opposite cortex. Radiocarpal and midcarpal arthroscopy is now performed to check for screw cutout. The rigidity of fracture fixation is assessed by palpating the fragments with a 1-mm hook probe or Freer elevator. After screw insertion, the guidewire is again driven distally if necessary to allow wrist extension and the fracture site is inspected arthroscopically. If rigid fixation has not been achieved, Slade et al have recommended pinning the distal fragment to the capitate (Fig. 18-24A-G).[107] This locks the midcarpal row and reduces fracture site motion, especially with short proximal or distal fragments where only a few screw threads cross the fracture site.

VOLAR APPROACH

Screw fixation of the scaphoid through a volar approach is hindered by the trapezium that prevents a straight-line approach to the central axis of the scaphoid. There is the

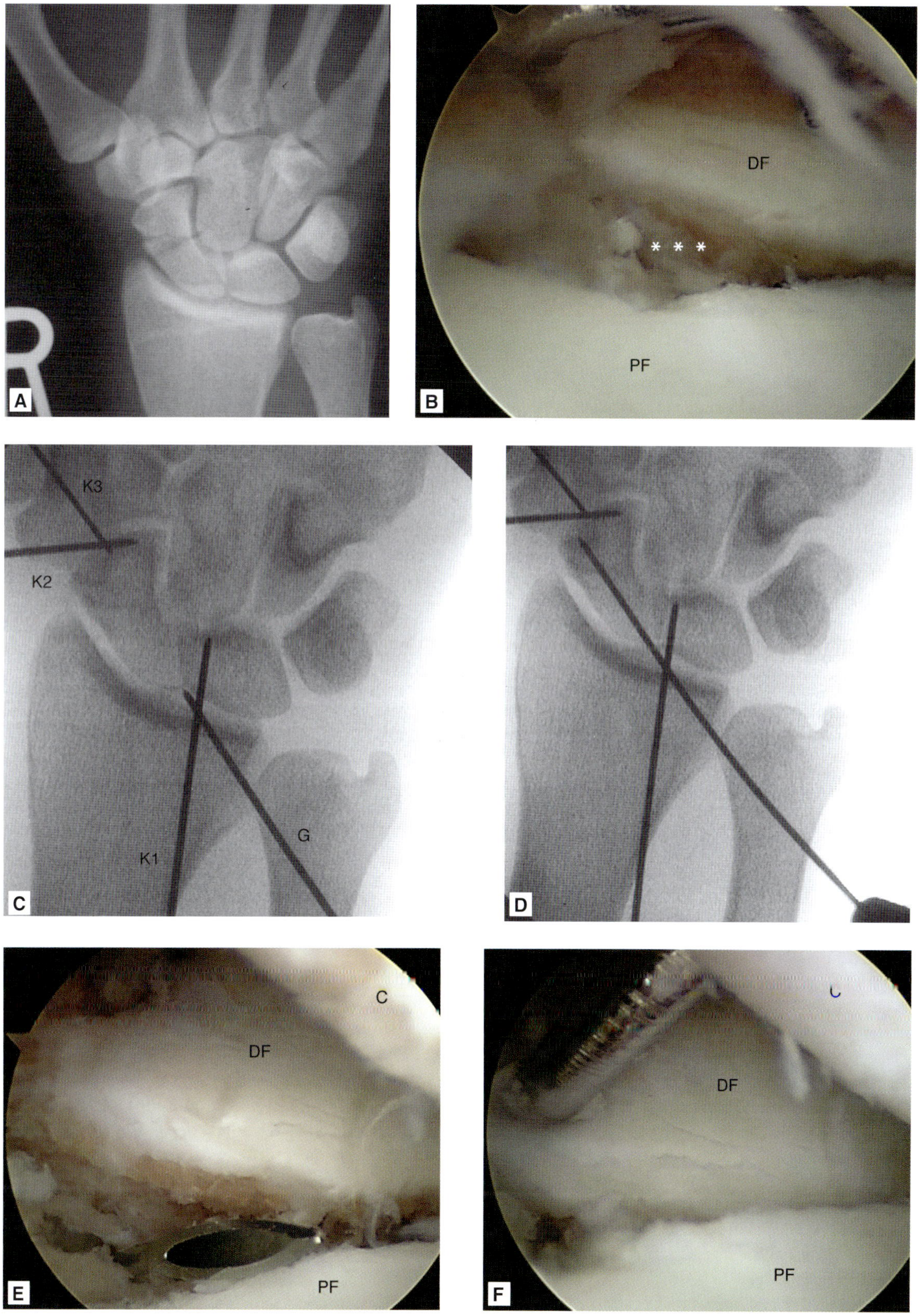

FIGURE 18-24 Arthroscopic-assisted scaphoid fixation. **A.** AP x-ray view of a comminuted scaphoid waist fracture. **B.** Arthroscopic view from the MCU portal. DF, distal scaphoid fragment; PF, proximal scaphoid fragment. **C.** Targeting K-wires are used for guidewire placement. **D.** Following insertion of the central guidewire. **E.** Fracture site is localized with a 22-gauge needle. C, capitate; DF, distal scaphoid fragment; PF, proximal scaphoid fragment. **F.** Percutaneous K-wires are used to lock the distal scaphoid fragment to the capitate.

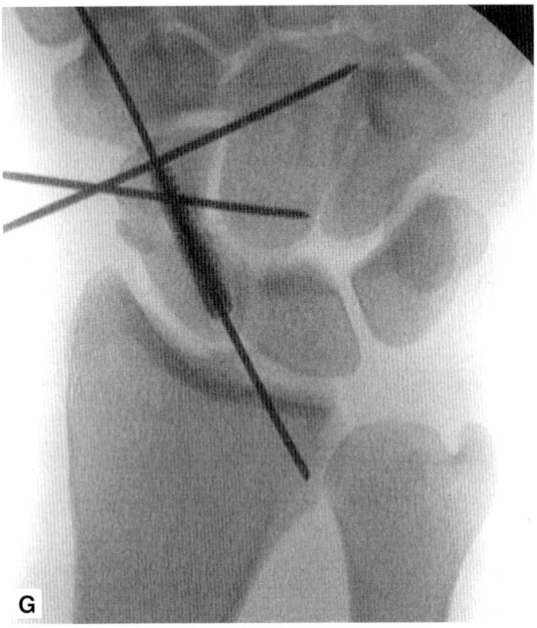

FIGURE 18-24 (*Continued*) **G.** AP x-ray following screw insertion.

added risk of screw cutout through the concave volar surface of the scaphoid or through the dorsoulnar aspect of the proximal pole. The volar technique has an advantage in that the articular defect from the entry site is limited to the radial edge of the ST joint, but a disadvantage is the limited area for screw insertion. Furthermore, an overly long screw will impinge on the ST joint and lead to osteoarthritis. Using a Herbert-Whipple screw, Menapace et al defined the safe starting point to be 4 to 5 mm from the volar prominence of the tubercle as measured from the lateral x-ray.[108]

Haddad and Goddard described volar percutaneous scaphoid fixation method using a cannulated screw.[109] The patient is placed supine on an operating table with the arm in traction. The hand is suspended by the thumb alone in a single Chinese finger trap with no countertraction. This position extends the scaphoid and ulnar deviates the wrist to improve access to the distal pole of the scaphoid. Importantly it permits free rotation of the hand throughout the operation and the scaphoid remains in the center of the x-ray field throughout. The proposed entry point of the guidewire is infiltrated with 2 cm^3 of 2% lidocaine and 1:200,000 adrenaline. The use of a tourniquet is optional.

The image intensifier C-arm is turned to a horizontal position and positioned so that the wrist is in the central axis. With the image intensifier in this position, it is then possible to screen the scaphoid continuously around the axis of the radial column. K-wires can be inserted and used as joysticks to manipulate the fragments into position as necessary. The quality of the reduction can then be checked radiographically and if necessary arthroscopically without disturbing the overall setup. The guidewire entry point is located using a 12-gauge IV needle introduced on the anteroradial aspect of the wrist just radial to and distal to the scaphoid tuberosity, and the needle is used to lever the distal pole of the scaphoid more radial to facilitate screw insertion. The forearm is rotated under fluoroscopy to line up the needle along the long axis of the scaphoid in all planes so that the guidewire exits the proximal pole just radial to the SL junction. The entry point can be changed by up to 1 mm by rotating the IV cannula. The guidewire is then inserted through the needle and drilled across the fracture site under fluoroscopy, stopping just short of the proximal pole. A small incision is made over the guidewire, followed by screw insertion. The length of the screw is determined using a second guidewire of the same length up the distal cortex of the scaphoid and undersized by 4 mm. The guidewire is then advanced through the proximal pole to exit on the dorsal aspect of the wrist to minimize the risk of inadvertent withdrawal, followed by reaming and screw insertion.

The postoperative dressing is changed at 1 week. Although some authors allow immediate and unrestricted motion, I prefer to immobilize the wrist in a short arm thumb spica cast for 6 to 8 weeks. When there is apparent union on the plain x-ray views, a longitudinal CT scan is performed to confirm that there is bridging callus on at least 3 cuts. Wrist motion and progressive strengthening exercises are then instituted.

HYBRID TECHNIQUE

Pirela-Cruz et al described a hybrid technique for a Herbert B-2 fracture with a standard size cannulated Acutrak screw.[110] They inserted a double-ended guidewire percutaneously, which is advanced out through the volar side at the tuberosity of the scaphoid until the guidewire is located within the proximal pole. The authors were usually able to obtain a satisfactory dorsal central position without drilling through the trapezium. The wrist was then placed into extension and ulnar deviation and the guidewire is advanced into the radius to prevent dislodgement after the length of the screw is determined. The scaphoid was reamed to within 2 to 3 mm of the proximal and a screw was inserted under fluoroscopic control.

ARTHROSCOPIC BONE GRAFTING

Ho recently described a technique of arthroscopic-assisted bone grafting of scaphoid nonunions.[111] The arthroscope is inserted in the MCU portal while the MCR portal is used for instrumentation. The proximal nonunion site is best seen from the STT-U portal that is radial to the extensor carpi radialis brevis tendon and ulnar to the EPL tendon, slightly distal to MCR portal. Loose implants (if present) are exchanged with a larger screw or multiple K-wires. Care is taken to preserve any intact cartilage or pseudocapsule over the nonunion site to avoid subsequent graft protrusion into the radiocarpal joint. Cancellous bone graft is tightly impacted into the nonunion site through an arthroscopic cannula. Ho's series included 37 patients with established symptomatic nonunions and 6 delayed unions with an average age of 28.7 years (range, 14-53 years). The median duration of symptoms was 8 months (range, 1-192 months). There were 5 distal third, 24 midthird, and 14 proximal third fractures with 5 cases of previous failed surgery and 10 cases with MRI evidence of avascular necrosis. Cannulated screws were used in 20 cases and multiple K wires in 23 cases. The average follow-up was 38.3 months (range, 5-103 months). The overall union rate was 90.7% (39/43). The average time to radiologic union was 12.2 weeks (6-24 weeks). Poor intraoperative bleeding of the proximal scaphoid still permitted union in 7 out of 10 cases while brisk bleeding was associated with union in 29 out of 30 cases. At the final follow-up, 27 patients were pain free while the average VAS in the remaining 16 patients was 2.53.

Complications

Screw length is often difficult to accurately determine by measuring a second K-wire that is placed parallel to the guidewire, due to interposition of soft tissue and obstruction by the edge of the trapezium. I keep the screw sterile in its package and superimpose it over the scaphoid under fluoroscopy to gauge the proper length. Penetration of the dorsal–radial surface of the scaphoid, which is exacerbated by any angular or humpback deformity aspect of the proximal pole, is common and can be minimized by using the pronated oblique views and undersizing the screw. Failure to bury the screw head will lead to impingement of the ST approach and eventual osteoarthritis. Screw cutout of the tuberosity can sometimes be salvaged by using an open technique and creating a gliding trough in the trapezium, switching to a smaller-diameter screw, and levering the tuberosity volarly with an elevator. Oblique insertion of the screw may lead to delayed union. Bending of the guidewire will impede drilling and tapping and may cause the cannulated screw driver to break. If this is recognized, the guidewire should be replaced rather than trying to force it.

Outcomes

Martinache and Mathoulin reviewed their results of a series of 37 acute scaphoid fractures that were treated by percutaneous screw insertion with an arthroscopic assist. There were 22 undisplaced and 15 displaced fractures.[112] In all the cases the use of wrist arthroscopy allowed the authors to check the quality of the reduction and the screw position. Bony union was achieved in all of the cases, within a median time of 62 days (range, 45-80). The functional recovery of the operated wrists was reported to be good with an average return to work at 21 days following the surgery.

Slade and Gillon recently reported a consecutive series of 234 fractures treated with percutaneous screw fixation using a dorsal approach.[113] The cases included 108 scaphoid nonunions (10 with a humpback deformity) and 126 acute injuries composed of 65 proximal pole fractures, 67 grossly displaced fractures, 12 trans-scaphoid perilunate dislocations, 4 trans-scaphoid transcapitate fractures, and 10 combined scaphoid and distal radius fractures. In each case arthroscopy was used to verify the quality of the reduction. CT scans confirmed that 125/126 acute fractures and 98/108 nonunions healed. The study demonstrated the utility of arthroscopy that aided the fracture reduction in 67 displaced fractures in addition to the 10 humpback deformities.

Concomitant soft tissue injuries are common. Caloia et al performed an arthroscopic examination on 24 patients with acute scaphoid fractures who were treated with percutaneous screw fixation through a dorsal approach.[46] The mean age was 32 years (range, 17-75 years). Fifteen of the 24 patients had an associated ligamentous or chondral injury. In a similar study, Shih et al reviewed 15 patients with an acute scaphoid fracture treated by percutaneous screw fixation under an arthroscopic control.[114] Two patients had a partial SL ligament tear; 4 had LT ligament tears that were debrided and K-wired. Five patients had a TFCC tear and 6 patients had chondral fractures. There were also 5 patients with injuries to the RSC ligament or LRL. At the 28-month follow-up all of the fractures had healed. Using the modified Mayo wrist score, 11 patients had excellent results and 4 had good results. These soft tissue injuries negatively impact the outcomes following treatment for the scaphoid fracture. Wong et al studied 52 patients with scaphoid fractures who were treated with percutaneous screw fixation.[115] All of the patients had wrist arthrograms and 22 underwent arthroscopy. Eighteen patients were found to have additional soft tissue injures that included 4 SL ligament tears, 8 LT ligament tears, 2 combined tears, and 3 TFCC tears. There was a noticeable difference in the outcomes in that the median modified Mayo wrist score was 95 in the patients without any associated ligament injuries as compared with a score of 85 in patients with associated ligament injuries. Jørgsholm et al published their experience with 41 patients, aged 38 years (14-71), with 11 displaced and 18 nondisplaced scaphoid waist fractures.[116] Twenty-nine patients (70%) had partial (19) or complete (10) SL ligament tears, 8 had LTIL tears, 11 had TFCC tears, and there were 8 complete and 7 partial tears of the dorsal capsule. These associated soft tissue injuries can affect the outcome.

TRANS-SCAPHOID PERILUNATE DISLOCATION

There has been some recent work into the use of arthroscopy and trans-scaphoid perilunate fracture–dislocations (Fig. 18-25A-F). Wong and Ip reviewed the results in 21 patients with a mean age of 29 years who underwent a closed reduction of the carpus, percutaneous screw fixation of the scaphoid fracture, and multiple K-wire fixation of the carpal dissociation.[117] There was a 95% union rate with a mean time of 16 weeks. The radiographic alignment of the carpus was satisfactory in 17/21 cases. The average Mayo wrist score was 80 with 3 excellent and 2 poor results. There was 1 patient with an asymptomatic DISI deformity. Two

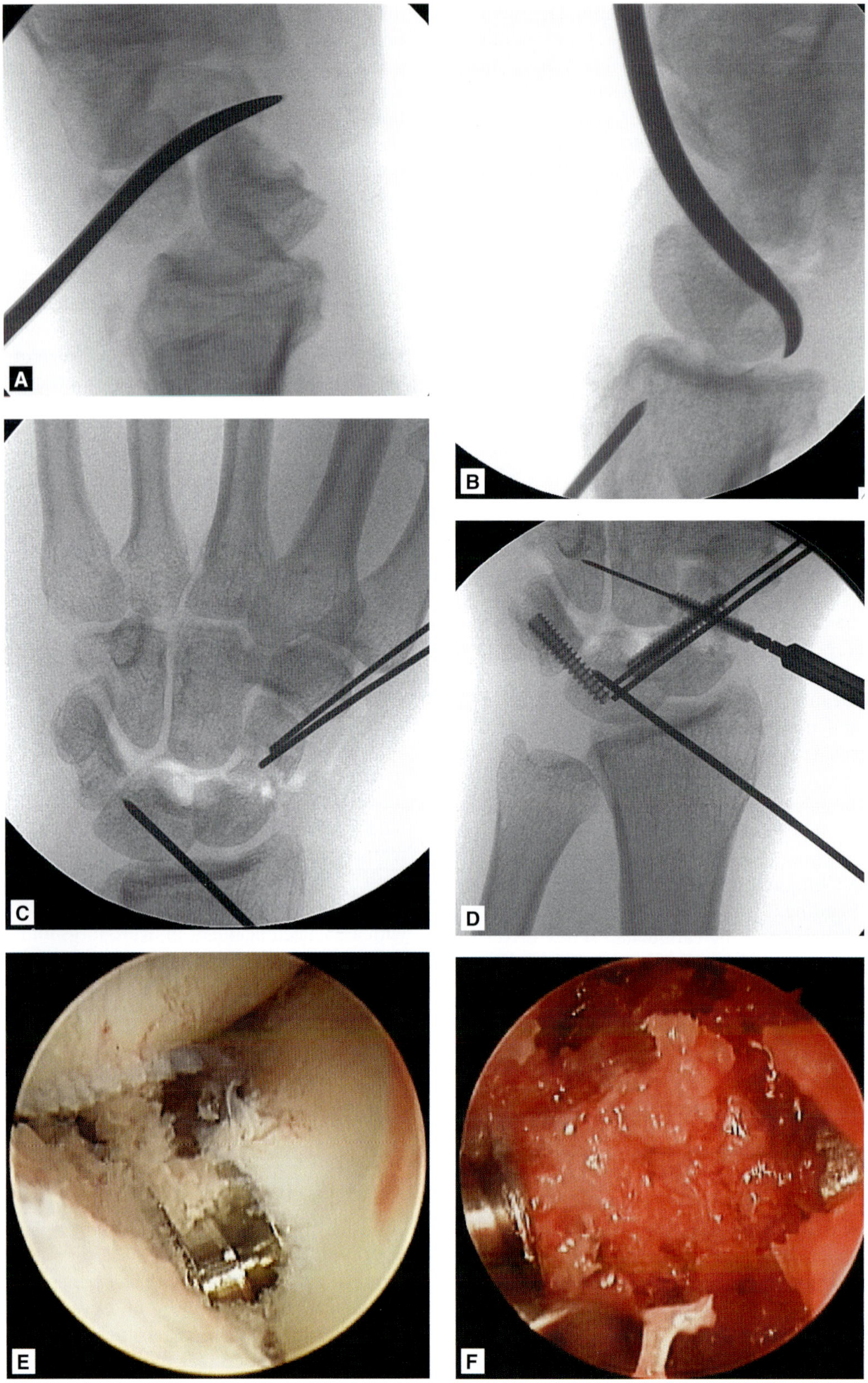

FIGURE 18-25 Arthroscopic-assisted trans-scaphoid perilunate fracture–dislocation. **A.** Lateral x-ray view of percutaneous insertion of a Freer elevator. **B.** Following midcarpal reduction. Note the preplaced dorsal K-wire in the distal radius. **C.** Lunate reduction is captured with the radioscaphoid K-wire and volar guidewires are inserted in the distal scaphoid fragment. **D.** Following screw fixation of the scaphoid fracture and screw fixation of the scaphocapitate and lunotriquetral joints. **E.** View of the scaphoid fracture from the STT portal demonstrating exposed screw threads. **F.** Following arthroscopic bone grafting through the MCR portal.

patients had radiographic evidence of midcarpal arthritis. One patient with a scaphoid nonunion required revision surgery and bone grafting. Kim et al treated 20 patients with an average age of 37.3 years (range, 19-57 years) who had an acute dorsal perilunate dislocation (5) or fracture–dislocation (15) with an arthroscopic scaphoid screw insertion at a median interval of 3.9 days (range, 1-20) from the time of injury, followed by K-wiring of the carpus for 10 weeks. At a mean follow-up of 31.2 months (range, 18-61 months), the mean flexion was 51° (25-70), mean extension 53° (30-70), radial deviation 17° (10-26), and ulnar deviation 30° (18-42). The mean DASH score was 18 (1-36) and PRWE score 30 (5-52). According to modified Mayo wrist scores there were 3 excellent, 8 good, 87 fair, and 2 poor results. Six patients had a concomitant SL ligament injury (Geissler II/III). Three had concomitant fractures (olecranon, hip, patellar/calcaneal). Nonunion developed in 2 patients with a trans-scaphoid perilunate injury; 1 of the 2 underwent scaphoid excision and midcarpal fusion.

Chou et al studied 24 patients treated by percutaneous screw (3.0-mm AO cannulated in 13 patients, Herbert-Whipple screw in 11 patients) within 7 days of the injury and closed reduction and carpal fixation with a 2.0-mm axial K-wire inserted across the capitolunate joint for 8 weeks.[118] Twenty-three patients (96%) achieved scaphoid union at a mean time of 18 weeks (range, 14-28 weeks). There was 1 nonunion, 1 required styloidectomy, and 1 required screw removal. At an average follow-up of 45 months (range, 25-67 months), the mean flexion was 78° ± 5°, extension 66° ± 10°, pronation 87° ± 5°, supination 75° ± 8°, radial deviation 30° ± 9°, and ulnar deviation 37° ± 5°. Grip strength averaged 28.3 ± 6 kg and the pain VAS averaged 21 (range, 16-25). The average Modified Mayo score was 83 (range, 65-93). There were 4 excellent, 17 good, and 3 fair results.

REFERENCES

1. Abrams RA, Petersen M, Botte MJ. Arthroscopic portals of the wrist: an anatomic study. *J Hand Surg Am*. 1994;19:940–944.
2. Mackinnon SE, Dellon AL. The overlap pattern of the lateral antebrachial cutaneous nerve and the superficial branch of the radial nerve. *J Hand Surg Am*. 1985;10:522–526.
3. Steinberg BD, Plancher KD, Idler RS. Percutaneous Kirschner wire fixation through the snuff box: an anatomic study. *J Hand Surg Am*. 1995;20:57–62.
4. Martin CH, Seiler JG 3rd, Lesesne JS. The cutaneous innervation of the palm: an anatomic study of the ulnar and median nerves. *J Hand Surg Am*. 1996;21:634–638.
5. Slutsky DJ. The use of a volar ulnar portal in wrist arthroscopy. *Arthroscopy*. 2004;20:158–163.
6. Slutsky DJ. Clinical applications of volar portals in wrist arthroscopy. *Tech Hand Up Extrem Surg*. 2004;8:229–238.
7. Kraan MC, Reece RJ, Smeets TJ, Veale DJ, Emery P, Tak PP. Comparison of synovial tissues from the knee joints and the small joints of rheumatoid arthritis patients: implications for pathogenesis and evaluation of treatment. *Arthritis Rheum*. 2002;46:2034–2038.
8. Chen C, Chandnani VP, Kang HS, Resnick D, Sartoris DJ, Haller J. Scapholunate advanced collapse: a common wrist abnormality in calcium pyrophosphate dihydrate crystal deposition disease. *Radiology*. 1990;177:459–461.
9. Donich AS, Lektrakul N, Liu CC, Theodorou DJ, Kakitsubata Y, Resnick D. Calcium pyrophosphate dihydrate crystal deposition disease of the wrist: trapezioscaphoid joint abnormality. *J Rheumatol*. 2000;27:2628–2634.
10. Wilczynski MC, Gelberman RH, Adams A, Goldfarb CA. Arthroscopic findings in gout of the wrist. *J Hand Surg Am*. 2009;34:244–250.
11. Adolfsson L, Frisen M. Arthroscopic synovectomy of the rheumatoid wrist. A 3.8 year follow-up. *J Hand Surg Br*. 1997;22:711–713.
12. Adolfsson L. Arthroscopic synovectomy of the wrist. *Hand Clin*. 2011; 27:395–399.
13. Culp R, Osterman A, Kaufmann RA. Wrist arthroscopy: operative orocedures. In: Green DP, Hotchkiss RN, Pederson WC, Wolfe SW, eds. *Green's Operative Hand Surgery*. Philadelphia: Elsevier Inc; 2005:781–803.
14. Bain GI, Roth JH. The role of arthroscopy in arthritis. "Ectomy" procedures. *Hand Clin*. 1995;11:51–58.
15. Whipple TL. The role of arthroscopy in the treatment of scapholunate instability. *Hand Clin*. 1995;11:37–40.
16. Bain GI, Begg M. Arthroscopic assessment and classification of Kienbock's disease. *Tech Hand Up Extrem Surg*. 2006;10:8–13.
17. Menth-Chiari WA, Poehling GG, Wiesler ER, Ruch DS. Arthroscopic debridement for the treatment of Kienbock's disease. *Arthroscopy*. 1999;15:12–19.
18. Menth-Chiari WA, Poehling GG. Preiser's disease: arthroscopic treatment of avascular necrosis of the scaphoid. *Arthroscopy*. 2000; 16:208–213.
19. Osterman AL, Raphael J. Arthroscopic resection of dorsal ganglion of the wrist. *Hand Clin*. 1995;11:7–12.
20. Ho PC, Griffiths J, Lo WN, Yen CH, Hung LK. Current treatment of ganglion of the wrist. *Hand Surg*. 2001;6:49–58.
21. Rizzo M, Berger RA, Steinmann SP, Bishop AT. Arthroscopic resection in the management of dorsal wrist ganglions: results with a minimum 2-year follow-up period. *J Hand Surg Am*. 2004;29:59–62.
22. Mathoulin C, Hoyos A, Pelacz J. Arthroscopic resection of wrist ganglia. *Hand Surg*. 2004;9:159–164.
23. Kang L, Akelman E, Weiss AP. Arthroscopic versus open dorsal ganglion excision: a prospective, randomized comparison of rates of recurrence and of residual pain. *J Hand Surg Am*. 2008;33:471–475.
24. Edwards SG, Johansen JA. Prospective outcomes and associations of wrist ganglion cysts resected arthroscopically. *J Hand Surg Am*. 2009;34:395–400.
25. Povlsen B, Tavakkolizadeh A. Outcome of surgery in patients with painful dorsal wrist ganglia and arthroscopic confirmed ligament injury: a five-year follow-up. *Hand Surg*. 2004;9:171–173.
26. Langner I, Krueger PC, Merk HR, Ekkernkamp A, Zach A. Ganglions of the wrist and associated triangular fibrocartilage lesions—a prospective study in arthroscopically-treated patients. *J Hand Surg Am*. 2012;37:1561–1567.
27. Lee SK, Gargano F, Hausman MR. Wrist arthrofibrosis. *Hand Clin*. 2006;22:529–538 [abstract vii].
28. Verhellen R, Bain GI. Arthroscopic capsular release for contracture of the wrist: a new technique. *Arthroscopy*. 2000;16:106–110.
29. Hattori T, Tsunoda K, Watanabe K, Nakao E, Hirata H, Nakamura R. Arthroscopic mobilization for contracture of the wrist. *Arthroscopy*. 2006;22:850–854.
30. Luchetti R, Atzei A, Fairplay T. Arthroscopic wrist arthrolysis after wrist fracture. *Arthroscopy*. 2007;23:255–260.
31. Geissler WB, Freeland AE, Savoie FH, McIntyre LW, Whipple TL. Intracarpal soft-tissue lesions associated with an intra-articular fracture of the distal end of the radius. *J Bone Joint Surg Am*. 1996;78:357–365.
32. Slutsky D. Current innovations in wrist arthroscopy. *J Hand Surg Am*. 2012;37:1932–1941.
33. Elsaidi GA, Ruch DS, Kuzma GR, Smith BP. Dorsal wrist ligament insertions stabilize the scapholunate interval: cadaver study. *Clin Orthop Relat Res*. 2004:152–157.
34. Short WH, Werner FW, Green JK, Sutton LG, Brutus JP. Biomechanical evaluation of the ligamentous stabilizers of the scaphoid and lunate: part III. *J Hand Surg Am*. 2007;32:297–309.
35. Rosenwasser MP, Miyasajsa KC, Strauch RJ. The RASL procedure: reduction and association of the scaphoid and lunate using the Herbert screw. *Tech Hand Up Extrem Surg*. 1997;1:263–272.

36. Hausman M. Arthroscopic reduction and association of the scaphoid and lunate. In: Slutsky DJ, Nagle DJ, eds. *Techniques in Hand and Wrist Arthroscopy*. Philadelphia: Elsevier Inc; 2007.
37. Slutsky DJ. Volar portals in wrist arthroscopy. *J Am Soc Surg Hand*. 2002;2:225–232.
38. Danoff JR, Karl JW, Birman MV, Rosenwasser MP. The use of thermal shrinkage for scapholunate instability. *Hand Clin*. 2011;27:309–317.
39. Goldberg SH, Carroll RE, Riansuwan K, Rosenwasser MP. Arthroscopic treatment of scapholunate ligament tears. In: Slutsky DJ, Nagle DJ, eds. *Techniques in Hand and Wrist Arthroscopy*. Philadelphia: Elsevier Inc; 2007.
40. O'Meeghan CJ, Stuart W, Mamo V, Stanley JK, Trail IA. The natural history of an untreated isolated scapholunate interosseus ligament injury. *J Hand Surg Br*. 2003;28:307–310.
41. Darlis NA, Weiser RW, Sotereanos DG. Partial scapholunate ligament injuries treated with arthroscopic debridement and thermal shrinkage. *J Hand Surg Am*. 2005;30:908–914.
42. Darlis NA, Kaufmann RA, Giannoulis F, Sotereanos DG. Arthroscopic debridement and closed pinning for chronic dynamic scapholunate instability. *J Hand Surg Am*. 2006;31:418–424.
43. Mathoulin CL, Dauphin N, Wahegaonkar AL. Arthroscopic dorsal capsuloligamentous repair in chronic scapholunate ligament tears. *Hand Clin*. 2011;27:563–572, xi.
44. White NJRD, Crow SA, Swart E, Rosenwasser MP. Reduction and association of the scaphoid and lunate (RASL): long-term follow-up of a reconstruction technique for chronic scapholunate dissociation. *J Hand Surg Am*. 2010;35:16–17.
45. Aviles AJ, Lee SK, Hausman MR. Arthroscopic reduction-association of the scapholunate. *Arthroscopy*. 2007;23:105.e101–105.
46. Caloia M, Caloia H, Pereira E. Arthroscopic scapholunate joint reduction. Is an effective treatment for irreparable scapholunate ligament tears? *Clin Orthop Relat Res*. 2012;470:972–978.
47. Hirsh L, Sodha S, Bozentka D, Monaghan B, Steinberg D, Beredjiklian PK. Arthroscopic electrothermal collagen shrinkage for symptomatic laxity of the scapholunate interosseous ligament. *J Hand Surg Br*. 2005;30:643–647.
48. Shih JT, Lee HM. Monopolar radiofrequency electrothermal shrinkage of the scapholunate ligament. *Arthroscopy*. 2006;22:553–557.
49. Battistella F, Golano P, Taverna E. Arthroscopic thermal shrinkage for scapholunate injuries. In: Slutsky DJ, Nagle DJ, eds. *Techniques in Hand and Wrist Arthroscopy*. Philadelphia: Elsevier Inc; 2007.
50. Ruch DS, Poehling GG. Arthroscopic management of partial scapholunate and lunotriquetral injuries of the wrist. *J Hand Surg Am*. 1996;21:412–417.
51. Weiss AP, Sachar K, Glowacki KA. Arthroscopic debridement alone for intercarpal ligament tears. *J Hand Surg Am*. 1997;22:344–349.
52. Slutsky D. Incidence of dorsal radiocarpal ligament tears in the presence of other intercarpal derangements. *Arthroscopy*. 2008;24:526–533.
53. Slutsky D. Arthroscopic repair of dorsoradiocarpal ligament tears. *Arthroscopy*. 2005;21:1486e1481–1486e1488.
54. Lichtman DM, Bruckner JD, Culp RW, Alexander CE. Palmar midcarpal instability: results of surgical reconstruction. *J Hand Surg Am*. 1993;18:307–315.
55. Goldfarb CA, Stern PJ, Kiefhaber TR. Palmar midcarpal instability: the results of treatment with 4-corner arthrodesis. *J Hand Surg Am*. 2004;29:258–263.
56. Lichtman DM, Culp RW, Joshi A. Palmar midcarpal instability. In: McGinty E, ed. *Operative Arthroscopy*. Philadelphia: Lippincott Williams & Wilkins; 2003:737–742.
57. Mason WT, Hargreaves DG. Arthroscopic thermal capsulorrhaphy for palmar midcarpal instability. *J Hand Surg Eur*. 2007;32:411–416.
58. Ishii S, Palmer AK, Werner FW, Short WH, Fortino MD. An anatomic study of the ligamentous structure of the triangular fibrocartilage complex. *J Hand Surg Am*. 1998;23:977–985.
59. Kauer JM. The articular disc of the hand. *Acta Anat (Basel)*. 1975;93:590–605.
60. Kleinman WB. Stability of the distal radioulna joint: biomechanics, pathophysiology, physical diagnosis, and restoration of function what we have learned in 25 years. *J Hand Surg Am*. 2007;32:1086–1106.
61. Adams BD, Samani JE, Holley KA. Triangular fibrocartilage injury: a laboratory model. *J Hand Surg Am*. 1996;21:189–193.
62. Haugstvedt JR, Berger RA, Nakamura T, Neale P, Berglund L, An KN. Relative contributions of the ulnar attachments of the triangular fibrocartilage complex to the dynamic stability of the distal radioulnar joint. *J Hand Surg Am*. 2006;31:445–451.
63. Lindau T, Adlercreutz C, Aspenberg P. Peripheral tears of the triangular fibrocartilage complex cause distal radioulnar joint instability after distal radial fractures. *J Hand Surg Am*. 2000;25:464–468.
64. Palmer AK. Triangular fibrocartilage complex lesions: a classification. *J Hand Surg Am*. 1989;14:594–606.
65. Tay SC, Tomita K, Berger RA. The "ulnar fovea sign" for defining ulnar wrist pain: an analysis of sensitivity and specificity. *J Hand Surg Am*. 2007;32:438–444.
66. Szabo RM. Distal radioulnar joint instability. *J Bone Joint Surg Am*. 2006;88:884–894.
67. Tomaino MM. Ulnar impaction syndrome in the ulnar negative and neutral wrist. Diagnosis and pathoanatomy. *J Hand Surg Br*. 1998;23:754–757.
68. Bille B, Harley B, Cohen H. A comparison of CT arthrography of the wrist to findings during wrist arthroscopy. *J Hand Surg Am*. 2007;32:834–841.
69. Trumble TE, Gilbert M, Vedder N. Isolated tears of the triangular fibrocartilage: management by early arthroscopic repair. *J Hand Surg Am*. 1997;22:57–65.
70. Moskal MJ, Savoie FH 3rd, Field LD. Arthroscopic capsulodesis of the lunotriquetral joint. *Clin Sports Med*. 2001;20:141–153, ix–x.
71. Reiter A, Wolf MB, Schmid U, et al. Arthroscopic repair of palmer 1B triangular fibrocartilage complex tears. *Arthroscopy*. 2008;24:1244–1250.
72. Estrella EP, Hung LK, Ho PC, Tse WL. Arthroscopic repair of triangular fibrocartilage complex tears. *Arthroscopy*. 2007;23:729–737, 737.e1.
73. Tatebe M, Horii E, Nakao E, et al. Repair of the triangular fibrocartilage complex after ulnar-shortening osteotomy: second-look arthroscopy. *J Hand Surg Am*. 2007;32:445–449.
74. Yao J, Lee AT. All-arthroscopic repair of palmer 1B triangular fibrocartilage complex tears using the FasT-Fix device. *J Hand Surg Am*. 2011;36:836–842.
75. Osterman AL. *Arthroscopic Treatment of Radial-sided TFCC Lesions*. International Wrist Investigator's Workshop. New York: ASSH; 2004.
76. Nakamura T. Radial sided tears of the triangular fibrocartilage. In: del Piñal F, Mathoulin C, Luchetti R, eds. *Arthroscopic Management of Distal Radius Fractures*. Heidelberg: Springer-Verlag; 2010:89–98.
77. Ruch DS, Yang CC, Smith BP. Results of acute arthroscopically repaired triangular fibrocartilage complex injuries associated with intra-articular distal radius fractures. *Arthroscopy*. 2003;19:511–516.
78. Atzei A, Rizzo A, Luchetti R, Fairplay T. Arthroscopic foveal repair of triangular fibrocartilage complex peripheral lesion with distal radioulnar joint instability. *Tech Hand Up Extrem Surg*. 2008;12:226–235.
79. Amrami KK, Felmlee JP. 3-Tesla imaging of the wrist and hand: techniques and applications. *Semin Musculoskelet Radiol*. 2008;12:223–237.
80. Slutsky DJ. Arthroscopic evaluation of the foveal attachment of the triangular fibrocartilage. *Hand Clin*. 2011;27:255–261.
81. Atzei A, Luchetti R. Foveal TFCC tear classification and treatment. *Hand Clin*. 2011;27:263–272.
82. Mikic ZD. Age changes in the triangular fibrocartilage of the wrist joint. *J Anat*. 1978;126:367–384.
83. Viegas SF, Ballantyne G. Attritional lesions of the wrist joint. *J Hand Surg Am*. 1987;12:1025–1029.
84. Tomaino MM, Elfar J. Ulnar impaction syndrome. *Hand Clin*. 2005;21:567–575.
85. Wnorowski DC, Palmer AK, Werner FW, Fortino MD. Anatomic and biomechanical analysis of the arthroscopic wafer procedure. *Arthroscopy*. 1992;8:204–212.
86. Osterman AL, Terrill RG. Arthroscopic treatment of TFCC lesions. *Hand Clin*. 1991;7:277–281.
87. Slutsky DJ. Distal radioulnar joint arthroscopy and the volar ulnar portal. *Tech Hand Up Extrem Surg*. 2007;11:38–44.
88. Shin AY, Weinstein LP, Berger RA, Bishop AT. Treatment of isolated injuries of the lunotriquetral ligament. A comparison of arthrodesis, ligament reconstruction and ligament repair. *J Bone Joint Surg Br*. 2001;83:1023–1028.
89. Bernstein MA, Nagle DJ, Martinez A, Stogin JM Jr, Wiedrich TA. A comparison of combined arthroscopic triangular fibrocartilage complex debridement and arthroscopic wafer distal ulna resection versus arthroscopic triangular fibrocartilage complex debridement and ulnar shortening osteotomy for ulnocarpal abutment syndrome. *Arthroscopy*. 2004;20:392–401.

90. Viegas SF, Wagner K, Patterson R, Peterson P. Medial (hamate) facet of the lunate. *J Hand Surg Am.* 1990;15:564–571.
91. Viegas SF, Patterson RM, Hokanson JA, Davis J. Wrist anatomy: incidence, distribution, and correlation of anatomic variations, tears, and arthrosis. *J Hand Surg Am.* 1993;18:463–475.
92. Harley BJ, Werner FW, Boles SD, Palmer AK. Arthroscopic resection of arthrosis of the proximal hamate: a clinical and biomechanical study. *J Hand Surg Am.* 2004;29:661–667.
93. Nakamura T, Cooney WP 3rd, Lui WH, et al. Radial styloidectomy: a biomechanical study on stability of the wrist joint. *J Hand Surg Am.* 2001;26:85–93.
94. Weiss ND, Molina RA, Gwin S. Arthroscopic proximal row carpectomy. *J Hand Surg Am.* 2011;36:577–582.
95. Ruch DS, Chang DS, Poehling GG. The arthroscopic treatment of avascular necrosis of the proximal pole following scaphoid nonunion. *Arthroscopy.* 1998;14:747–752.
96. Ruch DS, Papadonikolakis A. Resection of the scaphoid distal pole for symptomatic scaphoid nonunion after failed previous surgical treatment. *J Hand Surg Am.* 2006;31:588–593.
97. Dicpinigaitis P, Wolinsky P, Hiebert R, Egol K, Koval K, Tejwani N. Can external fixation maintain reduction after distal radius fractures? *J Trauma.* 2004;57:845–850.
98. del Piñal F, Garcia-Bernal FJ, Pisani D, Regalado J, Ayala H, Studer A. Dry arthroscopy of the wrist: surgical technique. *J Hand Surg Am.* 2007;32:119–123.
99. Mehta JA, Bain GI, Heptinstall RJ. Anatomical reduction of intra-articular fractures of the distal radius. An arthroscopically-assisted approach. *J Bone Joint Surg Br.* 2000;82:79–86.
100. Doi K, Hattori Y, Otsuka K, Abe Y, Yamamoto H. Intra-articular fractures of the distal aspect of the radius: arthroscopically assisted reduction compared with open reduction and internal fixation. *J Bone Joint Surg Am.* 1999;81:1093–1110.
101. Ruch DS, Vallee J, Poehling GG, Smith BP, Kuzma GR. Arthroscopic reduction versus fluoroscopic reduction in the management of intra-articular distal radius fractures. *Arthroscopy.* 2004;20:225–230.
102. Varitimidis SE, Basdekis GK, Dailiana ZH, Hantes ME, Bargiotas K, Malizos K. Treatment of intra-articular fractures of the distal radius: fluoroscopic or arthroscopic reduction? *J Bone Joint Surg Br.* 2008;90:778–785.
103. del Piñal F, Garcia-Bernal FJ, Delgado J, Sanmartin M, Regalado J, Cerezal L. Correction of malunited intra-articular distal radius fractures with an inside-out osteotomy technique. *J Hand Surg Am.* 2006;31:1029–1034.
104. del Piñal F, Cagigal L, Garcia-Bernal FJ, Studer A, Regalado J, Thams C. Arthroscopically guided osteotomy for management of intra-articular distal radius malunions. *J Hand Surg Am.* 2010;35:392–397.
105. Chan KW, McAdams TR. Central screw placement in percutaneous screw scaphoid fixation: a cadaveric comparison of proximal and distal techniques. *J Hand Surg Am.* 2004;29:74–79.
106. Heinzelmann AD, Archer G, Bindra RR. Anthropometry of the human scaphoid. *J Hand Surg Am.* 2007;32:1005–1008.
107. Slade JF 3rd, Geissler WB, Gutow AP, Merrell GA. Percutaneous internal fixation of selected scaphoid nonunions with an arthroscopically assisted dorsal approach. *J Bone Joint Surg Am.* 2003;85-A(suppl 4): 20–32.
108. Menapace KA, Larabee L, Arnoczky SP, Neginhal VS, Dass AG, Ross LM. Anatomic placement of the Herbert-Whipple screw in scaphoid fractures: a cadaver study. *J Hand Surg Am.* 2001;26:883–892.
109. Haddad FS, Goddard NJ. Acute percutaneous scaphoid fixation. A pilot study. *J Bone Joint Surg Br.* 1998;80:95–99.
110. Pirela-Cruz MA, Battista V, Burnette S, Hansen T. A technical note on percutaneous scaphoid fixation using a hybrid technique. *J Orthop Trauma.* 2005;19:570–573.
111. Ho PC. Arthroscopic bone grafting in scaphoid non union & delayed union. In: Slutsky DJ, Slade JF III, eds. New York: Thieme; 2010: 131–143.
112. Martinache X, Mathoulin C. Percutaneous fixation of scaphoid fractures with arthroscopic assistance. *Chir Main.* 2006;25(suppl 1): S171–S177.
113. Slade JF 3rd, Gillon T. Retrospective review of 234 scaphoid fractures and nonunions treated with arthroscopy for union and complications. *Scand J Surg.* 2008;97:280–289.
114. Shih JT, Lee HM, Hou YT, Tan CM. Results of arthroscopic reduction and percutaneous fixation for acute displaced scaphoid fractures. *Arthroscopy.* 2005;21:620–626.
115. Wong TC, Yip TH, Wu WC. Carpal ligament injuries with acute scaphoid fractures—a combined wrist injury. *J Hand Surg Br.* 2005;30: 415–418.
116. Jørgsholm P, Thomsen NO, Bjorkman A, Besjakov J, Abrahamsson SO. The incidence of intrinsic and extrinsic ligament injuries in scaphoid waist fractures. *J Hand Surg Am.* 2010;35:368–374.
117. Wong TC, Ip FK. Minimally invasive management of trans-scaphoid perilunate fracture–dislocations. *Hand Surg.* 2008;13:159–165.
118. Chou YC, Hsu YH, Cheng CY, Wu CC. Percutaneous screw and axial Kirschner wire fixation for acute transscaphoid perilunate fracture dislocation. *J Hand Surg Am.* 2012;37:715–720.

Scaphoid Fractures and Nonunions

19

Nathan Coleman, MD
Stephen Kennedy, MD
Jerry Huang, MD

RATIONALE AND BASIC SCIENCE PERTINENT TO THE PROCEDURES

The scaphoid has an important role in normal wrist mechanics, with ligament attachments that bridge the proximal and distal carpal rows. High shearing and bending loads make it susceptible to fracture, with scaphoid fractures accounting for 60% to 70% of carpal bone fractures.[1–5]

When disrupted by fracture, the scaphoid is at risk of nonunion and osteonecrosis. Eighty percent of its surface is covered by cartilage, leaving little surface for arterial supply, and it is bathed in synovial fluid. A dorsal branch of the radial artery enters the dorsal ridge and supplies 70% to 80% of the scaphoid proximally. Volar branches supply the distal 20%, with collateral circulation from the anterior interosseous artery.[6] The proximal pole is dependent on its intramedullary blood supply. Nonunion rates for scaphoid fractures depend on displacement and location, ranging from 5% for minimally displaced (<1 mm) to 92% for displaced proximal pole fractures.[7,8] Nonunion leads to altered carpal mechanics and progressive arthrosis that can result in chronic pain and decreased function.

Multiple features have been used to determine treatment for fractures and nonunions of the scaphoid. These include fracture location, displacement, and orientation, as well as comminution, deformity, instability, and evidence of delayed union.[9–12] Delayed union may vary from early cystic resorption to nonunion and pseudarthrosis.[12] Anatomic reduction, direct bone contact, and minimization of motion allow for optimal healing of scaphoid fractures and nonunions. Depending on the patient, fracture characteristics, and time from injury, treatment may be operative or nonoperative. Multiple surgical approaches can be used for fixation of scaphoid fractures, including open or percutaneous and volar or dorsal.

INDICATIONS

Indications for Cast Immobilization

Acute, nondisplaced fractures of the scaphoid waist or distal pole, without deformity or bone loss, are treated well with cast immobilization. The choice of immobilization is debated, but studies show that a short arm cast with the thumb free may not be significantly different from a long arm thumb spica cast.[13] We generally use a short arm thumb spica cast. The patient is followed clinically and radiographically, with cast changes and x-rays at 6-week intervals. Union typically takes 10 to 12 weeks, and often longer if the fracture is more proximal or if the presentation is delayed. Cast immobilization continues until there is radiographic evidence of complete bony union. In some cases, CT scans can be performed to confirm union. Nearly all nondisplaced scaphoid waist fractures will heal by 12 weeks with appropriate immobilization.[3,4]

Indications for Operative Management of Scaphoid Fracture

A scaphoid waist fracture with displacement of more than 1 mm is often cited as an indication for internal fixation. Fracture displacement, in terms of translation, angulation, or gapping, which is visible on plain radiographs, is an indication for surgery. Since proximal pole fractures may take more than 6 months to heal with cast immobilization, acute proximal pole fractures have become another indication for surgery. Other indications include a trans-scaphoid perilunate fracture–dislocation, concomitant distal radius fracture, or delayed presentation (>3 weeks) of a nondisplaced fracture with no prior treatment. Earlier return to sports in a high-level professional athlete is a relative indication as well as patients with claustrophobia or financial hardship who cannot tolerate cast immobilization.

Percutaneous techniques are ideal for acute waist fractures that are nondisplaced or minimally displaced and easily reducible, with minimal resorption or humpback deformity.[14] This has the advantage of minimal injury to the blood supply and avoidance of capsular ligament disruption.[15] Percutaneous treatment has been shown to result in faster healing time, reduced immobilization, and decreased time off work for labor-type occupations.[3,16] However, fracture reduction can be more challenging, with an increased risk of iatrogenic injury to tendons, nerves, and vessels.[17,18]

Most minimally displaced waist fractures can be treated with dorsal or volar percutaneous techniques, and the choice often has much to do with familiarity or preference. Central placement of the screw in the proximal fragment offers significant biomechanical advantage.[19] Central screw placement along the long axis of the scaphoid is more reliable with dorsal insertion compared with volar approach. Jeon et al evaluated 41 patients with an acute scaphoid fracture at an average of 30 months, who had percutaneous fixation via either the volar approach or the dorsal approach, at an average of 30 months after the surgery.[20] The volar approach was used in 19 patients and the dorsal approach in 22 patients. By using a computerized digital image program, the screws showed no significant difference between the 2 groups in the posteroanterior and lateral views; however, screws in the dorsal approach group were observed to be more parallel to the long axis of the scaphoid in the semipronated oblique view. The screws in the dorsal approach group were positioned more perpendicular to the fracture lines of the scaphoid compared with those of the volar approach group for all 3 different radiographic views. There was no statistically significant difference between the 2 treatment groups regarding fracture healing. The dorsal percutaneous technique can offer better control and fixation of proximal pole fractures, whereas the volar technique is well suited for more distal fractures. Volar percutaneous and open techniques often require some drilling and/or bone removal from the trapezium, and this may increase the radiographic evidence of scaphotrapezial arthritis.

Scaphoid waist and distal fractures can also be treated through an open volar approach.[9] For proximal third fractures, particularly the proximal pole, an open dorsal approach allows for evaluation of the fracture and proximal pole bone quality, as well as localization of the guidewire starting point. If there is avascularity of the proximal pole, a vascularized bone graft can be considered, as well as Kirschner wire fixation rather than screw fixation to avoid fragmentation.

Comminuted scaphoid waist fractures, delayed unions, and nonunions with humpback deformities are indications for autogenous bone grafting, using distal radius or iliac crest.

CONTRAINDICATIONS

Patient factors may limit the benefit of operative management, such as multiple medical comorbidities with high perioperative risks, low-demand patients, or patients with short life expectancy from terminal illness. Active infection precludes surgery.

Advanced arthrosis of the radioscaphoid and midcarpal joints, that is, a scaphoid nonunion advanced collapse (SNAC) wrist, is a contraindication, particularly in later stages, as the patient may be better served by salvage procedures such as proximal row carpectomy or scaphoidectomy and intercarpal fusion. Contraindications to the percutaneous fixation include irreducible fractures, fracture nonunions with deformity and bone loss, pseudarthrosis, osteonecrosis, and presence of radiocarpal or midcarpal arthrosis.[3]

SURGICAL TECHNIQUE

Dorsal Percutaneous Technique

No traction is needed for this technique. The wrist is flexed, slightly pronated, and ulnarly deviated (see Fig. 19-1). The starting point for K-wire insertion is the apex of the proximal pole at its most proximal and ulnar aspect. Inserting the guidewire by hand with the wrist flexed will offer the most control and ease with posteroanterior fluoroscopic imaging. Drive the K-wire down the central axis of the scaphoid, confirming its path with biplanar fluoroscopy. Avoid multiple passes with the K-wire by confirming your trajectory as the guidewire is being advanced. Measure the screw length and subtract 4 to 5 mm for optimal length. Advance the K-wire distally exiting at the radial base of the thumb (often through the trapezium). Make a small 1-cm incision at the insertion point dorsally. Spread with a hemostat to ensure that the extensor tendons are clear of the screw path (see Fig. 19-2). Ream over the wire to 2 mm short of the distal cortex, taking care to avoid penetrating the far cortex. Insert your compression screw of choice. Confirm its location with fluoroscopy.

Volar Percutaneous Technique

Under fluoroscopic guidance identify the scaphotrapeziotrapezoid (STT) joint. Insert a 0.045-in Kirschner wire through the skin to the distal tuberosity of the scaphoid. Take care to be colinear with the central axis of the scaphoid in both the sagittal and coronal planes. Once the starting point is confirmed, drive the Kirschner wire proximally across the fracture and stop once contact with the proximal pole subchondral bone is made. Alternatively, a 14-gauge angiocatheter needle can be used to localize the starting point and used as a cannula for the guidewire.[21,22] Make a small incision adjacent to the guidewire volarly and protect the superficial palmar branch of the radial artery. Measure the length of compression screw needed by using a depth gauge and subtract 4 to 5 mm to allow for adequate countersinking of the screw without distracting the fracture site. Prior to reaming, advance the guidewire so it exits dorsally in the wrist proximally. Ream over the guidewire and insert the compression screw. Confirm screw placement with live fluoroscopy.

Open Volar Approach

The skin incision overlies the distal flexor carpi radialis (FCR) tendon and is then extended radially in an oblique angle toward the base of the thumb, approximately 3 to 4 cm long. The superficial palmar branch of the radial artery may

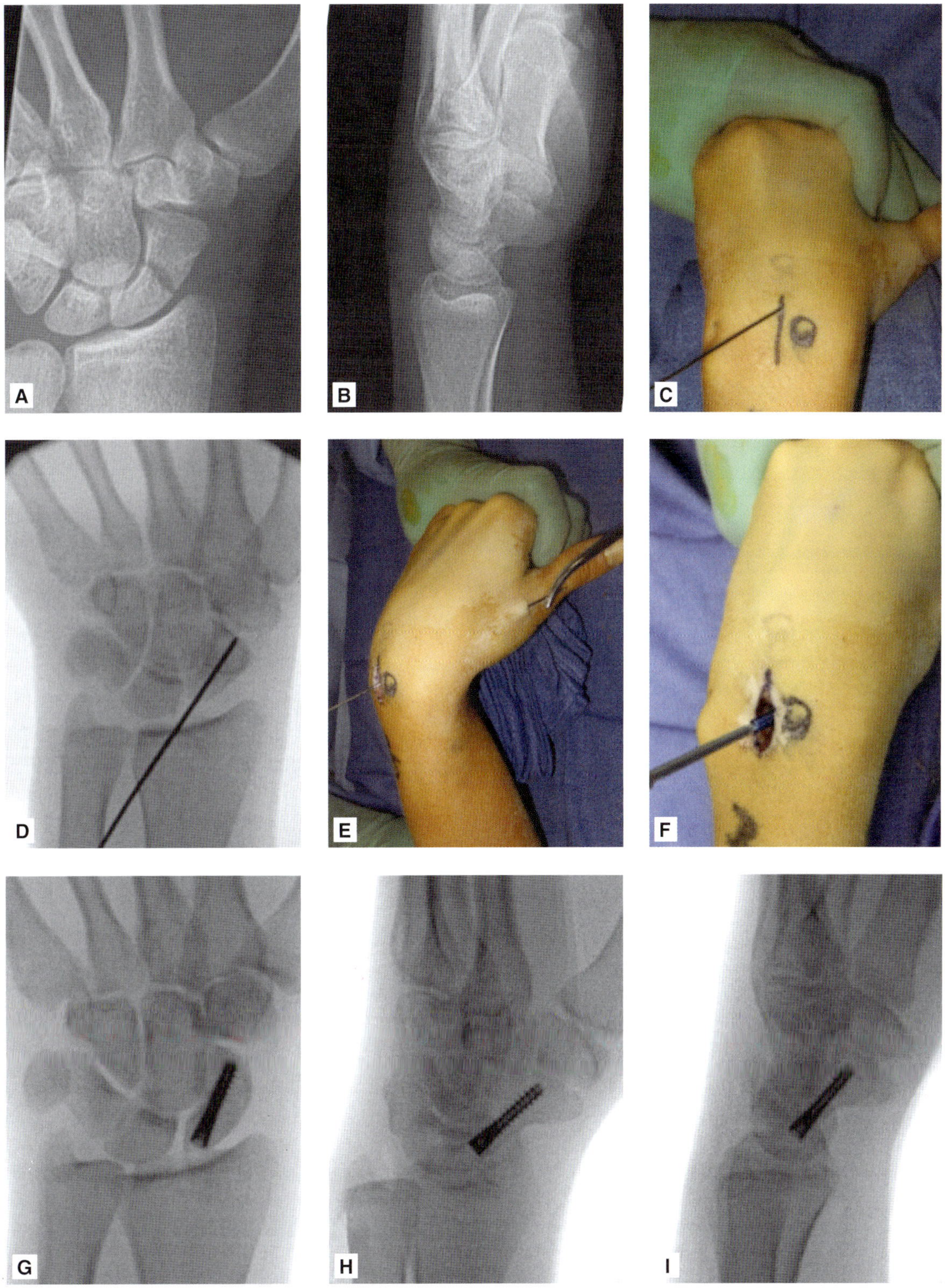

FIGURE 19-1 Operative procedure for dorsal percutaneous technique. **A** and **B.** Preoperative radiographs show minimal displacement and mild resorption at the fracture site. **C.** The start point is identified with the wrist in flexion and ulnar deviation. **D.** The position is checked on C-arm fluoroscopy in at least 2 planes and driven from the proximal fragment into the far cortex and the length is measured. Four to 5 mm is subtracted for the screw length. **E.** The wire is driven through the cortex, trapezium, and skin and clamped to avoid shear, rotation, or migration. The cannulated reamer is passed over the guidewire without passing through the far cortex. **F.** The screw is inserted, capsule repaired, and skin sutured. **G** to **I.** Postoperative radiographs showing central screw placement without penetration and satisfactory alignment of the scaphoid.

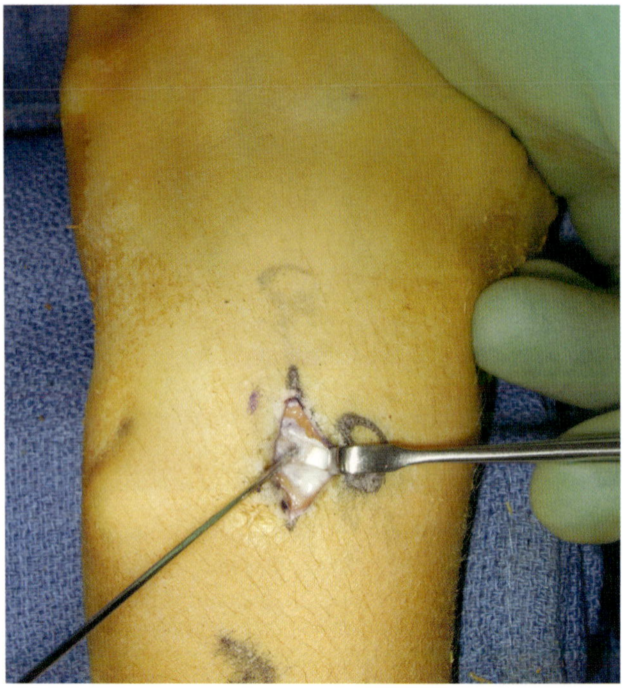

FIGURE 19-2 Intraoperative demonstration of proximity of tendon structures in the dorsal percutaneous technique. The extensor pollicis longus tendon sheath is immediately adjacent to the guide pin. Injury can be avoided by making a small dorsal incision prior to pin placement or spreading with a hemostat to avoid injury.

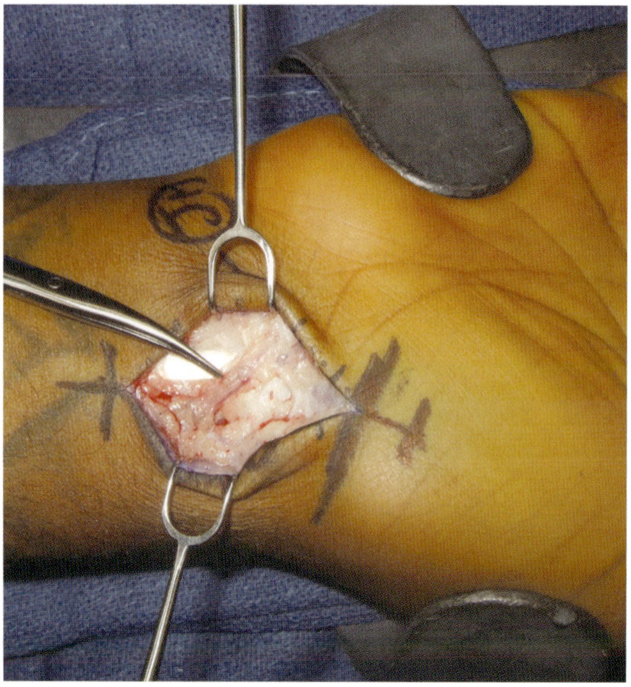

FIGURE 19-3 The volar approach to the scaphoid incision. Also seen is the superficial palmar branch of the radial artery, which may pass through the field of dissection.

be in the surgical field, and this should be protected as possible (see Fig. 19-3). Dissection is carried down through the FCR tendon sheath and the tendon is retracted to expose the base of the tendon sheath. Incise the deep tendon sheath to expose the volar wrist capsule deep to it. The wrist capsule includes the radioscaphocapitate ligament, which crosses the scaphoid waist. Sharp longitudinal division allows for later repair, and the proximal portion should be spared as possible to support the proximal pole. Enter the joint and visualize the scaphoid. Debride the facture site. In the case of a nonunion, it is important to debride all fibrous tissues from the nonunion site to allow intraosseous blood flow after bone grafting and repair.

Fracture reduction can bc achieved manually by extension and ulnar deviation of the wrist, with the use of dental picks or by inserting 0.062-in K-wires as manipulative devices into the fracture fragments (see Figs. 19-4 and 19-5). The lunate can be used to control the proximal fragment if joysticks are used. The distal fragment needs to be extended, supinated, and ulnarly deviated and the proximal fragment flexed to achieve reduction. Bone graft may be inserted at this point to ensure adequate bony contact and restoration of the scaphoid length. The lateral volar angulation of the scaphoid should be around 24°, with >45° being abnormal.[23] Place derotation K-wires to hold the fracture reduction once achieved. Confirm reduction with biplanar fluoroscopy. A rongeur can be used to excise the volar trapezium to expose the appropriate starting point for a guidewire (Fig. 19-4). Insert the guidewire volar to dorsal through the central axis of the scaphoid. Ream, insert the compression screw, and confirm screw position with fluoroscopy. Repair the radiocarpal joint capsule and radioscaphocapitate ligament with 3-0 absorbable sutures.

Open Dorsal Approach

Make a 3- to 4-cm incision beginning proximally over Lister's tubercle, and extending distally in line with the middle finger metacarpal, taking care to protect the branches of the superficial radial nerve. Incise the retinaculum and retract the extensor pollicis longus (EPL) tendon radially along with the extensor carpi radialis brevis and longus (ECRB, ECRL) tendons with ulnar retraction of the finger extensors. Incise the wrist joint capsule through a T-capsulotomy. Flex and ulnarly deviate the wrist to expose the proximal pole of the scaphoid. Debride the fracture or nonunion site bone graft as needed, and fix with multiple K-wires or a headless screw. If multiple passes are made with the guidewire, upsizing to a 0.062-in K-wire prior to drilling may be necessary to ensure accurate screw path.[24] Anchoring guidewires in the far cortex before reaming helps to avoid shearing the wire. Passing guidewires out through skin on both sides facilitates easy removal in the event the wire breaks. Use a soft tissue protector when reaming to avoid damage to the extensor tendons.

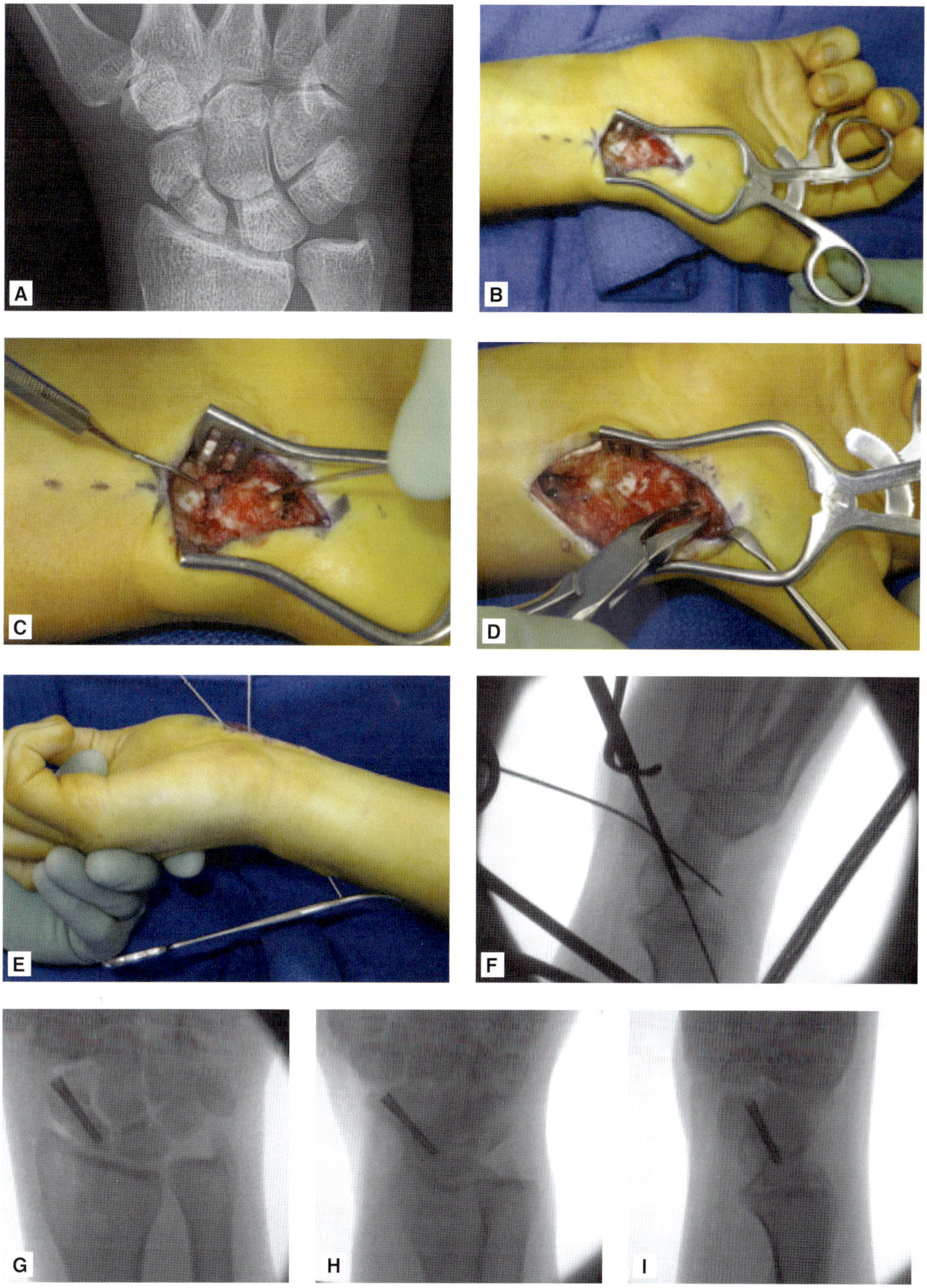

FIGURE 19-4 The open volar approach for established scaphoid nonunion, treated with internal screw fixation and packed cancellous radial autograft. **A.** Preoperative AP radiograph. **B.** The volar approach to the scaphoid. **C.** Joystick manipulation and the dental pick are used to manipulate and debride the nonunion. **D.** A small portion of volar trapezium is excised to gain access for the guide pin. **E.** The guide pin is inserted to the proximal cortex, measured, and then passed through the dorsal skin. This is done for easy removal of the guide pin in the infrequent event the guide pin breaks. The derotation wire is used to flex the scaphoid and gain access for the central guidewire. **F.** The cannulated reamer is passed over the guide pin, while the derotation wire is used to continue to flex the scaphoid, and the screw is inserted. **G** to **I.** Screw position is confirmed on multiplanar imaging, including PA, oblique, and lateral.

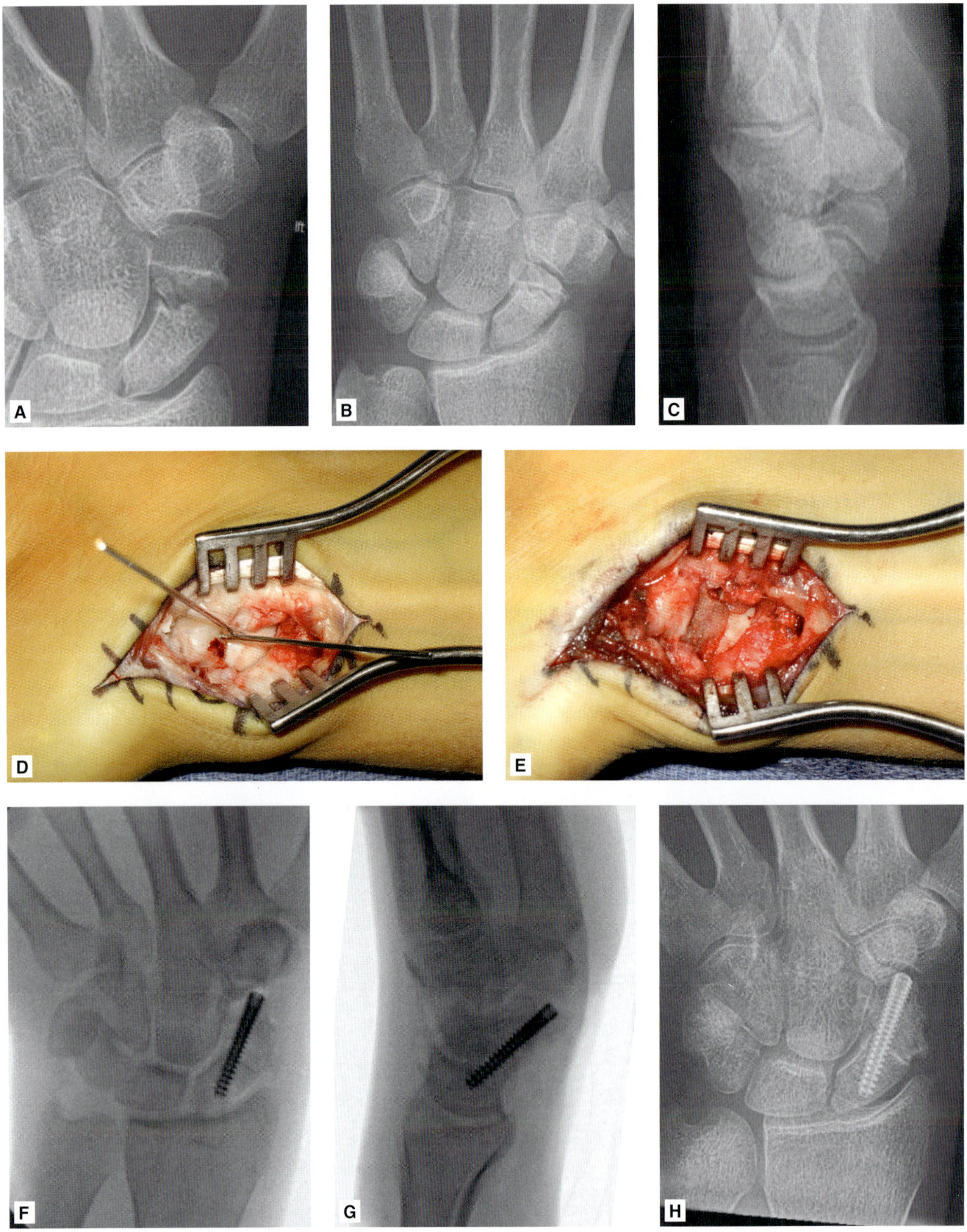

FIGURE 19-5 The open volar approach with structural graft for humpback deformity. **A-C.** Preoperative imaging of the scaphoid nonunion and flexion deformity. **D.** Joystick manipulation and debridement. **E.** Impacted corticocancellous autograft. **F** and **G.** Fluoroscopy images with the screw in place. **H.** Three months postoperative, with clinical and radiographic healing.

Humpback Deformity

A scaphoid nonunion with a humpback deformity is exposed through a volar approach. Insertion of 0.045-in Kirschner wires as joysticks in the proximal and distal poles allows for better visualization and correction of the flexion deformity (see Fig. 19-5). Fluoroscopic imaging is used to assess the degree of deformity of the scaphoid and position of the lunate, and a required size of bone graft. A caliper or a cut paper ruler is invaluable in measuring the dimensions of bone graft. A structural graft can be harvested from the volar aspect of the distal radius by extending the dissection proximally and elevating the pronator quadratus, or a tricortical graft can be obtained from the iliac crest. Aguilella and Garcia-Elias recently described harvesting a structural bone graft from the anterolateral corner of the distal radial metaphysis.[25]

The block is sized and shaped to fill the defect in the scaphoid. The graft is then press-fit into the defect followed by insertion of a derotation 0.045-in K-wire, reaming, and insertion of a headless cannulated screw. A small 0.045-in K-wire can be inserted across the waist to capture and buttress the volar aspect of the bone graft (see Fig. 19-6). This may also be left in place while the fracture heals to prevent translation and volar extrusion of the bone graft.

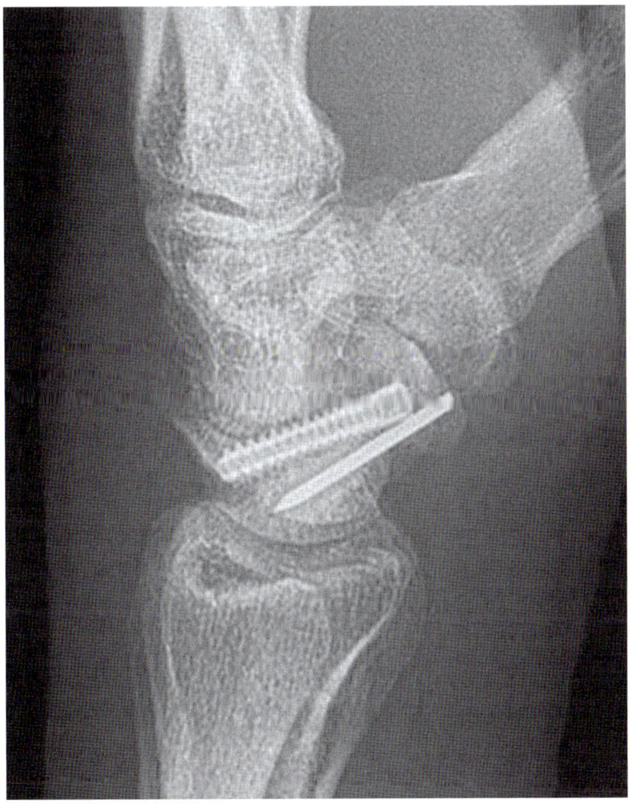

FIGURE 19-6 A volar Kirschner wire is used as a buttress in another patient to maintain the position of corticocancellous graft, in addition to the screw fixation in cancellous bone.

COMPLICATIONS

Complications of operative management of scaphoid fractures include articular screw penetration, loss of fixation, malunion, nonunion, proximal pole osteonecrosis, as well as the general risks of surgery such as infection or anesthetic risks. Percutaneous techniques reduce recovery time and complications, but carry the risk of iatrogenic tendon, nerve, and arterial injury. Vinnars et al reported an increased prevalence in radiographic signs of osteoarthritis involving the STT joint at a mean follow-up of 10 years in 75 patients who had undergone internal fixation via a volar approach of a minimal displaced scaphoid fracture using a Herbert screw.[26] A recent study by Geurts et al of 34 patients who underwent volar percutaneous fixation of acute scaphoid waist fractures via a transtrapezial approach, however, showed no evidence of symptomatic STT arthritis at a mean follow-up of 6.1 years.[27]

OUTCOMES

Modi et al performed a systematic review of the outcome-based literature comparing internal fixation with cast treatment for scaphoid fractures. This review included 3 randomized controlled trials (RCTs) and 2 retrospective reviews specifically comparing percutaneous fixation with cast treatment. This group found that there was a trend toward earlier union, earlier return of grip strength and ROM, and earlier return to work for those who underwent percutaneous fixation.[28] The review by Modi et al also included 3 RCTs comparing ORIF and cast immobilization. Open treatment had similar short-term results to percutaneous treatment methods, allowing for earlier return to work, less time to union, and improved function. Vinnars et al and Davis et al found, in manual laborers, that the total cost of internal fixation was less than that of cast treatment.[26,29] Bond et al found that with percutaneous screw fixation, time to union averaged 7 weeks compared with 12 weeks for cast immobilization, and average time until return to work was 7 weeks earlier.[30] Vinnars et al showed no difference in long-term outcomes at a mean of 10 years, except with a trend toward increased incidence of scaphotrapezial joint arthritis in the operatively treated group.[31]

REFERENCES

1. Suh N, Benson EC, Faber KJ, MacDermind J, Grewal R. Treatment of acute scaphoid fractures: a systematic review and meta-analysis. *Hand*. 2010;5:345–353.
2. Wolf JM, Dawson L, Mountcastle SB, Owens BD. The incidence of scaphoid fracture in a military population. *Injury*. 2009;40:1316–1319.
3. Geissler WB, Adams JE, Bindra RR, Lanzinger WD, Slutsky DJ. Scaphoid fractures: what's hot, what's not. *J Bone Joint Surg Am*. 2012;94(2):169–181.
4. Ring D, Jupiter JB, Herndon JH. Acute fractures of the scaphoid. *J Am Acad Orthop Surg*. 2000;8:225–231.
5. Moritomo H, Murase T, Goto A, Oka K, Sugamoto K, Yoshikawa H. In vivo three-dimensional kinematics of the midcarpal joint of the wrist. *J Bone Joint Surg Am*. 2006;88-A(3):611–621.

6. Gelberman RH, Menon J. The vascularity of the scaphoid bone. *J Hand Surg Am.* 1980;5(5):508–513.
7. Szabo RM, Manske D. Displaced fractures of the scaphoid. *Clin Orthop Relat Res.* 1988;230:30–38.
8. Steinmann SP, Adams JE. Scaphoid fractures and nonunions: diagnosis and treatment. *J Orthop Sci.* 2006;11:424–431.
9. Russe O. Fracture of the carpal navicular: diagnosis, non-operative treatment, and operative treatment. *J Bone Joint Surg Am.* 1960;42:759–768.
10. Cooney WP, Dobyns JH, Linscheid RL. Fractures of the scaphoid: a rational approach to management. *Clin Orthop Relat Res.* 1980;140:90–97.
11. Herbert TJ, Fisher WE. Management of the fractured scaphoid using a new bone screw. *J Bone Joint Surg Br.* 1984;66-B:114–123.
12. Geissler WB, Slade JF. Fractures of the carpal bones. In: Wolfe SW, Hotchkiss RN, Pederson WC, Kozin SH, eds. *Green's Operative Hand Surgery. Sixth Edition.* Philadelphia, PA: Elsevier Churchill Livingstone; 2011 [chapter 18].
13. Clay NR, Dias JJ, Costigan PS, Gregg PJ, Barton NJ. Need the thumb be immobilised in scaphoid fractures? A randomised prospective trial. *J Bone Joint Surg Br.* 1991;73:828–832.
14. Merrell G, Slade J. Technique for percutaneous fixation of displaced and nondisplaced acute scaphoid fractures and select nonunions. *J Hand Surg Am.* 2008;33A:966–973.
15. Wozasek GE, Moser KD. Percutaneous screw fixation for fractures of the scaphoid. *J Bone Joint Surg Br.* 1991;73:138–142.
16. Gutow AP. Percutaneous fixation of scaphoid fractures. *J Am Acad Orthop Surg.* 2007;15:474–485.
17. Kamineni S, Lavy CB. Percutaneous fixation of scaphoid fractures. *J Hand Surg Br.* 1999;24-B(1):85–88.
18. Weinberg AM, Pichler W, Grechenig S, Tesch NP, Heidari N, Grechenig W. The percutaneous antegrade scaphoid fracture fixation—a safe method? *Injury.* 2009;40(6):642–644.
19. McCallister WV, Knight J, Kaliappan R, Trumble TE. Central placement of the screw in simulated fractures of the scaphoid waist. *J Bone Joint Surg Am.* 2003;85-A(1):72–77.
20. Jeon IH, Micic ID, Oh CW, Park BC, Kim PT. Percutaneous screw fixation for scaphoid fracture: a comparison between the dorsal and the volar approaches. *J Hand Surg Am.* 2009;34(2):228–236.
21. Haddad FS, Goddard NJ. Acute percutaneous scaphoid fixation: a pilot study. *J Bone Joint Surg Br.* 1998;80:95–99.
22. Zlotolow DA, Knutsen E, Yao J. Optimization of volar percutaneous screw fixation for scaphoid waist fractures using traction, positioning, imaging, and an angiocatheter guide. *J Hand Surg Am.* 2011;36(5):916–921.
23. Trumble TE, Gilbert M, Murray LW, Smith J, Rafijah G, McCallister WV. Displaced scaphoid fractures treated with open reduction and internal fixation with a cannulated screw. *J Bone Joint Surg Am.* 2000;82-A(5):633–641.
24. Slade JF III, Gutow AP, Geissler WB. Percutaneous internal fixation of scaphoid fractures via an arthroscopically assisted dorsal approach. *J Bone Joint Surg Am.* 2002;84(suppl 2):21–36.
25. Aguilella L, Garcia-Elias M. The anterolateral corner of the radial metaphysis as a source of bone graft for the treatment of scaphoid nonunion. *J Hand Surg Am.* 2012;37:1258–1262.
26. Vinnars B, Ekenstam FA, Gerdin B. Comparison of direct and indirect costs of internal fixation and cast treatment in acute scaphoid fractures: a randomized trial involving 52 patients. *Acta Orthop.* 2007;78(5):672–679.
27. Geurts G, van Riet R, Meermans G, Verstreken F. Incidence of scaphotrapezial arthritis following volar percutaneous fixation of nondisplaced scaphoid waist fractures using a transtrapezial approach. *J Hand Surg Am.* 2011;36:1753–1758.
28. Modi CS, Nancoo T, Powers D, Ho K, Boer R, Turner SM. Operative versus nonoperative treatment of acute undisplaced and minimally displaced scaphoid waist fractures—a systematic review. *Injury.* 2009;40:268–273.
29. Davis EN, Chung KC, Kotsis SV, Lau FH, Vijan S. A cost/utility analysis of open reduction and internal fixation versus cast immobilization for acute nondisplaced mid-waist scaphoid fractures. *Plast Reconstr Surg.* 2006;117(4):1223–1235.
30. Bond CD, Shin AY, McBride MT, Dao KD. Percutaneous screw fixation or cast immobilization for nondisplaced scaphoid fractures. *J Bone Joint Surg Am.* 2001;83-A(4):483–488.
31. Vinnars B, Pietreanu M, Bodestedt A, Ekenstam FA, Gerdin B. Nonoperative compared with operative treatment of acute scaphoid fractures: a randomized clinical trial. *J Bone Joint Surg Am.* 2008;90-A(6):1176–1185.

20

Pedicled Vascularized Bone Grafts for Scaphoid Nonunion

David J. Slutsky, MD

INTRODUCTION

The emergence of vascularized bone grafts (VBGs) has changed the treatment of scaphoid nonunion. Their use can lead to a faster rate of union, and improve the viability of the proximal pole. They can also provide an alternative to a salvage procedure with previously failed conventional bone grafting. A variety of pedicled grafts from the dorsal and volar aspects of the distal radius have been described, as well as a pedicled graft from the thumb metacarpal. This chapter will describe these grafts along with their attributes and potential uses.

The emergence of vascularized bone grafts (VBGs) has changed the treatment of scaphoid nonunion. Their use can lead to a faster rate of union, and improve the viability of the proximal pole. They can also provide an alternative to a salvage procedure with previously failed conventional bone grafting. A variety of pedicled grafts from the dorsal and volar aspects of the distal radius have been described, as well as a pedicled graft from the thumb metacarpal. Free VBGs provide an additional option but will not be discussed in this chapter.

INDICATIONS

The following are some general indications for the use of VBGs, although it is of note that some authors use this type of graft for any scaphoid nonunion:

1. Avascular necrosis (AVN) of the proximal pole
2. Symptomatic proximal pole nonunion
3. Displaced proximal pole fractures
4. Failed traditional bone grafting

ABSOLUTE CONTRAINDICATIONS

The following constitute contraindications to the use of pedicle flaps based on the radius and thumb metacarpal:

1. Radiocarpal and midcarpal arthritis due to scaphoid nonunion advanced collapse (SNAC) wrist, stage II/III, that is, radiocarpal/midcarpal arthritis
2. Damage to the radial artery, first dorsal metacarpal artery (FDMA), or dorsal carpal arch

Relative contraindications to the procedure include previous surgery on or injury to the dorsal aspect of the wrist or distal radius, which might impair the blood supply to the dorsal capsule. Proceed carefully in smokers.

VBG WITH 1,2 INTERCOMPARTMENTAL SUPRARETINACULAR ARTERY (ICSRA)

In 1991 Zaidemberg et al described a pedicled VBG source from the dorsoradial aspect of the radius based on an ascending irrigating branch of the radial artery.[1] His group reported a 100% union rate in 11 patients with a scaphoid nonunion treated with this graft, at an average time to union of 6.2 weeks. The blood supply to the dorsal aspect of the carpus has been extensively described by Sheetz et al.[2] They described a number of pedicles from which potential VBGs may be harvested from the dorsum of the distal radius. The most common of these pedicles is the 1,2 ICSRA (aka ascending irrigating branch of the radial artery).

Anatomy

The 1,2 ICSRA branches from radial artery at an average of 1.9 mm proximal to the styloid (−6.3 to 3.2 mm). The internal diameter of the vessel averages 0.30 mm (0.14-0.58). The pedicle length averages 22.5 mm (15-31). The graft is located at 1 mm (8-18) proximal to articular surface where it incorporates largest number of perforators.

Pros/Cons

This graft can be used as an onlay graft to act as a vascular pedicle or a structural strut graft to maintain the scaphoid length. It has a constant artery with a long pedicle. Because it is rotated 180°, the pedicle is vulnerable to kinking. Dissection of the pedicle can be tedious and impingement and thrombosis of the pedicle over the radial styloid can occur over the radial styloid when attempting to pass the graft volarly. If this is attempted, it is prudent to perform a limited radial styloidectomy to decrease tension on the pedicle and facilitate volar passage.

Surgical Approach

The procedure is done under loupe magnification. The arm is elevated for 2 minutes rather than exsanguinated in order to visualize the arterial pedicle. The arm is abducted 90° with a proximal tourniquet inflated to 250 mm Hg. An S-shaped dorsoradial incision is made starting distally over the scaphoid, curving proximally over the fourth extensor compartment. The skin and subcutaneous tissue are elevated as a single layer over the extensor compartment while protecting the superficial radial nerve branches. The 1,2 ICSRA can be identified running proximally and superficially down a longitudinal ridge that separates the first and second extensor compartments. Two parallel longitudinal incisions are made at least 5 mm apart along the radial and ulnar sides of the 1,2 ICRSA. The bone graft is outlined over the radial metaphysis 1.5 to 2.0 cm proximal to the radial styloid after retracting the extensor pollicis brevis (EPB) and abductor pollicis longus (APL) radially and the extensor carpi radialis longus (ECRL) and brevis ulnarly.

A longitudinal capsulotomy is now made over the scaphoid and the nonunion is exposed. An undisplaced fibrous nonunion is curetted to remove all fibrous tissue, taking care not to destabilize the fragments. When there is an avascular proximal, the necrotic bone should be removed down to the subchondral bone supporting the articular surface. While keeping the wrist flexed, 1 volar guidewire and 1 dorsal K-wire are placed down the longitudinal scaphoid axis under fluoroscopic control. When the VBG is used as an onlay graft, a small (2.5-3.2 mm) cannulated headless screw is first inserted over the volar guidewire in order to provide provisional fixation of the nonunion and so as to not interfere with the VBG onlay (Fig. 20-1A-E). The dorsal K-wire is advanced distally and prepositioned in the distal fragment in preparation for capturing the onlay graft. A 1 cm^2 defect is outlined with an osteotome at right angles to the nonunion site and removed.

A slightly oversized graft, centered over the 1,2 ICSRA pedicle, is then osteotomized to a depth of 8 mm on its radial, ulnar, and distal aspects after the pedicle is ligated at the proximal edge. The distal portion of the pedicle is mobilized subperiosteally off the dorsal surface of the radius along with a cuff of retinaculum. A curved osteotome is then placed at the proximal osteotomy site and used to gently pry the graft from the radial metaphysis. The pedicle with its periosteal and retinacular cuff is completely separated from the radius and joint capsule. The graft is rotated 180° and press-fit into the dorsal defect over the nonunion site and held in place by driving the dorsal K-wire proximally. The capsule is closed without any compression or tension on the pedicle. The tourniquet can be released to check flap vascularity at this point and achieve hemostasis prior to skin closure. Postoperatively the wrist is immobilized in a thumb spica splint that is changed to a cast until there are radiographic signs of union that is confirmed by a CT scan at 3 to 4 months.

In the case of scaphoid collapse a useful technique is to volar flex the wrist until the lunate is corrected to a neutral alignment with respect to the radius. A 0.045-in K-wire is driven from the radius into the corrected lunate. The wrist is then brought into extension. A second 0.045-in K-wire can then be placed from the distal pole into the capitate to maintain the reduction of the distal pole prior to placement of the bone graft.

Outcomes

Chang et al[3] reported on the use of the 1,2 ICSRA VBG in 50 scaphoid nonunions in 49 patients. The average age was 24 years (range 14-66 years). The duration of the scaphoid nonunion averaged 23 months (range, 2-156 months). The average follow-up was 7.8 months (range, 2-49 months). Thirty-four scaphoid nonunions healed at an average of 15.6 weeks after surgery (range, 8-40 weeks). Prior surgery did not affect the outcomes in that 7/11 with prior surgery and 27/37 without prior surgery healed. The presence of AVN was a highly significant factor with a union rate of only 50% (12/24) regardless of whether previous surgery had been performed. The presence of a humpback deformity was also a poor prognostic factor for union. The authors concluded that scaphoid nonunions with severe bone loss due to a humpback deformity and patients with severe scapholunate dissociation and/or small or collapsed proximal fragments should be treated with other means. Waitayawinyu et al[4] had better outcomes in 30 patients with scaphoid nonunions (19 waist, 11 proximal poles with AVN) and no prior surgery who were treated with the 1,2 ICSRA graft. Their procedure differed in that a radial styloidectomy was routinely performed in order to diminish tension on the pedicle and all nonunions were stabilized with a cannulated screw.

The union rate was 93% (28/30 nonunions) with an average time to union of 5.1 months. The 2 failures had the highest scapholunate angle and went on to eventual union 11 and 13 months after conventional bone grafting.

VOLAR CARPAL ARTERY VASCULARIZED BONE GRAFT

Anatomy

This VBG was initially described by Kuhlmann et al[5] and recently popularized by Mathoulin et al.[6] The VBG is harvested from the volar ulnar metaphysis of the distal radius. It is nourished by the volar carpal artery that has a diameter of 0.5 to 1.0 mm. This artery originates from the radial artery at

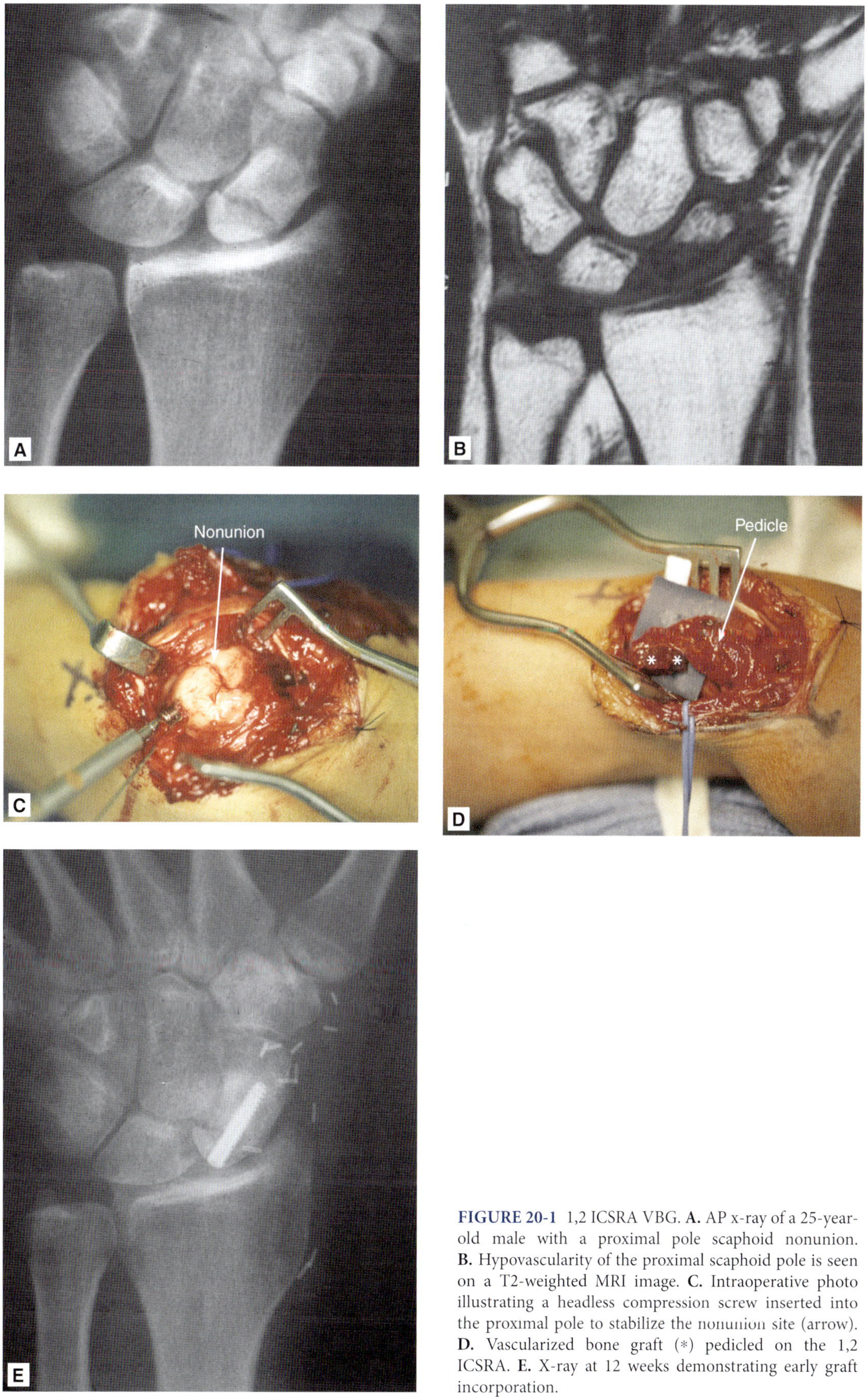

FIGURE 20-1 1,2 ICSRA VBG. **A.** AP x-ray of a 25-year-old male with a proximal pole scaphoid nonunion. **B.** Hypovascularity of the proximal scaphoid pole is seen on a T2-weighted MRI image. **C.** Intraoperative photo illustrating a headless compression screw inserted into the proximal pole to stabilize the nonunion site (arrow). **D.** Vascularized bone graft (*) pedicled on the 1,2 ICSRA. **E.** X-ray at 12 weeks demonstrating early graft incorporation.

the level of the radial styloid, and then traverses the palmar aspect of the distal radius along the distal edge of pronator quadratus (PQ). It forms a "T"-shaped anastomosis with the anterior interosseous artery. The average pedicle length is 3 cm (2-4.6 cm).[7]

Pros/Cons

This VBG has a long pedicle that is consistently present and harvesting the volar carpal artery does not interfere with the dorsal blood supply. It is ideal for scaphoid nonunions with a humpback deformity since the volar approach provides good access to the nonunion site for debridement and simplifies the insertion of a volar wedge-shaped graft to restore scaphoid height. It is a small graft, however, and technically difficult to raise. It cannot be used for nonunions of the distal one third. Since it is immediately adjacent to the radiocarpal joint, there is the risk of fracture into the radiocarpal joint or the sigmoid notch.

Surgical Approach

A 6-cm volar radial longitudinal incision is made under tourniquet control to expose the distal radius extending over the base of the thumb. The plane between the flexor carpi radialis and the radial artery is developed and an oblique capsulotomy is performed to expose the volar scaphoid. Fibrous scar tissue is debrided and necrotic bone at the fracture site is curetted until healthy bone is identified and punctate bleeding is seen. The scaphoid fragments are pried apart with an osteotome and pulled out to length with thumb traction. The bony defect is now measured. Transverse K-wires from the scaphoid fragments to the lunate and capitate can be used to temporarily maintain the reduction. If a dorsal intercalated segmental instability (DISI) deformity is present, the lunate can be flexed to neutral and held with a dorsal K-wire through the radius. The scaphoid fragments are then stabilized with longitudinal K-wires or a headless screw, which is placed as dorsally as possible for graft insetting.

The bone graft is harvested by flexing the wrist to relax the flexor tendons and the distal border of the PQ muscle is exposed. Parallel incisions are made 1 cm proximal to the distal border of the PQ and 2 to 3 mm distal to it. A scalpel and periosteal elevator are then used to detach a strip of the PQ muscle and periosteum that contains the volar carpal artery. The bone graft is harvested from the volar ulnar metaphysis. The radial border of the bone graft is first osteotomized using a 1-cm osteotome. The proximal and distal borders of the bone graft are then osteotomized in an oblique direction to form a wedge shape followed by the ulnar border. The bone graft is levered from the distal radius taking care to protect the pedicle. The distal strip of PQ muscle can be dissected as far laterally as the radial artery to allow a pedicle length of up to 5 cm (Fig. 20-2A-D). The graft is rotated and positioned within the scaphoid defect and held with a second prepositioned longitudinal K-wire. Any bone gaps may be filled with additional cancellous bone graft harvested from the distal radius. The position of the screw and fragments is checked fluoroscopically. The joint capsule is repaired while protecting the pedicle. The wrist is immobilized for a minimum of 6 weeks and an average of 10 weeks followed by wrist motion exercises.

Outcomes

Mathoulin and Fairbank[8] reported the largest series of 102 patients with scaphoid nonunions who were treated with this graft, aged 31 years (15-61). One-third of the patients had previous failed surgery. Twenty percent involved the proximal pole and 80% were waist fractures. Fifty-nine cases were Herbert stage D2; 43 were stage D. The median delay to surgery was 12.5 months (4-120), with a mean length of follow-up of 29 months. Union was achieved in 94% of the patients, with an average time to union of 9.5 weeks. Wrist flexion and extension improved by 22%, radial deviation by 40%, and ulnar deviation by 30%. Grip strength improved from 54% to 92%. The postoperative modified Mayo wrist score was good or excellent in 89%.

Dailiana et al[9] reported on a much smaller series of 9 waist nonunions. There was a 22-month delay to surgery with a mean follow-up of 24 months. One hundred percent union was achieved between 6 and 12 weeks. The Mayo modified wrist score increased from 63 to 92 with 5 excellent and 4 good results.

CAPSULAR-BASED VBG

Anatomy

This VBG, which was described by Sotereanos et al,[10] is an axial pattern flap based on fourth extracompartment artery (ECA) of the dorsal carpal arch, which extends between the anterior or postinterosseous artery proximally and the dorsal carpal arch or fifth ECA distally. The average pedicle diameter is 0.4 mm. The pedicle length ranges between 1 and 2 cm and easily reaches the proximal one-third of the scaphoid.

Pros/Cons

The VBG is based on a constant artery and the flap is easy to dissect. The graft only needs to rotate 10° to 30° on the pedicle to reach the scaphoid that lowers the risk of arterial kinking. A disadvantage is that it has a relatively short pedicle; hence, the graft is only useful for proximal one-third nonunions. It can be used as an onlay graft only and there is the risk of a radiocarpal articular fracture.

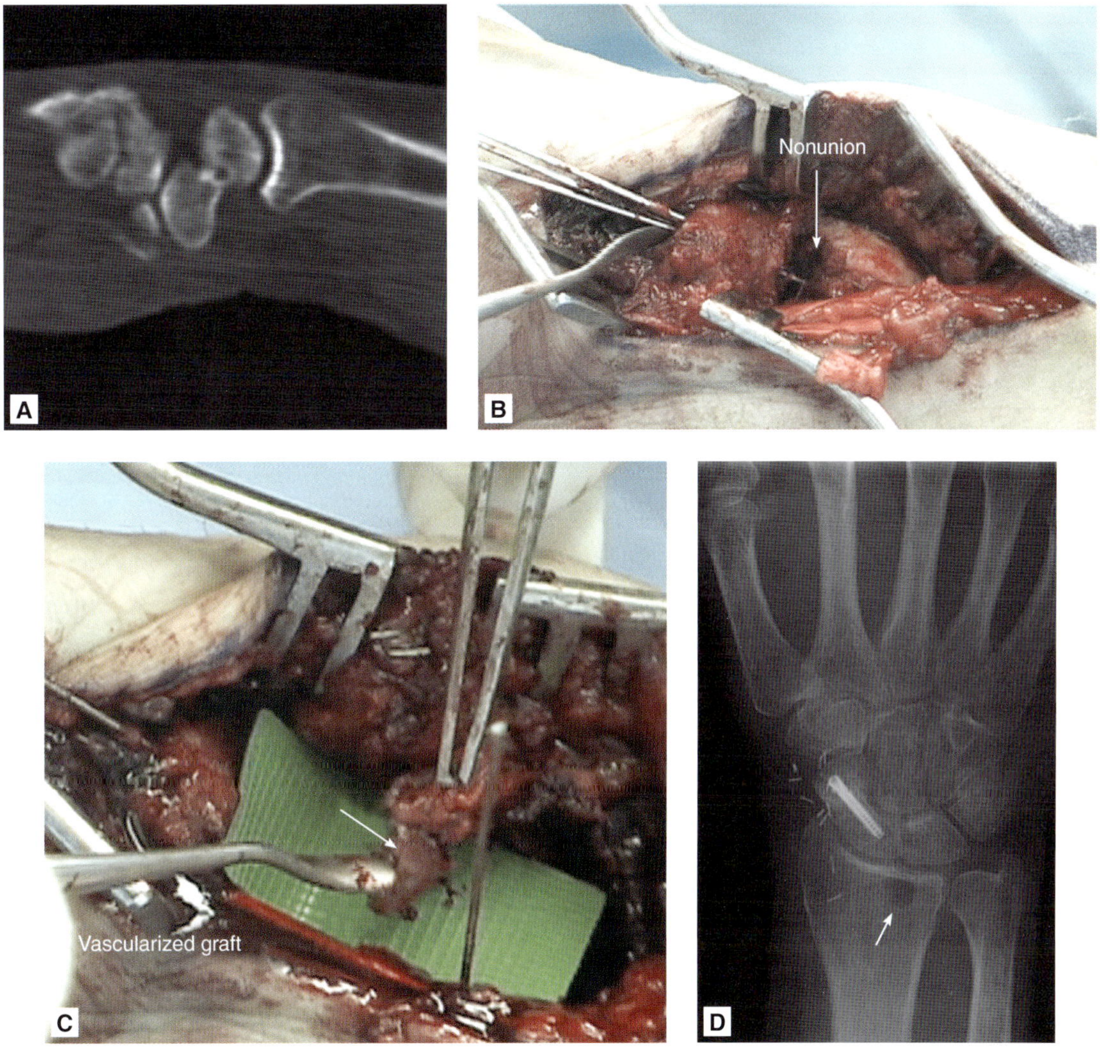

FIGURE 20-2 Volar carpal VBG. **A.** Lateral CT scan demonstrating a scaphoid waist nonunion with volar collapse. **B.** Volar aspect of the right wrist showing the scaphoid nonunion site is distracted, with preplaced K-wires in the distal pole (upper left). **C.** Volar VBG (arrow) is elevated on the volar carpal artery pedicle held by the forceps. **D.** AP x-ray of the healed nonunion. Note the donor-site defect in the volar ulnar metaphysis (arrow).

Surgical Approach

A dorsal incision is made under tourniquet control, just ulnar to Lister's tubercle. The fourth dorsal compartment is partially released to expose the wrist capsule and the distal radius. The extensor pollicis longus tendon is identified and retracted radially and the extensor digitorum communis tendons are retracted ulnarly. A trapezoidal capsular flap is outlined that is 2 cm in length and it widens from 1 cm at the bone block to 1.5 cm at its distal base. A 1 × 1 cm capsular-based vascularized distal radius graft, approximately 7 mm deep, is harvested from the distal aspect of the dorsal radius just ulnar and distal to Lister's tubercle using osteotomes. A 2- to 3-mm ridge of the distal radial cortex is left intact to minimize the risk of propagation onto the articular cartilage of the radiocarpal joint. The capsular flap is outlined sharply with a knife and elevated along with the bone graft in a proximodistal direction. Care should be taken to prevent detachment of the dorsal scapholunate ligament.

The scaphoid nonunion is now exposed. Two 1.0-mm Kirschner wires are inserted from the proximal pole of the scaphoid oriented toward the base of the thumb, with the wrist flexed. One of these serves as a guidewire for a cannulated screw and the other as an antirotation wire. Care is taken to place the guidewire for the screw perpendicular to the fracture site and as volar as possible, while maintaining sufficient purchase of the proximal and distal fragments. This guidewire should be also in a slight ulnar position so there is enough space for a bone anchor. The length of the screw is determined by measuring it next to an intact K-wire, followed by drilling and insertion of a headless cannulated screw or 2 K-wires. Once the fracture nonunion is secured, the nonunion site is debrided with a small curette, and a dorsal trough is created across the nonunion site taking care to avoid destabilizing the fragments. If the proximal pole fragment is too small to accommodate a trough, the graft can be inset into the excavated cavity of the proximal fragment. The bone graft is rotated 10° to 30° and inset into the trough. Sotereanos uses a bone anchor inserted just radial to the cannulated screw in the floor of the trough to tie down the VBG with 3-0 suture to prevent graft extrusion (Fig. 20-3A-E). After wound closure a short arm thumb spica cast is applied for 6 weeks followed by a splint until union.

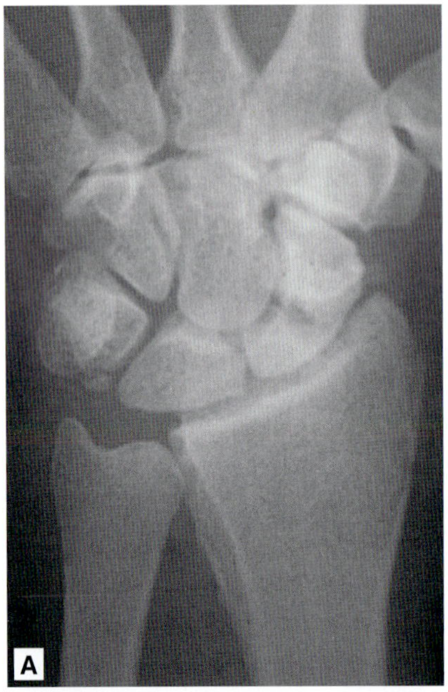

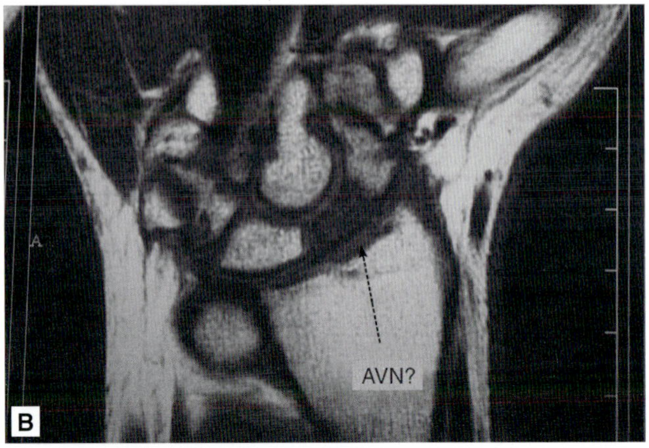

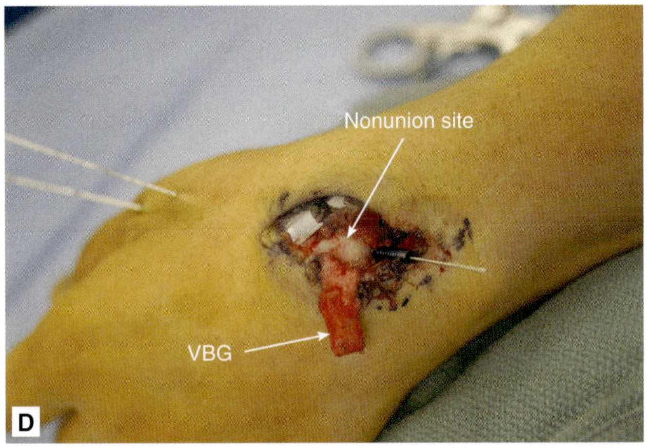

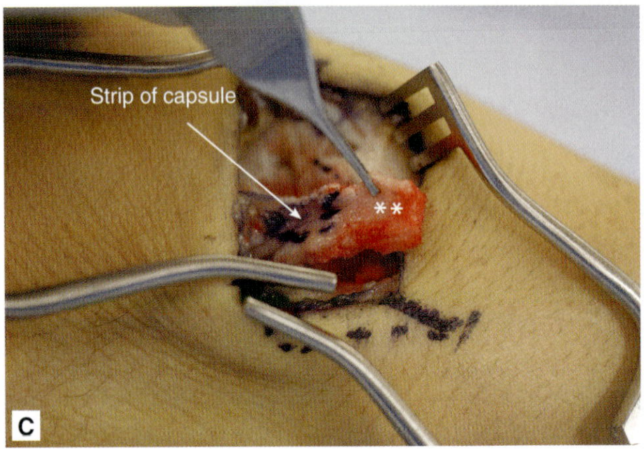

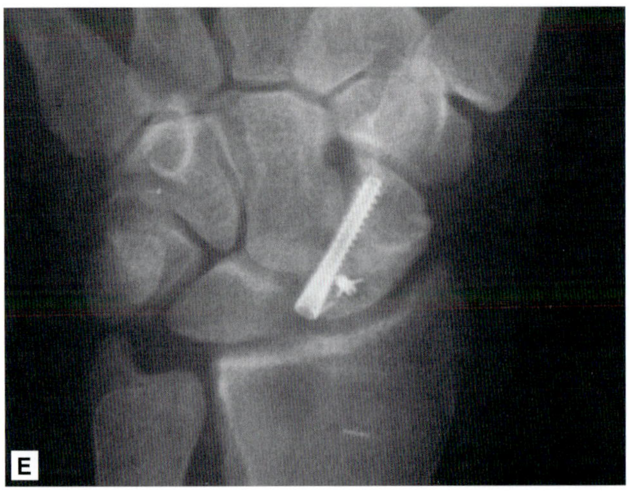

FIGURE 20-3 Dorsal capsular-based VBG. **A.** Nonunion at the junction of the proximal/middle third of the scaphoid. **B.** Hypovascularity of the proximal scaphoid pole is seen on a T2-weighted MRI image. **C.** Dorsal view of a left wrist showing a vascularized bone graft (*) pedicled on a strip of dorsal capsule (arrow). **D.** Intraoperative photo illustrating the proximity of the capsular graft (VBG) to the nonunion site while a headless compression screw is inserted into the proximal pole to stabilize the nonunion site. **E.** AP x-ray demonstrating the relative ulnar position of the headless screw and the bone anchor that is used to prevent graft extrusion.

Outcomes

Sotereanos et al[10] reported on their experience with this VBG in 13 patients, 10 of whom had AVN. The minimum follow-up was 1 year. Union was achieved in 10/13 patients by 13 weeks (range 6-23) weeks. Eight of the 10 patients with AVN went on to union. Wrist flexion averaged 45° versus 32° preoperatively, and extension averaged 68° versus 44°. The mean grip strength was 81% postoperatively versus 64% preoperatively.

VASCULARIZED THUMB METACARPAL GRAFT

Anatomy

This VBG, as described by Bertelli et al,[11] is based on the radial branch of the FDMA. The average vessel diameter is 1 mm. The pedicle arises from the radial artery 5 to 10 mm proximal to the trapeziometacarpal joint and continues along radial third of the dorsal side of the thumb metacarpal. The VBG is harvested from the metacarpal head giving a pedicle length of approximately 50 mm.

Pros/Cons

The pedicle can be quite long and is based on a constant artery. It can be used as an onlay or structural graft. The pedicle is rotated 180° that can lead to kinking. It has a large donor-site defect that can lead to fracture and it is technically difficult.

Surgical Approach

A nonunion that involves the distal pole or waist of the scaphoid is approached from the palmar aspect. The surgical incision is made over the flexor carpi radialis and along the junction of the palmar and dorsal skin over the thenar eminence. Once the nonunion is identified, all nonviable bone and fibrous tissue is removed. The wrist is flexed to correct the dorsal deviation of the lunate, and the lunate is temporally pinned to the radius. Then, the wrist is extended and ulnar deviated, and the bone defect measured.

The VBG is harvested by opening the EPB tendon sheath and retracting the EPB ulnarwards. The FDMA is identified and followed to the metacarpal head. A trapezoidal bone graft is harvested that is centered on the FDMA. Two fascial incisions are performed, 3 mm ulnar and radial to the FDMA. The radial incision is made along the margins of the APL. The fascial plane, which contains the FDMA and venae comitantes, is dissected off the periosteum. A VBG that is 10 mm long, 5 mm wide, and 3 mm in depth is elevated with osteotomies. This corresponds to one-third to two-thirds of the metacarpal head. A 2-cm wide tunnel down to the tendinous insertion of the APL is created. The graft then is passed underneath the EPB and APL and passed in a palmar direction toward the scaphoid defect. The VBG is placed transversally in the bone defect and press-fit into place. The vascular pedicle lies radially. The scaphoid is fixed with 2 K-wires, excluding the graft. The vascular pedicle then is inspected to detect any kinks, compression, or tension. The capsular flaps are loosely approximated and the subcutaneous layer and skin sutured.

A nonunion of the proximal pole is approached dorsally. A vertical incision along Lister's tubercle allows access to the nonunion, which is resected with a drill. A cavity is created in the proximal pole, creating 2- to 3-mm thick ulnar and radial columns. The cavity then is extended along the scaphoid dorsal rim. The scaphoid is fixed with 2 K-wires that pass from the scaphoid dorsal rim into the radial and ulnar proximal pole columns. The VBG is harvested through a separate thumb incision, matching the dimensions of the cavity. The graft is designed as distal as possible near the metacarpal head to provide a longer pedicle. A large tunnel is dissected down to the wrist extensors. The graft is passed over the radial artery and under the second extensor compartment toward the scaphoid defect. Additional cancellous graft from the radius is packed into the scaphoid defect. The thumb VBG is placed over the cancellous graft layer and impacted into the proximal pole-dorsal rim cavity. The capsular flaps are loosely approximated and the wound is closed. A below-elbow cast, including the thumb, is used for 8 to 12 weeks or until signs of union.

Outcomes

The series of Bertelli et al[12] included 57 scaphoid nonunions, 27 of which were present for more than 5 years. Twenty cases involved the proximal pole. The ages ranged from 18 to 51 years. Union was achieved in 53/57 patients (93%) at 12 months. The pinch and grip improved by an average of 20%. Wrist motion improved by 10% to 15%. The pain levels decreased by 70%. They did note that the functional results were better for nonunions that had been present for less than 2 years.

REFERENCES

1. Zaidemberg C, Siebert JW, Angrigiani C. A new vascularized bone graft for scaphoid nonunion. *J Hand Surg Am.* 1991;16:474–478.
2. Sheetz KK, Bishop AT, Berger RA. The arterial blood supply of the distal radius and ulna and its potential use in vascularized pedicled bone grafts. *J Hand Surg Am.* 1995;20:902–914.
3. Chang MA, Bishop AT, Moran SL, Shin AY. The outcomes and complications of 1,2-intercompartmental supraretinacular artery pedicled vascularized bone grafting of scaphoid nonunions. *J Hand Surg Am.* 2006;31:387–396.
4. Waitayawinyu T, McCallister WV, Katolik LI, Schlenker JD, Trumble TE. Outcome after vascularized bone grafting of scaphoid nonunions with avascular necrosis. *J Hand Surg Am.* 2009;34:387–394.
5. Kuhlmann JN, Mimoun M, Boabighi A, Baux S. Vascularized bone graft pedicled on the volar carpal artery for non-union of the scaphoid. *J Hand Surg Br.* 1987;12:203–210.

6. Mathoulin C, Haerle M, Vandeputte G. Vascularized bone graft in carpal bone reconstruction. *Ann Chir Plast Esthet.* 2005;50:43–48.
7. Haerle M, Schaller HE, Mathoulin C. Vascular anatomy of the palmar surfaces of the distal radius and ulna: its relevance to pedicled bone grafts at the distal palmar forearm. *J Hand Surg Br.* 2003;28:131–136.
8. Mathoulin C, Fairbank SM. The volar carpal artery vascularized bone graft for scaphoid nonunion. In: Slutsky DJ, Slade J III, eds. *The Scaphoid.* New York, Stuttgart: Thieme Medical Inc; 2010:225–231.
9. Dailiana ZH, Malizos KN, Zachos V, et al. Vascularized bone grafts from the palmar radius for the treatment of waist nonunions of the scaphoid. *J Hand Surg Am.* 2006;31:397–404.
10. Sotereanos DG, Darlis NA, Dailiana ZH, Sarris IK, Malizos KN. A capsular-based vascularized distal radius graft for proximal pole scaphoid pseudarthrosis. *J Hand Surg Am.* 2006;31:580–587.
11. Bertelli JA, Tacca CP, Rost JR. Thumb metacarpal vascularized bone graft in long-standing scaphoid nonunion—a useful graft via dorsal or palmar approach: a cohort study of 24 patients. *J Hand Surg Am.* 2004;29:1089–1097.
12. Bertelli JA, Tacca CP, Rost JR. Thumb metacarpal vascularized bone grafts. In: Slutsky DJ, Slade J III, eds. *The Scaphoid.* New York, Stuttgart: Thieme Medical Inc; 2010:232–242.

Acute Perilunate Dislocations and Fracture–Dislocations

21

Guillaume Herzberg, MD, PhD

INTRODUCTION

Perilunate dislocations and fracture–dislocations (PLD-PLFD) are high-energy carpal injuries.[1] They belong to the group of carpal dislocations (Fig. 21-1) that include also radiocarpal, carpometacarpal, and axial dislocations/fracture–dislocations.[2] Most typically PLD-PLFD result from a fall from a height in young males in their second or third decade. They represent only 7% of all carpal injuries.[3] For this reason, there are few series in the literature but still a large number of case reports.[4–6] Diagnosis of the path of the injury is of paramount importance because surgical repair should address each component of that "trauma line."[7] During the last years, there has been a great deal of literature regarding new aspects of their diagnosis and treatment. In the past, there were as many as 25% missed perilunate injuries. This is not the case anymore thanks to medical education and we will focus on acute perilunate injuries. Despite the severity of the injury, very acceptable results can be obtained in most cases if an appropriate treatment is provided at the acute period. There is evidence in the literature that closed reduction and cast is not a reliable treatment and should not be recommended.[8,9] Series using closed reduction and cast to treat PLD-PLFD have an unacceptable failure rate in terms of quality of reduction and outcome.[10] But a poor surgical treatment at the acute stage leads also to an irreparable situation with severe functional sequelae and posttraumatic arthritis.[2,7] Because these are very rare injuries, each surgeon's experience is limited. This is why surgeons should be prepared to understand any form of PLD-PLFD. Only an understanding of the whole extent of the path of injury will allow appropriate repairs. The purpose of this chapter is to provide a comprehensive update about these rare and complex injuries.

DIAGNOSIS AND CLASSIFICATION

Ninety percent of PLD-PLFD are closed injuries.[11–13] A typical open PLD-PLFD shows the lunate partially or totally extruded through a palmar wound.[14,15] Closed PLD-PLFD seen at the acute period usually show painful deformity and swelling of the wrist. Paresthesia in the median nerve territory is observed in about 1 of 3 cases and this finding should be recorded and followed. A comprehensive classification of perilunate injuries is based on plain and traction radiographs (Fig. 21-2). CT scan may be helpful in some difficult cases (Fig. 21-3) or in unusual variants in order to provide a focus on unclear radiographic features.

Standard PA and lateral radiographs are obtained in emergency. The PA view shows a marked derangement of the proximal carpal row with significant loss of carpal height, carpal bone overlaps, intercarpal gaps, and breaks in Gilula proximal row lines. The lateral view shows the main defining feature of PLD-PLFD, that is, complete volar or most often dorsal dislocation of the lunate from the capitate. The lunate itself may be partially or completely dislocated from the radius most often in a volar direction. Because any carpal dislocation may sustain several chronological sequences in its displacement (eg, forceful extension followed by carpal bone dislocation/enucleation from a reverse movement plus compression) and because partial spontaneous reduction may occur, there is no parallelism between the initial radiological displacement and the pathology.

Ten-pound PA traction radiographs under anesthesia or analgesia are invaluable in providing a thorough understanding of the path of the injury because they eliminate bone overlapping and suggest which ligaments are torn and which fractures should be fixed. The lateral traction views show the amount of reduction that is obtained.

Standard and traction radiographs define the path of trauma and the amount of displacement of the capitate and lunate. The injury line may be strictly perilunar in a pure ligamentous PLD or lesser arc of Johnson[16] or may have fractured the radial styloid, scaphoid, capitate, or triquetrum in the many PLFD variants of the greater arc of Johnson. The injury progresses most often from radial to ulnar as described by Mayfield[17] but occasionally from ulnar to radial as described by Viegas et al.[18–20] In most perilunar injuries, the proximal row is interrupted on each side of the lunate either through the perilunate joints or through the bones.

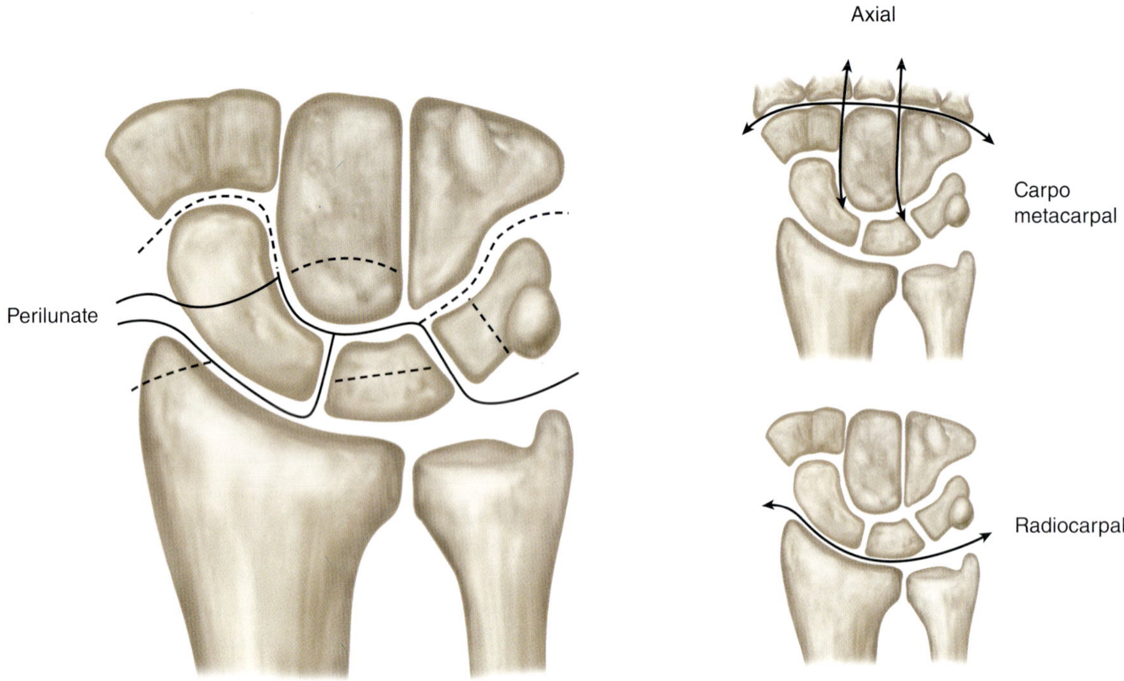

FIGURE 21-1 The 4 types of carpal dislocations.

The capitate displacement may be dorsal from the lunate in more than 90% with a volar lunate dislocation from the radius as an end stage, or sometimes palmar with a dorsal lunate dislocation as an end stage. In the most severe PLD-PLFD the lunate and/or the proximal scaphoid may be free of any ligamentous connections. This should be suspected from the initial radiographs. The consequences are important since the surgeon will have to choose between excision and reposition of the enucleated carpal bone(s). Associated avulsion or compression "chip" fractures (radial or ulnar styloid ...) are frequent. One of them is an osteochondral fracture of the head of the capitate. In a dorsal PLD-PLFD, it is a consequence of the impact of the dorsal lip of the lunate against the head of the capitate at the time of the dislocation. Depending on its size and its depth, an osteochondral fracture of the capitate may have a significant pejorative impact in terms of early midcarpal posttraumatic arthritis.

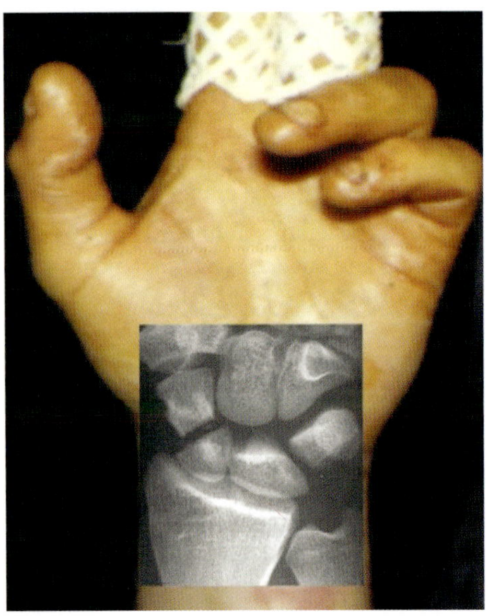

FIGURE 21-2 PA traction radiographs are very helpful to delineate the path of the injury.

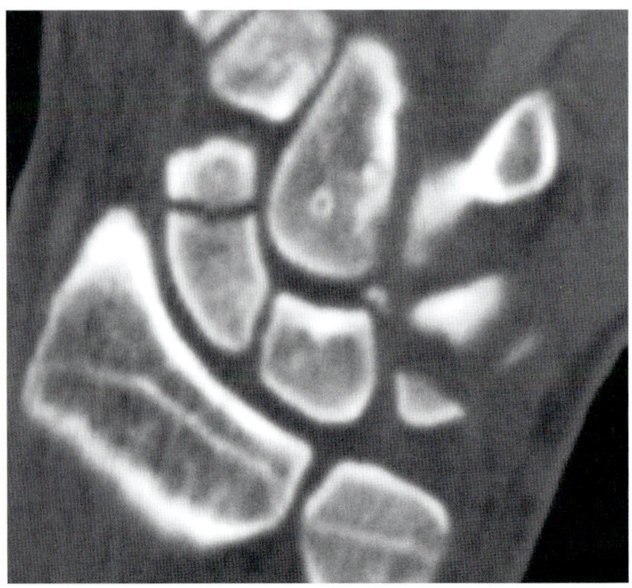

FIGURE 21-3 CT scan may be helpful in some difficult cases but should not be systematic.

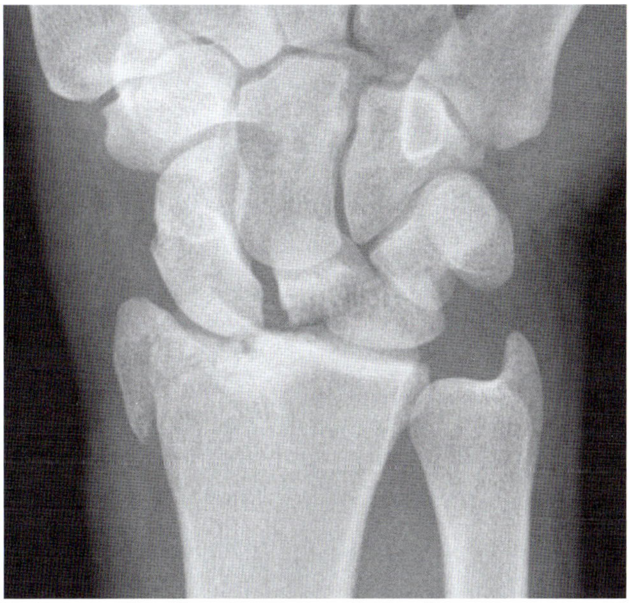

FIGURE 21-4 Unusual translunate perilunate dislocation variant.

The most frequent types of PLD PLFD are the dorsal trans-scaphoid type (about two thirds) and the dorsal PLD type (about one third).[21] Other PLD-PLFD are classified as variants and virtually every combination of injury is possible. This is why so many case reports of unusual types of PLD-PLFD are found in the literature. A new type of translunate perilunate injury was recently identified by Bain et al.[22-25] These authors identified in several patients a translunate arc of dislocation as depicted in Figure 21-4. The lunate may not be salvageable in most cases, which implies the choice of proximal row carpectomy in emergency. Due to the possibility of spontaneous reduction of any PLD-PLFD, one should discuss this diagnosis when faced with an injury of the proximal row apparently not dislocated but presenting with some chip fractures in the midcarpal joint.[26] This is especially true if the energy of the accident of this particular patient is known to have been severe.

TREATMENT AND OUTCOMES

Open Reduction and Internal Fixation

There is evidence in the literature to support early operative treatment of these complex highly unstable injuries whatever their type may be.[27-29] Not all PLD-PLFD have the same severity in terms of displacements and fractures. The injury being perilunate along a lesser or greater arc with virtually any possible combinations, the goal is to anatomically repair the bones and ligaments of the proximal row.

The median nerve is immediately at risk whatever the severity of the injury. This is due to increased carpal tunnel pressure from dislocated bones with or without secondary hematoma. This is why immediate closed reduction of the capitate–lunate joint using progressive distraction (10 lb) under anesthesia or analgesia is recommended by most authors.[30] This allows for traction radiographs as mentioned above and classification of the injury according to the path of the trauma and the direction of displacement. In the vast majority of cases gross reduction of the midcarpal joint by closed maneuvers is successful. In that situation, surgery for anatomic reduction and fixation of the carpal bones can be performed within 24 to 48 hours. If necessary, a CT scan may be performed during this period.

The surgeon should proceed directly to surgery in 2 situations: first of all, in the very rare situation where the midcarpal joint is irreducible by closed means due to soft tissue interposition; second, the surgeon should proceed to immediate ORIF in some particular PLD-PLFD variants where the lunate, the proximal scaphoid, or the head of the capitate is completely enucleated.

The best surgical approach(es) to achieve the above-mentioned goals is still controversial. There is evidence in the literature that different surgical approaches may lead to satisfactory repairs and outcomes. A specific strategy for each individual case will allow choosing the best approach, each of them having its advantages and drawbacks. A limited or extended dorsal approach has a potential for exposing and fixing all the proximal row bones and joints. A limited or extended palmar Russe approach shows the scaphoid well and may provide a view to the torn palmar ligaments lesions, but the palmar cutaneous branch of the median nerve may be at risk in that situation. Combining the approaches improves visualization by definition but increases postoperative fibrosis and stiffness. Overall, surgical approach(es) according to a "surgical strategy" should give a good view at the whole extent of the pathology and be as mini-invasive as possible. This is why arthroscopic treatment of these injuries is emerging.

When a classic ORIF is chosen, a large radial styloid fracture associated with the perilunar injury is well seen and fixed through a dorsal approach. A scaphoid fracture may be well seen and treated through a volar or a dorsal approach. The fixation will use a headless screw whenever possible to optimize quality of fixation and time of healing. However, some very unstable comminuted scaphoid fractures still require the use of K-wires. Well-placed K-wires are better than 1 poor screw. Cancellous bone grafting from the distal radius may be necessary.

A scapholunate dissociation is well seen through a dorsal approach, but some advocate the use of combined palmar approaches for its treatment. Repair may use bone anchors and K-wires or cerclage wire. Combined scaphoid fracture and scapholunate dissociation may be encountered in PLD-PLFD.[31] Combining scaphoid fracture fixation and scapholunate ligament repair is the preferred method.

A capitate fracture is well seen and fixed through a dorsal approach. It may be part of Fenton syndrome with rotation of the detached head fragment or may involve the body of the capitate. A palmarly dislocated capitate head requires a volar CT approach.

A lunotriquetral dissociation is well seen from dorsal. Its repair can be done from dorsal. One or 2 K-wires should stabilize the joint. A triquetral fracture is well seen and fixed from dorsal with 1 screw or 2 K-wires. An associated fracture of the lunate[32] is best seen and fixed through a palmar carpal tunnel approach.

For enucleations of carpal bones[33,34] or part of carpal bones (lunate with or without the proximal scaphoid, proximal scaphoid itself, or head of the capitate) reposition and fixation should be the first choice with inclusion into the anatomic repair of the whole injury. A second choice may be a proximal row carpectomy at the acute stage, but this has to be discussed with the patient before the operation. There is evidence in the literature that the outcome of carpal bone reposition results more often in osteointegration than in necrosis despite the obvious lack of vascularity.[35]

In dislocations of the lunate, usually in a palmar direction there are few ligamentous connections left (short radiolunate ligament). There is a risk for ulnar translation of the carpus[36] that can be prevented by inserting a radiolunate K-wire.[37]

When an osteochondral fracture of the capitate is seen, it should be classified according to Outerbridge and recorded in the patient's chart as it may explain later capitolunate arthrosis.

In a recent series of 25 dorsal trans-scaphoid PLFD with a mean follow-up of 45 months,[38] all the scaphoid fractures had screw fixation through a dorsal approach. The dorsal part of the lunotriquetral ligament was repaired using a bone anchor inserted into the lunate and the LT joint was stabilized with K-wires. All scaphoids healed in 16 weeks on average. No arthritis was found in any patient at a follow-up comprised between 25 and 79 months. At the last follow-up examination, 88% of patients were able to return to their preinjury occupation. The arc of flexion–extension averaged 113° and grip strength averaged 80% of the uninjured side. In another series of 14 dorsal trans-scaphoid PLFD with a mean follow-up of 8 years,[39] all the scaphoid fractures had fixation through a dorsal approach followed by uneventful healing. The average Mayo score was 79%. The arc of flexion–extension averaged 112° and grip strength averaged 79% of the uninjured side. The clinical results were very similar to the previously mentioned study, but 92% of the wrists had midcarpal arthritis at a follow-up comprised between 40 and 160 months. There was no correlation between this arthritis and the clinical result.

In a recent series of 22 dorsal PLD with a mean follow-up of 49 months,[40] a combined dorsal and volar approach with intraosseous scapholunate wiring technique was used. The dorsal part of the lunotriquetral ligament was repaired using a bone anchor and the LT joint was stabilized with K-wires. At follow-up the scapholunate angle was maintained compared with the postsurgery angle (48°). At the last follow-up examination, 45% of patients were able to return to their preinjury occupation. The arc of flexion–extension averaged 106° and grip strength averaged 77% of the uninjured side.

Arthroscopically Assisted Reduction and Internal Fixation

As stated above, the extent of the pathology in PLD-PLFD may vary depending on the energy of the injury. Long-term posttraumatic arthrosis after PLD-PLFD is the rule[41] as depicted in an example shown in Figure 21-5. In PLD-PLFD without dislocation of the lunate, arthroscopic treatment may be a satisfactory new option as a mini-invasive approach in order to minimize postoperative stiffness and arthrosis.[10,42–47] Although technically demanding, and provided that the surgeon uses a dry technique with automatic washouts (Fig. 21-6), it allows a complete and excellent visualization of the carpal joints and fractures (Fig. 21-7). Arthroscopy is particularly helpful in showing osteochondral fractures (Fig. 21-8), loose bodies (Fig. 21-9), as well as detailed views of fracture lines (Fig. 21-10). Combined with fluoroscopy it allows internal fixation of fractures and K-wire stabilization of the carpal bones (Figs. 21-11 and 21-12). It is a modern and more efficient version of percutaneous pinning of PLD-PLFD[48] and relies on the fact that pinning the carpal bones

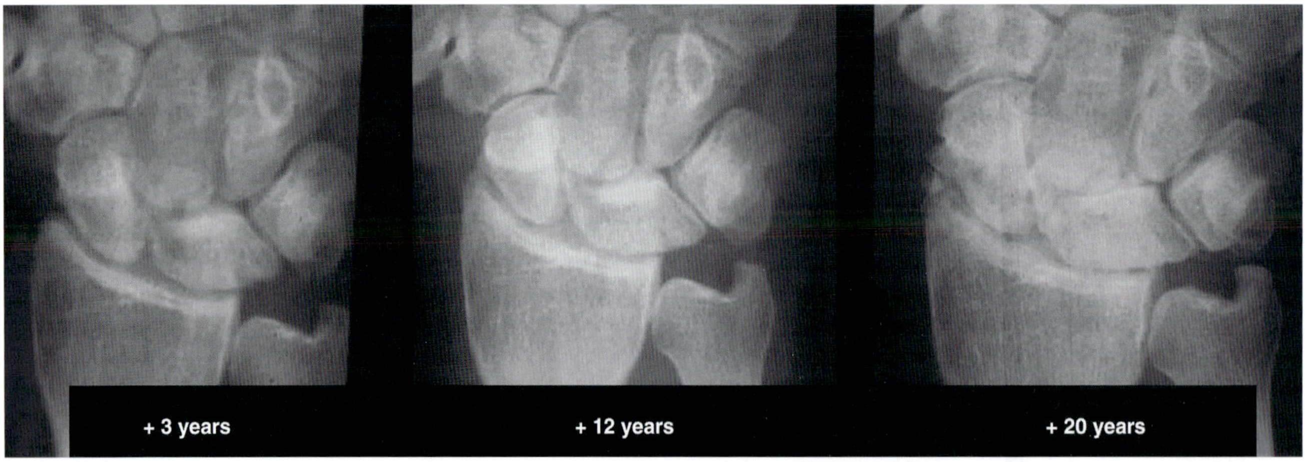

FIGURE 21-5 Perilunate injury after surgical treatment at the acute stage. Note the progression of arthrosis over the years.

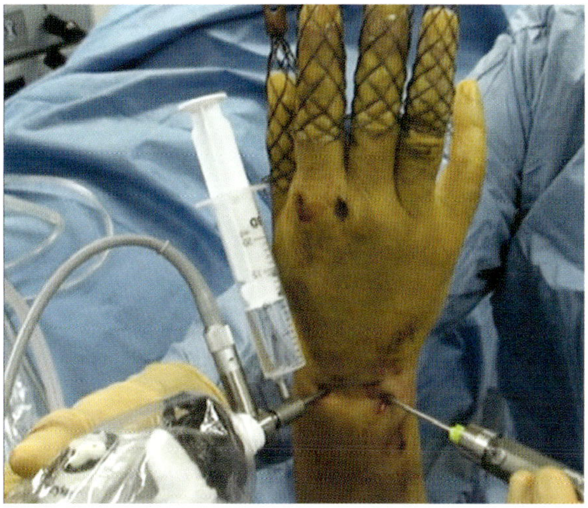

FIGURE 21-6 Dry arthroscopy combined with automatic washouts to clear the view and avoid wrist swelling.

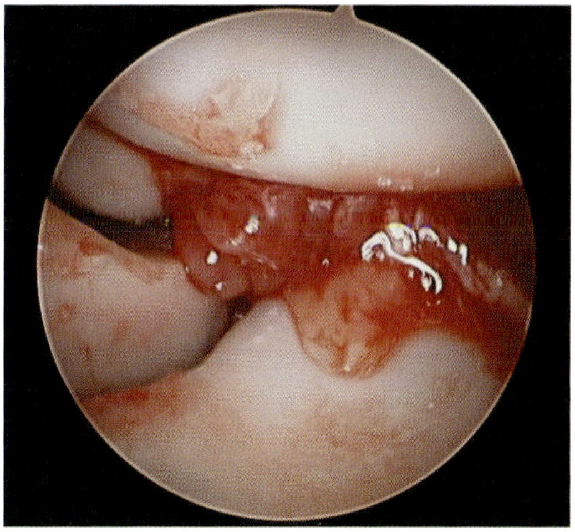

FIGURE 21-7 Dry arthroscopic midcarpal view of an acute perilunate dislocation from midcarpal radial portal. Note the complete lunotriquetral dissociation.

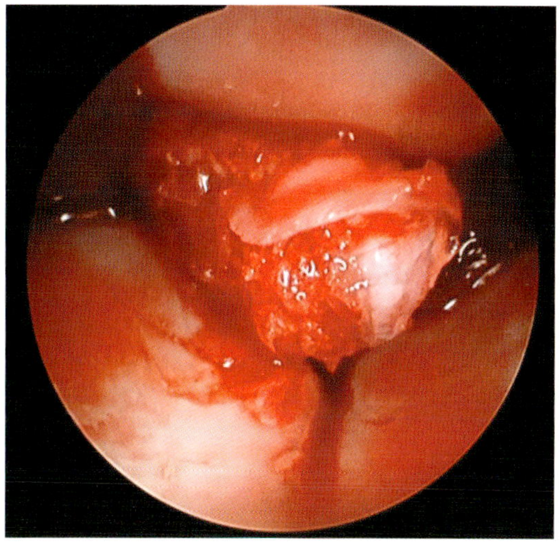

FIGURE 21-9 Dry arthroscopic radiocarpal view of an acute perilunate dislocation from 6R portal. Note the large free osteochondral fracture.

in anatomic position at the acute phase should allow for satisfactory intercarpal ligament healing.[7]

CONCLUSIONS

Most PLD-PLFD are closed high-energy injuries, now rarely missed at the acute stage. They produce a disruption of the "carpal ring" described by Lichtman resulting in a severe acute traumatic carpal instability. PLD-PLFD essentially disrupt the proximal row. They may produce enucleation(s) of carpal bones (or part of them) that represent end stages, generally produced by a sequential mechanism. Regarding the pathology, a myriad of combinations is possible. Ideally each dissociation spot, whether it is a fracture or an intercarpal

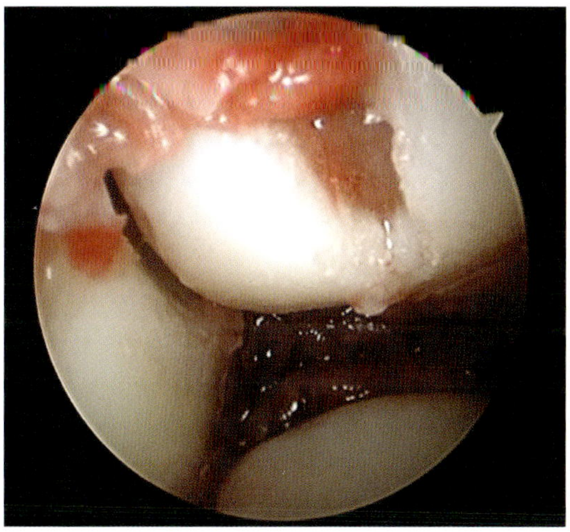

FIGURE 21-8 Dry arthroscopic midcarpal view of an acute perilunate dislocation from midcarpal radial portal. Note the severe osteochondral fracture on the head of the capitate.

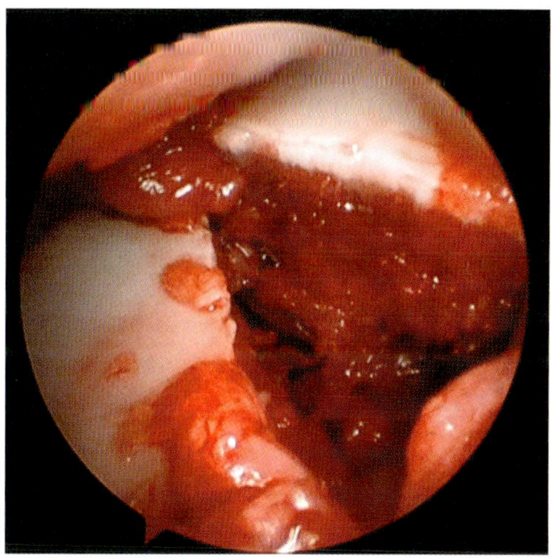

FIGURE 21-10 Dry arthroscopic midcarpal view of an acute transscaphoid perilunate dislocation from midcarpal radial portal. The scaphoid fracture line can be seen and debrided as needed.

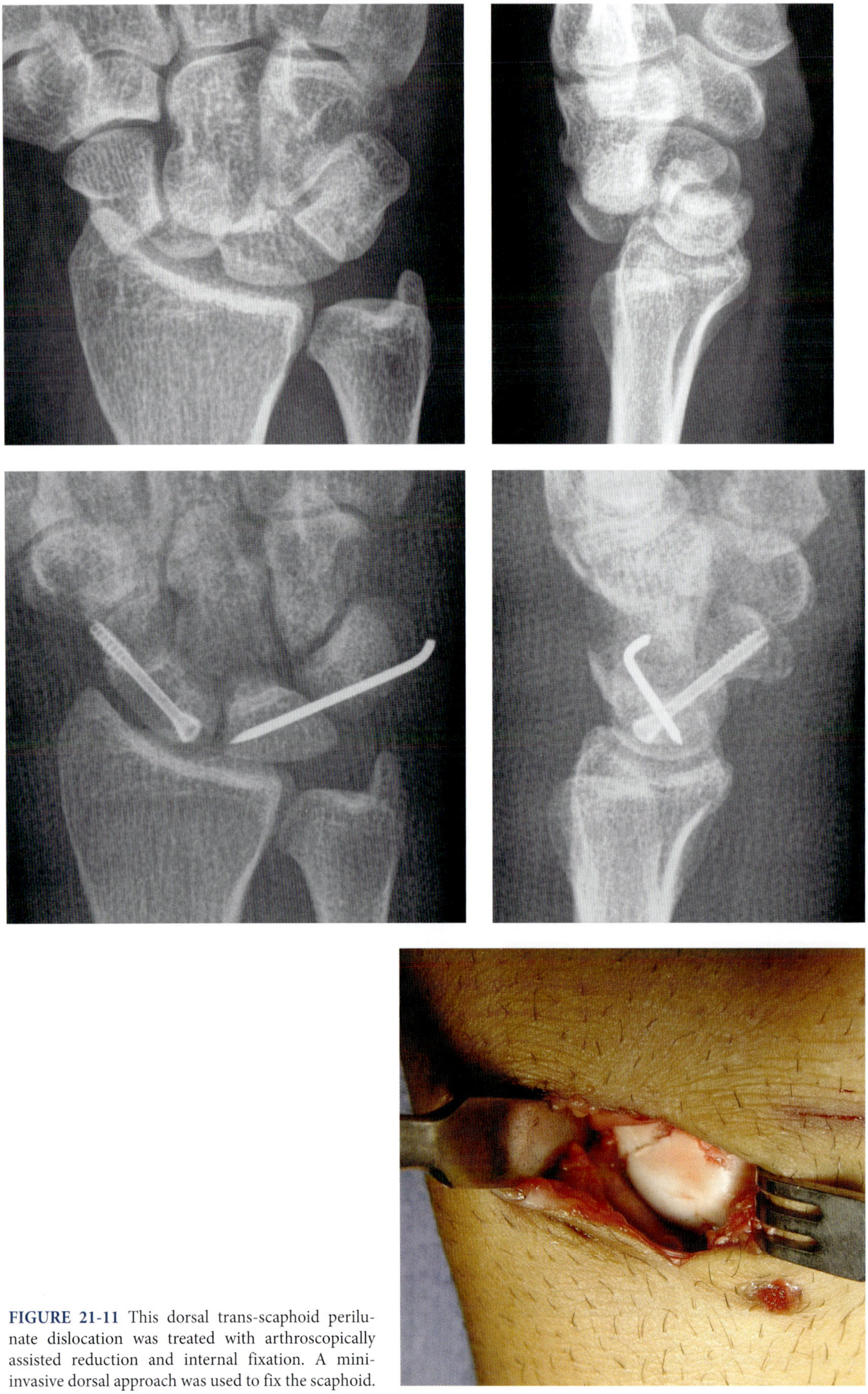

FIGURE 21-11 This dorsal trans-scaphoid perilunate dislocation was treated with arthroscopically assisted reduction and internal fixation. A mini-invasive dorsal approach was used to fix the scaphoid.

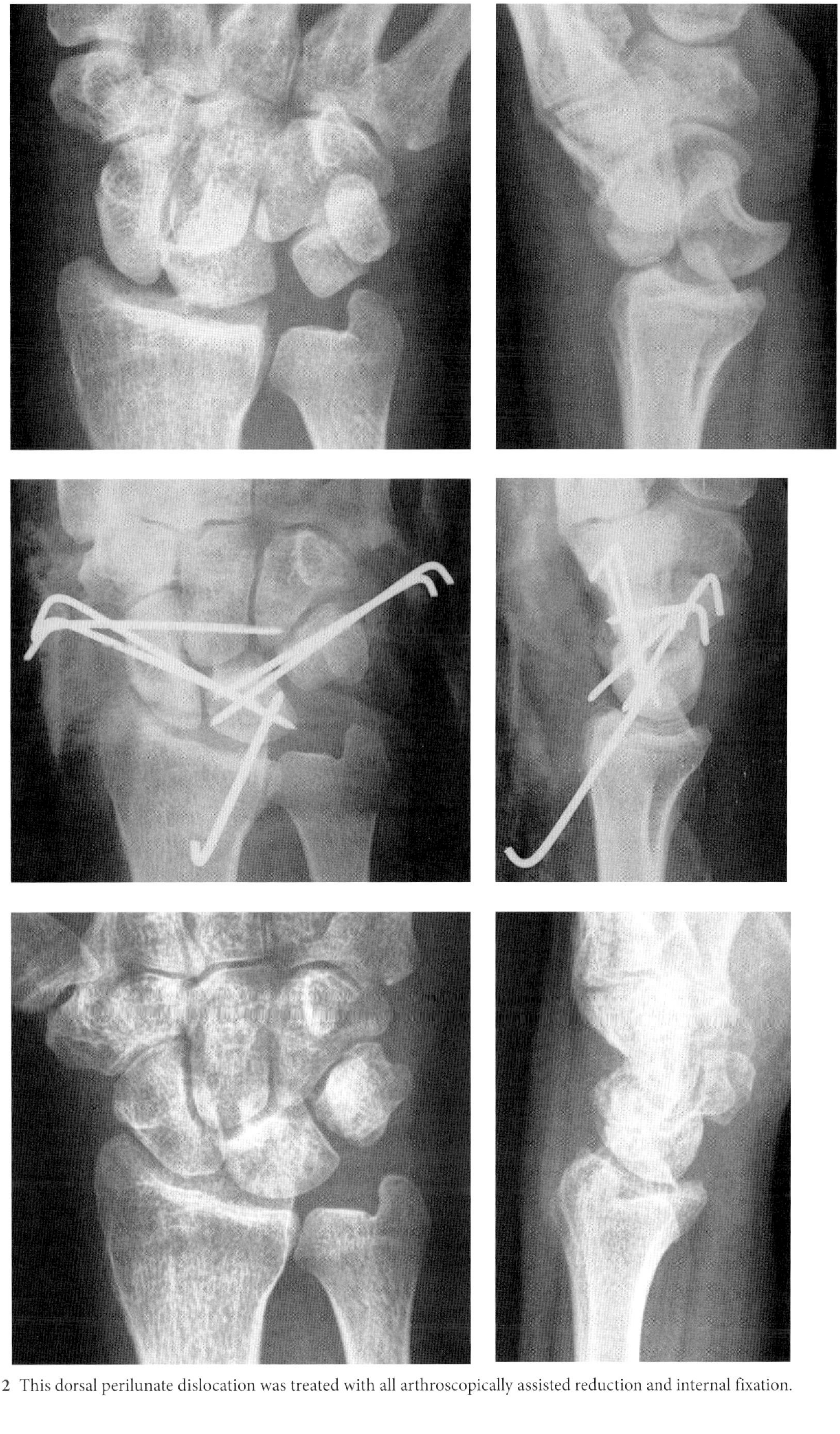

FIGURE 21-12 This dorsal perilunate dislocation was treated with all arthroscopically assisted reduction and internal fixation.

separation, should be addressed by the surgical repair in order to restore the normal anatomy. This is why accurate recognition of the path of the injury is of paramount importance because surgical repair should address each component of that "trauma line." Considering the impressive number of publications about variants of PLD-PLFD, it is virtually impossible to make exhaustive treatment recommendations. Understanding the paths of carpal dislocations from appropriate radiographs and considering that both rows should be scrutinized in order to diagnose combined variants will allow appropriate treatment at the acute stage. ORIF remains the gold standard, but arthroscopically assisted treatment is emerging for the least severe types of perilunate injuries. A combination of arthroscopy and mini-invasive approach may be a safe and modern approach trying to minimize the normal tissue injury related to exensive open approaches.

REFERENCES

1. Mulligan MT, Trumble TE. Trans-scaphoid perilunate dislocations. In: Slutsky DJ, ed. *The Scaphoid*. New York: Thieme; 2011:144–151.
2. Herzberg G. Perilunate fracture dislocations. In: Cooney WP, ed. *The Wrist. Diagnosis and Operative Treatment*. 2nd ed. Lippincott: Wolters Kluwer; 2010:550–578.
3. Dobyns JH, Linscheid RL. Carpal instability classification and historical perspective. In: Cooney WP, ed. *The Wrist. Diagnosis and Operative Treatment*. 2nd ed. Lippincott: Wolters Kluwer; 2010:608–616.
4. Chalidis BE, Dimitriou CG. Palmar dislocation of the scapholunate bone–ligament–bone complex. *J Hand Surg Eur Vol*. 2010;35(4):322.
5. Lee BJ, Kim SS, Lee SR, Jin JM, Yoon MG, Moon MS. Palmar scaphoid dislocation associated with dorsal perilunate dislocation: case report. *J Hand Surg Am*. 2010;35:726–731.
6. Sabat D, Dabas V, Suri T, Wangchuk T, Sural S, Dhal A. Trans-scaphoid trans capitate trans hamate fracture of the wrist: case report. *J Hand Surg Am*. 2010;35:1093–1096.
7. Herzberg G. Perilunate and axial carpal dislocations and fracture–dislocations. *J Hand Surg Am*. 2008;33:1659–1668.
8. Adkison JW, Chapman MW. Treatment of acute lunate and perilunate dislocations. *Clin Orthop Relat Res*. 1982;(164):199–207.
9. Apergis E, Maris J, Theodoratos G, Pavlakis D, Antoniou N. Perilunate dislocations and fracture–dislocations. Closed and early open reduction compared in 28 cases. *Acta Orthop Scand Suppl*. 1997;275: 55–59.
10. Weil WM, Slade JF, Trumble TE. Open and arthroscopic treatment of perilunate injuries. *Clin Orthop Relat Res*. 2006;445:120–133.
11. Redjal HR, Rafijah GH. Perilunate injuries of the wrist. In: Slutsky DJ, Osterman AL, eds. *Fractures and Injuries of the Distal Radius and Carpus. The Cutting Edge*. Philadelphia: Saunders Elsevier; 2010:425–435.
12. Sauder DJ, Athwal GS, Faber KJ, Roth JH. Perilunate injuries. *Hand Clin*. 2010;26:145.
13. Stanbury SJ, Elfar JC. Perilunate dislocation and perilunate fracture–dislocations. *J Am Acad Orthop Surg*. 2011;19(9):554–562.
14. Tolo ET, Shin AY. Fracture dislocations of the carpus. In: Trumble TE, Budoff JE, eds. *Hand Surgery. Update IV*. Rosemont, IL: ASSH; 2007:271–294.
15. Razafimahandry HJC. Luxation ouverte trans scapho rétrolunaire du carpe avec avulsion antébrachiale du semi lunaire et du fragment scaphoidien. *Chir Main*. 2009;28:113–115.
16. Johnson RP. The acutely injured wrist and its residuals. *Clin Orthop Relat Res*. 1980;(149):33–44.
17. Mayfield JK. Patterns of injury to carpal ligaments: a spectrum. *Clin Orthop Relat Res*. 1984;(187):36–42.
18. Viegas SF, Patterson RM, Peterson PD, et al. Ulnar-sided perilunate instability:an anatomic and biomechanic study. *J Hand Surg Am*. 1990;15:268–278.
19. Chin A, Garcia-Elias M. Combined reverse perilunate and axial-ulnar dislocation of the wrist: a case report. *J Hand Surg Eur Vol*. 2008;33E:672.
20. van Leuwen DH, Buijze GA, Ring D. Ulnar to radial dorsal fracture–dislocations of the wrist: a report of 2 cases. *J Hand Surg Am*. 2012;37(3):500–502.
21. Budoff JE. Treatment of acute lunate and perilunate dislocations. *J Hand Surg Am*. 2008;33:1424.
22. Bain GI, McLean JM, Turner PC, Sood A, Pourgiezis N. Translunate fracture with associated perilunate injury: 3 case reports with introduction of the translunate arc concept. *J Hand Surg Am*. 2008;33:1770–1776.
23. Briseño MR, Yao J. Lunate fractures in the face of a perilunar injury: an uncommon and easily missed pattern. *J Hand Surg Am*. 2011;37(1):63–67.
24. Enoki NR, Sheppard JE, Taljanovic MS. Transstyloid, translunate fracture–dislocation of the wrist: case report. *J Hand Surg Am*. 2008;33:1131–1134.
25. Reichel LM, Bell BR, Michnick SM, Reitman CA. Radial styloid fractures. *J Hand Surg Am*. 2012;37(8):1726–1741.
26. Christodoulou L, Palou CH, Chamberlain ST. Proximal row transcarpal fracture from a punching injury. *J Hand Surg Br*. 1999;24: 744–746.
27. Yao J, Jagadish A. Carpus: perilunate and greater arc injuries. In: Slutsky DJ, ed. *Principles and Practice of Wrist Surgery*. Philadelphia: Saunders Elsevier; 2010:473–484.
28. Kremer T, Wendt M, Riedel K, Sauerbier M, Germann G, Bickert B. Open reduction for perilunate injuries—clinical outcome and patient satisfaction. *J Hand Surg Am*. 2010;35:1599–1606.
29. Martinage A, Dréant N, Monteil MC, Chignon-Sicard B, Balaguer T, Lebreton E. Luxations et fractures-luxations périlunaires du carpe. *Chir Main*. 2008;27:31.
30. Murray PM. Trans scaphoid perilunar injuries: treatment and outcomes. In: Shin AY, ed. *Scaphoid Fractures. AAOS Monographs*. Rosemont, IL: American Academy of Orthopaedic Surgeons; 2007: 73–84.
31. Schadel-Hopfner M, Junge A, Böhringer G. Scapholunate ligament injury occurring with scaphoid fracture—a rare coincidence? *J Hand Surg Br*. 2005;30B:137.
32. Yakoubi M. Fracture luxation retrolunaire du carpe avec fracture du lunatum. Une nouvelle forme clinique; A propos d'une observation. *Chir Main*. 2007;26:247.
33. Domeshek LF, Harenberg PS, Rineer CA, Hadeed JG, Marcus JR, Erdmann D. Total scapholunate dislocation with complete scaphoid extrusion: case report. *J Hand Surg Am*. 2010;35:69–71.
34. Durand S, MacQuillan A, Delpit X. Isolated scaphoid fracture with anterosuperior dislocation of the proximal fragment. *Chir Main*. 2011;30(4):298–301.
35. Papadonikolalis A, Mavrodontidis AN, Zalavras C, Hantes M, Soucacos PN. Trans-scaphoid volar lunate dislocation. *J Bone Joint Surg Am*. 2003;85A:1805–1808.
36. Song D, Goodman S, Gilula LA, Wollstein R. Ulnocarpal translation in perilunate dislocations. *J Hand Surg Eur Vol*. 2009;34E:388.
37. Herzberg G. Acute dorsal trans-scaphoid perilunate dislocations: open reduction and internal fixation. *Tech Hand Upper Extrem Surg*. 2000;4:2–13.
38. Knoll VD, Allan C, Trumble TE. Trans-scaphoid perilunate fracture dislocations: results of screw fixation of the scaphoid and lunotriquetral repair with a dorsal approach. *J Hand Surg Am*. 2005;30: 1145–1152.
39. Herzberg G, Forissier D. Acute dorsal trans-scaphoid perilunate fracture–dislocations: medium term results. *J Hand Surg Br*. 2002;27B:498–502.
40. Trumble TE, Verheyden J. Treatment of isolated perilunate and lunate dislocations with combined dorsal and volar approach and intraosseous cerclage wire. *J Hand Surg Am*. 2004;29: 412–417.
41. Forli A, Courvoisier A, Wimsey S, Corcella D, Moutet F. Perilunate dislocations and trans-scaphoid perilunate fracture–dislocations: a retrospective study with minimum ten-year follow-up. *J Hand Surg Am*. 2010;35:62–68.
42. Geissler WB, Hammit MD. Arthroscopic aided fixation of scaphoid fractures. *Hand Clin*. 2001;17:575–588.

43. Jeon IH, Kim HJ, Min WK, Cho HS, Kim PT. Arthroscopically assisted percutaneous fixation for trans-scaphoid perilunate fracture dislocation. *J Hand Surg Eur Vol.* 2010;35(8):664–668.
44. Kim JP, Lee JS, Park MJ. Arthroscopic reduction and percutaneous fixation of perilunate dislocations and fracture dislocations. *Arthroscopy.* 2012;28(2):196–203.e2.
45. Park MJ, Ahn JH. Arthroscopically assisted reduction and percutaneous fixation of dorsal perilunate dislocations and fracture–dislocations. *Arthroscopy.* 2005;21:1153.
46. Savoie FH, Grondel RJ. Arthroscopy for carpal instability. *Orthop Clin North Am.* 1995;26:731.
47. Slade JF, Gillon T. Retrospective review of 234 scaphoid fractures and nonunions treated with arthroscopy for union and complications. *Scand J Surg.* 2008;97:280–289.
48. Chou YC, Hsu YH, Cheng CY, Wu CC. Percutaneous screw and axial Kirschner wire fixation for acute transscaphoid perilunate fracture dislocation. *J Hand Surg Am.* 2012;37(4):715–720.

Salvage Procedures for the Wrist

Lara Just-Kovac, MD
Michael Sauerbier, MD, PhD

22

The wrist is one of the most complex joints in the body and because of its remarkable range of motion it is vulnerable to injuries such as ligamentous sprains or fractures.[1–4]

If acute injuries such as a scaphoid fracture or scapholunate dissociation are left untreated, a characteristic pattern of progressive degenerative changes may occur, which have been termed scaphoid nonunion advanced collapse (SNAC) wrist and scapholunate advanced collapse (SLAC) wrist.

Watson and Ryu classified the severity of degenerative changes (SLAC and SNAC wrist) in stages.[5] Stage 1 SLAC involves degeneration of the radial styloid–scaphoid articulation.

Stage 2 includes the entire radioscaphoid joint. Stage 3 involves capitolunate (CL) degeneration, whereas stage 4 involves the radiolunate articulation, but this stage is uncommon. Similar to SLAC arthritis, stage 1 SNAC involves the radial styloid–scaphoid joint. Stage 2 includes progressive degeneration of the radioscaphoid articulation between the distal pole and the radial styloid and scaphocapitate (SC) degeneration. Stage 3 involves CL degeneration and progression of the radioscaphoid and SC degeneration. The articulation between the proximal pole of the scaphoid and the radius is generally spared (Fig. 22-1A and B).

The standard surgical technique in stage 1 SNAC involves bone grafting of scaphoid and internal fixation of the scaphoid nonunion line with a radial styloidectomy. In stage 1 SLAC wrist a scapholunate ligament reconstruction is performed in combination with a radial styloidectomy. Stage 2 in both instances can be treated with a proximal row carpectomy (PRC) or a midcarpal arthrodesis combined with a scaphoid excision. In stage 3 SLAC and SNAC wrist there is capitate arthrosis; therefore, a PRC is not an option and some type of midcarpal arthrodesis with scaphoid excision is commonly performed.

Viegas et al[6] classified the injury of lunotriquetral (LT) ligament tears into 3 stages. Stage 1 is a partial or complete disruption of the LT interosseous ligament without clinical and/or radiographic evidence of a dynamic or static palmar intercalated segment instability (PISI). Stage 2 is a complete disruption of the LT interosseous ligament with clinical and/or radiographic evidence of a dynamic VISI deformity. Stage 3 is a complete disruption of the LT interosseous with a static VISI deformity.

There are a variety of surgical procedures that can be used for salvage of the arthritic wrist, which will be discussed below.

RADIAL STYLOIDECTOMY

Radial styloidectomy is an early salvage procedure that may provide short-term relief of mechanical pain from radial styloid impingement. It is an acceptable alternative to more aggressive procedures in patients with low functional demands or those who wish to defer more definitive treatment by means of a proximal carpectomy or limited wrist fusion. Radial styloid impingement due to a SLAC or SNAC stage 1 is a common indication, and has been observed following a scaphotrapezial trapezoid (STT) or SC fusion.

The main risk following a radial styloidectomy is ulnar translocation of the carpus. Nakamura et al observed significantly increased radial translation with ulnar and palmar carpal displacement after 6- and 10-mm radial styloidectomies and therefore recommended a styloidectomy of no more than 3 to 4 mm.[7] Patients who do not have an intact radioscaphocapitate ligament are at risk for ulnar translocation and are not candidates for this procedure, especially if a PRC is contemplated. Ulnar translocation is a frequent sequela of long-standing rheumatoid disease; hence, any patient with chronic wrist involvement is a poor candidate for this procedure.

A 3-cm incision was made over Lister's tubercle protecting branches of the superficial radial nerve. The third and fourth extensor compartments are elevated and a capsulotomy is performed. Approximately 3 to 4 mm of the radial styloid is removed with an osteotome. Postoperatively the patient is splinted for the first week followed by progressive wrist motion and strengthening. There are few clinical studies reporting the results of an isolated styloidectomy.

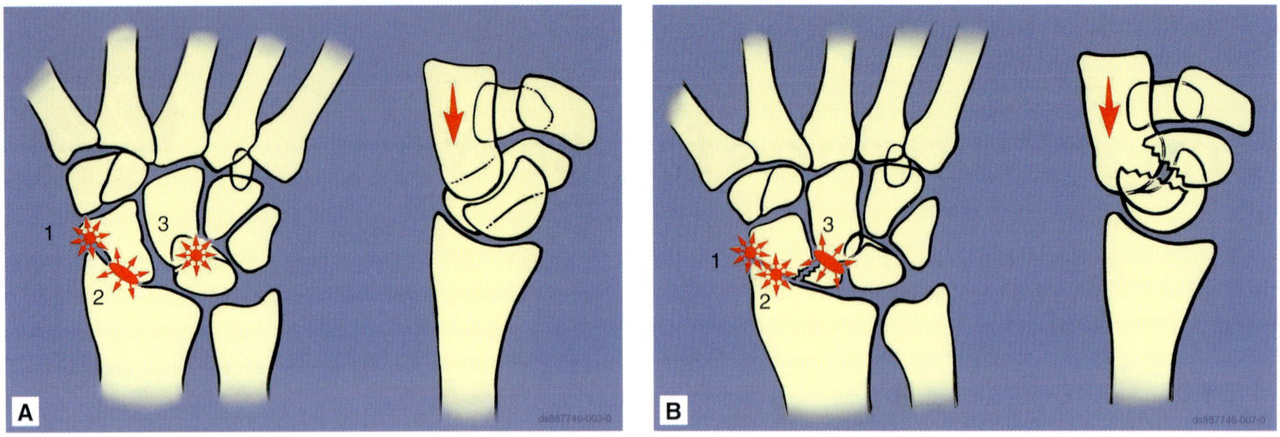

FIGURE 22-1 **A** and **B.** Evaluation of SLAC and SNAC wrist in stages 1 to 3.

SCAPHOCAPITATE ARTHRODESIS

In 1946, Sutro[8] first described a SC arthrodesis for the treatment of patients with a scaphoid nonunion. Pisano et al[9] recommended a SC arthrodesis in advanced Kienböck disease, chronic scapholunate instability, and chronic scaphoid nonunions. Several biomechanical studies have been published that demonstrate that a SC fusion unloads the lunate by shifting the load to the radioscaphoid joint. Horii et al demonstrated unloading of the radiolunate joint by 12%, whereas the radioscaphoid forces increased by 9%.

A scaphoid capitate fusion is indicated in arthrosis of the scaphotrapeziotrapezoid joint and chronic scapholunate dissociation or degenerative changes have occurred.

This procedure can only be used with a normal radioscaphoid joint and is therefore contraindicated with SLAC and SNAC wrist stages 1, 2, and 3.

The branches of the radial sensory nerve are identified and protected. The distal termination of the posterior interosseous nerve can be excised at the surgeon's discretion. The radiocarpal and intercarpal articular cartilage surfaces are carefully inspected for significant arthrosis. The status of the lunate is evaluated in Kienböck's disease. In case of a chronic scaphoid nonunion the proximal fragment may be left in place to increase the fusion surface area. The adjacent articular surfaces of the scaphoid and capitate are removed. The ideal radioscaphoid angle is between 30° and 57° based on a cadaver study[10] and the SC joint is stabilized with 2 guidewires. Cancellous bone graft is then packed into the SC interval. There are several options for final fixation including Kirschner wires, screws, staples, or even small plates. We prefer using cannulated scaphoid screws (Fig. 22-2A and B). The screw is best placed from the lateral (radial) aspect of waist of the scaphoid into the medial/distal part of the capitate to avoid necrosis of the head of the capitate.

Occasionally a radial styloidectomy may be performed in situations of radial styloid impingement. Prior to wound closure, final radiographs are obtained to evaluate hardware placement, the radioscaphoid angle, and alignment of the fusion. The wrist is immobilized in a splint with slight wrist extension for about 6 weeks after operation.

Sennwald and Ufenast performed a SC arthrodesis in 11 patients with Kienböck disease with a median age of 26 years. Ten patients had grade III and 1 had grade II disease by the Lichtman classification. The lunate was left in situ and a SC arthrodesis was performed with 2 lag screws and corticocancellous bone graft. At an average follow-up of 36 months 10 patients had complete pain relief and 1 had persistent pain. The average loss of the flexion/extension arc was 52%.[11]

Pisano et al examined 17 patients at 16 to 57 months (average, 23.4 months) after a SC arthrodesis. Indications for the surgery included scapholunate instability, isolated arthrosis, chronic scaphoid nonunion, and Kienböck disease. SC fusion with autogenous bone grafting was used to bridge carpal spaces. Two patients had nonunion of the SC arthrodesis, which required reoperation. Seven patients experienced persistent pain with heavy use; of these, 2 changed occupations and 1 remains disabled. Compared with the nonoperated side, SC fusion reduced the wrist extension an average of 28°, flexion 40°, radial deviation 14°, and ulnar deviation 14°. The greatest loss was of radial deviation. Static grip reached an average of 74% of the nonoperated side. More recently Delétang et al reported their experience with 31 patients who were treated with an SC fusion for chronic scapholunate instability. At an average follow-up of 5 years the average wrist motion was 41° in flexion and 39° in extension. Radial–ulnar deviation was 43°. Strength was 32.5 kg. The DASH score was 27% and the PRWE was 25%. Fifty percent of the wrists were pain-free at rest. Ninety-four percent of patients were satisfied with the procedure. Seventy-eight percent of patients had returned to their occupation. Radiographic analysis revealed that consolidation was obtained at 10.1 weeks. The postoperative radioscaphoid angle was 55° with good radioscaphoid congruence. There was no osteoarthritis in the radioscaphoid joint in 84% of the cases. The nonunion rate was 13%.[9,12]

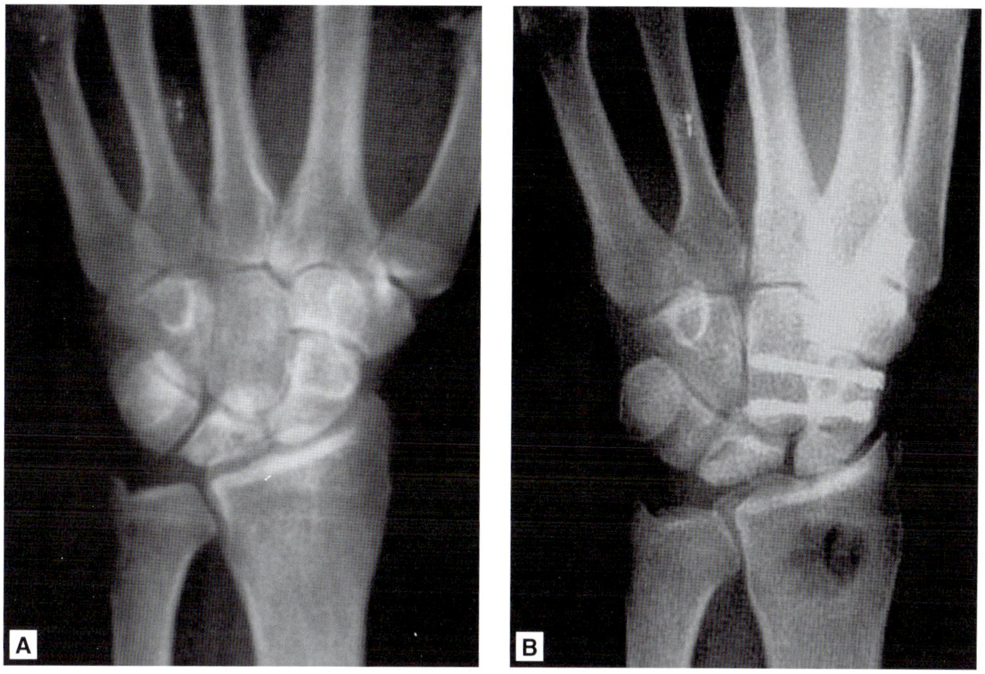

FIGURE 22-2 A 30-year-old male patient with Kienböck disease stage 3a (**A**). Scaphocapitate arthrodesis with 2 cannulated screws 6 months postoperatively (**B**).

FOUR-CORNER ARTHRODESIS

Watson and Ryu[5] popularized the wrist salvage procedure of scaphoid excision and arthrodesis of the capitate, lunate, triquetrum, and hamate, which is known as a 4-corner arthrodesis (FCA).

Unlike a SC fusion this can be performed when there is radioscaphoid and CL osteoarthritis. It is indicated in SLAC and SNAC stages 2 and 3 and for severe midcarpal instability.

This procedure can only be used with a normal radiolunate joint and is therefore contraindicated when there is degenerative arthrosis between the radius and lunate. Other contraindications are Kienböck disease and a wrist with ulnar translocation of the carpus.

A dorsal approach is performed through an S-shaped centered incision over Lister's tubercle. A radially based flap consisting of skin and subcutaneous tissue incorporating the superficial radial nerve is developed. The third extensor compartment is opened and the extensor pollicis longus tendon and muscle is retracted radially. The second and fourth compartments are left intact and elevated subperiosteally from the radius. The distal termination of the posterior interosseous nerve is excised proximal to the fourth compartment. A ligament-sparing capsulotomy as described by Berger et al is performed by elevating the capsule off its insertion into the triquetrum while making an oblique incision along the course of dorsal radiocarpal ligament and the distal intercarpal ligament that are preserved (Fig. 22-3).[13] The scaphoid is excised with the aid of an osteotome and a rongeur. The remaining

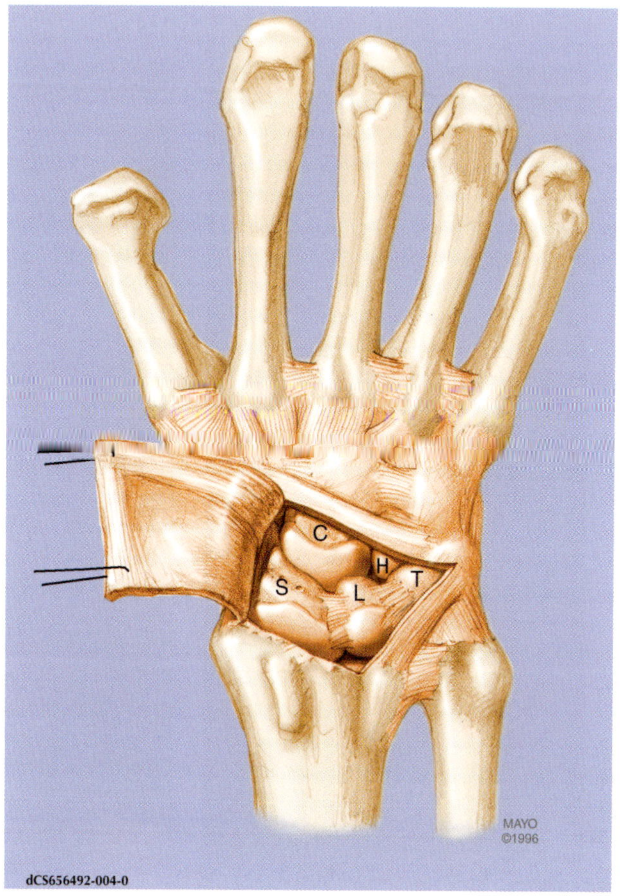

FIGURE 22-3 Ligament-sparing capsulotomy from a dorsal approach.

cartilage of the adjacent joint surfaces of the capitate, lunate, hamate, and triquetrum is completely removed down to bleeding cancellous bone. A K-wire is placed in the lunate and used as a joystick to correct the extended and ulnar deviated position. Two 1.5-mm K-wires are inserted into the capitate in a distal to proximal direction and advanced until they protrude slightly from the head of the capitate.

Cancellous bone graft from either the radius or the iliac crest is inserted between the capitate, lunate, hamate, and triquetrum. The 2 K-wires are then advanced into the lunate. One or two 1.5-mm K-wires are used to stabilize the hamate to the triquetrum. Finally the K-wires between radius and lunate are removed.

The wrist is immobilized in a circular forearm plaster cast for an average of 6 weeks. The K-wires are removed at approximately 12 weeks.

More recently we have been using a special locking plate for this type of partial fusion (Medartis AG, Basel, Switzerland; Fig. 22-4A-G). The plate is available in 2 sizes and offers 2 rows for implantation of the screws. The inner part has 4 holes for compression of the carpal bones, the outer part 8 holes for locking screws. Each of the fused 4 bones can be fixed with 2 screws. The main advantage of this new device is that immobilization can be very short because of the stable fixation of the fused 4 bones. The patients are mobilized after 3 weeks of casting.

Several fixation techniques as staples, Kirschner wires, screws, and plates have been used to achieve fusion. Kirschner wire fixation has been proven effective, but requires a period of 6 to 8 weeks of cast immobilization to provide bony fusion. One of the first circular plates was the Spider plate (Spider Limited Wrist Arthrodesis System; Kinetikos Medical, Inc, San Diego, CA). One study however reported a significantly higher complication rate and lower union rate in a series of 16 patients using circular plate fixation for FCA as compared with previously published techniques.[14] Nine out of the 16 patients (56%) had complications, including nonunion (25%), delayed union (6%), dorsal impingement (25%), radial styloid impingement (6%), and broken screws (13%). This particular paper is more reflective of the surgical technique and learning curve of the surgeon rather than the implant per se. Merrell et al (the inventors of the plate) reviewed the outcomes in a consecutive cohort of 28 patients who underwent a standardized FCA with a second-generation circular plate and distal radius bone grafting for a diagnosis of SLAC, SNAC, or midcarpal arthrosis.[15] At an average follow-up of 46 months, the wrist range of motion averaged 45% of the uninjured side (average extension, 35°; average flexion, 26°). Grip strength averaged 82% of the uninjured side. The mean visual analog scale pain and activity scores were 2.3/10 and 2.4/10. Radiographs demonstrated union of the primary CL fusion mass in all of the cases. There was 1 case of

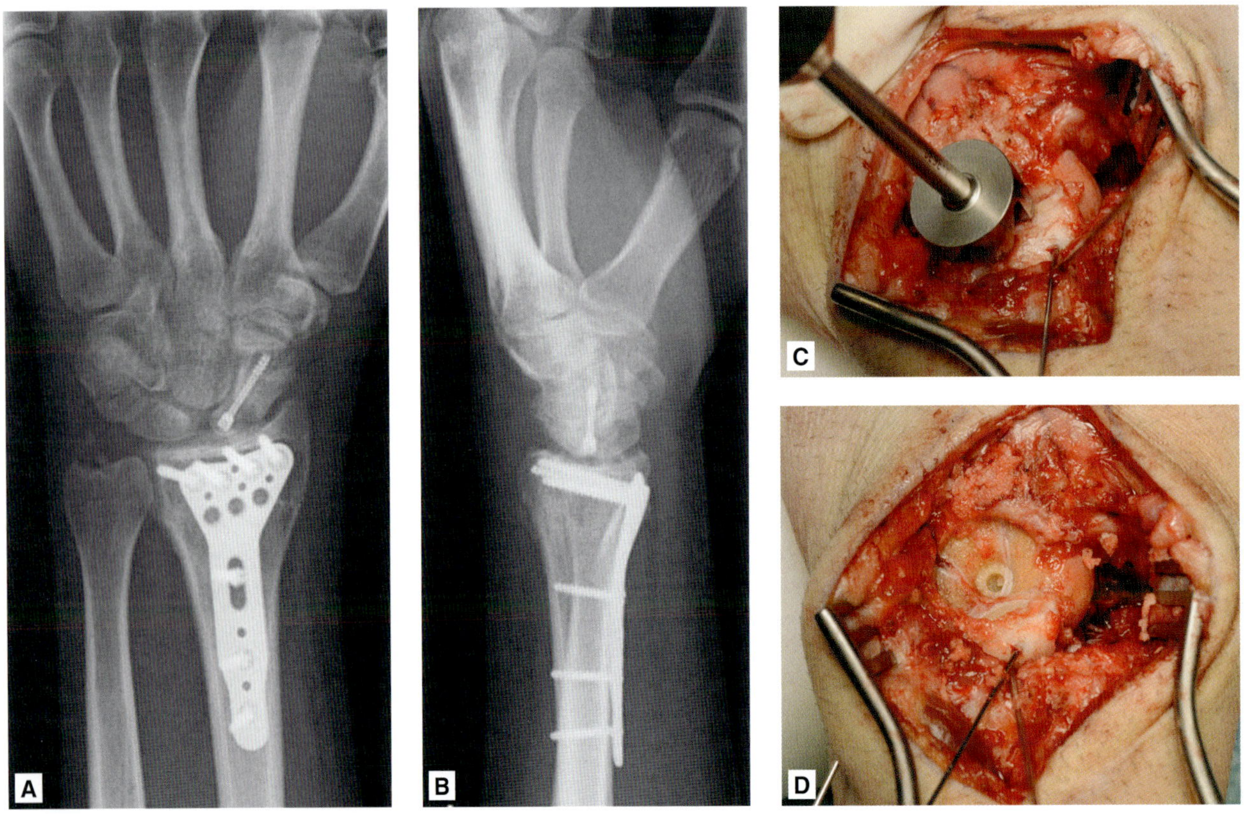

FIGURE 22-4 **A** and **B.** X-ray of a 35-year-old patient with a SNAC wrist following nonunion after scaphoid reconstruction of left wrist pa/lateral. **C** and **D.** Creation of a hole underneath the bony surface of lunate, capitate, hamate, and triquetrum with a special drilling device of the locking plate.

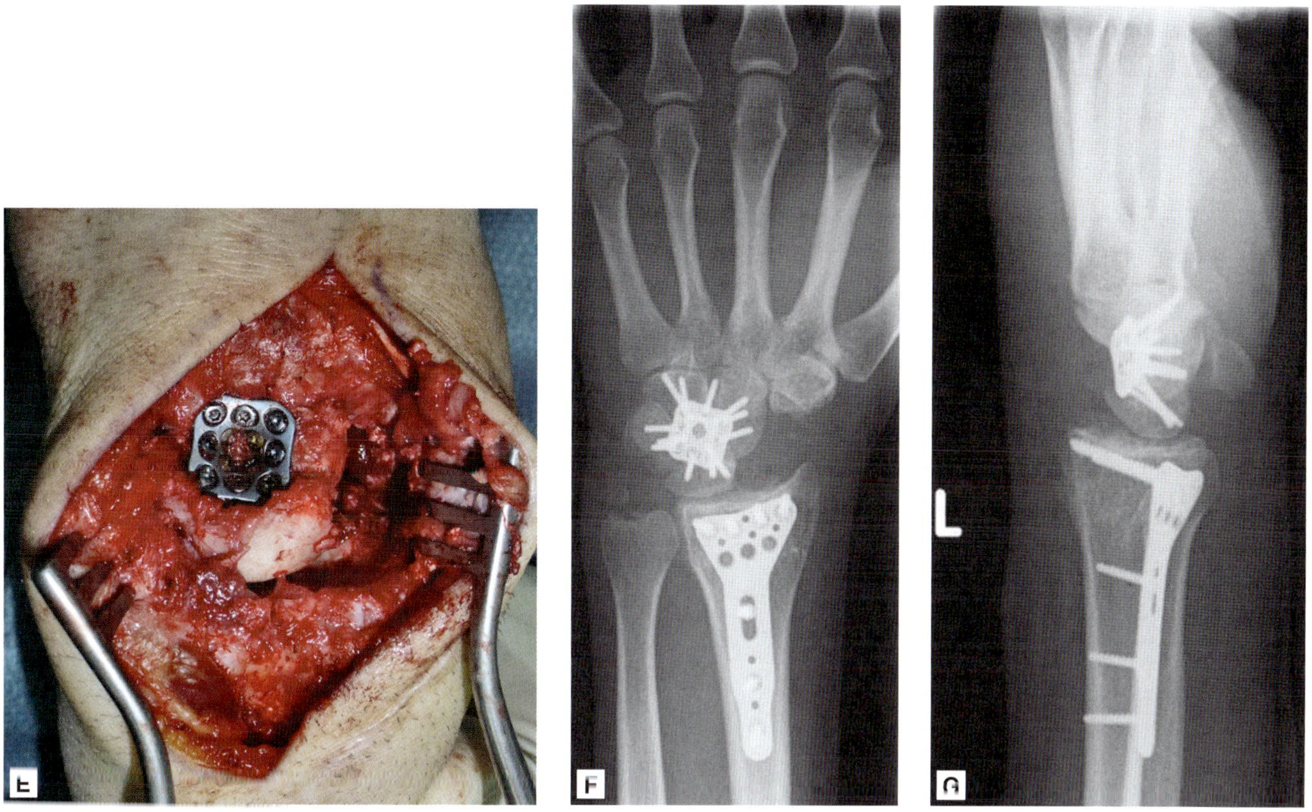

FIGURE 22-4 (*Continued*) **E.** Implantation of the locking plate with compression screws (yellow) as well as locking screws (blue) (Medartis AG). **F** and **G.** Postoperative x-ray pa/lateral after implantation of the locking plate. Physiotherapy for the wrist joint starts at 3 weeks postoperatively. The immobilization can be abandoned at this time.

peritriquetral nonunion and 1 case of asymptomatic loss of radiolunate joint space, 1 screw back-out in 1 case, and the plate broke in 1 case. Two patients underwent reoperation, 1 for radial styloid impingement pain and the other for lack of flexion.

Gupta et al[16] recently described successful 4-corner fusion in 6 patients using a cervical H-plate. Ozyurekoglu and Tuncer[17] reported a midcarpal arthrodesis technique using percutaneous, transmetacarpal headless compression screws using the scaphoid as a bone graft.

Krimmer et al reviewed 26 patients following a midcarpal fusion at an average follow-up of 14 months and demonstrated an average increase in the grip strength of 23%, whereas the wrist motion decreased by 33% to 40%.[18] In an older series from 1994 Krakauer et al compared the outcomes of 6 different reconstructive procedures for stages 2 and 3 SLAC wrist in 55 cases followed for an average of 50 months. Scaphoid excision and intercarpal arthrodesis was performed in 31 cases: FCA in 23 cases and CL arthrodesis in 8 cases. PRC was performed in 12 cases, radioscapholunate arthrodesis in 5 cases, radioscaphoid arthrodesis in 3 cases, and primary total wrist arthrodesis in 4 cases. There were 4 of 8 nonunions in the CL arthrodesis group compared with 2/23 in the FCA group. A PRC preserved wrist mobility to a greater degree, with a flexion–extension arc of 71°.[19]

More recently Sauerbier et al reviewed 31 male patients (average 41 years) who were treated for SNAC or SLAC wrist with midcarpal arthrodesis. At a mean follow-up of 15 months the pain was reduced by 50%, grip strength improved to 60% of the opposite side, and active range of motion averaged 50% of the contralateral wrist. Four patients required a total wrist arthrodesis for a nonunion.[20] Bain and Watts reviewed 31 patients at a minimum of 10 years of follow-up; there was no significant change in pain, wrist function, satisfaction, or arc of motion between 1 and 10 years after surgery. Two of 35 patients had to be converted to a total wrist arthrodesis for ongoing pain.[21] Krimmer et al compared the functional outcome following 4-corner fusion and total wrist fusion for SNAC and SLAC pathologies. According to the DASH score and the modified Mayo wrist score there were significantly better results for the 4-corner fusion than for the total wrist arthrodesis.[22–24]

SCAPHOTRAPEZIAL TRAPEZOID ARTHRODESIS

The STT arthrodesis was introduced by Witt[25] in 1956, Peterson and Lipscomb in 1967, and popularized by Watson in the 1980s.[26–28]

The indications for STT arthrodesis include primary arthrosis or instability of the scaphotrapeziotrapezoid joint and chronic scapholunate dissociation and SLAC stage 1.[29]

Further indications include Kienböck disease stages 3a and b when there is an intact radioscaphoid joint because the STT arthrodesis shifts the load from the radioulnar to the radioscaphoid column (Fig. 22-5).[30–33]

Contraindications include radioscaphoid and midcarpal arthrosis such as SNAC and SLAC stages 3 and 4.

A dorsal S-shaped incision over the STT joint is made and a radially based skin and subcutaneous flap containing the superficial branch of the radial nerve is elevated from the extensor retinaculum. The second and third extensor compartments are opened and the extensor pollicis longus tendon

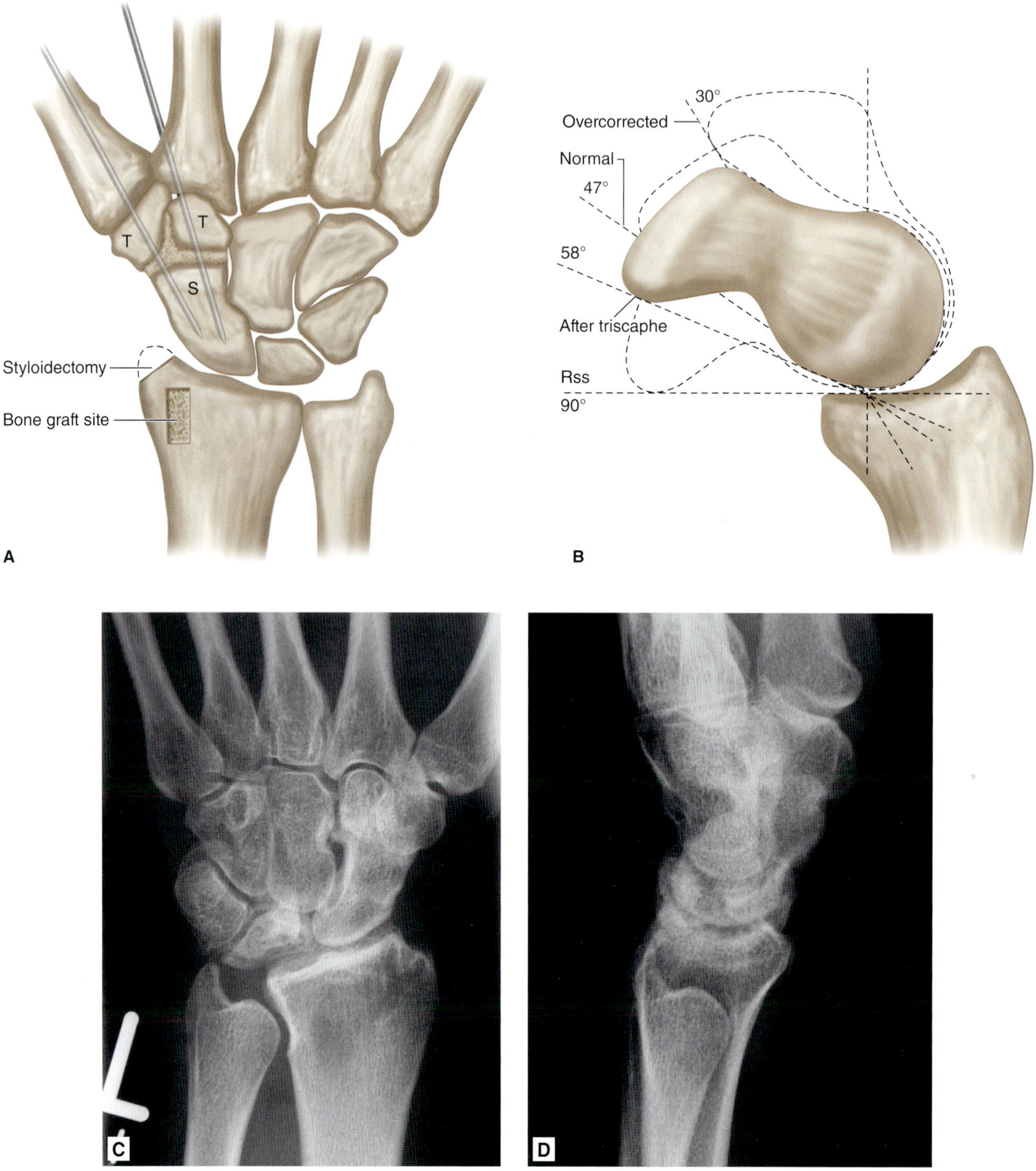

FIGURE 22-5 **A.** Technique with K-wire fixation and radial styloidectomy for a STT arthrodesis. **B.** Recommended radioscaphoid position with an angle between approximately 40° and 60°. **C** and **D.** A 28-year-old patient with a bony consolidated STT arthrodesis due to Kienböck disease.

and muscle is retracted radially. The posterior interosseous nerve is resected proximal to the fourth compartment. The capsule of the STT joint is opened with a transverse incision. The remaining cartilage of the adjacent joint surfaces of the distal scaphoid, trapezium, and trapezoid is completely removed with a rongeur or osteotome. 1.5-mm K-wires are inserted in the trapezium and trapezoid from a neck dorsal distal. The radioscaphoid angle is set at between 40° and 60° and corticocancellous bone from the distal radius is inserted into the remaining gap. Then the K-wires are advanced into the scaphoid and buried subcutaneously. A radial styloidectomy is now routinely performed because of the likelihood of radial styloid impingement.

The wrist is immobilized in a forearm cast for 6 weeks; K-wire removal is performed after 10 weeks. A locking plate (Medartis AG, Basel, Switzerland) has recently been developed for an STT fusion.

In a meta-analysis by Larsen et al, there was a 14% nonunion rate of 385 scaphotrapezium-trapezoid arthrodeses.[34] Kleinman and Carroll reviewed 47 wrists in 46 patients over a 10-year period and noted a complication rate of 52%.[35] Failure to attain perfect scaphoid reduction consistently resulted in persistent incapacitating pain. Radial styloid–scaphoid impingement was effectively treated by simple styloidectomy. Carpal osteomyelitis, lunate avascular necrosis, pin-tract infection, progressive medial carpal translation, and intractable pain without arthrosis were some of the more common complications. Watson et al examined 28 cases of Kienböck disease treated with scaphotrapeziotrapezoid arthrodesis at an average follow-up period of 51 months. Of these wrists, 9 required late lunate excision for pain and limited motion; however, only 3 patients in the entire series required further wrist salvage procedures (wrist arthrodesis, PRC). The wrist range of motion averaged 48° in extension, 52° in flexion, 11° in radial deviation, and 27° in ulnar deviation. Using a subjective pain relief rating scale, patients reported excellent results in 12 cases, good results in 9, fair results in 4, and poor results in 2.[28] Sauerbier et al reviewed the results of 26 patients with stage 3 of Kienböck disease treated with STT arthrodesis at a mean follow up of 35 months. The fusion healed in 25 patients at an average period of 7 weeks. Pain was reduced to 72% of the preoperative values at rest and 60% with stress. Active wrist range of motion was 65% of extension/flexion and 50% of radial/ulnar deviation on average compared with the contralateral hand. The average DASH score was 24.8; the Mayo and Krimmer wrist scores averaged 66 and 67.8 points, respectively,[36] compared with the other side. Meier et al treated 111 patients with an STT fusion. Indications included chronic SL dissociation (n = 15), primary STT arthrosis (n = 11), advanced Kienböck disease (n = 84), and 1 dislocation of the trapezium. At an average follow-up of 4 years (range, 2-8 years), the average wrist flexion/extension was (ROM) 81% of the preoperative value and 68% of the preoperative radial and ulnar deviation. The VAS were reduced to 76% (nonstress) and 55% (stress). The average grip strength improved to 65% of the contralateral side. The average modified Mayo wrist score was 66 points: 71 points for STT OA, 62 points in Kienböck disease, and 60 points in SL dissociation. The average DASH score was 27 points.[29]

SCAPHOCAPITOLUNATE (SCL) ARTHRODESIS

Hom and Ruby[37] proposed unacceptable high nonunion rates in scapholunate arthrodesis in 1991. There have not been any improvement in complication rates in recent years and this fusion is no longer recommended.

The SCL arthrodesis is an alternate treatment option in which the majority of the scaphoid is maintained to maximize physiological loading across the radiocarpal joint. A radial styloidectomy as well as a partial resection of the distal scaphoid can also be added in cases of painful radioscaphoid impingement.

Use the universal dorsal approach. The terminal branch of the posterior interosseous nerve is identified and resected. A dorsal longitudinal incision is then made through the third extensor compartment and the dorsal wrist capsule, extending into the radiocarpal and midcarpal joints. The scaphoid is examined. If 90% of the cartilage of the scaphoid fossa is well preserved, Fernandez recommends keeping the scaphoid in SLAC and SNAC wrists and proceeding with the SCL arthrodesis. Otherwise, a 4CF or PRC is considered. The distal fragment of the scaphoid is then excised in a piecemeal fashion, preserving the anterior capsule and ligaments. The cartilage and subchondral bone of the scapholunate, proximal SC, and CL articulations are removed. Any DISI deformity should be corrected while aligning the carpus for percutaneous pinning. Cancellous graft is inserted between the surfaces and pins (guidewires) should be placed across the CL, the scapholunate, and SC joints. Cannulated screws can be then used for final fixation. If the proximal scaphoid fragment is too small to maintain an intact rim of cartilage-to-cartilage contact with the capitate radially, an additional corticocancellous bone strut can be inserted into the radial aspect of the capitate and the radial aspect of the proximal scaphoid fragment to maintain support and prevent collapse of the scaphoid fragment. The wrist is immobilized for 6 weeks in a plaster forearm cast.

The success rate of scapholunate arthrodesis is low, regardless of the fixation technique. There is an unacceptably high rate of nonunion and clinical failure.[37] In 2003, in a follow-up study of 9 patients wrist motion was preserved within the functional range, extension to an average of 46° (range, 35°-60°), palmar flexion 41° (range, 40°-60°), radial deviation of 17° (range, 10°-25°), and ulnar deviation 34° (range, 30°-45°). Grip strength averaged 63% (range, 25-100) and pinch grip 70% (range, 43-100) of the unaffected side.[38]

In a 26-month follow-up, Chantelot et al[39] analyzed the functional results. They noticed a loss of range of motion of between 20% and 40%, especially for radial tilt and flexion. The grip strength was improved; all patients except 1 had residual pain.

Rotman et al performed a SCL fusion on 21 patients with an average age of 31 years for chronic SL dissociation or a scaphoid nonunion.[40] The operative procedure was done through a dorsal approach, with the use of autogenous bone grafting and Kirschner wire fixation. At an average follow-up of 28 months 81% healed after the primary procedure. The wrist motion averaged 35° of extension, 30° of flexion, 10° of radial deviation, and 20° of ulnar deviation. Grip strength averaged 70% of the uninvolved side. Pain was significantly reduced in 80% of the patients. Sixteen of 20 patients were able to return to work. The radiographic examination at final follow-up showed mild degenerative changes at the radiocarpal joint in 2 patients.

Klausmeyer et al recently reported their results in 20 patients who underwent an SCL arthrodesis, and radial styloidectomy.[41] The patients' ages ranged from 27 to 75 years (average age 62 years). Seven patients were treated for SNAC wrists, 12 patients for SLAC wrists, and 1 for degenerative joint disease following a transscapho-transcapitate perilunar dislocation. Sixteen patients had Herbert screw fixation and 4 had Spider plate fixation. All patients had autologous bone graft used for the arthrodesis. The mean follow-up was 4.6 years (range 2-9.6 years). Nineteen of 20 arthrodeses healed at an average of 9.6 weeks. One patient was reoperated 8 months after the initial operation with salvage of the SCL arthrodesis with a Spider plate with an adequate result. Postoperatively, the mean active flexion–extension arc was 70° and the radioulnar deviation arc was 23°. Pain decreased in all patients, 13 of whom were pain-free postoperatively. The average postoperative DASH score was 24 from 44 preoperatively. Radiographically, there was no radiolunate or radioscaphoid OA.

CAPITOLUNATE ARTHRODESIS

Scaphoid excision and FCA has been an accepted motion-preserving therapy for the degenerative wrist.[42–45] Recently there has been support for isolated CL arthrodesis with excision of the scaphoid and also the triquetrum.[46,47] The excision of the triquetrum is supposed to have advantages in reduction of the lunate, decreases the potential for ulnocarpal abutment (in ulnar positive wrists), and avoids late pisotriquetral arthritis. CL arthrodesis also improved motion, even though it has not been clinically observed. Cohen et al[48] showed, in a biomechanical study using a wrist motion simulator, decreased pressure ulnocarpal in resection of the triquetrum in isolated CL arthrodesis. But there was no significant change in radiolunate contact area after triquetral excision. In agreement with Scobercea et al, Cohen et al[48] are concerned about the routine excision of the triquetrum.

CL arthrodesis is used in degenerative arthritis that follows scapholunate instability or scaphoid pseudarthrosis. Another indication is an isolated destroyed CL joint after fracture. A comparable and more often used alternative is the 4-corner fusion.

The arthrosis of radiolunate joint as well as ulnar impaction syndrome is a contraindication for CL arthrodesis.

A dorsal S-shaped incision is performed. A radially based skin and subcutaneous flap is made, containing the superficial branch of the radial nerve. The third extensor compartment is opened and the extensor pollicis longus tendon and muscle is retracted radially. The second and fourth compartments are elevated subperiosteally from the radius. A segment of the posterior interosseous nerve is excised proximal to the fourth compartment. The capsule is opened with a radial-based flap, preserving the dorsal ligaments.

Then excision of the proximal part of scaphoid follows. The distal part of the scaphoid has to be trimmed to a trapezoid size to increase the distance from the radial scaphoid. Provisionally a K-wire from scaphoid to capitate may be forwarded. To further enlarge the distance to the scaphoid a radial styloidectomy (3 mm) can be performed. After exposing the CL joint, resection of the cartilage with interposition of a bone graft is carried out. Another Kirschner wire is placed between lunate and capitate. Very important is now to check range of extension and flexion of wrist. For stable fixation the Kirschner wires are replaced with headless compressive screws. A cast immobilization for 6 to 8 weeks is recommended.

Siegel and Ruby[49] reviewed the literature and compared different types of intracarpal fusion. The lunocapitate arthrodesis had higher incidence of nonunion than 4-corner fusion (35% vs 4%), and also higher rates of complications (62% vs 26%). Calandruccio et al[46] reported comparable fusion rates and range of motion to 4-corner fusion. Gatson et al[47] observed retrospectively no differences in grip strength, union rate, patient satisfaction, or need for revision surgery. Ferreres et al[50] reported in an 8- to 12-year follow-up with 17 patients a DASH score of 7.7 points (range 0-45), with only 1 case scoring over 40 points. According to the Mayo wrist score, there were 1 excellent, 5 good, 8 satisfactory, and 3 poor functional results, with an average score of 68 points (range 50-90).

LUNOTRIQUETRAL ARTHRODESIS

LT ligamentous instability is a common pathology for ulnar-sided wrist pain. Ambrose and Posner described an "ulnar snuffbox test" in which the examiner puts pressure on the ulnar aspect of the triquetrum to verify LT and pisotriquetral pathology.[51] There are plenty of differential diagnoses such as distal radioulnar joint disease, extensor and flexor carpi ulnaris tendinitis, etc. For further diagnostic, stress views may demonstrate dynamic dissociation (stage 2 in the classification[6]).

Indications for LT joint arthrodesis are symptomatic unstable dissociation of the LT joint and LT joint degenerative disease. In case of positive variance of the ulna producing an impaction syndrome, an osteotomy of the ulna may be performed additionally.

The LT joint is exposed through a transverse dorsal ulnar incision centered over the joint. The capsule is incised transversely to expose the LT joint. The adjacent articular surfaces of the lunate and triquetrum are removed with a rongeur to expose cancellous bone. Rims of the opposing cortical edges are left intact to preserve relationship of the 2 bones. Best results are achieved in removing the articular surfaces of lunate and triquetrum in a biconcave way. The implanted bone graft harvested from the radius or iliac crest can be packed into the recesses of the concave spaces and displacement is so prevented. Two guidewires are positioned into the ulnar aspect of the triquetrum and driven into the lunate. After x-ray control the guidewires are replaced through cannulated screws (Fig. 22-6). Immobilization is needed in a forearm plaster cast for 6 to 8 weeks.

Previously, Guidera et al[52] achieved primary LT arthrodesis fusion using cancellous bone graft and K-wires in all 24 patients. Postoperative wrist flexion/extension averaged 77%/80% of unaffected side. Pain relief had been good or very good in 83%. Bishop and coworkers compared LT reconstruction using a distally based strip of the tendon of extensor carpi ulnaris, LT repair, and LT arthrodesis after isolated LT injury. The mean follow-up was 9.5 years. Of the LT arthrodesis, 40.9% developed nonunion and 22.7% developed ulnocarpal impaction. The probability of not requiring further surgery at 5 years was 68.6% for reconstruction, 23.3% for repair, and 21.8% for arthrodesis. The DASH score for the arthrodesis group was 29.9, for the reconstruction group 19.7, and for the repair group 20.5. There was no significant difference. Objective improvements in strength and movement, and subjective indicators of pain relief and satisfaction were significantly higher in the LT repair and reconstruction groups than in those undergoing arthrodesis.[53]

RADIOCARPAL ARTHRODESIS

Radiolunate (Radioscapholunate) Arthrodesis

The radioscapholunate fusion already was introduced in 1955 by Watson-Jones and Gordon and King in 1961[54] for post-traumatic radiocarpal arthrosis. It has been the last option in SLAC and SNAC stage 2. Nowadays the RSL arthrodesis is a reasonable option when the articular surfaces of the distal radius, proximal scaphoid, and/or proximal lunate are compromised, especially after distal radius fractures. But reports of these operations are known only anecdotally.

Garcia-Elias et al[55] reported in 2005 the distal scaphoidectomy as an additional option to the RSL arthrodesis to retain more motion in extension, flexion, ulnar deviation, and radial deviation of the wrist and help prevent secondary midcarpal arthrosis.

In a few circumstances of SNAC pathology the proximal row might translocate ulnarly to such a degree that less than 50% of its articular surface remains in contact with the lunate fossa of the distal radius. In these cases a 4-corner fusion might have difficulties for a proper realignment and the radioscapholunate arthrodesis can help out.

The midcarpal joint must be carefully assessed for degenerative disease either in plain radiographs or with arthroscopy.

Midcarpal arthrosis is the absolute contraindication for RSL fusion as well as ulnar impaction syndrome.

A dorsal S-shaped incision is performed. As in most wrist procedures, a radially based skin and subcutaneous flap is made, containing the superficial branch of the radial nerve. The third extensor compartment is opened and the extensor pollicis longus tendon and muscle is retracted radially. The

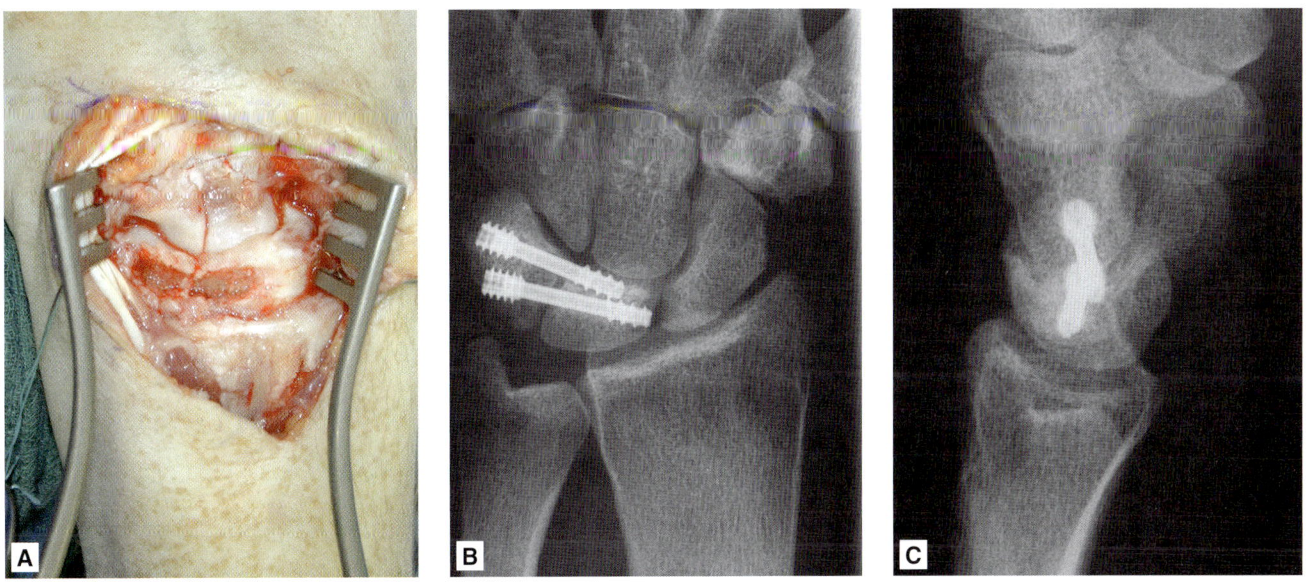

FIGURE 22-6 **A.** Intraoperative view for preparation of lunotriquetral arthrodesis due to instability. The lunate and the triquetrum (or corticocancellous strut) are ready to be inserted. **B** and **C.** Pa/lateral x-ray after LT arthrodesis with a 2-screw fixation technique.

second and fourth compartments are elevated subperiosteally from the radius. The compartments are not supposed to be opened. A segment of the posterior interosseous nerve is excised proximal to the fourth compartment. The capsule is opened in line with the dorsal radiotriquetral ligament with a distally based flap. The carpus is exposed and the radiocarpal joint checked for arthritic changes. If there is arthrosis in both joints, a RSL fusion cannot be performed and an alternative salvage procedure such as a total wrist arthrodesis or a total wrist arthroplasty should be considered.

After the removal of cartilage from radius, lunate, and scaphoid, according to the amount of resected surface, the gap is filled with corticocancellous bone of the radius or iliac crest (Fig. 22-7). Next are performed reduction of the bones in normal anatomical alignment (reduction out of DISI of the lunate if necessary) and a stabilization with K-wires.

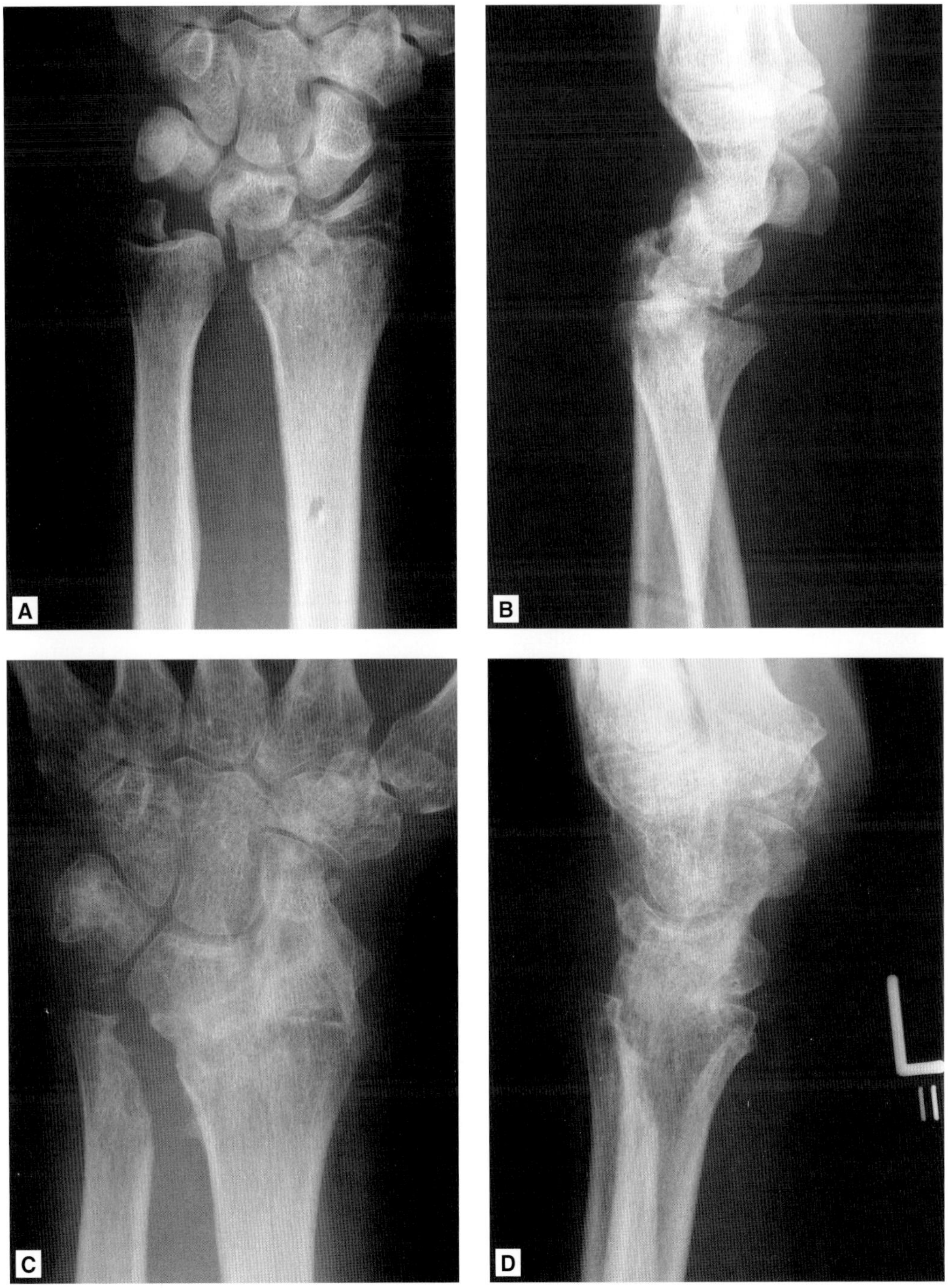

FIGURE 22-7 **A** and **B.** Complete destruction of the left radiocarpal joint and instability of the DRUJ in a 46-year-old male patient after a distal radius fracture and operation elsewhere. **C** and **D.** X-rays pa/lateral 6 months after an RSL arthrodesis and a Bowers hemiresection arthroplasty.

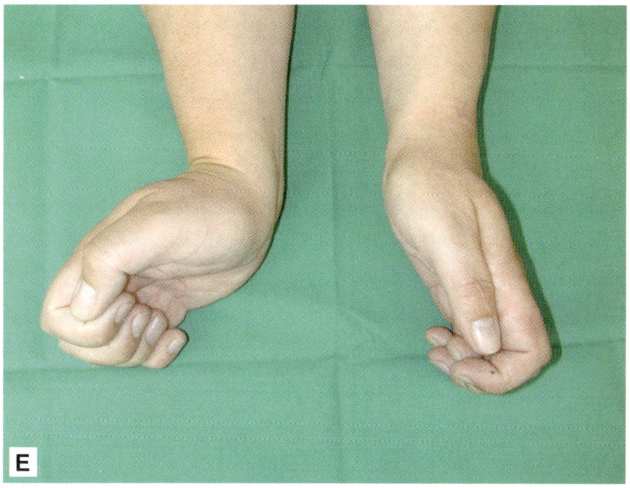

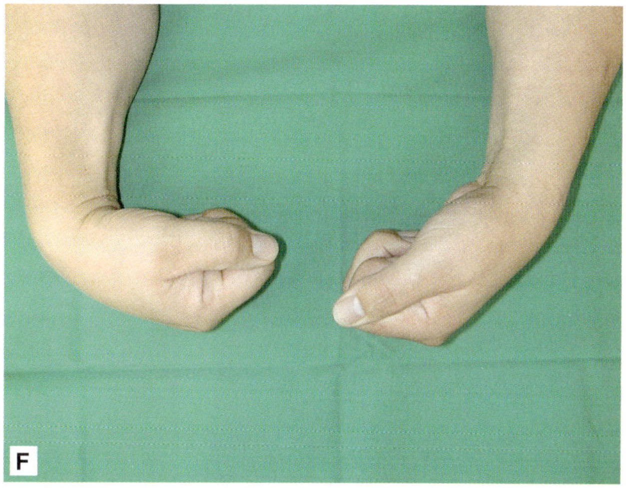

FIGURE 22-7 (*Continued*) **E** and **F.** The extension/flexion of the wrist joint reached 35/0/35°.

The ideal angle between radius and scaphoid should be 50° of flexion, while the lunate should be in neutral position.

Garcia-Elias et al[55] reported in 2005 the distal pole excision of the scaphoid as an additional option to retain more motion and help prevent secondary midcarpal arthrosis. The average postoperative ranges of motion were 32° of flexion and 35° of extension. Two patients exhibited secondary midcarpal degenerative joint disease. These results were significantly better compared with those previously published about RSL arthrodesis alone without resection of the distal scaphoid in terms of residual pain and decrease of wrist radial deviation and flexion.

The wrist is immobilized in a circular forearm plaster cast with inclusion of the proximal phalanx of the thumb for an average of 8 weeks.

In early times there have been many studies reporting high complication rates such as nonunion of the arthrodesis, early progressive arthritis, or persistent pain.[19,56]

In a recent study,[57] 73 patients were retrospectively evaluated, being treated by radioscapholunate fusion. The nonunion rate was high (21%). Ninety-seven percent of the patients showed satisfactory results even though functional limitation and residual pain existed. Arthrosis was found in 51%, mostly without affecting the clinical outcome. In a long-term follow-up the clinical outcome for radiolunate arthrodesis was good, with a mean visual analog score of 2 out of 10 for pain, mean grip strength of 13 kg, and mean range of flexion–extension of 60°. Outcomes as measured by questionnaires were good. The average DASH score was 41 points.[58]

In our department both techniques are not used in SNAC wrist. However, an RSL fusion should always be considered in cases with isolated radiocarpal arthrosis instead of a total wrist fusion. Recently we started using a special RSL-locking plate with a low-profile design (Medartis AG, Basel, Switzerland). The preliminary cases seem to be promising because immobilization is only necessary for 3 to 4 weeks (Fig. 22-8).

Proximal Row Carpectomy

PRC is an effective treatment option for degenerative or posttraumatic osteoarthritis of the wrist. It involves excision of the scaphoid, lunate, and triquetrum, and relies on the articulation of the remaining capitate from the distal row to articulate with the lunate fossa.

Being a contraindication for PRC, Tang and Imbriglia recently described a new technique of resurfacing the capitate in capitate arthrosis. They reported on 8 patients with capitate arthrosis who underwent a PRC. Using a bone graft harvested from the resected carpals, they did osteochondral resurfacing of the capitate. At 18-month follow-up, results compared favorably with traditional PRC.[59]

Placzek et al reported in 8 patients PRC with capitate head resection and dorsal capsular interposition. In 1-year follow-up they found pain relief in 75% of patients, but no improvement in ROM or grip strength was found.[60]

PRC is indicated in stage 2 SLAC/SNAC if shorter immobilization is indicated and static grip strength is not as important as it is for heavy manual worker.[59,61] In that case 4-corner fusion would be gold standard. PRC gives the best motion but may be associated with painful narrowing of the radiocapitate joint in the long term. Another indication is Kienböck disease stages 3a and b and in special cases stage 4.

Osteoarthritis of the capitate head and lunate fossa is traditionally a contraindication because of the expected narrowing of the radiocapitate joint.[19] Consequently, SNAC/SLAC stage 3 is an absolute contraindication for PRC and midcarpal arthrodesis may be treatment of choice.[62]

An S-shaped incision over the wrist is performed. A radially based skin and subcutaneous flap is made, containing the superficial branch of the radial nerve. The third extensor compartment is opened; the extensor pollicis longus tendon is retracted radially. The second and fourth compartments are elevated subperiosteally from the radius; a segment of the posterior interosseous nerve is excised proximal to the fourth

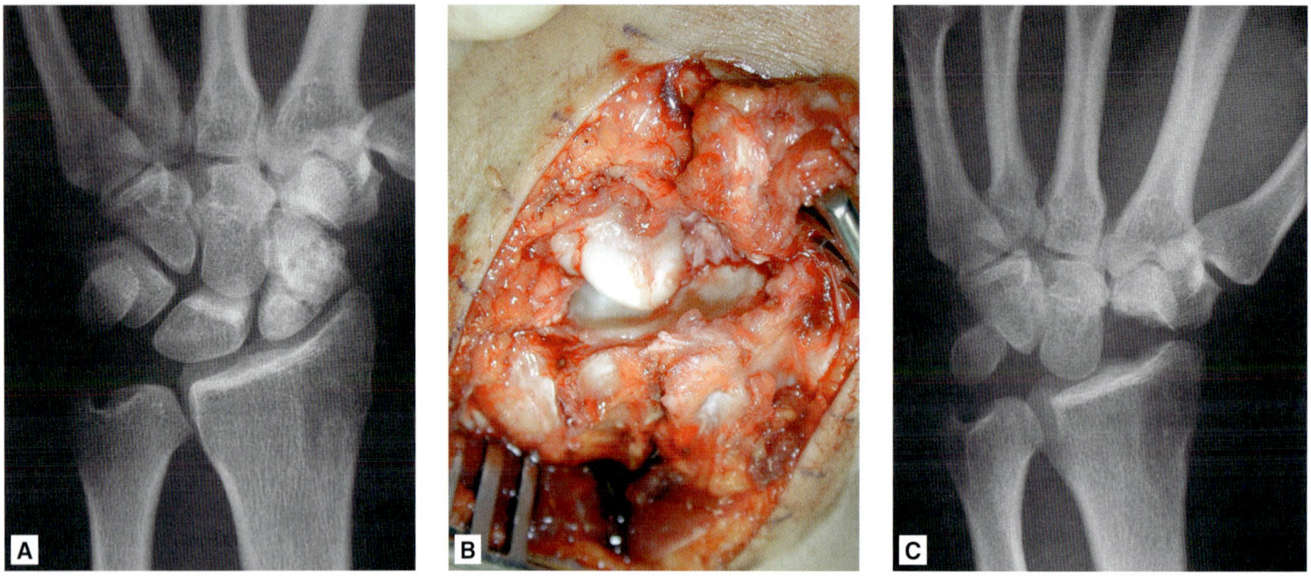

FIGURE 22-8 **A.** A 33-year-old female patient with arthroscopically confirmed SNAC wrist stage 2. **B.** Intraoperative view at the intact head of the capitate after removing the proximal row. **C.** Postoperative pa x-ray after PRC.

compartment. The capsule is opened with radial-based flap, preserving the dorsal ligaments.

To continue with the PRC, the cartilage of the capitate must be intact. Then the scaphoid, lunate, and triquetrum are excised with an osteotome and a rongeur. One should be sure not to damage the palmar capsule and wrist ligament. Under special circumstances additional radial styloidectomy is needed.

As soon as the proximal row is resected, the capitate will automatically articulate with the lunate fossa of the distal radius. The dorsal capsule of the wrist is closed tightly and the extensor retinaculum is closed including the sheath of the third extensor compartment within the EPL tendon.

The wrist is immobilized in a circular forearm plaster cast without inclusion of the metacarpal joints as well as the thumb for an average of 2 weeks for shrinking of the capsule. Then physiotherapy can be started.

After PRC 80% of the patients returned to their original occupation.[36]

Jebson et al reported visible radiocapitate degenerative changes in follow-up of 13 years.[63] Tränkle et al postulated postoperatively reduced pain in 87% of the patients and grip strength of 54% to the unaffected side; the DASH score was 27.8.[64] In 3 of 30 patients, Dacho et al reported visible radiocapitate degenerative changes at an average follow-up of 2 years, even though they were not associated with pain or loss of function.[61]

It can be concluded that PRC is a technically easy operation that preserves a satisfying ROM and pain relief.[65,66]

Richou et al evaluated a long-term clinical outcome study, where less pain in all 24 patients with PRC after an average of 116 months was reported. Eighty-three percent of the patients were satisfied. Grip strength averaged 78% of the contralateral site.[67]

Total Wrist Arthrodesis

Today several salvage procedures are available to treat delayed posttraumatic disorders of the wrist. Partial wrist fusions are supposed to stabilize the carpus and immobilize destroyed articulating surfaces while allowing motion in the unharmed parts of the wrist. The total wrist arthrodesis is the leading salvage procedure if also the partial fusions fail.

Field et al found a 25% incidence of "ulnar carpal pain" not otherwise specified following total wrist fusion.[68] The incidence of pisotriquetral dysfunction can be higher than literature, which suggests "ulnar carpal pain" could be due to pisotriquetral arthritis. Gatson et al do not recommend prophylactic excision of the pisiform, but patients undergoing wrist fusion should be assessed for pisotriquetral discomfort before surgery as physical examination and specific radiographs to look for degenerative changes. In a recent study Gatson et al reported a rarely documented complication of the total wrist arthrodesis: the pisotriquetral dysfunction resulting in degenerative changes.[69]

The main reason for total wrist arthrodesis includes the panarthrosis of the wrist and remaining pain after other midcarpal and carpal salvage procedures.

Using a straight dorsal approach from the third metacarpal bone to the distal radius, the second, third, and fourth extensor compartments are opened. The fourth compartment is subperiostally removed. The posterior interosseous nerve is resected if it is still untouched. The joint capsule is incised either with a radial-based flap or in a longitudinal manner. The cartilage of the radiocarpal as well as the affected intercarpal joints is removed with a rongeur or an osteotome. According to the amount of resected surface, the gap is filled with compression-resistant corticocancellous bone from the radius or under most circumstances from the iliac crest. The carpometacarpal joints should not be touched. Plate fixation is the standard technique for total wrist arthrodesis. In the last decade the AO wrist fusion plate was used by most hand surgeons.[70] The fusion plate is positioned from the proximal part of the third metacarpal bone till the distal dorsal radius, in 10° extension of the wrist. For further compression an additional screw can be placed into the capitate bone.

The wrist is immobilized in a circular forearm plaster cast without inclusion of the metacarpal joints for an average of 6 weeks. Recently we started the use of a new locking plate with a low-profile design (Medartis AG). The plate is available in 2 versions without bridging the CMC joint (long plate for regular wrist, short plate for arthrodesis after PRC; Fig. 22-9). Another type of this locking device is available in a longer version for bridging the CMC joint over the third metacarpal without fusion of the CMC. The plate may be used for wrist fusion under special circumstances such as rheumatoid arthritis, tumor resection, or other complicated wrist arthrodesis.

Nagy and Büchler recommended that the third carpometacarpal joint should not be included in the fusion mass. In 30 wrists where the third carpometacarpal joint was not included in the fusion, patients have been free of symptoms after plate removal. In comparison, 20 wrists that underwent third carpometacarpal joint arthrodesis had nonunion after plate removal.[71]

After reviewing the literature amazingly different results can be found. Watson et al have documented good pain relief and stable, functional wrists in a long-term follow-up.[72] However, there are up to 100% of complications reported in AO plate fusions such as nonunion, malalignment, infection, pain, hardware loosening, and tendon rupture.[73] Recent studies demonstrated that a total wrist arthrodesis does not always lead to complete pain relief.[70,74]

Kalb et al as well as Sauerbier et al showed remaining complaints after total wrist arthrodesis in patients with posttraumatic wrist arthrosis or Kienböck disease. Eighty percent of the patients complained about reduction of postoperative quality of life. Personal hygiene and washing the back may be pretty difficult with a fused wrist. Adey et al showed that 90% would elect to have a procedure that would improve wrist motion.[75] Bolano and Green[76] report of pain under stress in two thirds of the patients. Surprisingly most of the patients would undergo the procedure again.[70,74,77]

Sixty-four percent of the patients were complaining about persisting pain after total wrist arthrodesis.[75] Sauerbier et al supported these data by using the DASH score for comparison of total wrist arthrodesis and motion-preserving procedures.[70,74] The overall DASH score was 51.4. However, 70% of the patients returned to their original occupation.[74]

Regarding the ROM, performance of activities of daily life, and patient's satisfaction, the limited wrist arthrodesis

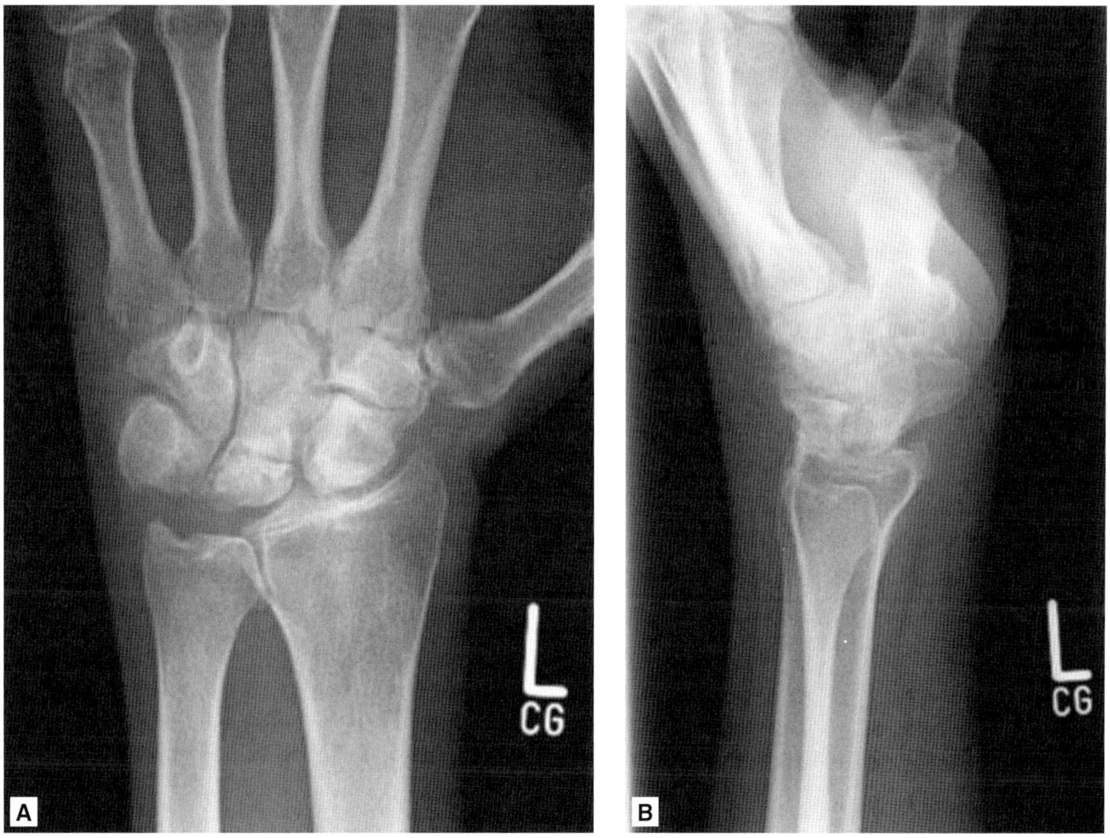

FIGURE 22-9 **A** and **B.** A 47-year-old gardener with wrist arthrosis.

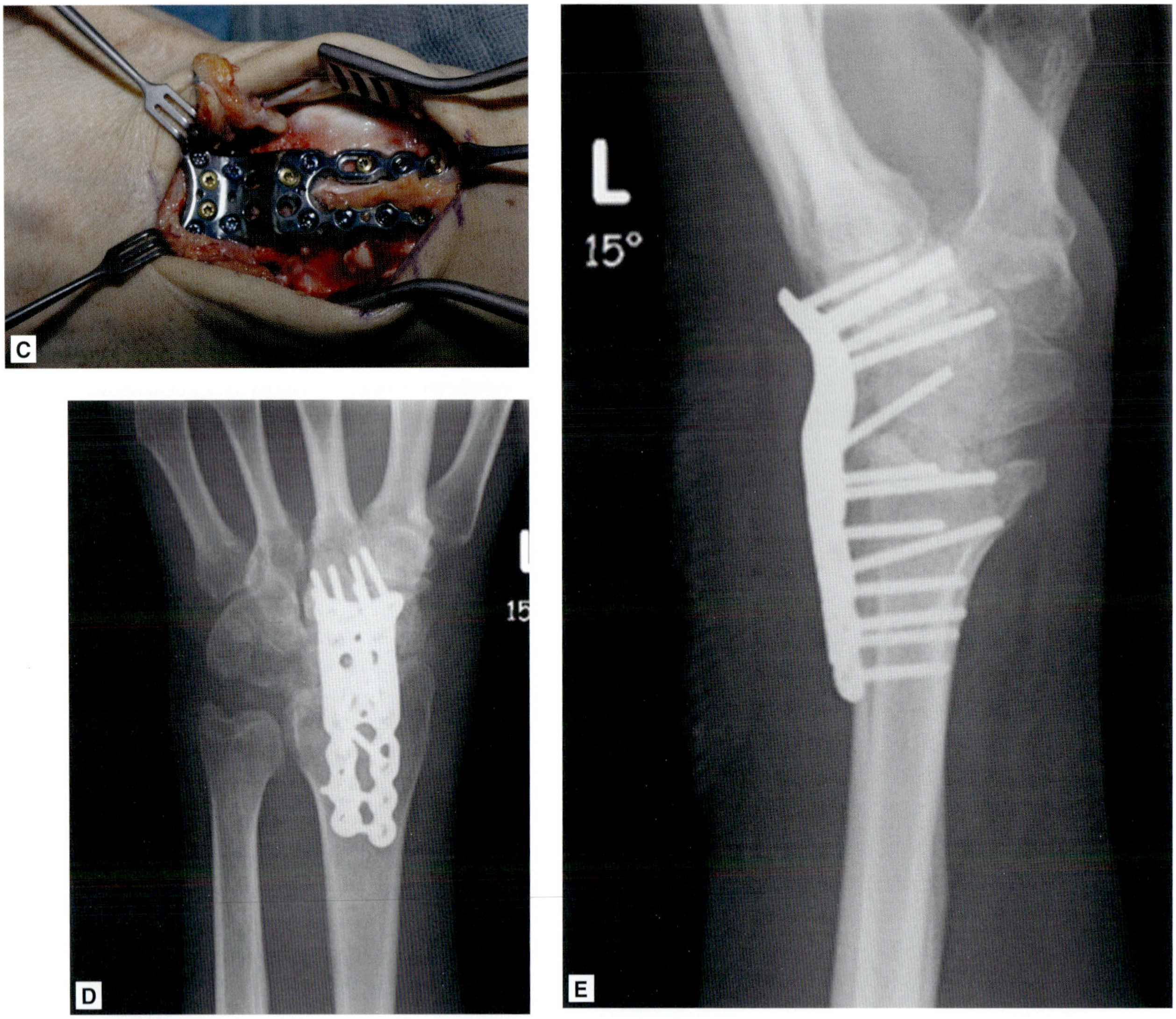

FIGURE 22-9 (*Continued*) **C** and **D.** Intraoperative view of the implanted locking device (Medartis AG, Basel, Switzerland). The CMC joint is spared. **E.** Postoperative x-ray lateral.

is superior to total wrist fusion.[24] The DASH score and ADL reports emphasize the data.[70] Total wrist arthrodesis should only be used for exceptional circumstances as last line of defense.

REFERENCES

1. Linscheid RL, Dobyns JH, Beabout JW, Bryan RS. Traumatic instability of the wrist: diagnosis, classification, and pathomechanics. *J Bone Joint Surg Am.* 1972;54:1612–1632.
2. Lichtman DM, Schneider JR, Swafford AR, Mack GR. Ulnar midcarpal instability—clinical and laboratory analysis. *J Hand Surg Am.* 1981;6:515–523.
3. International Wrist Investigators' Workshop Terminology Committee. Wrist: terminology and definitions. *J Bone Joint Surg Am.* 2002;84A(suppl 1):1–73.
4. Schmitt R, Stäbler A, Krimmer H. Karpale Instabilitäten. In: Schmitt R, Lanz U, eds. *Bildgebende Diagnostik der Hand.* Stuttgart: Thieme, Springer Verlag; 2004:261–284.
5. Watson HK, Ryu J. Evolution of arthritis of the wrist. *Clin Orthop Relat Res.* 1986;202;57–67.
6. Viegas S, Patterson R, Peterson P, et al. Ulnar sided perilunate instability: an anatomic and biomechanical study. *J Hand Surg Am.* 1990;15:268–278.
7. Nakamura T, Cooney WP 3rd, Lui WH, et al. Radial styloidectomy: a biomechanical study on stability of the wrist joint. *J Hand Surg Am.* 2001;26:85–93.
8. Sutro CJ. Treatment of nonunion of the carpal navicular bone. *Surgery.* 1946;20:536–540.
9. Pisano SM, Peimer CA, Wheeler DR, Sherwin F. Scaphocapitate intercarpal arthrodesis. *J Hand Surg Am.* 1991;16:328–333.
10. Minamikawa Y, Peimer CA, Yamaguchi T, Medige J, Sherwin FS. Ideal scaphoid angle for intercarpal arthrodesis. *J Hand Surg Am.* 1992;17:370–375.
11. Sennwald GR, Ufenast H. Scaphocapitate arthrodesis for the treatment of Kienbock's disease. *J Hand Surg Am.* 1995;20:506–510.
12. Delétang F, Segret J, Dap F, Dautel G. Chronic scapholunate instability treated by scaphocapitate fusion: a midterm outcome perspective. *Orthop Traumatol Surg Res.* 2011;97(2):164–171.
13. Berger RA, Bishop AT, Bettinger PC. New dorsal capsulotomy for the surgical exposure of the wrist. *Ann Plast Surg.* 1995;35:54–59.

14. Shindle MK, Burton KJ, Weiland AJ, Domb BG, Wolfe SW. Complications of circular plate fixation for four-corner arthrodesis. *J Hand Surg Eur Vol.* 2007;32(1):50–53.
15. Merrell GA, McDermott EM, Weiss AP. Four-corner arthrodesis using a circular plate and distal radius bone grafting: a consecutive case series. *J Hand Surg Am.* 2008;33(5):635–642.
16. Gupta RK, Chauhan DS, Singh H. Non-union scaphoid: four-corner fusion of the wrist. *Indian J Orthop.* 2010;44(2):208–211.
17. Ozyurekoglu T, Turker T. Results of a method of 4-corner arthrodesis using headless compression screws. *J Hand Surg Am.* 2012;37(3):486–492.
18. Krimmer H, Sauerbier M, Vispo-Seara JL, Schindler G, Lanz U. Advanced carpal collapse (SLAC-wrist) in scaphoid pseudarthrosis. Therapy concept: medio-carpal partial arthrodesis. *Handchir Mikrochir Plast Chir.* 1992;24(4):191–198.
19. Krakauer JD, Bishop AT, Cooney WP. Surgical treatment of scapholunate advanced collapse. *J Hand Surg Am.* 1994;19(5):751–759.
20. Sauerbier M, Bickert B, Tränkle M, Kluge S, Pelzer M, Germann G. Surgical treatment possibilities of advanced carpal collapse (SNAC/SLAC wrist). *Unfallchirurg.* 2000;103(7):564–571.
21. Bain GI, Watts AC. The outcome of scaphoid excision and four-corner arthrodesis for advances carpal collapse at a minimum of ten years. *J Hand Surg Am.* 2010;35(5):719–725.
22. Cooney WP, Bussey R, Dobyns JH, Linscheis RL. Difficult wrist fractures. *Clin Orthop Relat Res.* 1987;213:136–147.
23. Germann G, Wind G, Harth A. The DASH (Disability of Arm–Shoulder–Hand) Questionnaire—a new instrument for evaluating upper extremity treatment outcome. *Handchir Mikrochir Plast Chir.* 1999;31: 149–152.
24. Krimmer H, Wiemer P, Kalb K. A comparison of functional outcome following limited and total fusion of the wrist. *Handchir Mikrochir Plast Chir.* 2000;32:360–374.
25. Witt AN. Schädigungen der Gelenke des Daumenstrahls und ihre Behebung. *Chirurg.* 1956;27:193–199.
26. Peterson HA, Lipscomb PR. Intercarpal arthrodesis. *Arch Surg.* 1967;95(1):127–134.
27. Watson HK. Limited wrist arthrodesis. *Clin Orthop Relat Res.* 1980;149:126–136.
28. Watson HK, Monacelli DM, Milford RS, Ashmead D IV. Treatment of Kienböck's disease with scaphotrapezio-trapezoid arthrodesis. *J Hand Surg Am.* 1996;21:9–15.
29. Meier R, Prommersberger KJ, Krimmer H. Scapho-trapezio-trapezoid arthrodesis (triscaphe arthrodesis). *Handchir Mikrochir Plast Chir.* 2003;35(5):323–327.
30. Horii E, Garcia-Elias M, Bishop AT, Cooney WP, Linscheid RL, Chao EY. Effect on force transmission across the carpus in procedures to treat Kienböck's disease. *J Hand Surg Am.* 1990;15:393–400.
31. Gupta RK, Tuennerhoff HG, Haussmann P. STT-arthrodesis versus radial shortening osteotomy for Kienböck's disease. *Handchir Mikrochir Plast Chir.* 2003;35(5):328–332.
32. Lichtman DM, Degnan GG. Staging and its use in the determination of treatment modalities for Kienböck's disease. *Hand Clin.* 1993;9(3):409–416.
33. Hohendorff B, Mühldorfer-Fodor M, Kalb K, van Schoonhoven J, Prommersberger KJ. STT arthrodesis versus proximal row carpectomy for Lichtman stage IIIB Kienböck's disease: first results of an ongoing observational study. *Arch Orthop Trauma Surg.* 2012;132(9): 1327–1334.
34. Larsen CF, Jakoby RA, McCabe SJ. Nonunion rates of limited carpal arthrodesis: a meta-analysis of the literature. *J Hand Surg Am.* 1997;22:66–73.
35. Kleinman WB, Carroll C 4th. Scapho-trapezio-trapezoid arthrodesis for treatment of chronic static and dynamic scapho-lunate instability: a 10-year perspective on pitfalls and complications. *J Hand Surg Am.* 1990;15(3):408–414.
36. Sauerbier M, Tränkle M, Erdmann D, Menke H, Germann G. Functional outcome with scaphotrapeziotrapezoid arthrodesis in the treatment of Kienböck's disease stage III. *Ann Plast Surg.* 2000;44(6):618–625.
37. Hom S, Ruby LK. Attempted scapholunate arthrodesis for chronic scapholunate dissociation. *J Hand Surg Am.* 1991;16:334–339.
38. Zubairy AI, Jones WA. Scapholunate fusion in chronic symptomatic scapholunate instability. *J Hand Surg Br.* 2003;28(4):311–314.
39. Chantelot C, Becquet E, Leconte F, Lahoude-Chantelot S, Prodomme G, Fontaine C. Scaphocapitate arthrodesis for chronic scapholunate instability: a retrospective study of 13 cases. *Chir Main.* 2005;24(2):79–83.
40. Rotman MB, Manske PR, Pruitt DL, Szerzinski J. Scaphocapitolunate arthrodesis. *J Hand Surg Am.* 1993;18(1):26–33.
41. Klausmeyer M, Fernandez D, Caloia M. Scaphocapitolunate arthrodesis and radial styloidectomy. *J Wrist Surg.* 2012;1:47–54.
42. Cohen MS, Kozin SH. Degenerative arthritis of the wrist: proximal row carpectomy versus scaphoid excision and four-corner fusion. *J Hand Surg Am.* 2001;26:94–104.
43. Gill DRJ, Ireland DCR. Limited wrist arthrodesis for the salvage of SLAC wrist. *J Hand Surg Br.* 1997;22B:461–465.
44. Tomaino MM, Miler RJ, Cole I, Burton RI. Scapholunate advanced collapse wrist: proximal row carpectomy or limited wrist arthrodesis with scaphoid excision. *J Hand Surg Am.* 1994;19:134–142.
45. Wyrick JD, Stern PJ, Kiefhaber TR. Motion-preserving procedures in the treatment of scapholunate advanced collapse wrist: proximal row carpectomy versus four-corner arthrodesis. *J Hand Surg Am.* 1995;20:965–970.
46. Calandruccio JH, Gelberman RH, Duncan SFM, Goldfarb CA, Pae R, Gramig W. Capitolunate arthrodesis with scaphoid and triquetrum excision. *J Hand Surg Am.* 2000;25:824–832.
47. Gatson RG, Greenberg JA, Baltera RM, Mih A, Hastings H. Clinical outcomes of scaphoid and triquetral excision with capitolunate arthrodesis versus scaphoid excision and four-corner arthrodesis. *J Hand Surg Am.* 2009;34:1407–1412.
48. Cohen MS, Werner FW, Sutton LG, Short WH. Scaphoid excision and midcarpal arthrodesis: the effect of triquetral excision—a biomechanical study. *J Hand Surg Am.* 2012;37(3):493–499.
49. Siegel JM, Ruby LK. A critical look at intercarpal arthrodesis: review of the literature. *J Hand Surg Am.* 1996;21:717–723.
50. Ferreres M, Garcia-Elias M, Plaza R. Long-term results of lunocapitate arthrodesis with scaphoid excision for SLAC and SNAC wrists. *J Hand Surg Eur Vol.* 2009;34:603–608.
51. Ambrose L, Posner M. Luno-triquetral and midcarpal instability. *Hand Clin.* 1992;8:653–668.
52. Guidera PM, Watson HK, Dwyer TA, Orlando G, Zeppieri J, Yasuda M. Lunotriquetral arthrodesis using cancellous bone graft. *J Hand Surg Am.* 2001;26(3):422–427.
53. Shin AY, Weinstein LP, Berger RA, Bishop AT. Treatment of isolated injuries of the lunotriquetral ligament. A comparison of arthrodesis, ligament reconstruction and ligament repair. *J Bone Joint Surg Br.* 2001;83(7):1023–1028.
54. Gordon LH, King D. Partial wrist arthrodesis for old un-united fractures of the carpal navicular. *Am J Surg.* 1961;102:460–464.
55. Garcia-Elias M, Lluch A, Ferreres A, Papini-Zorli I, Rahimtoola ZO. Treatment of radiocarpal degenerative osteoarthritis by radioscapholunate arthrodesis and distal scaphoidectomy. *J Hand Surg Am.* 2005;30(1):8–15.
56. Nagy L, Buechler U. Long-term results of radioscapholunate fusion following fractures of the distal radius. *J Hand Surg Br.* 1997;22(6):705–710.
57. Muehldorfer M, Hohendorff B, Prommersberger KJ, Van Schoonhoven J. Medium term results after radioscapholunate fusion for posttraumatic osteoarthritis of the wrist. *Handchir Mikrochir Plast Chir* 2009;41(3):148–155.
58. Raven EE, Ottink KD, Doets KC. Radiolunate and radioscapholunate arthrodeses as treatments for rheumatoid and psoriatic arthritis: long-term follow-up. *J Hand Surg Am.* 2012;37(1):55–62.
59. Tang P, Imbriglia JE. Osteochondral resurfacing (OCRPRC) for capitate chondrosis in proximal row carpectomy. *J Hand Surg Am.* 2007;32:1334–1342.
60. Placzek JD, Boyer MI, Raaii F, Freeman DC, Gelberman RH. Proximal row carpectomy with capitate resection and capsular interposition for treatment of scapholunate advanced collapse. *Orthopedics.* 2008;31:75.
61. Dacho A, Sauerbier M, Germann G, Baumeister S. Comparison of proximal row carpectomy and midcarpal arthrodesis for the treatment of scaphoid nonunion advanced collapse (SNAC-wrist) and scapholunate advanced collapse (SLAC-wrist) in stage II. *J Plast Reconstr Aesthet Surg.* 2008;61(10):1210–1218.
62. Sauerbier M, Berger RA. Limited wrist arthrodesis. In: Weiss AP, Hastings H II, eds. *Surgery of the Arthritic Hand and Wrist.* Philadelphia: Lippincott Williams & Wilkins; 2002:121–139.

63. Jebson PJ, Hayes EP, Engber WD. Proximal row carpectomy: a minimum 10-year follow-up study. *J Hand Surg Am.* 2004;28:561–569.
64. Tränkle M, Sauerbier M, Blum K, Bickert B, Germann G. Proximal row carpectomy: a motion-preserving procedure in the treatment of advanced carpal collapse. *Unfallchirurg.* 2003;106(12):1010–1015.
65. Kremer T, Sauerbier M, Trankle M, Dragu A, Germann G, Baumeister S. Functional results after proximal row carpectomy to salvage a wrist. *Scand J Plast Reconstr Surg Hand Surg.* 2008;42(6):308–312.
66. Baumeister S, Germann G, Dragu A, et al. Functional results after proximal row carpectomy (PRC) in patients with SNAC-/SLAC-wrist stage II. *J Plast Reconstr Aesthet Surg.* 2008;61(10):1210–1218.
67. Richou J, Chuinrd C, Moineau G, Hanouz N, Hu W, Le Nen D. Proximal row carpectomy: long-term results. *Chir Main.* 2010;29(1):10–15.
68. Field J, Herbert TJ, Prosser R. Total wrist fusion. *J Hand Surg Br.* 1996;21:429–433.
69. Gatson RG, Lourie GM, Floyd WE 3rd, Swick M. Pisotriquetral dysfunction following limited and total wrist arthrodesis. *J Hand Surg Am.* 2007;32(9):1348–1355.
70. Sauerbier M, Kania NM, Kluge S, Bickert B, Germann G. Initial results of treatment with the new AO wrist joint arthrodesis plate. *Handchir Mikrochir Plast Chir.* 1998;31:260–265.
71. Nagy L, Büchler U. AO-wrist arthrodesis: with and without arthrodesis of the third carpometacarpal joint. *J Hand Surg Am.* 2002;27:940–947.
72. Watson HK, Weinzweig J, Guidera PM, Zeppieri J, Ashmead D. One thousand intercarpal arthrodesis. *J Hand Surg Br.* 1999;24:307–315.
73. Zachary SV, Stern PJ. Complications following AO/ASIF wrist arthrodesis. *J Hand Surg.* 1995;20A:339–344.
74. Sauerbier M, Tränkle M, Linsner G, Bickert B, Germann G. Midcarpal arthrodesis with complete scaphoid excision and interposition bone graft in the treatment of advanced carpal collapse (SNAC/SLAC wrist): operative technique and outcome assessment. *J Hand Surg Br.* 2000;25:341–345.
75. Adey L, Ring D, Jupiter JB. Health status after total wrist arthrodesis for posttraumatic arthritis. *J Hand Surg Am.* 2005;30(5):932–936.
76. Bolano LE, Green DP. Wrist arthrodesis on post-traumatic arthritis: a comparison of two methods. *J Hand Surg Am.* 1993;18:786–791.
77. Kalb KH, Ludwig A, Tauscher A, Landleitner B, Wiemer P, Krimmer H. Treatment outcome after surgical arthrodesis. *Handchir Mikrochir Plast Chir.* 1999;31:253–259.

Soft Tissue Coverage of the Carpus

Günter Germann, MD, PhD

23

INTRODUCTION

Sensibility, strength, dexterity, and aesthetics of the hand play an important role in the appearance and the overall impression of a person, since the hand is our most visible "contact zone" secondary only to the face. Soft tissue injuries of the forearm with exposed tendons, bones, or joints are therefore a major reconstructive challenge.

Advances in anatomy instrumentation and innovative microsurgical techniques have significantly changed the soft tissue reconstruction of the upper extremity. Continual refinements in the design and harvesting of flaps have led to improved aesthetic and functional results for both microsurgical free flaps and regional flaps.

A 1-stage reconstruction of the extremity is now the accepted standard, including tendon transfers, bone reconstruction, or nerve grafting, at the same time as the soft tissue coverage.[1]

Based on these changes the current concept of reconstruction consists of custom tailored solutions to match the individual profile of the patient—as minimal as possible but as complex as necessary. In certain situations a free flap might be the method of choice, whereas in other cases a simple skin graft may suffice. In cases where a complex procedure is the first choice the reconstructive ladder is replaced by the "reconstructive elevator."[2,3]

RELEVANT ANATOMY

There are 2 venous systems: a deep system consisting of paired or single venae comitantes accompanying the arteries and a superficial, large-caliber cutaneous system.

The radial artery lies deep to the brachioradialis muscle in the proximal half of the forearm and lateral to the flexor carpi radialis (FCR) tendon at the distal radius and gives off fasciocutaneous and septocutaneous perforators in the snuffbox, which are feeding a variety of flaps. The ulnar artery is larger than the radial artery, lies between the flexor carpi ulnaris (FCU) and the flexor digitorum profundus muscles, and gives off the common interosseous artery in the proximal forearm, which divides into the anterior and posterior interosseous arteries. The anterior interosseous artery runs along the ventral aspect of the interosseous membrane (IOM) and sends skin perforators that supply the skin of the distal two thirds of the forearm. It divides near the wrist into 2 terminal branches that join the anterior and dorsal networks and anastomose with the posterior anterior artery near the ulnar head to form an arterial loop. The posterior interosseous artery (PIA) penetrates the IOM to run along the dorsal aspect of the IOM, distal to the supinator muscle and proximal to the ulnar head in the intermuscular septum between the extensor carpi ulnaris and extensor digiti minimi muscle. The cutaneous perforators supply the extensor side of the proximal two thirds of the forearm.

The dorsal ulnar artery branch arises from the ulnar artery 2 to 6 cm proximal to the pisiform, and supplies the FCU muscle, the pisiform, and the skin along the ulnar side of the forearm before joining the dorsal carpal arch.

The 4 main arteries contribute to the vascular wrist system and build a palmar and dorsal network of transverse arches. There are 2 palmar (superficial palmar and deep palmar arch) and 3 transverse dorsal carpal arches (basal metacarpal arch, dorsal intercarpal arch, and dorsal radiocarpal arch) that are formed by the radial, ulnar, and interosseous anterior arteries. The PIA is less important for the supply of the wrist.[4–6]

CHOICE OF FLAPS—RECONSTRUCTIVE STRATEGY

All of the flaps are raised under tourniquet control and loupe magnification.

The choice of flap is dependent on the site and complexity of the defect, the available reconstructive options, and the patient anatomy.[1–3,7]

Regional and Distant Flaps

Regional flaps can be divided into several types of flaps:

1. Axial flaps based on forearm arteries, which include the septocutaneous and radial fascial forearm flap, the ulnar artery flap, and the posterior interosseous flap
2. Perforator flaps based on perforating vessels arising from the larger arteries or the carpal arch such as the distal ulnar perforator flap ("Becker flap"), distal radial perforator flaps ("free style flaps"), and proximally pedicled DCA flaps (for smaller defects)

GROIN FLAP

The groin flap can be raised as a pedicled or free flap. The pedicled version is a very reliable flap that can be raised swiftly. A free flap is characterized by its short pedicle and small vessel diameters thus limiting the versatility of the flap. Even in patients with a higher body mass index (BMI) the groin flap mostly provides reasonably thin cutaneous tissue. Flap dimensions are up to 10 × 25 cm.[8]

Indications

Defects of palmar and dorsal aspects of the carpus and the distal forearm.

Soft tissue coverage when a secondary procedure, that is, toe transfer is planned. Advantages include the fact that a large flap is possible and the donor site is inconspicuous with minimal morbidity. Disadvantages include the fact that it is pigmented, has a short pedicle, is very often bulky that may require a secondary defatting, and, if used as a pedicled flap, requires immobilizing the hand in a dependent position that can lead to upper extremity stiffness.

Contraindications

Need for early physical therapy after complex injuries.

Older patients where shoulder immobilization may be inappropriate.

Anatomy

The flap is supplied by the superficial circumflex iliac artery that is 0.8 to 1.8 mm in diameter and 1.5 to 2.0 cm long. The flap is drained by the deep and superficial veins that are 2.0 to 3.0 cm in diameter and 2.5 to 4.0 cm long. The flap is usually nonsensate, but it can be innervated by incorporating the T12 intercostal branches. The venous drainage is quite variable. The groin area is drained by the superficial epigastric vein (SEV), the superficial circumflex iliac vein (SCIV), and the associated venae comitantes. These veins drain into either the saphenous bulb or the femoral.

Surgical Technique

The flap should be designed so that one third is above and two thirds below the inguinal ligament. The pedicled flap is harvested under loupe magnification from the lateral border near the anterior superior iliac spine above the fascia. The vessels are dissected up to the medial border of the sartorius. The medial part can be tubed to allow more flexibility when inserting the flap. When used as a free flap, sometimes a medial dissection after Doppler identification of the course of the vessels may be helpful.

The fascia of the sartorius muscle is sometimes in immediate proximity to the vessels and can be included to avoid injury to the vessels. The vein and artery do not always run together. Care has to be taken to trace both vessels to their origin from the femoral vessels. If the artery appears too small, a small cuff of the femoral artery can be taken in rare cases to facilitate the vascular anastomosis.

Complications are rare in the pedicled groin flap. Distal necrosis may occur and can usually be solved by reinsetting of the flap. More common is tearing out of the flap when the patient tries to move the hand, and the hand is not sufficiently secured.

Additional complications can occur when the flap is divided; therefore, I would recommend following the principle of "cut and run," meaning division of the flap without immediate insetting.

When the flap is too long, distal venous congestion may occur. Tubing of the proximal part may also impair the distal perfusion.

This frequently results in partial necrosis of the flap. We prefer to leave a generous distal portion at the defect site and debulk it at the time of pedicle division. Within a few days it becomes apparent which parts of the flap may not survive so that the vital parts can be safely inserted to close the defect definitively.

Although we still consider the groin flap a valuable option, it has to be emphasized that usually 4 to 5 surgical procedures are required to reach a final result. Not all of them require general anesthesia, but it may take up to more than 1 year until debulking and contouring is completed, which is an argument in favor of free tissue transfers in some cases despite the potential risks.

REGIONAL FLAPS

Proximal Dorsal Metacarpal Artery (DMCA) Flaps

These flaps are based on the metacarpal arteries arising from the dorsal carpal arch.[4–6,9,10]

INDICATIONS

Smaller defects around the wrist that can be reconstructed with a reverse proximal pedicle flap.

CONTRAINDICATIONS

Defects that are too large for this type of flaps.

Injuries to the dorsal carpus with potential disruption of the feeding vessels especially in cases of previous skin graft over the dorsal wrist.

SURGICAL TECHNIQUE

The flap design is centered over the course of the vessel that has been identified and marked by Doppler examination. The flap dissection starts distally in the web space to achieve a wide arc of rotation and includes the fascia of the interosseous muscle to be sure that that artery is included. The flap dissection then proceeds proximally until the necessary arc of rotation is secured.

Advantages include a versatile flap design and primary closure of the donor site.

The disadvantages include need for a meticulous dissection especially when the intertendinous connections obstruct the view and the flap is only suitable for small defects.

Complications are rare. The most important tip for dissection is to identify the palmar–dorsal perforator in the web space to trace the artery proximally. The fascia of the interosseous muscle should be included.

A potential pitfall is the handling of the intertendinous connections. In our practice it has proven to be useful to divide those and reattach them later. Sometimes it can be even helpful to include a muscle cuff to secure the pedicle.

Indications for these flaps are rare and we have only used these flaps on a few occasions. However, it still is a good option, when small defects cannot be reconstructed with a local rotation flap.

Radial Forearm Flap

The "classic" radial forearm flap in all its modifications is based on the radial artery that has to be sacrificed for this flap. It can be used as a distally based pedicle flap for coverage of ipsilateral carpal or distal forearm defects, or as a free flap for coverage of contralateral palmar defects. It can be also raised as a fascial flap, either pedicled or free. Flap dimensions can be up to 8 × 20 cm.[11,12]

INDICATIONS

This includes defects around the wrist, flow-through flap reconstruction (as a free flap), and coverage of palmar defects (as a fascia flap).

CONTRAINDICATIONS

Donor-site defects in younger female patients can be unsightly. Severe arterial disease, heavy smokers, or severe diabetes.

ANATOMY

This flap is supplied by the radial artery and its perforators with a vessel diameter of 3 to 4 mm and it is drained by the 2 venae comitantes with a diameter of 3 to 5 mm and superficial veins. The pedicle length is up to 15 cm. The flap can be innervated by incorporating the lateral antebrachial cutaneous nerve.

SURGICAL TECHNIQUE

The flap design is centered over the course of the vessel that has been identified by Doppler preoperatively. Flap harvest is performed under tourniquet control. The radial artery is identified distally so that the pedicle can be securely traced. The flap is then incised circumferentially. The dissection proceeds subfascially toward the pedicle. I usually start from the ulnar side, but this is not mandatory. Care has to be taken to preserve the septal connection including the perforating vessels supplying the skin island. After the flap is completely raised, the tourniquet is let down and flap perfusion is checked. Then a vascular clamp is applied to the inflow from the proximal artery. Flap perfusion should be still normal for a couple of minutes before the proximal artery is ligated and the flap can be rotated into the defect. A primary closure of the donor site can be performed with narrow donor-site defects, whereas wider defects usually need full-thickness or thick split-thickness skin grafts (Fig. 23-1A-C).

In case of a free flap transfer we also temporarily occlude the distal pedicle to ensure sufficient flap perfusion before pedicle division.

Fascial flaps are raised using the same technique except that the incision is centered over the vessel and the dissection proceeds from there toward the edges of the outlined flap dimensions. Advantages of this flap include the ability to reconstruct large defects; the pedicle is long and reliable for wide arc of rotation; it experiences a free flap; it can be harvested as a complex flap including tendon and bone; and it is a thin flap even in obese patients. Disadvantages include the need to sacrifice each artery, along with a conspicuous donor site with the risk of tendon exposure distally if a skin graft does not take completely.

Complications are rare. The most frequent complications include distal venous congestion and incomplete take of the skin graft for the donor site.

Several considerations should be kept in mind. The arc of rotation should not be too acute to avoid venous kinking. The flap should be designed 10% larger than the defect to prevent undue tension of the flap edges. The paratenon of the flexor tendons, especially of the FCR, should be preserved to provide a better wound bed for the skin graft. Distally it is important to dissect around the tendons of the FCR and brachioradialis to harvest the septum with the vascular pedicle.

Most publications stress the importance of a positive Allen test to make sure that the vascular arch between ulnar artery and radial artery is intact. Personal experience and those of others have shown that in cases of doubt the dissection can be started proximally and ends 4 to 5 cm proximal to the wrist. There are multiple connections around the wrist that still provide sufficient distal inflow to facilitate a

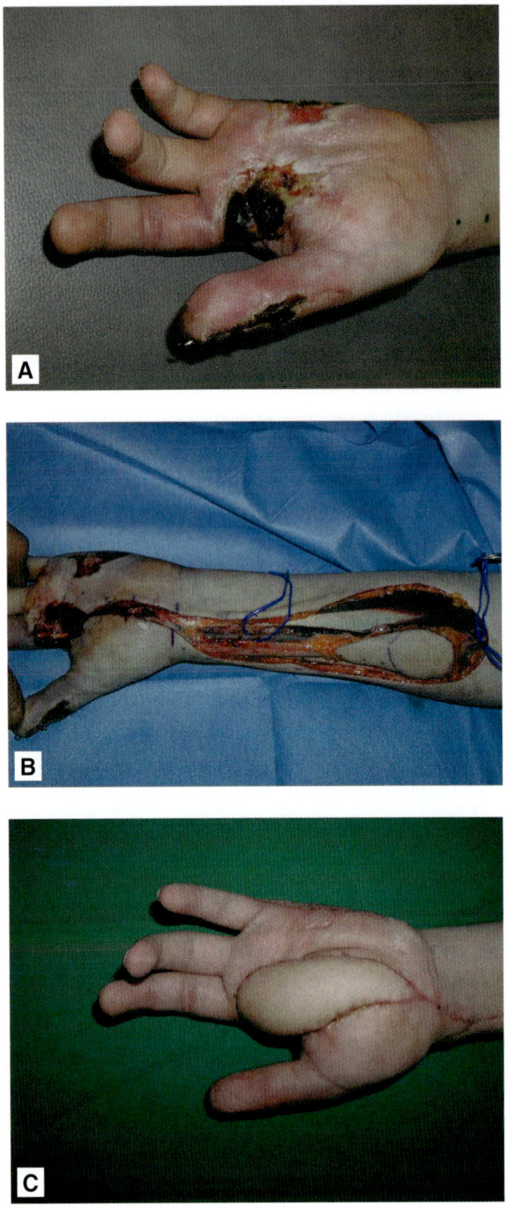

FIGURE 23-1 **A.** Contact burn to the thumb and the web space. **B.** A classic radial forearm flap is raised. The skin island is designed in a way that allows primary closure of the donor site to reduce donor-site morbidity. **C.** The flap has healed completely but shows the typical postoperative swelling that usually dissolves within 12 weeks.

pedicled radial forearm flap. Our experiences with this flap are excellent and it remains a workhorse for us.

ULNAR ARTERY FLAP ("BECKER FLAP")

Anatomy

The ulnar artery flap, in contrast to the radial forearm flap, is based on a strong perforator vessel that is approximately 1.5 mm in diameter, with accompanying veins of up to 1 mm in diameter that originate from the ulnar artery 3.5 to 4 cm proximal to the wrist crease and pass under the ulnar aspect of the FCU tendon.

The flap is centered over the ulnopalmar aspect of the forearm. Flap dimensions can reach 4 to 6 × 20 to 24 cm. The flap is not innervated.[13]

Indications

This flap is indicated for defects of the palmar and dorsal aspects of the wrist, and dorsum of the hand in addition to selected defects in the palm, which require contouring.

Contraindications

The flap was indicated with a history of blunt trauma or lacerations to the ulnar wrist that may damage the pedicle. The conspicuous donor site may preclude this flap in female patients.

Surgical Technique

The flap is outlined over the course of the ulnar artery on the ulnar–palmar aspect of the forearm. The dissection starts distally by incising the flap and identifying the perforator vessel passing under the FCU tendon. As soon as this vessel is identified, the incision is extended palmarly exposing the ulnar neurovascular bundle. The flap includes the fascia of the FCU, which is peeled off the muscle. The dissection proceeds distally after the ulnar border of the flap has been incised. The flap is thin so the perforator vessel arborizing in the subcutaneous layer can be recognized.

There are 2 ways of rotating the flap into the defect. One is to leave the most distal part of the flap (distal to the entrance of the perforator) intact that leaves a small dog ear after the flap has been rotated into the defect. This may help prevent kinking of the pedicle. Other authors raise the flap as a propeller flap by isolating the pedicle and tracing back to its exit point underneath the FCU tendon. This increases the arc of rotation and prevents the necessity of secondary debulking. Advantages include the fact that it is a long, narrow flap with a wide arc of rotation, the donor site can be closed primarily in many cases, it is a reliable flap due to the consistent vascular anatomy, and it does not require sacrifice of a major artery.

Disadvantages include the fact there is a dog ear at the pivot point, and wider flaps may need skin grafting of the donor site.

Complications, Tips, and Tricks

The Becker flap does not have many inherent complications. The vascular supply is robust and constant. We have also designed this flap in some cases with a cutaneous tail by extending the distal portion of the flap to facilitate donor-site closure.

For smaller defects, the flap can be raised as a fascial flap.

We have performed this flap on a few occasions and found it to be very valuable as an alternative when other options are not available, or are not considered to be best suited for defects of both aspects of the wrist and hand.

POSTERIOR INTEROSSEOUS ARTERY FLAP

Anatomy

The PIA flap is usually raised as a distally based pedicle flap. It can be harvested in rare cases as a proximally based pedicled rotation flap or a free flap based on the proximal outflow.

The flap is centered over the course of the posterior interosseous vessels where they penetrate through the IOM proximal to the wrist. The PIA is 0.8 to 1.2 mm in diameter at this point and is accompanied by 2 concomitant veins. It runs proximally between the tendons of the ECU and the EDM. The flap dimensions can be as large as 6 × 15 cm and is usually not innervated.[14]

Indications

Indications include defects of the wrist area or the dorsum of the hand, defects in the first web space after release of burn contractures, and reconstruction of the first web space in congenital hand deformities.

Contraindications

The flap was contraindicated with open trauma to the dorsal wrist area with the possibility of injury to the PIA and [illegible] a risk of interfering with the radial motor branches during flap dissection.

Surgical Technique

The flap is outlined over the ulnar–dorsal aspect of the proximal forearm. The point where the PIA penetrates through the IOM is determined by Doppler examination. The dissection starts by identifying the tendons of the ECU and EDM bordering the septum containing the perforating vessels, which can be traced to their exit point from the IOM.

The dissection then proceeds proximally, taking care to preserve the integrity of the septum and to constantly check the course of the ECU and EDM. The fascia of the muscles is peeled off and included with the septum. At some point the vascular pedicle runs directly on the periosteum of the ulna so that many authors recommend including a strip of periosteum from the ulna to help prevent injury to the pedicle.

The flap is then dissected until the first motor branches of the posterior interosseous nerve are encountered. In selected cases, 1 of the motor branches can be divided to increase the pedicle length. The dissection stops at this point. A microvascular clamp is applied to the proximal artery and the tourniquet is released to check flap perfusion. If flap is well perfused, it is rotated into the defect (Fig. 23-2A-E).

Donor-site closure can be achieved primarily, when the defect is smaller than 6 cm, but most frequently it requires a skin graft.

The PIA flap raises frequently discussions between supporters and opponents of this flap. Venous congestion is frequently observed but apparently resolves in the majority of cases. One way to avoid this could be to leave a wider strip of fascia distally that contains small venous branches which drain into other vessels that the pedicle veins.

The arc of rotation is also important to avoid venous congestion. Any sharp angle should be avoided. Any tissue available around the pedicle may also support venous drainage.

Proximal injury to motor branches of the radial nerve poses the greatest danger. They have to be identified during dissection and spared. However, in some cases of absolute necessity, 1 of these branches may have to be divided to reach the planned flap length and arc of rotation.

In these cases one should consider this pedicle more proximally until the vessel diameter reaches a caliber that is suitable for microanastomoses, and then raising this as a free flap.

It is of utmost importance to identify the ECU and EDM tendon before starting the dissection, since it is very easy to slip into the wrong dissection plane between the "wrong" muscles.

Our experience is mixed. We encountered some form of venous congestion in many flaps, but lost only 1 due to persistent venous congestion. However, the flap is not one of our preferred flaps, but after taking the precautions described above it still is a valuable option for the right indication.

FREE FLAPS

Fascial Flaps

Fascial flaps have gained increasing popularity in reconstruction of defects in the hand, on the palmar side as well as for the dorsum of the hand. They provide thin and supple tissue that provides a perfect gliding surface for the underlying tendons, but possesses sufficient durability to withstand pressure loads during gripping. They are usually simultaneously combined with split-thickness skin grafts for epidermal reconstruction.

There is a choice of fascial flaps available. The superficial tempoparietal fascia flap (TPF) has the most inconspicuous donor site with only a small risk of limited alopecia along the incision line. However, the veins of the vascular pedicle may

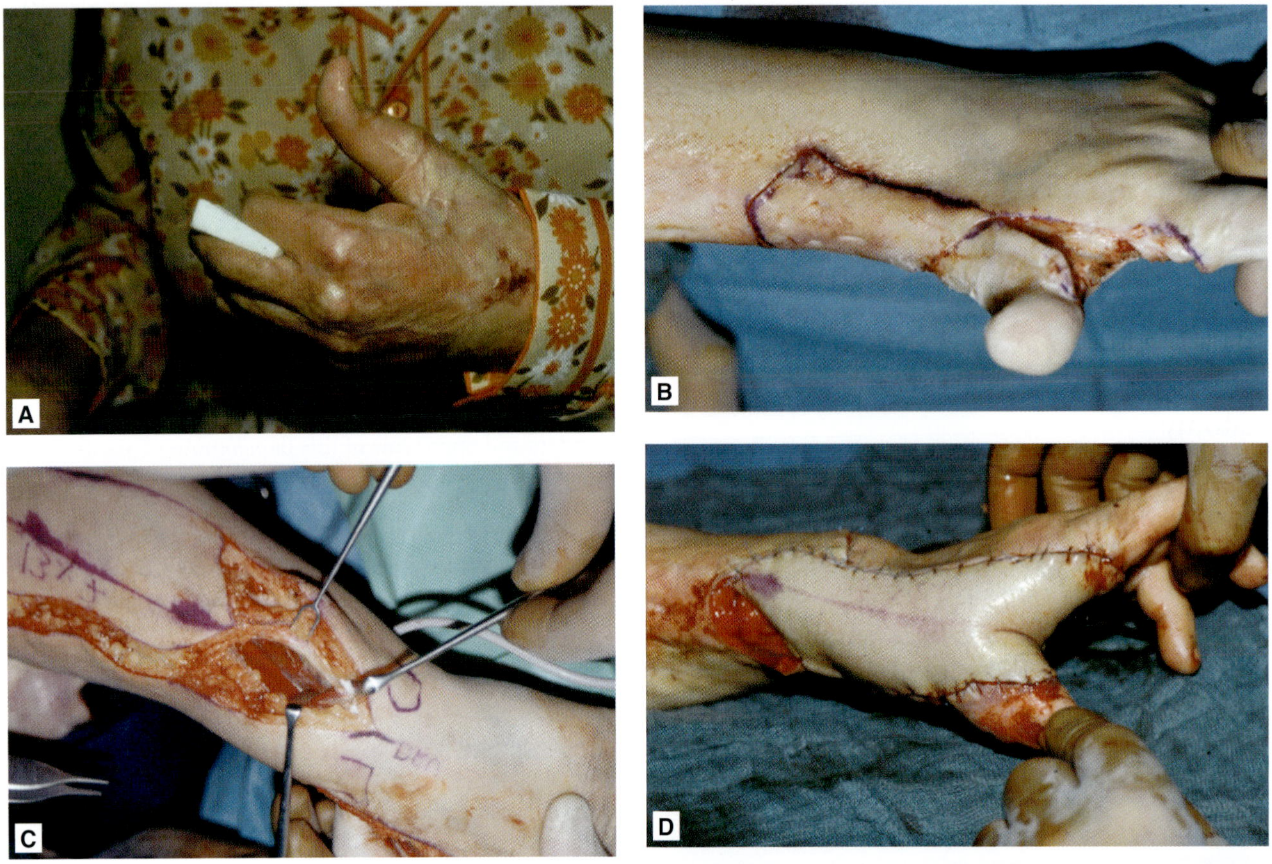

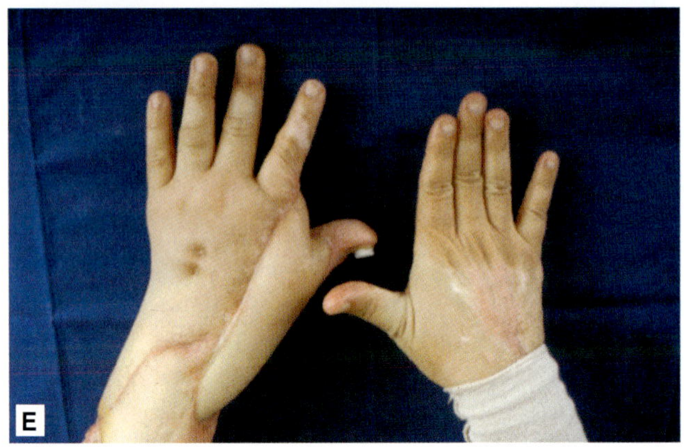

FIGURE 23-2 **A.** Burn contracture of the first web space with severe functional impairment. **B.** The contracture is released from the web space to the distal area of the dorsoradial forearm. **C.** A posterior interosseus flap (PIA) has been raised based on the vascular arcade running in the intermuscular septum. **D.** The flap fits perfectly into the defect. **E.** Postoperatively the flap shows some swelling, which is usually treated by lymph drainage and compression garments.

be very small or even absent. Other fascial flaps suited for the upper extremity are the serratus anterior fascial (SAF) flap, the radial forearm fascia (RFF) flap, the lateral arm fascia flap, and the anterolateral thigh fascial flap. This chapter will discuss only the TPF and the SAF flap.[15]

Tempoparietal Fascia Flap (TPF)

ANATOMY

The TPF is not an innervated flap based on the superficial temporal artery (STA) running on the fascial layer under the skin. The STA has a diameter of 1 to 1.5 mm and the venae comitantes have a diameter of 0.8 to 1.5 mm. They supply the superficial fascial layer as well as the deeper layer. Both can be raised together, if a composite transfer is indicated. It is ideally suited for situations where thin, supple coverage with no bulk is required. Flap dimensions can reach 8 × 12 cm.[13]

INDICATIONS

This flap is suitable for defects of the palm, dorsum of the hand, and wrist.

CONTRAINDICATIONS

The flap is not indicated when there is an injury to the donor site.

SURGICAL TECHNIQUE

The flap is based on the superficial temporal vessel. The vessels run on the surface of the flap, which makes the dissection more complicated than in many standard flaps. Care has to be taken to stay in the right dissection plane. Preinjection of the incision line with local anesthesia + epinephrine helps to keep the T- or Y-shaped incision bloodless. The flap is then raised in the plane between the hair follicles and the fascial surface containing the easily visible pedicle. The pedicle is traced back as much as possible in the pretragal area to increase the vessel diameter.

Flap dimensions are then outlined on the flap and incised. The remaining flap harvest is easy since there is a bloodless plane underneath the superficial leaf.

Hemostasis should be meticulous to allow complete take of the split-thickness skin graft.

The most frequent complications include oozing from small capillaries leading to hematoma formation under the skin graft, and the loss of the most distal flap portion. We recommend oversizing the flap dimensions and waiting for approximately 20 minutes before microsurgical transfer. Monitoring the flap perfusion with fluorescent angiography might be helpful to determine jeopardized flap areas.

The incision should be oblique to avoid alopecia. Injection of local anesthesia in the dissection plane may facilitate the flap harvest ("hydrodissection"). Ideally the skin graft is taken from the scalp, so the entire reconstructive procedure can be performed with no visible donor site, which is not found in any other flap.

The TPF has proven to be a very valuable tool in reconstructing defects in the hand and around the wrist. Although it is thin and supple, it is robust and allows secondary procedures under the flap. Especially in the palm, the TPF provided an excellent coverage with respect to grip pattern and perfect gliding surfaces for tendons. It has become one of the standard flaps, especially in view of the almost invisible donor site.

Serratus Fascia Flap

ANATOMY

The serratus fascia flap is overlying the serratus muscle. It provides excellent fascial tissue that is thin, supple, and still mechanically stable. It is based on the thoracodorsal artery that is 1.5 to 3 mm and the thoracodorsal vein that is 2 to 3.5 mm. The flap can be innervated by the long thoracic nerve. Flap dimension can reach 10 × 15 cm.[15]

INDICATIONS

The serratus fascia flap is indicated for defects of the palm, dorsum of the hand, and wrist.

CONTRAINDICATIONS

It is contraindicated with injuries to the donor site such as previous thoracic surgery or a laceration of the thoracodorsal vascular pedicle.

SURGICAL TECHNIQUE

The flap is usually raised with the patient in a lateral position. The incision is along the anterior border of the latissimus dorsi muscle. Raising the anterior border gives access to the serratus anterior muscle and the overlying fascia. The vessel runs on top of the fascia originating proximally from the thoracodorsal vascular bundle. This allows an extremely long pedicle that can be traced back to the subscapular trunk. The long pedicle with large-caliber vessels allows for microanastomoses remote from the zone of injury.

During the dissection, care has to be taken that the long thoracic nerve is preserved and holes in the fascia have to be avoided. In our experience the serratus fascia is slightly thinner than the TPF and therefore prone to perforations during dissection. This may lead to loss of tissue immediately adjacent to the perforated areas.

The flap is dissected from distal to proximal toward the thoracodorsal vascular bundle. Usually the branches to the latissimus dorsi have to be divided, if a long pedicle is required.

We recommend harvest of the skin graft from the scalp to minimize donor-site morbidity. A 1-stage skin graft transfer is recommended; therefore, careful hemostasis is mandatory.

As in the TPF, the most frequent complications are oozing from small capillaries leading to hematoma formation under the skin graft, and the loss of the most distal flap portion. We also recommend oversizing the flap and waiting for approximately 20 minutes before microsurgical transfer. Care should be taken not to lacerate the long thoracic nerve to avoid winging of the scapula by preserving the lower slips of the serratus muscle.

We consider the TPF and the SAF to be almost equivalent in their properties, although the SAF tissue is a little more delicate. The scar at the donor site makes it a second option in most cases; however, the scar can be usually hidden under clothing. If the defect requires a slightly larger flap, the SAF would be our prime choice.

CUTANEOUS/FASCIOCUTANEOUS FLAPS

The selection of cutaneous flaps depends predominantly on the profile of the patient and the body constitution. Flaps for the carpus and the dorsum of the hand have to be thin and pliable, whereas flaps for forearm or upper arm reconstruction can be a little bulkier.

Lateral Arm Flap

ANATOMY

This flap represents our first choice for smaller defects. The donor site is negligible; the scar can usually be hidden. Donor defects up to 6 to 8 cm can be closed primarily. If this flap is found to be thick, it can be thinned out intraoperatively. The flap is based on the recurrent branch of the radial artery that has a diameter of 1.0 to 1.5 mm. The vena comitans has a diameter of 0.8 to 1.5 mm. The flap can be innervated with a branch of the radial nerve.[16,17]

INDICATIONS

The lateral arm flap is indicated for defects of the palm, dorsal hand, wrist, and first web space.

CONTRAINDICATIONS

The flap is contraindicated if the patient's upper arm is too bulky and in cases where the donor site cannot be closed primarily, especially in female patients.

SURGICAL TECHNIQUE

The flap is designed over the groove between the flexor and extensor muscle groups in the upper arm. The dissection usually starts distally by identifying the septum between triceps and the elbow flexor muscles and the radial nerve that reduces the risk of injury to the nerve during dissection. After identification of the septum including the vascular pedicle that runs close to the periosteum, the dissection continues from the medial aspect along the septum down to the periosteum of the humerus. The pedicle length is 6 to 8 cm.

The pedicle is released from the septum and the dissection proceeds cephalad. The pedicle dives under the insertion of the deltoid muscle but can be traced under the muscle when the diameter of the vessels is considered too small.

Several modifications are possible. The flap can be extended toward the elbow that changes the shape of the flap from a more triangular pattern to a flat thin flap. A segment of humerus can be raised with the flap, if a complex defect has to be reconstructed, and the flap can be innervated by inclusion of a branch of the radial nerve (Fig. 23-3A-D).

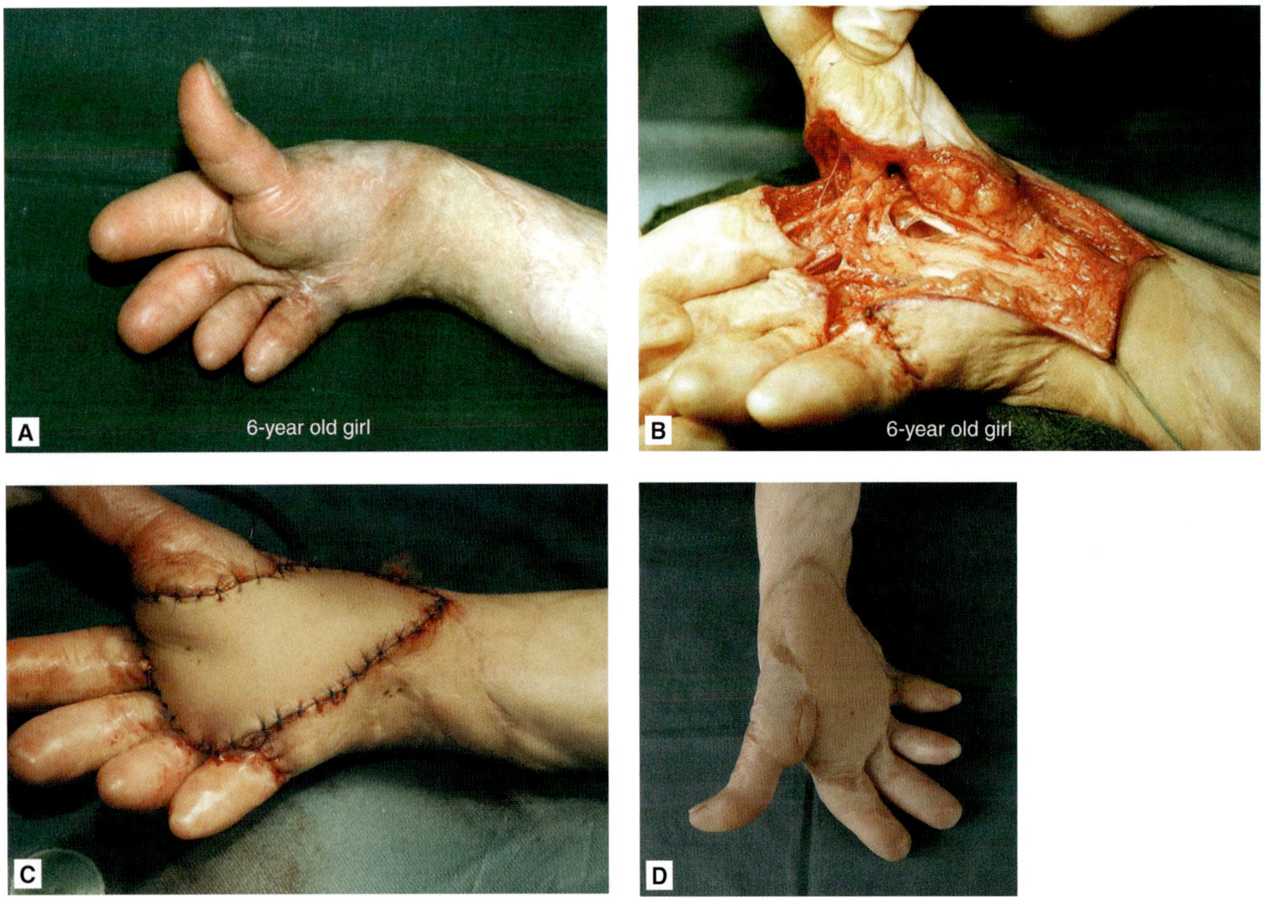

FIGURE 23-3 **A.** Severe burn contracture in a 6-year-old girl. **B.** Situation after contracture release with complex defect in the web space. **C.** A lateral arm flap with its triangular shape fits perfectly into these types of defect. **D.** Stable result 3 years postoperatively.

Possible complications of the lateral arm flap are a temporary weakness of radial nerve–innervated muscles, detachment of the vascular pedicle, not a proper release from the humerus, and laceration of the radial nerve.

Early identification of the radial nerve during the beginning of the dissection may avoid any problem during the further course of the procedure.

The vessel diameter is similar to the diameter of the gracilis vessels. Sometimes the pedicle has to be pursued further cephalad to obtain adequate vascular dimensions for microsurgery.

The lateral arm flap has become one of our standard tools in hand reconstruction. One of the disadvantages is the triangular shape of the flap, which sometimes needs secondary corrective procedures. The donor scar can usually be hidden under clothing and there are no remote donor sites.

Anterior Lateral Thigh (ALT) Flap

ANATOMY

The flap is based on the descending branch of the circumflex femoral artery that is 1.5 to 2.5 mm in diameter. The venae comitantes are 1.5 to 2.5 mm in diameter. The flap is usually not innervated.

The ALT flap is preferred for larger defects. Even in individuals in whom a thick subcutaneous layer is found, the thigh region does not necessarily have the same properties. The ALT flap is suitable for large defects and can be raised with strips of fascia (TFL) or muscle segments (rectus femoris/vastus lateralis) for the reconstruction of more complex defects. A long pedicle permits microanastomoses remote from the zone of injury that adds to the reliability of the flap.[18,19]

INDICATIONS

The flap is indicated for larger defects of the wrist area and forearm.

CONTRAINDICATIONS

The flap is contraindicated if the subcutaneous layer in the thigh is too bulky.

SURGICAL TECHNIQUE

The perforator vessel scan can be mapped preoperatively by Doppler. A line is drawn from the iliac crest to the lateral femoral condyle. Most perforators are found along this line. The flap is centered over the vascular axis, and dissection starts proximally to identify the perforator vessels.

The flap is then incised circumferentially and additional perforators are identified. The flap is raised above the fascia; only a small cuff of fascia is left around the exit points of the perforators. In more than 60% the course of the vessels is intramuscular that makes the dissection tedious. Numerous small vessels have to be clipped or coagulated during dissection, until the circumflex femoral artery is reached. When the vessels run in an intermuscular septum, dissection is faster and safer.

The flap can be harvested including a strip of tendon from the TFL aponeurosis or a muscle segment, if a bone cavity has to be sealed.

The most dire complication is the injury to the vascular pedicle during dissection. Early identification of the pedicle helps to avoid this risk.

The flap can be thinned during the dissection, but this requires considerable experience and should not be performed by surgeons starting with this type of flaps.

The donor site can usually be closed primarily in flaps intended for upper extremity reconstruction. If closure proves to be difficult, generous mobilization helps to achieve primary closure (Fig. 23-4A-C).

The ALT flap has become our workhorse in lower extremity reconstruction, but is rather infrequently used in the carpal area. However, in thin patients, it may be a valuable option, when other solutions are not available or are not considered suitable.

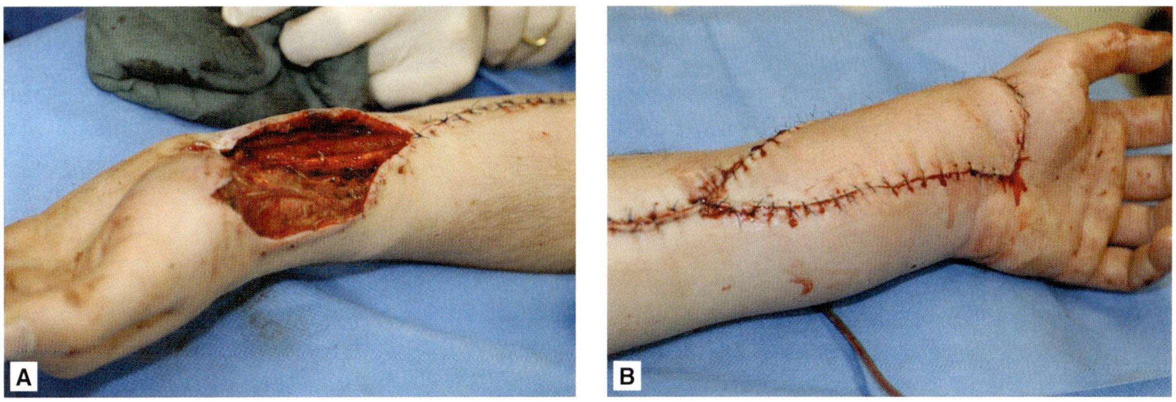

FIGURE 23-4 **A.** A 24-year-old cook. Defect after debridement of a severe soft tissue infection following an injury with an oyster knife. **B.** Free parascapular flap. Arterial end-to-side anastomosis to radial artery, venous end-to-end anastomosis to cephalic vein.

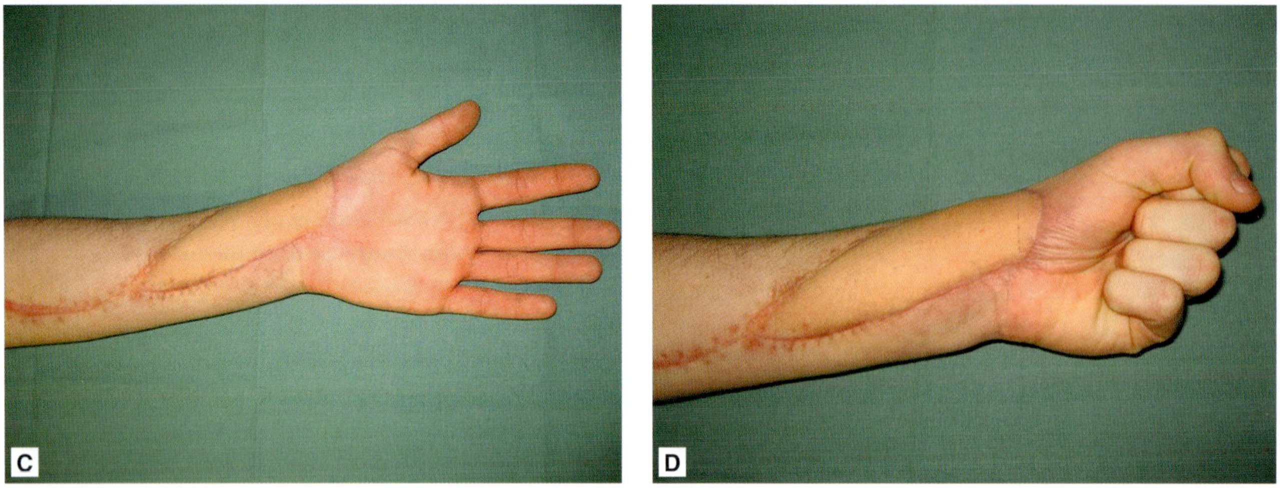

FIGURE 23-4 (*Continued*) **C** and **D.** Excellent aesthetic long-term result.

The scapular/parascapular flap is the alternative for mid-size–large defects. It offers more variability than the ALT flap, since it can be raised as a composite flap with bony, muscle, and skin components. The donor site frequently demonstrates some widening of the scar, but can be hidden under clothing.[20]

The use of the radial forearm flap has decreased significantly in recent years, although it is the easiest flap to raise. Because of its conspicuous donor site, it should be limited to rare indications or patients who do not put too much emphasis on the aesthetic appearance of the donor site.

REFERENCES

1. Germann G, Sherman R, Levin LS. *Decision Making in Reconstructive Surgery—Upper Extremity.* New York: Springer; 1999.
2. Levin LS, Germann G. *Atlas of the Hand Clinics: Local Flap Coverage About the Hand.* Philadelphia: WB Saunders; 1998.
3. Engel H, Germann G. Advanced concepts in vascularised tissue transfer in the hand. In: Siemionow MZ, ed. *Tissue Surgery, New Techniques in Surgery Series.* Vol. 1. 2006:23–40.
4. Arria P, Gilbert A. Lambeaux des arteres interossueses dorsales de la main. In: Gilbert A, Masquelet AG, hentz VR, eds. *Les lambeaux artériels pédiculés du membre supérieur, Monographie du groupe d'études de la main.* 1990.
5. Salmon M. *Les artéres de la peau.* Paris: Masson; 1912.
6. Spalteholz W. Die Verteilung der Blutgefässe in der Hand. *Arch Anat Med Phys.* 1893:1–54.
7. Germann G. Principles of flap design for surgery of the hand. *Atlas Hand Clin.* 1998;3:33–57.
8. McGregor IA, Jackson IT. The groin flap. *Br J Plast Surg.* 1972;25:3.
9. Hrabowski M, Kloeters O, Germann G. Reverse homodigital dorsoradial flap for thumb soft tissue reconstruction: surgical technique. *J Hand Surg Am.* 2010;35:659–662.
10. Early MJ, Milner R. Dorsal metacarpal flaps. *J Hand Surg Br.* 1987;40:333–341.
11. Gang RK. The radial forearm flap for reconstruction of the upper extremity. *J Hand Surg Br.* 1990;15:84–88.
12. Swanson E, Boyd JB, Manktelow RT. The radial forearm flap: reconstructive applications and donor site defects in 35 consecutive patients. *Plast Reconstr Surg.* 1990;85:258–266.
13. Becker C, Gilbert A. Le lambeau cubital. *Ann Chir Main.* 1988;7:136–142.
14. Zancolli EA, Angrigiani C. Posterior interosseus island forearm flap. *J Hand Surg Br.* 1988;13:130–135.
15. Flügel A, Kehrer A, Heitmann C, Germann G, Sauerbier M. Coverage of soft tissue defects of the hand with free fascial flaps. *Microsurgery.* 2005;25:47–53.
16. Katsaros J, Schusterman M, Beppu M, Banis JC, Acland RC. The lateral upper arm flap: anatomy and clinical application. *Ann Plast Surg.* 1984;12:489–500.
17. Akinci M, Ay S, Kamiloglu S, Ercetin O. Lateral arm free flaps in the defects of the upper extremity—a review of 72 cases. *Hand Surg.* 2005;10:177–185.
18. Engel H, Gazyakan E, Cheng MH, Piel D, Germann G, Giessler G. Customized reconstruction with the free anterolateral thigh perforator flap. *Microsurgery.* 2008;28:489–494.
19. Sauerbier M, Unglaub F. Perforator flaps in the upper extremity. *Clin Plast Surg.* 2010;37:667–676.
20. Nassif T, Vidal L, Bovet JL, Baudet J. The parascapular flap: a new cutaneous microsurgical flap. *Plast Reconstr Surg.* 1982;69:591–600.

24

Nerve Compression Syndromes at the Wrist

David J. Slutsky, MD

NERVE PHYSIOLOGY

The connective tissue of nerves includes the outer epineurial layer, which contains loosely woven collagen fibers and elastin. The epineurium protects the nerve from compression and stretch and therefore tends to be thicker in places that experience repetitive shear force such as the cubital tunnel at the elbow. The perineurium separates groups of fascicles and constitutes a diffusion barrier, which protects the axons from infection and chemical insult. The perineurium is relatively unyielding, which allows for a positive endoneurial pressure. This same property can lead to a minicompartment syndrome when the endoneurial pressure increases. The individual axons are surrounded by the endoneurium that provides support and a framework for regeneration of nerve fibers after injury.

The nerve cell membrane is composed of a lipid bilayer that has a hydrophilic (water loving) and a hydrophobic end. This leads to an ionic separation across the nerve axon that results in a charge separation. Although there are a number of charged proteins, the electrical gradients are mostly due to the difference in concentrations between sodium (Na^+) and potassium (K^+) ions. Minute changes in these concentrations lead to a change in the membrane potential even though there is relatively little actual ion flow.

The interior of the axon has a charge of approximately −90 mV, with a relatively greater concentration of K^+ ions with respect to the outside. There is a passive leak of K^+ ions out and Na^+ ions in, which causes the interior of the axon to become less negative with regards to the outside. There is an ATP-dependent Na^+/K^+ pump that imports K^+ and exports Na^+ in a ratio of 2 K^+ for every 3 Na^+. This maintains the normal resting membrane potential, and prevents spontaneous depolarization. Since maintaining the ionic charge separation across the membrane requires energy, this mechanism stops when the energy supply is interrupted. In other words, local nerve ischemia will prevent depolarization. This is one of the mechanisms for the conduction block that occurs with nerve compression.

Depolarization is an all or none phenomenon and cannot be stopped once it starts. In unmyelinated nerves, the Na^+ channels are spread out along the membrane and there is sequential depolarization along the membrane, that is, each section of the membrane must be depolarized in turn. This leads to slow conduction velocities in the range of 10 to 15 m/s.

In myelinated nerves, there is also a relative paucity of Na^+ channels except at the internodes. The current flows down the axon, stopping only at the nodes of Ranvier. Depolarization thus jumps from node to node (saltatory conduction) rather than sequentially depolarizing each section of the membrane. This markedly speeds up the conduction velocities, which are in the range of 90 to 100 m/s.

The electrical resistance to current flow varies inversely with diameter. Larger nerves conduct faster than smaller nerves. In order to survive, organisms must be able to react quickly to their environment; hence, nerve conduction must be fast. In complex organisms with billions of axons, increasing the nerve diameter is not a viable option. Myelination solves this problem by increasing impulse conduction without the need to increase the fiber diameter. The result of myelination is a 50 times decrease in nerve diameter with a 4 times increase in the conduction velocity.[1]

Nerve Compression

In early nerve compression the symptoms are of a vascular nature. The initial changes occur at the blood–nerve barrier. Fluid shifts that occur with limb position result in endoneurial edema.[2] There is no lymphatic drainage of the endoneurial space; hence, endoneurial edema clears slowly. The edema cuts off the blood supply by pinching off the arterioles that course through the perineurium obliquely.[3] This impairs the Na^+/K^+ exchange pump that is ATP dependent. This ultimately results in a reversible metabolic conduction block, which leads to paresthesiae.[4]

The dramatic relief of symptoms that sometimes occurs following surgical decompression also suggests an ischemic etiology to compression neuropathies. The mechanical source of compression may obstruct venous return resulting in segmental anoxia, capillary vasodilation, and edema.

The edema compounds the compressive effects, and leads to abnormal axonal and cellular exchange. Surgical release at this early stage generally yields good results. Prolonged compression, however, results in intraneural fibrosis, after which nerve recovery is less likely to occur after decompression.

Nerves are viscoelastic and as such must undergo significant changes in length in order to accommodate the myriad combination of joint positions. Nerves have a longitudinal blood supply that is reinforced periodically by segmental perforators. They are surrounded by a vascularized gliding layer that facilitates the nerve gliding that accompanies joint movement. Chronic compression leads to inflammation and secondary fibrosis that disrupts this gliding layer, ultimately leading to nerve tethering. Any compressive neuropathy therefore frequently has a component of traction neuropathy as well. Traction alone can cause conduction block. Nerves can only elongate by 8% until there is a disruption of the blood supply.[5] Traction therefore leads to nerve ischemia with secondary impairment of the Na^+/K^+ pump, which culminates in a conduction block. This is clinically manifested as numbness or paresthesia.

The foundation underlying many of the provocative tests for nerve compression exploits the relative nerve ischemia by transiently increasing the nerve insult through manual pressure, awkward joint positioning, and/or traction to elicit numbness or paresthesiae in the distribution of that specific nerve. A knowledge of the normal nerve course and topographic anatomy is thus essential.

Electrodiagnostic Studies

Ancillary testing cannot replace a detailed history and thorough examination of the upper limb, but they can provide a means for staging the degree of neuropathy and for ruling out more generalized disorders that may masquerade as a focal neuropathy.

Nerve fibers show varying susceptibility to compression.[6] The large fibers are more vulnerable to compression and ischemia. The neurophysiology of electrical recording is such that the recording electrode will detect activity in the largest myelinated fibers first, since these fibers conduct at the fastest rates and have a lower depolarization threshold than the small unmyelinated nerves. Latency and conduction velocity depend on the time that transpires from stimulation of the nerve to the first recording. If only a fraction of the large, thickly myelinated fibers remain and transmit impulses, the recorded latency and conduction velocity remains normal because the recording electrode mostly detects the fastest fibers.[7] The electrical conduction in smaller, thinly myelinated or nonmyelinated nerves is much slower and hence not usually detected in a routine nerve conduction study (NCS). Large myelinated and small unmyelinated fibers can be affected differently. Connective tissue changes follow with focal nerve fiber changes. The large myelinated nerves undergo segmental demyelination, while the small unmyelinated nerves undergo degeneration and regeneration. Normal fascicles are adjacent to abnormal fascicles. The NCS only tests the faster conducting fibers. This explains the seeming paradox of the patient who has established carpal tunnel syndrome but yet normal electrodiagnostic studies. It is the worst fascicles that produce symptoms, but it is the best fascicles that account for the normal nerve conduction studies.[8]

With early compression the symptoms are intermittent, and the edema is reversible. When there are constant symptoms, there is usually myelin damage and/or chronic endoneurial edema. This demyelination is responsible for the slowing of nerve conduction. If the compression continues, some of the axons will die. If there are fewer nerve fibers, the size of the electrical charge will be smaller, leading to smaller amplitudes. When there is sensory or motor loss, there is usually degeneration of nerve fibers. Despite the restoration of neural blood flow following nerve decompression, remyelination of the axon is often incomplete, which accounts for persistently abnormal nerve conduction even though the patient may be without symptoms.[9]

QUANTITATIVE SENSORY TESTING (QST)

QST is reportedly more sensitive than the NCS since only 25% of the large myelinated nerve fibers need to be conducting normally in order to yield a normal nerve conduction test. A-β fibers are the fibers of the peripheral nerve that allow the skin to feel the sensation of touch. Nerve density is defined as the number of nerve fibers per square millimeter. The nerve threshold is the minimum amount of force necessary to cause the touch receptors to fire. With nerve degeneration it is more difficult to distinguish 2 points from 1 point. Static and moving 2-point discrimination (2PD) typically test the innervation density. Threshold tests would include vibrometry and Semmes Weinstein monofilament testing (SWT). Vibrometry is relatively insensitive to early changes and is not commonly used. Semmes Weinstein testing involves placing nylon filaments of varying thickness on the skin until the filament is seen to deflect. The test is repeated with varying-diameter filaments until the threshold is determined. Abnormal SWT is consistent with nerve demyelination.

Dellon and coworkers developed the pressure-specified sensory device (PSSD) that tests 1-point static (1PS) and 2-point static (2PS) and 1-point moving (1PM) and 2-point moving (2PM) discrimination. 2PS is the first to go with nerve degeneration; 1PM is the first to return with nerve regeneration. The authors have likened an increased pressure threshold to increased distal latency or decreased conduction velocity as no nerve fibers have died yet, but are just demyelinated. When 2PD changes, this is indicative that nerve fibers are dying and it is analogous to a decrease in amplitude.[10,11]

Classification of Nerve Injury

PHYSIOLOGIC CONDUCTION BLOCK

Lundborg and Dahlin described a physiologic conduction block that is due to either intraneural ischemia or a metabolic (ionic) conduction block, with little or no fiber pathology.[4] Intraneural ischemia impairs the ATP-dependent Na^+/K^+ pump that stops any nerve impulse transmission. An example of this would be the reversible compression of the sciatic nerve that one may experience with prolonged sitting at a movie theater. Sensory and motor conduction across the compressed segment is blocked by this loss of circulation, but immediately recovers once the compression is released. With more prolonged ischemia intraneural edema develops; hence, recovery occurs over days or weeks. Axonal transport is also energy dependent; hence, extended ischemia may affect the nerve cell body function and viability. Irreversible nerve fiber damage does occur if the ischemia lasts more than 6 to 8 hours.[3]

NEURAPRAXIA

The nerve connective tissue remains intact, but there is focal demyelination, which allows current leakage. The time for the action potential to reach threshold at successive nodes is consequently prolonged. Partial lesions demonstrate slowing due to the loss of faster conducting fibers or demyelination of surviving fibers. The more protracted the compression, the slower the nerve conduction velocity (NCV) due to repeated episodes of demyelination and subsequent remyelination. More extensive demyelination results in complete conduction block. The most apparent finding on the EMG is reduced recruitment, due to a reduced number of motor unit potentials firing more rapidly than normal.[12] The clinical correlate is that of muscle weakness without denervation, but fibrillation potentials may occasionally be seen.

DISTAL MEDIAN NEUROPATHY

Carpal Tunnel Syndrome

ANATOMY

The carpal tunnel is open-ended proximally and distally, but behaves like a closed compartment physiologically and maintains its own distinct tissue fluid pressure levels. It is a fibro-osseous canal that is bounded by the concave arch of the carpal bones dorsally, and the flexor retinaculum (FR) palmarly. The hook of the hamate, triquetrum, and pisiform form the ulnar border, while the radial border consists of the scaphoid, trapezium, and the fascial septum overlying the FCR. The FR consists of 3 zones: a proximal zone that is continuous with the deep forearm fascia, a central zone that is composed of the transverse carpal ligament (TCL), and a third zone that consists of the aponeurosis between the thenar and hypothenar muscles.[13] The median nerve at the wrist has approximately 30 fascicles. The motor recurrent branch often consists of 2 fascicles that are situated in a volar position, with the various sensory groups in the radial, ulnar, and dorsal positions. The motor branch can be separated from the main trunk without harm for up to 100 mm proximal to the thenar muscles.[14] The sensory fibers travel within the common digital nerves to the thumb, and index and middle fingers, as well as the communicating branch to the third web space.

PATHOPHYSIOLOGY

There are 2 potential sites of compression anatomically. The first is at the proximal edge of the TCL, where compression may be produced by acute wrist flexion. This accounts for the positive Phalen test (wrist flexion test) in CTS. The second is adjacent to the hook of the hamate, where an hourglass deformity of the median nerve may be seen. In this case the patient will have a positive median nerve compression (Durkan) test but a negative Phalen test.[15] Compression within the carpal tunnel may also result from any lesion that takes up space within the canal such as flexor tenosynovitis, hematoma, palmar carpal dislocation, distal radius fractures, tumors, and ganglia. Although many cases have been attributed to a nonspecific synovitis, synovial biopsies typically fail to show evidence of inflammation. They do reveal edema and vascular sclerosis, which may by themselves be secondary to compression rather than the primary event.

HISTORY

The patient will typically complain of numbness and paresthesia in the median nerve distribution. Initially the symptoms occur at night due to a combination of wrist flexion during sleep and fluid shifts that occur with the horizontal position, which increases the carpal canal pressure. In this early stage of nerve compression the symptoms are of a vascular nature, which culminate in endoneurial edema. With early compression the symptoms are intermittent, and the edema is reversible. As the symptoms progress they become more frequent during the day and are precipitated by gripping and pinching activities as well as those tasks requiring repetitive wrist flexion. When there are constant symptoms, there is usually myelin damage and/or chronic endoneurial edema.[16]

PHYSICAL EXAMINATION

CTS represents a constellation of signs and symptoms in which no 1 test absolutely confirms its diagnosis. A positive Tinel sign may be present over the median nerve at the wrist, and produces paresthesia in the thumb and radial 2.5 digits. Phalen test consists of passive wrist flexion for 1 minute, which, when positive, produces subjective paresthesia in a median nerve pattern. This is best performed with the elbows extended since simultaneous wrist and elbow flexion may reproduce ulnar nerve symptoms as well. Direct compression of the nerve or the Durkan test is thought to be more sensitive. Szabo et al found that if a patient had an abnormal hand diagram, abnormal sensibility by SWT testing, a positive Durkan test, and night pain, the probability of having CTS was 0.86. If all 4 of these conditions were normal, the probability of having CTS was 0.0068.[15]

ELECTRODIAGNOSTIC STUDIES

The NCS can yield useful information, but the severity of the preoperative nerve conduction deficit does not provide significant data for prediction of the final outcome or return to work after carpal tunnel release (CTR). There are some caveats for nerve conduction studies in CTS. First, sensory abnormalities usually occur before motor abnormalities. In other words, the distal sensory latencies often slow before the distal motor latency (DML). This is not surprising since 94% of the axons in the median nerve at the wrist level are sensory.[17] The sensory nerve axons are larger than the motor axons and hence more susceptible to compression. If the DML is abnormal in the presence of normal sensory nerve action potentials (SNAPs), extra care must be taken to rule out anterior horn cell disease or a C8 radiculopathy, although isolated recurrent motor branch compression has been reported.[18] Second, the nerve conduction studies may not return to normal following decompression due to retrograde fiber degeneration or incomplete remyelination, even in the presence of a full clinical recovery.

Median Nerve Motor Studies. The recording electrode is placed at the midpoint of the abductor pollicis brevis (APB), and the reference electrode is placed over the APB insertion at the thumb MP joint.[19] A ground plate is applied to the dorsum of the hand. The first stimulus (S1) is applied 8 cm proximal to the recording electrode (E-1). Across-elbow conduction is performed by stimulating the median nerve in the antecubital fossa above the elbow (S2). If conduction in the arm is desired, a third stimulus site (S3) is applied in the axilla, 10 to 12 cm proximal to S2. Typical normal values include a DML >4.2 milliseconds, amplitude >4.0 MV, and forearm NCV >48 m/s. (Normal values may vary according to the lab.)

Median Nerve Sensory Studies. Antidromic studies are popular since the digital nerves are closer to the skin, which results in larger waveforms than orthodromic studies. Ring electrodes placed 3 to 4 cm apart are applied to the thumb, index, middle, and ring fingers. The median nerve is stimulated at the wrist: 10 cm proximally for the thumb and 14 cm for the digits. Comparative latencies have become more prevalent because different sensory nerves can be compared in the same digit under the same conditions of temperature, digit circumference, and skin conductivity. This tends to minimize recording pitfalls. Comparative latencies are taken from radial sensory nerve recordings from the thumb and from the ulnar digital nerve to the ring. Normal values include peak latencies of less than 3.5 milliseconds, with <0.5 milliseconds between radial–median and median–ulnar comparative latency differences.

Since the NCV is calculated over the length of the nerve, focal conduction defects tend to be normalized. Measuring the transcarpal latency directly can aid in the detection of this focal conduction slowing. A direct recording of the conduction across the TCL prevents any slowing in this area from being normalized by the faster conduction of the median nerve proximal to the TCL. The transcarpal conduction reflects the median nerve conduction directly underneath the transcarpal ligament. The median nerve is stimulated 14 cm from the ring electrode, and the latency is recorded. The median nerve is then stimulated 7 or 8 cm proximal to the ring electrode and the latencies are subtracted. When a distance of 7 cm is used, a normal latency is less than 1.7 milliseconds. With an 8-cm distance the latency should be less than 2.2 milliseconds.

A median midpalmar orthodromic latency can provide the same information. This is performed by stimulating the median nerve in the second interspace, and recording the mixed nerve response at the wrist 8 cm proximally. Normal values are less than 2.2 milliseconds. Segmental stimulation in 1-cm increments across the carpal canal has also been reported.

The incidence of type I errors (false-positive) increases with multiple sensitive tests. This had led some investigators to devise a comparative sensory index (CSI).[20] This consists of the sum of the thumb median–radial difference, the ring median–ulnar difference, and the median-ulnar midpalmar orthodromic difference. A normal value is <1.0 milliseconds. The CSI is more sensitive and more specific, since it hinges on 3 parameters, which diminishes the technical error associated with making the diagnosis on 1 specific test. The CSI is also temperature independent, since all of the nerves are examined under identical local condition of conductivity, temperature, and digit circumference.

QUANTITATIVE SENSORY TESTING

Static 2PD testing remains normal in mild cases. With more severe and/or longer-standing median nerve compression, the 2PD becomes abnormal, that is, >5 mm in variable combinations of the thumb, index, middle, and radial ring fingers. Loss of protective sensation occurs when the 2PD is >15 mm, and >25 mm correlates with complete anesthesia. 2PD is relatively insensitive in picking up changes as compared with testing using the PSSD. In CTS, testing of the index pulp may initially show an abnormal 2PS pressure threshold. With progression one sees a widening of the 2PS distance, followed by an abnormal 1PS threshold.

Weber and Rude evaluated 54 patients with carpal tunnel syndrome including 26 control subjects comparing nerve conduction studies with PSSD testing.[26] The NCV test had a sensitivity of 80% and specificity of 77%, whereas the PSSD testing had a sensitivity of 91% and specificity of 82%. The difference was not statistically different however. I performed a prospective side-by-side comparison of NCS and PSSD testing in 64 patients (94 tests) with clinical signs and symptoms of CTS.[27] Twelve of these patients then underwent a CTR and were tested again at 4 to 6 months. Clinical improvement was gauged by relief of symptoms, absent provocative tests, and at least a 1.04 improvement in the Brigham CTS questionnaire. Both the NCS and PSSD were roughly comparable in terms of sensitivity and specificity.

When combined, however, 88/94 cases of CTS were detected, including 14 patients who had symptoms of CTS but negative clinical signs.

NONOPERATIVE MANAGEMENT

Nonoperative therapy includes splinting the wrist in a neutral position, steroid injections, and management of any underlying systemic diseases. Steroid injection offers transient relief to 80% of patients, but only 20% will be symptom free 12 months later. Those most likely to benefit from conservative management have had symptoms for less than 1 year, only intermittent numbness, normal 2PD, <1- to 2-millisecond prolongation of distal motor and sensory latencies, and no motor findings. Forty percent of this group will remain symptom free for longer than 12 months.[21]

Surgical Indications

1. *Mild CTS*: Failed trial of conservative treatment with splints, NSAIDs, and activity modification for at least 1 month. No sensory or motor loss, nocturnal symptoms, and/or transient paresthesia only with prolonged gripping or pinching. No thenar wasting, no change in 2PD. May have a prolonged 2PS. There may be normal NCS, increased CSI, or slowing of distal median SNAPs but with a normal DML. Normal EMG.
2. *Moderate CTS*: Failed trial of splinting and/or cortisone injections. Frequent daytime symptoms even without gripping. May have abnormal 2PS and 1PS, 2PD <15 mm. No wasting of ABP but may have weak abduction. NCS may show slowing of distal SNAPs. DML slowing of <1 to 2 milliseconds, but no drop in amplitude. Normal EMG.
3. *Severe CTS*: No indication for conservative treatment. Frequent to constant symptoms. Abnormal 2PS, 1PS, 2PD >15 mm. Slowed to absent SNAPs, prolonged DML with amplitude loss. EMG shows membrane instability, decreased recruitment, and fibs/psw.
4. Acute CTS secondary to distal radius fracture, bleeding disorder, burn, or other cause of massive swelling.

Contraindications

1. Untreated hypothyroidism, diabetes, or other metabolic neuropathy.

SURGICAL TECHNIQUE

The procedure is performed under tourniquet control. A 3- to 5-cm incision is made in the palm parallel to the thenar crease and in line with the ring finger axis in order to protect the palmar cutaneous branch of the median and ulnar nerves. Tenotomy scissors are used to spread down to the palmar aponeurosis. This is divided exposing the TCL. The TCL is divided from distal to proximal. A hemostat may be used to protect the median nerve. The skin is retracted and the deep FR is divided under direct vision for an additional 2 cm. The nerve and tendons are retracted to the radial side and the floor of the canal is inspected for any masses. The recurrent motor branch is inspected and decompressed separately if necessary. The same considerations apply when using a mini-incision technique (Fig. 24-1A-E). The tourniquet is released and hemostasis is obtained. The wound is closed with 4-0 nylon mattress sutures after injection of local anesthetic.

POSTOPERATIVE CARE

Finger motion begins immediately, which also aids in median nerve excursion. A below-elbow splint is applied for comfort for the first week followed by desensitization and progressive strengthening.

ANCILLARY PROCEDURES

In advanced cases of nerve compression, internal neurolysis and epineurotomy have been described. No significant differences were found in comparisons of patients with and without this procedure; hence, they are no longer recommended.[22] Small finger numbness due to coexistent Guyon canal compression often improves after CTR alone since MRI studies have demonstrated an increase in the volume of Guyon canal after a CTR.[23] Routine tenosynovectomy does not provide better results than CTR alone and is mostly recommended with associated proliferative tenosynovitis from some other cause such as rheumatoid arthritis or granulomatous infection.[24] Ketchum did a comparison of open CTR, CTR with flexor tenosynovectomy, and tenosynovectomy alone. He noted a significant decrease in pillar pain and earlier return to work in the isolated synovectomy group.[25]

COMPLICATIONS

Pillar pain is an oft-cited complication. The cause of this is murky and the treatment is debatable. This has been the impetus for procedures that range from z-plasty lengthening of the TCL to mini incision and endoscopic techniques. Injury to the palmar cutaneous branch of the median nerve is a cause of persistent scar tenderness and led to the plea for a more ulnar-based incision. Blind release of the TCL, which was commonplace in the 1960s, occasionally resulted in laceration to the deep motor branch. Injury to branches of the superficial palmar arch are repaired or tied off as indicated. Median nerve anomalies or altered anatomy may lead to inadvertent nerve laceration. Any recognized fascicular lacerations should be repaired under microscopic magnification immediately or as soon as they are recognized postoperatively since this will maximize the chances for recovery. Acute infection is treated aggressively with antibiotic treatment and/or drainage as necessary. Wound coverage problems with exposed tendons or nerve may be covered with pedicled or free flaps. Causalgia should be treated with stellate blocks and aggressive therapy including edema control and dynamic finger splinting.

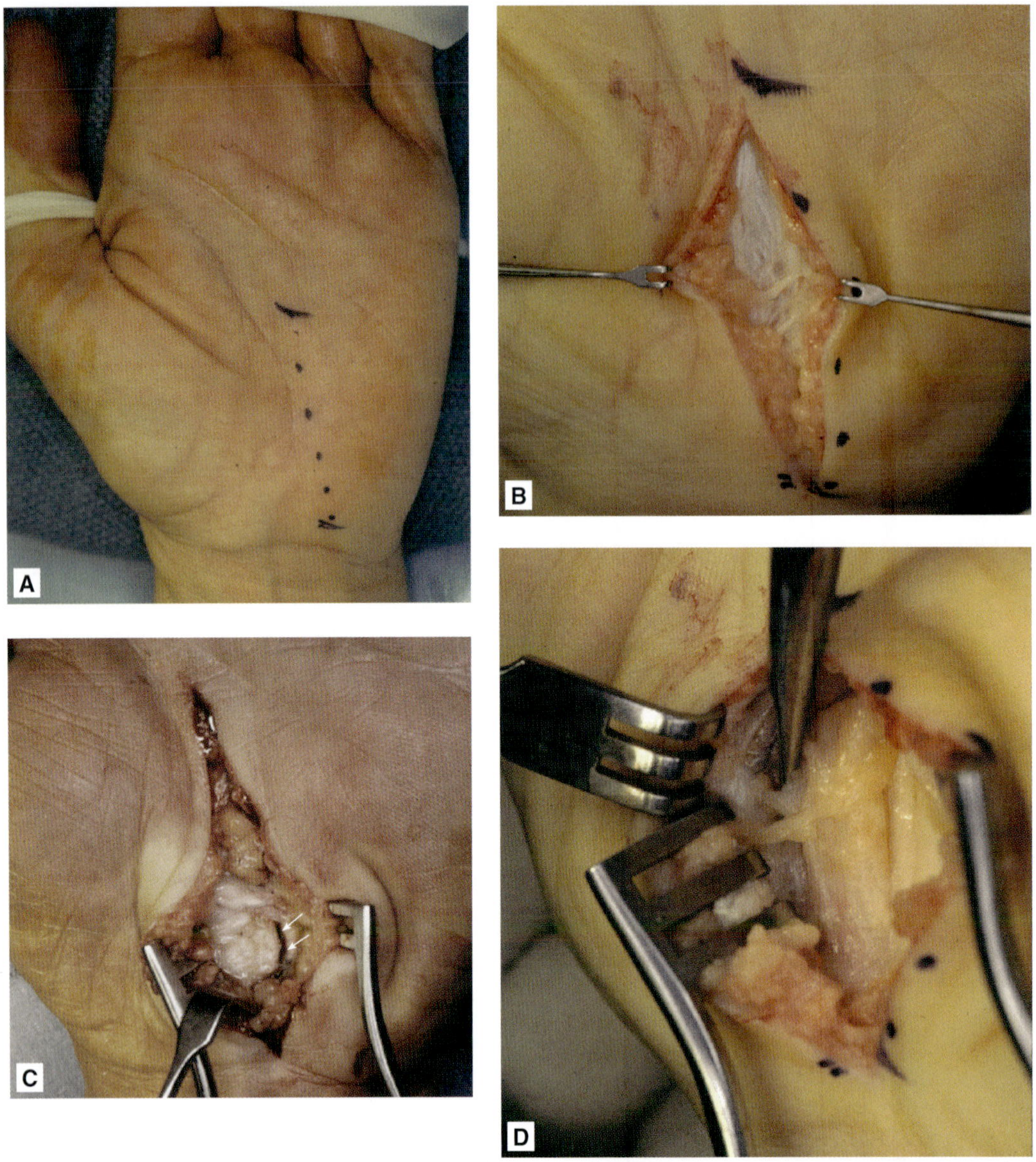

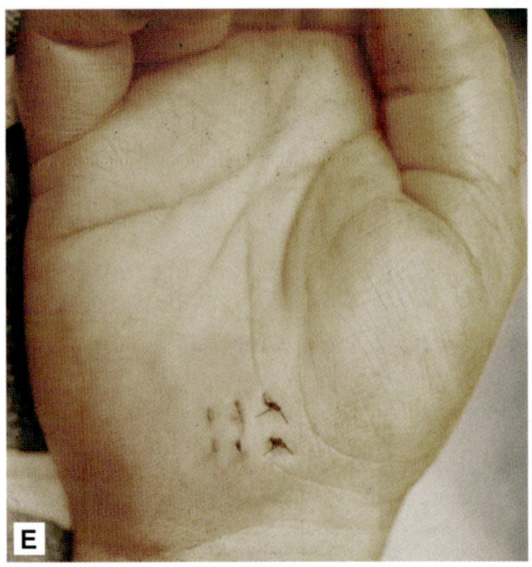

FIGURE 24-1 Carpal tunnel release. **A.** The standard carpal tunnel incision is parallel to the thenar crease along the ring finger axis to avoid injury to the palmar cutaneous branches of the median and ulnar nerves. **B.** The palmar aponeurosis is identified by the longitudinally oriented fibers. **C.** The fibers of the transverse carpal ligament (TCL) are transversely oriented. Arrows are pointing to a partial incision in the ligament. **D.** Release of the TCL exposes the median nerve. The tip of the scissors is behind the recurrent motor branch. **E.** Mini-incision technique.

OUTCOMES

Open median nerve decompression leads to symptomatic relief in the majority of patients.[26–28] When there is clinical evidence of demyelination, patients should be instructed of the possibility of residual symptoms and delayed improvement. After open CTR, patients typically regain their preoperative baseline grip strength within 3 months, and pinch strength within 6 weeks. Mini-incision open techniques have similar outcomes but carry a higher risk of incomplete TCL release.

Endoscopic Carpal Tunnel Release

SURGICAL INDICATIONS

The indications for endoscopic carpal tunnel release (ECTR) are the same as for an open release.[29] The patient should have the appropriate symptoms and signs of carpal tunnel syndrome and have failed a trial of conservative treatment with splinting, NSAIDs, and activity modification.

CONTRAINDICATIONS

Absolute contraindications include any distortion of the carpal canal due to tumor, previous surgery, carpal fracture/dislocation, or malunion of the radius. A loss of wrist extension of more than 20° to 30° from either bony fusion or wrist contracture would hamper this procedure by impeding the correct placement of the endosocope. Unfamiliarity with the regional anatomy is another contraindication.

Relative contraindications abound and are not universally agreed upon. Flexor tendon thickening due to synovial hyperplasia or adhesions from previous flexor tendon repairs will complicate the procedure. Recurrent or persistent carpal tunnel syndrome following a previous release often includes a component of traction neuropathy due to scar that may thwart attempts at ECTR. Suspicion of separate entrapment of the recurrent motor branch requires an open procedure.

SURGICAL TECHNIQUE (AGEE METHOD)

The use of the Agee endoscope (MicroAire, Charlottesville, Virginia) is integral to this procedure. A 2.7-mm 30° angle arthroscope along with a fiber-optic light source and camera setup is interfaced with the Agee system. The patient is positioned in the supine position with the arm abducted and lying on an arm board. The procedure is performed under tourniquet control after limb exsanguination. My preference is to use a general anesthetic due to the not infrequent difficulties with instrumentation including fogging of the camera lens (which can be minimized by warming the scope in saline). Regional and local anesthesia are acceptable alternatives.

A number of anatomical landmarks are identified and outlined with a marking pen to guide placement of the scope. The hook of the hamate, flexor carpi ulnaris (FCU), and pisiform are palpated and drawn on the skin. It is vital to keep the scope radial to the hamate hook at all times in order to prevent inadvertent penetration of Guyon canal. A straight line is drawn connecting the longitudinal axis of the ring finger with a transverse line across the proximal wrist crease. The palmaris longus (PL) tendon (if present) is traced. The dissection should stay medial to the PL that protects the median nerve. A 2-cm transverse incision is placed in the proximal wrist crease between the PL and pisiform. As the surgeon's comfort level increases this incision can be placed in the distal wrist crease, although there is more subcutaneous fat to contend with. The plane between the subcutaneous fat and the deep forearm fascia or FR is identified and developed. A distally based U-shaped flap of the FR is elevated by making 2 parallel incisions approximately 1 cm apart and 1 to 2 cm long through the deep fascia between the FCU and PL/median nerve. The incisions are then connected by a proximal transverse cut. Care is taken to avoid penetration of the underlying flexor synovium to lessen unwitting tendon laceration. The distally based flap is elevated with a skin hook while developing the plane between the superficial flexor tendon synovium and the undersurface of the TCL. Establishing this plane is crucial in circumventing improper scope placement.

At this point, the wrist is hyperextended over 2 folded towels. The hamate hook finder or which consists of a small dilator is gently inserted superficial to the flexor tendons in line with the ring finger. With proper placement the dilator will abut against the hook of the hamate by sweeping it in an ulnar direction. If there is no obstruction to ulnar passage of the dilator, then it should be removed and reinserted; otherwise there is the dire risk of injury to the ulnar nerve and artery. Two incrementally sized dilators are then gently inserted to enlarge the gliding path for the scope. The distal tip of the dilators can be easily palpated in the midpalm by levering the tip palmarwards. Multiple passes of the dilators increase the risk of a median neuropraxia, especially in small wrists. The soft tissue elevator is then inserted and used to gently scrape any synovium from the undersurface of the TCL. While the assistant maintains the wrist in hyperextension, the tip of the Agee endoscope is then gently inserted into the canal. The surface line marking the axis of the ring finger is used as a guide. The shiny transverse fibers of the undersurface of the TCL should now come into view. Oftentimes fogging of the scope, fluid from fatty tissue, or synovial remnants will block the view. In this event, the scope should be removed and defogged and the synovial elevator used once more. Since the scope is often colder than the carpal canal, keeping the scope in warm water until just before use may minimize the fogging. The distal edge of the TCL must be completely visualized. This can be identified by a change of the transverse fibers to an ill-defined fat pad, which contains the superficial palmar arch and the common digital branch to the third web space. Ballottement of the fat pad can aid in the demarcation zone. The hook blade should not be engaged until the distal edge is well seen. It is prudent to start the blade 2 to 3 mm from the distal edge on the first pass. The hook blade is then maintained upright while the scope is slowly withdrawn proximally, keeping the blade in sight at all times. The scope is then reinserted to visualize the cut. The TCL is under tension and will usually split apart allowing identification of the muscle fibers of the overlying palmaris brevis, or the longitudinally oriented fibers of the palmar aponeurosis. A second pass may be made at this point to release the distalmost fibers of the TCL. The scope is then removed (Fig. 24-2A-F).

The proximal skin flap is then retracted to allow visualization of the deep FR. Tenotomy scissors are used to divide the retinaculum for an additional 2 cm. The scope is then reinserted into the carpal canal, and the tourniquet is deflated. Pulsatile bleeding is suggestive of an injury to the superficial

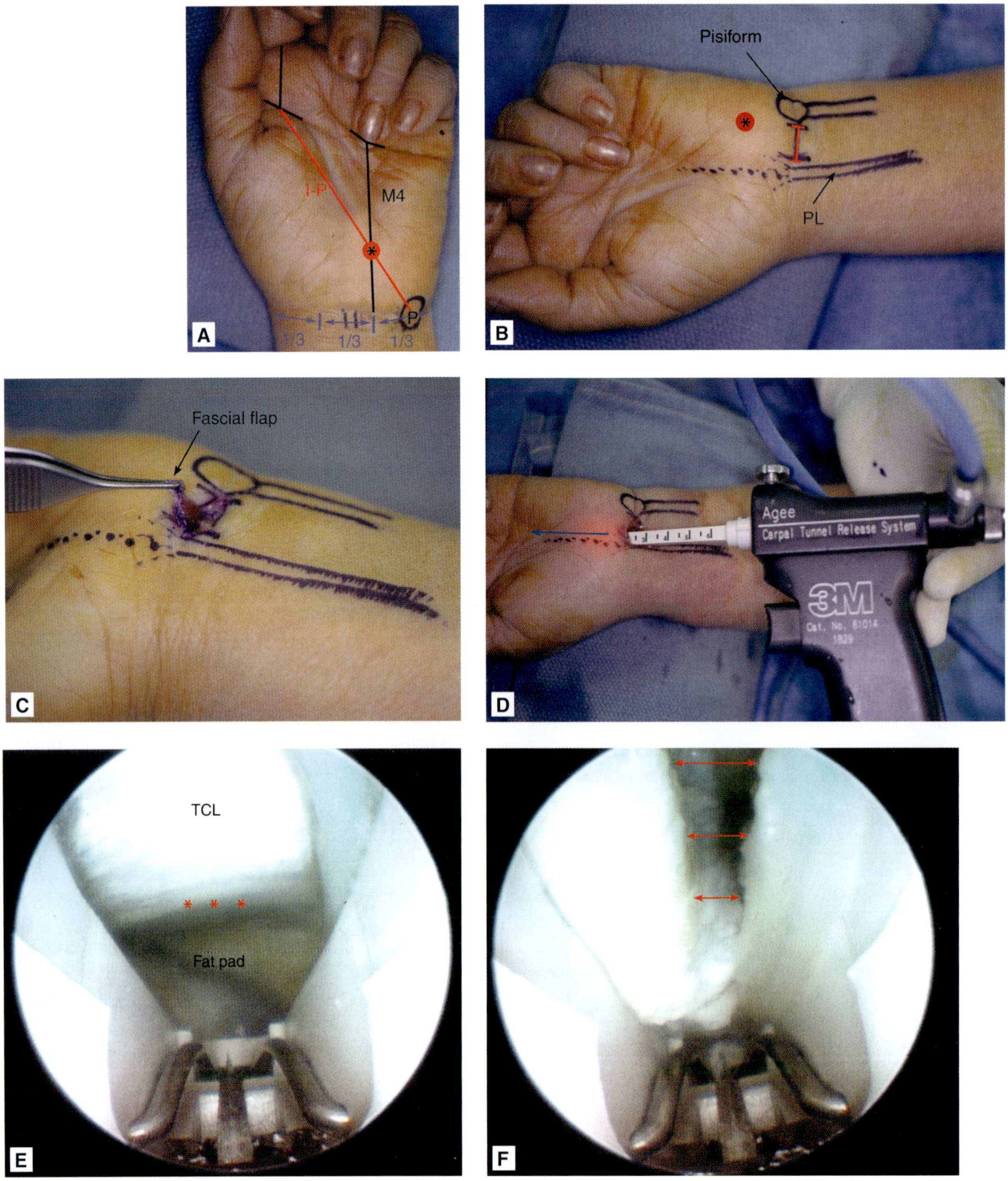

FIGURE 24-2 Endoscopic carpal tunnel release. **A.** Landmarks for locating the hamate hook (*). I-P, index pisiform line; M4, fourth metacarpal line; P, pisiform. **B.** Skin incision at distal wrist crease (in red). **C.** Outlining a distally based fascial flap. **D.** Insertion of the Agee endoscope that is aligned with the ring finger axis. **E.** View through the endoscope of the white undersurface of the transverse carpal ligament (TCL). The appearance of the midpalmar fat pad demarcates the distal edge of the TCL (*). **F.** After complete release of the TCL. Note the increased separation of the ligament edges (arrows) with exposure of the palmar brevis, which denotes a complete ligament release.

palmar arch, which is then explored through an open incision. Digital nerve injury cannot be recognized by any means, but a high level of suspicion and due diligence will dictate the need for exploration. It is possible for the mesoneurial tissue surrounding the median nerve to become interposed between the scope and the undersurface of the TCL. It will not have the appearance of nerve tissue and lead to a false sense of safety, but it can be drawn in by the hook blade, which may lead to a partial or complete median nerve laceration. If there is any doubt, the scope should be removed and the field cleared as described above. If the view cannot be improved, then conversion to an open procedure is necessary. The wound is infiltrated with Marcaine and closed with an absorbable subcuticular suture and steri-strips.

POSTOPERATIVE CARE

The patient is placed in a large bulky hand dressing with a volar wrist splint for comfort. Finger motion begins immediately, which also results in nerve excursion. The splint is removed at 1 week and the patient is started on a home wrist range of motion program. The sutures are removed at 2 weeks and light gripping exercises are instituted.

COMPLICATIONS

There have been significant and devastating complications reported, which are often related to poor scope placement or inadequate visualization of the TCL. This includes partial and complete median nerve lacerations, common digital nerve lacerations, and injuries to the superficial palmar arch.[30] I have noted a neurapraxia of the third common digital nerve branch in small female patients with small carpal canals that has lasted up to 6 months. Flexor tendon lacerations have also been reported. If there is anything less than complete visualization, the procedure should be converted to an open CTR. Placing the scope in Guyon canal due to inadequate identification of the hook of the hamate has resulted in ulnar nerve and artery lacerations.[31] Incomplete release of the TCL is commonly reported and is a major criticism of this technique.[32]

OUTCOMES

Agee et al carried out a 10-center randomized prospective multicenter study of endoscopic release using this technique. For patients in the device group with 1 affected hand, the median time for return to work was 21.5 days less than that for the control group.[33] Another large multicenter prospective study of 192 cases demonstrated, at least in the short term, that the patients treated with the endoscopic method had significantly greater grip strength, pinch strength, and hand dexterity. The open technique resulted in greater scar tenderness during the first 3 months after surgery as well as a longer time until the patients could return to work.[34]

Everyone is not in agreement on this point though. In a small study of 25 patients with bilateral carpal tunnel syndrome who underwent an endoscopic release by the Agee technique on 1 hand and open release on the other, the investigators found no significant advantages in terms of return of grip strength, manual dexterity, or sensation.[35] Foucher and coworkers examined their initial experience with this technique in 95 hands at 4.5 years.[36] Seventy-two percent of hands were free of symptoms and 94% were described by the patients as functionally normal. Seventeen hands (out of 27) with residual or recurrent symptoms were examined. Nine hands (9 patients) were only partially improved (mean 6.7 on a 10-point scale) and in 8 hands (7 patients), some symptoms had recurred after a mean delay of 3.8 years.

DISTAL ULNAR NEUROPATHY

Anatomy

The ulnar tunnel or Guyon canal is approximately 4 cm in length, which begins at the proximal edge of the carpal transverse ligament and ends at the fibrous arch of the hypothenar arch. It is bounded medially by the pisiform, and radially by the hamate hook. The floor consists of the carpal transverse ligament and the roof consists of the continuation of the deep forearm fascia, that is, the volar carpal ligament. The ulnar nerve has 15 to 25 fascicles at the wrist. It can be clearly divided into a volar sensory component and a dorsal motor component. At the wrist, the ulnar nerve passes over the TCL, medial to the ulnar artery, through Guyon canal. The deep motor branch is given off at the pisiform and passes underneath a fibrous arch to lie on the palmar surface of the interossei. It crosses the palm deep to the flexor tendons, to terminate in the adductor pollicis and ulnar head of the flexor pollicis brevis.

Pathophysiology

The standard teaching divides the sites of compression in Guyon canal into 3 zones. In zone I, nerve compression leads to mixed motor and sensory symptoms. In zone II, symptoms are purely sensory, and in zone III, symptoms are purely motor and restricted to muscles innervated by the deep ulnar motor branch.[37] Two sites of entrapment distal to the abductor digiti minimi have also been described.[38] In these cases the ADM will be preserved while there is weakness and wasting of the intrinsics.

History

The patient may also present with complaints of numbness and tingling of the small and/or ring finger. The dorsoulnar aspect of the hand however is not affected. The patient may give a history of repetitive percussion using the hypothenar eminence that may occur with autobody technicians, martial artists, and Kodo drummers. Bicyclists who ride for extended periods in the crouch position may entrap the deep motor branch against the hamate hook while grasping the handlebars. A history of Raynaud disease symptoms should alert one to the possibility of ulnar artery thrombosis.

Physical

There are no characteristic findings of ulnar tunnel entrapment per se. A Tinel sign may be present at the wrist but not the elbow unless there is an associated cubital tunnel entrapment. Intrinsic atrophy may also occur in chronic compression, but the FCU and the FDP are not affected. There should be a negative Tinel sign at the elbow and a negative elbow flexion test. If there is an associated ulnar artery aneurysm, there may be a palpable thrill and an audible bruit. With ulnar artery thrombosis, the Allen test will be positive for ulnar artery occlusion. With an associated fracture of the hook of the hamate, there will be localized tenderness in the palm, 1 cm radial and 1 cm distal to the pisiform. Ancillary testing such as ultrasound, CT, angiography, and MRI may be employed to aid in the diagnosis of these associated entities.

Electrodiagnostic Studies

The usual nerve conduction studies are inadequate at assessing ulnar nerve entrapment in the palm. Short segment incremental study (SSIS) is a sensitive and specific way to assess the deep motor branch since focal conduction abnormalities also tend to be normalized over the distance between the ADM and the FDI.[39] The ulnar nerve is stimulated in 1-cm increments from 3 to 4 cm proximal and distal to the wrist crease. Abnormal values include a >0.5-millisecond jump or a >120% drop in amplitude. When this is combined with FDI conduction and interosseous-latency differences, the diagnostic yield increases.

Quantitative Sensory Testing

The 2PS to the small finger is the first to go, followed by an abnormal 1 PS. The dorsoulnar carpus should remain normal unless there is an associated C8-T1 radiculopathy.

Nonoperative Treatment

The mainstay of treatment is activity modification. Bicyclists should avoid riding in the crouch position with their hands low on the handlebars since this is a recognized precipitant of symptoms, and change their hand position frequently. Autobody repair technicians, martial artists, and Kodo drummers should avoid repetitive percussion on the ulnar border of their palm. Wrist splinting and cortisone injections have no role in this condition.

SURGICAL INDICATIONS

Intrinsic wasting and/or sensory loss are a sine qua non for decompression. The presence of a mass-occupying lesion also mandates surgical treatment. Ulnar artery thrombosis or aneurysm may be treated with ulnar artery repair or ligation.

CONTRAINDICATIONS

Ulnar motor and/or sensory disturbances due to more proximal causes preclude a distal release. Ulnar sensory disturbances in CTS were a common indication for release in the 1980s, but have now become an infrequent indication for the release of Guyon canal since the majority of patients experience improvement following a CTR.[40]

Surgical Technique

The ulnar nerve is identified proximal to the distal wrist crease between the FCU and the flexor tendons through a curving incision that crosses the wrist obliquely, and bisects the interval between the pisiform and the hook of the hamate. The ulnar nerve is followed distally as the volar carpal ligament is released. The ulnar artery is inspected for thrombosis or aneurysm. The fibrous arch of the hypothenar muscles is incised and the floor of the canal is explored for masses, fibrous bands, or anomalous muscles. With entrapment in the palm, the deep motor branch is followed distally as it traverses the palm lying on the interosseous fascia, deep to the flexor tendons and superficial palmar arch. The dissection is completed as the motor branch ends in the muscle belly of the adductor pollicis (Fig. 24-3A-D).

Complications

These are mostly related to injury to the branches of the ulnar nerve or artery. Injury to the palmar cutaneous branches of the ulnar nerve or the nerve of Henle (if present) may result in scar tenderness and hypoesthesia. Uncommonly injury to the pisiform ligament complex can result in instability of the pisotriquetral joint.[41]

Outcomes

Clinical recovery is seen in the majority of patients when the ulnar nerve entrapment is due to a space-occupying lesion.[12] Motor recovery is less predictable when compared with sensory recovery, especially when the compression is due to a fibrotic hypothenar arch or of a long-standing nature.

SUPERFICIAL RADIAL NERVE ENTRAPMENT

Anatomy

The radial sensory nerve exits from under the brachioradialis approximately 5 cm proximal to the radial styloid and bifurcates into a major volar and a major dorsal branch at

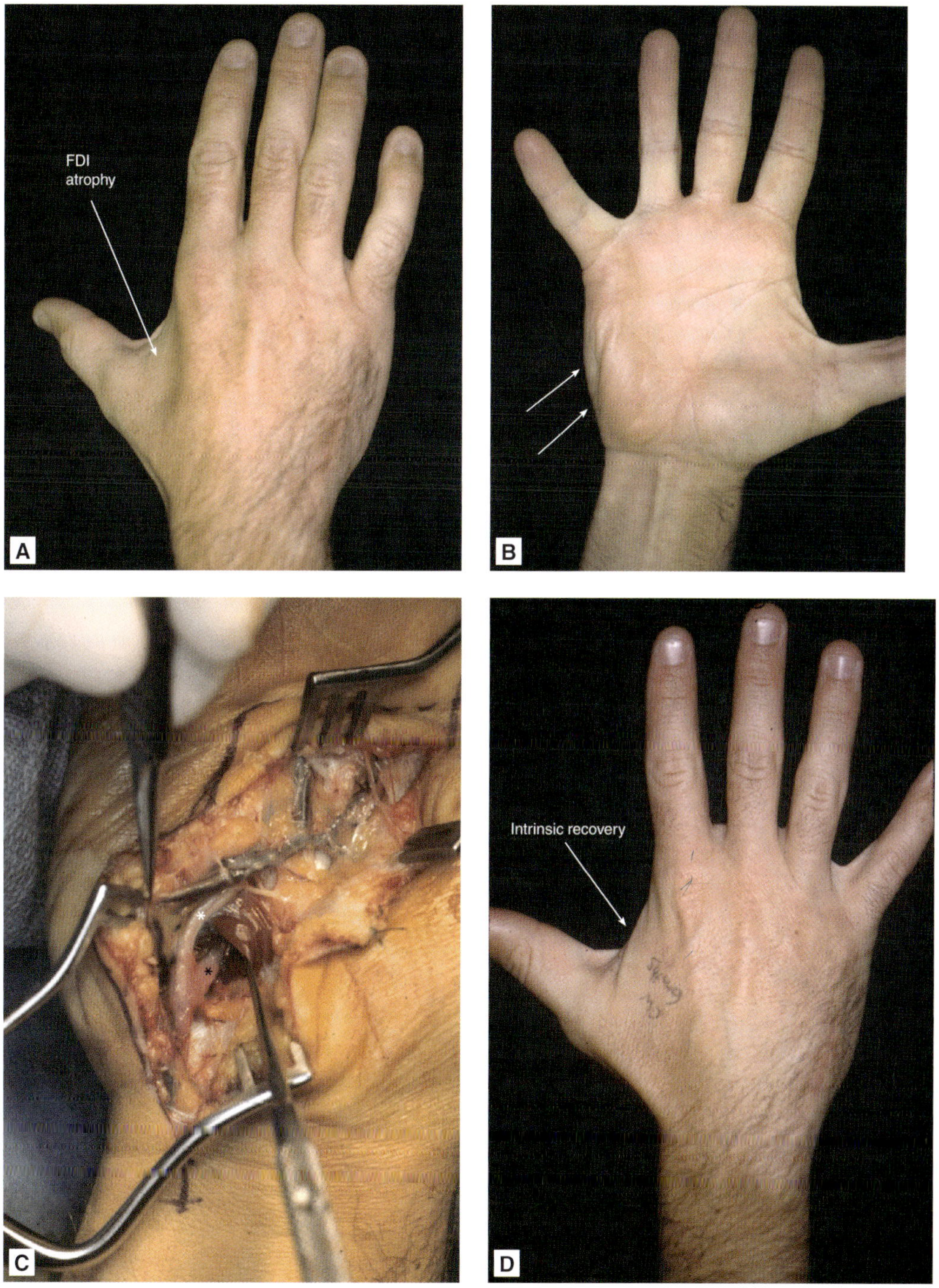

FIGURE 24-3 Distal ulnar neuropathy. **A** and **B.** Preoperative photographs of attempted index finger abduction. Note the marked wasting of the first, second, and third dorsal interossei, but the normal bulk of the abductor digiti minimi (arrows). **C.** Intraoperative view following an ulnar nerve decompression in Guyon canal as it splits into a superficial sensory branch (white asterisk) and deep motor branch (*) that passes under the hypothenar arch. **D.** Six months after operation. Note the normal bulk of the dorsal interossei and the active index finger abduction.

a mean distance of 4.2 cm proximal to the radial styloid. It then moves distally where it supplies sensation to the dorsum of the thumb, the first web space, and the dorsoradial aspect of the carpus, extending up to the index and middle fingers.

Pathophysiology

The superficial radial nerve (SRN) can be injured in the distal forearm or at the wrist by tight bracelets or watch bands, handcuffs, radius fractures, lacerations, venous cutdown, and blunt trauma. The SRN may also be entrapped as it exits the fascia between the tendons of the BR and ECRB.

History

Pertinent history may include compressive or crushing forearm injuries, work activities requiring frequent pronation and wrist hyperextension, and associated illnesses, such as diabetes. Symptoms included altered sensibility over the dorsoradial aspect of the hand and dorsoradial cutaneous pain with ulnar flexion of the wrist or with gripping and pinching.

Physical

Physical examination includes altered touch perception, moving 2PD >15 mm, static 2PD that is 5 mm greater than the contralateral first web space, a positive Tinel sign over the SRN, and aggravation of the patient's symptoms with forced forearm pronation and wrist ulnar flexion.[43]

Quantitative Sensory Testing

The patients will have an abnormal 2PS and possibly 1PS over the dorsum of the first web.

Electrodiagnostic Studies

The distal radial sensory latency may be normal even in the presence of abnormal forearm conduction. This commonly occurs with nerve entrapment due to segmental conduction velocity slowing. In more advanced cases slowing or a complete block of the distal SRN occurs. If the response is absent, it is difficult to localize the lesion.

SURGICAL INDICATIONS

A failure to improve following conservative treatment with avoidance of repetitive wrist deviation and tight bands or jewelry is an appropriate reason.

CONTRAINDICATIONS

De Quervain tenosynovitis often includes a component of SRN irritation and should be treated before considering SRN decompression.

Surgical Technique

A 2-cm incision is made approximately proximal to the radial styloid. The SRN is identified as it exits from underneath the tendon of the brachioradialis. The overlying fascia is split while care is taken not to disturb the nerve.

Outcomes

Dellon and MacKinnon reported on a group of 51 patients with complaints related to entrapment of the superficial sensory branch of the radial nerve. Seven (37%) of 19 patients were treated with nonoperative modalities after a mean of 28 months from the onset of symptoms or their injuries were improved. Of the 32 patients treated with surgery there was excellent subjective improvement in 37%, good subjective improvement in 49%, and fair subjective improvement in 6%, and 8% were not improved.[43]

Complications

The complications for each procedure are similar. They include wound problems related to infection, skin healing, tender scars due to injured cutaneous nerves, hematoma, and iatrogenic injury due to rough nerve handling and/or retraction. These can be minimized by meticulous hemostasis, gentle nerve handling, and precise surgical technique. Stiffness can occur and is minimized by early joint mobilization. The incidence of residual symptoms is predicated by the preoperative degree of nerve injury.

REFERENCES

1. Waxman SG. Determinants of conduction velocity in myelinated nerve fibers. *Muscle Nerve*. 1980;3:141–150.
2. Rydevik B, Lundborg G. Permeability of intraneural microvessels and perineurium following acute, graded experimental nerve compression. *Scand J Plast Reconstr Surg*. 1977;11:179–187.
3. Lundborg G. Ischemic nerve injury. Experimental studies on intraneural microvascular pathophysiology and nerve function in a limb subjected to temporary circulatory arrest. *Scand J Plast Reconstr Surg Suppl*. 1970;6:3–113.
4. Lundborg G, Dahlin LB. The pathophysiology of nerve compression. *Hand Clin*. 1992;8:215–227.
5. Clark WL, Trumble TE, Swiontkowski MF, Tencer AF. Nerve tension and blood flow in a rat model of immediate and delayed repairs. *J Hand Surg Am*. 1992;17:677–687.
6. Dahlin LB, Shyu BC, Danielsen N, Andersson SA. Effects of nerve compression or ischaemia on conduction properties of myelinated and non-myelinated nerve fibres. An experimental study in the rabbit common peroneal nerve. *Acta Physiol Scand*. 1989;136:97–105.
7. Brumback RA, Bobele GB, Rayan GM. Electrodiagnosis of compressive nerve lesions. *Hand Clin*. 1992;8:241–254.
8. Dellon A. Pitfalls in interpretation of electrophysiological testing. In: Gelberman RH, ed. *Operative Nerve Repair and Reconstruction*. Philadelphia: J.B. Lippincott Company; 1991:185–196.
9. Eversmann WW Jr, Ritsick JA. Intraoperative changes in motor nerve conduction latency in carpal tunnel syndrome. *J Hand Surg Am*. 1978;3:77–81.
10. Tassler PL, Dellon AL. Correlation of measurements of pressure perception using the pressure-specified sensory device with electrodiagnostic testing. *J Occup Environ Med*. 1995;37:862–866.
11. Rosenberg D, Conolley J, Dellon AL. Thenar eminence quantitative sensory testing in the diagnosis of proximal median nerve compression. *J Hand Ther*. 2001;14:258–265.
12. Trojaborg W, Sindrup EH. Motor and sensory conduction in different segments of the radial nerve in normal subjects. *J Neurol Neurosurg Psychiatry*. 1969;32:354–359.
13. Cobb TK, Dalley BK, Posteraro RH, Lewis RC. Anatomy of the flexor retinaculum. *J Hand Surg Am*. 1993;18:91–99.

14. Williams HB, Jabaley ME. The importance of internal anatomy of the peripheral nerves to nerve repair in the forearm and hand. *Hand Clin.* 1986;2:689–707.
15. Szabo RM, Slater RR Jr, Farver TB, Stanton DB, Sharman WK. The value of diagnostic testing in carpal tunnel syndrome. *J Hand Surg Am.* 1999;24:704–714.
16. Mackinnon SE, Dellon AL. Experimental study of chronic nerve compression. Clinical implications. *Hand Clin.* 1986;2:639–650.
17. Lundborg G, Gelberman RH, Minteer-Convery M, Lee YF, Hargens AR. Median nerve compression in the carpal tunnel—functional response to experimentally induced controlled pressure. *J Hand Surg Am.* 1982;7:252–259.
18. Bennett JB, Crouch CC. Compression syndrome of the recurrent motor branch of the median nerve. *J Hand Surg Am.* 1982;7:407–409.
19. Dumitru D. *Electrodiagnostic Medicine.* Philadelphia: Hanley and Belfus Inc; 1995:47–584.
20. Robinson LR, Micklesen PJ, Wang L. Optimizing the number of tests for carpal tunnel syndrome. *Muscle Nerve.* 2000;23:1880–1882.
21. Gelberman RH, Aronson D, Weisman MH. Carpal-tunnel syndrome. Results of a prospective trial of steroid injection and splinting. *J Bone Joint Surg Am.* 1980;62:1181–1184.
22. Gelberman RH, Pfeffer GB, Galbraith RT, et al. Results of treatment of severe carpal-tunnel syndrome without internal neurolysis of the median nerve. *J Bone Joint Surg Am.* 1987;69:896–903.
23. Silver MA, Gelberman RH, Gellman H, Rhoades CE. Carpal tunnel syndrome: associated abnormalities in ulnar nerve function and the effect of carpal tunnel release on these abnormalities. *J Hand Surg Am.* 1985;10:710–713.
24. Shum C, Parisien M, Strauch RJ, Rosenwasser MP. The role of flexor tenosynovectomy in the operative treatment of carpal tunnel syndrome. *J Bone Joint Surg Am.* 2002;84-A:221–225.
25. Ketchum LD. A comparison of flexor tenosynovectomy, open carpal tunnel release, and open carpal tunnel release with flexor tenosynovectomy in the treatment of carpal tunnel syndrome. *Plast Reconstr Surg.* 2004;113:2020–2029.
26. Weber RA, Rude MJ. Clinical outcomes of carpal tunnel release in patients 65 and older. *J Hand Surg Am.* 2005;30:75–80.
27. Slutsky DJ. Use of nerve conduction studies and the pressure-specified sensory device in the diagnosis of carpal tunnel syndrome. *J Hand Surg Eur Vol.* 2009;34(1):60–65.
28. Boyd KU, Gan BS, Ross DC, et al. Outcomes in carpal tunnel syndrome: symptom severity, conservative management and progression to surgery. *Clin Invest Med.* 2005;28:254–260.
29. Slutsky D. Agee endoscopic carpal tunnel release. In: Slutsky DJ, Nagle DJ, eds. *Techniques in Hand and Wrist Arthroscopy.* Philadelphia: Elsevier Inc; 2007.
30. Murphy RX Jr, Jennings JF, Wukich DK. Major neurovascular complications of endoscopic carpal tunnel release. *J Hand Surg Am.* 1994;19:114–118.
31. Luallin SR, Toby EB. Incidental Guyon's canal release during attempted endoscopic carpal tunnel release: an anatomical study and report of two cases. *Arthroscopy.* 1993;9:382–386 [discussion 81].
32. Varitimidis SE, Herndon JH, Sotereanos DG. Failed endoscopic carpal tunnel release. Operative findings and results of open revision surgery. *J Hand Surg Br.* 1999;24:465–467.
33. Agee JM, McCarroll HR Jr, Tortosa RD, et al. Endoscopic release of the carpal tunnel: a randomized prospective multicenter study. *J Hand Surg Am.* 1992;17:987–995.
34. Trumble TE, Diao E, Abrams RA, Gilbert-Anderson MM. Single-portal endoscopic carpal tunnel release compared with open release: a prospective, randomized trial. *J Bone Joint Surg Am.* 2002;84-A:1107–1115.
35. Schonauer F, Varma S, Belcher HJ. Endoscopic carpal tunnel release: practice in evolution. *Scand J Plast Reconstr Surg Hand Surg.* 2003;37:360–364.
36. Erhard L, Ozalp T, Citron N, Foucher G. Carpal tunnel release by the Agee endoscopic technique. Results at 4 year follow-up. *J Hand Surg Br.* 1999;24:583–585.
37. Shea JD, McClain EJ. Ulnar-nerve compression syndromes at and below the wrist. *J Bone Joint Surg Am.* 1969;51:1095–1103.
38. Wu JS, Morris JD, Hogan GR. Ulnar neuropathy at the wrist: case report and review of literature. *Arch Phys Med Rehabil.* 1985;66:785–788.
39. McIntosh KA, Preston DC, Logigian EL. Short-segment incremental studies to localize ulnar nerve entrapment at the wrist. *Neurology.* 1998;50:303–306.
40. Rayan GM, Jameson BH, Chung KW. The pisotriquetral joint: anatomic, biomechanical, and radiographic analysis. *J Hand Surg Am.* 2005;30:596–602.
41. Foucher G, Berard V, Snider G, Lenoble E, Constantinesco A. Distal ulnar nerve entrapment due to tumors of Guyon's canal. A series of ten cases. *Handchir Mikrochir Plast Chir.* 1993;25:61–65.
42. Zoch G, Meissl G, Millesi H. Results of decompression of the ulnar nerve in Guyon's canal. *Handchir Mikrochir Plast Chir.* 1990;22:125–129.
43. Dellon AL, Mackinnon SE. Radial sensory nerve entrapment in the forearm. *J Hand Surg Am.* 1986;11:199–205.

25

Distal Anterior Interosseous Nerve Transfer for Intrinsic Reanimation

Collier S. Pace, MD
Michael B. Wood, MD

INTRODUCTION

Nerve transfers have grown in popularity over the past several decades for reconstruction of peripheral nerve lesions. These procedures were initially used to treat injuries of the brachial plexus, but have since evolved to treat lesions at various levels of the upper and lower extremities.[1] In general, a nerve transfer should be considered when other methods of reconstruction, such as direct repair and tendon transfer, are known to have suboptimal outcomes. Ulnar nerve lesions proximal to the forearm and occasionally lesions of the median nerve in the midforearm are 2 examples of such injuries. Both of these injuries result in significant functional deficits related to the loss of intrinsic muscle function and fingertip sensibility.

In regards to high ulnar nerve injuries in adult patients, clinical experience shows there is rarely significant recovery of intrinsic muscle function following a direct neurorrhaphy or nerve graft reconstruction.[2] In such a situation a poor outcome is likely due to the long distance the axons must travel to reach their target motor end plates. Additionally, the ulnar nerve at the elbow is made up of both sensory and motor fascicles; therefore, the fascicular mismatch following a primary repair leads to misdirection of the axons. The same is true for median nerve injuries in the middle and proximal thirds of the forearm, especially when a long nerve graft is required. Based on rat studies, axons advance at 1 to 3 mm per day following a nerve laceration, whereas the motor end plates degenerate by 1% per week; therefore, at 1 year the nerve can only grow 350 mm and there is an approximate 50% loss of end plates; hence, any further delay in reinnervation leads to irreversible intrinsic muscle fibrosis.[3] Sensory end organs, on the other hand, can be reinnervated for a longer period of time since there is no motor end plate and the sensory end organs remain viable for years. One may see a recovery of protective sensibility following repair of a proximal nerve injury even after years.[4]

In order to restore hand function after a high ulnar nerve or proximal forearm median nerve injury, there are a number of ancillary procedures that can augment the functional recovery, including a dermadesis, tenodesis or capsulodesis for clawing, arthrodesis, and a variety of tendon transfers. These procedures often do not provide an ideal functional result, or require sacrifice of another muscle group that can further impede the function of an already limited hand.[5,6] As a consequence, the distal anterior interosseous nerve (DAIN) transfer has emerged as an additional option for intrinsic muscle reconstruction. The DAIN can be transferred to the deep motor branch (DMB) of the ulnar nerve or the thenar branch (TB) of the median nerve, depending on the site of injury.

The reported results to date suggest that DAIN transfer is an excellent treatment consideration for these difficult injuries and fulfills many of the principles that have been developed for successful nerve transfer surgery (see Table 25-1). Specifically, the DAIN lies in close proximity to the target musculature in the hand, consists almost entirely of motor axons, and is of adequate caliber to match the 2 recipient nerves mentioned above. The first clinical application of this procedure was performed by Wang and Zhu in 1979 and published in 1997.[7] There have since been several studies documenting good functional results with minimal donor-site morbidity.[8-11]

INDICATIONS

DAIN transfer is used to reanimate the intrinsic muscles of the hand. As stated above, the most common indication for this procedure is a proximal ulnar nerve injury. A high ulnar nerve injury typically results in denervation of the 2 most ulnar flexor digitorum profundus (FDP) muscles, the flexor carpi ulnaris (FCU) muscle, the hypothenar muscles, the palmar and dorsal interosseous muscles, and the adductor pollicis muscle. The FDP and FCU function will often recover to some degree following a primary nerve repair, since their motor end plates are close to the site of injury. Therefore, the primary goal of a DAIN transfer is to restore function to the ulnar innervated intrinsic muscles of the hand.

TABLE 25-1: Principles of Nerve Transfer Surgery

1. The donor nerve must be functional. This should be confirmed preoperatively by physical examination, and/or intraoperatively by direct nerve stimulation
2. A predominantly motor nerve should be used
3. Sacrifice of the donor nerve should result in minimal functional loss
4. The target fascicles of the recipient nerve should be able to be readily identified and isolated
5. Direct and tension-free coaptation should be possible without the use of a nerve graft
6. Nerve transfer should ideally occur within 6 months of the initial injury
7. There should be an adequate match in donor and recipient nerve caliber and number of axons

TABLE 25-2: Indications and Contraindications for Distal Anterior Interosseous Nerve Transfer

Indications	Contraindications
• Isolated ulnar nerve injury proximal to the forearm • Injury to the median nerve distal to the branch of the AIN	*Absolute* • Greater than 12- to 18-month delay following injury • The DAIN axons have been damaged at any level • The recipient fascicle has been damaged and precludes accurate coaptation or regeneration • Evidence of motor reanimation from primary repair *Relative* • The ulnar nerve lesion is in the distal or middle third of the forearm and amenable to primary repair • The ulnar nerve lesion is at or below the elbow in a young patient

An additional, though less common, indication for DAIN nerve transfer is a median nerve injury in the forearm just distal to the takeoff of the AIN. It is important, however, to verify that the distal AIN is indeed intact. Additionally, with a distal median nerve injury a primary neurorrhaphy may reach the APB end plates sooner than a DAIN transfer. Moreover, an opponensplasty provides reasonable function. Because of this, a DAIN transfer is a less common indication in a low median nerve palsy.

CONTRAINDICATIONS

Absolute Contraindications

If a prolonged period of time has passed since the initial injury, there may not be a benefit to performing nerve transfer. A DAIN transfer should be done within 6 months of injury with an upper limit of 12 months.[12]

Damage to the DAIN axons precludes the use of this transfer. If there is still concern regarding the viability of the AIN after physical examination, an MRI may be used to compare the mass of pronator quadratus (PQ) with the contralateral side. Electromyographic studies may be useful as well. In uncertain cases, direct DAIN stimulation at the time of surgery may be necessary to confirm satisfactory function.

Extensive damage to the distal motor fascicles constitutes another contraindication.

Finally, in the case of a previous high ulnar nerve repair, one should ascertain that there is no evidence of recovery of motor function. This can be challenging to discern, as the innervation pattern of upper extremity musculature does not always fit the "textbook" description. The innervation patterns of the FCU and FDP can vary in terms of their contributions from the ulnar and median nerves.[13,14] Furthermore, the presence of Martin-Gruber and Riche-Cannieu anastomoses can also complicate the hand examination. Electromyographic studies can help clarify this.

Relative Contraindications

Ulnar nerve lesions in the middle or distal thirds of the forearm that are amenable to primary repair will likely not benefit from DAIN transfer. If these lesions are repaired in a timely manner, the functional gains may be superior with direct coaptation or nerve graft reconstruction of the injured nerve. This is because the coaptation site of the DAIN to the ulnar DMB fascicles may not be substantially closer to the hand intrinsic motor end plates than would be the case with an orthotopic neurorrhaphy.

When the ulnar lesion is in the proximal third of the forearm, the age of the patient and the degree of injury may help dictate the reconstruction. A nerve transfer should not be performed in a young patient with a clean nerve transection that can be repaired primarily, due to the more favorable outcomes reported in younger age groups (Table 25-2).[2]

PREOPERATIVE CONSIDERATIONS

The patient should be fully recovered from their initial trauma prior to proceeding with nerve transfer. Adequate vascular supply should be confirmed in the upper extremity, especially if major blood vessels were damaged in the initial injury. All wounds from the original injury should be well healed. Ideally, hand therapy should be started preoperatively to ensure the hand is as supple as possible prior to nerve transfer.[12]

SURGICAL TECHNIQUE

The patient should be positioned supine with the injured upper extremity abducted to 90° on a hand table. A pneumatic tourniquet should be placed about the proximal arm, and a nerve stimulator and operating microscope should be available in the room.

There are several considerations that go into planning the incision. The incision will be dependent on whether the DMB or TB has been chosen as the recipient nerve. Additionally, if there is an exploratory component of the procedure to assess the level of injury, or if ancillary procedures are planned concomitantly, these must be incorporated into the incision design and placement. A decision must be made prior to beginning the procedure whether the donor or recipient nerve will be approached first. This is important because after inflation of the tourniquet there is a limited amount of time in which intraoperative nerve stimulation is possible to determine nerve function. The description of this procedure in past works varies in regards to which nerve should be approached first.[12,15,16] The surgeon should assess the overall extent of the injury and decide whether intraoperative testing of either the donor or recipient nerve would be necessary or helpful. In most patients if intraoperative stimulation is indicated, it is to confirm adequate function of the DAIN.

Distal Anterior Interosseous Nerve Transfer to the Deep Motor Branch of the Ulnar Nerve

An incision is made approximately 3 to 4 cm distal to the wrist flexor crease at the level of the Kaplan's cardinal line in line with the fourth web space. The incision is continued proximally across the wrist in a zigzag manner, crossing directly over Guyon canal just radial to the pisiform. It is continued proximally to the junction of the middle and distal thirds of the forearm, keeping slightly ulnar to the midline.

The dissection is then deepened through the antebrachial fascia between the FCU and the finger flexor tendons. Care should be taken to protect the median nerve, which is adherent to the undersurface of the flexor digitorum superficialis (FDS), as well as the ulnar neurovascular structures beneath the FCU. The FDS and FDP tendons are retracted radially to expose the PQ muscle, the interosseous membrane, the AIN, and the anterior interosseous artery and veins. The DAIN typically enters the PQ approximately 5 to 10 cm proximal to the ulnar styloid.[17] The AIN is isolated from the vessels and secured with a small-caliber vessel loop. Intraoperative nerve stimulation is then performed to assess the AIN viability prior to transfer.

The nerve is then traced distally within the substance of the PQ muscle until it bifurcates or trifurcates, which is typically at the level of the proximal third or half of the muscle. It is then sharply transected at this level.

After isolating the donor nerve, attention is then turned toward preparation of the recipient fascicles. The ulnar nerve should be isolated from the ulnar artery and veins and secured with a vessel loop. Care should be taken to protect the dorsal cutaneous sensory branch during this dissection. The contents of Guyon canal are exposed by dividing the palmaris brevis and the volar carpal ligament. The superficial branch of the ulnar nerve should be visible beneath the palmaris brevis and superficial to the hypothenar muscles. The DMB will lie deep to the pisohamate ligament, radial to the hook of hamate.[18]

The motor fascicles are separated from the sensory fascicles from distal to proximal. Any interfascicular connections can be safely divided up to the midforearm level. MacKinnon and coworkers prefer to trace the fascicle visually until the midforearm before physically separating the fascicles.[16]

The DMB should not be divided until sufficient length has been gained to permit a tension-free coaptation to the DAIN with the wrist extended 30° and the fingers extended.

The DAIN is passed deep to the flexor tendons and coapted to the DMB with 10-0 epineural sutures using an operating microscope. If the wrist cannot be extended to 30° without undue tension on or disruption of the coaptation site, the wrist should be splinted in neutral or an interposition nerve graft using the lateral antebrachial cutaneous nerve can be used, but this will likely result in poorer outcomes.

The tourniquet is then released and hemostasis obtained. The volar carpal ligament and antebrachial fascia are not repaired and the wound is closed in layers.

Distal Anterior Interosseous to the Thenar Branch of the Median Nerve

When DAIN transfer is used for thenar reanimation, the surgical approach to the donor nerve is essentially unchanged, but the distal incision is oriented more radially to allow for visualization of the TB. Care should be taken to avoid injury to the palmar cutaneous branch of the median nerve. The transverse carpal ligament is divided completely and an interfascicular dissection is performed, isolating the TB fascicles from the sensory fascicles. The remainder of the operation, in addition to the postoperative care, is identical to that described above.

POSTOPERATIVE REHABILITATION

The postoperative immobilization should be individualized. In most patients the wrist is splinted in neutral position with the MP joints flexed and IP joints extended for 3 weeks. If the neurorrhaphy site was under any significant tension, the wrist is immobilized in mild flexion for 4 weeks followed by progressive mobilization. In a young or potentially noncompliant patient a long arm cast is applied for 3 weeks to protect the repair. Signs of intrinsic reinnervation typically occur between 6 and 9 months, often initially evidenced by intrinsic muscle contraction during forearm pronation. Over time, motor reeducation should occur spontaneously with activities of daily living. If this does not occur, formal hand therapy may be required, including the use of biofeedback and functional electrical stimulation.

If there is no clinical evidence of reinnervation by 10 to 12 months postoperatively, EMG is performed. If there is evidence of reinnervation, hand therapy is continued. If

TABLE 25-3: Summary of Published Outcomes of Distal Anterior Interosseous Nerve Transfer

Study	Number of Patients	Outcome Measure	Results
Wang and Zhu[7,a]	14	British Medical Research Council Grade	Grade 5—3 patients Grade 4—6 patients Grade 3—3 patients Grade 2—2 patients
Battiston and Lanzetta[8,b]	7	Highet-Zachary scale and lateral pinch and grip strength as a percentage of the contralateral side	Excellent—1 patient[c] Good—5 patients Poor—1 patient
Haase and Chung[10]	2	Clinical examination	Clinical signs of reinnervation in both patients
Novak and Mackinnon[9]	8	Preoperative and postoperative lateral pinch and grip strength	Mean lateral pinch improved from 2.2 to 13.8 lb, and mean grip strength improved from 8.8 to 61.2 lb
Flores[11,b]	5	Highet-Zachary scale	All patients achieved a "good" result

[a]A portion of these procedures were transfers of the DAIN to the TB. Additionally, a nerve graft was used for each case.
[b]Concomitant nerve transfers were performed in each of these studies for improvement in sensory function.
[c]This patient was 11 years old.

there is no electromyographic evidence of reinnervation by 1 year postoperatively, it is likely the procedure has failed and alternative treatment considerations, including tendon transfers, should be discussed with the patient.

COMPLICATIONS

Complications from DAIN transfer are rare, and the minimal donor-site morbidity makes this procedure an attractive initial option for treating high ulnar nerve injuries. There is no apparent loss of pronation strength, and no special risk of infection or hematoma.

OUTCOMES

The literature on outcomes of this procedure mostly consists of small retrospective case series (Table 25-3).[7–11] Additionally, the outcome measures vary a great deal from study to study. This makes it challenging to assess the true results of this relatively uncommon procedure.

An additional benefit of this procedure that we have observed is the prevention of and reversal of intrinsic muscle atrophy, since the lack of soft tissue bulk provided by the intrinsics may make power grip uncomfortable. Figures 25-1 to 25-6 demonstrate the postoperative result from a DAIN to DMB nerve transfer at 7 years of follow-up. The patient was a 20-year-old male who sustained a complete, sharp transection of the left ulnar nerve 12 cm proximal to the elbow. He underwent a direct repair at the time of injury and a follow-up DAIN to DMB transfer 8 months later. Return of function was demonstrated 16 months after the initial injury and 8 months after the nerve transfer procedure. Reanimation was first noted by contraction of the ulnar innervated lumbrical muscles while pronating the forearm. Function continued to improve over several years and the patient is now a surgical resident physician.

In conclusion, the DAIN to DMB nerve transfer should be considered as a reconstructive option for an isolated high

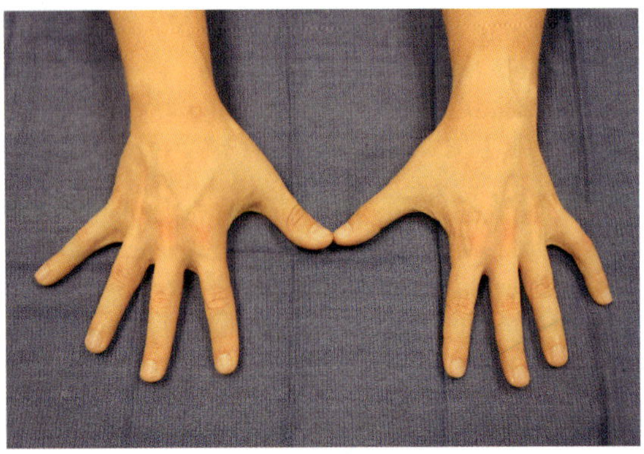

FIGURE 25-1 Finger abduction, dorsal view, 84 months post left DAIN to DMB transfer. Note some residual claw deformity of left small finger.

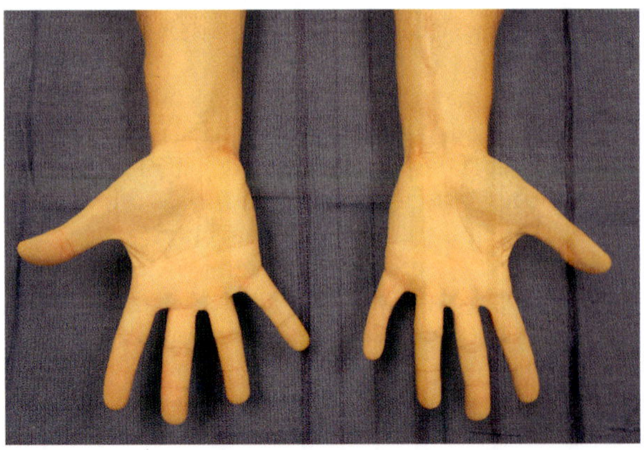

FIGURE 25-2 Finger abduction, palmar view, patient above.

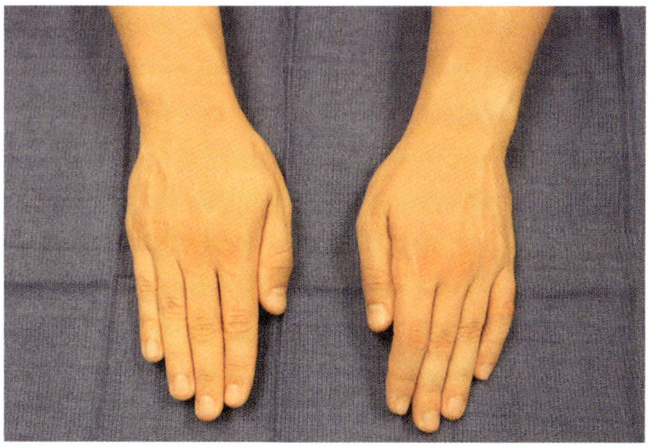

FIGURE 25-3 Finger adduction, dorsal view, patient above.

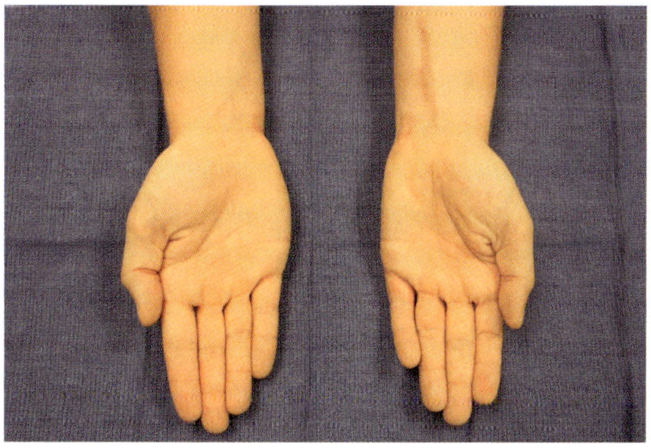

FIGURE 25-4 Finger adduction, palmar view, patient above.

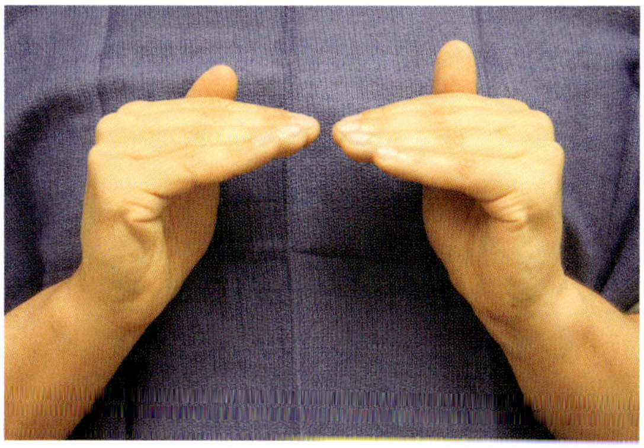

FIGURE 25-5 Intrinsic plus positioning demonstrating function of the lumbrical muscles, patient above.

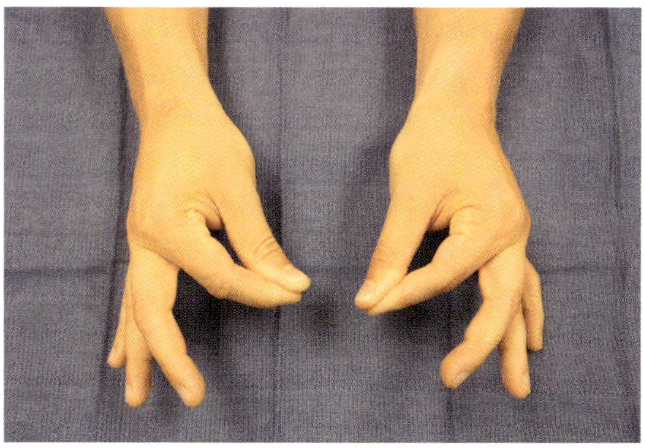

FIGURE 25-6 Fingertip pinch demonstrating the absence of a Froment sign.

ulnar nerve injury. The donor-site morbidity is negligible and the functional outcomes are predictable and preclude the need for further surgery provided the procedure is carried out in a timely manner. Additionally, other reconstructive options, such as tendon transfers, are still available in the event of a poor outcome.

REFERENCES

1. Mackinnon SE, Novak CB. Nerve transfers. New options for reconstruction following nerve injury. *Hand Clin*. 1999;15:643–666.
2. Gaul JS. Intrinsic motor recovery—a long term study of ulnar nerve repair. *J Hand Surg Am*. 1982;7:502–508.
3. Kobayashi J, Mackinnon SE, Watanabe O, et al. The effect of duration of muscle denervation on functional recovery in the rat model. *Muscle Nerve*. 1997;20:858–866.
4. Wood MB. Treatment of irreparable nerve damage in the hand. In: Slutsky DJ, Hentz VR, eds. *Peripheral Nerve Surgery*. Philadelphia: Churchill Livingstone; 2006:109–114.
5. Anderson GA. Ulnar nerve palsy. In: Green DP, Hotchkiss RN, Pederson WC, Wolfe SW, eds. *Green's Operative Hand Surgery*. Philadelphia: Churchill Livingstone; 2005:1161–1196.
6. Tse R, Hentz VR. Tendon transfer procedures for low and high ulnar nerve injury. In: Chung KC, ed. *Operative Techniques: Hand and Wrist Surgery*. Philadelphia: Saunders/Elsevier; 2008:371–398.
7. Wang Y, Zhu S. Transfer of a branch of the anterior interosseous nerve to the motor branch of the median and ulnar nerve. *Chin Med J Engl*. 1997;110:216–219.
8. Battiston B, Lanzetta M. Reconstruction of high ulnar nerve lesions by distal double median to ulnar nerve transfer. *J Hand Surg Am*. 1999;24A:1185–1191.
9. Novak CB, Mackinnon SE. Distal anterior interosseous nerve transfer to the deep motor branch of the ulnar nerve for reconstruction of high ulnar nerve injuries. *J Reconstr Microsurg*. 2002;18:459–464.
10. Haase SC, Chung KC. Anterior interosseous nerve transfer to the motor branch of the ulnar nerve for high ulnar nerve injuries. *Ann Plast Surg*. 2002;49:285–290.
11. Flores LP. Distal anterior interosseous nerve transfer to the deep ulnar nerve and end-to-side suture of the superficial ulnar nerve to the third common palmar digital nerve for treatment of high ulnar nerve injuries. *Arq Neuropsiquiatr*. 2011;69:519–524.
12. Tai CY, Tung TH, Myckatyn TM, Mackinnon SE. Distal anterior interosseous nerve transfer for ulnar motor reinnervation. In: Chung KC, ed. *Operative Techniques: Hand and Wrist Surgery*. Philadelphia: Saunders/Elsevier; 2008:497–504.
13. Ang GG, Rozen WM, Vally F, Eizenberg N, Grinsell D. Anomalies of the flexor carpi ulnaris: clinical case report and cadaveric study. *Clin Anat*. 2010;23:427–430.
14. Oh CS, Won HS, Lee KS, Chung IH, Kim SM. Anatomic variation of the innervation of the flexor digitorum profundus muscle and its clinical implications. *Muscle Nerve*. 2009;39:498–502.
15. Wood MB. Hand intrinsic muscle reanimation by transfer of the distal portion of the anterior interosseous nerve. *J Am Soc Surg Hand*. 2004;4:227–230.
16. Brown JM, Yee A, Mackinnon SE. Distal median to ulnar nerve transfers to restore ulnar motor and sensory function within the hand: technical nuances. *Neurosurgery*. 2009;65:966–978.
17. Tubbs RS, Custis JW, Salter G, Wellons JC, Blount JP, Oakes WJ. Quantitation of and superficial surgical landmarks for the anterior interosseous nerve. *J Neurosurg*. 2006;104:787–791.
18. Atkins SE, Logan B, Mcgrouther DA. The deep (motor) branch of the ulnar nerve: a detailed examination of its course and the clinical significance of its damage. *J Hand Surg Eur*. 2009;34E:47–57.

III

DISTAL RADIUS

Management of Distal Radius Fractures

David J. Slutsky, MD

26

Distal radius fractures (DRFs) occur as a consequence of trauma. There is a bimodal distribution with high-energy fractures occurring in younger people, mostly males, and low-energy fractures occurring in older persons, mostly females.[1] They are one of the most common fractures. In 2006 there were 195.2 fractures per 100,000 people.[2] At least $164,000,000 was spent on hospitalizations related to DRFs in 2000.[3]

ANATOMY

The articular surface of the radius is triangular, with the apex of the triangle at the radial styloid. It slopes in a volar and ulnar direction with a radial inclination of 23° (range 13°-30°), a radial length of 12 mm (range 8-18 mm), and an average volar tilt of 12° (1°-21°). The dorsal surface of the distal radius is convex and irregular, and it is covered by the 6 dorsal extensor compartments. The dorsal cortex is thin, which often results in comminution that can lead to an abnormal dorsal tilt. Lister's tubercle acts as a fulcrum for the extensor pollicis longus (EPL) tendon, which lies in a groove on the ulnar side of the tubercle. The volar side of the distal radius, which is covered by the pronator quadratus (PQ), is flat and makes a smooth curve that is concave from proximal to distal. A cartilaginous anteroposterior ridge divides the distal articular surface of the radius into a scaphoid facet and a lunate facet. The scaphoid fossa is triangular, whereas the lunate fossa is more quadrangular in shape. The triangular fibrocartilage complex (TFCC) originates on the ulnar rim of the lunate fossa and extends ulnarly to insert into the base of the ulnar styloid. The articulation of the ulnar head to the radius is not congruent, with the radius of curvature of the shallow sigmoid notch being slightly greater than that of the convexity of the ulna head. Only the brachioradialis (BR) tendon inserts onto the distal radius. The other wrist flexor or extensor tendons pass across the distal radius to insert on the carpal bones or the base of the metacarpals.

The dorsum of the radius is cloaked by the arborizations of the superficial radial nerve (SRN) and the dorsal cutaneous branch of the ulnar nerve (DCBUN). The SRN exits from under the BR approximately 5 cm proximal to the radial styloid and bifurcates into a major volar and a major dorsal branch at a mean distance of 4.2 cm proximal to the radial styloid. Either partial or complete overlap of the lateral antebrachial cutaneous nerve (LABCN) with the SRN occurs up to 75% of the time. The DCBUN arises from the ulnar nerve 6 cm proximal to the ulnar head and becomes subcutaneous 5 cm proximal to the pisiform. It crosses the ulnar snuffbox and gives off 3 to 9 branches that supply the dorsoulnar aspect of the carpus, small finger, and ulnar ring finger.

MECHANISM OF INJURY

Falling onto an outstretched hand is the most commonly cited mechanism of injury in DRFs. The mechanism typically involves a combination of axial loading, a bending moment, and either supination or pronation. The degree, direction, and extent of the applied load may cause further coronal or sagittal splits within the lunate or scaphoid facets. Increasing wrist extension at the time of impact could result in more dorsal comminution. Arthroscopic studies have revealed a high incidence of associated soft tissue injuries, which can impact the prognosis (Table 26-1). A recent computed tomographic (CT) study of 100 DRFs revealed that the fracture lines were significantly more likely to occur at the intervals between the ligament attachments than at the ligament attachments.[8] Common sites of fractures were the center of the sigmoid notch, between the short and long radiolunate ligaments, and the central and dorsal ulnar aspects of the scaphoid fossa. The authors postulated that either the ligament attachment sites might be strengthened by the ligamentous insertions or the ligaments might insert in regions of higher bone quality. These findings might explain why ligamentotaxis can be successful in reducing those articular rim fragments with a preserved ligament attachment. Central articular die-punch fragments are not reduced because of the lack of ligamentous attachments.

TABLE 26-1: Incidence of Soft Tissue Injuries with Distal Radius Fractures

	Type of DRF	% TFCC	% SLIL	% LTIL	% Extrinsic
Fontes	30 (intra- and extra-articular)	70	40	17	17
Geissler et al[4]	60 (intra-articular)	49	32	15	
Lindau et al[5]	50 (intra-articular)	78	54	16	
Richards et al[6]	118 (intra- and extra-articular)	35 (intra) 53 (extra)	21 (intra) 7 (extra)	7 (intra) 13 (extra)	
Mehta et al[7]	31 (intra- and extra-articular)	58	85	61	

BASIC FRACTURE HEALING

When a bone fractures, the stored energy is released. At low loading speeds the energy can dissipate through a single crack. At high loading speed the energy cannot dissipate rapidly enough through a single crack. Comminution and extensive soft tissue damage occur. Fractures that exhibit multiple fracture lines are thus inherently more unstable due to the greater energy absorption at the time of injury. The major factors determining the mechanical environment of a healing fracture include the rigidity of the selected fixation device, the fracture configuration, the accuracy of fracture reduction, and the amount and type of loading at the fracture gap. The fracture site stability may be artificially enhanced by a variety of external or internal means, which include cast treatment, pins, external fixation, intramedullary implants, and plates. Fracture healing under unstable or flexible fixation typically occurs by callus formation. This applies to cast treatment with or without supplemental pin fixation, as well as external fixation.

Four biomechanical stages of fracture healing have been defined: stage I—failure through original fracture site, with low stiffness; stage II—failure through original fracture site, with high stiffness; stage III—failure partially through original fracture site and partially through intact bone, with high stiffness; and stage IV—failure entirely through intact bone, with high stiffness.[9] These data help to determine the level of activity that is safe for patients with a healing fracture. The distal radius is composed largely of cancellous metaphyseal bone. Bone healing in cortical and cancellous bone is qualitatively similar, but the speed and reliability of healing is generally better in cancellous bone due to the comparatively large fracture surface. Extra-articular fractures are thought to be healed by 5 weeks after injury.[10]

For the purposes of rehabilitation of DRFs, stage I would roughly correspond to the initial 4 weeks or the soft callus phase. Protection of the fracture from excessive forces is needed to prevent shortening and angulation. Stage II would coincide with the 4- to 8-week time period. The period beyond 8 weeks would represent stages III and IV where the fracture has clinically united and can tolerate progressive loading.[11]

FRACTURE SITE FORCES

Movement of the bone fragments depends on the amount of external loading, stiffness of the fixation device, and the stiffness of the tissue bridging the fracture.

The physiologic forces with wrist motion have been estimated to lie between 88 and 135 N (1 lb of force = 4.48 N).[12] Eighty-two percent of the loads across the wrist are transmitted through the distal radius.[13] Cadaver studies have demonstrated that for every 10 N of grip force, 26 N is transmitted through the distal radius metaphysis. Given that the average male grip force is 463 N or 105 psi, this would imply that up to 2410 N of force could be applied to the distal radius during power gripping.[14] Rikli et al measured the in vivo dynamic intra-articular pressures under local anesthesia in the radio-ulnocarpal joint of a healthy volunteer.[15] With the forearm in neutral rotation, the forces ranged from 107 N with wrist flexion to 197 N with wrist extension. The highest forces of up to 245 N were seen with the wrist in radial deviation and the forearm in supination. Moss et al showed that in a cadaver study with AO/ASIF type C2 fractures the average failure load for a volar plate with a 7–distal screw construct was 139 N (±78) versus 108 N (±18) for a 4-screw construct before failure, which was defined as 2 mm or more of displacement of any fracture fragment.[16] External fixators compress as much as 3 mm under a 729-N load.[17] As a general guide, the grip forces during therapy should therefore remain under 140 N (36 psi) during the initial 4 weeks in order to prevent a failure of fixation. Either type of fixation, however, provides enough stability to institute immediate wrist motion. Newer-generation locking volar plates are stronger and may tolerate higher loading conditions, but fracture site settling will still occur.

RADIOGRAPHIC STUDIES

The initial x-rays should include a standard posteroanterior, lateral, and oblique view. Traction views can help distinguish an intra-articular from an extra-articular fracture. The posterior–anterior (PA) view should be taken with the elbow and shoulder at 90° and the forearm in neutral rotation, which standardizes the assessment of the ulnar variance. A true lateral x-ray is taken with the forearm in neutral rotation and

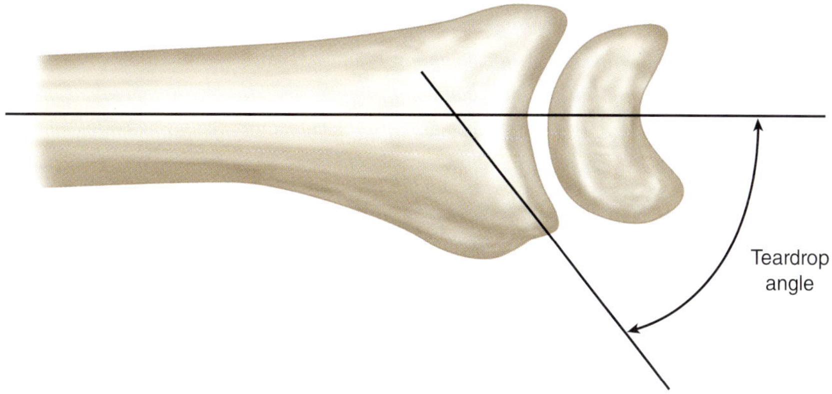

FIGURE 26-1 The teardrop angle is measured between a line drawn down the longitudinal axis of the radial shaft with a line drawn down the center of the teardrop.

with the volar aspects of the pisiform and distal pole of the scaphoid overlapped.[18] A 10° to 20° lateral inclined view where the beam is directed from distal radial to proximal ulnar provides a true lateral view of the ulnar two thirds of the articular surface, which is normally at an inclination of about 10°. This is especially important following volar plating, to assess whether the ulnarmost subchondral screws penetrate the joint surface.[19] A 45° pronated oblique view can be used to assess the distal radioulnar joint (DRUJ) congruency since it profiles the dorsal ulnar cortex that supports the dorsal lunate articular facet and forms the dorsal margin of the sigmoid notch.

Medoff outlined some useful radiographic relationships. He described the teardrop, which is a dense, U-shaped outline seen at the distal end of the radius on the lateral view.[20] It is formed from the confluent outlines of the distal shaft and distal radial ridge, and terminates in the volar rim of the lunate facet. The thickness of the cortical bone that forms the base of the teardrop is noted to be significantly greater than the thickness of the dorsal cortical bone and reflects the greater loading forces that normally occur along the volar surface of the radius. The teardrop angle is determined by measuring the angle between a line extended along the longitudinal axis of the radial shaft and a line that is drawn down the center of the teardrop (Fig. 26-1). The normal angle is 70°. Depression of the teardrop angle below 45° is indicative of a sagittal split of the articular surface. The volar ulnar fragment arises because of impaction of the lunate into the lunate facet, which is then driven by the carpus into dorsiflexion. Medoff also observed that with a wrist in neutral on the 10° lateral x-ray, a line extended from the volar cortex of the radial shaft should be nearly collinear with the center axis of rotation of the proximal pole of the capitate.[20] Fractures with volar or dorsal displacement result in translation of the carpus with the capitate migrating volar or dorsal to this line. The AP distance is the point-to-point distance between the corner of the dorsal rim and the corner of the volar rim on the lateral view. In a series of 20 patients with DRFs treated in Hawaii, an increase in the AP distance of more than 21 mm in men and 19 mm in women was correlated with a sagittal split with a separate dorsal ulnar and volar ulnar fragment.

The variations in the height of Lister's tubercle and in the depth of the EPL groove are considerable. The triangular shape of the dorsal cortex can obscure the determination of screw protrusion through the dorsal cortex, which can potentially lead to EPL rupture. A CT study of 30 cadaver forearms and wrists revealed that the size of Lister's tubercle varied from 1.4 to 6.6 mm (average 3.3 mm) in height radial to the tubercle, and the depth of the EPL groove varied from 0.6 to 3.2 mm (average 1.6 mm).[21] Joseph and Harvey described a dorsal tangential view (horizon view) in which the wrist is hyperflexed and the beam is directed along the long axis of the radius to detect dorsal screw protrusion (Fig. 26-2).

CT with sagittal and coronal reconstructions is valuable for operative decision making in intra-articular fracture patterns. CT is particularly helpful in die-punch fractures (fractures with a central depression of the articular surface), volar lip fractures, and fractures involving the scaphoid facet. The axial view is useful to assess the congruency of the sigmoid notch.

CLASSIFICATION

A number of different classification systems for DRFs have been described but are no longer in widespread use. The Frykman classification system focused on the intra-articular extension of the fracture and involvement of the DRUJ and the ulnar styloid. The Mayo classification emphasized the extent of articular involvement, whereas the Melone classification highlighted the "die-punch" lunate facet fracture. Trumble et al[22] recommended identifying the following clinical/radiographic features: (i) displacement—dorsal versus volar, (ii) comminution—<50% or only involving 1 cortex versus >50% or involving 2 or more cortices, (iii) articular involvement—intra-articular versus extra-articular, (iv) ulna involvement—styloid, head, neck, DRUJ dislocation, or radial head injury, and (v) associated soft tissue injuries—intercarpal ligament injuries, including scapholunate and lunotriquetral ligament tears, or injuries to the TFCC.

The AO classification, with its 27 categories, is primarily useful for broad anatomic categorization of large numbers of

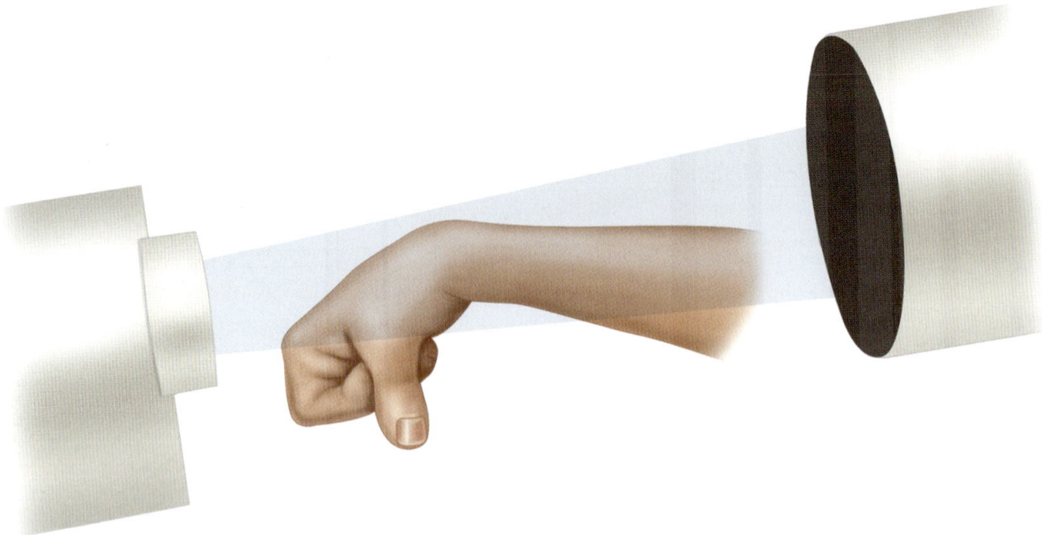

FIGURE 26-2 Diagram of wrist position for the horizon view to detect dorsal screw protrusion.

fractures for trauma registries and research purposes. A-type fractures are extra-articular fractures that spare the articular surface. B-type partial intra-articular fractures spare a portion of the articular surface that remains in continuity with the metaphysis and can result in volar lip, dorsal lip, radial styloid, and medial corner fractures, whereas impaction injuries can cause die-punch fractures. C-type fractures are composed of complex articular fractures where none of the articular surface remains in continuity with the metaphysis.

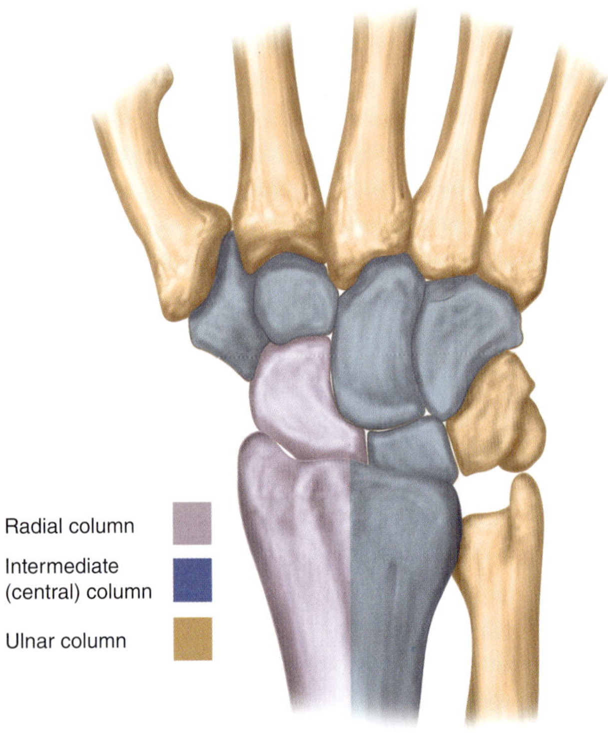

FIGURE 26-3 Three-column model of the distal part of the radius.

The fractures can be divided into those with a dorsal or volar pattern and a direct impaction fracture with or without comminution. The fracture pattern can be a T or Y split of the articular surface or both. Metaphyseal comminution may involve greater than 50% of the diameter of the metaphysis on any radiographic view and involve 2 or more of the cortices. Rikli and Regazzoni introduced the 3-column concept in which the distal radius is divided into medial, intermediate, and lateral columns (Fig. 26-3).[23] This theory emphasizes that the lateral, or radial, column is an osseous buttress for the carpus and is an attachment point for the intracapsular ligaments; the primary function of the intermediate column is load transmission; and the medial, or ulnar, column serves as an axis for forearm and wrist rotation as well as a post for secondary load transmission. This classification is the basis for the fragment-specific fixation technique. Medoff expanded on this concept and described 5 basic fracture components: the radial column, ulnar corner, dorsal wall, free intra-articular, and volar rim (Fig. 26-4).[20]

TREATMENT OF DISTAL RADIUS FRACTURES

The American Academy of Orthopedic Surgeons (AAOS) developed an evidence-based distal radius clinical practice guideline based on a systematic literature review.[24] Of the 2625 abstracts that were screened, 73 met the criteria for inclusion. Each recommendation in this guideline summary is accompanied by a grade indicating the strength of the recommendation (Table 26-2). The guidelines are summarized in Table 26-3. It is apparent that the current literature does not have a sufficient number of evidence-based studies to answer many of the questions posed by the AAOS work group, but the hope is that this will improve when the guidelines are revisited.

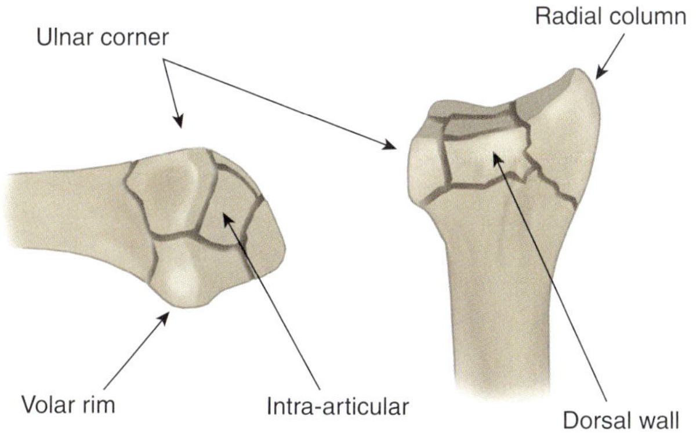

FIGURE 26-4 Medoff classification of intra-articular distal radius fractures.

Indications for Closed Treatment

The fractures of the distal radius best suited for nonoperative treatment are undisplaced and minimally displaced stable extra-articular fractures and selected undisplaced intra-articular fractures. Patients with nondisplaced extra-articular or simple intra-articular fractures can be treated by casting without manipulation. Fractures with any displacement and loss of radial length, radial inclination, or palmar tilt should be reduced to improve the alignment and stability of the fracture.

Contraindications

Fractures that will likely require surgical treatment include (i) redisplaced fractures, (ii) dorsal tilt greater than 20° that cannot be corrected with a closed reduction, (iii) intra-articular step or gap of greater than 1 mm, and (iv) more than 3 mm of radial shortening.

TECHNIQUE OF CLOSED REDUCTION

Colles fractures with dorsal angulation are the most common and occur from a fall on an outstretched hand with supination of the forearm. The reduction can be performed under a hematoma block or Bier block. They are reduced by initially hyperextending the wrist to disengage the distal fragment, longitudinal traction to restore the length, and then volar translation and pronation of the distal fragment. Acute fractures can be initially immobilized in a volar and dorsal splint or sugar tong splint with the wrist in approximately 30° of flexion, pronation, and ulnar deviation, and then converted to a short arm cast in 1 to 2 weeks after the acute swelling has resolved. The choice of a long arm or short arm cast has not been definitively resolved, but it does not appear to affect the outcome. Smith fractures with volar angulation are less common and occur with pronation of the hand during a torsional injury. These fractures are reduced in forearm supination and wrist extension, but they are usually unstable and require internal fixation. Immediate finger motion is instituted following reduction, along with tendon gliding exercises and edema control (see the section "Rehabilitation").

X-rays are taken at weeks 1, 2, 3, and 6. Any signs of carpal tunnel compression must be addressed as described below. One must be diligent for signs of a delayed EPL rupture, which is more common with undisplaced fractures. Cast immobilization cannot prevent fracture site settling and cannot control a significant intra-articular step-off.

Percutaneous Pinning

EXTRAFOCAL PINNING

Percutaneous K-wire fixation is indicated in fractures that can be initially reduced by closed reduction but are unstable due to comminution. Weil and Trumble showed that young patients with displaced extra-articular DRFs and minimal comminution can be treated by percutaneous pin fixation alone, whereas patients over 55 years of age and younger patients with comminution involving 2 or more surfaces of the radial metaphysis or >50% of the metaphyseal diameter require bridging fixation in addition to percutaneous pin fixation.[25] The K-wires (0.045-0.062 in) can be inserted into the radial styloid, between the first and second compartments, just ulnar to the second compartment, through Lister's tubercle and into the dorsal ulnar corner of the distal radius

TABLE 26-2: AAOS Guidelines: Strength of Recommendations

Strength	Overall Quality of Evidence	Description of Evidence
Strong	Good	Level I evidence from more than 1 study with consistent findings for recommending for or against the intervention or diagnostic
Moderate	Fair	Level II or III evidence from more than 1 study with consistent findings, or Level I evidence from a single study for recommending for or against the intervention or diagnostic
Weak	Poor	Level IV or V evidence from more than 1 study with consistent findings, or Level II or III evidence from a single study for recommending for or against the intervention or diagnostic
Inconclusive	None or conflicting	The evidence is insufficient or conflicting and does not allow a recommendation for or against the intervention or diagnostic
Consensus	No evidence	There is no supporting evidence. In the absence of reliable evidence, the work group is making a recommendation based on their clinical opinion considering the known harms and benefits associated with the treatment

TABLE 26-3: AAOS DRF Guidelines

1. We are unable to recommend for or against performing nerve decompression when nerve dysfunction persists after reduction
Strength of recommendation: inconclusive
2. We are unable to recommend for or against casting as definitive treatment for unstable fractures that are initially adequately reduced
Strength of recommendation: inconclusive
3. **We suggest operative fixation for fractures with postreduction radial shortening >3 mm, dorsal tilt >10°, or intra-articular displacement or step-off >2 mm as opposed to cast fixation**
Strength of recommendation: moderate
4. We are unable to recommend for or against any 1 specific operative method for fixation of distal radius fractures
Strength of recommendation: inconclusive
5. We are unable to recommend for or against operative treatment for patients over age 55 with distal radius fractures
Strength of recommendation: inconclusive
6. We are unable to recommend for or against locking plates in patients over the age of 55 who are treated operatively
Strength of recommendation: inconclusive
7. **We suggest rigid immobilization in preference to removable splints when using nonoperative treatment for the management of displaced distal radius fractures**
Strength of recommendation: moderate
8. The use of removable splints is an option when treating minimally displaced distal radius fractures
Strength of recommendation: weak
9. We are unable to recommend for or against immobilization of the elbow in patients treated with cast immobilization
Strength of recommendation: inconclusive
10. Arthroscopic evaluation of the articular surface is an option during operative treatment of intra-articular distal radius fractures
Strength of recommendation: weak
11. Operative treatment of associated ligament injuries (SLIL injuries, LT, or TFCC tears) at the time of radius fixation is an option
Strength of recommendation: weak
12. Arthroscopy is an option in patients with distal radius intra-articular fractures to improve diagnostic accuracy for wrist ligament injuries, and CT is an option to improve diagnostic accuracy for patterns of intra-articular fractures
Strength of recommendation: weak
13. We are unable to recommend for or against the use of supplemental bone grafts or substitutes when using locking plates
Strength of recommendation: inconclusive
14. We are unable to recommend for or against the use of bone graft (autograft or allograft) or bone graft substitutes for the filling of a bone void as an adjunct to other operative treatments
Strength of recommendation: inconclusive
15. In the absence of reliable evidence, it is the opinion of the work group that distal radius fractures that are treated nonoperatively be followed by ongoing radiographic evaluation for 3 weeks and at cessation of immobilization
Strength of recommendation: consensus
16. We are unable to recommend whether 2 or 3 Kirschner wires should be used for distal radius fracture fixation
Strength of recommendation: inconclusive
17. We are unable to recommend for or against using the occurrence of distal radius fractures to predict future fragility fractures
Strength of recommendation: inconclusive
18. We are unable to recommend for or against concurrent surgical treatment of distal radioulnar joint instability in patients with operatively treated distal radius fractures
Strength of recommendation: inconclusive
19. **We suggest that all patients with distal radius fractures receive a postreduction true lateral x-ray of the carpus to assess DRUJ alignment**
Strength of recommendation: moderate
20. In the absence of reliable evidence, it is the opinion of the work group that all patients with distal radius fractures and unremitting pain during follow-up be reevaluated
Strength of recommendation: consensus
21. A home exercise program is an option for patients prescribed therapy after distal radius fracture
Strength of recommendation: weak
22. In the absence of reliable evidence, it is the opinion of the work group that patients perform active finger motion exercises following diagnosis of distal radius fractures
Strength of recommendation: consensus
23. **We suggest that patients do not need to begin early wrist motion routinely following stable fracture fixation**
Strength of recommendation: moderate
24. In order to limit complications when using external fixation, it is an option to limit the duration of fixation
Strength of recommendation: weak
25. We are unable to recommend against overdistraction of the wrist when using an external fixator
Strength of recommendation: inconclusive
26. **We suggest adjuvant treatment of distal radius fractures with vitamin C for the prevention of disproportionate pain**
Strength of recommendation: moderate
27. Ultrasound and/or ice are options for adjuvant treatment of distal radius fractures
Strength of recommendation: weak
28. We are unable to recommend for or against fixation of ulnar styloid fractures associated with distal radius fractures
Strength of recommendation: inconclusive
29. We are unable to recommend for or against using external fixation alone for the management of distal radius fractures where there is depressed lunate fossa or 4-part fracture (sagittal split)
Strength of recommendation: inconclusive

INTRAFOCAL PINNING (KAPANDJI TECHNIQUE)

Intrafocal percutaneous pinning of the distal radius was described by Kapandji using 0.062-in K-wires.[26] Under fluoroscopy the K-wires are driven into the radial styloid fracture site to restore radial inclination and the dorsal fracture line to restore the palmar tilt. The pins are levered to correct the deformity and then redirected proximally before advancing them across the opposite cortex in both the posteroanterior and lateral planes. Three to 4 pins are used and the wrist is immobilized in a short arm cast for 6 weeks, or an external fixator is used as described above.

OUTCOMES

There is no recent literature on this technique. One randomized prospective study compared 50 patients with an extra-articular distal radial fractures that were treated by closed reduction and casting as compared with Kapandji pinning in 48 patients.[27] At a mean follow-up of 1 year using the Cooney score, 74% in the closed reduction and plaster cast group achieved an excellent to good result compared with 75% in the Kapandji pinning group. No statistically significant differences could be found between the 2 groups in terms of maintenance of reduction and the functional outcome.

Intramedullary Fixation

INDICATIONS

1. Unstable extra-articular DRFs that cannot be maintained with closed reduction
2. Simple intra-articular fractures

CONTRAINDICATIONS

1. Complex intra-articular fractures
2. Metaphyseal-diaphyseal comminution with proximal extension

SURGICAL TECHNIQUE

This will vary depending on the specific implant that is used, but the surgical approach shares common features. A closed reduction of the fracture is performed and held with percutaneous K-wires through the styloid and dorsally between the fourth and fifth extensor compartments. A 3-cm midline longitudinal incision is made centered over the tip of the radial styloid. Branches of the SRN are identified and mobilized. The periosteum between the first and second dorsal extensor tendons is elevated and a cortical window is made using an awl under fluoroscopic control, approximately 5 mm proximal to the tip of the styloid, to prevent penetration of the articular surface. A small canal finder is inserted into the intramedullary canal along the radial cortex. Progressively larger broaches are inserted and advanced across the fracture site. The implant is mounted on the external jig and gently inserted aiming medially so that no part of the nail is protruding above the radial cortex until the distal locking screw is just underneath the subchondral bone. The distal locking screws are inserted into the nail, taking care to avoid penetrating the sigmoid notch. Any fine-tuning of the fracture position is performed followed by insertion of the proximal locking screws through small incisions.

OUTCOMES

There are a few published studies using this type of device. Nishiwaki et al reviewed 31 patients with a mean age of 67 years (range, 51-85 years) with 1 AO type A2, 24 type A3, and 4 type C2 distal radial fractures. At a 1-year follow-up the active range of motion of the injured wrist relative to that on the uninjured side averaged 95% of flexion, 95% of extension, 93% of ulnar deviation, 91% of radial deviation, 99% of pronation, and 99% of supination. The mean grip strength was 96% of that on the uninjured side. According to the modified Mayo wrist score, there were 20 excellent and 9 good results. The mean DASH score was 4.8 points. The average radial inclination was 25°, volar tilt 11°, radial length 10 mm, and the ulnar variance was +1 mm. A loss of reduction occurred in 2 patients.[28]

External Fixation

LIGAMENTOTAXIS

External fixation of DRFs may be used in a bridging or nonbridging manner. Bridging external fixation of DRFs typically relies on ligamentotaxis to both obtain and maintain a reduction of the fracture fragments. As longitudinal traction is applied to the carpus, the tension is transmitted mostly through the radioscaphocapitate and long radiolunate ligaments to restore the radial length. In a similar vein, pronation of the carpus can indirectly correct the supination deformity of the distal fragment. Ligamentotaxis has a number of shortcomings when applied to the treatment of displaced intra-articular fractures. Since ligaments exhibit viscoelastic behavior, there is a gradual loss of the initial distraction force applied to the fracture site through stress relaxation (Fig. 26-5A and B). The immediate improvement in radial height, inclination, and volar tilt is significantly decreased by the time of fixator removal. In a series of 70 cases, Dicpinigaitis et al observed a loss of reduction of volar tilt for up to 6 months after external fixation in 34 of the patients, despite the use of adjuvant pinning.[29] The initial deformity, patient age, use of bone graft, and duration of external fixation were not predictors of loss of reduction.

Traction does not correct the dorsal tilt of the distal fracture fragment. This is because the stout volar radiocarpal ligaments are shorter and they pull out to length before the thinner dorsal radiocarpal ligaments exert any traction.[30] Excessive traction may actually increase the dorsal tilt. A dorsally directed vector is still necessary to restore the normal volar angulation. This is usually accomplished by applying manual thumb pressure over the dorsum of the distal fragment. With intra-articular fractures, ligamentotaxis reduces the radial styloid fragment, but for the above reasons it does not reduce a depressed lunate fragment. When there is a sagittal split of the medial fragment, traction causes the volar medial fragment to rotate that often necessitates an open reduction (Fig. 26-6A and B). External fixation cannot control radial translation and cannot be used with an unstable DRUJ.

BIOMECHANICAL CONSIDERATIONS FOR EXTERNAL FIXATION

Increasing the rigidity of the fixator does not appreciably increase the rigidity of fixation of the individual fracture

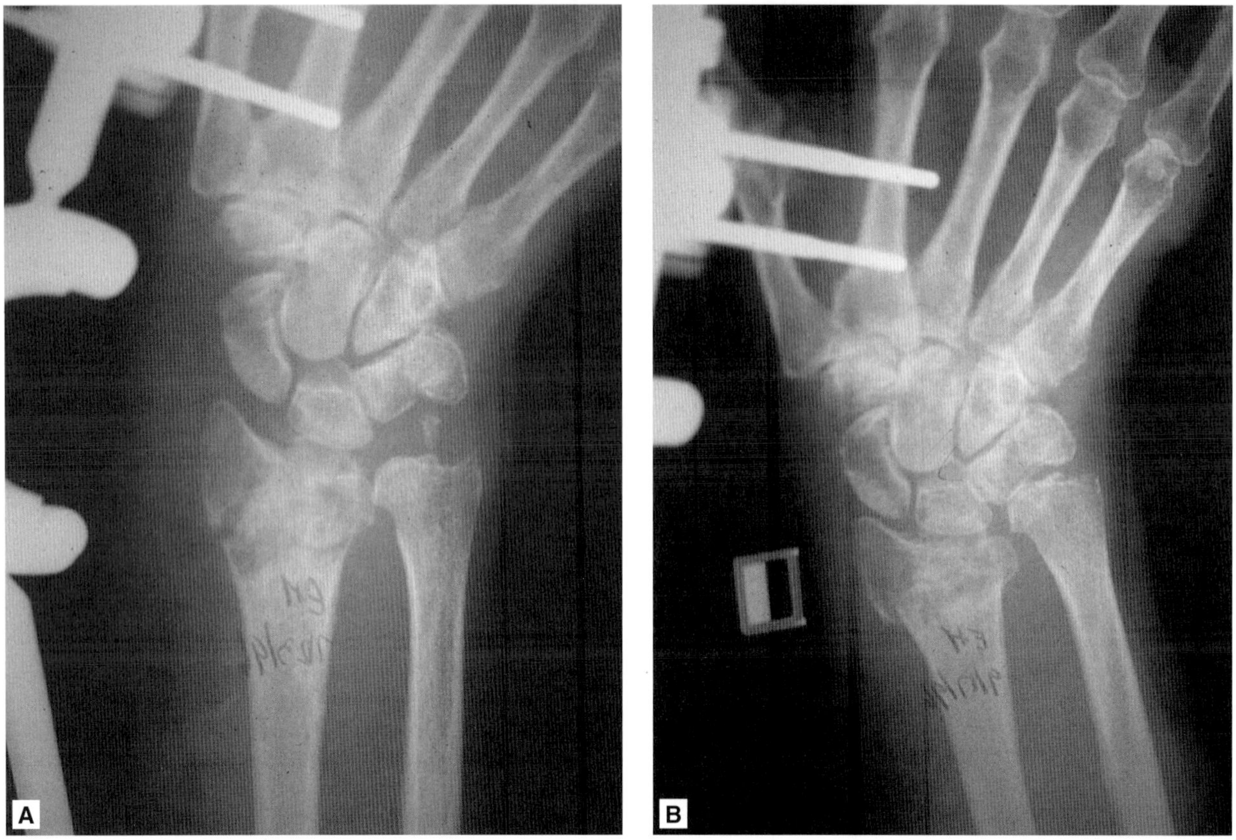

FIGURE 26-5 **A.** Initial reduction of a comminuted intra-articular distal radius fracture. Note the amount of carpal distraction. **B.** Marked radial shortening at 6 weeks in the fixator due to stress relaxation.

fragments.[12] There are a number of ways, however, in which to augment the stability of the construct. After restoration of radial length and alignment by the external fixator, percutaneous pin fixation can lock in the radial styloid buttress and support the lunate fossa fragment.[31] A fifth radial styloid pin attached to the frame of a spanning AO (Synthes, Paoli, Pennsylvania) external fixator prevents a loss of radial length through settling.[32] The addition of a dorsal pin attached to a sidebar easily corrects the dorsal tilt found in many DRFs. K-wire fixation enhances the stability of external fixation. Supplemental K-wire fixation is more critical to the fracture fixation than the mechanical rigidity of the external fixator itself. Stabilizing a fracture fragment with a nontransfixing K-wire that is attached to an outrigger is just as effective as a K-wire that transfixes the fracture fragments.[12]

BRIDGING EXTERNAL FIXATION

As compared with conventional plate fixation, bridging external fixation may be used in a temporary manner or it may be used for definitive management of the DRF. If there is difficulty regaining supination, Hanel and coworkers recommend immobilizing the patient in a long arm splint in supination in-between wrist motion exercises.[33] The fixator is typically removed in the office at 6 weeks.

TEMPORARY EXTERNAL FIXATION: INDICATIONS

1. Initial management of severe grade open fractures with extensive soft tissue loss
2. Temporizing measure to resuscitate a polytraumatized patient
3. Pending transfer to a tertiary referral facility for definitive fracture management
4. For complex fractures to both aid in the provisional fracture reduction and allow a better CT evaluation of the fracture characteristics prior to double-plate fixation

DEFINITIVE EXTERNAL FIXATION: INDICATIONS

1. Unstable extra-articular DRFs
2. Two-part and selected 3-part intra-articular fractures without displacement
3. Combined internal and external fixation

CONTRAINDICATIONS

Bridging external fixation should not be used as the sole method of stabilization in the following situations:

1. Ulnar translocation due to an unstable DRUJ
2. Intra-articular volar shear fractures (Barton, reverse Barton)

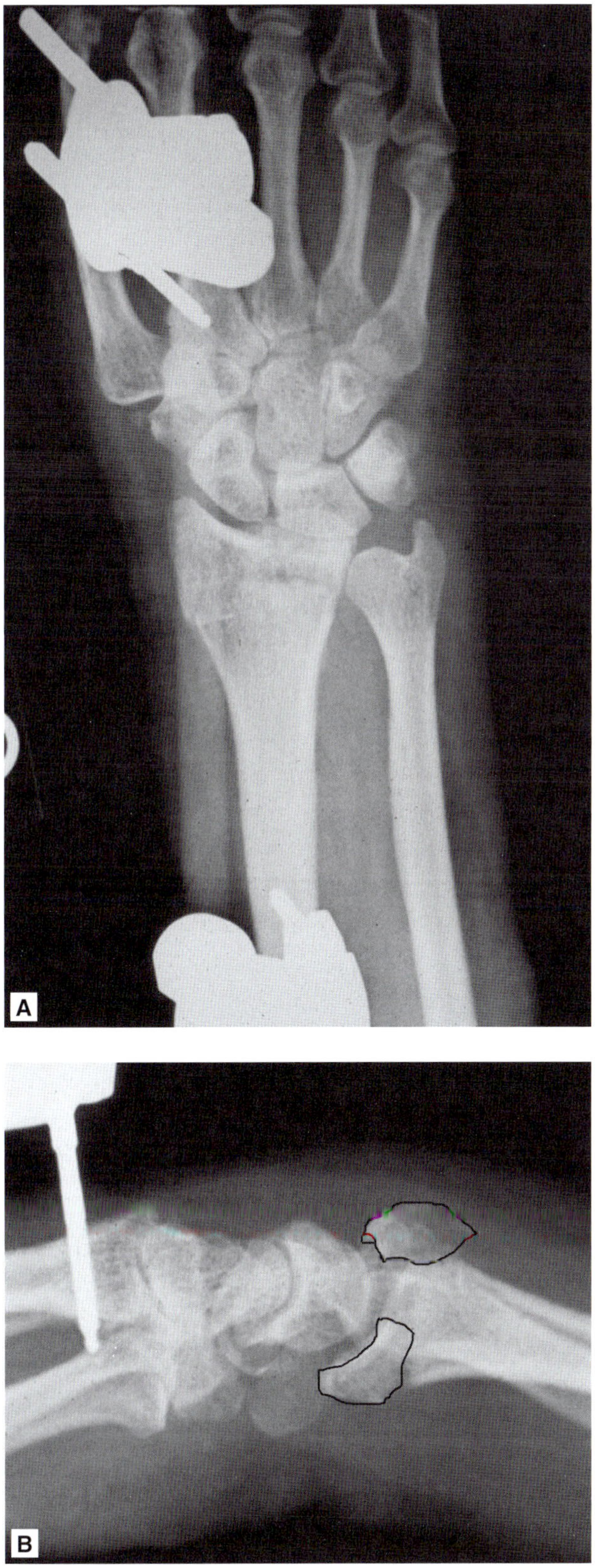

FIGURE 26-6 Four-part intra-articular fracture. **A.** Anteroposterior view reveals restoration of the radial height and apparent congruency of the joint with ligamentotaxis. **B.** Close-up of a lateral view reveals the sagittal split and increased rotation of the palmar medial fragment (outlines).

3. Disrupted volar carpal ligaments/radiocarpal dislocations
4. Marked metaphyseal comminution
5. Combined index and middle finger metacarpal fractures due to the interference with distal pin site placement

SURGICAL TECHNIQUE

Open pin insertion is necessary to prevent cutaneous nerve and tendon injury. When inserting the dorsal pins, it is important to engage the volar ulnar lip of the distal radius where the bone density is highest, especially in osteopenic bone.

The proximal pins are placed at the junction of the proximal and middle thirds of the radius. At this level the radius is covered by the tendons of extensor carpi radialis longus (ECRL) and extensor carpi radialis brevis (ECRB) as well as the extensor digitorum communis (EDC). The proximal pins can be inserted in the standard midlateral position by retracting the BR tendon and the SRN, in the dorsoradial position between the ECRL and ECRB, or dorsally between the ECRB and EDC, which carries less risk of injury to the SRN.

COMPLICATIONS

Fixator loosening with loss of fracture position can be avoided by periodically checking and tightening the fixator connections. Fixator failure by itself is uncommon, but many commercially available fixators are approved for single use only due to the risk of unrecognized material fatigue or failure of any locking ball joints. Pin site complications include infection, loosening, and interference with extensor tendon gliding. The risk of injury to branches of the SRN mandates open pin site insertion. Bad outcomes associated with external fixation are often related to overdistraction. One biomechanical study documented the effect of distraction of the wrist on metacarpophalangeal (MCP) joint motion. More than 5 mm of wrist distraction increases the load required for the flexor digitorum sublimus (FDS) to generate MCP joint flexion for the middle, ring, and small fingers. For the index finger, however, as much as 2 mm of wrist distraction significantly increases the load required for flexion at the MCP joint.[34] Many cases of intrinsic tightness and finger stiffness that are attributed to reflex sympathetic dystrophy are a consequence of prolonged and excessive traction that can be prevented by limiting the duration and amount of traction and instituting early dynamic MP flexion splinting even while in the fixator (Fig. 26-7).

The degree and duration of distraction correlates with the amount of subsequent wrist stiffness.[35] Distraction, flexion, and locked ulnar deviation of the external fixator encourage pronation contractures. Distraction also increases the carpal canal pressure, which may predispose to acute carpal tunnel syndrome.[36] Metaphyseal defects should be grafted to diminish bending loads and to allow fixator removal after 6 weeks that minimizes the fixator-related complications.

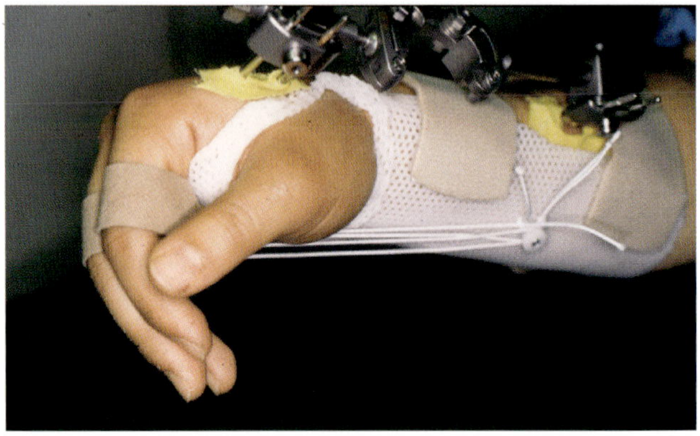

FIGURE 26-7 Dynamic MP flexion splinting in combination with external fixation.

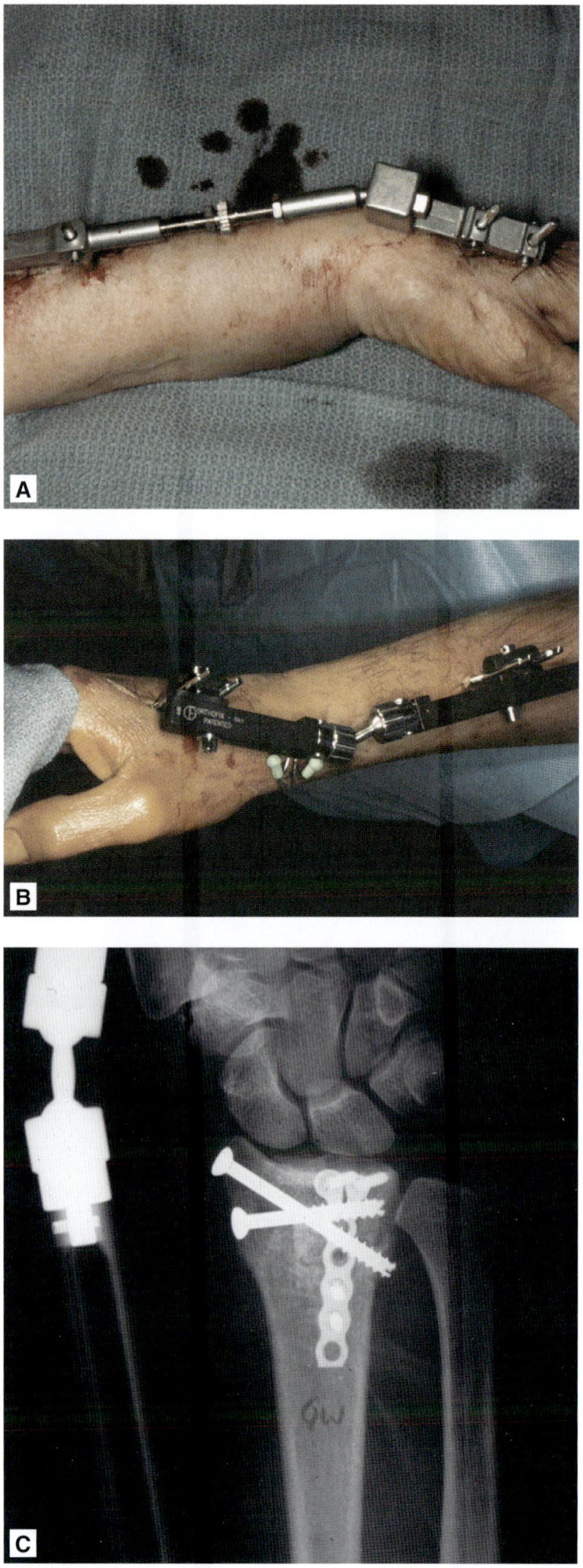

FIGURE 26-8 A. Improper application of an external fixator with marked wrist flexion. B. Proper fixator application with wrist in neutral and adjuvant pinning to maintain the fracture reduction. C. ORIF of the volar medial fragments combined with bridging external fixation.

Augmented External Fixation

The use of supplemental K-wire fixation can expand the indications for external fixation. As noted above, K-wire fixation not only enhances the reduction of the fracture fragments but also increases the rigidity of the entire construct. Many authors have stressed the importance of using the external fixator as a neutralization device rather than a traction device. Ligamentotaxis is used to obtain a reduction of the fracture fragments, which is then captured with percutaneous K-wire fixation. The traction on the fixator can then be reduced, which allows positioning of the wrist in neutral or slight extension. This serves to reduce extensor tendon tightness and facilitates finger motion. In 4-part fractures where there is a sagittal split of the medial fragment, longitudinal traction accentuates the palmar translation and rotation of the volar medial fragment. Dorsal to volar K-wire placement carries the risk of injury to the volar neurovascular bundles especially with K-wire migration. For these reasons any sagittal split of the articular surface typically requires open treatment (Fig. 26-8A-C).

INDICATIONS

1. Intra-articular radial styloid fractures[37]
2. Three 3-part intra-articular fractures
3. Following percutaneous reduction of a depressed lunate fragment
4. Arthroscopic-aided reduction of DRFs

CONTRAINDICATIONS

1. Marked metaphyseal comminution
2. Volar/dorsal intra-articular shear fractures

Nonbridging External Fixation

Nonbridging fixation does not rely on ligamentotaxis and it allows early wrist motion. Newer fixator designs have expanded the application of this technique.[38]

INDICATIONS

1. Redisplaced extra-articular fractures following an initially acceptable closed reduction
2. Fractures with ≥2 mm of radial shortening and ≥15° of dorsal tilt following a closed reduction, especially if there is comminution of 2 or more cortices[43]
3. Selected cases of undisplaced or reducible 2- and 3-part intra-articular fractures of the distal radius provided there is good bone density and a stable DRUJ

CONTRAINDICATIONS

1. When the distal fragment is too small for pin placement. At least 1 cm of intact volar cortex is required for pin purchase.
2. Volar shear fractures.
3. In children with open epiphyses.

SURGICAL TECHNIQUE

The technique is similar to bridging external fixation, with the use of a tourniquet and intraoperative fluoroscopy. I prefer to use a custom external fixator with a dorsal outrigger (Fig. 26-9A-J), although an AO delta frame external fixator (Mathys Medical Ltd, Bettlach, Switzerland) can be applied in a nonbridging manner as described by Gradl et al.[39] Two dorsal 3.0-mm pins are inserted in the distal fragment through separate longitudinal incisions. The pins can be placed on either side of Lister's tubercle or the EPL tendon, as well as between the EDC and the extensor digit minimi (EDM). The starting position of the pin should be approximately halfway between the fracture and the radiocarpal joint. A temporary K-wire can be used to gauge the proper angle. The first pin is inserted through Lister's tubercle parallel to the joint surface in the lateral plane until it engages the volar cortex. The second dorsal pin is inserted in a similar manner but on the ulnar side of the EPL or EDC tendons. The dorsal tilt is corrected by levering the pins distally until the normal volar inclination has been restored. The fixator frame is then applied and tightened.

In the case of intra-articular fractures the radial styloid fragment is reduced with ligamentotaxis using a traction tower under fluoroscopic control. An arthroscopic-aided reduction can be performed at this time (Fig. 26-10A-I). Any excessive supination or radial translation of the distal fragment is corrected prior to pin insertion. The styloid may be held with a provisional 0.062-in K-wire. An oblique 3.0-mm pin is then hand drilled at approximately 45° angle from the tip of the radial styloid across the fracture site to engage the ulnar cortex of the proximal fragment. The pin is fastened to a single pin clamp attached to the distal fixator arm. A more proximal pin clamp is used as a drill guide for insertion of a horizontal styloid pin to both fixate and provide subchondral support for the lunate fragment. The K-wire can be removed or left in place for added support as necessary. Next 2 proximal pins are inserted in the midradius using the double pin clamp as a drill guide. The dorsal tilt can be corrected by using a Freer elevator inserted percutaneously in the fracture site after the radial styloid reduction. Two dorsal 3.0-mm pins are inserted in the distal fragment through separate longitudinal incisions as described for the extra-articular

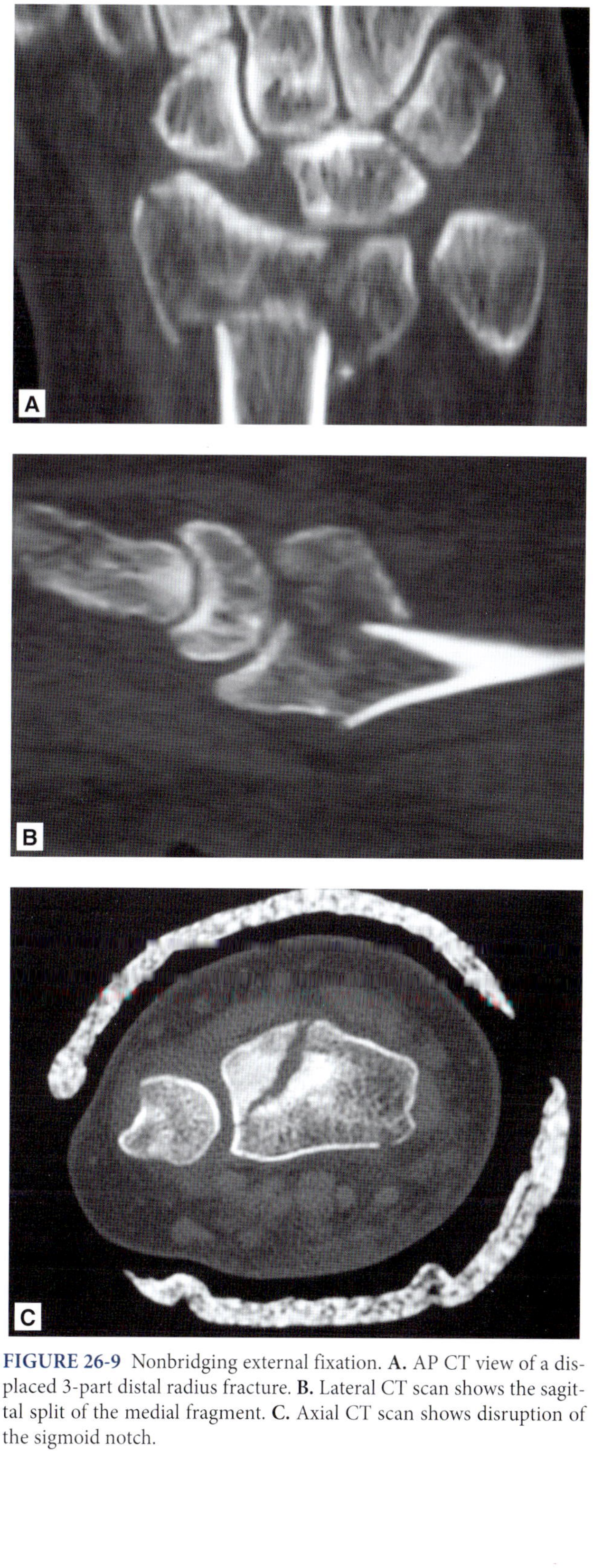

FIGURE 26-9 Nonbridging external fixation. **A.** AP CT view of a displaced 3-part distal radius fracture. **B.** Lateral CT scan shows the sagittal split of the medial fragment. **C.** Axial CT scan shows disruption of the sigmoid notch.

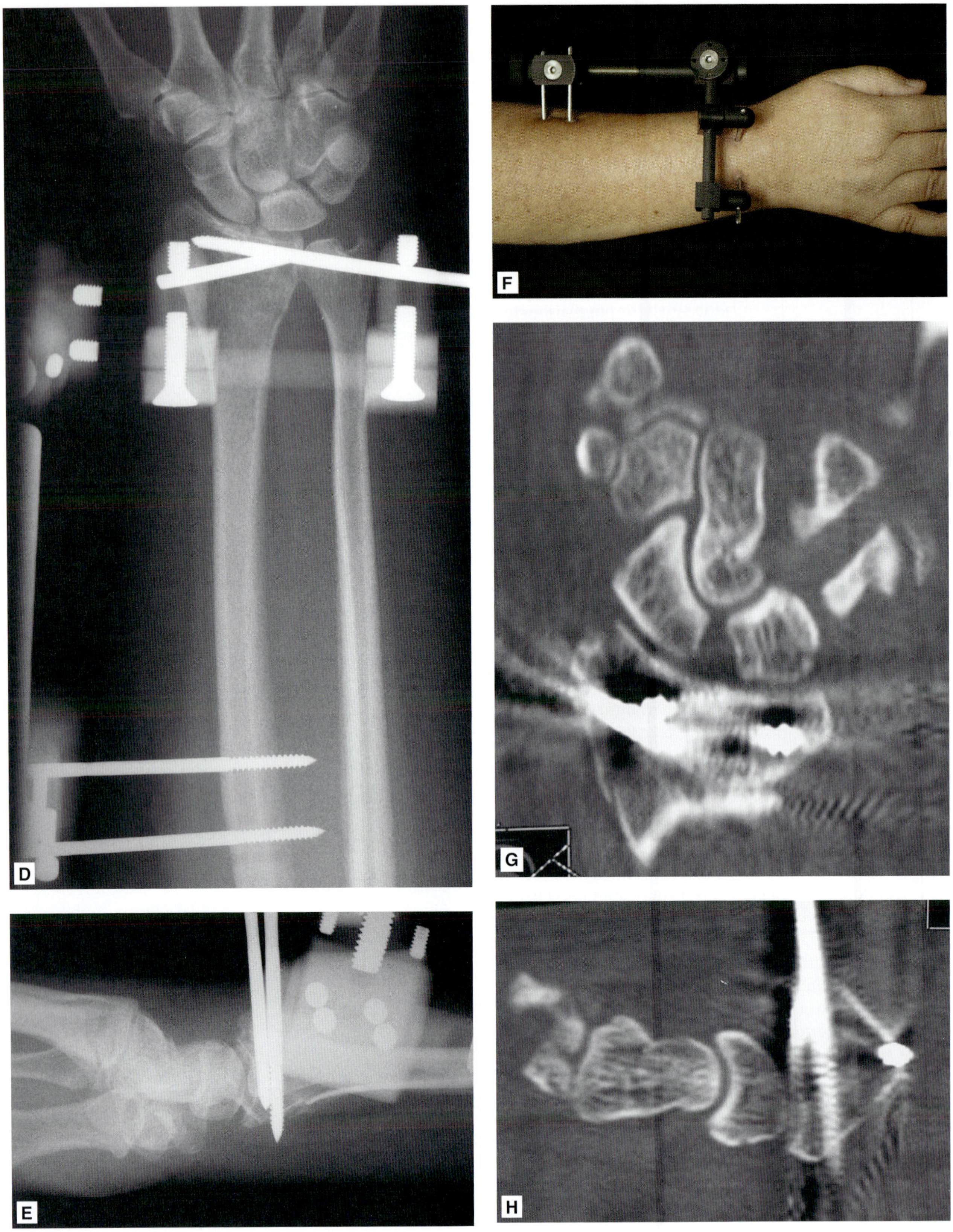

FIGURE 26-9 (*Continued*) **D.** Application of a nonbridging external fixator. **E.** Reduction of sagittal split. **F.** Clinical appearance. **G** and **H.** CT scans show the anatomic reconstruction of the joint space.

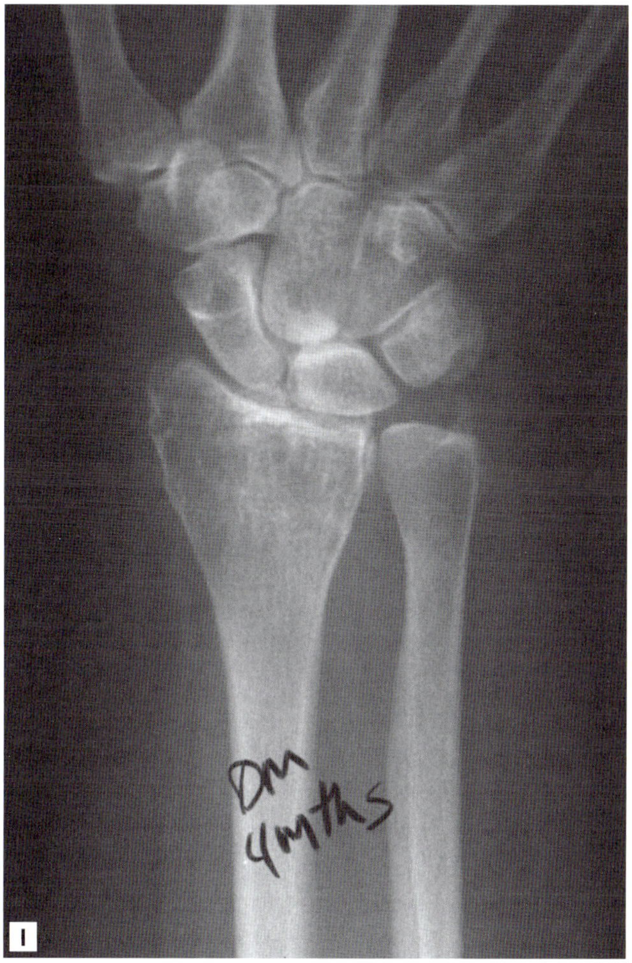

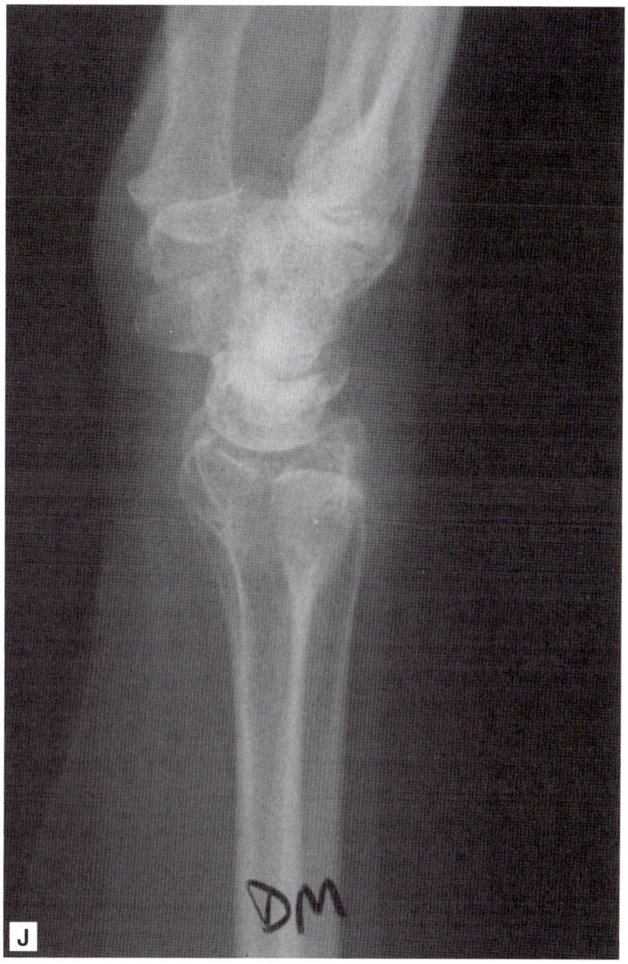

FIGURE 26-9 (*Continued*) **I** and **J.** Anteroposterior and lateral view at 4 months.

fractures. The first 3.0-mm pin is inserted through Lister's tubercle parallel to the joint surface in the lateral plane until it engages the volar cortex. The dorsal sidearm is positioned parallel to the joint space. A single pin clamp attached to the dorsal sidearm is fastened to this pin, and then both are locked in place. After the 2 proximal pins are inserted in the midradius, a distractor unit is used to lengthen the fixator until the volar tilt of the articular surface has been restored. An additional dorsal pin is inserted on the ulnar side of the EPL or EDC tendons using the second single pin clamp on the outrigger bar as a drill guide. The radial styloid pins are then inserted.

COMPLICATIONS

The immediate complications include injury to branches of the SRN or dorsal cutaneous branches of the ulnar nerve. Loss of fixation due to poor pin placement or interference with extensor tendon gliding can be minimized by careful technique and open rather than percutaneous pin insertion. Pin pullout due to fracture of the distal fragment can occur if the distal fragment is too small or osteopenic, or if the reduction is too vigorous. If this occurs, the fixator can be converted to a bridging construct. An incomplete reduction is also possible, especially with nascent malunions. The use of many standard external fixator frames applied in a nonbridging manner can result in articular incongruity. Overreduction of the fracture can also occur, especially when there is volar comminution. Late collapse after fixator removal can occur in osteopenic bone that often requires subchondral support beyond the 6 weeks of fixator application. Due to the risk of late collapse, adjuvant internal fixation with locking plates is advised in elderly and osteopenic patients since fracture site settling may occur for up to 6 months.[29]

COMBINED FIXATION

Combined fixation can be performed with the fixator applied in either a bridging or a nonbridging mode. Joint bridging fixation is indicated when there is central comminution to help unload the articular fragments, but it can also be used to obtain the reduction and regain radial length in osteopenic bone or in fractures that are more than 4 weeks old, to

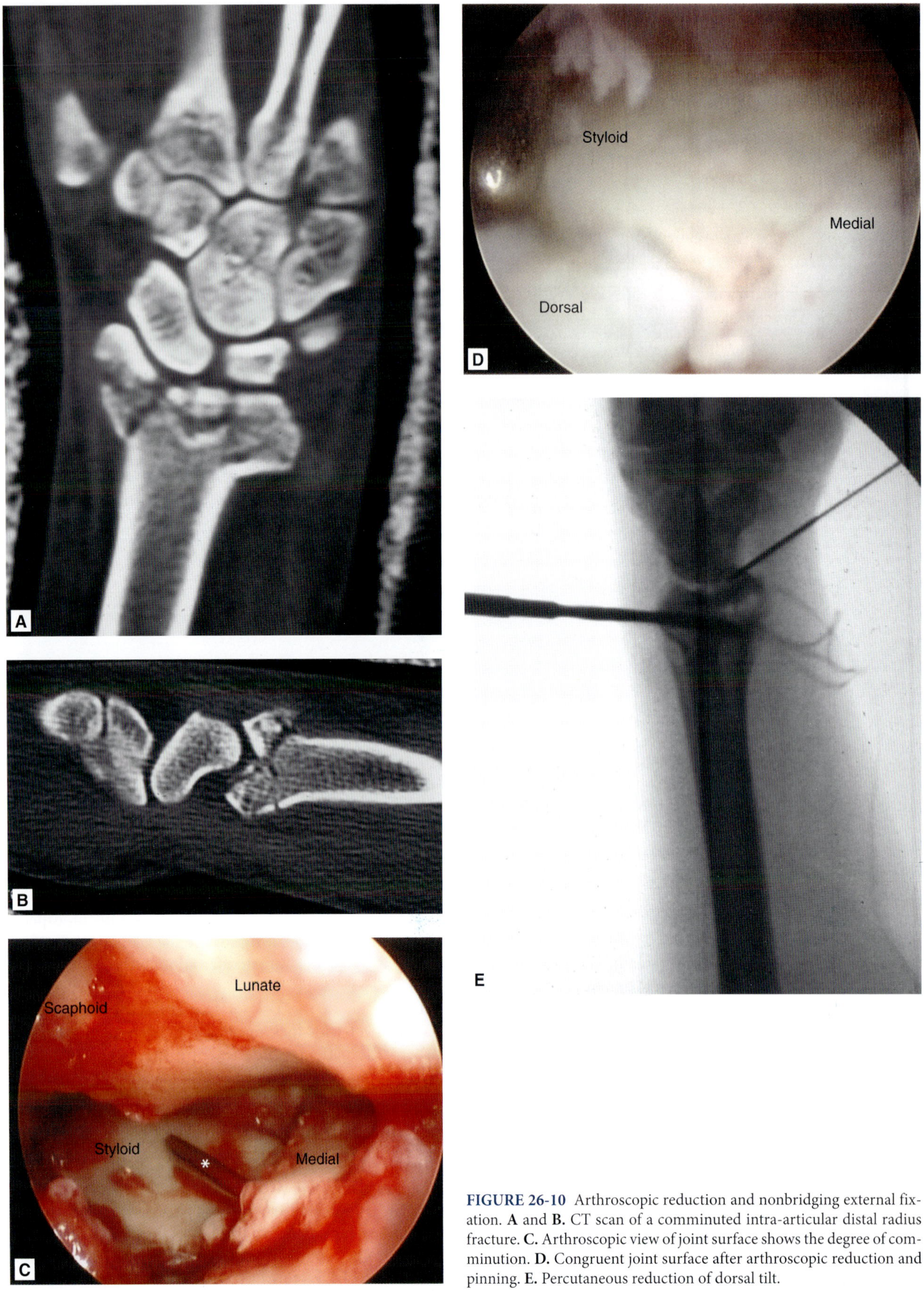

FIGURE 26-10 Arthroscopic reduction and nonbridging external fixation. **A** and **B.** CT scan of a comminuted intra-articular distal radius fracture. **C.** Arthroscopic view of joint surface shows the degree of comminution. **D.** Congruent joint surface after arthroscopic reduction and pinning. **E.** Percutaneous reduction of dorsal tilt.

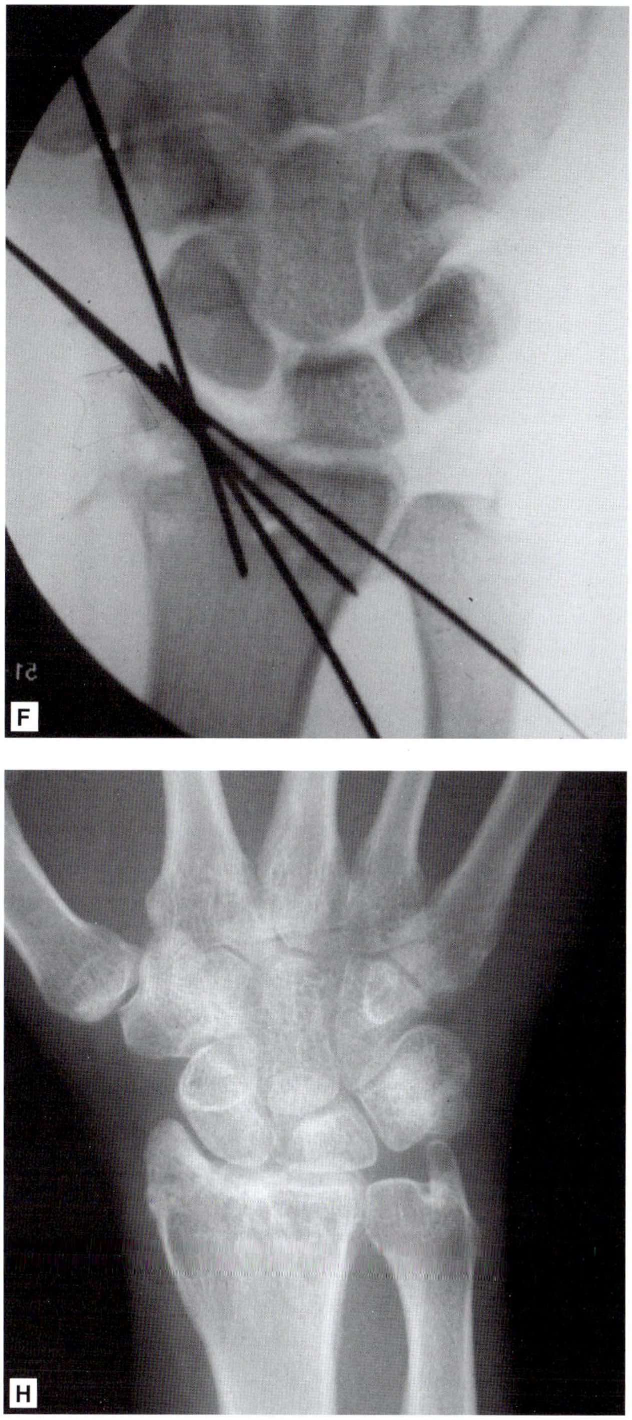

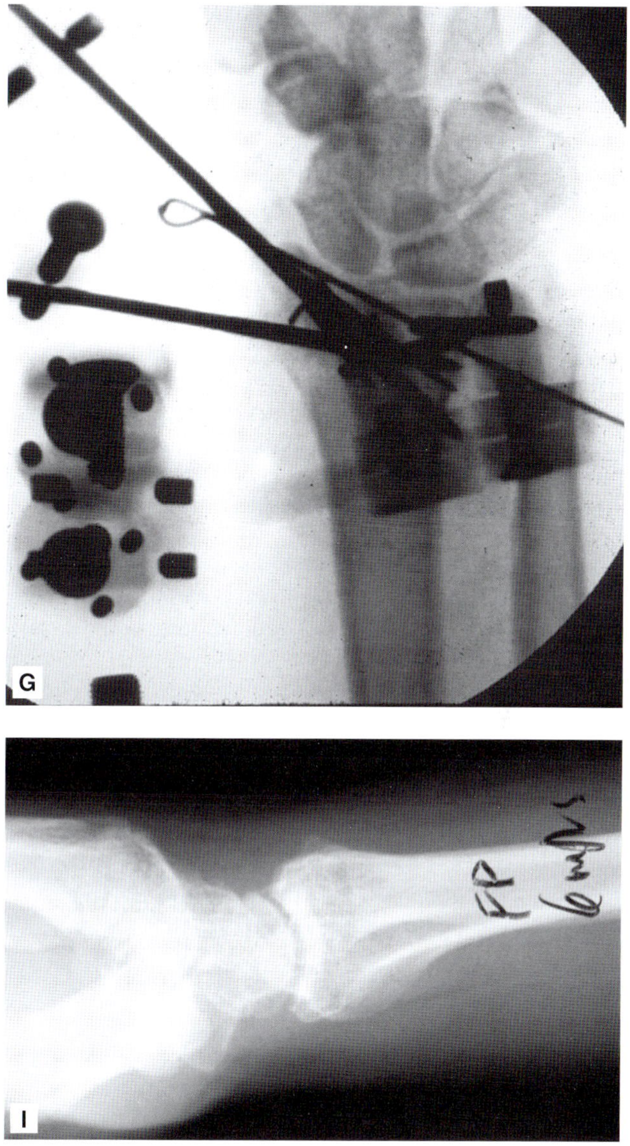

FIGURE 26-10 (*Continued*) **F.** Fluoroscopic appearance after reduction and pinning. **G.** Application of nonbridging external fixator. **H.** Result at 6 months with restored radial height and tilt. **I.** Congruent joint space with neutral lateral tilt.

minimize the levering of the articular fragments that can lead to further comminution.

OUTCOMES

Harley and coauthors reviewed 50 patients younger than 65 years of age with mostly AO-ASIF C2 and C3 DRFs who were randomized to treatment with percutaneous pinning and casting or augmented external fixation.[36] They found that the use of augmented external fixation did not improve the mean radial length, radial angulation, or volar tilt. There were no significant differences in the mean DASH scores, total range of motion, or grip strength. Kreder et al compared the results of open reduction and internal fixation (ORIF) versus external fixation and pinning.[33] A total of 179 adult patients with displaced intra-articular fractures of the distal radius were randomized to receive indirect percutaneous reduction and external fixation (n = 88) or ORIF (n = 91). There was no statistically significant difference in the radiological restoration of anatomic features or the range of movement between the groups at 2 years. The patients who underwent indirect reduction and percutaneous fixation however had a more rapid return of function and a better functional outcome than those who underwent ORIF, provided that the intra-articular step and gap deformity were minimized. Margaliot et al performed a meta-analysis of 46 articles with 28 (917 patients) external fixation studies and 18 (603 patients) internal fixation studies. They did not detect a clinically or statistically significant difference in pooled grip strength, wrist range of motion, radiographic alignment, pain, and physician-rated outcomes between the 2 treatment arms. There were higher rates of infection, hardware failure, and neuritis with external fixation and higher rates of tendon complications and early hardware removal with internal fixation. Considerable heterogeneity was present in all of the studies that adversely affected the precision of the meta-analysis.

With regards to nonbridging external fixation, Gradl et al examined 25 consecutive patients with fractures of the distal radius who were treated with nonbridging external fixation for 6 weeks.[39] The stepwise surgical technique comprised a preliminary joint bridging construction for reduction, insertion of 3 to 4 K-wires in the distal fragment that were attached to a dorsal outrigger bar parallel to the fracture line, and lastly the removal of the joint bridging part. At a 2-year follow-up all fractures united with an average palmar tilt of 0° and an articular step-off of ≤2 mm. A loss of radial length occurred in 4 patients where only 3 K-wires were inserted in the distal fragment. No radial shortening was seen in fractures with 4 K-wires inserted in the distal fragment. The average wrist extension was 55° and flexion of 64° without significant differences between extra- and intra-articular fractures. McQueen performed a prospective study of 641 patients with unstable fractures of the distal radius treated with external fixation. Fifty-nine percent of these cases were treated with nonbridging external fixation, mostly in AO type A3.2 and C2.1 fractures. Patients treated with nonbridging external fixation had statistically significant better radiological results throughout the period of review. In particular, this technique consistently restored the volar tilt and carpal alignment. Radiological improvement was mirrored by functional improvement. Most functional indices were statistically better at an early stage, whereas wrist flexion and grip strength remained significantly better at the final review. Complication rates were similar between the 2 groups.[40] In a follow-up study of 546 of these patients it was noted that fractures treated with bridging external fixation had a 6 times increased risk of dorsal malunion (P <.001) and a 2.5 times increased risk of radial shortening (P <.001) compared with nonbridging techniques.[41]

Plate Fixation

The advent of locking plate technology has revolutionized the treatment of DRFs, especially in osteopenic bone. The anatomy of the fracture will dictate whether a volar or dorsal or combined approach is necessary. It is the surgeon's discretion as to whether a locking volar plate or fragment-specific plates are used. Rather than advocating a specific implant, the general principles for reduction and fixation of a DRF will be discussed.

INDICATIONS

1. Postreduction radial shortening ≥3 mm, dorsal tilt >10°, or intra-articular displacement or step-off ≥2 mm
2. ≥2 mm of articular step-off or gap
3. Volar/dorsal intra-articular shear fractures
4. Three- and 4-part intra-articular fractures
5. Marked metaphyseal comminution

CONTRAINDICATIONS

1. Very small radial column fragments
2. Very distal volar fracture line (volar rim fractures), especially following radiocarpal fracture dislocation

SURGICAL TECHNIQUE

Dorsal Plating. Access to the dorsal aspect of the distal radius is required to address dorsal wall and ulnar corner fragments, as well as impacted free articular fragments (Fig. 26-11A-D). A longitudinal or S-shaped incision is made centered over Lister's tubercle. The EPL is identified distally and traced proximally to the third dorsal compartment that is released. Cutaneous nerve branches are mobilized and protected. The extensor retinaculum can be released in a Z-fashion and used to provide plate coverage. The extensor tendons of the fourth compartment are then elevated off the dorsal capsule, or the compartment is opened to allow retraction of the tendons to the radial or ulnar side as necessary. A dorsal capsulotomy can be performed to evaluate the articular surface. It is useful to retract the thin dorsal cortical fragments in a book-like fashion to expose the articular surface. A dental probe and Freer elevators are used to elevate and align the articular fragments, which are then held with subchondral 0.035- and 0.045-in Kirschner wires and supported with subchondral bone graft. The dorsal cortical fragments are pushed back down into place and 1 or two 2.0-mm/2.4-mm low-profile dorsal locking plates are used to hold the reduction. Any retained K-wires can be cut and bent percutaneously or buried. The EPL and, if desired, the extensor tendons are transposed dorsal to the retinaculum that is used for plate coverage.

Volar Plating. The surgical approach is between the flexor carpi radialis (FCR) tendon and the radial artery, as popularized by Orbay and Fernandez.[42] A curved or longitudinal incision is made directly along the FCR tendon, which is then retracted ulnarly to protect the median nerve. The incision can be extended distally along the border of the thenar eminence after dividing the superficial communicating

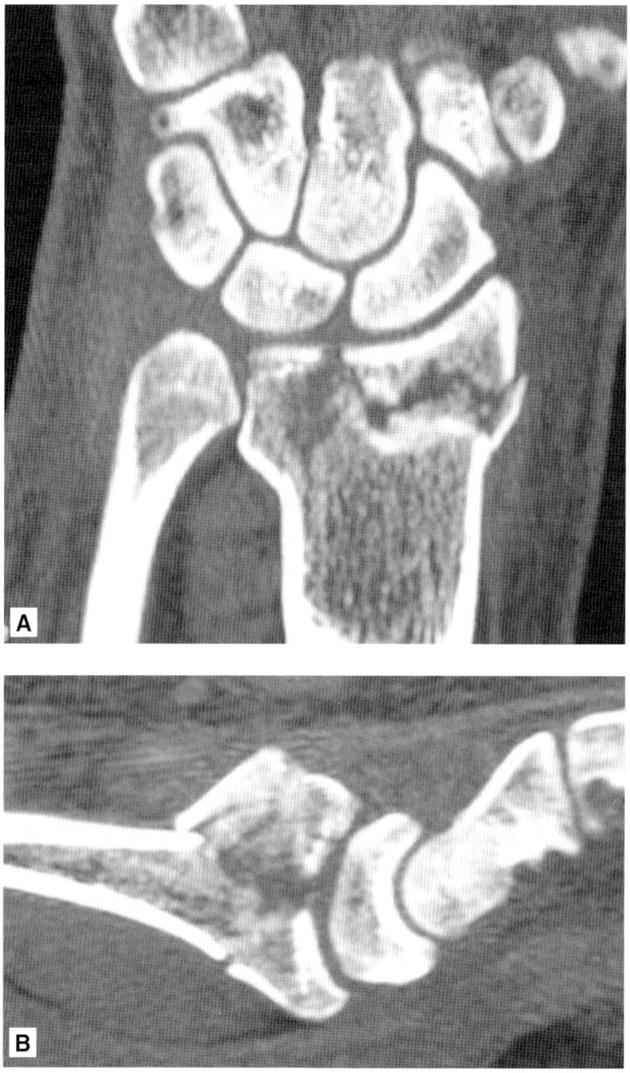

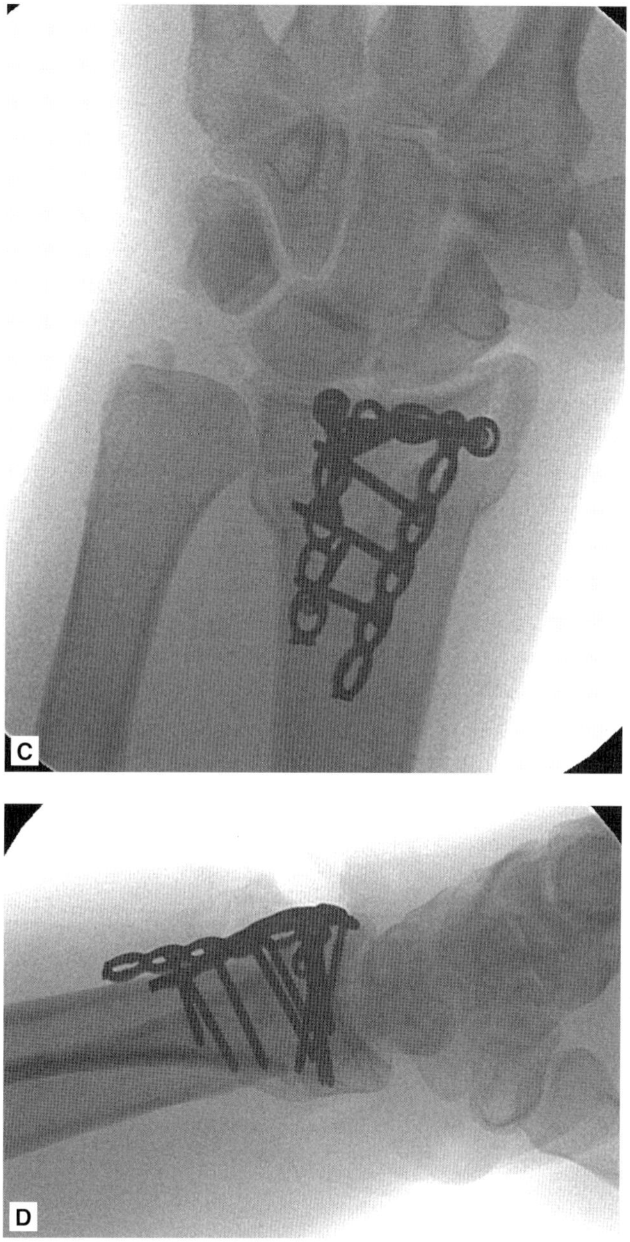

FIGURE 26-11 **A.** Four-part intra-articular fracture. **B.** Lateral x-ray shows displacement of dorsal fragments. **C.** Application of 2.0-mm locking plates. **D.** Congruent joint reduction.

branch of the radial artery to release the FCR attachments to the trapezium. The PQ muscle is released 1 to 2 mm beyond the distal margin of the muscular fibers through the fibrous tissue proximal to the volar capsular ligaments, which they have termed the intermediate fibrous zone. The PQ is then elevated subperiosteally from the volar cortex, leaving a small cuff radially for reattachment if desired. The BR tendon, which is a major deforming force on the radial styloid fragment, is completely detached from the radial column along with release of the first dorsal compartment. Care is taken to avoid injury to the tendons in the first dorsal compartment and branches of the SRN. A large key elevator can be hooked into the sigmoid notch and used to retract the flexor tendons ulnarly to gain access to the volar medial fragments. Fracture reduction should be meticulous, but an anatomic restoration of the metaphyseal fragments does not guarantee an anatomic reduction of the articular surface. If there is any doubt, a dorsal capsulotomy or an arthroscopic assessment of the articular surface is warranted (Fig. 26-12A-D). The edge of each fragment should be cleaned back to a sharp surface to facilitate cortical apposition. Forceful leverage of the fracture can cause further fragmentation and can be avoided by using temporary external fixation with a distractor. Large volar rim fragments can be stabilized with a locking volar plate, but smaller fragments have to be keyed in separately with small Kirschner wires before plate application. The fractured volar rim of the lunate fossa is found on the ulnar aspect of the distal radius and is critical for stability of the radiocarpal

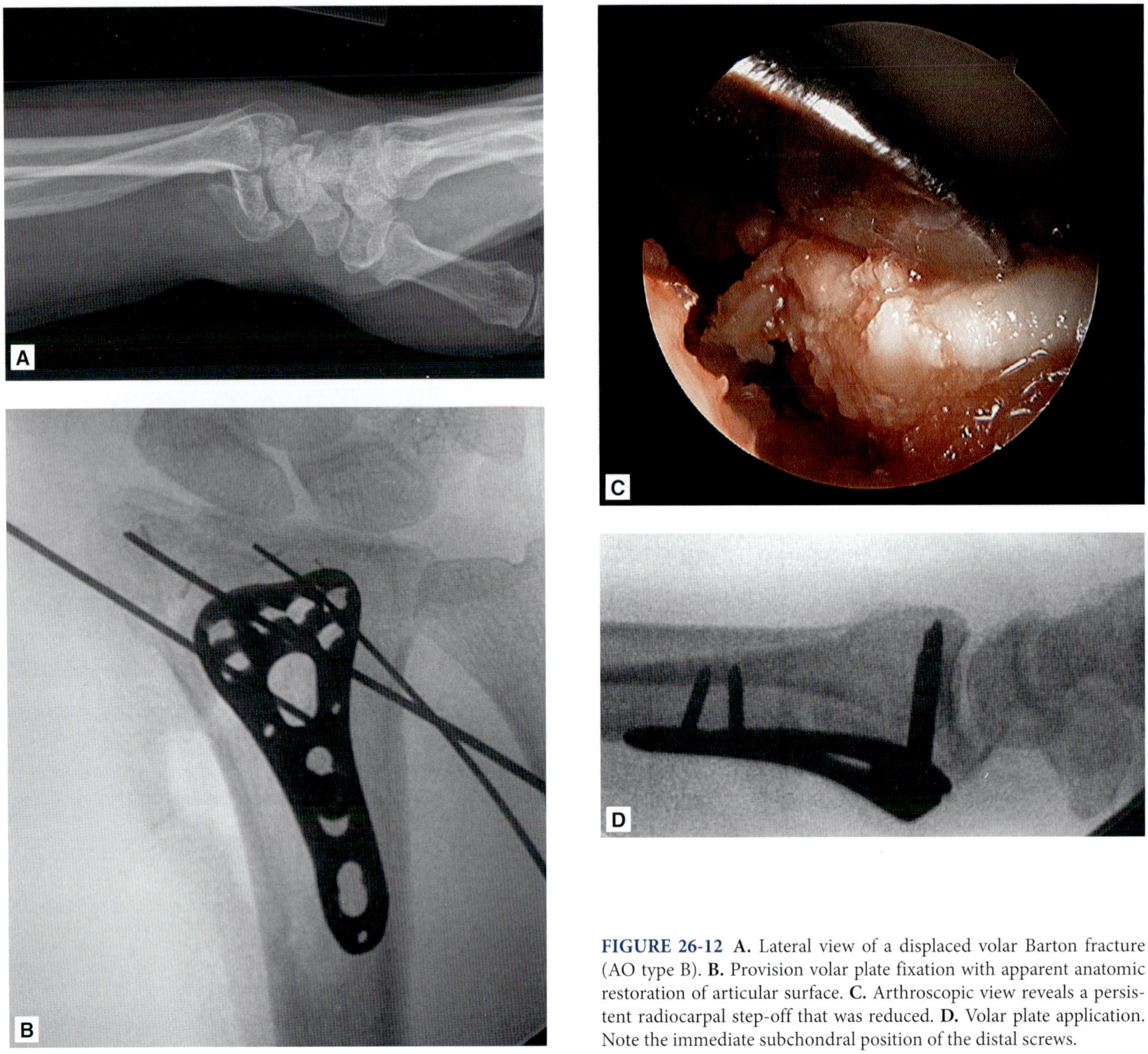

FIGURE 26-12 **A.** Lateral view of a displaced volar Barton fracture (AO type B). **B.** Provision volar plate fixation with apparent anatomic restoration of articular surface. **C.** Arthroscopic view reveals a persistent radiocarpal step-off that was reduced. **D.** Volar plate application. Note the immediate subchondral position of the distal screws.

joint. Failure to control this fragment can result in volar dislocation of the carpus. Very distal fragments cannot be controlled with a plate and can be treated with screws, K-wires, or tension band fixation. In some cases a separate volar ulnar approach is necessary. A longitudinal incision is made along the ulnar edge of the flexor tendons. It can be extended distally with release of the carpal tunnel (Fig. 26-13A-E). The ulnar nerve and artery are identified deep to the flexor carpi ulnaris tendon. The flexor tendons are retracted radially to expose the volar rim of the distal radius and the DRUJ. The origin of the PQ muscle on the ulna is incised and reflected radially to expose the volar medial fragment. The volar rim fragment is stabilized first, followed by a dorsal approach to elevate the depressed fragments. Bone grafting and internal fixation with Kirschner wires or a dorsal buttress plate are added to stabilize the articular fragments (Fig. 26-14A-E).

Orbay and Fernandez reported favorable outcomes with volar fixed-angle fixation of dorsally displaced DRFs.[42] They noted that the concave surface of the volar radius is limited distally by a transverse ridge or watershed line. Distal to the watershed line, the radius slopes in a dorsodistal direction and receives the proximal attachments of the volar wrist capsule and the volar capsular ligaments. This ridge lies approximately 2 mm from the joint line on its ulnar aspect and 10 to 15 mm on its radial aspect. They recommended that any implant should not project distal to the watershed line to avoid impingement and possibly rupture of the flexor tendons. In 1 cadaver study the contact pressure on the flexor pollicis longus significantly increased under loading when the distal plate edge was placed distal to the watershed line with the wrist in 30° and 60° of extension even when the fracture was anatomically reduced.[43]

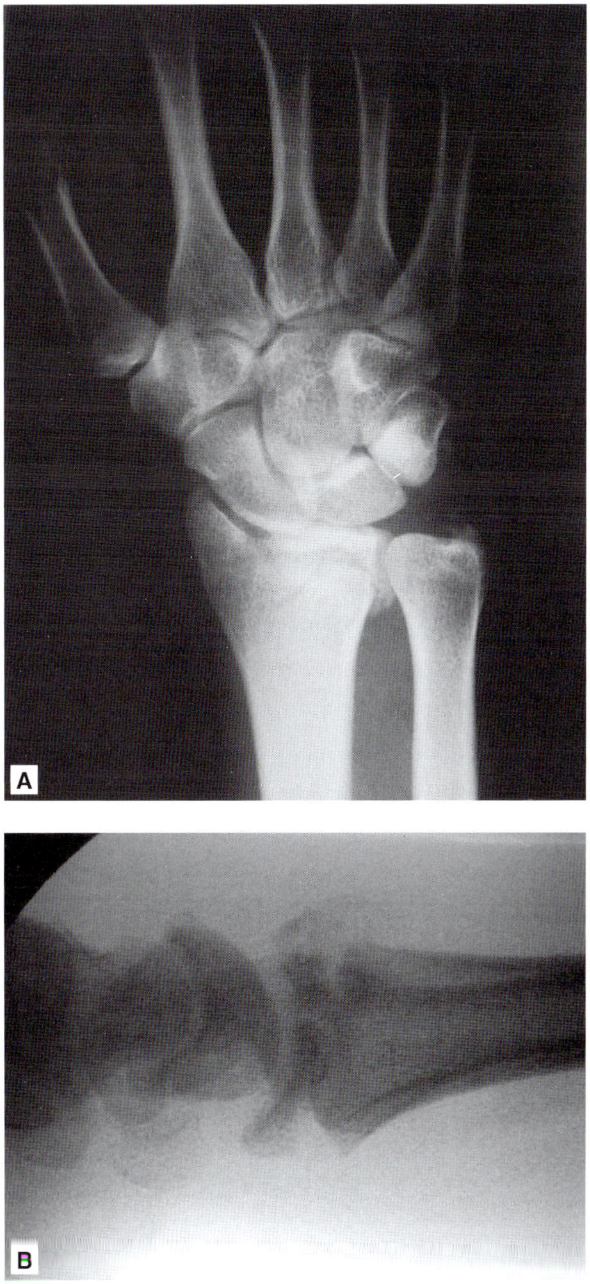

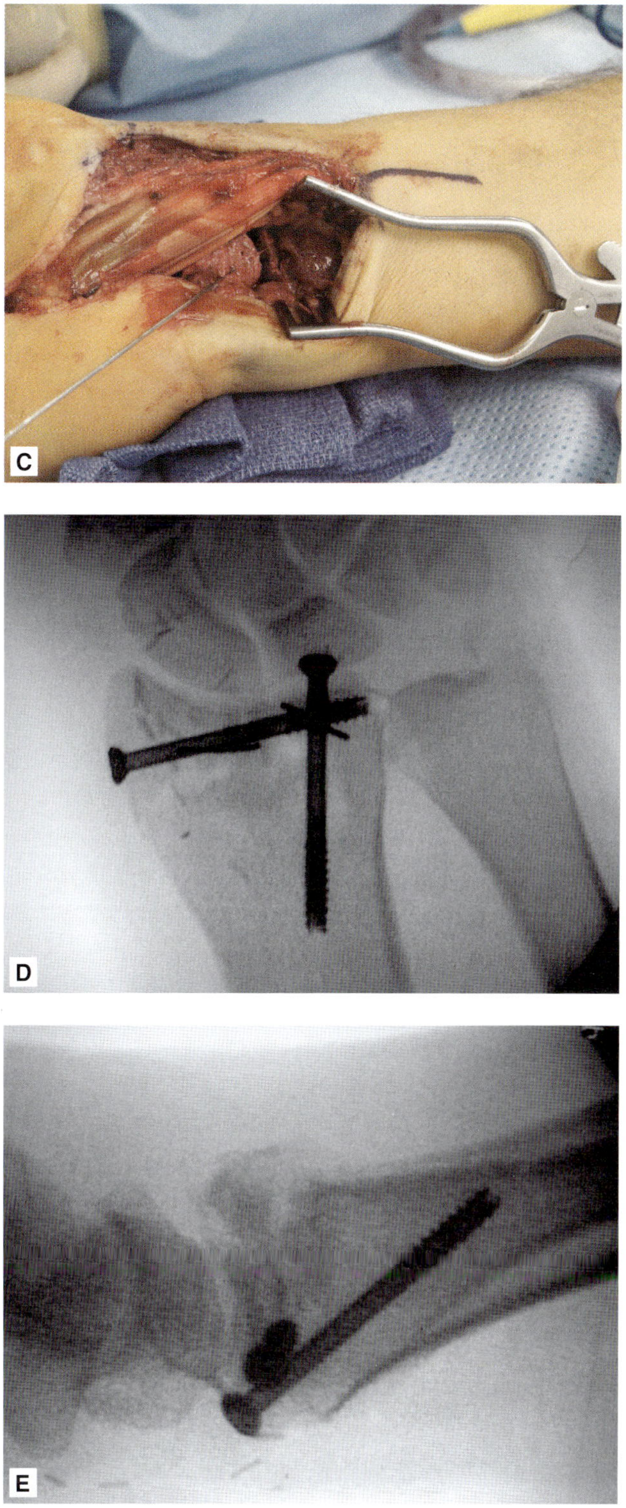

FIGURE 26-13 Extended carpal tunnel approach. **A.** AP view of a volar rim fracture. **B.** The small size of the distal fragment precludes plate fixation. **C.** Extended carpal tunnel approach with retraction of the flexor tendons exposes the lunate fossa and volar medial fragment. **D.** Screw fixation of the displaced radial styloid and volar medial fragment. **E.** Lateral view demonstrates a congruent reduction of the articular surface.

Orbay and coworkers described an intrafocal reduction technique where the proximal shaft is pronated out of the way after release of the BR tendon in order to access the dorsal aspect of the fracture.[44] This maneuver allows debridement of the fracture hematoma or callus and release of the dorsal fibrous tissue in order to regain radial length. It is helpful to insert the more ulnar screws perpendicular or even angled slightly proximal relative to the plate and then perform a 20° lateral x-ray to ensure there is no penetration of the articular surface. The more radial screws are then inserted with the radial styloid screw angled distally toward the tip since the bulk of the styloid bone is dorsal and radial. Dorsomedial

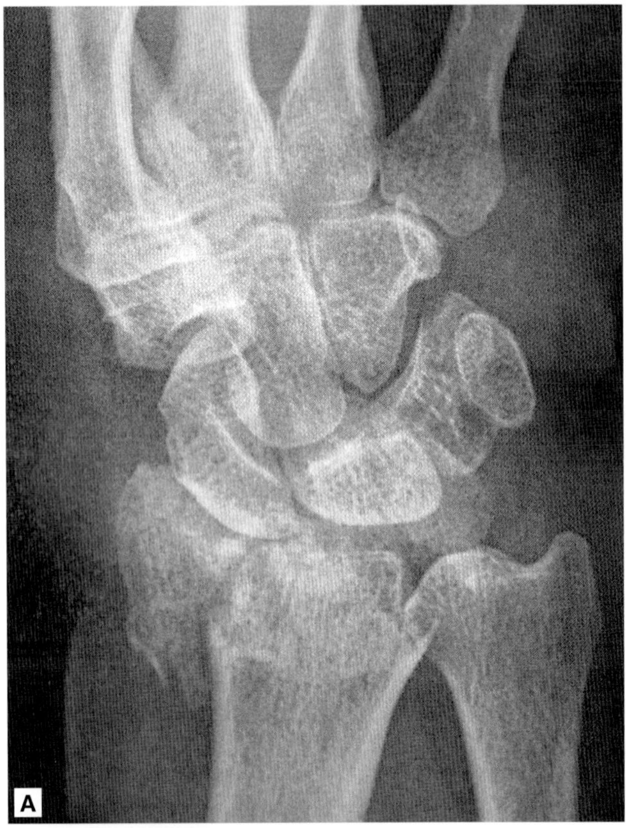

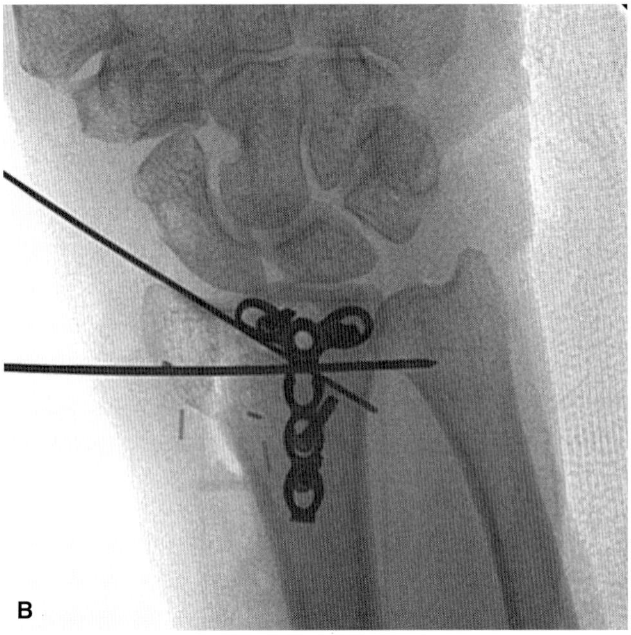

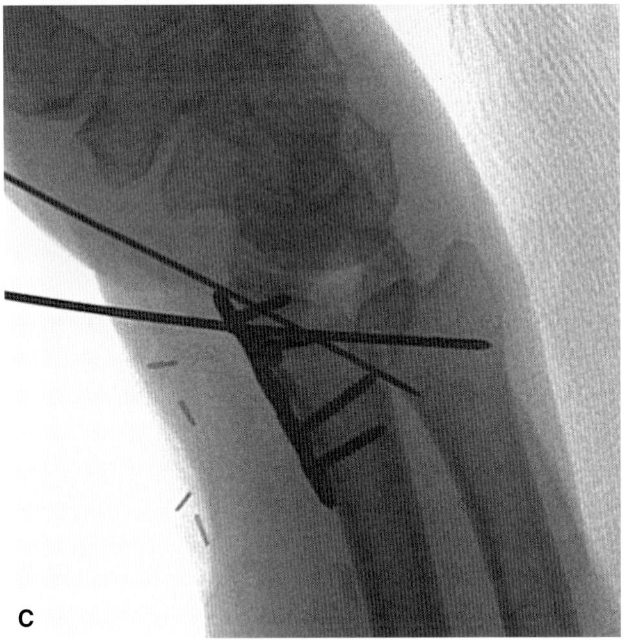

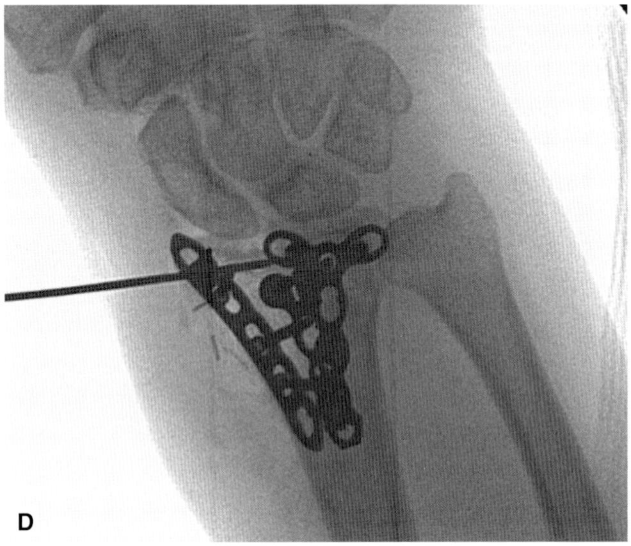

FIGURE 26-14 **A.** Comminuted intra-articular fracture in a 70-year-old osteopenic patient. **B.** Fixation of the volar medial fragment with a 2.0-mm locking plate. **C.** Note that the screws only capture the volar medial rim. **D.** Individual fixation of radial styloid and dorsal medial fragment.

fragments are often associated with a coronal plane split in the DRUJ. They can be difficult to reduce from a volar approach and difficult to capture with a single peg through a volar implant. A small dorsal incision directly over the interval between the fourth and fifth extensor compartments can be used to aid in reducing this fragment, which can then be captured with a volar locking screw inserted through the implant. It is prudent to undersize the locking screws by 2 to 4 mm to prevent past pointing and extensor tendon impingement, since the screw tip does not need to engage the dorsal cortex. Wall et al showed that locked unicortical distal screws of at least 75% length produce construct stiffness similar to

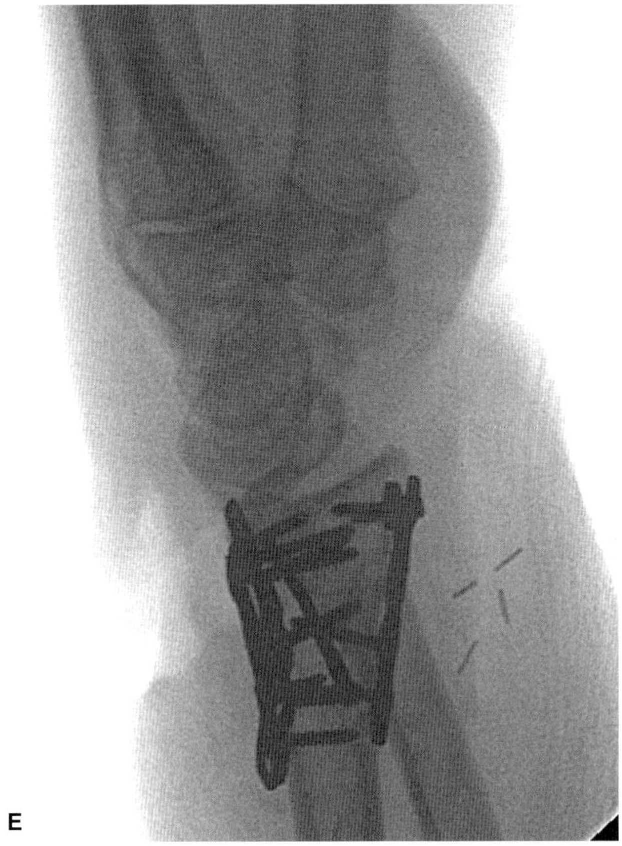

FIGURE 26-14 *(Continued)* **E.** Oblique view demonstrates a congruent radiocarpal joint.

bicortical fixation.[45] The screws should also be placed as subchondral as possible due to the fracture site settling that occurs. In a biomechanical study, Drobetz et al demonstrated that the rigidity of the plate construct is significantly higher in radiuses that the distal screws were placed close to the subchondral zone and that the amount of radial shortening after cyclic loading correlated significantly with the distance the distal screws were placed proximal to the subchondral zone.[46] Martineau et al performed a biomechanical evaluation of locking screw and locking smooth peg configurations following volar plate fixation of AO C3 intra-articular DRFs in 16 anatomic radius models. They found that constructs with subchondral locking screws inserted into the ulnar side of the lunate fragment were significantly stronger as opposed to smooth locking pegs.[47]

REDUCTION TECHNIQUES

Ross and coworkers have described a number of reduction techniques that are applicable to volar locking plates.[48] The plate may be applied to the volar aspect of the radius in the desired position and temporarily fixed to the proximal radial shaft with Kirschner wires. At least 1 distal screw is then inserted to achieve tangential subchondral support of the dorsal half of the articular surface but not locked. A drill can then be passed through an adjacent screw hole and used as a lever to correct the dorsal tilt, which is then maintained by locking the first screw. If further correction is necessary, the plate can be secured distally first so that the shaft of the plate is elevated off the radius. A bone reduction clamp is then used to reduce the shaft of the plate to the shaft of the radius that corrects the dorsal angulation. A sagittal gap between the scaphoid and lunate fossae can be closed by manipulating the fragments with K-wires or drill guides inserted through the distal plate, which are then substituted by locking screws. If there is a loss of radial angulation, then the plate may be applied with the proximal end directed ulnarward so that when the plate is realigned onto the proximal shaft, the radial angulation will be corrected. Radial length can be restored by loosening the proximal screw in the sliding hole and pushing the plate distally, and then retightening.

Radial translation must be corrected since this can affect the DRUJ and restrict forearm rotation. The proximal sliding hole screw is loosened slightly and forms a pivot point for the correction. A bear claw bone holder can then be positioned with 1 limb over the ulnar border of the radius just proximal to the fracture line and 1 limb over the radial side of the plate or through 1 of the holes on the plate. When the clamp is tightened, progressive ulnar translation of the distal fragment will occur using the proximal screw as a pivot point. Once satisfactory translation has been achieved, the proximal screw is tightened.

Benson and Medoff[49] described a radial palmar approach for application of a radial styloid implant (Fig. 26-15A-D). Typically, a 7-cm linear incision is made starting at the radial styloid moving proximally, just radial to the radial pulse. Longitudinal blunt dissection is carried out through the subcutaneous fat, and the numerous branches of the radial sensory nerve and the termination of the LABCN are identified and retracted. The first extensor compartment is next identified and released to mobilize the abductor pollicis longus and extensor pollicis brevis tendons either dorsally or palmarly for exposure of the fracture segments, and to expose the BR tendon, which is divided. The extensor pollicis brevis usually has a separate subsheath that can be released. They recommend leaving the last centimeter of the first extensor compartment sheath intact to reduce the likelihood of tendon subluxation postoperatively. The plane of dissection is volar to the radial artery, first extensor compartment, and radial sensory branches.

OUTCOMES

Volar plate fixation can ensure an anatomic reduction as compared with casting, but this does not necessarily correlate with patient-rated outcomes in older age groups. In 1 prospective study, 73 patients aged 65 years of age or older with displaced and unstable distal radial fracture were randomized to ORIF with a volar locking plate ($n = 36$) or closed reduction and cast immobilization ($n = 37$).[50] Grip strength, dorsal radial tilt, radial inclination, and radial shortening were all significantly better in the operative treatment group

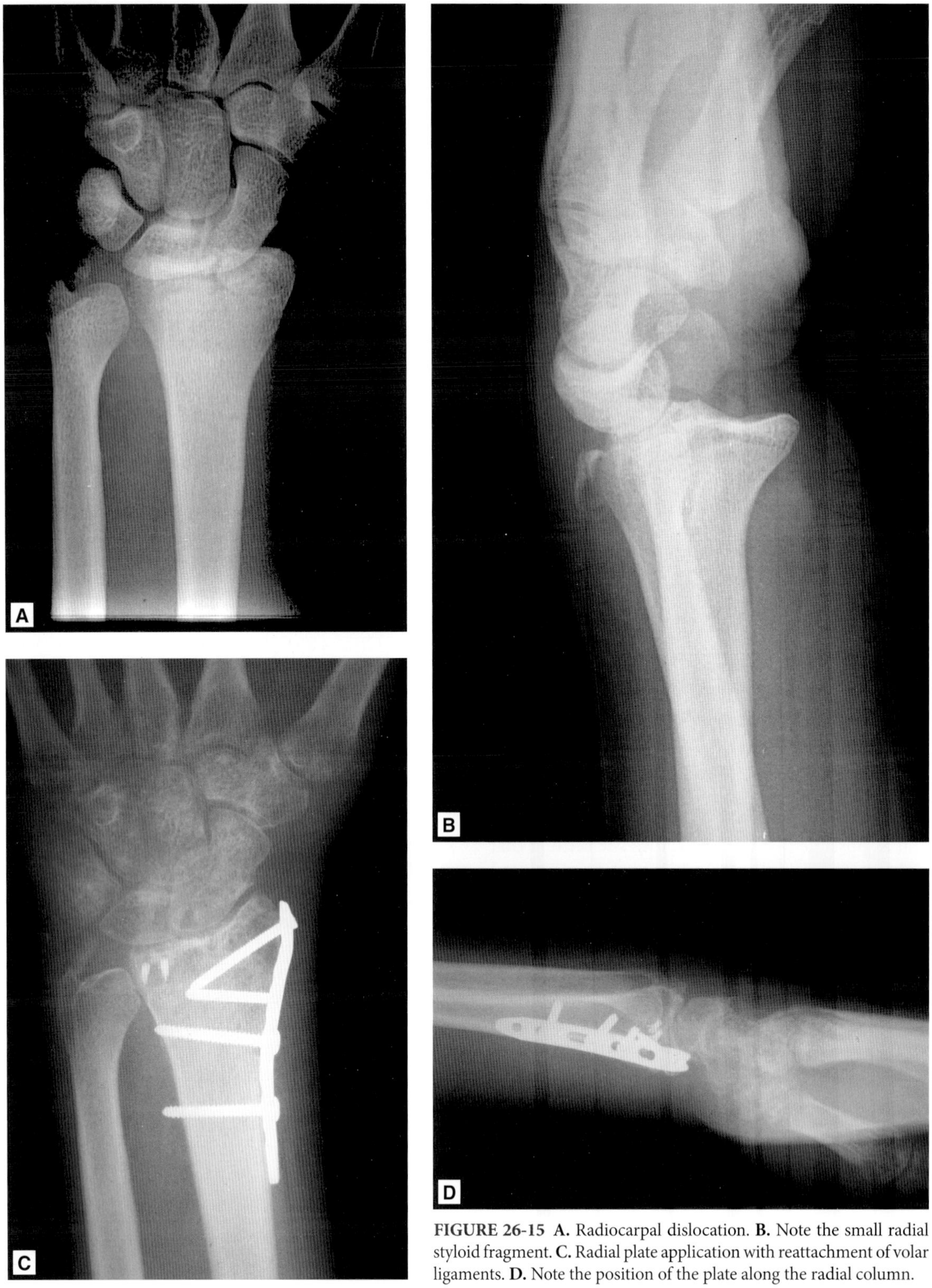

FIGURE 26-15 **A.** Radiocarpal dislocation. **B.** Note the small radial styloid fragment. **C.** Radial plate application with reattachment of volar ligaments. **D.** Note the position of the plate along the radial column.

at 1 year (P <.05). There were however no significant differences between the groups in terms of the range of motion, pain levels, PRWE, and DASH scores at 1 year. The number of complications was significantly higher in the operative treatment group (13 compared with 5, P <.05).

Chou et al reviewed the results of 41 patients who underwent internal fixation of AO C3 fractures with 2.4-mm titanium locking plates. Patients in group 1 ($n = 22$) were treated with dorsal locking plates, and those in group 2 ($n = 19$) with volar locking plates. No significant difference was noted between the 2 groups in terms of radial inclination, volar tilt, and ulnar variance, and wrist motion at 1 year.[51]

Chung et al reviewed 55 patients with DRFs treated with volar locked plates, who were divided into 2 age-based cohorts consisting of 20 to 40 years of age (30 patients) and >60 years (25 patients).[52] In the young age group there were 11 type A, 5 type B, and 14 type C fractures as compared with the older age group with 13 type A, 3 type B, and 9 type C fractures. At the 1-year follow-up there was no statistically significant difference in the Michigan Hand Questionnaire scores, Jebsen-Taylor test, or grip strengths. There were 5 complications in each group.

Grewal et al randomized 53 patients with DRFs who failed closed reduction and casting to ORIF with dorsal pi plates (n = 9) or volar locked plates (n = 18) versus external fixation and percutaneous pinning (n = 26).[53] The groups were comparable except that the PRWE detected higher pain and disability with external fixation before surgery that may have indicated a more severe initial injury. At the 1-year follow-up the PRWE scores were significantly lower for patients treated with ORIF compared with those with external fixation, with the best outcomes observed with volar locking plates. There were no significant differences in the DASH scores, ROM, or grip strengths.

Jupiter and Marent-Huber conducted a multicenter prospective study of 150 patients with a mean age of 51 years with DRFs stabilized with 2.4-mm locking plates. Of these, 102 had AO type C intra-articular fractures. There was a ≤2-mm step-off in 20 patients, and a >2-mm step-off in 5 patients. A loss of reduction occurred in 2 patients. Twenty-seven percent of the patients showed an increase of at least 1 grade in radiographic signs of arthritis at 2 years. The mean Gartland and Werley score improved significantly from 4 points at 6 months to 2 points at 2 years. The mean DASH score changed from a preinjury baseline of 2 to 7 points at 2 years (P <.0001).[54]

Bone Graft and Bone Substitutes

The standard teaching has been to bone graft any areas of metaphyseal comminution. This notion has been recently challenged and is largely surgeon preference. Myriad bone graft substitutes are used with increasing frequency, but evidence medicine is lacking to support their use. Handoll and Watts performed a Cochrane database search on the use of bone grafts and substitutes in DRFs.[55] Ten heterogeneous trials involving 874 adults with generally unstable fractures were grouped into 6 comparisons. Four trials (239 participants) found that the implantation of autogenous bone graft (1 trial), Norian SRS (calcium sulfate bone substitute—2 trials), and methyl methacrylate cement (1 trial) improved the anatomic outcomes compared with plaster cast alone; and 2 found it improved function. One trial (323 participants) comparing Norian SRS versus plaster cast or external fixation found no difference in functional or anatomic outcomes at 1 year. One trial (48 participants with external fixation) found that autogenous bone graft did not significantly change the outcome. One trial (93 participants with dorsal plate fixation) found autografts slightly improved wrist function compared with allogeneic bone material but with an excess of donor-site complications. The authors concluded that bone scaffolding materials may improve the anatomic outcome compared with plaster cast alone, but there was otherwise insufficient evidence to draw any other conclusions. The AAOS distal radius work group came to similar conclusions. They were unable to recommend for or against the use of supplemental bone grafts or substitutes when using locking plates, or for filling of a bone void as an adjunct to other operative treatments (Table 26-3).[24]

COMPLICATIONS

There are myriad potential complications. Finger and thumb flexor tendon ruptures have been reported, especially with distal plate placement. The extensor tendon and especially the EPL are prone to irritation or rupture due to past pointing of the distal screws following locked volar plate application. Loss of fixation of the volar lunate facet fragment is a disastrous complication that may require repeat surgery and can lead to persistent volar subluxation of the carpus.[44] This can also occur with subsidence of dorsoulnar fragments. Subsidence is common in osteopenic bone, which highlights the need to place the distal screws in a subchondral position.

One recent study compared the complication rates in 100 patients with 104 DRFs treated with low-profile dorsal nonlocking plates (n = 57) or volar locking plates (n = 47).[56] The mean age for the dorsal group was 51 years (range, 19-85 years) and mean age for the volar group was 56 years (range, 19-84 years). Of the fracture types, there were 22 AO type A fractures, 2 type B fractures, and 33 type C fractures in the dorsal plating group as compared with 5 AO type A fractures, 10 type B fractures, and 32 type C fractures in the volar plating group. At a mean follow-up by phone interview of 44 ± 21 months 18 patients (8 dorsal, 10 volar) experienced complications. In the dorsal plate group there were 1 failure of reduction, 6 patients with hardware discomfort, and 3 patients with tendon irritation, which required plate removal in 3 cases and screw removal in 3 cases, but no cases of neuropathy. In the volar plate group there were 1 failure of reduction, 7 patients with plate removal for hardware discomfort, and 1 case of an FPL tendon rupture. There were 3 cases of a median nerve palsy treated with a carpal tunnel release and 1 case of ulnar nerve palsy treated with a neurolysis. There were no significant differences in the rate of complications with respect to age and plate location.

Distraction Plating

INDICATIONS

High-energy fractures of the distal radius with extensive metaphyseal comminution can be difficult to treat by conventional methods. Hanel et al described the use of this technique in polytraumatized patients in order to allow immediate weight bearing through the injured wrist to assist with mobilization.[57]

The bridge plate acts as an internal fixator and depends on ligamentotaxis for fracture reduction (Fig. 26-16A-C). Since the original series the indications have been expanded to include the following:

1. Unstable DRFs associated with polytrauma to assist with weight bearing
2. Bilateral DRFs with severe comminution extending into the diaphysis
3. Combined complex injuries requiring extensive soft tissue and bony reconstruction

CONTRAINDICATIONS

1. Active infection
2. Inadequate soft tissue coverage
3. Circulatory instability precluding the administration of general or regional block anesthesia

SURGICAL TECHNIQUE

A 4-cm longitudinal incision is first made over the dorsal aspect of the middle finger metacarpal with retraction of the extensor tendon mechanism. A 2.7-mm Synthes locking bridge plate or 2.4-mm Synthes mandibular plate (Synthes, Inc, West Chester, Pennsylvania) is placed over the skin. Fluoroscopic imaging is used to determine the placement of the second incision, which is made over the dorsoradial aspect of the proximal radius, at least 4 cm proximal to the most proximal extent of the fracture line, to allow for placement of at least 3 cortical screws. The dissection is carried down to the shaft, adjacent to the BR, taking care to protect branches of the SRN. A third incision is made, centered over Lister's tubercle, and the EPL tendon is retracted. A scalpel is used to develop the plane between the fourth dorsal compartment of the extensor tendons and the dorsal periosteum and joint capsule. The plate is then passed in a retrograde fashion from the distal wound along the floor of the finger extensor tendons to the middle finger metacarpal. The fracture is provisionally reduced with traction, followed by

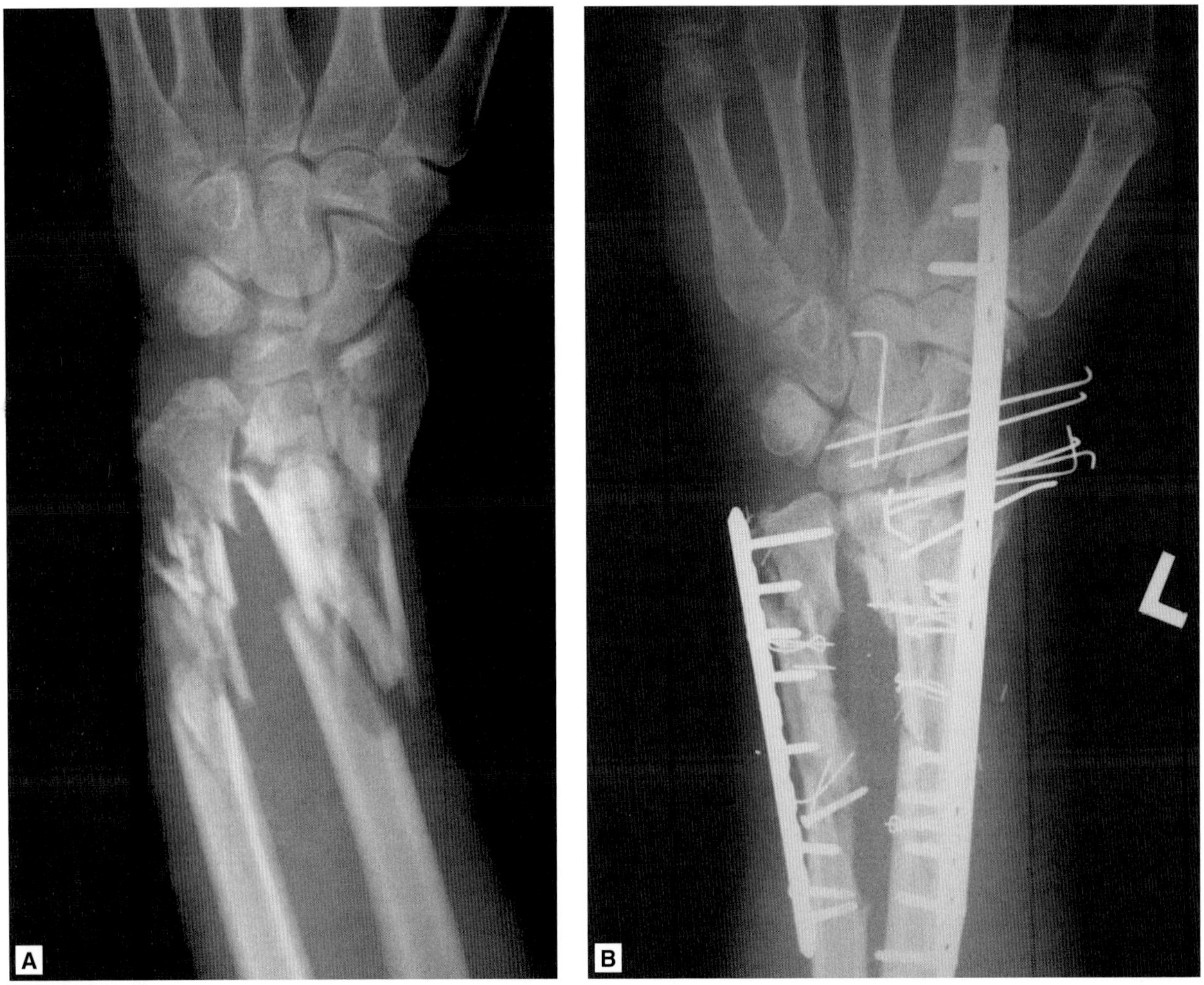

FIGURE 26-16 **A.** Markedly comminuted fracture of the radius and ulna. **B.** Distraction plating with adjuvant pin fixation of a lunate fracture, SL ligament injury, and ORIF of the ulnar.

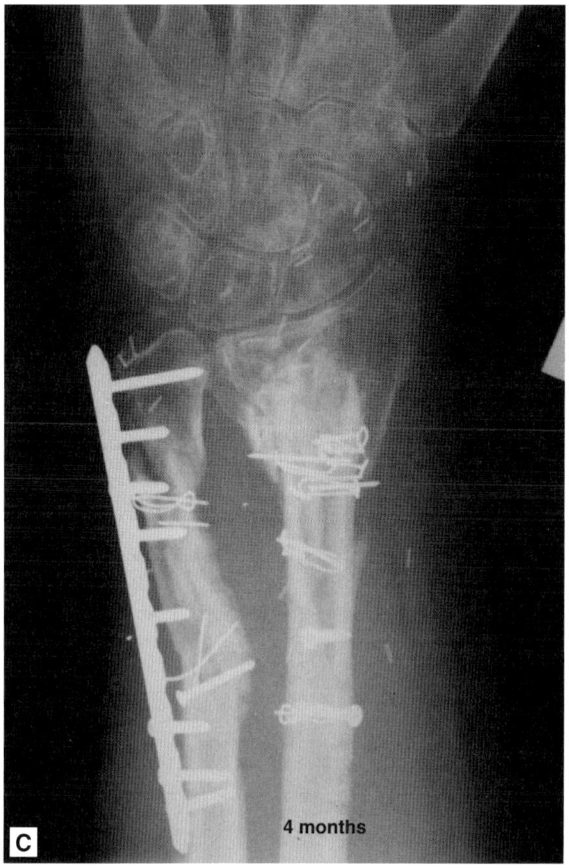

FIGURE 26-16 (*Continued*) **C.** Maintenance of radial height and articular surface after bridge plate removal.

centering the plate over the middle finger metacarpal distally and the radial shaft proximally. The plate is secured to the metacarpal distally with a single screw. Traction is reapplied followed by fixation with cortical screws proximally. Radiocarpal separation of ≥5 mm is avoided to prevent overdistraction. Supplemental fixation of articular fragments with Kirschner wires and small screws can be added (Fig. 26-16A-C). In addition, a 3.5-mm screw placed into the subchondral bone beneath the lunate fossa may help prevent collapse. Alternatively, the plate can be applied to the index finger metacarpal with passage of the plate through the floor of the second dorsal compartment in a retrograde fashion.

COMPLICATIONS

In a retrospective study of 144 fractures, Hanel et al reported wound healing complications in 2, hardware failure in 5, 2 malunions, 2 nonunions, 2 infections, 1 EPL rupture, and 2 extensor tendon adhesions requiring a tenolysis.[58]

OUTCOMES

Richard et al reported their results in 33 patients over 60 years of age with comminuted DRFs treated with internal distraction plating. At the final follow-up, all fractures had healed with a mean radial inclination of 20°, a mean palmar tilt of 5°, and a mean positive ulnar variance of 0.6 mm. The mean values for wrist motion included 46° flexion, 50° extension, 79° pronation, and 77° supination. The mean DASH score was 32. Ruch et al treated 22 with a distraction plate for a comminuted distal radial fracture using a 3.5-mm ASIF plate.[59] The articular surface was anatomically reduced and was secured with Kirschner wires or screws and 11/22 were bone grafted. The plate was removed after fracture healing at an average of 124 days with an average palmar tilt of 4.6°, an average ulnar variance of 0°, and an average radial shortening of 2 mm. Wrist flexion averaged 57°, extension 65°, pronation 77°, and supination 76°. The average DASH score was 11.5 points at an average follow-up of 24.8 months. According to the Gartland-Werley rating system, there were 14 excellent results, 6 good results, and 2 fair results.

Distal Radioulnar Joint Instability

DRUJ stability must be assessed as a part of the management of a DRF since this can adversely affect the outcomes. One CT study showed that persistent volar subluxation of the ulnar head restricted forearm pronation, whereas persistent dorsal subluxation restricted supination.[60] Loss of supination significantly impacts patient-rated outcomes.[61] Internal fixation can often correct any initial DRUJ instability through the restoration of the bony anatomy. Persistent instability however can occur in a number of situations. Failure to capture the dorsomedial fragment that makes up the dorsal margin of the sigmoid notch can result in dorsal subluxation of the carpus. This can also occur with volar radioulnar ligament avulsion. There have been numerous recent reports of good outcomes following nonoperative treatment of basistyloid fractures when associated with a DRF, provided the DRUJ is stable.[62-64] A fracture through the base of the ulnar styloid with foveal detachment of the TFCC can occur. If the DRUJ is persistently unstable however following ORIF of the DRF, with noticeable clunking during forearm compression and passive rotation, then the ulnar styloid fracture should undergo internal fixation. DRUJ instability should also be suspected if there is inordinate difficulty in correcting the radial translation of the distal fragment since the lack of restraint by the foveal fibers combined with a loss of the stabilizing effect of the radioulnar ligaments attached to the displaced ulnar styloid allows radial translocation of the distal fragment (Fig. 26-17A-D). A 2-cm incision just volar to the ECU provides excellent exposure of the ulnar styloid, which lies dorsally with the forearm in pronation. The styloid fracture can be stabilized with 0.035-mm K-wires, supplemented by a 22-gauge tension band wire. Alternatively, the fracture can be repaired with a cannulated screw or a bone anchor.

Rehabilitation

One must keep in mind that the soft tissue envelope greatly influences the final functional result, even though all of the

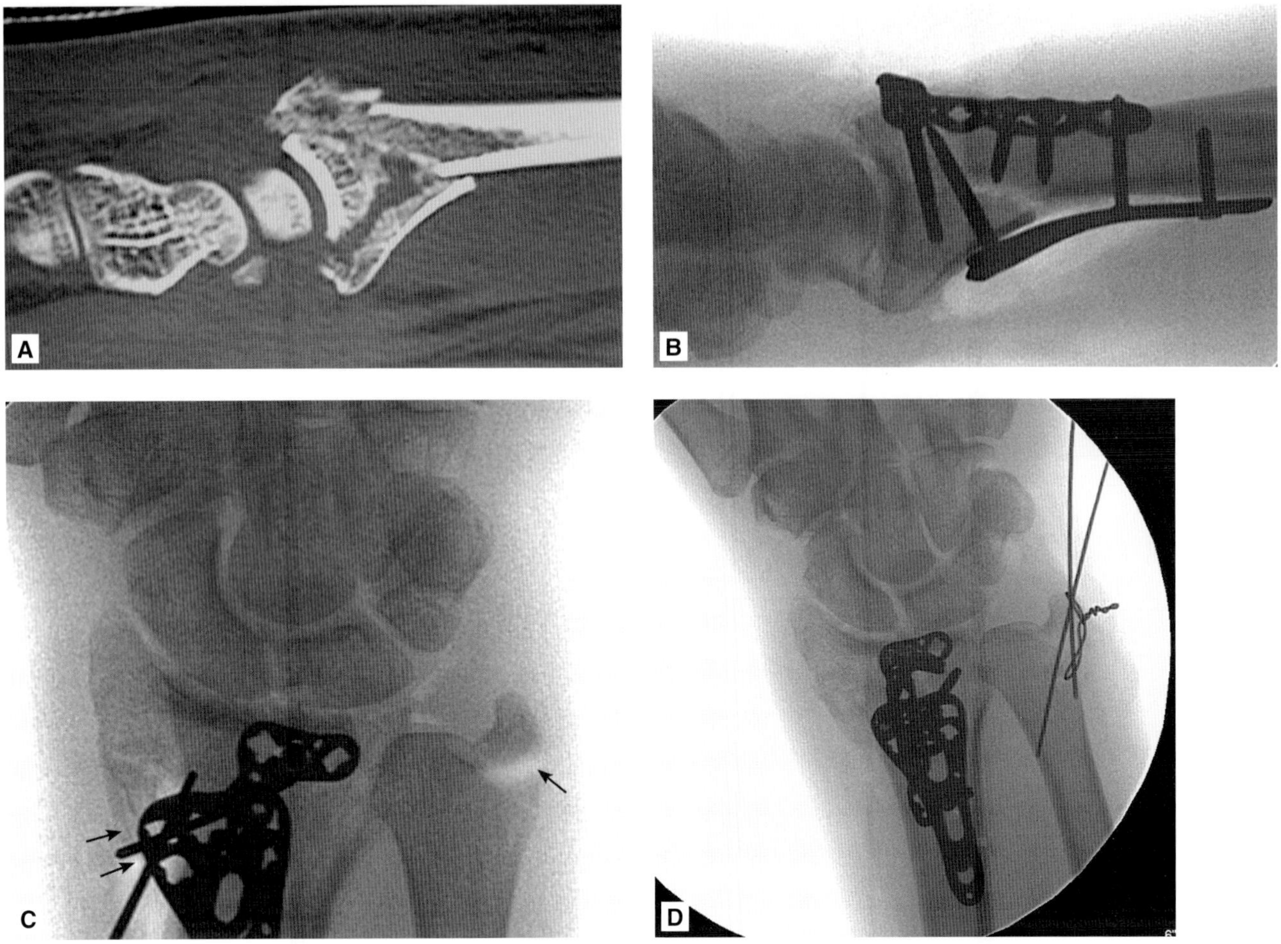

FIGURE 26-17 DRF and DRUJ instability. **A.** Intra-articular fracture with central comminution and depression. **B.** Lateral view following plate fixation showing a congruent radiocarpal articular surface. **C.** Persistent radial subluxation of fracture (double arrow) with persistent ulnar styloid displacement (single arrow) and DRUJ "clunking" with forearm rotation. **D.** Tension band fixation of ulnar styloid corrects the radial translation and DRUJ instability.

initial attention may be focused on the fracture position. The inflammatory cascade that results in edema, pain, and joint stiffness must be treated aggressively and concomitantly with the bony injury.

Immediate finger motion is crucial. One long-term outcome study of Colles fractures showed the only factors that influenced patient dissatisfaction at 10 years were loss of radial height and finger stiffness.[65]

EDEMA FLUID

Simple hand edema is a collection of water and electrolytes. Inflammatory edema however consists of a highly viscous exudate that contains fibrinogen. In many instances the fibrin network is resorbed by about 7 to 10 days. Other times the fibrinogen is polymerized into fibrin, which becomes a lattice work for invading fibroblasts. The fibroblasts produce collagen, which, if the part is immobilized, forms a randomly oriented, dense interstitial scar that obliterates the normal gliding surfaces. Edema restricts finger motion by increasing the moment arms of skin on the extensor side and by direct obstruction on the flexor side. The work needed to effect a joint angle change is dependent on the product of the tissue pressure and the volumetric change during angulation. This requires an increase in the muscular force that is necessary to bend a swollen finger. Compression, repeated finger flexion, and dynamic splinting redistribute this fluid to areas with lower tissue pressure. This allows the skin to lie closer to the joint axis, which decreases the effort needed for finger flexion.

Treatment for acute edema begins immediately with elevation, ice, and Coban wrap to reduce finger edema. Subacute and chronic management techniques include active and passive range of motion exercises, manual edema mobilization such as retrograde massage, and compression dressings and garments. Contrast baths, electrical stimulation, and the use of a Jobst intermittent compression unit have also been used.

To allow flexor tendons to glide to their maximum potential, the 3 basic fist positions are performed as part of a tendon gliding exercise program: straight fist, full fist, and hook fist. Synergistic wrist and finger motion increases passive flexor tendon excursion by generating forces that pull the tendon through the pulley system. A finger rehabilitation protocol is outlined in Table 26-4.[11]

FRACTURE SITE STABILITY

For the purposes of rehabilitation it is useful to consider the stability of the DRF site in 3 phases, consisting of low, intermediate, and high fracture site rigidity, which will in turn guide the therapist as to the loads that can be placed across the fracture site.[11] When internal or external fixation is used, the loads placed on the fracture site may be adjusted accordingly (Table 26-5). The following procedure-specific protocol can be used as a general guide depending on the type of fixation:

Cast treatment:
- Weeks 1 to 6: finger rehabilitation protocol
- Weeks 6 to 8 (after cast removal): phase I wrist exercises
- Weeks 8 to 10: phase II wrist exercise
- ≥10 weeks: phase III wrist exercises

Intrafocal pinning:
- Weeks 1 to 6: finger rehabilitation protocol
- Weeks 6 to 8 (after pin removal): phase I exercises
- Weeks 8 to 10: phase II exercises
- ≥10 weeks: phase III wrist exercises

Bridging external fixator:
- Weeks 1 to 6: finger rehabilitation protocol
- Weeks 6 to 8 (after fixator removal): phase I wrist exercises
- Weeks 8 to 10: phase II wrist exercises
- ≥10 weeks: phase III wrist exercises

Nonbridging external fixator:
- Weeks 1 to 6: finger rehabilitation protocol; phase I wrist exercises
- Weeks 6 to 10 (after fixator removal): phase II wrist exercises
- ≥10 weeks: phase III exercises

Volar/dorsal plating:
- Weeks 1 to 4: finger rehabilitation protocol; phase I wrist exercises
- Weeks 4 to 8: phase II wrist exercises
- ≥8 weeks: phase III exercises

Formal therapy however does not necessarily improve the average wrist motion or patient-related outcome scores. Souer et al studied the effect of formal occupational therapy 6 months after volar plate fixation of DRFs versus patients who performed independent exercises.[66] At 6 months, there was a significant difference in mean wrist extension (55° vs 62°), ulnar deviation (82% vs 93%), mean supination (84° vs 90°), mean grip strength (81% vs 92%), and mean Mayo score, in the patients who were prescribed independent exercises. There were no differences in the DASH score at any time point.

TABLE 26-4: Finger Rehabilitation Protocol

Days 1-7
Individual passive and active finger and thumb motion
Gentle active finger flexion/extension
Gentle active finger PIP and DIP joint blocking
Thumb opposition and flexion/extension exercises
Intrinsic tightness stretching exercises
Aggressive edema management
Tendon gliding exercises
Weeks 2-4
Dynamic MCP flexion splint if passive MCP flexion <40°
Dynamic PIP flexion splint if passive PIP flexion <60°
Switch to PIP flexion strap after >80° of passive PIP flexion achieved
Dynamic PIP and DIP flexion strap if passive DIP flexion <40°
Intrinsic tendon tightness: dynamic PIP flexion splint with MCP blocked in full extension
Extrinsic extensor tendon tightness: dynamic PIP/DIP flexion strap while in dynamic MCP flexion splint
Extrinsic flexor tendon tightness: add static PIP/DIP extension splints while in dynamic MCP extension splint; incrementally increase wrist extension if wrist is cleared for motion
Weeks 4-8
Add static progressive PIP flexion splint at night if flexion is still <60°
Add static progressive MCP flexion splint at night if flexion is still <40°
Dynamic/static progressive PIP extension splint if PIP flexion contracture >30°
Dynamic/static progressive MCP extension splint if MCP flexion contracture >30°
Dynamic/static progressive thumb opposition splint if opposition >2 cm from fifth MCP joint
For resistant cases, consider dynamic splinting 30-60 min 2 to 3 times per day, combined with static progressive splinting 4-8 h at night
After week 8
Home splinting until motion plateaus

TABLE 26-5: Wrist Rehabilitation Protocol

Phase I: low fracture site rigidity
Custom or noncustom below-elbow splint
Gentle active and passive wrist flexion/extension, radial/ulnar deviation, pronation/supination
Phase II: intermediate fracture site rigidity
Dynamic/static progressive wrist flexion splinting if passive wrist flexion <30°
Dynamic/static progressive wrist extension splinting if passive wrist extension <30°
Dynamic/static progressive supination splinting if passive supination <60°
Dynamic static progressive pronation splinting if passive pronation <60°
Incorporate light functional activities and light strengthening
Phase III: high fracture site rigidity
Progress strengthening exercises and functional activities as tolerated
Home splinting until motion plateaus

Factors Influencing the Outcome of Distal Radius Fractures

There are myriad factors affecting the clinical result following a DRF.[67] Most of these predictions are based on the radiographic findings, although the surrounding soft tissue envelope as well the intracarpal ligaments has a marked influence.

ANATOMIC PREDICTORS OF FRACTURE INSTABILITY

Fracture instability may be defined as an inability to resist displacement after an anatomic reduction. In a now classic paper, Lafontaine et al identified a number of risk factors that were associated with redisplacement of a DRF despite an initial satisfactory reduction. These included the presence of dorsal tilt ≥20°, comminution, intra-articular involvement, an associated fracture of the ulna, and age greater than 60 years. If 3 or more of these factors were present, there was a high likelihood of fracture collapse.[68] Advanced age influences fracture instability due to the associated osteopenia. In patients over 60 years old, Leone et al found that the degree of radial shortening, volar tilt, the amount of dorsal comminution, and advanced age were predictive of early or late failure. An unexpected finding was that one third of undisplaced fractures occurred in patients over 65 years of age.[69] Nesbitt et al determined that age was the only statistically significant predictor of secondary displacement.[70] After obtaining an acceptable initial closed reduction, those patients who were more than 60 years of age had 4 times the risk for 4-week failure over those younger than age 60 years. The risk for displacement increased as age increased. Due to the risk of late collapse, adjuvant internal fixation with locking plates should be considered in elderly and osteopenic patients.

ANATOMIC PREDICTORS OF OSTEOARTHRITIS (OA)

Articular congruity is paramount in the development of posttraumatic OA. In another classic paper Knirk and Jupiter retrospectively reviewed 43 intra-articular fractures in 40 young adults (mean age, 27.6 years) that were treated at Mass General Hospital, with a mean follow-up of 6.7 years. Since most of the fractures (38/43) were treated with older, nonrigid fixation methods that were popular at that time including cast or pins and plaster, there was a high incidence of residual intra-articular incongruity. Knirk and Jupiter noted that radiographic evidence of arthritis was present in 8/8 of the fractures whose articular incongruity was 2 mm or more, in contrast to only 2/19 of the fractures that healed with a congruous joint. OA was found in 22/24 of the patients who had any step-off whatsoever.[71] Catalano et al studied 21 patients under the age of 45 years who had undergone internal fixation of displaced intra-articular fractures.[72] At an average of 7.1 years, osteoarthrosis of the radiocarpal joint was radiographically apparent in 16 wrists (76%). A strong association was found between the development of osteoarthrosis of the radiocarpal joint and residual displacement of articular fragments at the time of bony union ($P < .01$). They revisited 16 of these patients at 15 years. Arthrosis was present in 13/16 of the wrists and there was an additional 67% reduction of the joint space.[73] The predictive value of these studies is that articular incongruity following a DRF is the most significant factor in the development of radiocarpal OA. Articular displacement that is identified on the initial injury films thus warrants a more aggressive surgical approach.

PREDICTORS OF RESIDUAL IMPAIRMENT

The landmark paper by Gartland and Werley was instrumental in establishing the link between the anatomic restoration of a DRF and the functional outcome.[74] This finding has been corroborated by many studies since then. Aro and Koivunen looked at the outcomes in 92 patients over the age of 55 years. They noted that even minor axial shortening of the radius following a Colles fracture affected the outcome. The functional end result was unsatisfactory in 4% of the patients with an acceptable anatomic result, in 25% of the patients with radial shortening of 3 to 5 mm, and in 31% of the patients with shortening of more than 5 mm.[75] Combined deformities are also significant. Trumble et al showed that axial compression of ≥2 mm and dorsal angulation of ≥15° adversely affect the end results.[76]

Malunion however does not always lead to a bad outcome. Grewal and MacDermid prospectively followed 216 patients with extra-articular DRFs for 1 year and assessed the patient-reported outcomes using the DASH and PRWE.[77] The overall alignment of the DRF was designated as "unacceptable" if the dorsal angulation was >10°, if the radial inclination was <15°, or if there was ≥3 mm of ulnar positive variance. Patients under the age of 65 demonstrated a very strong link between poor outcomes and the presence of malalignment of the distal radius. Patients 65 years and older showed no significant relationship between malalignment of the distal radius and patient reports of pain and disability. Based on relative risk, malalignment increased the risk of having a poor outcome (DASH >20 or PRWE >20) in all age groups. Using the DASH score, patients over the age of 65 however will experience 1 bad outcome for every 8 patients who present with unacceptable alignment. This contrasts with younger patients where 1 in 2 (based on the DASH) or 1 in 3 (based on the PRWE) will experience a poor outcome if left with a malaligned DRF.[51]

ULNAR WRIST PAIN

Ulnocarpal impingement and DRUJ incongruency are related to the amount of radial shortening and are a common cause of ulnar-sided wrist pain. One study of 109 Colles fractures treated with closed reduction and casting determined that the most important factor for predicting ulnar wrist pain was incongruity of the DRUJ due to residual dorsal angulation of the radius.[78] Others have found that an increase in the ulnar variance was the most important radiological parameter affecting outcome.[79]

PREDICTORS OF LOSS OF WRIST MOTION

Experimentally, radial shortening of 10 mm reduces forearm pronation by 47% and supination by 29%. Five millimeters of ulnar translation deformity results in an mean 23% loss of pronation.[80] Clinical experience has shown that axial compression of more than 2 mm and dorsal angulation exceeding 15° were directly related to diminished range of motion.[81] Comminution and intra-articular involvement also predispose toward a loss of movement. In a study of 169 DRFs in adults under the age of 50, fracture union with a step in the radiocarpal articular surface was associated with loss of wrist mobility and difficulty with fine dextrous tasks.[82] The predictive value of this evidence is that if a loss of motion is due to bony malalignment, prolonged therapy will be of no benefit.

REFERENCES

1. Chen NC, Jupiter JB. Management of distal radial fractures. *J Bone Joint Surg Am*. 2007;89:2051–2062.
2. Court-Brown CM, Caesar B. Epidemiology of adult fractures: a review. *Injury*. 2006;37:691–697.
3. Kakarlapudi TK, Santini A, Shahane SA, et al. The cost of treatment of distal radial fractures. *Injury*. 2000;31:229–232.
4. Geissler WB, Freeland AE, Savoie FH, et al. Intracarpal soft-tissue lesions associated with an intra-articular fracture of the distal end of the radius. *J Bone Joint Surg Am*. 1996;78:357–365.
5. Lindau T, Arner M, Hagberg L. Intraarticular lesions in distal fractures of the radius in young adults. A descriptive arthroscopic study in 50 patients. *J Hand Surg Br*. 1997;22:638–643.
6. Richards RS, Bennett JD, Roth JH, et al. Arthroscopic diagnosis of intra-articular soft tissue injuries associated with distal radial fractures. *J Hand Surg Am*. 1997;22:772–776.
7. Mehta JA, Bain GI, Heptinstall RJ. Anatomical reduction of intra-articular fractures of the distal radius. An arthroscopically-assisted approach. *J Bone Joint Surg Br*. 2000;82(1):79–86.
8. Mandziak DG, Watts AC, Bain GI. Ligament contribution to patterns of articular fractures of the distal radius. *J Hand Surg Am*. 2011;36:1621–1625.
9. White AA 3rd, Panjabi MM, Southwick WO. The four biomechanical stages of fracture repair. *J Bone Joint Surg Am*. 1977;59:188–192.
10. Vang Hansen F, Staunstrup H, Mikkelsen S. A comparison of 3 and 5 weeks immobilization for older type 1 and 2 Colles' fractures. *J Hand Surg Br*. 1998;23:400–401.
11. Slutsky DJ, Herman M. Rehabilitation of distal radius fractures: a biomechanical guide. *Hand Clin*. 2005;21:455–468.
12. Wolfe SW, Swigart CR, Grauer J, et al. Augmented external fixation of distal radius fractures: a biomechanical analysis. *J Hand Surg Am*. 1998;23:127–134.
13. Palmer AK, Werner FW. Biomechanics of the distal radioulnar joint. *Clin Orthop Relat Res*. 1984:26–35.
14. Putnam MD, Meyer NJ, Nelson EW, et al. Distal radial metaphyseal forces in an extrinsic grip model: implications for postfracture rehabilitation. *J Hand Surg Am*. 2000;25:469–475.
15. Rikli DA, Honigmann P, Babst R, et al. Intra-articular pressure measurement in the radioulnocarpal joint using a novel sensor: in vitro and in vivo results. *J Hand Surg Am*. 2007;32:67–75.
16. Moss DP, Means KR Jr, Parks BG, et al. A biomechanical comparison of volar locked plating of intra-articular distal radius fractures: use of 4 versus 7 screws for distal fixation. *J Hand Surg Am*. 2011;36:1907–1911.
17. Frykman GK, Peckham RH, Willard K, et al. External fixators for treatment of unstable wrist fractures. A biomechanical, design feature, and cost comparison. *Hand Clin*. 1993;9:555–565.
18. Yang Z, Mann FA, Gilula LA, et al. Scaphopisocapitate alignment: criterion to establish a neutral lateral view of the wrist. *Radiology*. 1997;205:865–869.
19. Boyer MI, Korcek KJ, Gelberman RH, et al. Anatomic tilt x-rays of the distal radius: an ex vivo analysis of surgical fixation. *J Hand Surg Am*. 2004;29:116–122.
20. Medoff RJ. Essential radiographic evaluation for distal radius fractures. *Hand Clin*. 2005;21:279–288.
21. Pichler W, Windisch G, Schaffler G, et al. Computer tomography aided 3D analysis of the distal dorsal radius surface and the effects on volar plate osteosynthesis. *J Hand Surg Eur Vol*. 2009;34:598–602.
22. Trumble TE, Culp RW, Hanel DP, et al. Intra-articular fractures of the distal aspect of the radius. *Instr Course Lect*. 1999;48:465–480.
23. Rikli DA, Regazzoni P. Fractures of the distal end of the radius treated by internal fixation and early function. A preliminary report of 20 cases. *J Bone Joint Surg Br*. 1996;78:588–592.
24. Lichtman DM, Bindra RR, Boyer MI, et al. American Academy of Orthopaedic Surgeons clinical practice guideline on: the treatment of distal radius fractures. *J Bone Joint Surg Am*. 2011;93:775–778.
25. Weil WM, Trumble TE. Treatment of distal radius fractures with intrafocal (kapandji) pinning and supplemental skeletal stabilization. *Hand Clin*. 2005;21:317–328.
26. Kapandji A. Intra-focal pinning of fractures of the distal end of the radius 10 years later. *Ann Chir Main*. 1987;6:57–63.
27. Stoffelen DV, Broos PL. Closed reduction versus Kapandji-pinning for extra-articular distal radial fractures. *J Hand Surg Br*. 1999;24:89–91.
28. Nishiwaki M, Tazaki K, Shimizu H, et al. Prospective study of distal radial fractures treated with an intramedullary nail. *J Bone Joint Surg Am*. 2011;93:1436–1441.
29. Dicpinigaitis P, Wolinsky P, Hiebert R, et al. Can external fixation maintain reduction after distal radius fractures? *J Trauma*. 2004;57:845–850.
30. Bartosh RA, Saldana MJ. Intraarticular fractures of the distal radius: a cadaveric study to determine if ligamentotaxis restores radiopalmar tilt. *J Hand Surg Am*. 1990;15:18–21.
31. Seitz WH Jr, Froimson AI, Leb R, et al. Augmented external fixation of unstable distal radius fractures. *J Hand Surg Am*. 1991;16:1010–1016.
32. Werber KD, Raeder F, Brauer RB, et al. External fixation of distal radial fractures: four compared with five pins: a randomized prospective study. *J Bone Joint Surg Am*. 2003;85-A:660–666.
33. Kreder HJ, Hanel DP, Agel J, et al. Indirect reduction and percutaneous fixation versus open reduction and internal fixation for displaced intra-articular fractures of the distal radius: a randomised, controlled trial. *J Bone Joint Surg Br*. 2005;87:829–836.
34. Papadonikolakis A, Shen J, Garrett JP, et al. The effect of increasing distraction on digital motion after external fixation of the wrist. *J Hand Surg Am*. 2005;30:773–779.
35. Kaempffe FA, Farbach J. A modified surgical procedure for cubital tunnel syndrome: partial medial epicondylectomy. *J Hand Surg Am*. 1998;23:492–499.
36. Harley BJ, Scharfenberger A, Beaupre LA, Jomha N, Weber DW. Augmented external fixation versus percutaneous pinning and casting for unstable fractures of the distal radius a prospective randomized trial. *J Hand Surg Am*. 2004;29(5):815–824.
37. Slutsky DJ. External fixation of distal radius fractures. *J Hand Surg Am*. 2007;32:1624–1637.
38. Slutsky DJ. Nonbridging external fixation of intra-articular distal radius fractures. *Hand Clin*. 2005;21:381–394.
39. Gradl G, Jupiter JB, Gierer P, et al. Fractures of the distal radius treated with a nonbridging external fixation technique using multiplanar k-wires. *J Hand Surg Am*. 2005;30:960–968.
40. McQueen MM. Non-spanning external fixation of the distal radius. *Hand Clin*. 2005;21:375–380.
41. Hayes AJ, Duffy PJ, McQueen MM. Bridging and non-bridging external fixation in the treatment of unstable fractures of the distal radius: a retrospective study of 588 patients. *Acta Orthop*. 2008;79:540–547.
42. Orbay JL, Fernandez DL. Volar fixation for dorsally displaced fractures of the distal radius: a preliminary report. *J Hand Surg Am*. 2002;27:205–215.
43. Tanaka Y, Aoki M, Izumi T, et al. Effect of distal radius volar plate position on contact pressure between the flexor pollicis longus tendon and the distal plate edge. *J Hand Surg Am*. 2011;36:1790–1797.
44. Harness NG, Jupiter JB, Orbay JL, et al. Loss of fixation of the volar lunate facet fragment in fractures of the distal part of the radius. *J Bone Joint Surg Am*. 2004;86-A:1900–1908.

45. Wall LB, Brodt MD, Silva MJ, et al. The effects of screw length on stability of simulated osteoporotic distal radius fractures fixed with volar locking plates. *J Hand Surg Am*. 2012;37:446–453.
46. Drobetz H, Bryant AL, Pokorny T, et al. Volar fixed-angle plating of distal radius extension fractures: influence of plate position on secondary loss of reduction—a biomechanic study in a cadaveric model. *J Hand Surg Am*. 2006;31:615–622.
47. Martineau PA, Waitayawinyu T, Malone KJ, et al. Volar plating of AO C3 distal radius fractures: biomechanical evaluation of locking screw and locking smooth peg configurations. *J Hand Surg Am*. 2008; 33:827–834.
48. Saw N, Roberts C, Cutbush K, et al. Early experience with the TriMed fragment-specific fracture fixation system in intraarticular distal radius fractures. *J Hand Surg Eur Vol*. 2008;33:53–58.
49. Benson LS, Medoff R. Fragment specific fixation of distal radius fractures. In: Slutsky DJ, Osterman AL, eds. *Fractures and Injuries of the Distal Radius and Carpus*. Philadelphia, Saunders/Elsevier; 2009.
50. Arora R, Lutz M, Deml C, et al. A prospective randomized trial comparing nonoperative treatment with volar locking plate fixation for displaced and unstable distal radial fractures in patients sixty-five years of age and older. *J Bone Joint Surg Am*. 2011;93:2146–2153.
51. Chou YC, Chen AC, Chen CY, et al. Dorsal and volar 2.4-mm titanium locking plate fixation for AO type C3 dorsally comminuted distal radius fractures. *J Hand Surg Am*. 2011;36:974–981.
52. Chung KC, Squitieri L, Kim HM. Comparative outcomes study using the volar locking plating system for distal radius fractures in both young adults and adults older than 60 years. *J Hand Surg Am*. 2008;33:809–819.
53. Grewal R, MacDermid JC, King GJ, et al. Open reduction internal fixation versus percutaneous pinning with external fixation of distal radius fractures: a prospective, randomized clinical trial. *J Hand Surg Am*. 2011;36:1899–1906.
54. Jupiter JB, Marent-Huber M. Operative management of distal radial fractures with 2.4-millimeter locking plates. A multicenter prospective case series. *J Bone Joint Surg Am*. 2009;91:55–65.
55. Handoll HH, Watts AC. Bone grafts and bone substitutes for treating distal radial fractures in adults. *Cochrane Database Syst Rev*. 2008:CD006836.
56. Yu YR, Makhni MC, Tabrizi S, et al. Complications of low-profile dorsal versus volar locking plates in the distal radius: a comparative study. *J Hand Surg Am*. 2011;36:1135–1141.
57. Hanel DP, Lu TS, Weil WM. Bridge plating of distal radius fractures: the Harborview method. *Clin Orthop Relat Res*. 2006;445:91–99.
58. Hanel DP, Ruhlman SD, Katolik LI, et al. Complications associated with distraction plate fixation of wrist fractures. *Hand Clin*. 2010;26:237–243.
59. Ruch DS, Ginn TA, Yang CC, et al. Use of a distraction plate for distal radial fractures with metaphyseal and diaphyseal comminution. *J Bone Joint Surg Am*. 2005;87:945–954.
60. Ishikawa J, Iwasaki N, Minami A. Influence of distal radioulnar joint subluxation on restricted forearm rotation after distal radius fracture. *J Hand Surg Am*. 2005;30:1178–1184.
61. Swart E, Nellans K, Rosenwasser M. The effects of pain, supination, and grip strength on patient-rated disability after operatively treated distal radius fractures. *J Hand Surg Am*. 2012;37:957–962.
62. Sammer DM, Shah HM, Shauver MJ, et al. The effect of ulnar styloid fractures on patient-rated outcomes after volar locking plating of distal radius fractures. *J Hand Surg Am*. 2009;34:1595–1602.
63. Souer JS, Ring D, Matschke S, et al. Effect of an unrepaired fracture of the ulnar styloid base on outcome after plate-and-screw fixation of a distal radial fracture. *J Bone Joint Surg Am*. 2009;91: 830–838.
64. Zenke Y, Sakai A, Oshige T, et al. The effect of an associated ulnar styloid fracture on the outcome after fixation of a fracture of the distal radius. *J Bone Joint Surg Br*. 2009;91:102–107.
65. Warwick D, Field J, Prothero D, et al. Function ten years after Colles' fracture. *Clin Orthop Relat Res*. 1993:270–274.
66. Souer JS, Buijze G, Ring D. A prospective randomized controlled trial comparing occupational therapy with independent exercises after volar plate fixation of a fracture of the distal part of the radius. *J Bone Joint Surg Am*. 2011;93:1761–1766.
67. Slutsky DJ. Predicting the outcome of distal radius fractures. *Hand Clin*. 2005;21:289–294.
68. Lafontaine M, Delince P, Hardy D, et al. Instability of fractures of the lower end of the radius: apropos of a series of 167 cases. *Acta Orthop Belg*. 1989;55:203–216.
69. Leone J, Bhandari M, Adili A, et al. Predictors of early and late instability following conservative treatment of extra-articular distal radius fractures. *Arch Orthop Trauma Surg*. 2004;124:38–41.
70. Nesbitt KS, Failla JM, Les C. Assessment of instability factors in adult distal radius fractures. *J Hand Surg Am*. 2004;29:1128–1138.
71. Knirk JL, Jupiter JB. Intra-articular fractures of the distal end of the radius in young adults. *J Bone Joint Surg Am*. 1986;68:647–659.
72. Catalano LW 3rd, Cole RJ, Gelberman RH, et al. Displaced intra-articular fractures of the distal aspect of the radius. Long-term results in young adults after open reduction and internal fixation. *J Bone Joint Surg Am*. 1997;79:1290–1302.
73. Goldfarb CA, Rudzki JR, Catalano LW, et al. Fifteen-year outcome of displaced intra-articular fractures of the distal radius. *J Hand Surg Am*. 2006;31:633–639.
74. Gartland JJ Jr, Werley CW. Evaluation of healed Colles' fractures. *J Bone Joint Surg Am*. 1951;33-A:895–907.
75. Aro HT, Koivunen T. Minor axial shortening of the radius affects outcome of Colles' fracture treatment. *J Hand Surg Am*. 1991;16: 392–398.
76. Trumble TE, Schmitt SR, Vedder NB. Factors affecting functional outcome of displaced intra-articular distal radius fractures. *J Hand Surg Am*. 1994;19:325–340.
77. Grewal R, MacDermid JC. The risk of adverse outcomes in extra-articular distal radius fractures is increased with malalignment in patients of all ages but mitigated in older patients. *J Hand Surg Am*. 2007;32:962–970.
78. Tsukazaki T, Iwasaki K. Ulnar wrist pain after Colles' fracture. 109 fractures followed for 4 years. *Acta Orthop Scand*. 1993;64: 462–464.
79. Geissler WB, Fernandez DL, Lamey DM. Distal radioulnar joint injuries associated with fractures of the distal radius. *Clin Orthop Relat Res*. 1996:135–146.
80. Bronstein AJ, Trumble TE, Tencer AF. The effects of distal radius fracture malalignment on forearm rotation: a cadaveric study. *J Hand Surg Am*. 1997;22:258–262.
81. Leung F, Ozkan M, Chow SP. Conservative treatment of intra-articular fractures of the distal radius—factors affecting functional outcome. *Hand Surg*. 2000;5:145–153.
82. Gliatis JD, Plessas SJ, Davis TR. Outcome of distal radial fractures in young adults. *J Hand Surg Br*. 2000;25:535–543.

Arthroscopic Treatment of Distal Radius Fractures

27

Francisco del Piñal, MD, PhD
Melissa Klausmeyer, MD

RATIONALE

Contrary to general belief, arthroscopic-assisted reduction in distal radius fractures can be done in an expeditious manner and with minimal OR resource consumption. In many cases of simple articular fractures, step-offs and gaps are present that can be corrected with the arthroscopic technique.[1–5] Use of the arthroscope in intra-articular distal radius fractures undoubtedly adds a level of complexity to the management of distal radius fractures. But it provides undeniable advantages as well: the ability to remove debris and hematoma, to see inside the joint with light and magnification, to directly manipulate intra-articular fragments, and to evaluate for concomitant ligamentous injury.

INDICATIONS

We use arthroscopy routinely for all displaced articular fractures of the distal radius that are scheduled for ORIF. We do not universally use the arthroscope in extra-articular fractures; in this case we limit the indication to active individuals with a suspicion of ligament injury or a major distal radioulnar joint (DRUJ) instability at the end of the radius fixation. Additionally, we use an arthroscope in distal extra-articular fractures where there is doubt about the location of the hardware, specifically to check for inadvertent placement of the screws in the joint space.

There is no age limit of the patients. The operation is scheduled as soon as possible in our practice, unlike many authors who recommend waiting 3 to 5 days to minimize bleeding of the fracture site and for avoiding major extravasation of fluid risking a compartment syndrome. The latter problem does not exist if the surgeon uses the dry arthroscopic technique.[6,7]

CONTRAINDICATIONS

Arthroscopic-assisted reduction is contraindicated with overt superficial infection. As stated above, we employ the dry technique to avoid the risk of compartment syndrome. If the wet technique is chosen, continuous fluid irrigation cannot be performed when there is marked capsular tearing, which would lead to extensive fluid extravasation and thus the risk of compartment syndrome. The dry technique is contraindicated when using thermal probes unless intermittent fluid irrigation is used.

SURGICAL TECHNIQUE

Before addressing the treatment of the fracture itself, the surgeon needs to be acquainted with the dry arthroscopic technique.[6–8] The technique can be summarized in the 3 basic rules:

1. The valve of the sheath of the arthroscope is kept open at all times to allow air circulation.
2. Suction of the shaver or burr is used only when aspiration is necessary, and left in the "off" position for the remainder of the operation. Otherwise, the contents of the joint will be stirred up by the suction, obscuring vision through the scope.
3. The joint is flushed with 5- to 10-mL aliquots of saline to clear debris and blood as needed.

The management of the severely comminuted articular fractures (more than 4 articular fragments or with free osteochondral fragments) is difficult and is not recommended until the surgeon and OR personnel have enough experience with the management of simple fractures. Finally, having the assistance of another surgeon is invaluable until one is familiar with the logistics of the operation, and it is essential in more complex fractures.

A systematic approach is fundamental in this "complex" operation. With slight modifications the operation can be summarized as follows: (a) temporary fixation of the articular fragments with Kirschner wires (K-wires) to a volar locking plate under fluoroscopic control; (b) arthroscopic fine-tuning of the reduction; (c) rigid articular fragment fixation under arthroscopic guidance; (d) triangular fibrocartilage complex (TFCC) and midcarpal exploration.

A flexor carpi radialis (FCR) approach is used to address the typical 4-part fracture. A 6-cm incision is made overlying the FCR. The tendon sheath is divided and the FCR is retracted ulnarly. The pronator quadratus is elevated from the fracture. The brachoradialis tendon is left undisturbed. A volar locking plate is provisionally applied and stabilized to the shaft of the radius by inserting a screw into the elliptical hole on the stem of the plate. This will allow some adjustment of the plate as needed. Next, the reduction of the distal fragments is done by traction and flexion. The dorsal fragments are manually compressed to the construct as the plate acts as a mold. Usually, several attempts and maneuvers are needed before the "best" provisional reduction is obtained, as judged by the fluoroscopic views and direct observation of the metaphyseal component of the fracture. Radial length, volar tilt, and radial inclination should be corrected and held with the aid of the plate. The articular fragments are then provisionally secured to the distal plate by inserting K-wires through the auxiliary holes and an additional proximal screw is inserted. No locking pegs are used at this stage.

At this point, we suspend the hand from a custom-made traction system with 7 to 10 kg of distraction.[9] A 2.7-mm/30° scope is used for most cases. Because of edema and the disrupted bony anatomy, it is slightly more difficult to establish the portals than in a standard arthroscopy case. However, with deep palpation, Lister's tubercle can be located as well as the joint space just distal to it. This guides the placement of the 3-4 portal. Small transverse incisions are used for each portal as they heal with minimal scarring and do not require suturing at the end of the operation. The entrance of the portal is enlarged with a mosquito clamp, and the scope is introduced and directed ulnarly to establish another portal for triangulation.

Use of the 4-5 portal is avoided to prevent interference with the reduction of the dorsoulnar radius. Instead, the 6R portal is the preferred ulnar portal for triangulation. This portal is established by palpating the proximal rounded surface of the triquetrum; the portal placement is just proximal to the triquetrum but as distal as possible. This avoids the TFCC that may be detached from the dorsal capsule or fovea and may impede the entrance into the radiocarpal joint. With the scope in the 3-4 portal, a 2.9-mm shaver is inserted into the 6R portal to aspirate blood and debris. The joint is irrigated with saline in 5- to 10-mL aliquots from a syringe attached to the valve of the scope. After the fragments that need to be mobilized are identified from the 3-4 view, the scope is swapped to 6R. The scope remains in 6R until the completion of the fixation. In this position, the scope rests on the ulnar head and the TFCC. If the scope is kept in the 3-4 (or 4-5) portal, it rests on the unstable dorsal distal radius; this can displace reduced fragments or impede their reduction (Fig. 27-1). Although the volar-radial portal is useful for addressing dorsal rim fragments,[10,11] we prefer to keep the scope in 6R, advance the scope volarly, and turn the lens dorsally to view the dorsal rim. This avoids changing portals and redisplacing volar fragments that are not yet rigidly fixed.

Except in the most complex cases, only 1 or 2 fragments will need to be addressed arthroscopically, and usually these fragments are depressed. Several authors recommend elevating these fragments by inserting an instrument into the

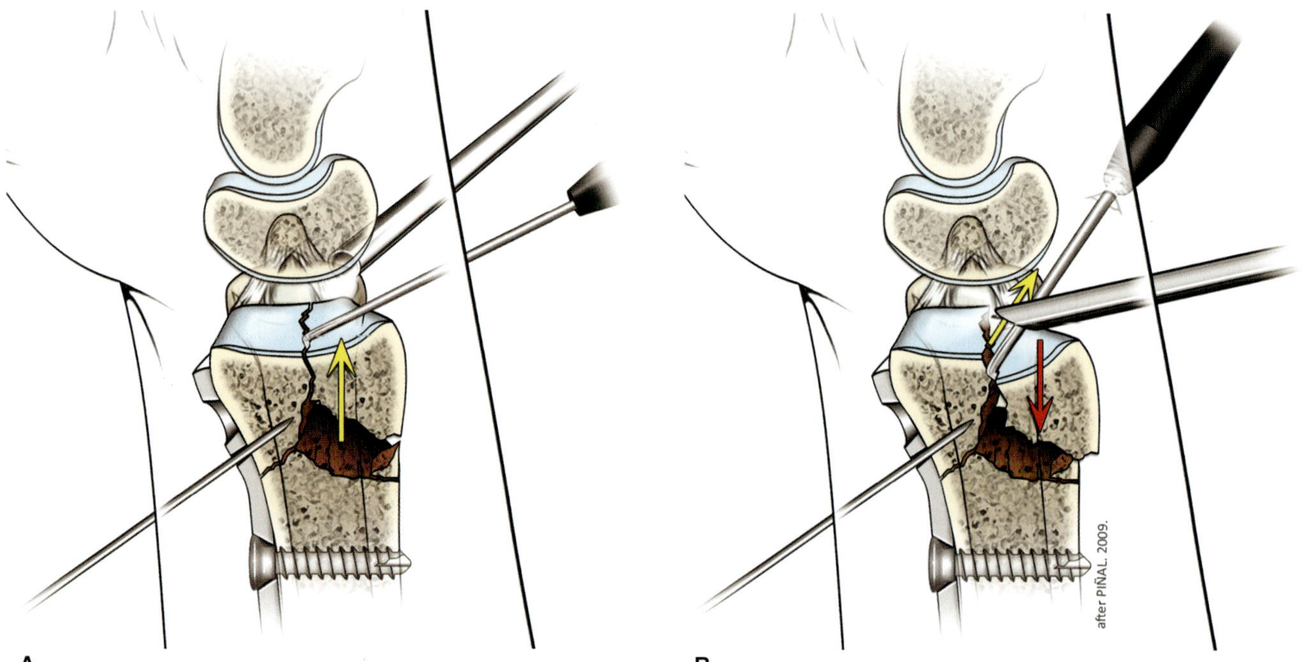

FIGURE 27-1 **A.** When the scope is place in 6R, it rests on the stable platform of the ulnar head. **B.** If the scope is placed in any other portal, it conflicts with the reduction (red and yellow arrows) and is unstable. (Copyright © 2011 by Dr Piñal.)

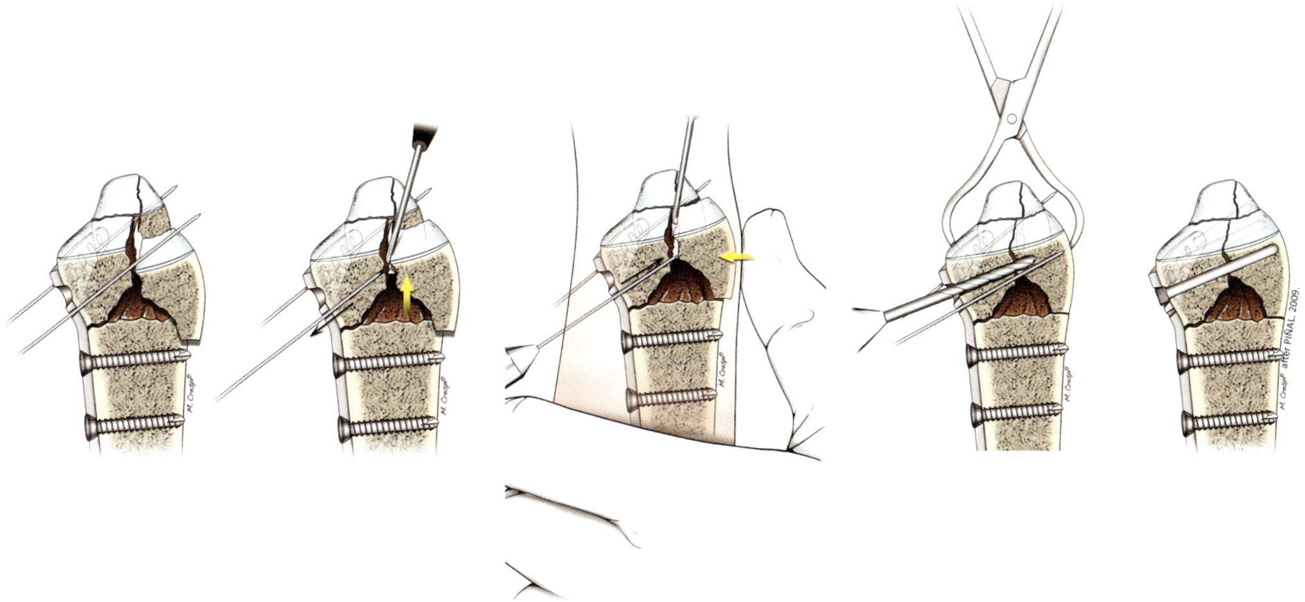

FIGURE 27-2 The preferred technique for reducing depressed dorsal fragments. The probe is used to assist in reduction, and tension is maintained on the construct while the distal screws are inserted. (Copyright © 2011 by Dr Piñal.)

metaphysis (proximal to the fragment) through an additional dorsal skin incision. Our preferred technique is to use a shoulder or knee probe in the 3-4 portal and hook the fragment to pull it distally (Figs. 27-2 and 27-3). The fragment is released from the provisional fixation by backing out the specific K-wire that secures it; then the fragment is slightly overreduced with the probe. At this point, the surgeon maintains the reduction by compressing it in a volar direction. The assistant surgeon then slowly readvances the K-wire into the dorsal cortex to capture the reduction, taking care not to impale the extensor tendons (or the other surgeon's thumb!). Once the joint is reduced, the locking pegs/screws are inserted. Those pegs/screws in critical positions are placed under arthroscopic control, since a loss of reduction may occur while drilling. This step may be facilitated by releasing the traction slightly to relax the flexor tendons, which are then retracted ulnarly. Smaller fragments can be held in position with the flat surface of a Freer elevator in order to avoid "crumbling" during drilling. Once the major articular fragments are stable to probe palpation, the hand is released from the traction and laid flat on the operating table for insertion of the remaining pegs and screws. A final arthroscopic survey is performed to ensure there is no hardware penetration of the articular surface.

Occasionally, the articular fragments are displaced distally and are prominent in the joint space. In this case, the traction is partially released, and the fragment is reduced by pushing it down with a Freer elevator. Pressure is applied with the surgeon's thumb or bone tenaculum to maintain reduction while the definitive fixation is performed. Small dorsal rim fragments do not need to be fixed to the plate as these fragments do not bear significant load. Large unstable dorsal

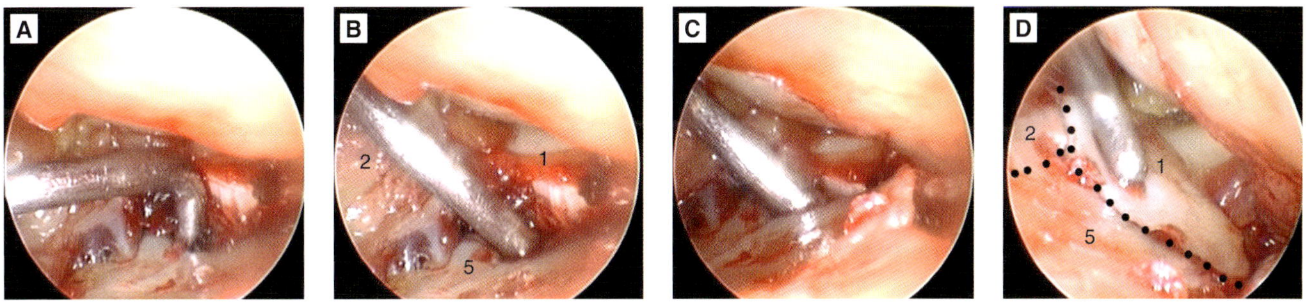

FIGURE 27-3 Reduction of a fragment in the scaphoid fossa. **A.** The 3-mm shoulder probe is used to estimate the step-off. **B.** The probe is placed under the depressed fragment. **C.** The probe is used to elevate the fragment. **D.** The fragment is leveled with the rest of the joint. (Scope is 6R, viewing a right wrist in the radial direction. (1) Volar rim of scaphoid fossa; (2) dorsal rim; (5) scaphoid fossa.) (Copyright © 2011 by Dr Piñal.)

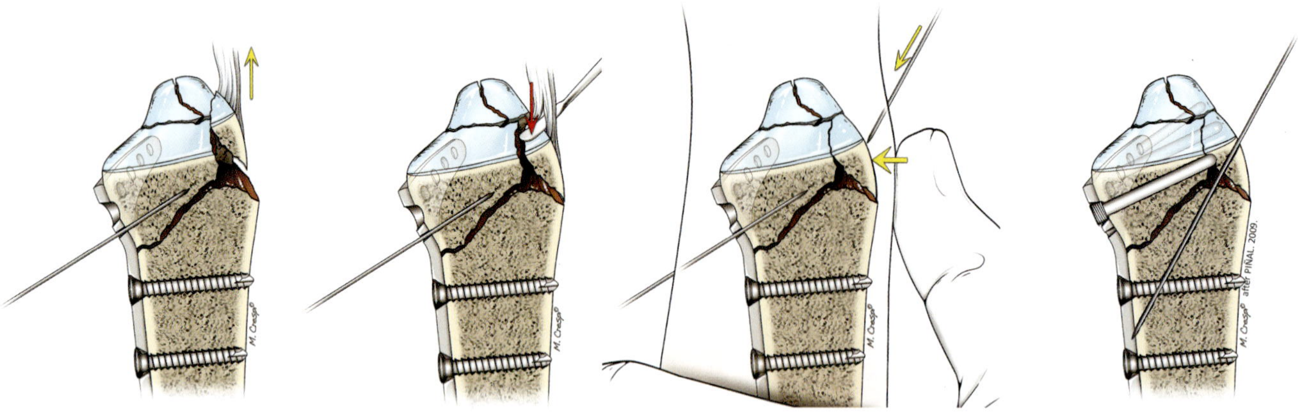

FIGURE 27-4 Technique of arthroscopic reduction of an elevated dorsal rim fragment. The Freer elevator is used to reduce the fragment while tension is maintained by the surgeon's thumb. (From del Piñal.[17] Copyright © 2009, with kind permission of Springer Science_Business Media.)

fragments can be fixed by the locking pegs/screws if large enough; otherwise K-wire fixation is used (Fig. 27-4). The K-wires are left protruding percutaneously and are removed in the office in 3 to 4 weeks. In order to avoid skin irritation, the patients are allowed wrist flexion but not extension until the K-wires are removed.

It is important to stress that large dorsal fragments that appear distally displaced in relation to the anterior fragments on fluoroscopy rarely are. In fact, usually it is the anterior fragment (often the volar-ulnar fragment) that remains dorsally rotated. Clues to help recognize this deformity include the absence of collapse in the dorsal cortex and the depression of Medoff's "teardrop angle" ($N = 70°$)[12] (Fig. 27-5). In these instances, the joint is reduced by derotating and elevating the anterior fragment to the level of the dorsal fragment rather than depressing the dorsal fragment (Fig. 27-5). This is performed in a similar manner to reduction of dorsally depressed fragments, but the K-wire should be completely

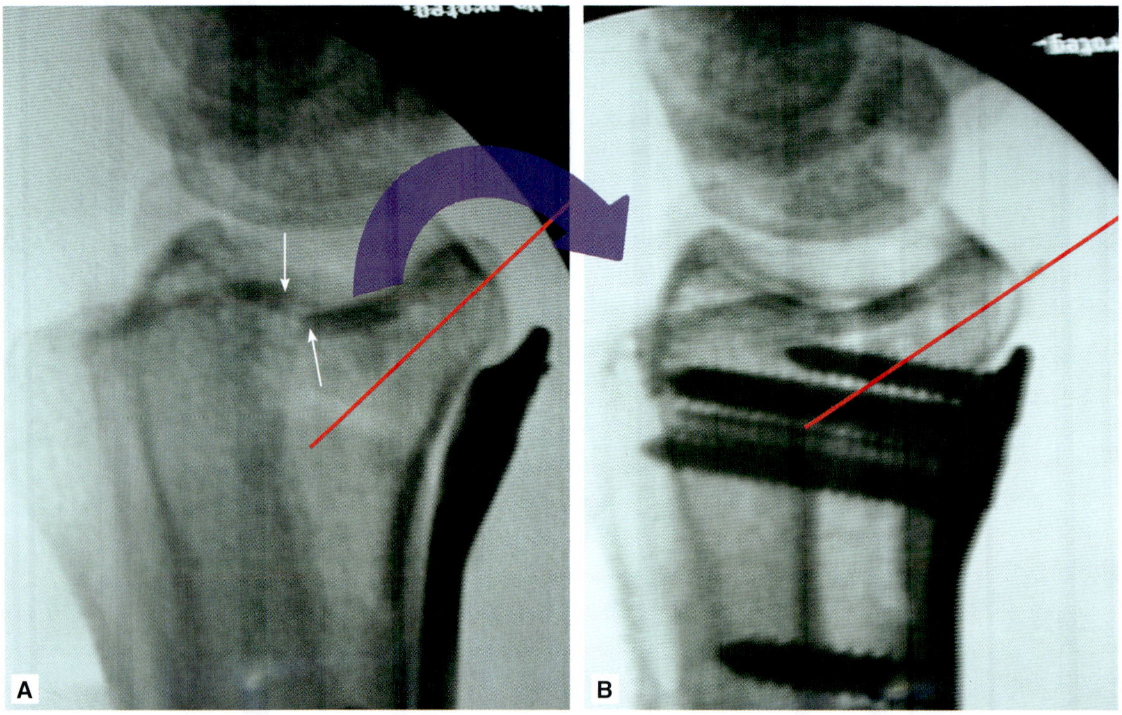

FIGURE 27-5 **A.** Fluoroscopic view of a pseudoelevated dorsal fragment with a step-off at the lunate facet (white arrows). Notice, however, that the dorsal cortex is restored without gaps and that the "teardrop angle" (red line) is slightly decreased. Both of these suggest a malrotated volar fragment. **B.** After the anteroulnar fragment was derotated, anatomic restoration of the lunate fossa was achieved (normal teardrop angle). (Copyright © 2011 by Dr Piñal.)

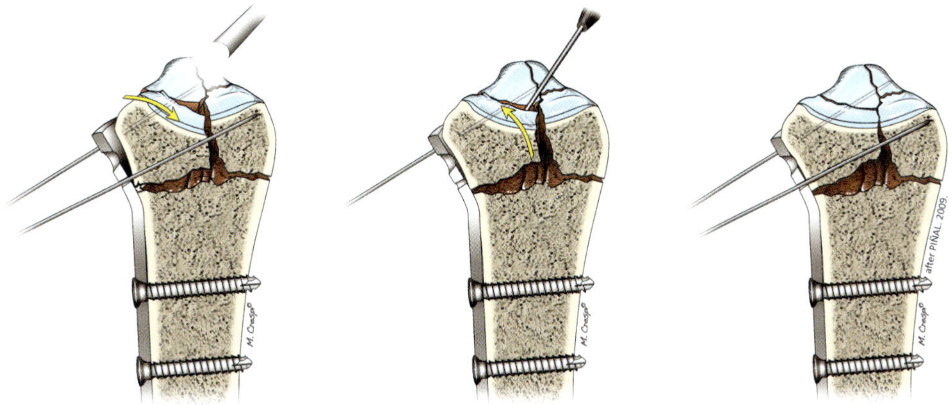

FIGURE 27-6 Preferred technique for reduction of an anterior malrotated fragment. The reduction requires the complete removal of the corresponding K-wire prior to manipulation of the fragment. (Copyright © 2011 by Dr Piñal.)

withdrawn before attempting to mobilize the anterior fragment (Figs. 27-6 and 27-7).

Free osteochondral fragments are at times extremely unstable and have a tendency to sink into the metaphyseal void after reduction. To prevent this, we support the fragments by inserting the distal layer of locking pegs in the plate to act as a hammock. The fragments are kept slightly overreduced and then impacted with a Freer elevator. Alternatively, they may be impacted by releasing the traction and using the corresponding carpal bone as a mold. A grasper may be necessary to manipulate a severely displaced fragment (Figs. 27-8 and 27-9).

In very comminuted fractures, displacement of some articular fragments will persist after fluoroscopic reduction. Backing out all of the K-wires and attempting to reduce and fix all of the mobile fragments at the same time is an impossible endeavor in our hands. We recommend a systematic approach beginning ulnarly and progressing radially in most cases (Fig. 27-10). With the scope in the 6R portal and resting on the ulnar head, the "keystone" lunate fossa is reduced first and stabilized by inserting 1 or 2 locking pegs/screws in the ulnar part of the plate. The radial portion of the joint is now addressed and fine-tuned under arthroscopic guidance followed by insertion of locking screws to stabilize the scaphoid fossa. A similar technique is also necessary when the metaphysis is too comminuted to support the articular fragments.

Management of TFCC injuries and concomitant ligamentous injuries[7,13] is beyond the scope of this chapter but may affect the outcome if not addressed.[14,15] This part of the operation is always performed after rigid fixation of the radius to prevent secondary displacement. Furthermore, DRUJ instability should be assessed only after the radius is reduced and stabilized.[16]

The joint is thoroughly flushed after completion of the procedure. Assessment of the midcarpal joint is performed. Then, the pronator quadratus is sutured to the brachioradialis tendon with 2 or 3 resorbable stitches. The volar skin incision is closed in a single layer with a subcuticular

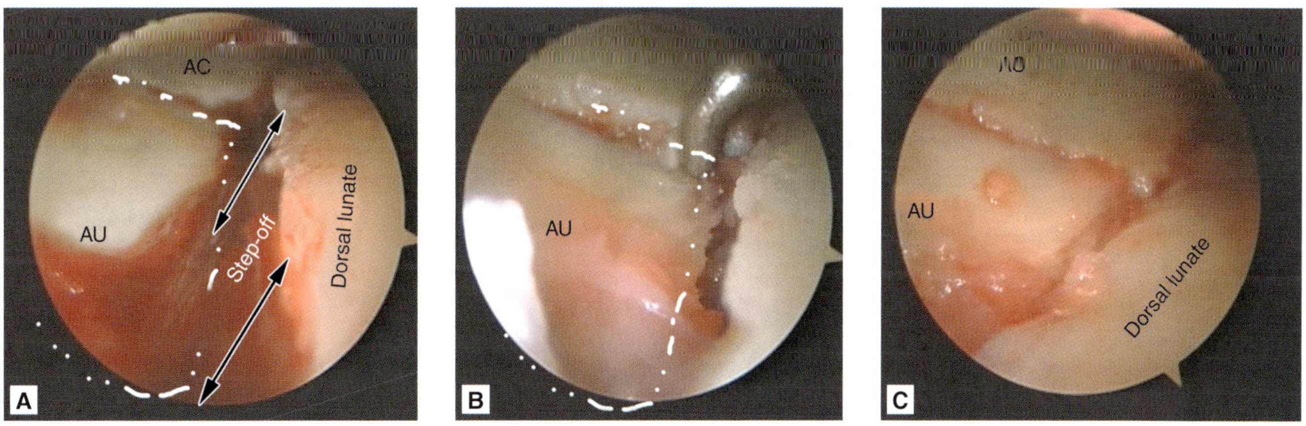

FIGURE 27-7 Correction of a pseudoelevated dorsal fragment. **A.** Although the dorsal lunate fossa fragment appears elevated with a step-off of approximately 3 mm, the displacement is actually due to malrotation of the anteroulnar fragment of the lunate fossa (AU). **B.** With a shoulder probe inserted through the 3-4 portal, the anterior fragment is derotated. **C.** The 2 volar components of the lunate fossa (AU and AC) are now level with the dorsal fragment. (Copyright © 2011 by Dr Piñal.)

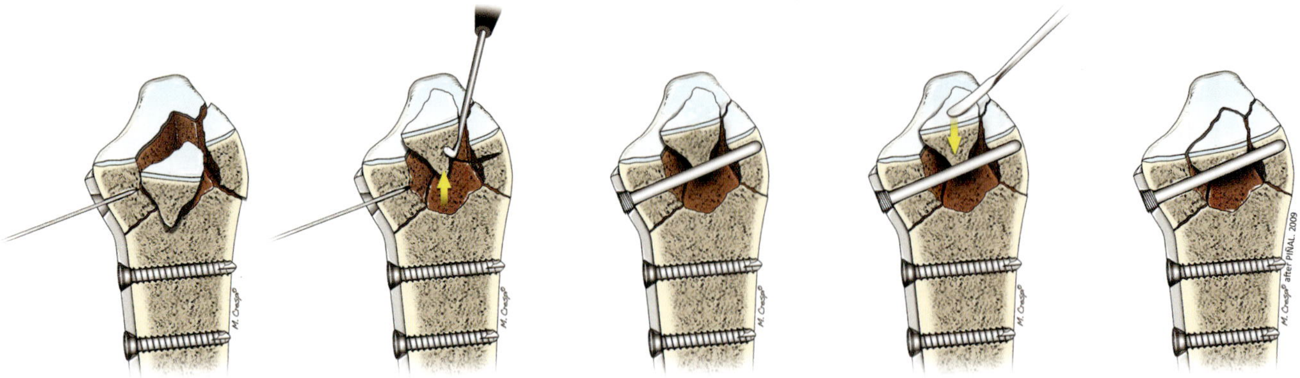

FIGURE 27-8 Preferred management of free osteochondral fragments. Temporary K-wire fixation is not sufficient to maintain reduction. Instead, a locking peg is inserted in the distal row of the plate and the fragment is impacted with a Freer elevator in order to completely reduce it. (Copyright © 2011 by Dr Piñal.)

3/0 nylon suture. The transverse portal incisions do not need to be sutured as they will heal with a minimal scar. A protective splint is provided and removed in 1 to 2 days. Self-directed active and assisted exercises are encouraged at that time. A removable plastic splint is fabricated and is worn only when the patient is at risk of further trauma. After 4 or 5 weeks, any limitation of arc of motion is addressed by assisted exercises under the supervision of a physiotherapist. Exceptions are made in those cases that required additional fixation for dorsal rim fixation with K-wires for which 3 weeks of extension blocking is required. Concomitant soft tissue injuries also modify the aftercare.

COMPLICATIONS

Dorsal soft tissue scarring may make repositioning of the depressed dorsal fragments impossible in as little time as 10 to 14 days. Forceful maneuvers to reduce the fragments may cause further fragmentation. If the surgeon notices that the fragments do not move easily, it is recommended to use a Freer elevator to bluntly release all the proximal periosteum and scarred soft tissues under arthroscopic control (Fig. 27-11).

With a severely comminuted intra-articular fracture with metaphyseal or diaphyseal comminution, it is possible to lose the extra-articular reduction while addressing the intra-articular component (Fig. 27-12A). This is a particular risk when the metaphyseal fragments are not substantial enough to support the K-wires that are used for the temporary articular reduction. When pressure is applied to the intra-articular fragments, the tenuous K-wire stabilization collapses, and the extra-articular reduction is lost since the comminuted metaphysis is not a reliable foundation on which to base the articular construct. Instead of performing the reduction proximally to distally (from diaphysis to metaphysis to epiphysis), we prefer a different approach: the "platform" technique. The plate is first applied to the diaphysis. Then, under fluoroscopy, the largest articular fragment

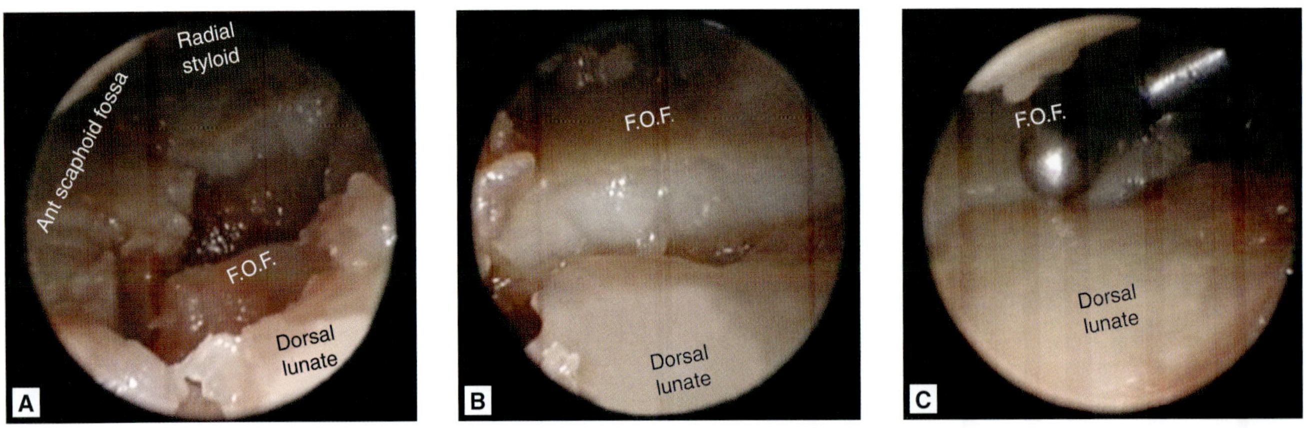

FIGURE 27-9 Corresponding arthroscopic view of Figure 27-8. **A.** A free osteochondral fragment (F.O.F.) sank into the metaphyseal void in the scaphoid fossa. After several attempts at reduction, the fragment did not have sufficient support to resist the stress of the probe. **B.** After a locking peg was inserted, a supporting hammock is created. The free osteochondral fragment is shown overreduced before it is leveled by the probe (**C**). (Copyright © 2011 by Dr Piñal.)

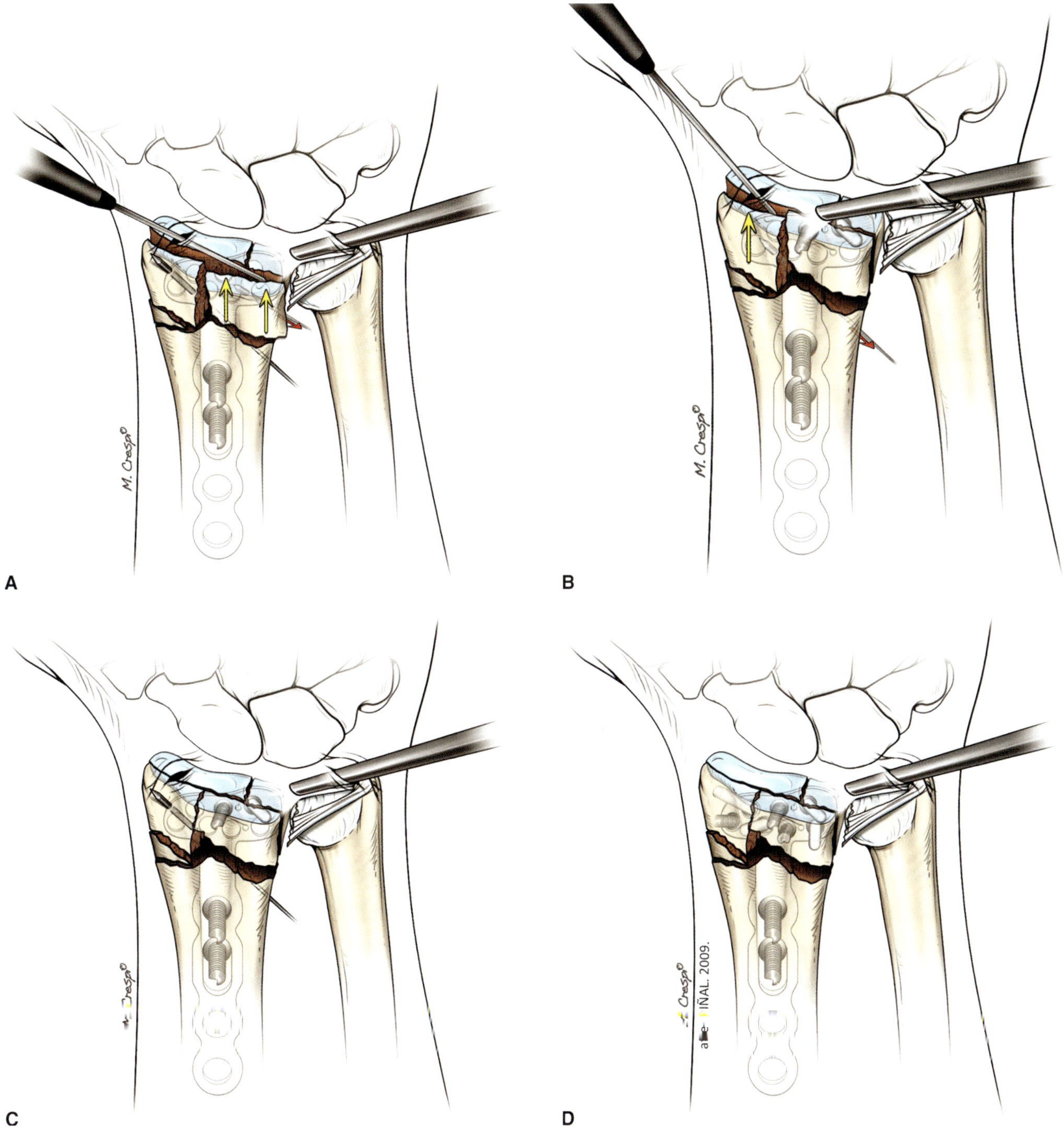

FIGURE 27-10 Preferred technique for reduction when several fragments remain displaced. **A.** The volar lunate fossa fragment (keystone) is reduced and (**B**) secured with locking screws. The reduction (**C**) and fixation (**D**) occur in an ulnar to radial direction. (From del Piñal.[17] Copyright © 2009, with kind permission of Springer Science+Business Media.)

is secured to the distal aspect of the plate with locking pegs/screws (Fig. 27-12B). This establishes the radial length. Next, under arthroscopy, the reduction and fixation continue with the remaining articular fragments. Once the articular "platform" is established, the metaphyseal fragments are reduced and the fixation is completed (Fig. 27-12C-F).

OUTCOMES

We have treated more than 200 articular distal radius fractures under arthroscopic control. We reviewed 19 of the most comminuted fractures.[17] They all had "explosion fractures": more than 5 articular fragments and/or a free

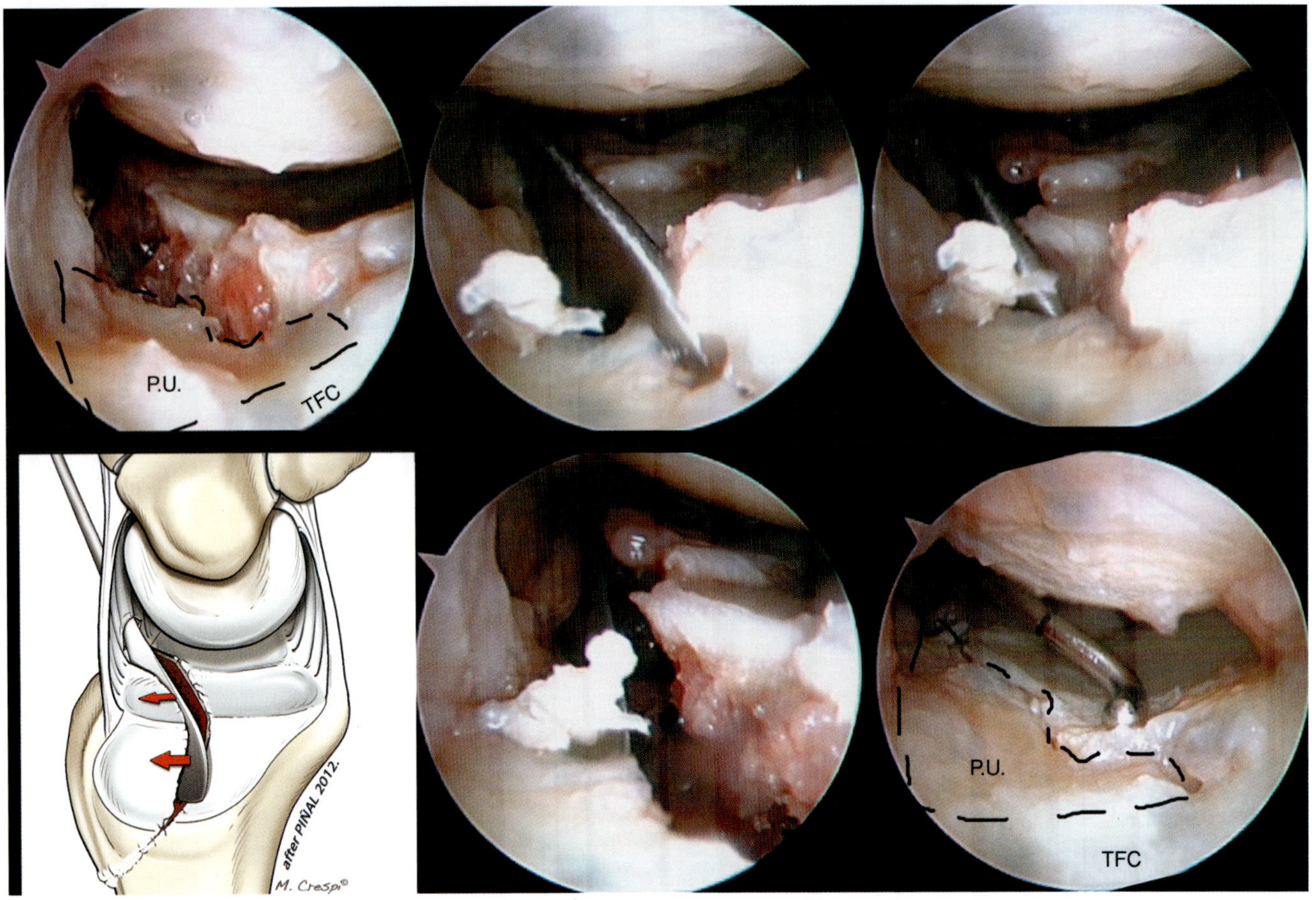

FIGURE 27-11 Two weeks after the injury this posteroulnar fragment (P.U.) was already healed in malposition and could not be reduced. A Freer elevator was introduced through 6R and the callus was broken. The fragment was aggressively manipulated with the Freer elevator in order for the soft tissues to yield and to permit anatomic reduction. (Copyright © 2012 by Dr Piñal.)

osteochondral fragment. The patients were evaluated clinically and radiographically at a minimum of 2-year follow-up. In 1 case the extra-articular reduction was lost, but in all other patients, the radiographic parameters were satisfactorily maintained. The average range of motion was 105° of flexion–extension; average grip strength was 85% of the contralateral side, and the average DASH score was 6. This study confirms that (dry) arthroscopy is feasible in the most severely articular comminuted C3 fractures. In a more recent case outside of the study group, 1 patient suffered collapse of the lunate fossa and required radiolunate arthrodesis.

Additionally, in a level 1 study, Doi et al compared conventional ORIF treatment of intra-articular distal radius fractures with arthroscopically assisted reduction. They found improved outcome for patients treated with an arthroscopically assisted procedure when measured with both the Gartland and Werley scoring system and that of Green and O'Brien.[18] The group that had an arthroscopically assisted procedure also had significantly better ranges of flexion–extension and radial–ulnar deviation of the wrist and grip strength ($P < .05$).

Varitimidis et al performed a level I trial comparing arthroscopic reduction and fixation of distal radius fracture combined with arthroscopic treatment of associated intracarpal and TFCC injuries with fluoroscopic reduction and fixation of the radius alone. In the arthroscopy group, the DASH scores were clinically important at the 3-month interval. Regardless of arthroscopy, the difference in function as determined by DASH scores was not relevant at 1 and 2 years postoperatively.[5] A weakness of the study included the possibility of preexisting carpal lesions and that the true incidence of carpal ligament lesions in the fluoroscopy group was unknown.

Ruch et al performed a retrospective study of 15 patients with comminuted intra-articular distal radius fractures who were treated with an arthroscopic reduction and external fixation and percutaneous pinning versus 15 patients who underwent a fluoroscopic reduction.[2] The patients who underwent the arthroscopic reduction had significantly improved supination compared with those who underwent the fluoroscopic reduction (88° vs 73°; $P = .02$) as well as better wrist extension (mean, 77° vs 69°; $P = .01$) and wrist flexion (mean, 78° vs 59°; $P = .02$). The radial length and the DASH scores were similar for both groups.

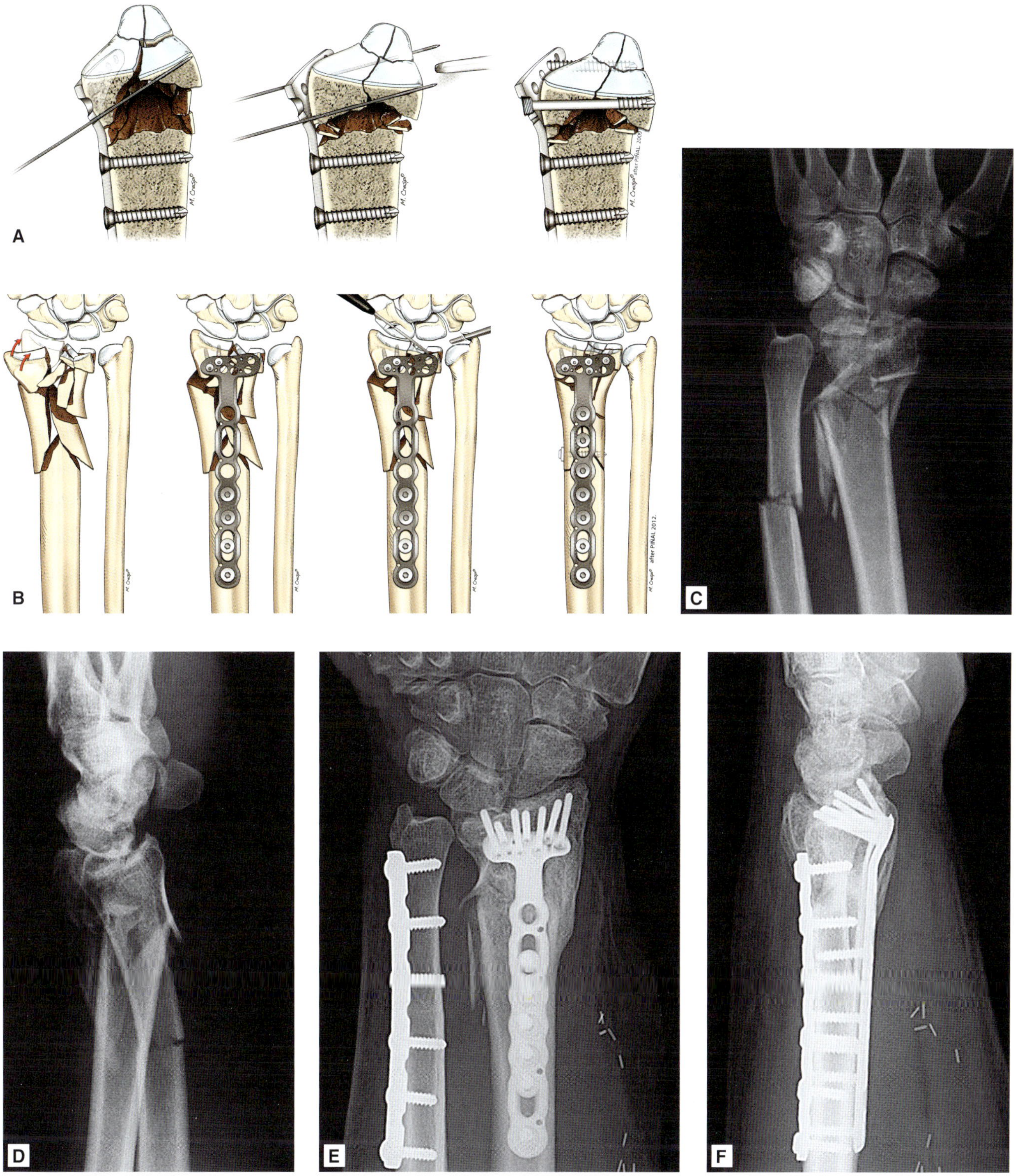

FIGURE 27-12 **A.** If the metaphysis is severely comminuted, the comminuted fragments will not support the temporary K-wire fixation, and secondary displacement may occur. In this scenario it is better to first create a stable articular surface. **B.** The length of the radius is restored by stabilizing the largest articular fragment with 2 pegs using fluoroscopy. The other articular fragments are then assembled to this stable base under arthroscopic control. **C-F.** Clinical case. Preoperative radiograms (left) of a C33 fracture in a manual laborer. Radiograms at 1 year (right) demonstrate that the length of the radius is maintained despite the severe comminution. (Copyright © 2012 by Dr Piñal.)

REFERENCES

1. Augé WK 2nd, Velázquez PA. The application of indirect reduction techniques in the distal radius: the role of adjuvant arthroscopy. *Arthroscopy*. 2000;16:830–835.
2. Ruch DS, Vallee J, Poehling GG, Smith BP, Kuzma GR. Arthroscopic reduction versus fluoroscopic reduction in the management of intra-articular distal radius fractures. *Arthroscopy*. 2004;20:225–230.
3. Edwards CC III, Harasztic J, McGillivary GR, Gutow AP. Intra-articular distal radius fractures: arthroscopic assessment of radiographically assisted reduction. *J Hand Surg Am*. 2001;26:1036–1041.
4. Lutsky K, Boyer MI, Steffen JA, Goldfarb CA. Arthroscopic assessment of intra-articular distal radius fractures after open reduction and internal fixation from a volar approach. *J Hand Surg Am*. 2008;33:476–484.
5. Varitimidis SE, Badekis GK, Dailiana ZH, Hantes ME, Bargiotas K, Malizos K. Treatment of intra-articular fractures of the distal radius: fluoroscopic or arthroscopic reduction? *J Bone Joint Surg Br*. 2008;90:778–785.
6. del Piñal F, García-Bernal FJ, Pisani D, Regalado J, Ayala H, Studer A. Dry arthroscopy of the wrist: surgical technique. *J Hand Surg Am*. 2007;32(1):119–123.
7. del Piñal F. Dry arthroscopy and its applications. *Hand Clin*. 2011;27:335–345.
8. del Piñal F. Technical tips for (dry) arthroscopic reduction and internal fixation of distal radius fractures. *J Hand Surg Am*. 2011;36:1694–1705.
9. del Piñal F, García-Bernal FJ, Delgado J, Sanmartín M, Regalado J, Cerezal L. Correction of malunited intra-articular distal radius fractures with an inside-out osteotomy technique. *J Hand Surg Am*. 2006;31:1029–1034.
10. Herzberg G. Intra-articular fracture of the distal radius: arthroscopic-assisted reduction. *J Hand Surg Am*. 2010;35:1517–1519.
11. Slutsky D. Wrist arthroscopy. In: Wolfe SW, Hotchkiss RM, Pederson WC, Kozin SH, eds. *Green's Operative Hand Surgery*. 6th ed. Philadelphia: Elsevier; 2011:709–741.
12. Medoff RJ. Essential radiographic evaluation for distal radius fractures. *Hand Clin*. 2005;21:279–288.
13. Geissler WB. Arthroscopically assisted reduction of intra-articular fractures of the distal radius. *Hand Clin*. 1995;11:19–29.
14. Forward DP, Lindau TR, Melsom DS. Intercarpal ligament injuries associated with fractures of the distal part of the radius. *J Bone Joint Surg Am*. 2007;89:2334–2340.
15. Lindau T, Adlercreutz C, Aspenberg P. Peripheral tears of the triangular fibrocartilage complex cause distal radioulnar joint instability after distal radial fractures. *J Hand Surg Am*. 2000;25:464–468.
16. Geissler WB, Fernandez DL, Lamey DM. Distal radioulnar joint injuries associated with fractures of the distal radius. *Clin Orthop Relat Res*. 1996;327:135–146.
17. del Piñal F. Treatment of explosion type distal radius fractures. In: del Piñal F, Mathoulin C, Luchetti C, eds. *Arthroscopic Management of Distal Radius Fractures*. Berlin: Springer Verlag; 2010:41–65.
18. Doi K, Hattori Y, Otsuka K, Abe Y, Yamamoto H. Intra-articular fractures of the distal aspect of the radius: arthroscopically assisted reduction compared with open reduction and internal fixation. *J Bone Joint Surg Am*. 1999:81:1093–1110.

28

Malunion and Nonunion of the Distal Radius

Jesse B. Jupiter, MD
Gertrude Gradl, MD

MALUNION

Rationale and Basic Science Pertinent to the Procedure

There has been a dramatic increase in internal fixation of distal radial fractures in the last decade, corresponding with the introduction of the volar locking plating system in 2000.[1,2] While some investigators have observed a substantial decrease in symptomatic malunions following plate fixation, reports have identified between 5% and 15% of patients having a loss of reduction and symptomatic deformity.[3-7]

Changes of carpal alignment in malunions of the distal radius lead to mechanical overload of the radiocarpal and midcarpal joints. This overload can cause ligament attenuation, synovitis, and progressive dynamic instability.[8,9]

Biomechanical studies demonstrated that a residual dorsal or palmar tilt of more than 20° alters load distributions in the radiolunate joint, while a radial shortening of more than 4 to 6 mm produces a positive ulnar variance, predisposing patients to develop ulnar impaction syndrome and triangular fibrocartilage complex lesions.[10,11]

Indications

We consider an osteotomy in patients with distal radius malunion and functional limitations of the forearm with pain or limitation of supination or pronation, loss of flexion or extension, or loss of grip strength. An extra-articular osteotomy is strongly considered in patients with subluxation of the radiocarpal joint or midcarpal instability. An intra-articular osteotomy is also indicated in patients with subluxation of the radiocarpal joint with coronal incongruity or in patients with an intra-articular step-off that is greater than 2 mm.

The ideal candidate includes highly motivated patients with clearly defined symptoms and a preoperative range of motion of no less than 70% of normal. Sedentary, low-demand, elderly patients who have few symptoms and adequate wrist function might not benefit from corrective surgery.

Although the correction of an extra-articular deformity can be safely delayed until the soft tissues offer an ideal surgical environment, and maximal residual function of the wrist has been regained, an intra-articular deformity should be dealt with as soon as possible, before irreversible articular damage occurs. There is no time limit on the osteotomy; rather, advanced osteoarthrosis is the limiting factor; hence, the osteotomy should not be delayed, especially if it leads to arthrosis. Jupiter and coworkers[13] compared the results of early and late osteotomies in 2 similar cohorts and concluded that early correction provided easier radial and DRUJ realignment because of the absence of soft tissue and capsular contractures. The need for structural iliac crest bone graft was diminished because the local nascent callus material was used to fill defects. They concluded that although the functional results are similar in both groups, early surgery resulted in considerably less total disability and an earlier return to work.

Contraindications

Infirmity and poor general health represent formal contraindications to performing a corrective osteotomy. Contraindications also include acceptable hand function despite the malunion, advanced degenerative articular changes, fixed carpal malalignment, limited functional capabilities, severe osteoporosis, or complex regional pain syndrome. Age is not a contraindication to surgery.

Surgical Technique

The required equipment depends on the implants that are used but always includes a small fragment set, an oscillating saw, and an image intensifier. Prophylactic antibiotics (eg, third-generation cephalosporin) are administered within 1 hour prior to surgical incision.

Depending on the need to harvest bone graft from the iliac crest, general or regional anesthesia is used. The patient is placed in a supine position with the forearm on a hand table. The affected arm and wrist as well as the iliac crest are prepped and draped in a standard sterile fashion. The extremity is exsanguinated with an Esmarch bandage, and a pneumatic tourniquet is inflated to 250 mm Hg.

- For dorsally displaced malunions, a dorsal approach has traditionally been used, but with the introduction of fixed-angle implants, it is also possible to use volar approaches. A dorsal exposure allows direct visualization of the articular surface through a dorsal capsulotomy. It is therefore useful for the treatment of extra- or intra-articular malunions associated with dorsal subluxation and simple articular malunions in the sagittal plane. The volar exposure is useful for volar malunions or articular malunions associated with volar subluxation. Use of a volar approach also allows easier correction of a malrotation, less risk of extensor tendon problems, and less requirement for structural bone graft.

DORSAL APPROACH

The dorsal approach was previously in vogue and has been well described.[12]

Preoperative x-rays are performed of the injured and normal sides so that when they are superimposed, they allow one to plan the osteotomy site and measure the angular deformity in the sagittal plane (lateral view) and the frontal plane (anteroposterior view). A 7-cm incision is made starting just distal to Lister's tubercle and moving proximally, incising the extensor retinaculum between the second and third extensor compartments. The extensor pollicis longus tendon is retracted radially and the extensors ulnarly. A small K-wire can be inserted into the radiocarpal joint to gauge the sagittal inclination of the articular surface. If a single angular correction is planned, the osteotomy cut has to be exactly parallel to the joint surface in the sagittal plane. If correction of radial inclination and malrotation is needed, the cut has to be aligned perpendicular to the distal fragment in both the sagittal and AP planes. Two threaded 2.5-mm K-wires are inserted subtending the angle of correction on both sides of the future osteotomy. These K-wires serve not only to guide intraoperative correction but also to manipulate and maintain the distal fragment in the correct position. The osteotomy is performed with an oscillating saw parallel to the distal K-wire, but leaving the volar cortex partially intact. The osteotomy is opened dorsally by flexing the wrist until both K-wires are parallel in the sagittal plane. The brachioradialis is released and the radial length is restored with use of a small laminar spreader. The correction can be temporarily maintained with the aid of a small external fixator. A corticocancellous iliac crest graft is shaped to fit into the defect and held with K-wires. If rotational correction is needed, 1 or 2 K-wires are inserted through the graft into the proximal fragment in the correct axial alignment, and then the distal fragment can be rotated (usually pronated) on the graft to the desired position. A dorsal locking 2.7-mm plate or two 2.4-mm plates can then be applied on the radial border between the wrist extensors and the first dorsal compartment, and dorsoulnarly under the fourth compartment, and then the K-wires are removed.

VOLAR APPROACH

A 7- to 8-cm longitudinal volar radial skin incision is made slightly radial to the flexor carpi radialis (FCR) tendon and the interval between the FCR and radial artery is identified and mobilized. The exposure is helped by release or lengthening of the brachioradialis as well as opening the first extensor compartment. Hohman retractors are placed on either side of the distal radius at the site of the proposed osteotomy.

A 0.6-mm smooth Kirschner wire is placed into the distal fragment parallel to the joint surface in the sagittal plane and perpendicular to the distal fragment in the frontal plane. A second wire is placed perpendicular to the shaft proximal to the site of deformity. The distal component of the plate is fixed temporarily to the distal radius. The drill holes for the most ulnar and radial fixed-angle screws of the proximal row of holes in the volar locking plate are prepared at this point. The plate is removed, and the osteotomy cut is performed from volar to dorsal through the old fracture site perpendicular to the axis of the radius in the anteroposterior plane and parallel to the joint surface in the sagittal plane. It may be preferable in some instances to perform the osteotomy with the plate in place. A bone clamp can be used to pronate the proximal shaft in order to expose the dorsal periosteum and callus that must be released in order to regain radial length, along with any dorsal osteophytes that can cause extensor tendon rupture. Next the plate is fixed to the distal fragment with screws using the predrilled holes. Correction in all 3 planes occurs simultaneously as the proximal part of the plate is progressively reduced to the radial shaft with a bone clamp.

If additional length is required, a laminar spreader can be placed in the osteotomy site to wedge it open. The stability of these fixed-angle devices maintains the radial length even in osteopenic bone. Ring et al showed that there is no need for an iliac crest structural corticocancellous bone graft, and the gap may be filled with morcellized autogenous bone grafts[23] or bone substitutes such as Norian SRS®[13] (Fig. 28-1A-L).

INTRA-ARTICULAR MALUNIONS

Corrective osteotomy of intra-articular malunions is appealing, since articular incongruity is directly associated with the development of radiocarpal arthrosis. A volar, dorsal, or combined approach can be used, depending on the anatomy of the malunion. With the volar approach, the joint is visualized through the osteotomy site, leaving the radiocarpal ligaments intact. With a dorsal approach, the joint is visualized through a capsulotomy. The previous fracture site is identified visually and with image intensification. Smooth 0.045-in K wires are inserted into fracture fragments to be used to "joystick" the fragments for reduction. A sharp osteotome or a small oscillating blade may be used to open the fracture site. If an oscillating blade is used, an incomplete cut is made and then completed with a sharp osteotome.

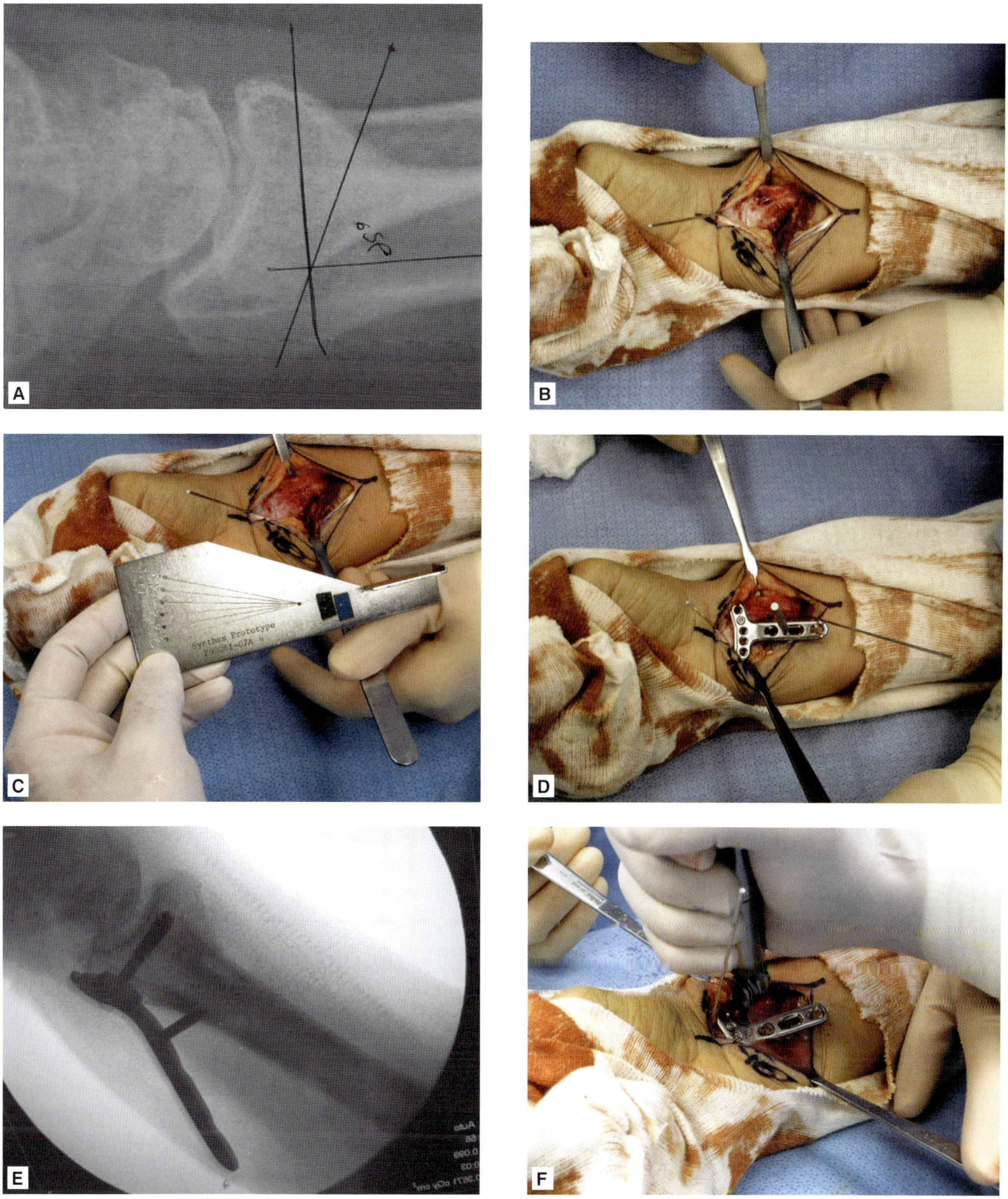

FIGURE 28-1 A dorsally displaced malunion of the distal radius in a 62-year-old woman. **A.** The radiological appearance of the deformity. **B.** A smooth Kirschner wire is inserted into the radiocarpal joint parallel to the dorsally angulated articular surface. **C.** Using a template will allow more precise placement of the proximal Kirschner wire into the radius. **D.** A distal locking screw secures the implant into the distal fragment. **E.** X-ray image confirms the position of the implant in the sagittal plane. A 12-mm screw has been placed in the most distal hole of the straight limb of the plate that will confirm a 25° correction. **F.** With the plate in place an osteotomy is created with a sagittal saw.

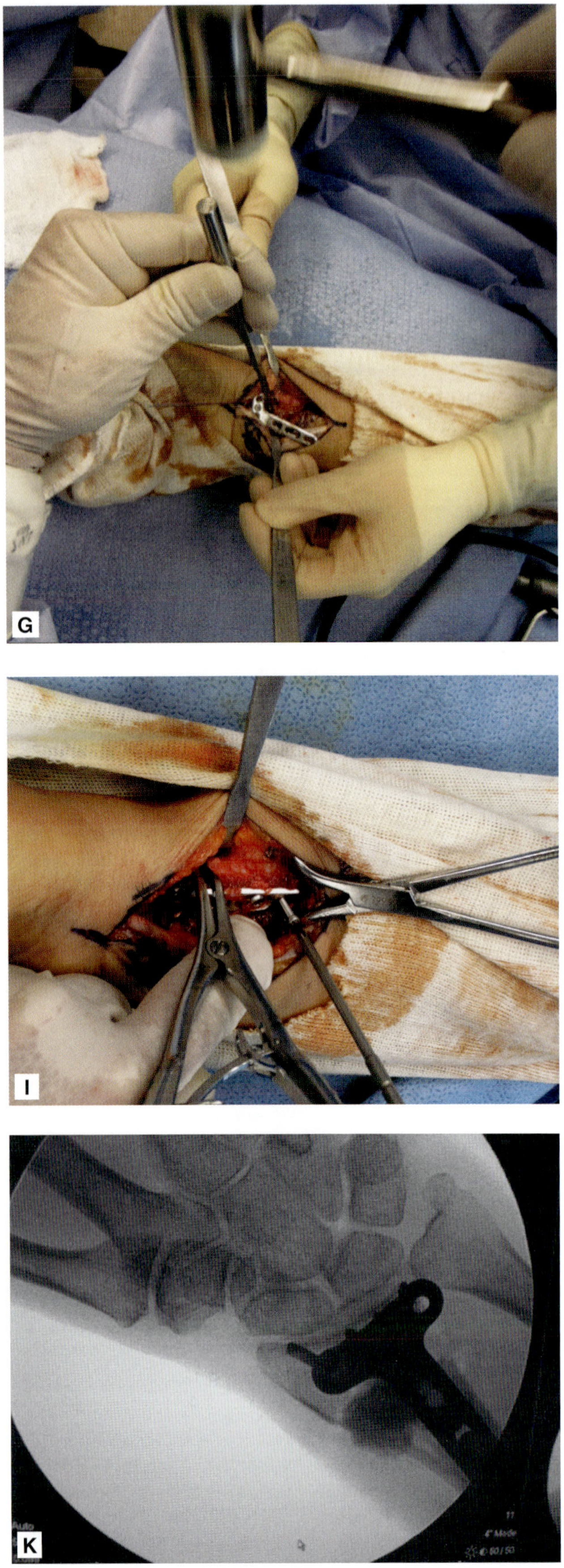

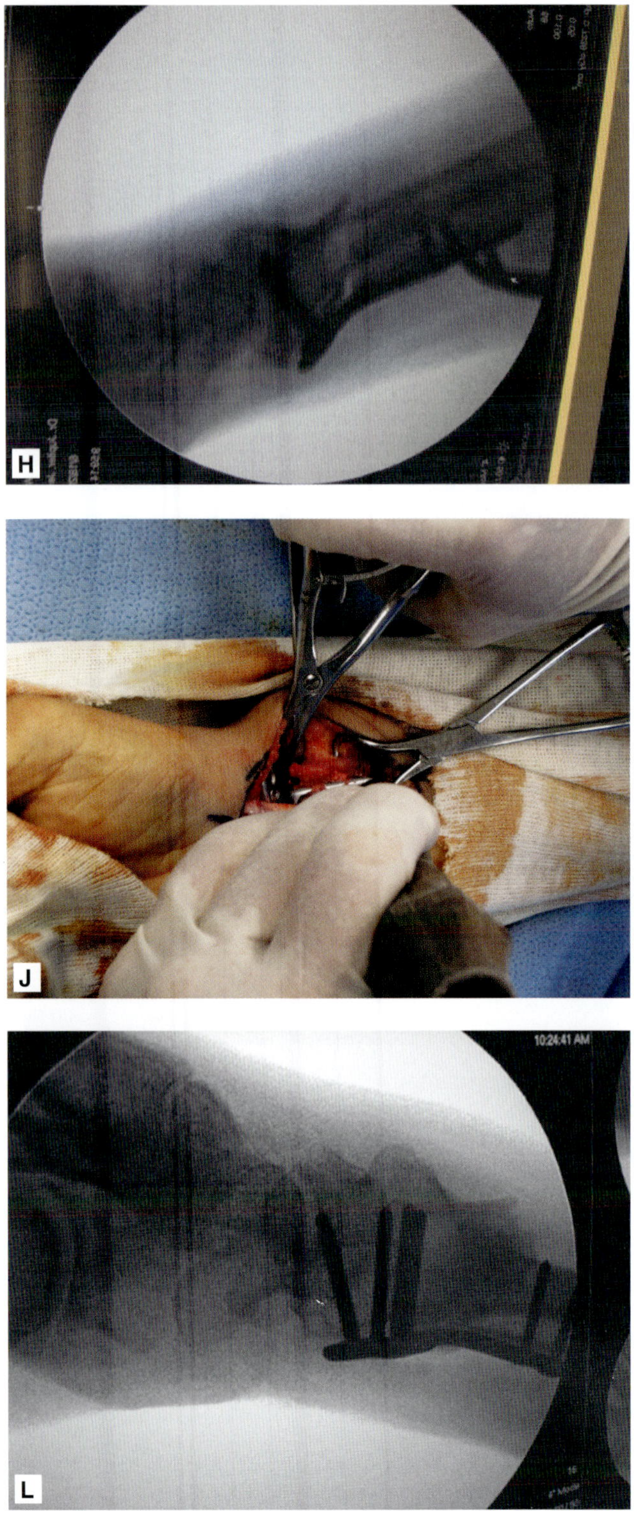

FIGURE 28-1 (*Continued*) **G.** The osteotomy can be safely completed with a thin bladed osteotome. **H.** The initial correction before lengthening. **I.** The laminar spreader is placed into the osteotomy to regain length. **J.** The proximal screws are now placed. **K.** The defect is filled with Norian SRS. **L.** Follow-up radiographs.

An osteotome or small Cobb elevator is then used to gently free the original fracture site and to mobilize the articular fragment into proper position. The fragments are manipulated using the previously placed wires and can be provisionally fixed by using either 0.045- or 0.062-in K wires. Another option is to use a mini-external fixator to hold the joysticks. A plate and screw construct is then applied.

DISTAL RADIOULNAR JOINT

The distal radioulnar joint must be considered with any distal radius osteotomy. The arthritic distal radioulnar joint can be treated with a Darrach, Sauvé-Kapandji, or Bowers hemiresection arthroplasty. We have had clinical success with the Darrach procedure with a Breen-Jupiter stabilization of the residual ulnar shaft using slips of the extensor and flexor carpi ulnaris.[14]

Complications

Complications include infection, wrist stiffness, persistent deformity, loss of reduction, nonunion, symptomatic hardware, hardware failure, tendon rupture, and persisting pain and disability on the ulnar side of the wrist.

Outcome

Sato et al[15] reported their results of 28 corrective osteotomies for volarly malunited distal radius with an average follow-up of 25 months (range, 12-60 months). Pain and wrist range of motion improved in all patients. The modified Mayo wrist score was excellent in 16 patients, good in 10 patients, and fair in 2 patients.

Lozano-Calderon et al[16] reviewed 22 patients with an average follow-up of 13 years (range 6-24 years) after corrective osteotomy for both extra- and intra-articular malunions. Grip strength averaged 71% of the unaffected side and active wrist motion was 79% of the opposite upper extremity. The DASH score averaged 16 points.

While multiple reports exist in the literature on the success of corrective osteotomy of malunion following nonoperative treatment,[17-19] there is a paucity of literature regarding the results after failed plate fixation as the primary fracture treatment. The first and senior author evaluated 18 patients (8 women, 10 men; mean age 41 years) at an average of 7 years (range 2-12 years) after osteotomy of a malunited fracture of the distal radius following failed internal fixation.

Wrist motion and pain improved with the operation in all cases. The average increase in grip strength was 27% (range, 0%-66%). The modified Mayo wrist score averaged 79 points (range, 50-100 points), with 12 excellent, 2 good, and 4 satisfactory results. The DASH score decreased from 59 points (range, 23-90) before the operation to 23 points (range, 1-51) at the time of follow-up. Using the Fernandez point score system there were 10 good, 2 fair, and 6 poor results. Final follow-up radiographs showed an average improvement in dorsal tilt of 17° (range, 8°-25°), an average improvement in volar tilt of 22° (range, 10°-32°), an improvement of 6° radial inclination (range, 22°-31°), and a decrease of 3.1 mm in ulnar variance (range, 2-11 mm).

NONUNION

Rationale and Basic Science Pertinent to the Procedure

Nonunion of the distal radius has been considered rare but is now being reported with increasing frequency.[20,21] This might be attributed to the increasing number of operatively treated fractures. Excessive distraction with an external fixator, unstable fixation, or premature active wrist motion may compromise healing.[20-22] Other factors associated with nonunion include infection, extensive comminution, concomitant fracture of the distal ulna, diabetes, smoking, and certain psychiatric disorders that affect patients' compliance.[23-25] Most nonunions are synovial. The wrist is usually deformed, unstable, and painful. Some patients have a severe radial deviation deformity. Operative treatment can improve upper limb function in patients with nonunion of the distal radius by either fusing the wrist or healing the fracture.

Indications

Patients with limited radiographic evidence of healing 4 months after the injury should be considered to have delayed healing and patients with limited radiographic evidence 6 months after the fracture should be considered to have fracture nonunion. An attempt to gain union and restore at least some amount of wrist motion should be made in active patients with high functional demands.

Contraindications

Infirm, debilitated, and demented patients with limited functional demands can be managed nonoperatively. Active or chronic infection must be eradicated prior to considering surgery. A wrist fusion should be considered if there is less than 5 mm of bone between the lunate facet of the distal radius articular surface and the fracture site.

Surgical Technique

Fernandez et al have outlined 2 important principles that include the concept of applying 2 plates in orthogonal planes and the use of fixed-angle plates. A wrist fusion however may still be necessary with very small distal fragments or for infirm patients where the goal is pain management.[23]

The fracture is approached through a volar Henry approach and any fibrous or synovial tissues are removed from the fracture site. The sclerotic fracture ends are freshened back to bleeding bone and the intramedullary canal is opened with a drill bit to facilitate the ingrowth of vessels. A small distractor can be used to restore length, along with a release of the brachioradialis, but it is often necessary to shorten or resect the distal ulna as well. The resected ulna can be used for bone graft. The fracture fragments are then held with temporary K-wire fixation and the distractor while 2 locking plates are applied at 90° to each other to maintain the reduction. Any bone defects are filled with autogenous cancellous bone (Fig. 28-2A-H).

Complications

In the face of a persistent nonunion the implants will eventually loosen or break. Limited motion, persistent pain, and progressive arthrosis may ultimately necessitate a wrist fusion.

Outcome

Segalman et al reported their results of 12 distal radius nonunions in 11 patients over a 24-year period. Nine fractures were considered to have insufficient metaphyseal bone to allow internal fixation; 6 of these fractures were treated with wrist arthrodesis and 3 patients were treated nonoperatively. Bony union was achieved in all operatively treated fractures.

Fernandez et al[21] reported 3 excellent, 4 good, 2 fair, and 1 poor result at an average of 3 years and 6 months after open reduction and internal fixation of an ununited fracture of the distal radius. All 10 fractures had healed within 3 months. The senior author compared 10 patients with a nonunion of the distal radius in whom the distal fragment had less than 5 mm of subchondral bone supporting the articular surface distal to the site of the nonunion with a group of 13 patients with a nonunion of the distal radius with a larger distal fragment.[20]

At an average follow-up of 28 months, union was achieved in all but 1 patient. Two patients required subsequent operations for distal radioulnar joint dysfunction. Both groups regained an extension–flexion arc of approximately 80°. Active forearm rotation was 140°. According to the Fernandez point score system, only 7 patients had good or excellent results reflecting the salvage nature of these procedures.

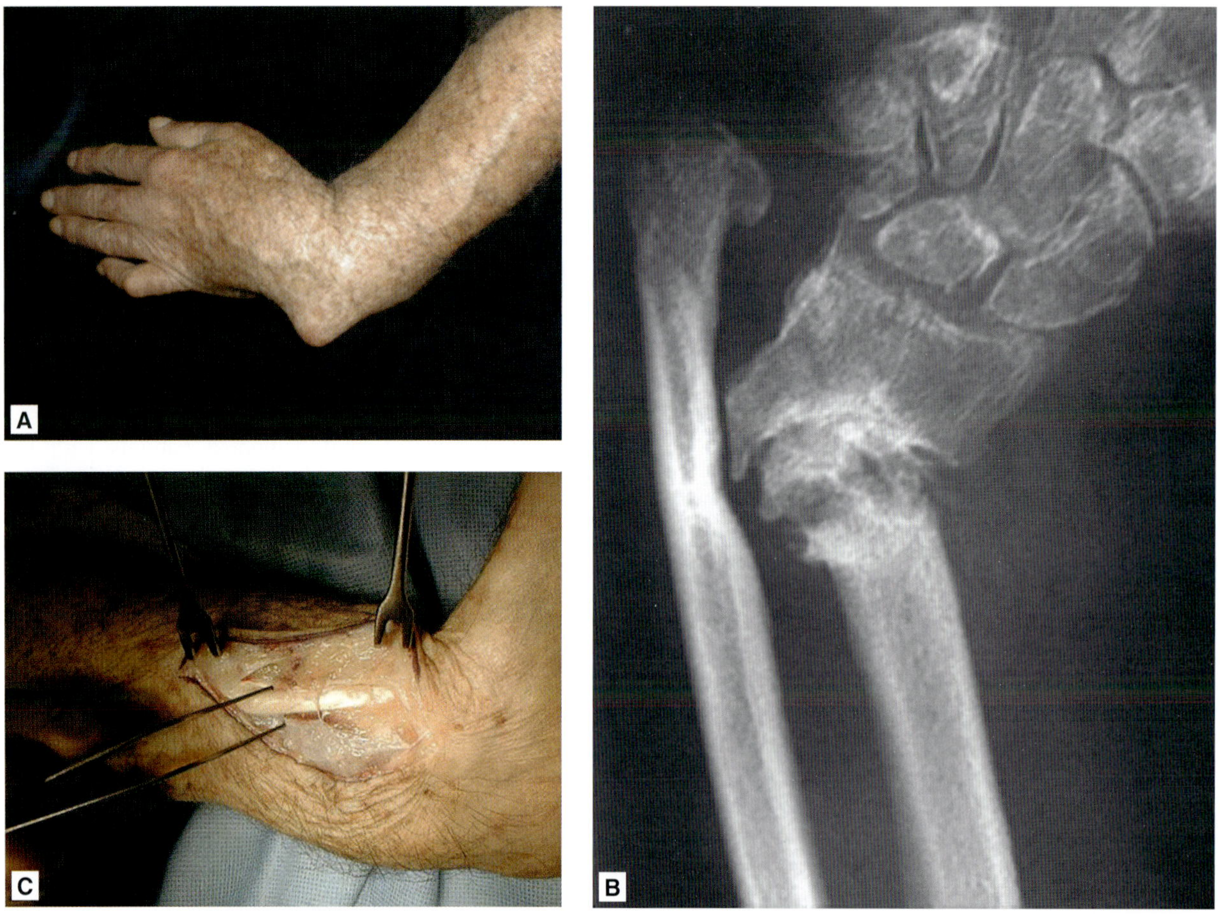

FIGURE 28-2 A long-standing nonunion with extreme shortening and deformity in a 60-year-old male. **A** and **B.** The clinical and radiological appearance of the deformity. **C.** A longitudinal radial-based incision.

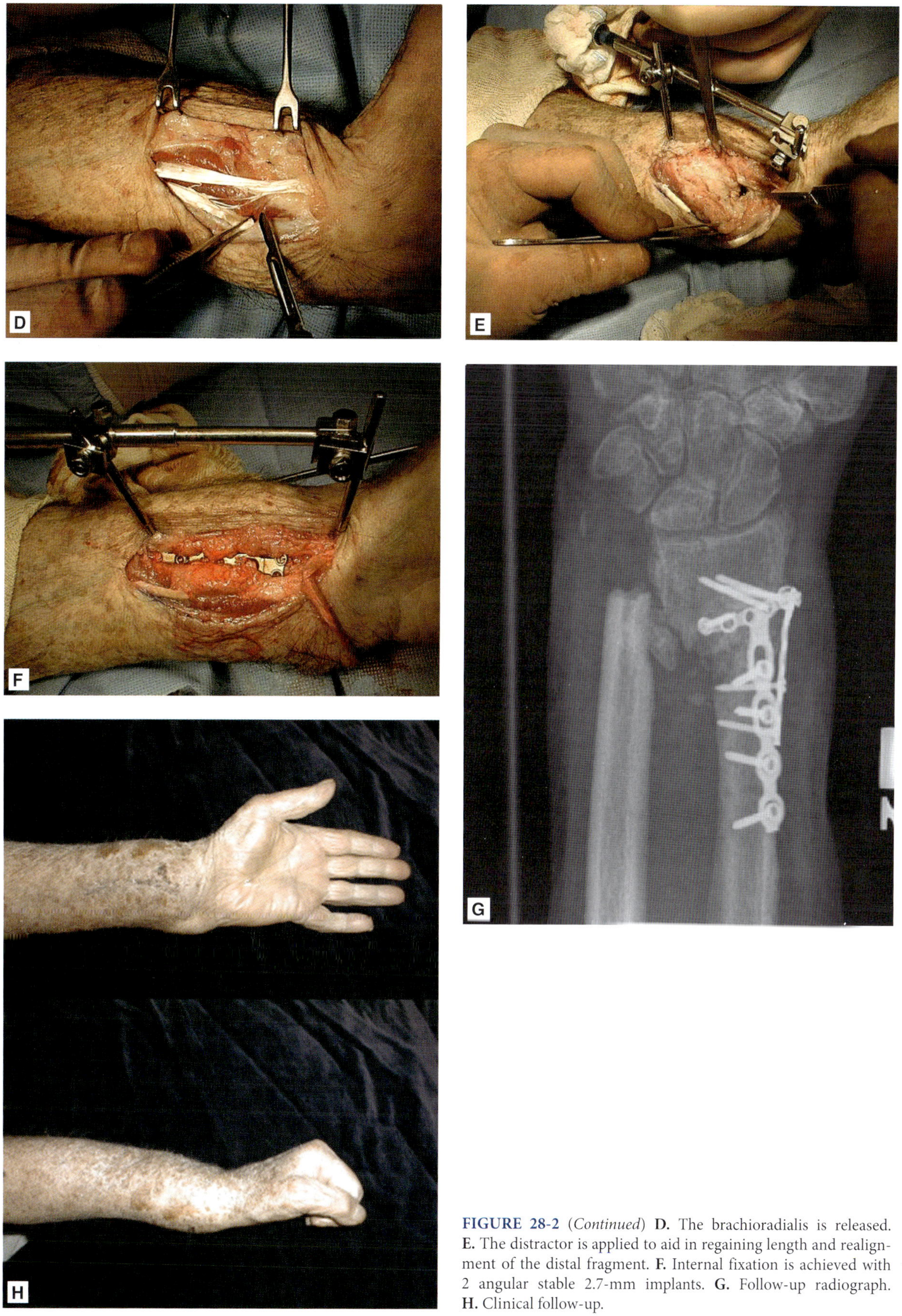

FIGURE 28-2 (*Continued*) **D.** The brachioradialis is released. **E.** The distractor is applied to aid in regaining length and realignment of the distal fragment. **F.** Internal fixation is achieved with 2 angular stable 2.7-mm implants. **G.** Follow-up radiograph. **H.** Clinical follow-up.

REFERENCES

1. Koval KJ, Harrast JJ, Anglen JO, Weinstein JN. Fractures of the distal part of the radius. The evolution of practice over time. Where's the evidence? *J Bone Joint Surg Am.* 2008;90:1855–1861.
2. Chung KC, Shauver MJ, Birkmeyer JD. Trends in the United States in the treatment of distal radial fractures in the elderly. *J Bone Joint Surg Am.* 2009;91:1868–1873.
3. Douthit JD. Volar plating of dorsally comminuted fractures of the distal radius: a 6-year study. *Am J Orthop.* 2005;34:140–147.
4. Chirpaz-Cerbat JM, Ruatti S, Houillon C, Ionescu S. Dorsally displaced distal radius fractures treated by fixed-angle volar plating: grip and pronosupination strength recovery. A prospective study. *Orthop Traumatol Surg Res.* 2011;97:465–470.
5. Hollevoet N. Effect of patient age on malunion of operatively treated distal radius fractures. *Acta Orthop Belg.* 2010;76:743–750.
6. Rozental TD, Beredjiklian PK, Bozentka DJ. Functional outcome and complications following two types of dorsal plating for unstable fractures of the distal part of the radius. *J Bone Joint Surg Am.* 2003; 85-A:1956–1960.
7. Harness NG, Jupiter JB, Orbay JL, Raskin KB, Fernandez DL. Loss of fixation of the volar lunate facet fragment in fractures of the distal part of the radius. *J Bone Joint Surg Am.* 2004;86-A:1900–1908.
8. Taleisnik J, Watson HK. Midcarpal instability caused by malunited fractures of the distal radius. *J Hand Surg Am.* 1984;9:350–357.
9. Park MJ, Cooney WP 3rd, Hahn ME, Looi KP, An KN. The effects of dorsally angulated distal radius fractures on carpal kinematics. *J Hand Surg Am.* 2002;27:223–232.
10. Pogue DJ, Viegas SF, Patterson RM, et al. Effects of distal radius fracture malunion on wrist joint mechanics. *J Hand Surg Am.* 1990; 15:721–727.
11. Kihara H, Palmer AK, Werner FW, Short WH, Fortino MD. The effect of dorsally angulated distal radius fractures on distal radioulnar joint congruency and forearm rotation. *J Hand Surg Am.* 1996;21:40–47.
12. Shea K, Fernandez DL, Jupiter JB, Martin C Jr. Corrective osteotomy for malunited, volarly displaced fractures of the distal end of the radius. *J Bone Joint Surg Am.* 1997;79:1816–1826.
13. Lozano-Calderon S, Moore M, Liebman M, Jupiter JB. Distal radius osteotomy in the elderly patient using angular stable implants and Norian bone cement. *J Hand Surg Am.* 2007;32:976–983.
14. Breen TF, Jupiter JB. Extensor carpi ulnaris and flexor carpi ulnaris tenodesis of the unstable distal ulna. *J Hand Surg Am.* 1989;14:612–617.
15. Sato K, Nakamura T, Iwamoto T, Toyama Y, Ikegami H, Takayama S. Corrective osteotomy for volarly malunited distal radius fracture. *J Hand Surg Am.* 2009;34:27–33, 33.e21.
16. Lozano-Calderon SA, Brouwer KM, Doornberg JN, Goslings JC, Kloen P, Jupiter JB. Long-term outcomes of corrective osteotomy for the treatment of distal radius malunion. *J Hand Surg Eur Vol.* 2010; 35:370–380.
17. Ring D, Prommersberger KJ, Gonzalez del Pino J, Capomassi M, Slullitel M, Jupiter JB. Corrective osteotomy for intra-articular malunion of the distal part of the radius. *J Bone Joint Surg Am.* 2005; 87:1503–1509.
18. Ring D, Roberge C, Morgan T, Jupiter JB. Osteotomy for malunited fractures of the distal radius: a comparison of structural and nonstructural autogenous bone grafts. *J Hand Surg Am.* 2002;27:216–222.
19. Prommersberger KJ, Van Schoonhoven J, Lanz UB. Outcome after corrective osteotomy for malunited fractures of the distal end of the radius. *J Hand Surg Br.* 2002;27:55–60.
20. Prommersberger KJ, Fernandez DL, Ring D, Jupiter JB, Lanz UB. Open reduction and internal fixation of un-united fractures of the distal radius: does the size of the distal fragment affect the result? *Chir Main.* 2002;21:113–123.
21. Fernandez DL, Ring D, Jupiter JB. Surgical management of delayed union and nonunion of distal radius fractures. *J Hand Surg Am.* 2001;26:201–209.
22. Segalman KA, Clark GL. Un-united fractures of the distal radius: a report of 12 cases. *J Hand Surg Am.* 1998;23:914–919.
23. Jain AK, Sinha S. Infected nonunion of the long bones. *Clin Orthop Relat Res.* 2005:57–65.
24. McKee MD, Waddell JP, Yoo D, Richards RR. Nonunion of distal radial fractures associated with distal ulnar shaft fractures: a report of four cases. *J Orthop Trauma.* 1997;11:49–53.
25. Smith VA, Wright TW. Nonunion of the distal radius. *J Hand Surg Br.* 1999;24:601–603.

Radiocarpal Dislocation

Christian Dumontier, MD
Philippe Saffar, MD

29

INTRODUCTION

Radiocarpal dislocations are rare injuries whose description and treatment still remain confusing. Dunn estimated that their frequency was 0.2% of all dislocations, while Moneim et al stated that they could represent 20% of all wrist injuries.[1,2]

Most of the 70 cases reported in the 19th century were not radiocarpal dislocations but intracarpal dislocations, epiphyseal injuries, or very displaced wrist fractures. Since 1901, few cases of radiocarpal dislocation have been reported and misdiagnosis is common. Dunn reported 6 cases in 1972.[1] However, 1 of his cases was a very comminuted distal radial fracture; 1 dislocation was secondary to an anterior marginal rim, and the other to a fracture of the posterior margin. In their review of 438 x-rays, Ilyas et al[3] found a radiocarpal dislocation in 2.7% of patients (12 cases, 10 with associated fracture).

Our review of literature in 1995 yielded 80 cases in the literature since 1921. There have been 3 series since then.[4–6] These injuries are associated with a spectrum of injury patterns. Dorsal dislocations are more common than volar dislocations with 10/2 ratio according to Ilyas et al, as compared with a 23/4 ratio in our series.[3,4] The soft-tissue disruption can lead to radiocarpal instability, resulting in ulnar translocation and multidirectional radiocarpal instability.

MECHANISM OF INJURY

The exact mechanism of radiocarpal dislocation is still unknown. From a literature review and our own experience of 27 cases, we postulated that the dislocation resulted from a combination of wrist hyperextension, frontal deviation, and a rotational movement.[4]

Other authors have postulated that posterior dislocations occur with wrist hyperextension, pronation, and radial deviation.[7–9] Hyperextension alone is unlikely to produce a radiocarpal dislocation[10] (Fig. 29-1).

CLASSIFICATION

Moneim et al[2] classified radiocarpal fracture–dislocations into 2 types based on the presence or absence of concurrent injury to the intercarpal joint. In a type I injury, the normal carpal anatomy is maintained, with dislocation of the radiocarpal joint. Type II injuries involve an associated scapholunate or lunotriquetral ligament injury in addition to the radiocarpal dislocation.

We introduced an anatomic classification based on the type of ligamentous injury.[4] The most important radiocarpal ligaments insert on the radial aspect of the anterior margin of the radius.

Group 1 injuries include pure ligamentous radiocarpal dislocations or dislocations with only a small cortical or radial styloid avulsion fracture (Fig. 29-2). In this group the volar radiocarpal ligaments are torn. This ligamentous tear was sometimes replaced by a chip fracture at the insertion site of the ligaments. Posteriorly, the ligamentous injury presented most often as a capsuloperiosteal avulsion similar to a Bankart lesion rather than a rupture of the dorsal radiocarpal ligaments.

Group 2 injuries include dislocations with a large radial styloid fracture fragment involving at least one-third of the scaphoid fossa of the distal radius (Fig. 29-3). However, in our cases, the radial styloid fragment was not larger than the scaphoid fossa and the fracture line was horizontal, not oblique that we believe is consistent with a traction or rotational injury rather than a compressive force. On the dorsal surface, the ligamentous injury represents more of a capsuloperiosteal avulsion than a tear of the dorsal radiocarpal ligaments. Group 1 dislocations consist of a global ligamentous injury, which have the potential for multidirectional instability and pose a greater management challenge than do group 2 injuries. In group 2 injuries, the radiocarpal ligaments remain attached to the fractured large radial styloid fragment.[11] Stability can more reliably be restored with secure anatomic fixation of the fracture.[12]

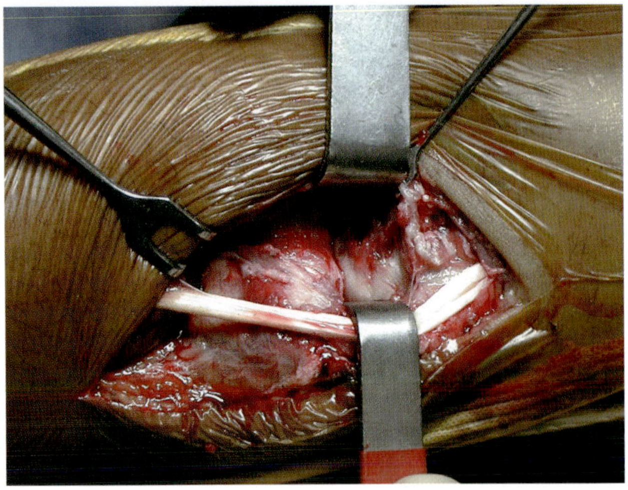

FIGURE 29-1 Preoperative view of an avulsion injury of the DRUJ in a pure radiocarpal dislocation. Most patients in the literature present with DRUJ lesion suggesting a rotational movement during injury.

CLINICAL PRESENTATION

The few series that are available suggest that these injuries are the result of severe high-energy trauma and that they occur most commonly in young men (males 87%, average 32 years, range 17-85). The patient typically presents with a painful, swollen, and deformed wrist. The most common mechanisms of injury are falls from a height, motor vehicle injuries, and industrial injuries.[2,6,10,13] Consequently, open wounds and associated injuries are common. In 1 series of open radiocarpal fracture–dislocations, an associated fracture or injury to other organ systems was found in every patient.[14] Recently Wang et al reported 3 cases of ipsilateral elbow and radiocarpal dislocation.[15]

Neurologic deficits of the injured extremity are common and are often associated with vascular insufficiency of the hand. Arterial occlusion secondary to the deformity may result in ischemia, which should be corrected by expeditious reduction of the joint with longitudinal traction. Neurologic injury is also common, particularly with open injuries.[12] The median nerve is more often involved than is the ulnar nerve. Less commonly, a radiocarpal dislocation may be associated with an irreducible distal radioulnar joint dislocation when soft tissue such as tendon or nerves or osteoarticular fragments become incarcerated within the joint.[4,7,16]

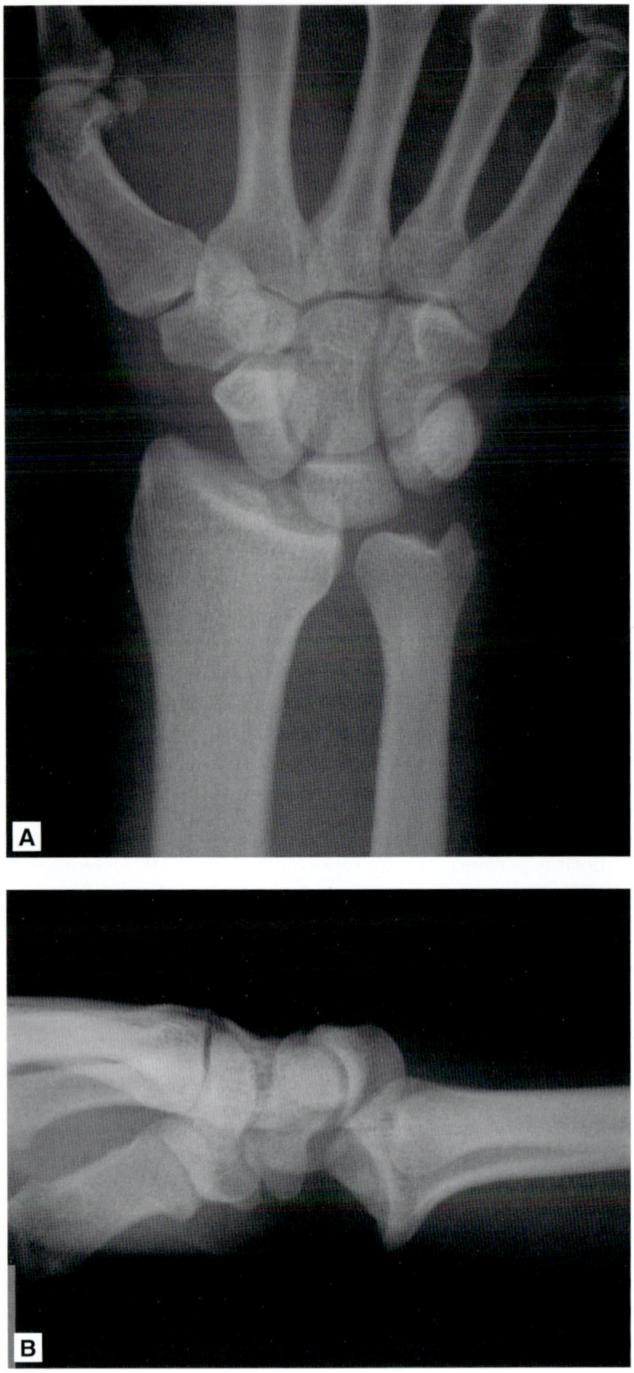

FIGURE 29-2 Pure radiocarpal dislocations are rare injuries with avulsion of ligaments from the radius. Most often these are posterior dislocations. **A.** AP view. **B.** Lateral view.

SURGICAL TREATMENT

As most cases are case reports, with short follow-up, no real consensus exists. Although closed reduction and cast immobilization have been reported to yield satisfactory results, we, as others, consider these injuries to be complex and unstable conditions that routinely warrant surgical reduction and fixation to attain a stable, concentric, and congruent wrist joint. All irreducible dislocations, open injuries, and cases involving neurovascular embarrassment require surgical treatment.

The steps in surgical treatment of radiocarpal fracture–dislocation are as follows[12]:

1. First, a provisional radiocarpal joint reduction is performed with longitudinal traction. An extensile volar

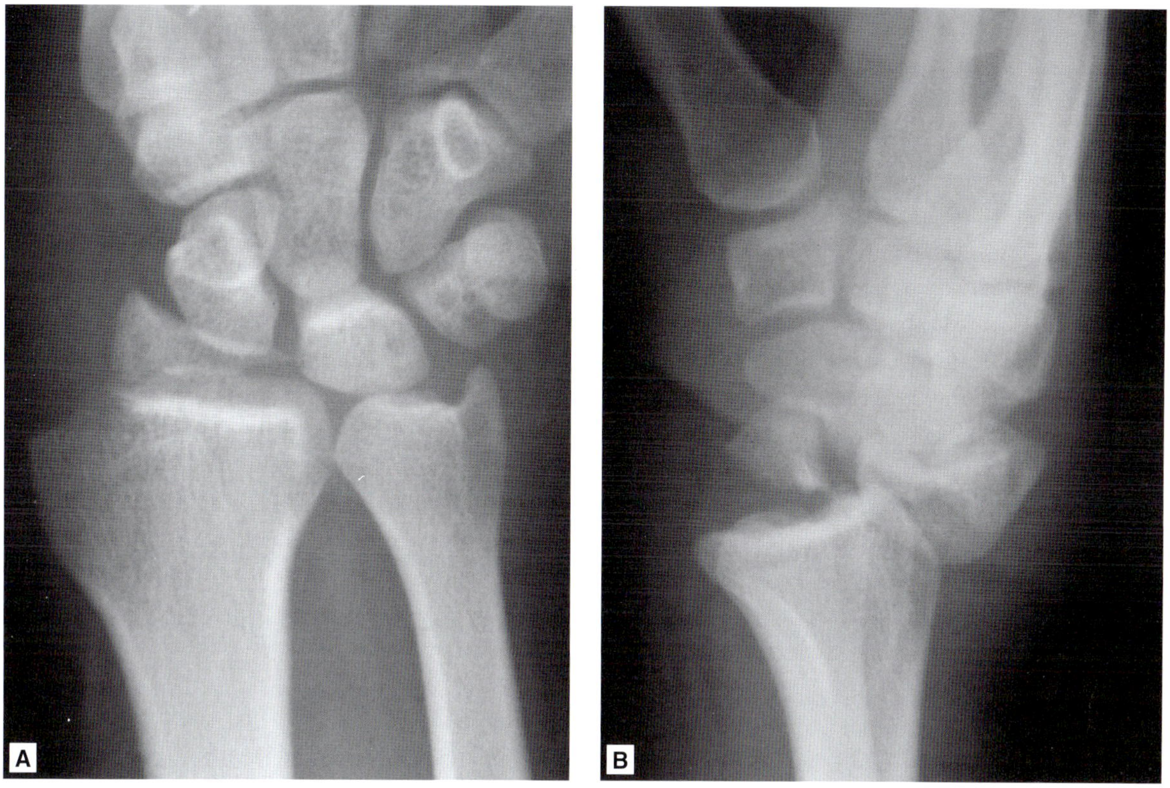

FIGURE 29-3 In group 2 radiocarpal dislocations, an associated fracture of the radial styloid is seen. However, in most patients, the fracture line is mostly horizontal and represents more of a rotational injury. **A.** AP view. **B.** Lateral view.

approach ulnar to the flexor tendons and median nerve is used so that both the carpal tunnel and Guyon canal can be decompressed as needed.

2. The radiocarpal joint is examined through the volar capsular site of disruption and debrided of any loose cartilage or bone fragments. Stay sutures or suture anchors are then placed in the area of capsular and ligament disruption but are not tied down.
3. Fluoroscopy is used to identify any carpal fractures or interosseous ligament injuries that are confirmed and treated through a separate dorsal incision.
4. If needed, the fractured radial styloid is accurately reduced and internally fixed with a Kirschner wire, a compression screw, or plate (Fig. 29-4). The stay sutures that were previously placed to repair the extrinsic volar ligaments are now tied. The origins of the short radiolunate and radioscaphocapitate ligaments are repaired in particular to avoid late volar subluxation or ulnar translocation, respectively. Reduction and stability of the fixation is confirmed both visually and radiographically. The ulnar column is exposed in the case of distal radioulnar joint instability and the ulnocarpal ligaments are reattached. Large ulnar styloid fractures require internal fixation with screws or tension band wiring. This procedure usually restores a concentric distal radioulnar joint. In the presence of persistent instability, the distal radioulnar joint is examined and evacuated of any interposed tissue, followed by repair of the ulnocarpal ligaments. Persistent instability can be addressed by pinning the distal radioulnar joint in midsupination.

Additional stability to the construct can be provided with the use of an external fixator or radiolunate pin.

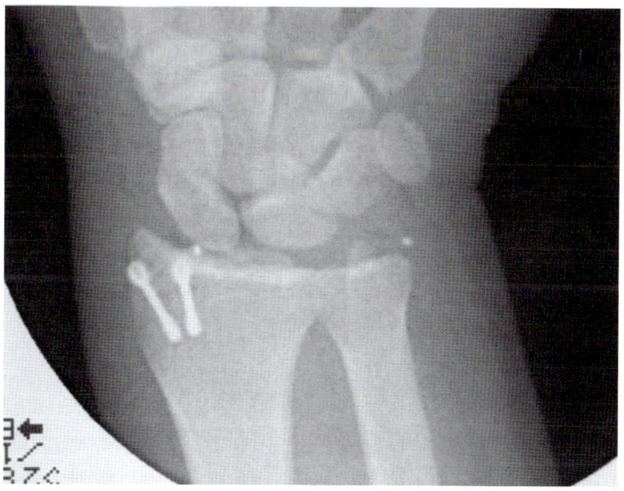

FIGURE 29-4 Screw fixation of the styloid fragment in a group 2 dislocation.

COMPLICATIONS

The most common complication following radiocarpal dislocation or fracture–dislocation is residual loss of motion and instability. On average, a patient can expect to lose 30% to 40% of total arc of wrist flexion/extension. The other major complication is posttraumatic arthritis related to residual articular step-off. Chronic radiocarpal and distal radioulnar instability or ulnar translation of the carpus are more common with group 1 injury patterns. Some patients may present with chronic anterior or ulnar translation when the gravity of the initial injury has been missed.[17] Less commonly, septic arthritis, tendon rupture, and hardware irritation have been reported.[4,12]

OUTCOME

Mudgal et al[6] reported on a series of 12 patients who presented with a radiocarpal fracture–dislocation. Four cases were open injuries, 7 had neurologic compromise, 2 had an intercarpal ligamentous injury, and 5 had an associated injury. Excluding patients with concomitant intercarpal injury, the mean wrist motion at the final follow-up consisted of 53° of extension, 59° of flexion, 82° of pronation, and 74° of supination. These results are consistent with the other large series in the literature, which indicate that an overall 30% to 40% decrease in total arc of wrist flexion–extension can be expected following successful open treatment.[4,5,14,18]

Three of 12 patients of series of Mudgal et al[6] and of Girard et al[5] had evidence of radiocarpal arthritis. Schoenecker et al[9] reported that 4 of the 6 patients in their series developed arthritis. Five out of 6 patients in the series by Le Nen et al[19] had some narrowing of their radiocarpal joint. Oberladstätter et al[18] reported 5 patients out of 8 having mild-to-moderate arthritis. We found that 3 of our 27 patients developed radiocarpal arthritis (Fig. 29-5).

Factors predictive of poor outcome include open injury, complete radiocarpal ligamentous avulsion, associated nerve injury, intercarpal ligamentous injury, and other body part injuries. Neurologic injuries are generally neurapraxic, and resolution can be expected with decompression. More severe nerve compression or stretch injuries result in an inconsistent neurologic recovery. Nyquist and Stern[14] reported on 10 cases of open radiocarpal fracture–dislocations in which all 10 were complicated by an associated injury and 7 involved neurologic compromise. At follow-up, all patients had variable and inconsistent recovery of sensibility.

In 2001 we published a series of 27 cases of recent radiocarpal dislocations. Four were volarly displaced and 23 dorsally. Twenty patients were males and 7 were females, with an average age of 32.3 years (18-58). Thirteen patients dislocated their right wrist, 13 their left wrist, and it was not detailed in 1 case. All dislocations were closed injuries and 17 patients presented with associated lesions. Only 3 patients had no associated lesions while medical data were lacking for 7 patients.

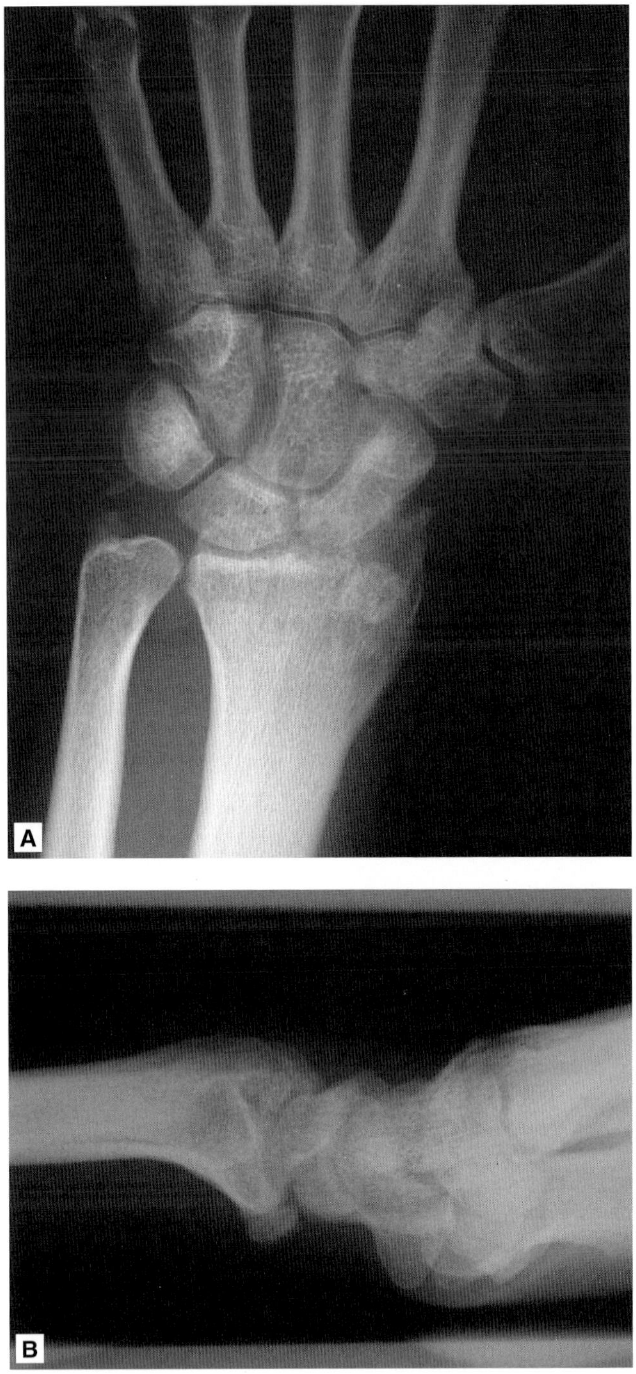

FIGURE 29-5 Early degenerative changes in a group 1 radiocarpal dislocation. **A.** Narrowing of the joint space. **B.** Ossification of the injured anterior ligaments is seen on the lateral view.

Fourteen patients presented at the time of injury with a distal radioulnar joint lesion: 1 patient presented with an irreducible distal radioulnar joint dislocation due to the interposition of the flexor digitorum profundus of the small finger. Four patients had a severe distal radioulnar joint instability that required radioulnar stabilization with K-wires. The other 9 patients had an ulnar styloid fracture.

Group 1 patients included 2 cases of pure dislocation: 1 anterior and 1 posterior who presented 4 days after trauma. Under anesthesia, these 2 cases proved to be highly unstable, with persistent subluxation and ulnar translocation after close reduction. Both cases required percutaneous K-wire stabilization. Two patients had a posterior radiocarpal dislocation with associated ulnar styloid fracture. One patient who was treated conservatively developed an ulnar translocation of the carpus while still in his cast. He refused further treatment and, at the 6-year follow-up, was still able to work as a garage mechanic.

Three patients had a dorsal radiocarpal dislocation with a fracture of only the tip of the radial styloid. Two developed a global carpal ulnar translocation while the other had an ulnar translocation of the carpus with a late development of an increased scapholunate gap.

Patients in group 2 presented with a radiocarpal dislocation and an associated fracture of the scaphoid fossa of the radius. We found that the configuration of the radial styloid fracture line was very horizontal and never extended ulnar to the scaphoid fossa. Posteriorly, the ligamentous injury presented most often as a capsuloperiosteal avulsion.

Three patients presented with anterior radiocarpal dislocation, of whom 2 had an associated fracture of the scaphoid fossa and 1 only chip fracture of the anterior margin of the radius. Seventeen patients presented with dorsal radiocarpal dislocation and a scaphoid fossa fracture.

Group 1 patients (n = 7) were reviewed at an average follow-up of 26.8 months. Four reported slight pain and 1 moderate pain. Pronation was 76°, supination 66°, wrist flexion 54°, wrist extension 54°, radial inclination 15°, and ulnar inclination 18°. The average grip strength was 35 kg. One patient was highly unstable at the time of injury. His carpus was fixed with K-wires and at a 16-month follow-up, his carpus remained stable under fluoroscopic evaluation. The 4 other patients developed an ulnar translocation of the carpus without scapholunate dissociation in 3 and with scapholunate dissociation in 1.

Group 2 patients (n = 20) were reviewed at an average follow-up of 53 months. Among the 13 patients available for follow-up, 6 reported no pain, 4 slight pain, and 2 moderate pain. Mean pronation was 62°, supination 75°, wrist flexion 50°, wrist extension 55°, radial inclination 21°, and ulnar inclination 38°. Average grip strength was 37 kg. Six patients presented with complications: 1 patient developed a K-wire infection and septic arthritis that was treated with splinting and intravenous antibiotics. She required a secondary distal ulna resection for DRUJ stiffness. One patient had a pronosupination deficit and was treated with a Sauvé-Kapandji procedure. Three patients developed posttraumatic arthritis due to the persistence of an articular step-off. One also had a secondary flexor tendon rupture. Another patient had a persistent chronic posterior subluxation of the carpus on x-rays.

CONCLUSION

Radiocarpal dislocations are rare and severe injuries. Classification in 2 groups helps to understand the best treatment option. In group 1, ligamentous injuries are more important and should be addressed to avoid instability. In group 2, adequate bony fixation provides stability. However, in both groups, the associated lesions may limit the functional recovery and should be addressed at the same time.

REFERENCES

1. Dunn AW. Fractures and dislocations of the carpus. *Surg Clin North Am.* 1972;52:1513–1538.
2. Moneim MS, Bolger JT, Omer GEJ. Radiocarpal dislocation—classification and rationale for management. *Clin Orthop.* 1985; 192:199–209.
3. Ilyas AM, Williamson C, Mugdal CS. Radiocarpal dislocation. Is it a rare injury? *J Hand Surg Eur Vol.* 2011;36(2):164–165.
4. Dumontier C, Meyer zu Reckendorf G, Sautet A, Lenoble E, Saffar P, Allieu Y. Radiocarpal dislocations: classification and proposal for treatment. A review of twenty-seven cases. *J Bone Joint Surg Am.* 2001;83: 212–218.
5. Girard J, Cassagnaud X, Maynou C, Bachour F, Prodhomme G, Mestdagh H. Luxation radiocarpienne: 12 cas et revue de la littérature [Radiocarpal dislocation: twelve cases and a review of the literature]. *Rev Chir Orthop Reparatrice Appar Mot.* 2004;90(5):426–433.
6. Mudgal CS, Psenica J, Jupiter JB. Radiocarpal fracture–dislocation. *J Hand Surg Br.* 1999;24:92–98.
7. Fernandez DL. Irreducible radiocarpal fracture–dislocation and radioulnar dissociation with entrapment of the ulnar nerve, artery and flexor profundus II-V. Case report. *J Hand Surg Am.* 1981;6:456–461.
8. Gerard Y, Schernberg F, Elzein F. Les luxations fractures postérieures de la radio-carpienne [Posterior radiocarpal fracture–dislocations]. *Rev Chir Orthop.* 1981;67:92–96.
9. Schoenecker PL, Gilula LA, Shively RA, Manske PR. Radiocarpal fracture dislocation. *Clin Orthop.* 1985;197:237–244.
10. Bilos ZJ, Pankovich AM, Yela S. Fracture dislocation of the radiocarpal joint. *J Bone Joint Surg Am.* 1977;59A:198–203.
11. Siegel DB, Gelberman RH. Radial styloidectomy: an anatomical study with special reference to radiocarpal intracapsular ligamentous morphology. *J Hand Surg Am.* 1991;16:40–44.
12. Ilyas AM, Mudgal CS. Radiocarpal fracture–dislocations. *J Am Acad Orthop Surg.* 2008;16:647–655.
13. Dumontier C, Lenoble E, Saffar P. Radiocarpal dislocations and fracture–dislocations. In: Saffar P, Cooney WP III, eds. *Fractures of the Distal Radius.* London, UK: Martin Dunitz; 1995:267–279.
14. Nyquist SR, Stern PJ. Open radiocarpal fracture–dislocations. *J Hand Surg Am.* 1984;9:707–710.
15. Wang GX, Zhu XJ, Wang ZG, Zhou HD. Operative treatment for adult patients with simultaneous fracture and dislocation of ipsilateral elbow and radiocarpal joint: 3 cases report. *Zhongguo Gu Shang.* 2012;25(4):345–347 [in Chinese].
16. Ayekoloye CI, Shah N, Kumar A, Kurdy N. Irreducible dorsal radiocarpal fracture dislocation with dissociation of the distal radioulnar joint: a case report. *Acta Orthop Belg.* 2002;68:171–174.
17. Freeland AE, Ferguson CA, McCraney WO. Palmar radiocarpal dislocation resulting in ulnar radiocarpal translocation and multidirectional instability. *Orthopedics.* 2006;29(7):604–608.
18. Oberladstätter J, Arora R, Dallapozza C, Smekal V, Rieger M, Lutz M. Sagittal wrist motion following dorsal radiocarpal fracture dislocations. *Handchir Mikrochir Plast Chir.* 2007;39:49–53.
19. Le Nen D, Riot O, Caro P, Lefevre C, Courtois B. Luxations-fractures de la radiocarpienne. Etude clinique de 6 cas et revue de la littérature. *Ann Chir Main Mbre Sup.* 1991;10:5–12.

IV

DISTAL RADIOULNAR JOINT

30

Causes and Management of Acute and Chronic Distal Radioulnar Joint Instability

Toshiyasu Nakamura, MD, PhD

CAUSES OF DISTAL RADIOULNAR JOINT INSTABILITY

Mechanism of Distal Radioulnar Joint Instability

The distal radioulnar joint (DRUJ) is a cylindrical joint consisting of the sigmoid notch of the radius, the head of the ulna, triangular fibrocartilage complex (TFCC), and the dorsal and palmar joint capsules.[1,2] The TFCC also consists of the articular disc, radioulnar ligament (RUL), ulnolunate ligament, ulnotriquetral ligament, meniscus homologue, and sheath floor of the extensor carpi ulnaris (ECU).[3,4] The RUL is considered the primary stabilizer of the DRUJ throughout forearm rotation.[4–6] It originates from the fovea of the ulna and the base of the ulnar styloid process, passes on the proximal surface of the TFCC, and is bifurcated into dorsal and palmar portions. The dorsal portion then attaches to the very dorsal edge of the sigmoid notch of the radius and the palmar portion attaches to the very palmar edges of the sigmoid notch of the radius (Fig. 30-1).[7,8]

The DRUJ has incongruity since the diameter of the sigmoid notch of the radius is larger than that of the ulnar head. This incongruity leads to slight dorsopalmar translation between the radius and ulna during pronation–supination motions (Fig. 30-2).[1,2] This DRUJ incongruity is more obvious in the neutral and palmar positions, while the DRUJ becomes taut likely due to balancing of the pronator quadratus (PQ) and ECU muscles in the supinated position.[2]

Some investigators defined DRUJ instability as a static dislocation or subluxation of the joint detected by CT,[9] even though patients with DRUJ dislocation are rarely reported. Clinically, patients with DRUJ instability do not clearly demonstrate dislocation of the DRUJ. They may often report a "click" or "slack" during forearm rotational movements.[10] The "click" or "slack" is probably due to a small abnormal translation or a "clunk-like" motion of the radius to the ulna during dynamic motion (Fig. 30-3).[10] Dislocation should represent the static situation rather than the dynamic.[9] Rupture of the entire or distal structure of the interosseous membrane (IOM) of the forearm and TFCC would be needed to produce static dislocation of the DRUJ; however, small abnormal movements between the radius and ulna within the DRUJ can occur at specific positions during dynamic forearm rotation to produce a case of "dynamic" DRUJ instability[10] (Fig. 30-3).

The precise mechanism of producing DRUJ instability has not yet been completely revealed. There are several factors that may influence DRUJ instability such as bony incongruity due to forearm bony malunion, altered axis of rotation, soft tissue injury of the TFCC and IOM, and dynamic factors producing muscle deficiency, primarily of the PQ and ECU.[10] Since the TFCC is a primary stabilizer for the DRUJ, a torn TFCC produces DRUJ instability. Avulsion of the RUL from the fovea of the ulna may induce severe DRUJ instability, because the ulnar fovea is the widest attachment area for the RUL (Fig. 30-1).[4,5,11]

Palmer[12] classified TFCC tears into traumatic (Class 1) and degenerative (Class 2) tears. Traumatic TFCC tears were also subclassified as central tears (1A), ulnar tears (1B), distal tears (1C), and radial tears (1D) based on the clinical patterns seen with radiocarpal arthroscopy.[12] Palmer 1B tears are also recognized as peripheral tears of the TFCC, which may be associated with an ulnar styloid fracture. This is because the TFCC attachment to the ulnar styloid had been reported initially in the 1980s and 1990s. As the TFCC is anchored to the ulnar fovea and base of the styloid, a hyperrotation force or dislocation force applied to the RUL from the ulnar head, such as in fall, may disrupt the RUL not only from the ulnar styloid but also from the fovea.[13,14]

A foveal detachment of the TFCC is clearly evident in clinical practice.[13,14] Atzei[15] recently subclassified the Palmer 1B tear into a distal component, a proximal component, or both (complete). An isolated foveal detachment is equivalent to a proximal component tear. A central slit tear (1A) does not demonstrate severe DRUJ instability. Radial avulsion (1D) of the TFCC, including both or either the

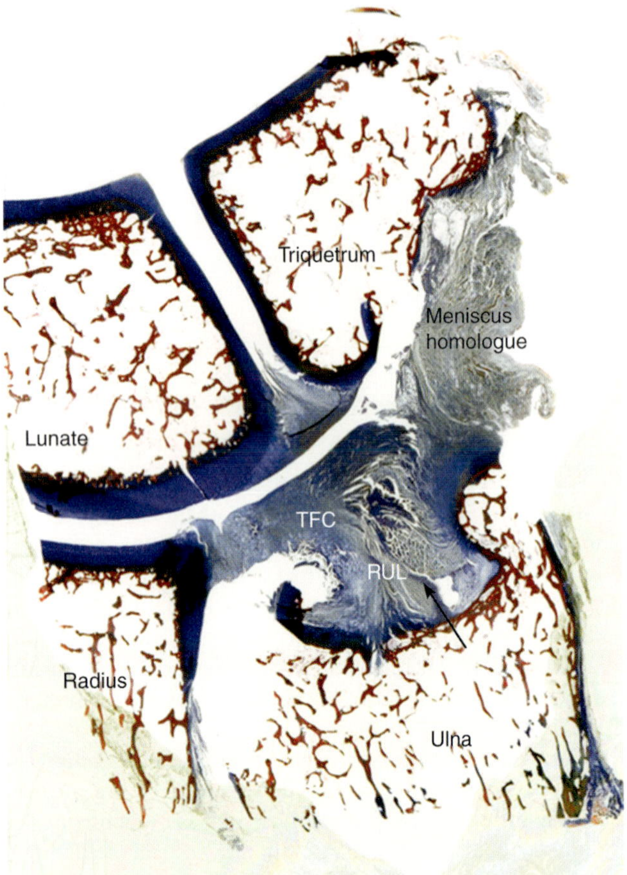

FIGURE 30-1 Histologic section of the DRUJ, consisting of the radius, ulna, lunate, triquetrum, triangular fibrocartilage (TFC), and radioulnar ligament (RUL). Vertical origin of the RUL from the wide area of the ulnar fovea is noted (arrow).

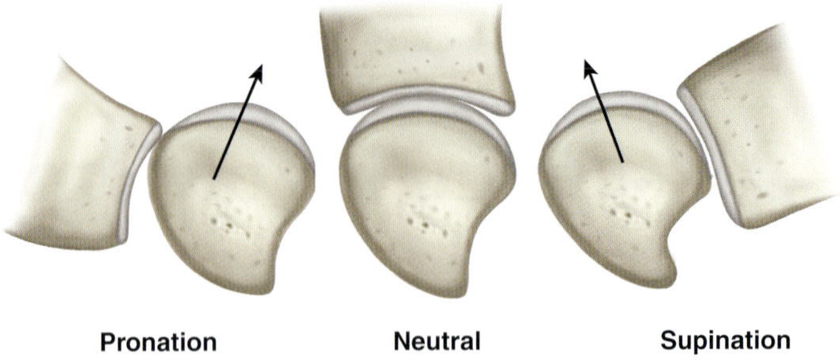

FIGURE 30-2 Illustration of the DRUJ during pronation–supination, which indicates slight dorsopalmar translation between the 2 bones during the pronation–supination motion.

dorsal or palmar rim (where the RUL passes), also reveals DRUJ instability,[16] while a radial tear inside the TFC, commonly seen in clinical practice, may not produce DRUJ instability.

The distal portion of the TFCC is like a hammock, which includes, surrounds, and supports the ulnar carpus, and is very stable with 2 tight anchors to the fovea. Once the anchors are disrupted, the hammock is unsteady. DRUJ stability can be achieved by reanchoring the RUL, with arthroscopic or open repair,[14] or reconstruction using the palmaris longus tendon.[17]

Clinical Evaluation of DRUJ Instability

There are several clinical or physical techniques used to assess DRUJ stability. These testing maneuvers include the

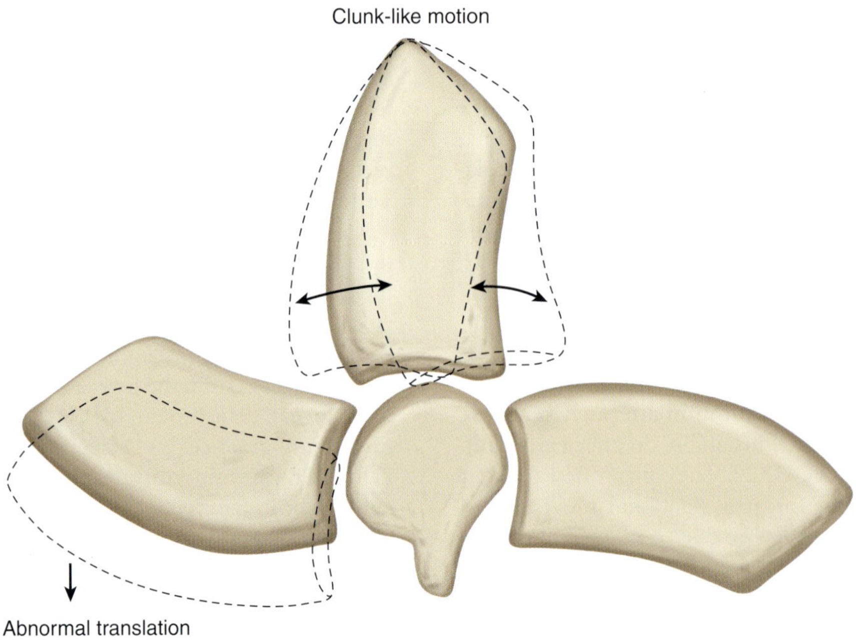

FIGURE 30-3 Schematic of mechanism of DRUJ instability indicating abnormal translation (arrow) or clunk-like motion (arrowheads).

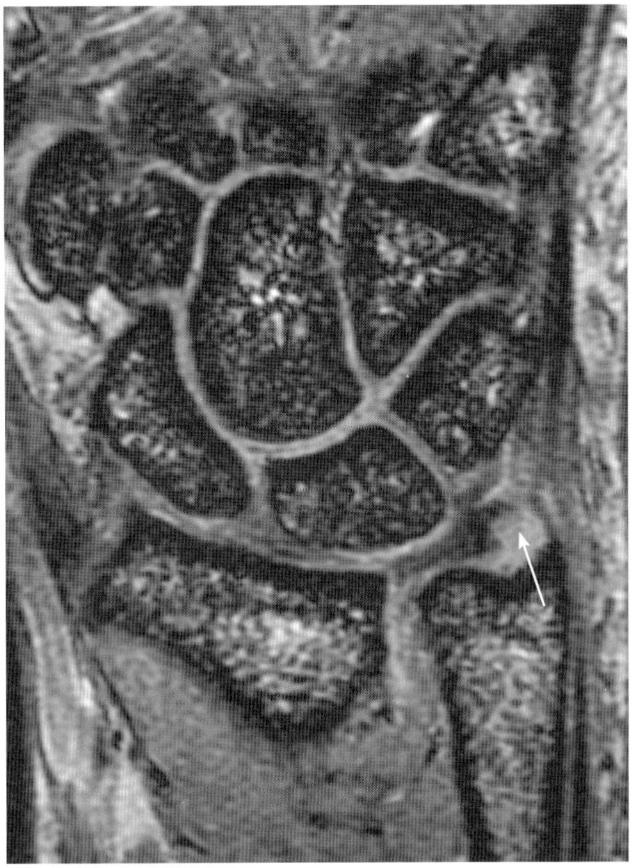

FIGURE 30-4 MRI of TFCC foveal detachment. Note the high-signal-intensity area at the fovea without a low-signal ligament structure (arrow).

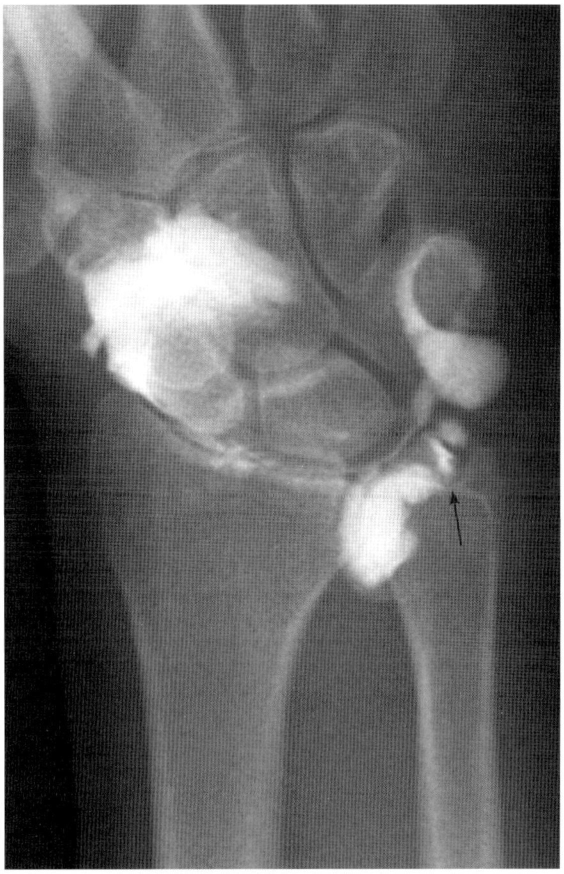

FIGURE 30-5 Arthrogram of foveal tear. Dye infiltrates to the fovea lesion of the TFCC that indicates a foveal avulsion (arrow).

ulnocarpal stress test, fovea sign, and DRUJ instability test. The ulnocarpal stress test is effective for assessing a TFCC tear. Tenderness on the palmar side of the base of the ulnar styloid is a positive foveal sign and suggests a foveal tear.[18] Tenderness of the dorsal aspect of the fovea may also indicate foveal detachment. The most reliable physical test for DRUJ instability is the ballottement test, in which dorsopalmar stability between the ulna and radius is examined in the neutral, pronated, and supinated positions.[14,19] There may not be a foveal tear when a firm "end point" is felt, which indicates ligamentous restraint. A complete foveal detachment would result in a situation in which no "end point" is found, demonstrating multidirectional DRUJ instability. A partial RUL tear would clinically present with a firm "end point" with increased excursion in either the dorsal or palmar direction. The piano-key sign, which presents as a floating ulnar head in the pronation position, may also help to diagnose a foveal avulsion.

MRI can clearly demonstrate a TFCC tear including foveal detachment (Fig. 30-4). An arthrogram also shows pooling of the dye at the fovea and inclusion of the dye between the TFCC and ulnar fovea when there is TFCC foveal detachment (Fig. 30-5), or dye infiltration into the proximal side of the TFCC.

Radiocarpal arthroscopy using a 1.9- to 2.7-mm arthroscope can successfully evaluate TFCC injuries. The 3-4 portal is used for the arthroscope and the 4-5 or 6R portal is used for the probe during the procedure. Associated soft tissue injury, such as scapholunate interosseous ligament tears, can be detected through radiocarpal arthroscopy. The distal surface of the TFCC can also be visualized during radiocarpal arthroscopy. In DRUJ instability patients, radiocarpal arthroscopy can only demonstrate the loss of the trampoline effect and the loss of peripheral tension (positive hook test[15]) in the disc in those with foveal disruption, since the TFCC is not continuously connected to the ulna.

This author recommends DRUJ arthroscopy for evaluation of the foveal origin of the RUL, which can directly visualize a TFCC rupture (Fig. 30-6). The DRUJ (distal) portal is just 5 mm proximal to the 6R portal, just ulnar to the extensor digiti minimi tendon and just distal to the head of the ulna. Saline is used to expand the DRUJ. Mosquito forceps divide the subcutaneous tissue, and then the tip of the mosquito forceps is advanced until it reaches the head of the ulna. The forceps are then used to gradually divide and penetrate the upper side of the DRUJ joint capsule and then to enter the joint. The mosquito forceps are next used to guide the 1.9-mm scope into the DRUJ.

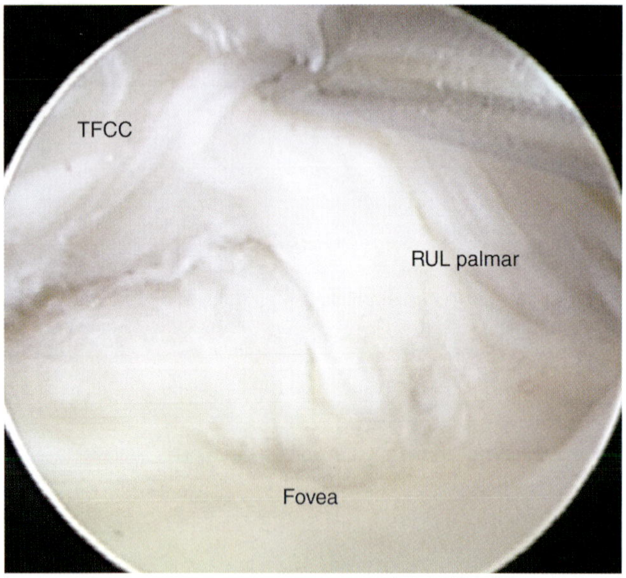

FIGURE 30-6 DRUJ arthroscopy offers direct visualization of the ulnar head, radial sigmoid notch, proximal surface of the TFCC, fovea, and RUL. This case shows an absence of the dorsal portion of the radioulnar ligament (RUL). The palmar portion of the RUL is intact.

The DRUJ space including the fovea area can easily be seen in cases of foveal detachment because the DRUJ is loose.[14] It is difficult to visualize the foveal area with DRUJ arthroscopy when the TFCC is completely attached to the ulna without any DRUJ instability, although the joint surface of ulnar head and sigmoid notch of the radius can easily be seen. Arthroscopy for DRUJ instability presents with several possible RUL findings, including: (1) complete foveal detachment, depicting an empty RUL, vacant ligament tissue surrounded by synovial tissue and fragile scarring; (2) partial avulsion on either the dorsal or palmar portion of the RUL, which indicates moderate DRUJ instability that has either a palmar or dorsal end point; (3) relaxation of the ligament corresponding to partial healing of a partial RUL tear, indicating mild DRUJ instability where the end points are obvious in both the palmar and dorsal directions, but the DRUJ is lax when compared with the contralateral side.[14]

INDICATION

We reserve arthroscopic repair for a relatively acute or new injury (up to 6 months after the initial injury), and complete or partial ulnar disruption of the TFCC at the fovea.[14] Younger patients (up to 50 years old) appear to be the best candidates for the arthroscopic procedure due to their greater RUL healing potential. An open repair technique is suitable when DRUJ arthroscopy visualization of the RUL indicates scar or synovial healing without ligament tissue. This open repair technique can be indicated for acute and chronic cases within 1 year after the initial injury. Refreshment of the fovea area can be done in an open fashion with the open technique, which is more secure and accurate than when done arthroscopically. Techniques described are suited for wrists with a neutral or minus variance. A certain shearing stress is expected to be present between the ulnar head and the sutured site of the TFCC, which may induce subsequent rupture of sutures in wrists with a positive ulnar variance. The positive ulna should be leveled into a neutral ulnar variance by an ulnar shortening procedure when open repair or reconstruction is indicated. This author prefers reconstruction (reattachment) of the TFCC using an ECU half-slip tendon when more than 1 year has passed since the initial injury, or if there is too much RUL destruction to allow for ligament repair.

CONTRAINDICATIONS

Contraindication for this technique includes massive and complete TFCC destruction, such as that found in patients with rheumatoid arthritis. Another contraindication is severe DRUJ degeneration or osteoarthritic change, which should be treated with a Sauvé-Kapandji reconstruction, or ulnar head resection.

TECHNIQUES

Arthroscopic Transosseous TFCC Repair

The underlying concept of this technique is based on the TFCC anatomical characteristics.[15] There is a line between the

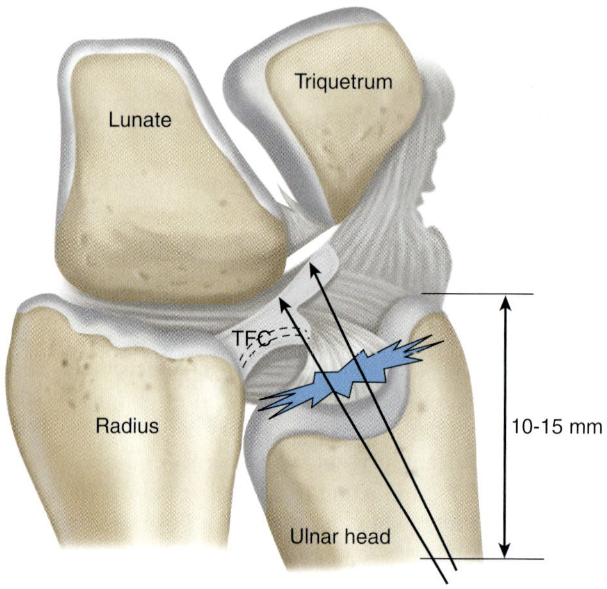

FIGURE 30-7 Basic concept of the arthroscopic transosseous TFCC repair. The line between the point on the ulnar cortex 10 to 15 mm proximal from the tip of the ulnar styloid (corresponding to the small ulnar prominence just proximal to the ulnar head) and ulnar half of the TFC passes through the fovea lesion theoretically. Theoretically the TFCC can be sutured to the fovea with an outside-in pullout technique if the stitches are introduced into this area.

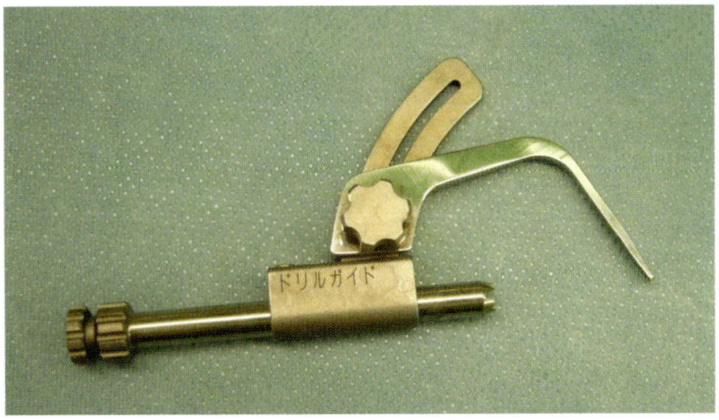

FIGURE 30-8 Original targeting device.

ulnar half area of the TFC, including the apex of the TFC, and a point that is 10 to 15 mm proximal from the ulnar styloid (corresponding to the point just proximal to the ulnar prominence) passing through the center of the fovea, which serves as the isometric point of the forearm rotation[5] (Fig. 30-7). The foveal area is debrided by a small shaver inserted from the DRUJ-ulnar portal after foveal detachment of the TFCC is confirmed by DRUJ arthroscopy. An original target device (Fig. 30-8; Nakashima Medical, Okayama, Japan) is inserted through the 4-5 or 6R portal and an approximately 1-cm longitudinal incision is made on the ulnar side of the ulnar cortex, at a point 10 to 15 mm proximal from the tip of the ulnar styloid, with the periosteum elevated. A small spike on the target device is set on the ulnar half of the TFC. Two separate small holes are made from the ulnar cortex with a 1.2-mm K-wire attached to the ulnar half of the TFC (Fig. 30-9). A 21-gauge injection needle, in which a 4-0 nylon loop stitch had been set, was then passed through 1 tunnel from the outside into the radiocarpal joint. This was then repeated through the other bone tunnel. Mosquito nonhook forceps from the 4-5 or 6R portal pulled out both loop stitches. Then,

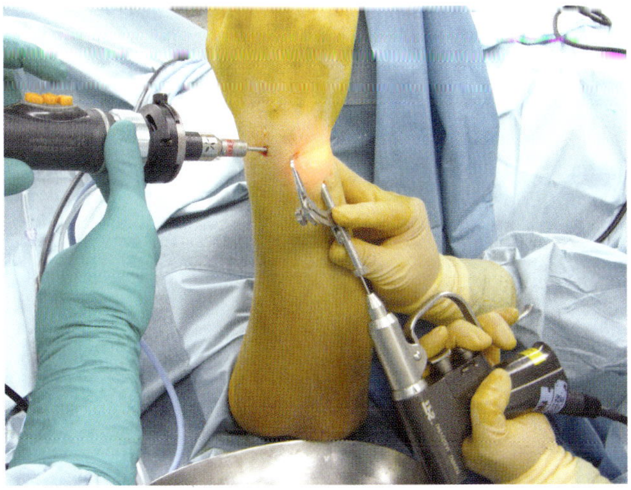

FIGURE 30-9 A 1.2-mm K-wire is drilled from ulnar side of the ulnar to the ulnocarpal joint using a target device.

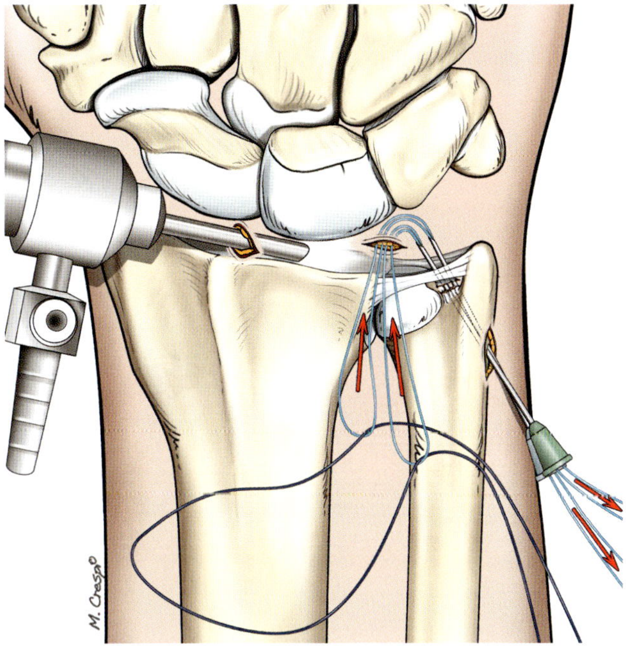

FIGURE 30-10 A 21-gauge needle with a 4-0 nylon loop stitch is passed from the ulnar cortex to the ulnar half of the TFC. This drawing indicates that 2 nonabsorbable 3-0 polyester stitches are introduced from the RC joint to the ulnar cortex with loop stitches.

2 nonabsorbable 3-0 polyester sutures (TiCron, Covidien, Mansfield, Massachusetts) were introduced from the RC joint to the ulnar cortex by loop stitches (Fig. 30-10) to make an outside-in pullout suture of the TFCC to the fovea. The TFCC was then tightly sutured to the ulnar fovea with this technique to restabilize the DRUJ (Fig. 30-11).

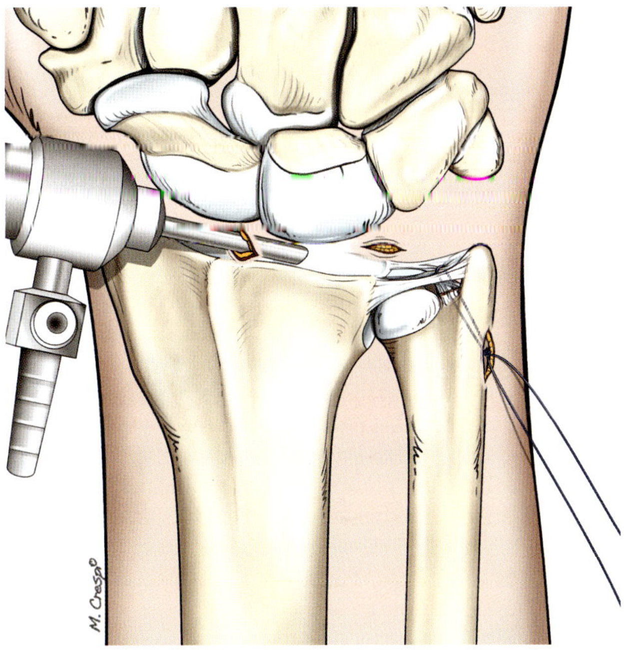

FIGURE 30-11 Diagram of arthroscopic TFCC transosseous repair.

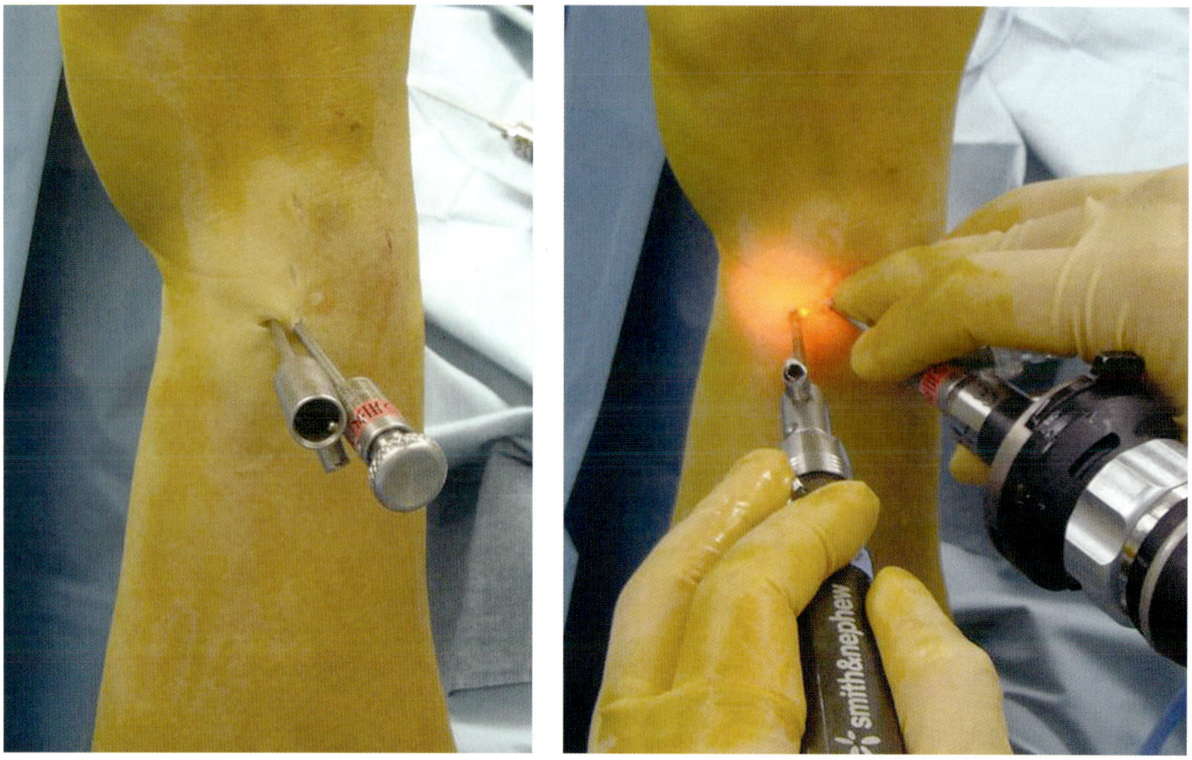

FIGURE 30-12 The shaver is inserted into the DRUJ through the DRUJ-ulnar portal.

One practical pitfall of this procedure is in refreshment of the fovea area through DRUJ arthroscopy. The ulnar portal is used for the DRUJ shaver, which is just 5 mm ulnar to the DRUJ (distal) portal. Care must be taken not to damage the arthroscope when the DRUJ-ulnar portal is made. Ideally, 2 trocars are prepared, 1 for the scope and 1 for the shaver. Before introducing the scope and shaver, 2 trocars are securely inserted into the DRUJ (Fig. 30-12). This author prefers open repair or reconstruction when DRUJ arthroscopy reveals less RUL healing potential, such as when there is severe scarring or synovial thickening without any ligamentous tissue.

TFCC Open Repair

A dorsal C-shaped skin incision is used extending from the 4-5 or 6R portal and the DRUJ portal. After the C-flap is elevated, the superficial sensory branches of the ulnar nerve need to be preserved. The sixth extensor compartment is opened and the ECU retracted. The dorsal DRUJ capsule is elevated from the ulnar head with a scalpel to expose the DRUJ after the radial ridge of the ECU sheath floor is released. A small ring elevator is inserted into the DRUJ to dislocate the ulnar head (Fig. 30-13), which is easily done if there is a foveal disruption of the TFCC.[13,14]

The condition of the RUL fibers can be assessed by pulling the distal remnant with a pair of forceps to determine whether

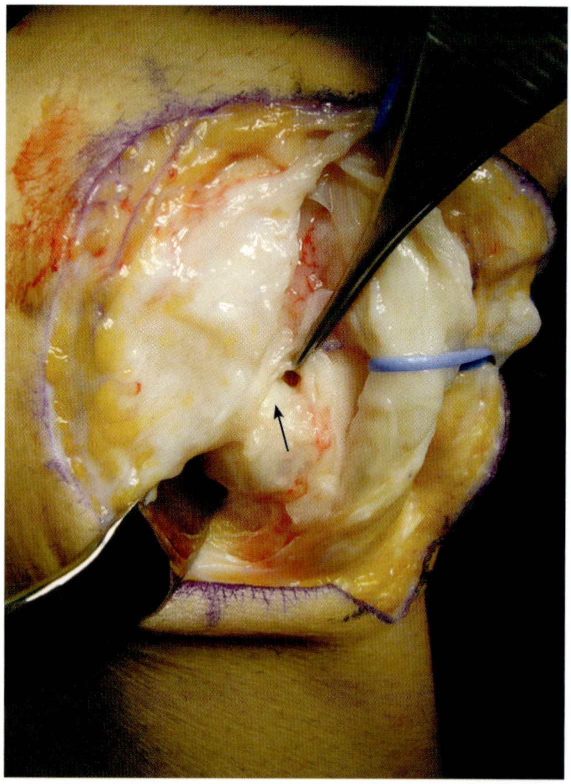

FIGURE 30-13 Opening of the DRUJ through the sixth compartment. The ring retractor is inserted to dislocate the ulnar head. The arrow indicates a TFCC avulsion at the fovea.

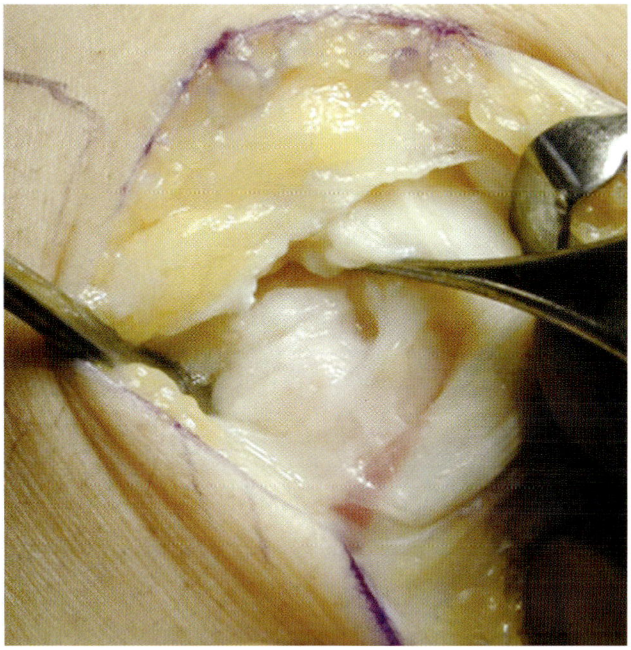

FIGURE 30-14 The RUL condition is checked with forceps.

it can be sutured (Fig. 30-14). The fovea region is debrided of scar tissue and 2 small holes are made with a 1.2-mm K-wire, as close to the center of the fovea as possible, which is an isometric point on the ulna during forearm rotation. Two 3-0 nylon or polyester sutures are passed through the first bone hole from the ulnar fovea to the lateral cortex of the ulna using 21-gauge needles. The disrupted RUL is sutured with a double 3-dimensional mattress and a locking suture technique (Figs. 30-15 and 30-16). The ECU is reduced to the sheath and then repaired. The dorsal DRUJ capsule is anatomically repaired with closure of the ECU sheath.

Practical tips of the open procedure include: (1) the opening site of the DRUJ; (2) precise positioning of the 2 bone tunnels; and (3) the suture method. This author prefers opening of the sixth compartment, which is the closest and most direct route to the fovea. Garcia-Elias recommended opening the fifth compartment; however, this incision must damage the dorsal area of the TFCC.[13] The 2 bone tunnels must be the closest to the center area of the fovea origin of the RUL. When the bone tunnels are made at an eccentric position, the range of forearm rotation should be reduced. This author recommends the double mattress anchoring method[13] on the ECU sheath floor for secure suturing, because the simple in–out technique through the disc has the potential risk of cutting through the stitches on the disc.

TFCC Reconstruction Using the ECU Half-slip Tendon

This reconstruction technique is suitable for a chronic (at least 6 months after the initial injury) or a severely or completely

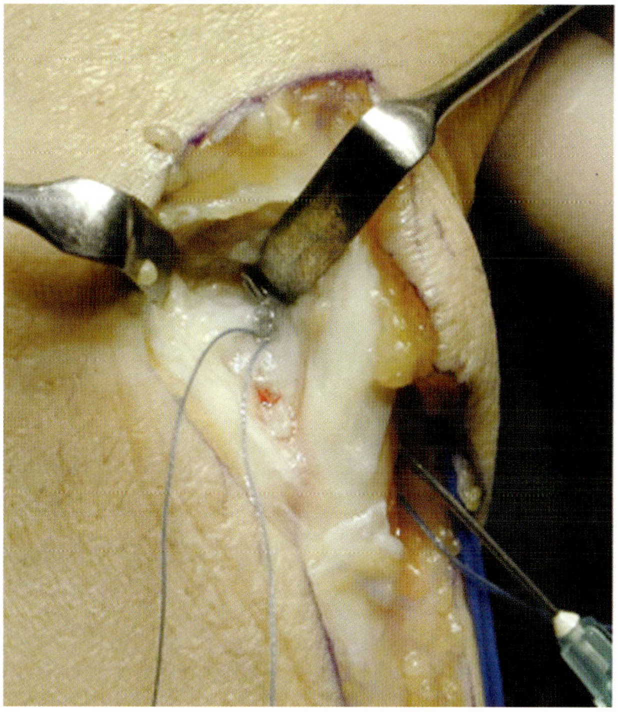

FIGURE 30-15 Two nonabsorbable 3-0 polyester sutures are introduced from the fovea to the ulnar cortex. The TFCC is tightly repaired to the fovea with an open pullout technique.

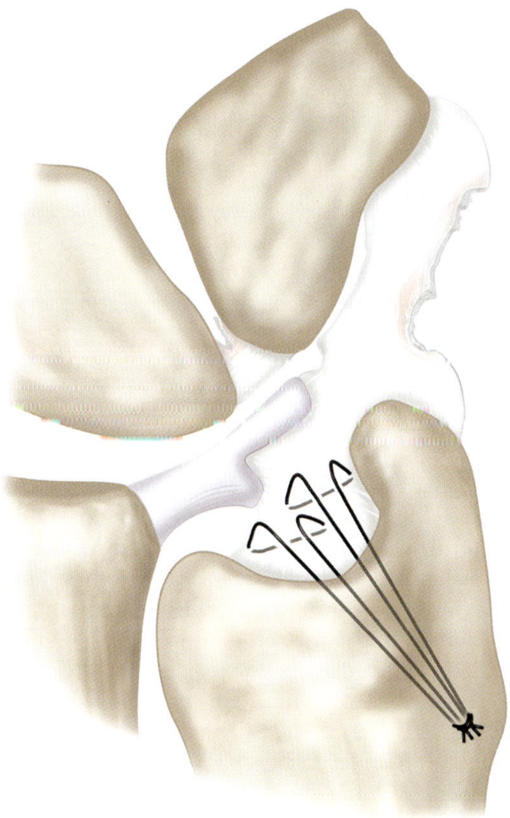

FIGURE 30-16 Diagram of an open transosseous TFCC repair. Solid lines represent the sutures.

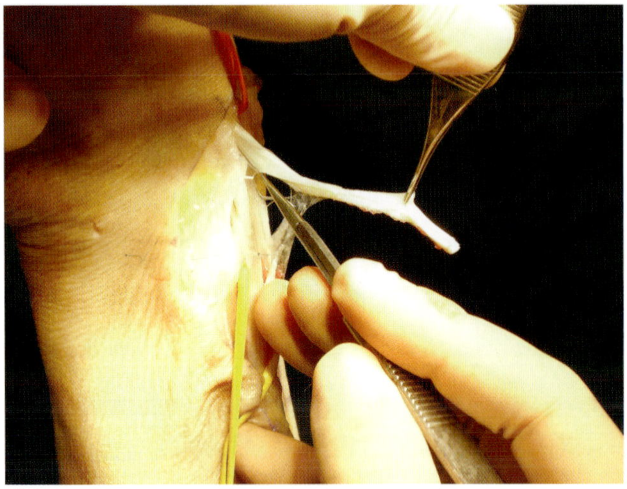

FIGURE 30-17 The first step of TFCC reattachment. The distally based half-slip of the ECU attaches the TFCC to the ulnar fovea.

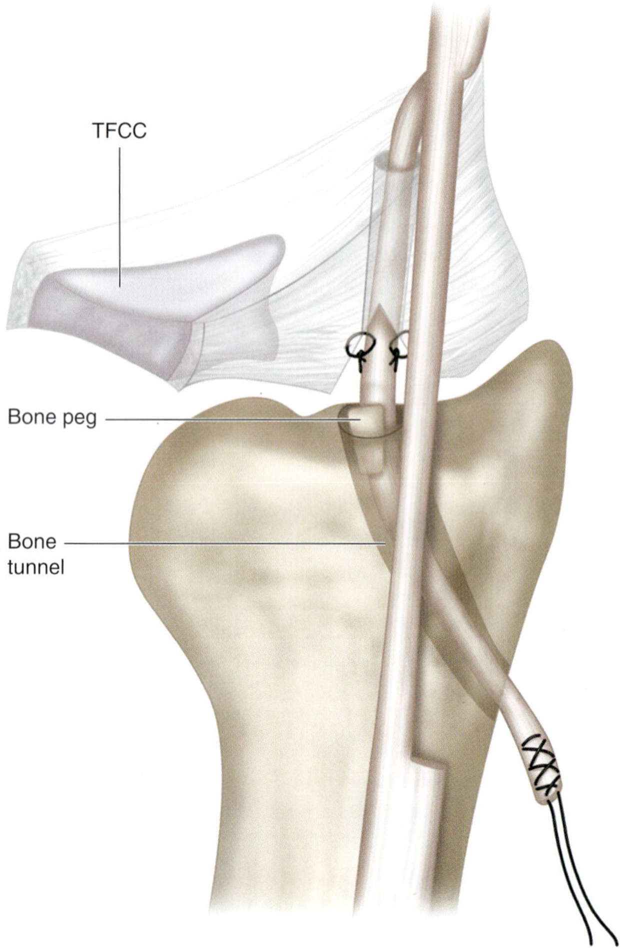

FIGURE 30-18 Illustration of the technique. The remnant TFCC is sutured to the ECU half-slip at the fovea. The ECU half-slip is passed to the ulnar tunnel made by a 2.5-mm diameter drill to the ulnar cortex. A small bone peg is already inserted to the bone tunnel at the fovea.

damaged TFCC at the ulnar fovea, all of which demonstrate severe DRUJ instability. The technique described is suited for wrists with the neutral or minus ulnar variance. Ulnar shortening is performed in wrists with a positive variance to be equalized to the neutral variance before reconstruction.

The same incision as for open repair through the sixth compartment is made to explore the DRUJ. A 3-cm longitudinal incision of the ECU sheath at the DRUJ is made and the ECU is dislocated outside. After the radial ridge of the ECU subsheath is longitudinally cut, the dorsal capsule of the DRUJ appears just beneath the ECU subsheath. Elevating the dorsal DRUJ capsule from the ulnar head by surgical knife opens the DRUJ. A small ring elevator is inserted into the DRUJ to dislocate the ulnar head.

The condition of the RUL fibers must be examined by pulling the distal remnant with the forceps to determine whether it can be sutured. Reattachment of the TFCC using the ECU half-slip is suitable when a severely damaged or fragile RUL is noted.

The fovea of the ulna is refreshed and scar tissue is removed to expose the bone marrow for TFCC reattachment. One bone tunnel is made with a 2.5-mm diameter drill from the center of the fovea to the ulnar cortex. The position of the bone tunnel at the fovea is as close to the center of the fovea as possible, which serves as an isometric point on the ulna during forearm rotation.[5] The distally based ECU half-slip tendon is harvested (Fig. 30-17), and then introduced into the TFCC from this distal small incision made at the radiocarpal joint level, passing through the TFCC, and attached to the DRUJ surface at the fovea (Fig. 30-18). The palmar portion of the RUL is sutured to the half-slip of the ECU tendon at the RUL origin. The ECU half-slip was subsequently anchored to the ulnar fovea with a small titanium interference screw to reattach the TFCC (Fig. 30-19). An additional horizontal mattress suture is used for closure of the 5-mm longitudinal incision at the dorsal portion of the RUL. The remaining ECU is reduced to the sheath, which is stitched back. The dorsal DRUJ capsule is automatically reset with closure of the ECU sheath.

POSTOPERATIVE COURSE

Two weeks of long-arm casting and a subsequent 3 weeks of short arm casting are necessary following arthroscopic or open TFCC repair and reconstruction using the ECU half-slip tendon. Active ROM exercises are initiated after removal of the cast at 5 weeks after the surgery. Passive ROM exercise with the aid of an occupational therapist may be needed if there is loss of forearm rotation at 7 weeks following the surgery. Full pronation–supination range can usually be achieved at 8 to 9 weeks after the operation followed by initiation of isometric muscle strengthening exercises with a weight up to 3 kg. The weight may be increased to 5 kg at 3 months following surgery. The patient may be back to normal sports activity levels 6 months after TFCC repair and 9 months after reconstruction.

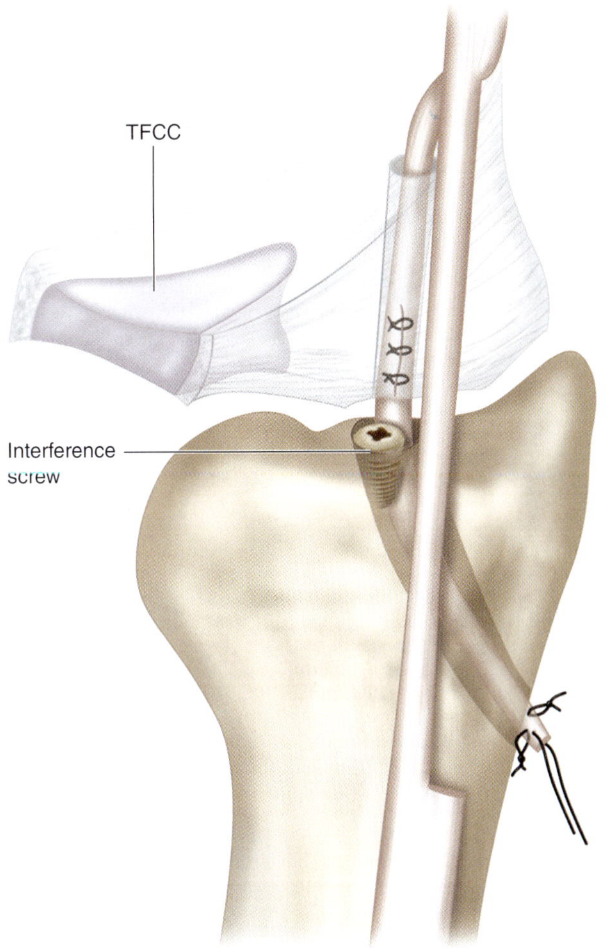

FIGURE 30-19 Schematic of the final step of TFCC reattachment. The small interference screw is set at the fovea to anchor the TFCC. The small longitudinal incision is sutured.

OUTCOMES

Arthroscopic Transosseous Repair

We treated 26 wrists with arthroscopic transosseous repair techniques. There were 14 males and 12 females, with a mean age of 28 years. The injured side included 13 right wrists and 13 left wrists. The time period between the initial injury and the surgery averaged 8 months (range, 1 month to 4 years). Ulnar variance was +2 mm in 5 wrists, +1 mm in 1 wrist, 0 mm in 18 wrists, and −1 mm in 2 wrists. The mean postoperative follow-up period was 3.5 years (range, 12-60 months). All cases demonstrated ulnar detachment at the fovea. Pain, range of forearm pronation–supination, and DRUJ instability were examined in all cases. The clinical evaluation system including relief of pain, range of pronation/supination, and DRUJ instability was used for DRUJ evaluations.[14]

Seventeen of 26 wrists indicated no pain after arthroscopic transosseous repair of the foveal TFCC detachment. Severe pain remained in 2 wrists. Recurrence of pain was found 8 to 12 months after the surgery in 4 wrists. Mild pain was noted in 3 wrists postoperatively at the final follow-up. There was no loss of range of rotation preoperatively and 25 wrists indicated full range of pronation and supination postoperatively, but 1 wrist displayed a 45° loss of supination postoperatively, following an open DRUJ release. DRUJ instability was found in all wrists preoperatively. There was no postoperative DRUJ instability in 19 wrists. Moderate-to-severe DRUJ instability was noted in 7 wrists. Final clinical results obtained included 15 excellent, 3 good, 4 fair, and 4 poor results with the DRUJ evaluating system.[14]

Open TFCC Repair

We treated 66 TFCC tears with an open transosseous repair. There were 36 males and 28 females, with a mean age of 31 years. The injured side included 37 right wrists, 25 left wrists, and 2 of these patients had bilateral injuries. The time period between the initial injury and the operation averaged 5 months (range, 0 months to 25 years). Ulnar variance was positive in 13, neutral in 50, and minus in 3 wrists. The follow-up period averaged 3 years (range, 2-9 years). Relief of pain, range of pronation/supination, and DRUJ stability were evaluated.[14]

Sixty among 66 wrists indicated no pain following open foveal repair of the TFCC. Severe pain remained in 2 wrists at final follow-up. There was no preoperative loss of forearm range of rotation, but 1 wrist showed a 45° loss of supination postoperatively. DRUJ instability was found in all wrists preoperatively, and postoperative DRUJ stability was achieved in 56 wrists. Moderate-to-severe postoperative DRUJ instability was noted in 4 wrists. The final clinical results obtained were 56 excellent, 6 good, 2 fair, and 2 poor with the open repair.

TFCC Reconstruction

Since 1998, we treated 29 wrists having ulnar detachment of the TFCC with our reconstruction technique using a half-slip of the ECU tendon. There were 19 right, 8 left, and 1 bilateral wrist patients with an average age of 34.8 years (range, 13-68). All complained preoperatively of ulnar-sided wrist pain and severe DRUJ instability. Neutral ulnar variance was present in 23 wrists and positive in 6 wrists. Ulnar shortening equalized the abutment before the reconstruction in the positive variance wrists. The time period from the initial injury to surgery was 1 month to 48 years.

Twenty-six wrists indicated no pain and slight pain remained in 3 wrists following surgery. Complete restabilization of the DRUJ was achieved in 26 wrists; however, there remained moderate DRUJ instability in 2 wrists postoperatively. Severe DRUJ instability remained in 1 wrist. There were 25 excellent results, 2 good results, 1 fair result, and 1 poor result.

DISCUSSION

Recent anatomical and biomechanical studies have advanced our knowledge of repair methods for TFCC foveal disruption.[5,7,8] The TFCC can be thought of as a hammock, which surrounds and supports the carpus with 2 tight anchors to the fovea corresponding to the dorsal and palmar portions of the RUL. Once both anchors are disrupted, the hammock is unsteady and unstable. DRUJ stability can be restored by reanchoring the RUL.[14] The direction of the sutures is best when they are placed parallel to the direction of the vertical RUL fibers.[7,8] Because of the isometric nature of the RUL,[5] the fibers must be attached to the center of the fovea.[13,14]

Avulsion of the TFCC from the fovea may induce DRUJ instability,[11] but the conventional arthroscopic capsular repair technique of the TFCC to the dorsal or ulnar joint capsule[20–22] does not reconstitute the foveal origin, where the RUL mainly arises. There are several papers on arthroscopic-assisted transosseous repair techniques of the TFCC. Atzei explored the foveal lesion arthroscopically and used a mini-incision to insert a bone anchor at the fovea.[15] Iwasaki and Minami[23] used a 2.9-mm drill hole made from the proximal ulnar cortex to the fovea under fluoroscopic control with a radiocarpal arthroscopically assisted suture of the TFCC to the ulnar periosteum. We also obtained excellent clinical results with arthroscopic transosseous repair techniques,[14] which reattach the TFCC into the fovea directly.

Open repair is a more reliable repair technique.[24–27] In this technique, refreshment of the fovea area is easy[13,14]; thus, it is indicated for chronic cases within 1 year of the initial injury. Although the incision is relatively longer than with arthroscopic repair, we obtained excellent clinical results than arthroscopic repair.

Our reconstruction technique using the ECU half-slip tendon for chronic, severe DRUJ instability cases produced excellent clinical results. There were several described reconstruction techniques using the palmaris longus tendon,[28,29] indicating invasive techniques for both the radius and ulna. Our reattachment technique has a real anatomical basis for the reattachment of the TFCC to the ulnar fovea, which resulted in excellent DRUJ stability and excellent clinical results.

REFERENCES

1. af Ekenstam F, Hagert CG. Anatomical studies on the geometry and stability of the distal radio ulnar joint. *Scand J Plast Reconstr Surg.* 1985;19:17–25.
2. af Ekenstam F, Hagert CG. The distal radio ulnar joint: the influence of geometry and ligament on simulated Colles' fracture. An experimental study. *Scand J Plast Reconstr Surg.* 1985;19:27–31.
3. Palmer AK, Werner FW. The triangular fibrocartilage complex of the wrist—anatomy and function. *J Hand Surg Am.* 1981;6:153–162.
4. Nakamura T, Yabe Y, Horiuchi Y. Functional anatomy of the triangular fibrocartilage complex. *J Hand Surg Br.* 1996;21:581–586.
5. Nakamura T, Makita A. The proximal ligamentous component of the triangular fibrocartilage complex: functional anatomy and three-dimensional changes in length of the radioulnar ligament during pronation and supination. *J Hand Surg Br.* 2000;25:479–486.
6. Schuind F, An KN, Berglund L, et al. The distal radioulnar ligaments: a biomechanical study. *J Hand Surg Am.* 1991;16:1106–1114.
7. Nakamura T, Yabe Y. Histological anatomy of the triangular fibrocartilage complex of the human wrist. *Ann Anat.* 2000;182: 567–572.
8. Nakamura T, Takayama S, Horiuchi Y, Yabe Y. Origins and insertions of the triangular fibrocartilage complex—a histological study. *J Hand Surg Br.* 2001;26:446–454.
9. Mino DE, Palmer AK, Levinsohn EM. The role of radiography and computerised tomography in the diagnosis of subluxation and dislocation of the distal radioulnar joint. *J Hand Surg Am.* 1983; 8:23–31.
10. Nakamura T, Berger RA, Fujita M, et al. Distal radioulnar joint instability during forearm rotation: effect of muscle loading. *J Jpn Soc Surg Hand.* 2002;18:306–311.
11. Haugstvedt JR, Berger RA, Nakamura T, Neale P, Berglund L, An KN. Relative contributions of the ulnar attachment of the triangular fibrocartilage complex to the dynamic stability of the distal radioulnar joint. *J Hand Surg Am.* 2006;31:445–451.
12. Palmer AK. Triangular fibrocartilage complex lesions: a classification. *J Hand Surg Am.* 1989;14:594–606.
13. Nakamura T, Nakao Y, Ikegami H, Sato K, Takayama S. Open repair of the ulnar disruption of the triangular fibrocartilage complex with double 3D-mattress suturing technique. *Tech Hand Up Extrem Surg.* 2004;8:116–123.
14. Nakamura T, Sato K, Okazaki M, et al. Repair of foveal detachment of the triangular fibrocartilage complex: open and arthroscopic transosseous techniques. *Hand Clin.* 2011;27:281–290.
15. Atzei A. New trends in arthroscopic management of type 1-B TFCC injuries with DRUJ instability. *J Hand Surg Eur Vol.* 2009;34: 582–591.
16. Nakamura T. Radial sided tear of the triangular fibrocartilage complex. In: Del Pinal F, Mathoulin C, Rucchetti L, eds. *Arthroscopic Repair of Fracture of the Distal Radius.* Berlin: Springer; 2010:89–98.
17. Adams BD. Anatomic reconstruction of the distal radioulnar ligaments for DRUJ instability. *Tech Hand Up Extrem Surg.* 2000;4:154–160.
18. Tay SC, Tomita K, Berger RA. The "ulnar fovea sign" for defining ulnar wrist pain: an analysis of sensitivity and specificity. *J Hand Surg Am.* 2007;32:438–444.
19. Moriya T, Aoki M, Iba K, Ozasa Y, Wada T, Yamashita T. Effect of triangular ligament tears on distal radioulnar joint instability and evaluation of three clinical tests: a biomechanical study. *J Hand Surg Eur Vol.* 2009;34:219–223.
20. Haugstvedt JR, Husby T. Results of repair of peripheral tears in the triangular fibrocartilage complex using an arthroscopic suture technique. *Scan J Plast Reconstr Surg.* 1999;33:439–447.
21. Lindau T, Adlercreutz C, Aspenberg P. Peripheral tears of the triangular fibrocartilage complex cause distal radioulnar joint instability after distal radius fractures. *J Hand Surg Am.* 2000;25:464–468.
22. Millants P, De Smet L, Van Ransbeeck H. Outcome study of arthroscopic suturing of ulnar avulsion of the triangular fibrocartilage complex of the wrist. *Chir Main.* 2002;21:298–300.
23. Iwasaki N, Minami A. Arthroscopically assisted reattachment of avulsed triangular fibrocartilage complex to the fovea of the ulnar head. *J Hand Surg Am.* 2009;34:1323–1326.
24. Hermansdorfer JD, Kleinman WB. Management of chronic peripheral tears of the triangular fibrocartilage complex. *J Hand Surg Am.* 1991;16:340–346.
25. Sennward GR, Lauterburg M, Zdravkovic V. A new technique of reattachment after traumatic avulsion of the TFCC at its ulnar insertion. *J Hand Surg Br.* 1995;20:178–184.
26. Chou KH, Sarris IK, Sotereanos DG. Suture anchor repair of ulnar sided triangular fibrocartilage complex tears. *J Hand Surg Br.* 2003;28:546–550.
27. Walker LG. Stabilization of the distal radioulnar joint after ulnar styloid nonunion using Mitek anchors. *Orthop Rev.* 1994;23:769–772.
28. Scheker LR, Belliappa PP, Acosta R, German DS. Reconstruction of the dorsal ligament of the triangular fibrocartilage complex. *J Hand Surg Br.* 1994;19:310–318.
29. Adams BD, Berger RA. An anatomic reconstruction of the distal radioulnar ligaments for posttraumatic distal radioulnar joint instability. *J Hand Surg Am.* 2002;27:243–251.

Distal Ulnar Head and Neck Fractures

David M. Brogan, MD
Brian J. Klika, MD
David G. Dennison, MD

31

RATIONALE AND BASIC SCIENCE

Ulnar head and neck fractures are typically associated with high-energy injuries involving damage to the distal radius, and they have been reported to occur with an incidence of 5.6% in 1 series of distal radius fractures.[1] Isolated injuries of the ulnar head or neck do occur but are very rare.[2–4] Biyani identified 4 main patterns of ulnar head and neck fractures, based on whether the fracture is intra-articular or extra-articular, has styloid involvement, or displays evidence of comminution (Fig. 31-1). Nonoperative treatment of displaced ulnar head and neck fractures can have relatively poor outcomes, with 1 series showing only 60% of patients achieving a good or excellent result[1] while several small series of ulnar head and neck fractures treated with plate fixation have shown promising results.[5–7] Herein, we will describe current options for surgical fixation of head and neck fractures of the ulna.

Distal Ulna Anatomy

To fully appreciate the implications of ulnar head and neck fractures on wrist function, one must understand the anatomy of the distal ulna and associated distal radioulnar joint (DRUJ). The distal aspect of the ulna has 3 main osseous components: the ulnar head, styloid, and fovea. The ulnar head can be further subdivided into the pole and seat. The pole of the ulna articulates with the triangular fibrocartilage complex (TFCC), while the seat of the ulna articulates with the sigmoid notch of the radius[8] (Fig. 31-2). The radius of curvature of the seat of the ulna is smaller than the sigmoid notch and the result of this difference in curvature is that only 20% of the DRUJ stability stems from the bony morphology.[9,10] Therefore, dynamic and static ligamentous stabilizers are required to maintain articular congruity. Three main structures are usually identified as being critical to DRUJ stability: (1) the TFCC; (2) the extensor carpi ulnaris (ECU) tendon and subsheath; and (3) the distal interosseous ligament (DIOL).[11]

The anatomy and biomechanics of the TFCC have been described by both Palmer and Werner.[12,13] The TFCC consists of the ulnolunate and ulnotriquetral ligaments, the ulnar collateral ligaments, and a central disc. The dorsal and volar edges of the TFCC essentially form the dorsal and volar radioulnar ligaments that stabilize the DRUJ. These ligaments originate from the dorsal and volar margins of the ulnar side of the lunate fossa and near the distal sigmoid notch. Both the dorsal and volar radioulnar ligaments attach in 2 locations on the distal ulna—the deep fibers into a broad, vertical space on the fovea and the superficial fibers to a narrower, more horizontal area on the base of the ulnar styloid.[10,14] It is thought by some that the foveal insertion of the radioulnar ligaments is more important for DRUJ stability[14] and this may explain why ulnar styloid fractures have varying effects on DRUJ instability.

Mechanism of Injury

Isolated ulnar head fractures can be classified into two categories—head fractures alone or head fractures with extra-articular ulnar involvement (such as the ulnar styloid).[15] The literature on these isolated injuries is limited to small case series, exemplifying their rare nature.[2,3,16] One proposed mechanism of an isolated ulnar head fracture is a direct blow to the ulna while in full supination.[2]

The more common mechanism of a distal ulnar fracture is a fall on the hand and wrist that also produces a distal radius fracture. The combination of these two fractures is significant due to the high likelihood of an associated ligamentous injury. To aid in the understanding of these fractures, Orbay proposed a classification system for ulnar-sided injuries that accompany distal radius fractures. The crux of this classification is the sequential loss of ligamentous stability with increasing severity of injury[11] (Fig. 31-3). In Type A, energy absorbed by the impact from the hand is transmitted to the carpal bones and subsequently to the distal radius. If the energy is not sufficient to break the ligamentous attachments of the distal radius, the radius fractures but remains

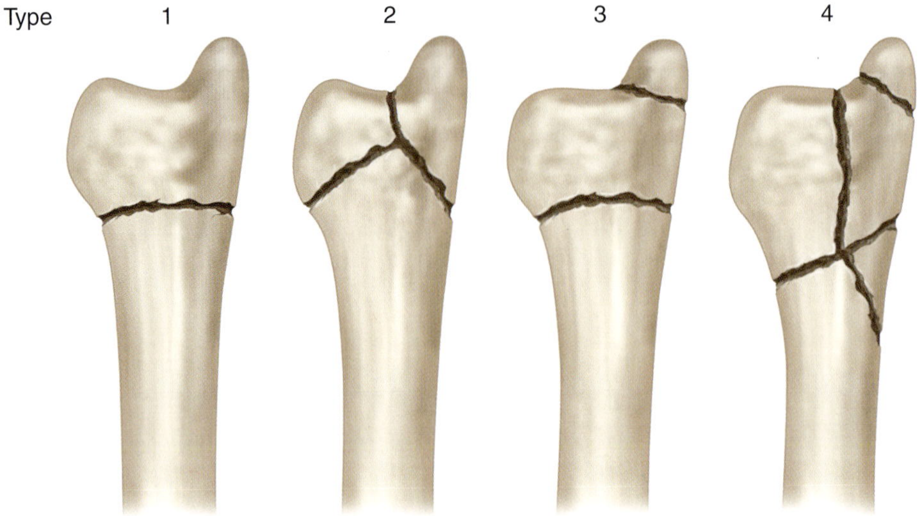

FIGURE 31-1 Biyani's classification system for distal ulnar fractures. (Reproduced with permission from Biyani et al.[1] Copyright Elsevier.)

nondisplaced. In Type B, a higher amount of energy causes rupture of the ligaments attaching the radius and ulna, with the TFCC and ECU subsheath rupturing first, often with an associated ulnar styloid fracture. This allows displacement of the distal radius fragment, but the DIOL often remains intact, likely because of its proximal attachment to the ulna. If this is the case, restoration of the bony architecture of the distal radius will restore the length–tension relationship of the DIOL and provide adequate stabilization of the DRUJ. In Type C, the displacement is so severe and the energy so great that the DIOL also ruptures, resulting in an unstable DRUJ requiring repair or reconstruction. This classification however has inherent variations depending on the presence and quality of the DIOL. In fact, there is an increasing awareness of the presence of anatomic variations in the DIOL (such as the distal oblique bundle [DOB])[17] and their importance on stability of the DRUJ.[18] For example, the absence of a DOB of the DIOL was found to be associated with a significant increase in DRUJ laxity in the neutral forearm position.[19]

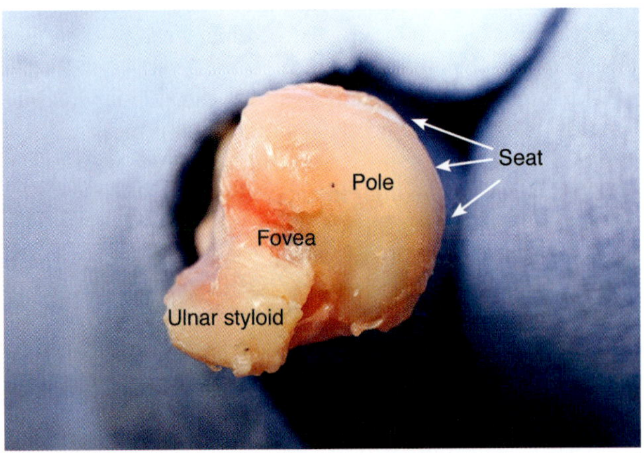

FIGURE 31-2 Axial view of a cadaveric dissection of the distal ulna demonstrating the head, pole, seat, and styloid process.

The decision for operative treatment relies on a global evaluation of the function and stability of the DRUJ. Injuries that produce instability or limitation of motion represent clear operative indications. A displaced fracture of the seat of the ulna could limit rotation or lead to arthritis and pain with forearm rotation. A fracture of the pole of the ulna may affect the TFCC or interfere with normal motion around the lunate and triquetrum, while a fracture through the fovea may disrupt the radioulnar ligaments and compromise DRUJ stability.

Ulnar Styloid Fractures

Much has been written about operative treatment of ulnar styloid fractures, particularly in the setting of distal radius fractures, but the variable results make the decision to treat these injuries controversial. Some authors have reported that fractures involving the ulnar styloid are associated with DRUJ instability,[20] particularly fractures involving the base of the styloid and those with displacement >2 mm.[21] Other authors have observed no evidence of increased instability in distal radius fractures with concomitant ulnar styloid fractures[22]; even nonunited proximal ulnar styloid fractures have been found to have no effect on wrist function or pain.[23] Our preference is to assess the DRUJ stability (measuring translation of the radius relative to the ulna in neutral rotation, pronation, and supination) after open reduction and internal fixation (ORIF) of the distal radius fracture, and then proceed with ulnar styloid fixation and/or foveal repair if instability is present.

INDICATIONS

The ideal candidates for ORIF of fractures of the ulnar head and neck are patients who have suffered a displaced fracture (Fig. 31-4) with good soft tissue around the fracture. This is

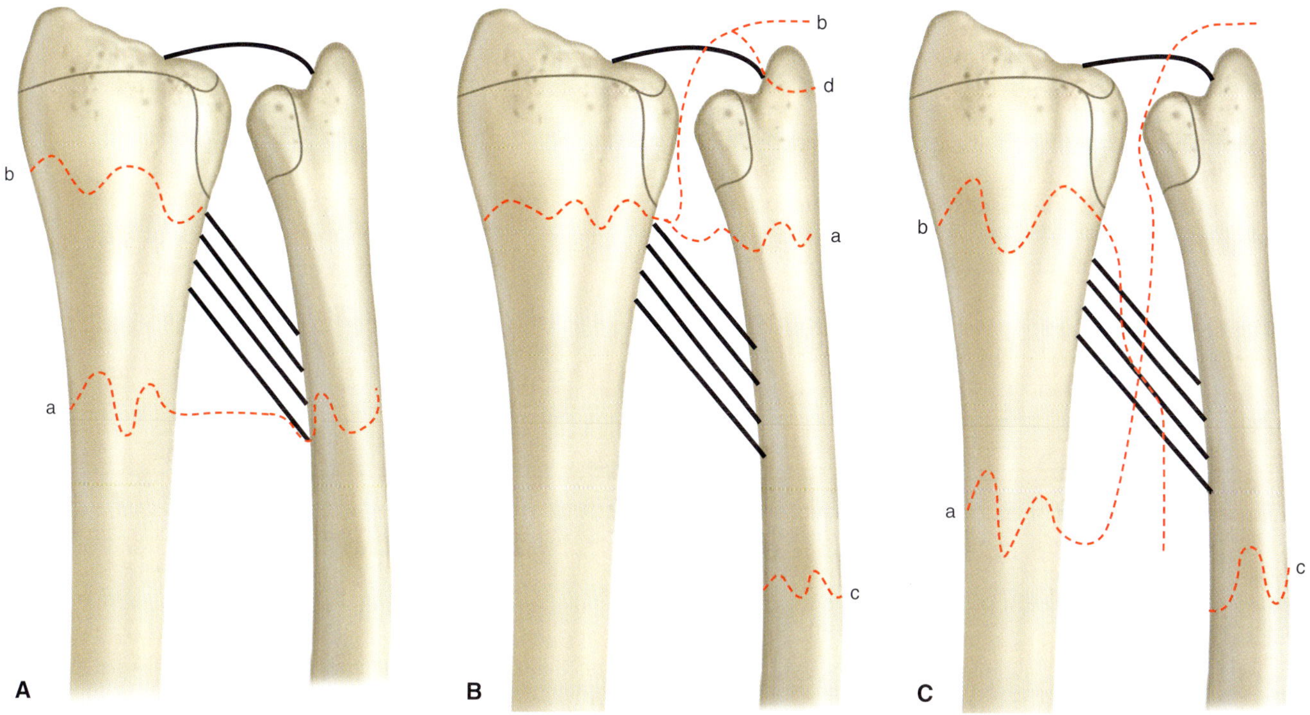

FIGURE 31-3 Orbay's system for sequential loss of ligamentous stability. **A.** Type A injury. This injury is found in minimally displaced distal radial fractures (fracture line b) and in fractures of both radius and ulna that occur just proximal to the distal interosseous ligament (fracture line a). **B.** Type B injury. Although rupture of the triangular fibrocartilage complex and the extensor carpi ulnaris tendon sheath occurs, the distal interosseous ligament remains intact. Distal radioulnar joint subluxation is corrected, and adequate stability is restored after anatomic reduction of the skeletal structures. The distal ulna and/or the ulnar styloid may fracture (fracture lines a, c, and d) or may not be fractured (line b). This is the concomitant DRUJ injury found in most displaced distal radial fractures. **C.** Type C injury. This is the concomitant DRUJ injury found in the Galeazzi fracture (fracture line a), fractures of the distal radius with radioulnar diastases (fracture lines b and c), and some high-energy comminuted distal radial and ulnar fractures. (Reproduced with permission from Orbay.[11] Copyright Elsevier.)

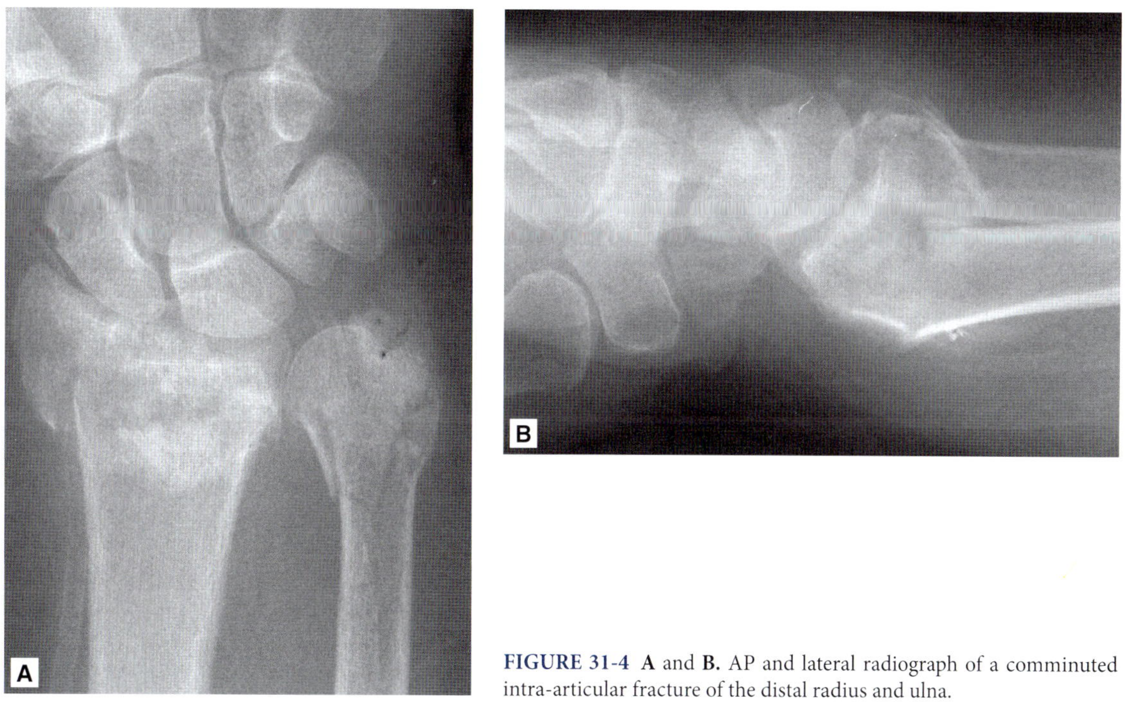

FIGURE 31-4 **A** and **B.** AP and lateral radiograph of a comminuted intra-articular fracture of the distal radius and ulna.

particularly important for patients with resulting incongruity of the DRUJ, as conservative management results in weaker grip and residual pain.[24] Criteria for considering operative treatment of the distal ulna include diaphyseal translation >1/3 or angulation >10°.[25,26] Patients with a complex fracture dislocation of the ulna (those in which reduction is blocked by interposed soft tissue) or articular displacement should undergo ORIF. DRUJ instability that persists following internal fixation of a distal radius fracture is also treated with ORIF.

There is no ideal age range for repair of the distal ulna; however, mild DRUJ instability will be better tolerated by elderly, low-demand patients. Open fractures are treated urgently. Combined, displaced fractures of the radius and ulna are ideally treated within the first few days after injury. The distal radius fracture should be fixed first as many distal ulnar fractures will be reduced, or considerably improved in alignment, following an anatomic reduction of the distal radius. Distal ulnar fractures that remain unstable or displaced, or that block forearm rotation, can then be reduced and stabilized.

CONTRAINDICATIONS

General contraindications include the patient's general medical state, an inadequate soft tissue envelope, and the presence of preexisting DRUJ arthritis. Severely comminuted fractures with complete or near-complete loss of the ulnar head articular surface are likely best served with a salvage technique such as arthroplasty or resection. Severe osteoporosis and poor bone quality may also present a challenge for stabilization of the fracture fragments with internal fixation. In severely comminuted fractures with poor bone quality, conservative treatment of the ulna with a later salvage procedure may be considered as well.

SURGICAL TECHNIQUE

Prior to surgery all radiographs and imaging are reviewed, paying particular attention to the obliquity of the DRUJ and the ulnar variance. Arthritis and cystic changes consistent with impaction should be identified as these findings may direct treatment. For instance, if findings for impaction are present, slight shortening of the ulna may be accomplished during ORIF. Similarly, if there is radiographic and symptomatic DRUJ arthritis, a resection or implant arthroplasty may be reasonable.

The patient is positioned supine with a well-padded nonsterile arm tourniquet. If the patient is intubated, the endotracheal tube should be on the opposite side of the injured arm. The arm is then prepared with usual sterile technique and draped with the distal arm, elbow, and forearm positioned in the center of the table (Fig. 31-5). The elbow can then be flexed to 90° to allow unrestricted access to the ulnar

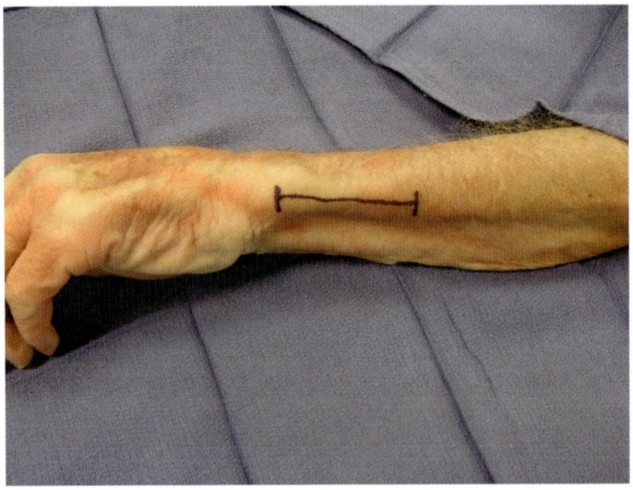

FIGURE 31-5 The hand, forearm, and elbow are prepped, draped, and centered in the middle of the table. The elbow may be flexed to 90° or the forearm pronated to allow direct access to the distal ulna.

aspect of the distal ulnar head and neck. A wrist traction tower with finger trap traction may be useful to hold the forearm in this position. Alternatively, the forearm may be pronated for dorsal exposure to the DRUJ if needed for an intra-articular fracture or for a foveal TFCC repair.

For unstable fractures or displaced fractures our preference is to use a Y-, T-, or L-shaped 2.0-mm locking plate (Fig. 31-6A and B). The exact choice of implant is dependent upon the configuration of the fracture fragments. Condylar blade plates and fragment-specific implants are also good options to achieve stable fixation.[6]

For fractures that can be reduced and stabilized from the direct ulnar approach, a longitudinal incision is made in the interval between the ECU and flexor carpi ulnaris (FCU). The dorsal sensory branch of the ulnar nerve (DSBUN) is identified and protected (Fig. 31-7). The extensor retinaculum is divided longitudinally and then the capsule and periosteum are incised while protecting the ECU tendon dorsally in the groove of the distal ulna.

Displaced ulnar head fractures that require open reduction are approached dorsally. The incision is placed over the DRUJ, the DSBUN is identified and protected, and then the fifth extensor compartment is identified and incised, releasing the tendon (Fig. 31-8A). The floor of the fifth compartment is incised with a transverse limb proximal to the dorsal radioulnar ligament, followed by a longitudinal incision placed about 2 mm from the sigmoid notch forming an "L"-shaped flap (Fig. 31-8B). Reflection of the flap provides wide access to the ulnar head (Fig. 31-8C). If a plate is needed for the neck fracture and exposure is needed for the head injury, a longer incision will allow for greater exposure to the DRUJ in addition to the ulnar exposure for plate application.

Following fracture reduction, temporary K-wires are inserted in a position that will not interfere with the planned plate position. The distal location of the plate is guided by a K-wire inserted from an ulnar to radial direction just beneath

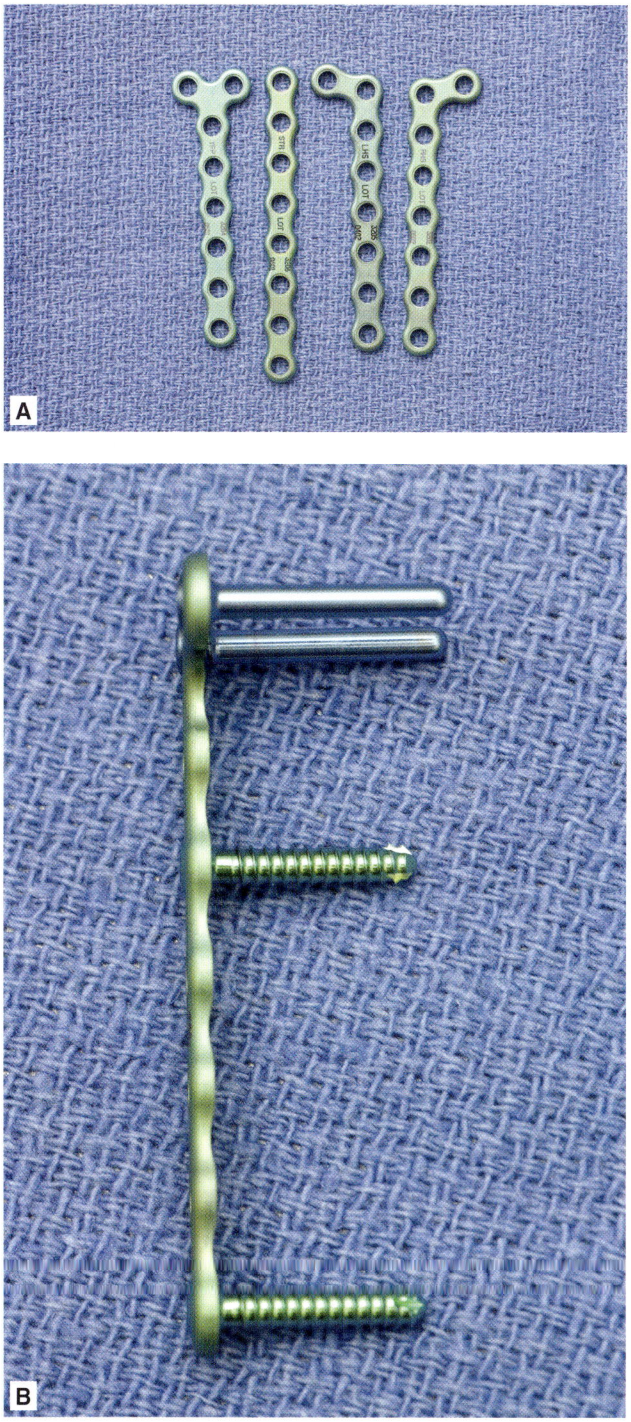

FIGURE 31-6 **A.** Locking plates are available in a variety of shapes; the selection of one is dictated by the fracture pattern. **B.** Lateral view of the locking plate shows the distal smooth pegs and more proximal screws.

the TFCC to mark the distal end of the ulna. The distal end of the plate is then positioned against this K-wire and the proximal portion centered on the ulna. The position is checked with fluoroscopy. A distal locking peg is inserted with the plate directly on the bone, taking care to ensure that the drill hole is unicortical and does not penetrate the opposite

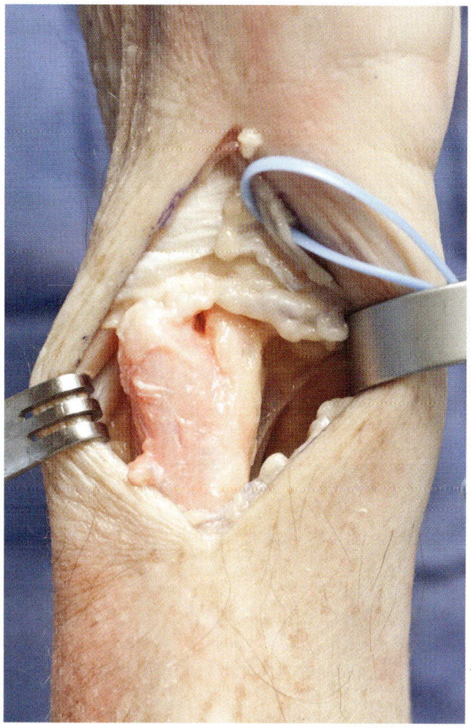

FIGURE 31-7 Cadaveric dissection demonstrating the direct ulnar approach. The dorsal sensory branch of the ulnar nerve is identified in the subcutaneous tissues and protected throughout the procedure. Splitting the interval between the extensor carpi ulnaris (ECU) and the flexor carpi ulnaris (FCU) provides adequate visualization of the ulnar head and neck.

subchondral bone. Once the peg or screw is inserted and locked to the plate, it is checked again to make sure it does not penetrate the ulnar head. This can be inspected with multiple fluoroscopic views along with careful examination of pronation and supination in an attempt to elicit any crepitus or block to motion. The plate is then initially secured to the ulna proximally with a nonlocked screw to compress the plate to the bone.

Following inspection of the provisional fixation, the remaining locking screws and pegs are inserted into the distal fragment. Two screws or pegs are often sufficient, while some larger fragments may allow additional pegs or screws. The angle of the second or third distal peg may be varied to capture other fragments as needed. Interfragmentary screw fixation outside of the plate may be used for articular fractures as well. If the plate is applied volarly, care must be taken to ensure that the plate does not affect pronation or supination and that the tips of the pegs do not interfere with the ECU tendon within the dorsal groove of the ulna. Fixation of the plate to the ulna proximally is completed by either locking screws or bicortical nonlocking screws[5] (Fig. 31-9). When basilar ulnar styloid fractures are also present, fixation can be obtained with a figure-of-eight suture around the plate or through the plate holes or a usual tension band technique through the bone. We prefer suture

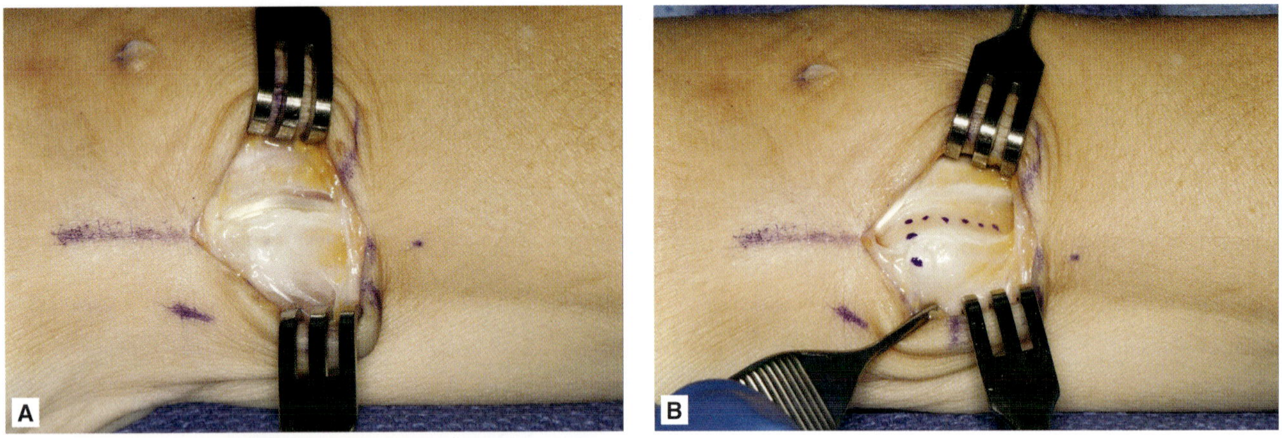

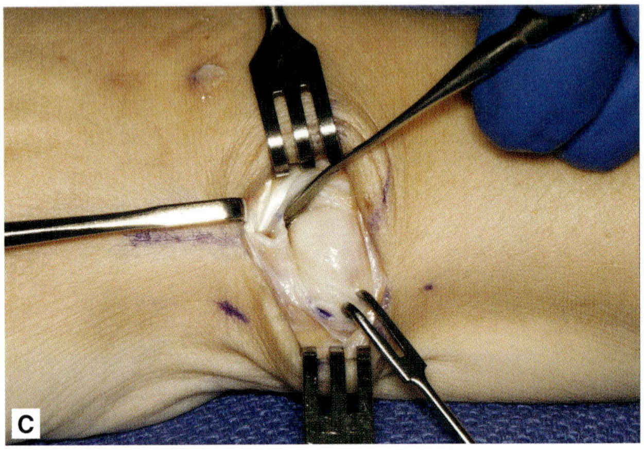

FIGURE 31-8 **A.** Dorsal approach to the ulnar head demonstrating an incision over the fifth extensor compartment with release of the tendon. **B.** Demarcation of an L-shaped incision through the floor of the fifth compartment. **C.** This approach allows wide access to the ulnar head for reduction of fractures.

(2-0 braided, undyed) instead of wire since little force is required to maintain the reduction of the styloid once the radius is reduced. Furthermore, this avoids the potential complication of broken hardware. Foveal repair of the TFCC may also be incorporated into the repair.

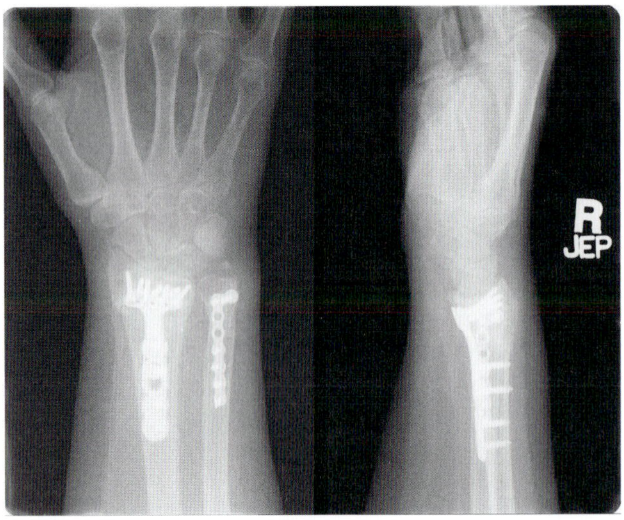

FIGURE 31-9 AP and lateral x-rays of the same fracture after ORIF of the distal radius and ulna. The patient achieved union of both fractures.

Closure is in layers with repair of capsular tissue and then repair of the extensor retinaculum over the hardware using buried knots with 4-0 suture. The patient is immobilized in a sugar-tong splint with the forearm in neutral rotation while immediate finger and shoulder range of motion exercises are initiated. Immobilization of the forearm is often continued for up to 3 weeks, but motion may be advanced to gentle active forearm rotation through a short arc of rotation (30° of pronation and supination) alternating with a resting long arm splint at 7 to 10 days if the patient is comfortable. Wrist and forearm motion are then advanced depending on the presence of a distal radius fracture. With stable fixation of the ulna and radius, motion may begin in most planes when comfortable. Pronation and supination are carefully monitored, advancing from an initial arc of 30° of pronation to 30° of supination. A short arm splint is then used and subsequently discontinued once 45° of pronation and 45° of supination are achieved. When soft tissue repairs have been required, initial splinting in neutral rotation may be required for 6 weeks.

Practical Tips

- Most distal ulnar fractures are associated with a distal radius fracture. Therefore, treatment should begin with reduction and stabilization of the radius first.

- Next, the reduction of the distal ulna and the stability of the fracture are examined. Unstable fractures or those with significant articular displacement are then reduced and stabilized.
- If an ulnar styloid fracture accompanies the ulnar head and neck fractures, the DRUJ is examined after the radius and ulnar fractures are reduced and stabilized. If instability is present, the styloid is also reduced and stabilized.

- When applying smaller plates, precontouring (AO technique) may be required to minimize gapping of the opposite cortex if compression is also applied across the fracture.
- Minimal soft tissue dissection is ideal to preserve the blood supply to the distal radius and ulna.
- The ulnar plate may be placed extraperiosteally to minimize soft tissue disruption.
- The initial distal fixation to the head and neck fragment allows the plate to assist with reduction of the ulnar shaft.
- Multiple fluoroscopic views must be obtained to make certain that there is no prominent hardware within the DRUJ, the ulnocarpal joint, or the ECU groove.

Potential Pitfalls

- The DSBUN must be identified and protected to prevent painful dysesthesias—K-wires and implants must not impinge or entrap the nerve.
- Positioning of the plate directly on the ulnar border may result in prominent hardware. Depending on the fracture pattern, the plate may be placed volarly with care taken to ensure that it does not interfere with pronation and supination.
- Fractures that include the diaphyseal ulna should be treated with standard plating techniques (3.5-mm LCDCP) for forearm fractures.
- The ECU groove should be inspected to ensure there is no hardware present within the sulcus.

Controversies

The optimal fixation for distal ulnar fractures has not been established. K-wire fixation of the distal ulna to the radius can be considered, although this technique remains challenging, may not provide adequate alignment or stability,[6] and has limited capability with osteoporotic bone.

An alternative method is condylar blade plate fixation as initially described by Ring et al.[6] In this technique, an ulnar incision is made utilizing the interval between the ECU and FCU. Provisional fixation is obtained with K-wires, followed by application of the plate to the medial ulna. The blade plate track is drilled, confirmed with fluoroscopy, and the plate is contoured to fit along the ulnar diaphysis. The screw adjacent to the blade is next inserted to bring the plate to the bone and the remaining proximal screws are inserted.

Another technique utilizing an intrafocal pin plate for distal ulnar fracture fixation has been described by Foster and Bindra.[7] The intrafocal pin plate consists of a long, S-shaped stem with a locking 1-hole or 2-hole plate. A 2-cm longitudinal skin incision is centered over the fracture site along the subcutaneous border of the ulna. Dissection proceeds between the FCU and ECU as described above. The pin is then inserted into the medullary cavity to its maximum depth (Fig. 31-10). Reduction is achieved and verified with fluoroscopy as the distal fragment is aligned with the proximal fragment. Locking screws are utilized in the plate to stabilize the distal fragment and prevent subsidence. The low-profile nature, locked screw capability, and minimal dissection requirement for this device make it a viable option in the osteoporotic, elderly patient.

Associated ulnar head articular fractures may be repaired with screws independent of a plate[3] and ulnar styloid fractures may be secured with a tension band configuration.

COMPLICATIONS

Complications following distal ulnar fractures have been described with both operative and nonoperative treatments. In patients undergoing nonoperative treatment of distal radius fractures with concomitant distal ulnar fractures, nonunion or malunion resulting in restricted supination and pronation may occur. Biyani et al[1] reported a nonunion incidence of 13% in their series of comminuted distal ulnar fractures.

McKee et al[27] reported on 4 cases of distal radial nonunions with associated distal ulnar shaft fractures. Of these 4 patients, there was concomitant ulnar nonunion in 3 cases. Sequelae from nonunion as well as malunion may include progressive deformity, pain, and loss of motion or function. Radial deviation of the hand and wrist as a result of malunion can lead to ulnar head prominence. Ulnar head prominence (ulnar positive variance) can lead to increased load across the ulnocarpal joint,[28] thus limiting motion or producing painful impaction. Similarly, excessive fracture callus formation and synostosis can greatly diminish forearm rotation and function.

Paresthesias, particularly in the distribution of the DSBUN, may be encountered postoperatively. Despite careful protection of the nerve throughout the procedure, retraction alone can often result in paresthesias. Most of these sensory deficits represent a neurapraxia and often recover by 3 months after surgery.[5] Malunion or hardware problems may cause pain or stiffness requiring revision or hardware removal.

OUTCOMES

We reported a retrospective review of 5 patients with a distal radius fracture who underwent locked plate fixation of a concomitant unstable distal ulnar fracture.[5] The average age was 52 years (range, 47-61 years) with an average follow-up

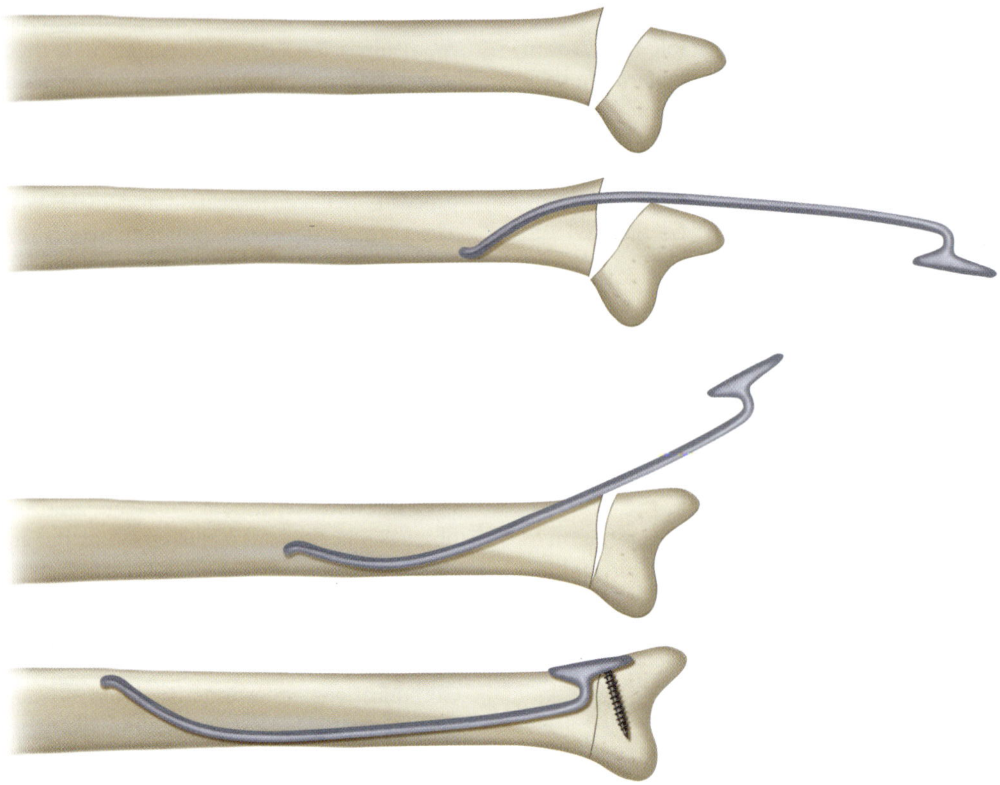

FIGURE 31-10 Diagram of fixation utilizing a pin plate. The intramedullary portion of the plate is threaded through the fracture site and the plate is turned 180° to allow reduction. Locking screws are then utilized to fix the plate to the distal fragment. (Reproduced with permission from Foster and Bindra.[7] Copyright Elsevier.)

of 11.6 months (range, 6-17 months). There were 2 open and 3 closed fractures. Fracture patterns reviewed in the study included 1 simple neck, 1 comminuted neck, 1 head, and 2 head and neck fractures of the distal ulna. All distal radius fracture implants were locked volar plates. All distal ulnar and distal radius fractures healed. The average postoperative wrist motion was: flexion 59°, extension 59°, pronation 67°, and supination 72°. The average grip strength was 97% of the opposite extremity. The ulnar variance averaged −0.4 mm (−2.5 to 1.5 mm), the average radial inclination was 20° (range, 18°-23°), and the average volar tilt was 8° (range, −2° to 12°). All DRUJs were stable. Using the modified Gartland and Werley rating score, there were 4 excellent results and 1 good result. No patient in the series required hardware removal.

Ring et al reviewed the results of condylar blade plate fixation of an unstable distal ulnar fracture associated with a distal radius fracture in 24 patients at an average follow-up of 26 months (range, 12-50 months).[6] There were 1 simple fracture of the ulnar neck, 20 comminuted fractures of the ulnar neck, and 3 fractures of the head and neck. The final average wrist motion was: 50° of flexion (range, 30°-80°), 52° of extension (range, 40°-90°), 76° of pronation (range, 45°-90°), and 70° of supination (range, 45°-90°). The grip strength averaged 64% of the uninjured extremity (range, 35%-100%). Radiographically the average palmar tilt of the distal articular surface of the radius was 8° (range, 0°-20°), ulnar inclination 21° (range, 15°-25°), with an ulnar positive variance of 1 mm (range, 0-4 mm). According to the modified Gartland and Werley score there were 6 excellent, 15 good, and 4 fair results. Two patients required repeat surgery for a nonunion and 7 required hardware removal.

For patients with severely comminuted ulnar head or neck fractures, restoration of the articular surface may not be possible. In this setting, salvage procedures should be considered. Satisfactory results have been shown for patients undergoing distal ulnar resection. Ruchelsman et al[29] reviewed 11 patients who underwent distal ulnar resection for comminuted distal ulnar fractures performed in conjunction with distal radial fixation. Postoperatively, the mean wrist flexion measured 53° and wrist extension measured 52°. The mean postoperative supination measured 77° and pronation measured 81°. The mean grip strength measured 90% of the contralateral side with 8 of 11 patients achieving equal contralateral grip strength. All distal radius fractures achieved union in their series and all patients experienced good to excellent results.[29]

REFERENCES

1. Biyani A, Simison AJ, Klenerman L. Fractures of the distal radius and ulna. *J Hand Surg Br.* 1995;20:357–364.
2. Jakab E, Ganos DL, Gagnon S. Isolated intra-articular fracture of the ulnar head. *J Orthop Trauma.* 1993;7(3):290–292.
3. Solan MC, Rees R, Molloy S, Proctor MT. Internal fixation after intra-articular fracture of the distal ulna. *J Bone Joint Surg Br.* 2003; 85(2):279–280.

4. Goikoetxea X, Garmilla I, Etxebarria I, Careaga M. Isolated intra-articular fracture of the distal ulna: a rare injury related to airbag deployment. *J Orthop Trauma.* 2006;20:292–294.
5. Dennison DG. Open reduction and internal locked fixation of unstable distal ulna fractures with concomitant distal radius fracture. *J Hand Surg Am.* 2007;32(6):801–805.
6. Ring D, McCarty LP, Campbell D, Jupiter JB. Condylar blade plate fixation of unstable fractures of the distal ulna associated with fracture of the distal radius. *J Hand Surg Am.* 2004;29(1):103–109.
7. Foster BJ, Bindra RR. Intrafocal pin plate fixation of distal ulna fractures associated with distal radius fractures. *J Hand Surg Am.* 2012;37(2):356–359.
8. Sharma A, Kumar A, Singh P. Anatomical study of the distal end of cadaveric human ulna: a clinical consideration for the management of distal radioulnar joint injuries. *Singapore Med J.* 2011;52(9):673–676.
9. Stuart PR, Berger RA, Linscheid RL, An KN. The dorsopalmar stability of the distal radioulnar joint. *J Hand Surg Am.* 2000;25(4):689–699.
10. Sammer DM, Chung KC. Management of the distal radioulnar joint and ulnar styloid fracture. *Hand Clin.* 2012;28(2):199–206.
11. Orbay JL. Ulnar head and styloid fractures. In: Slutsky DJ, ed. *Principles and Practice of Wrist Surgery*. 1st ed. Philadelphia: Saunders Elsevier; 2010 [chapter 15].
12. Palmer AK, Werner FW. The triangular fibrocartilage complex of the wrist: anatomy and function. *J Hand Surg Am.* 1981;6:153–162.
13. Palmer AK, Werner FW. Biomechanics of the distal radioulnar joint. *Clin Orthop Relat Res.* 1984;187:26–35.
14. Nakamura T, Takayama S, Horiuchi Y, Yabe Y. Origins and insertions of the triangular fibrocartilage complex: a histological study. *J Hand Surg Br.* 2001;26B:446–454.
15. Logan A, Lindau T. The management of distal ulnar fractures in adults: a review of the literature and recommendations for treatment. *Strategies Trauma Limb Reconstr.* 2008;3(2):49–56.
16. Tamura Y, Inoue G. Dislocation of the distal radioulnar joint associated with an intraarticular fracture of the ulnar head: report of two cases. *J Orthop Trauma.* 1998;12(1):68–70.
17. Noda K, Goto A, Murase T, Sugamoto K, Yoshikawa H, Moritomo H. Interosseous membrane of the forearm: an anatomical study of ligament attachment locations. *J Hand Surg Am.* 2009;34(3):415–422.
18. Moritomo H. The distal interosseous membrane: current concepts in wrist anatomy and biomechanics. *J Hand Surg Am.* 2012;37(7):1501–1507.
19. Kitamura T, Moritomo H, Arimitsu S, et al. The biomechanical effect of the distal interosseous membrane on distal radioulnar joint stability: a preliminary anatomic study. *J Hand Surg Am.* 2011;36(10):1626–1630.
20. Oskarsson GV, Aaser P, Hjall A. Do we underestimate the predictive value of the ulnar styloid affection in Colles fractures? *Arch Orthop Trauma Surg.* 1997;116(6):341–344.
21. May MM, Lawton JN, Blazar PE. Ulnar styloid fractures associated with distal radius fractures: incidence and implications for distal radioulnar joint instability. *J Hand Surg Am.* 2002;27:965–971.
22. Kim JK, Koh YD, Do NH. Should an ulnar styloid fracture be fixed following volar plate fixation of a distal radial fracture? *J Bone Joint Surg Am.* 2010;92(1):1–6.
23. Buijze GA, Ring D. Clinical impact of united versus nonunited fractures of the proximal half of the ulnar styloid following volar plate fixation of the distal radius. *J Hand Surg Am.* 2010;35(2):223–227.
24. Roysam G. The distal radio-ulnar joint in Colles' fractures. *J Bone Joint Surg Br.* 1993;75(1):58–60.
25. Tarr R, Garfinkel A, Sarmiento A. The effects of angular and rotational deformities of both bones of the forearm. *J Bone Joint Surg Am.* 1984;66(1):65–70.
26. Yasutomi T, Nakatsuchi Y, Koike H, Uchiyama S. Mechanism of limitation of pronation/supination of the forearm in geometric models of deformities of the forearm bones. *Biomechanics.* 2002;17(6):456–463.
27. McKee MD, Waddell JP, Yoo D, Richards RR. Nonunion of distal radial fractures associated with distal ulnar shaft fractures: a report of four cases. *J Orthop Trauma.* 1997;11(1):49–53.
28. Werner FW, Palmer AK, Fortino MD, Short WH. Force transmission through the distal ulna: effect of ulnar variance, lunate fossa angulation, and radial and palmar tilt of the distal radius. *J Hand Surg Am.* 1992;17:423–428.
29. Ruchelsman D, Raskin K, Rettig M. Outcome following acute primary distal ulna resection for comminuted distal ulna fractures at the time of operative fixation of unstable fractures of the distal radius. *Hand (N Y).* 2009;4(4):391–396.

32

DRUJ Arthroscopy

Andrea Atzei, MD
Riccardo Luchetti, MD

Arthroscopy of distal radioulnar joint (DRUJ) has only recently become more widespread.[1–3] Arthroscopic evaluation of the DRUJ represents an innovative tool of strategic importance for the diagnostic evaluation and treatment of this joint. It allows for the visualization of the articular cartilage, capsule, and the triangular fibrocartilage complex (TFCC).

This chapter will present the anatomy and biomechanics of the DRUJ, and the technique of DRUJ arthroscopy and discuss its indications and surgical applications.

INDICATIONS

The DRUJ is susceptible to traumatic and posttraumatic changes or inflammatory and degenerative disorders that can produce pain and functional impairment.

Arthroscopy allows for inspection of the articular surfaces of both the ulnar head and sigmoid notch.[4] Posttraumatic or degenerative cartilage defects, loose bodies, or osteophytes can be visualized and eventually treated. DRUJ synovitis, following traumatic or systemic inflammatory conditions (including gout and rheumatoid arthritis), can be evaluated and treated arthroscopically. Posttraumatic DRUJ stiffness can be treated by an arthroscopic arthrolysis as well.

DRUJ arthroscopy allows for the recognition and treatment of isolated detachment of the foveal insertion of the TFCC in which the capsular attachments are still preserved.[5] Through DRUJ arthroscopy, the avulsed radioulnar ligament (RUL) is debrided and the "vacant fovea" is freshened to permit repair via transosseous sutures or bone anchors. Likewise, in the early stages of ulnocarpal impaction (UCI), the central disc may present with only an isolated partial thickness tear on the proximal surface due to the local friction against the prominent ulnar head. Yet the distal surface maintains a normal appearance when viewed from the radiocarpal joint. DRUJ arthroscopy allows for proximal disc debridement and wafer resection of the ulnar head, preventing the complete disc resection required to perform the procedure through the ulnocarpal (UC) joint. In addition, more sophisticated salvage procedures for DRUJ posttraumatic or degenerative chondromalacia, like a Bowers resection arthroplasty or a Sauvé-Kapandji procedure, can be done arthroscopically.[6]

CONTRAINDICATIONS

There are no absolute contraindications to DRUJ arthroscopy. It is relatively contraindicated in an extremely small joint that would increase the risk of iatrogenic damage. Radiographic evidence of degenerative changes will alert the surgeon to this risk.

TECHNIQUE OF DRUJ ARTHROSCOPY

The patient is positioned supine under regional anesthesia, usually brachial plexus block, with the arm abducted under tourniquet control. The wrist is positioned vertically with the elbow flexed to 90°, as for a standard wrist arthroscopy. Finger traps are placed on the index and middle (or ring) fingers with 3 to 5 kg of traction using some type of traction tower.[7] In such a small and narrow joint, use of a wide-angle 1.9-mm arthroscope is preferred for the easy access and reduced risk of damage to the intra-articular structures. In our experience fluid distention of the DRUJ is not necessary, since it rarely improves the quality of view achieved by the simple joint distraction provided by the traction tower. Particularly if we expect to perform an arthroscopic procedure or an open surgical approach after arthroscopy, we prefer to use the "dry arthroscopy" technique.[7,8] Presently, we limit the use of saline to flush out the synovial liquid in intense DRUJ synovitis, and then the joint is dried with suction. During traditional "wet arthroscopy," the synovial fringes float in front of the scope and prevent good vision, especially in this narrow joint. DRUJ arthroscopy usually follows a previous arthroscopic survey of the radiocarpal and midcarpal joints. The traditional DRUJ portals are on the dorsal aspect of the wrist: proximal (P-DRUJ) and distal (D-DRUJ) DRUJ portals. Recently other 2 portals have been

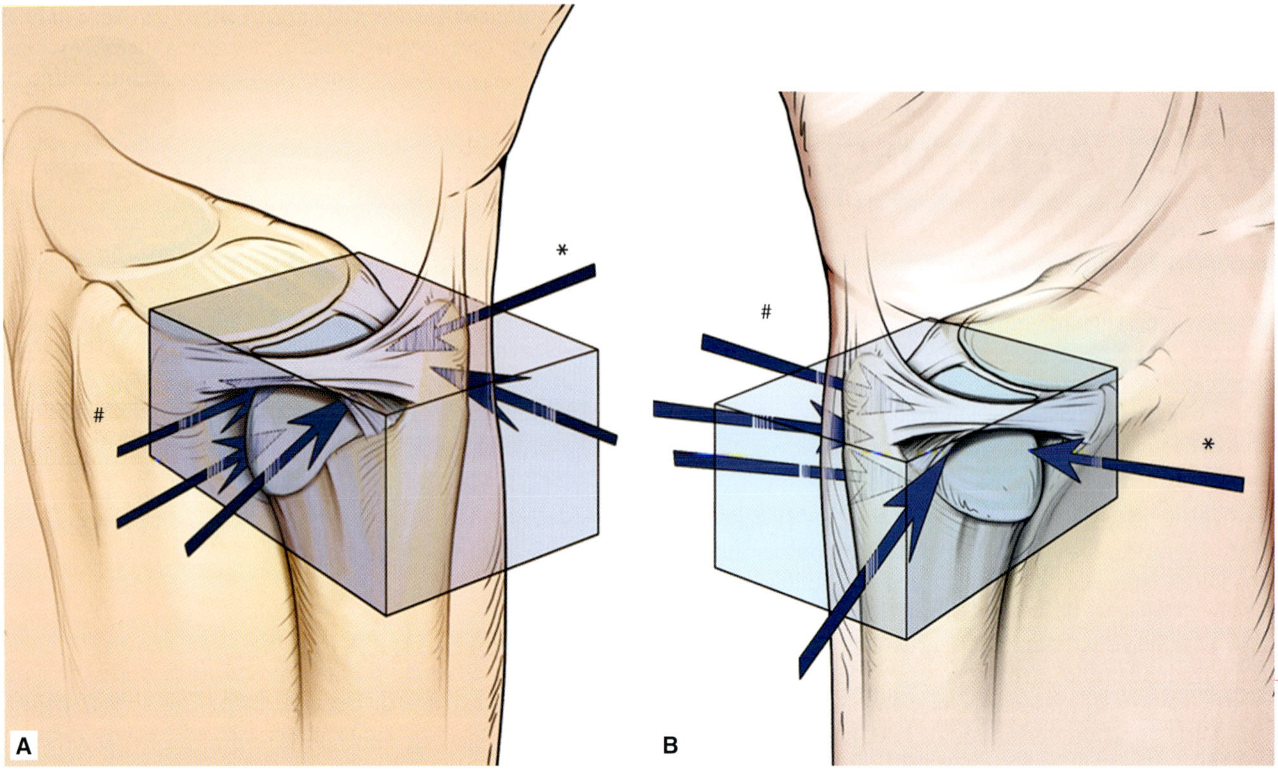

FIGURE 32-1 Drawings of arthroscopic portal to the DRUJ. **A.** Dorsal approach to the DRUJ with 3 portals: (#) preferred dorsal portal. **B.** Volar approach to the DRUJ with 2 portals: (*) preferred palmar portal.

described: the direct foveal (DF)[9] and the volar DRUJ portal.[3] The DF portal is immediately under the 6U portal and is used as a working portal about the foveal insertion of the TFCC. The volar DRUJ portal is located on the volar aspect of the wrist immediately ulnar to the edge of the flexor tendons and it is used for scope and instrument introduction (Fig. 32-1).

We prefer to start the DRUJ exploration through a dorsal portal that is located at a midpoint between the traditional P- and D-DRUJ portals (Fig. 32-2), in a triangular space that can be defined as the "medial soft corner," which is below the insertion of the TFCC on the radius, at the point where the distal profile of the ulnar head curves to parallel the sigmoid notch (Fig. 32-3). After a 22-gauge needle is inserted to confirm correct portal placement, a longitudinal skin incision is made and a mosquito is used to spread the subcutaneous tissues and penetrate the joint through the dorsal capsule, just below the TFCC and medial to the ulnar head. Care should be taken not to damage the extensor digiti minimi (EDM), running in the fifth dorsal compartment. The 1.9-mm arthroscope is introduced through a cannula with a blunt obturator. The arthroscope is short enough to be grasped while keeping the index finger in constant contact of the skin of the wrist in order to stabilize and control the minute movements of the scope within the joint. Full wrist supination allows easier access to the DRUJ through the dorsal portals (Fig. 32-4). We recommend starting joint exploration by rotating the scope, rather than moving its tip inside the joint. Three important structures should be assessed: (1) the surface of the ulnar head, (2) the deep TFCC fibers and their foveal insertion, and (3) the sigmoid notch. DRUJ exploration starts with the scope rotated ulnarwards to observe the ulnar head at the bottom (Fig. 32-5) and the TFCC ligament above. A 22-G needle, introduced from the area of the DF portal, may elevate the ligament to obtain a better vision of the ulnar part of the TFCC that curves proximally to insert onto the fovea (Fig. 32-6). The sigmoid notch (Fig. 32-7) is visualized by rotating the scope 180° radialwards and following the slope of the ulnar head that curves downward to face the radius. Wrist pronosupination is helpful for a thorough exploration of the opposing surfaces of the sigmoid notch and ulnar head (Fig. 32-8).

Accessory working portals are required for probe or instrument introduction. In our experience, the easiest portal to establish is the DF, which is located approximately 1 cm proximal to the 6U portal, just palmar to the ulnar styloid.[9] Portal placement can be confirmed by the introduction of a 22-G needle under arthroscopic surveillance. The wrist is positioned in full supination so that the dorsal sensory branch of the ulnar nerve (DSBUN) is displaced dorsally, the scalpel cuts the skin only, and the path to the capsule is prepared by gentle spreading of the subcutaneous tissues with a mosquito and a blunt trocar.

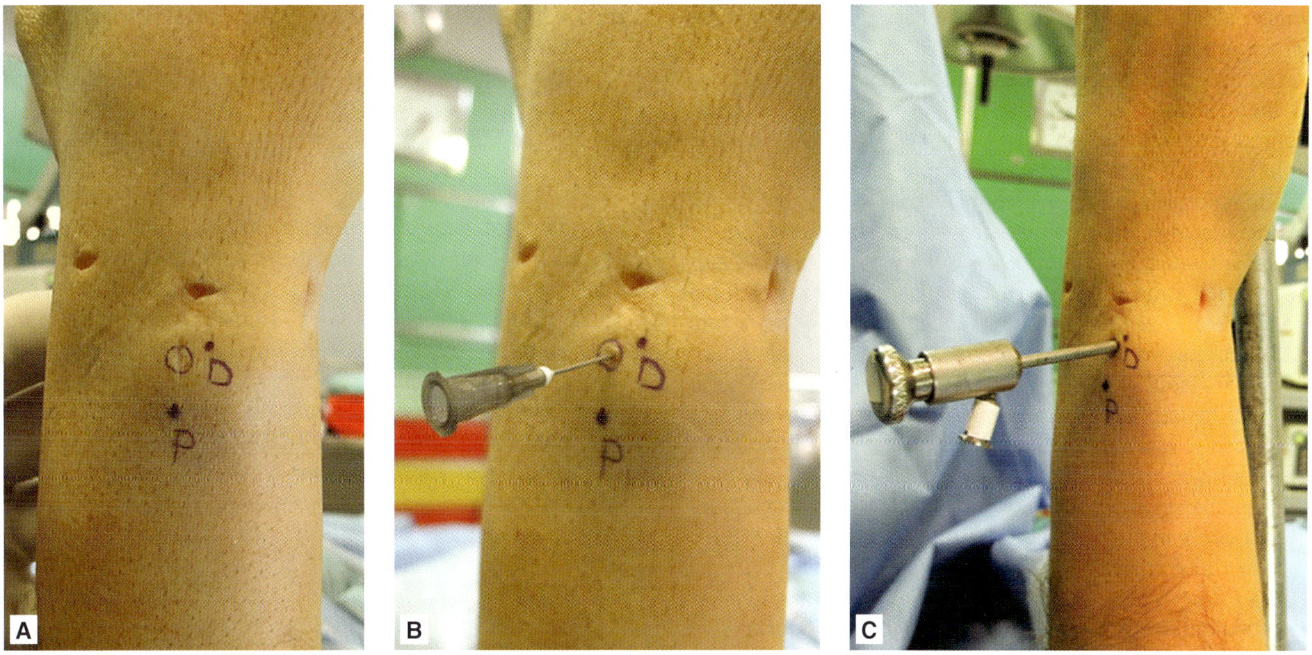

FIGURE 32-2 Clinical localization of the dorsal DRUJ portal by needle followed by introduction of the trocar.

The DRUJ volar portal is performed using a switching rod/trocar following a procedure similar to that proposed by Snyder for the creation of the anterior portal of the shoulder.[10]

The arthroscope is inserted through D-DRUJ portal and its tip is pushed against the anterior capsule below the TFCC ligament; then the scope is removed and a blunt trocar or switching rod is introduced into the cannula. It is pushed palmarward to perforate the capsule and tent the skin (Fig. 32-9A). In our experience, the ulnar neurovascular bundle has never been damaged in the execution of this technique. It is believed that the neurovascular structure is moved away by the gentle passage of the blunt trocar. A small stab wound is made over the tip of the trocar and the trocar and cannula are passed outside the skin (Fig. 32-9B). Then the trocar is removed and the cannula is used as a guide to introduce the probe or the shaver (full radius) into the joint (Fig. 32-10A and B). A standard shaver/burr or a small probe fits perfectly inside the cannula and the procedure is straightforward and safe (Fig. 32-11).

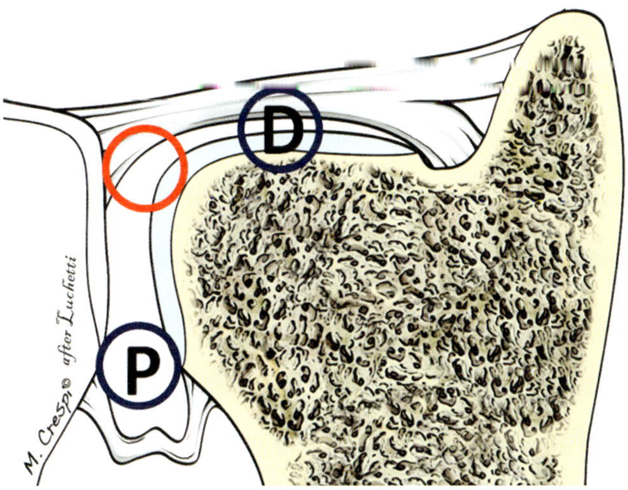

FIGURE 32-3 Anatomical drawings of the position of the preferred DRUJ portal.

The blunt tipped switching rod is necessary to switch the scope from the dorsal to the palmar side. The switching rod is introduced into the cannula protruding from the palmar portal. Then the cannula is removed from the dorsal portal to be introduced in the volar portal through the switching rod. Finally, the switching rod is removed to allow introduction of the scope to observe the joint from the palmar side (Fig. 32-12A and B).

SURGICAL PROCEDURES

Synovectomy and Loose Body Removal

These are the simplest and commonest procedures. Hypertrophic synovium is often found even in the healthy DRUJ and is localized mainly to the dorsal and volar edges of the sigmoid notch and close to the fovea. Use of a small shaver (1.9- or 2.5-mm full radius) is recommended. After resection of the pathologic synovitis, an injection of cortisone with carbocaine and epinephrine is suggested to reduce bleeding and postoperative pain.

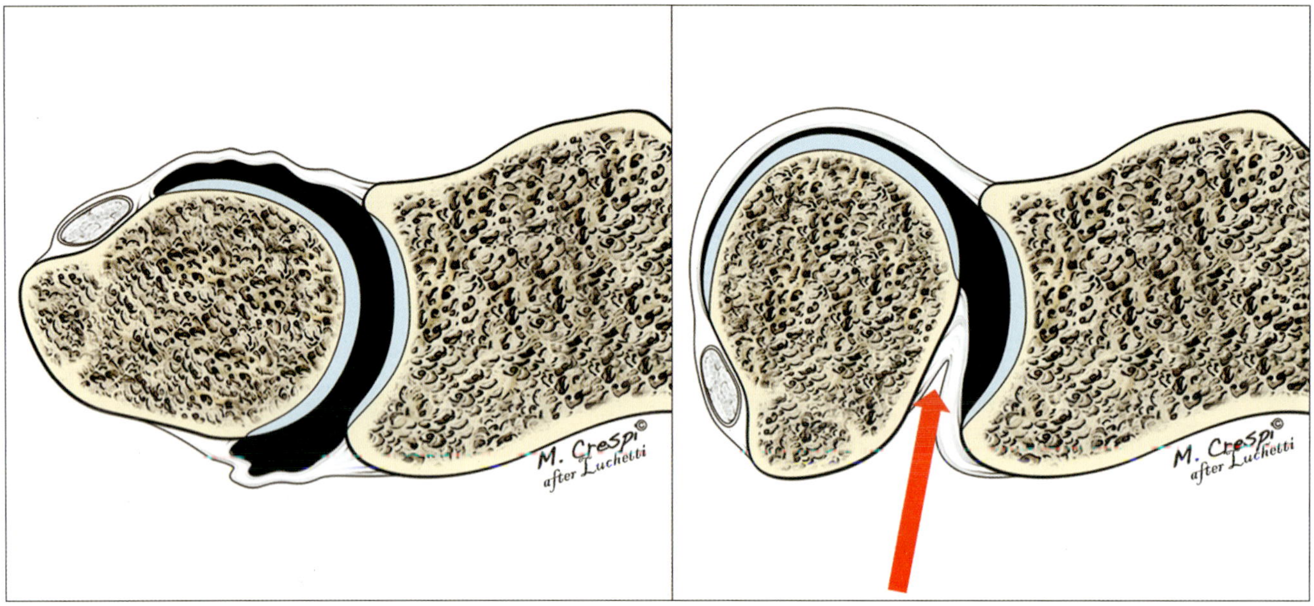

FIGURE 32-4 Drawing showing the introduction position of the arthroscope (red arrow) into the DRUJ: vision from the top.

Loose bodies should be searched for among synovial fringes close to the fovea and in the proximal pouch of the joint.

DRUJ Arthrolysis

A DRUJ arthrolysis usually follows a radiocarpal arthrolysis, but occasionally is performed as an isolated procedure.[11] The prerequisite that ensures a good result for DRUJ arthroscopic arthrolysis is the preservation of a normal articular surface. Stiffness is due to capsular retraction, intra-articular fibrotic bands, and synovitis that in turn make arthroscopy more difficult. Two situations are encountered: (a) TFCC intact and (b) TFCC damaged with central perforation.

a. When the TFCC is intact, it should be preserved and DRUJ arthrolysis is performed using dorsal and volar DRUJ portals. The scope is introduced in the preferred DRUJ dorsal portal and the instruments in the volar portal. At the beginning of the procedure, usually, fibrosis

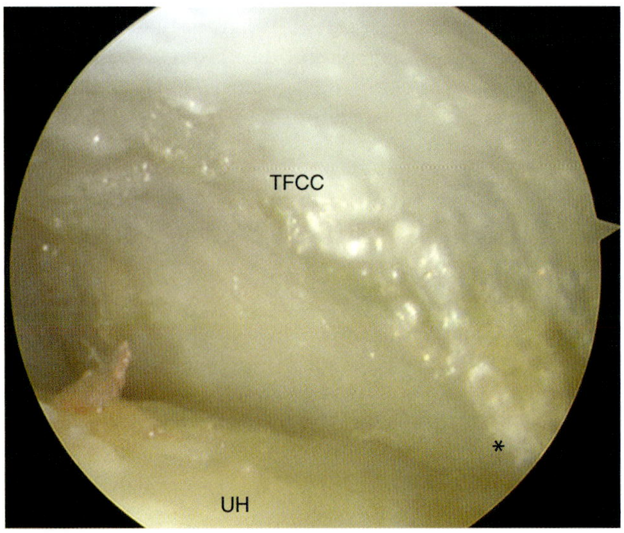

FIGURE 32-5 Arthroscopic image of the DRUJ: triangular fibrocartilage complex (TFCC) and ulnar head (UH).

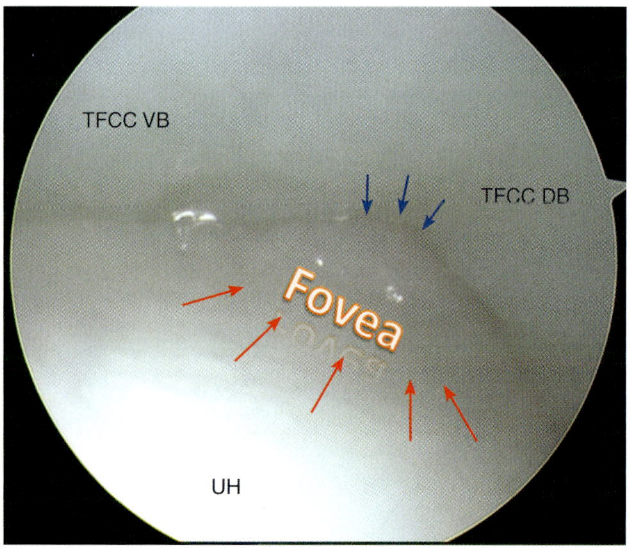

FIGURE 32-6 Arthroscopic image of the TFCC insertion (blue arrows) at the fovea (red arrows): volar branch of the TFCC (TFCC VB) and dorsal branch of the TFCC (TFCC DB).

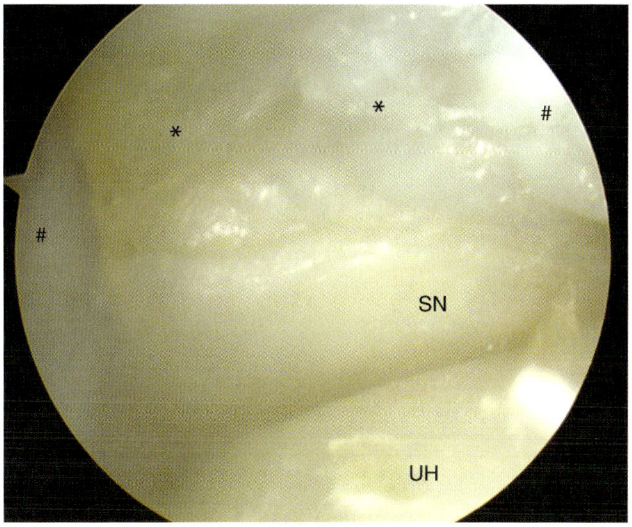

FIGURE 32-7 Arthroscopic images of the DRU joint: SN, sigmoid notch; UH, ulnar head; (*) central insertion of the TFCC; (#) radial insertion of the volar and dorsal branches of the TFCC.

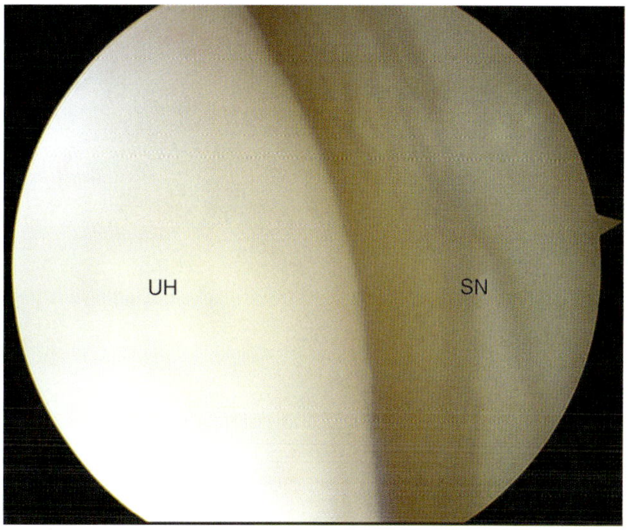

FIGURE 32-8 Arthroscopic images of the DRUJ: SN, sigmoid notch; UH, ulnar head.

does not permit good visualization and sometimes fluid is used to expand the joint and improve the vision. Once some vision is achieved and the tip of the instruments can be recognized, the fibrosis is progressively removed with a full radius resector or more aggressive motorized blade.

From the arthroscopic point of view, the DRUJ includes 2 spaces (Fig. 32-13): that which is between the TFCC ligament and the ulnar head, and the other between the ulnar head and the sigmoid notch. In a posttraumatic condition, both the spaces are involved. Fibrosis under

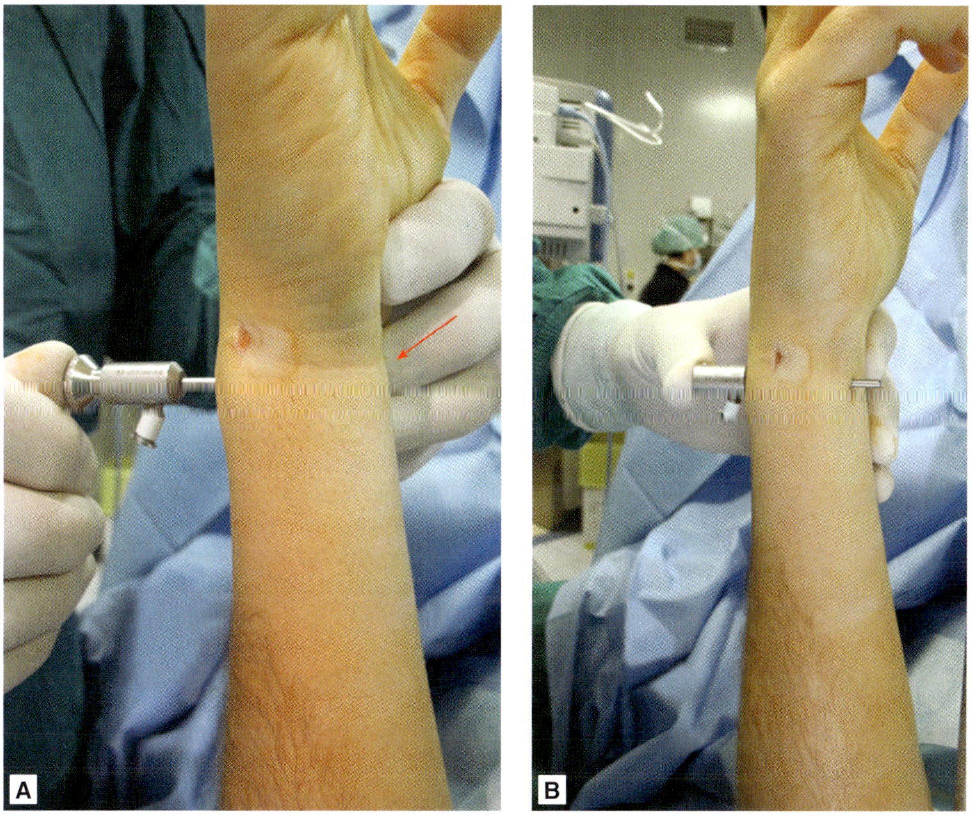

FIGURE 32-9 Technical procedure to perform the volar arthroscopic portal. **A.** Trocar perforated the volar capsule and tented the skin (red arrow). **B.** Trocar passed the skin through a short incision (volar portal).

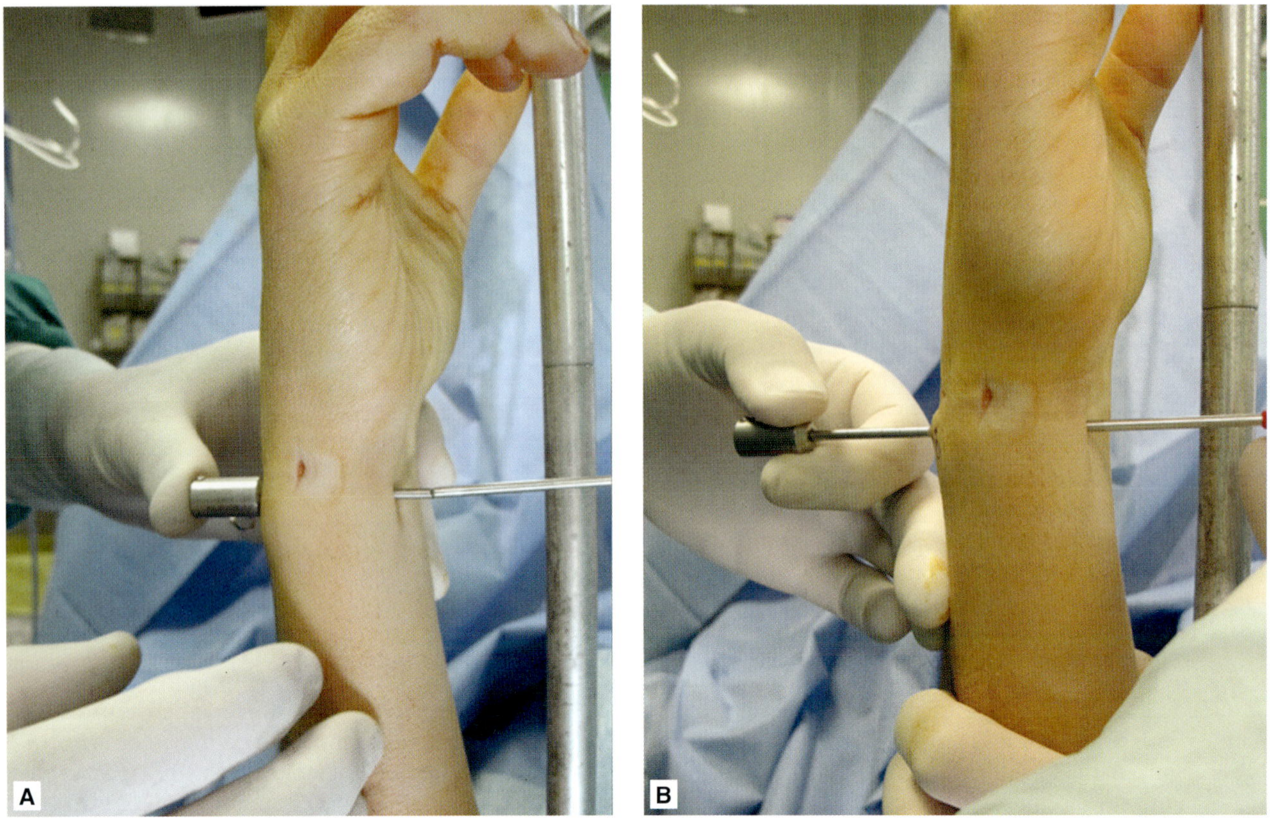

FIGURE 32-10 Technique of shaver introduction into the DRUJ through the volar portal. The trocar is used as a guide (**A**) to enter into the joint (**B**).

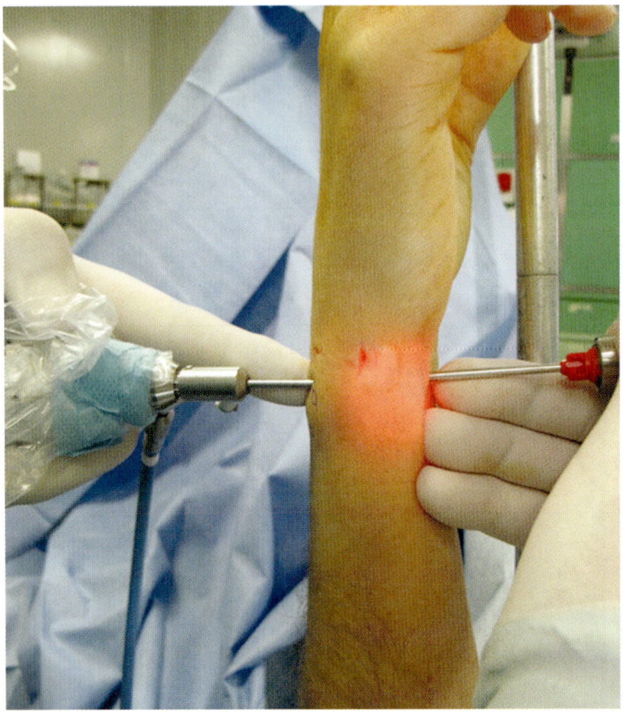

FIGURE 32-11 Position of arthroscope and shaver. The surgeon is positioned in front of the ulnar side of the wrist.

the TFCC precludes any visualization by arthroscopy, and in the absence of a central TFCC perforation good visualization is difficult. In these conditions, we suggest introducing a blunt dissector between the TFCC and the ulnar head, and gently dissecting the adhesions. It could also be done by shaving using the traditional dorsal portals or the DF portal. The second space, lying between the ulnar head and the sigmoid notch, is affected by contraction of the volar and dorsal capsule, which limits pronosupination. Fibrotic bands can be present between the 2 articular surfaces, as a result of a fracture involving 1 or both of them. Arthroscopic arthrolysis of this space starts with the scope in the distal dorsal portal and instruments in the proximal one. The dorsal and the volar capsule must be detached and/or resected (Fig. 32-14). An anterior capsulectomy improves supination and posterior capsulectomy improves pronation. To facilitate visualization and speed up this part of the procedure, a curved dissector is introduced into the joint from the proximal portal. By passing it from dorsal to volar, it is possible to detach the capsule from the margins of the sigmoid notch and cut the fibrotic bands. The radial and ulnar insertion of the TFCC ligament, as well as the articular surface of the ulnar head and sigmoid notch, must be preserved. Finally, after removing the wrist traction, gentle pronation and supination maneuvers are performed

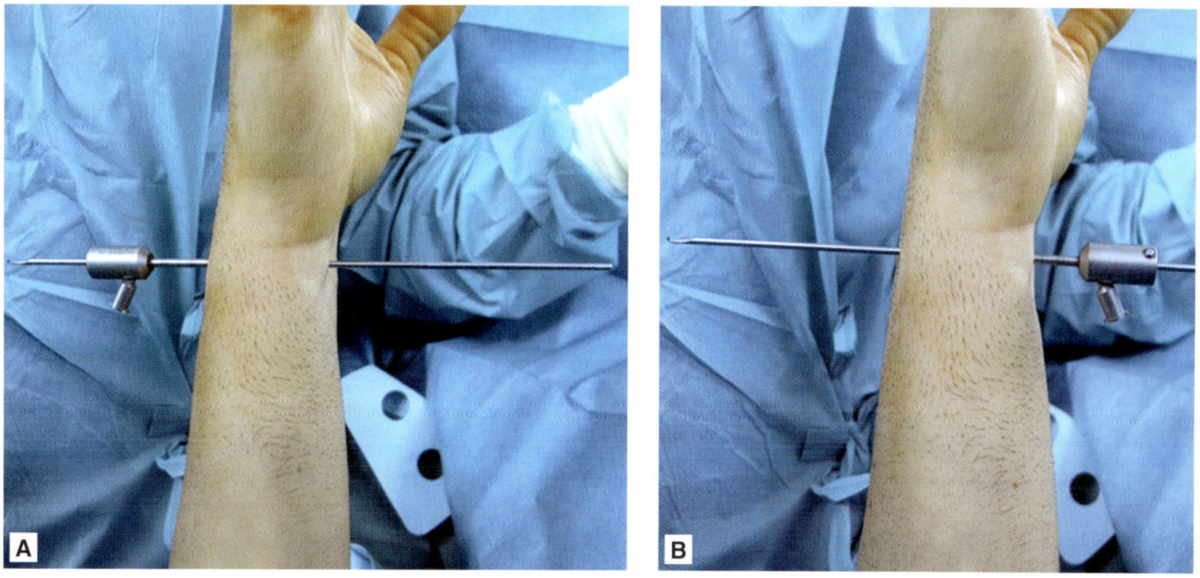

FIGURE 32-12 Technique of changing the position of the trocar from the dorsal (A) to the volar portal (B) using a switching rod.

to evaluate the amount of improvement in the range of motion (ROM).

b. When the TFCC has a central lesion, the arthrolysis can start using radiocarpal arthroscopy, using the 3-4 and 6R portals, for the scope and instruments. The TFCC perforation is enlarged as necessary to visualize the DRUJ. The procedure then proceeds by switching the scope to the 6R portal and introducing the motorized instrumentation and dissectors via the D-DRUJ portal. The fibrotic bands between the ulnar head and the sigmoid notch are resected and the volar and dorsal capsule detached as necessary. In this condition, an arthroscopic wafer resection is also required at the end of the procedure.

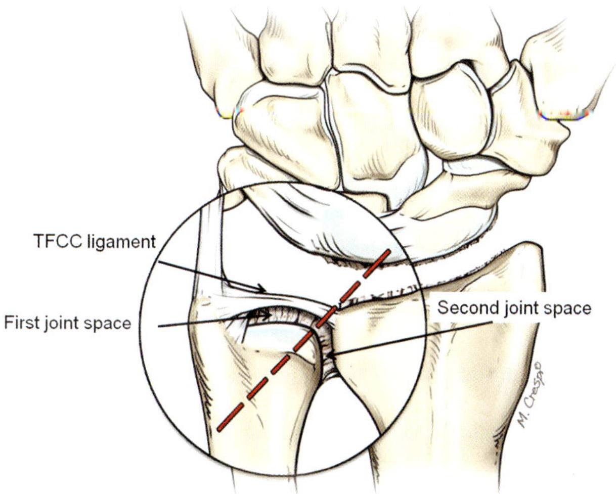

FIGURE 32-13 Drawings of DRUJ with adherences and fibrosis. The dotted red line divides the articular spaces: the superior space is under the TFCC ligament and the inferior is the proper articular space.

Reattachment of the Foveal Detachment of the TFCC

Isolated detachment of the foveal insertions of the TFCC is an uncommon form of TFCC peripheral tear that is associated with DRUJ instability, which is a type 3 tear according to Atzei-EWAS classification.[4] In this type of lesion the TFCC appears normal from the radiocarpal joint but there is a positive hook test, that is, the entire TFCC can be pulled radially and proximally with the hook probe. DRUJ arthroscopy is used to visualize the ruptured deep fibers and the "vacant fovea" (Fig. 32-15).

With the scope in the D-DRUJ portal, the TFCC can be elevated with a probe and the RUL remnants can be debrided with a shaver via the DF portal. Through the same portal, a burr can be used to "refresh" the foveal area and prepare for

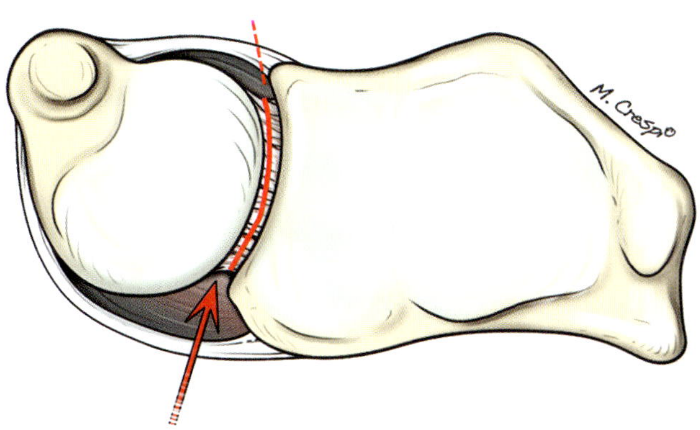

FIGURE 32-14 Drawing showing the technical procedure to resect the adherences between the ulnar head and the sigmoid notch (red line) through the volar approach (red arrow). Dorsal capsule is also resected (dotted red line).

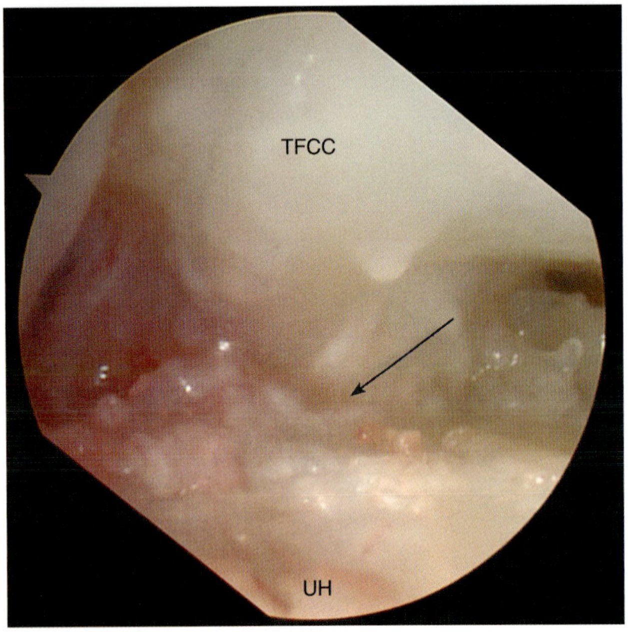

FIGURE 32-15 Arthroscopic image of the TFCC partial detachment from fovea insertion (black arrow).

reattachment of the foveal fibers. We prefer to use a 4-strand suture attached to a bone anchor, introduced through the DF portal, under arthroscopic control (Fig. 32-16A-C). Each suture is threaded through a 22-G Tuohy needle that is introduced via the DF portal under the RULs and pushed upward to pierce the ligament (Fig. 32-16D). Then the suture can be retrieved in the UC joint via the 6U portal. The sutures are placed in pairs, 1 for each branch of the RUL, and tied with a gliding knot and a knot pusher through the 6U portal. For an optimal healing, the knot pusher compresses the RUL against the bleeding fovea and no suture material is interposed between the healing surfaces. Postoperatively, the patient is placed in long arm or Münster-type thermoplastic splint for 4 weeks. Then wrist flexion/extension is started and progressive forearm rotation is allowed, but the splint is still worn between exercises until the sixth week. Progressive resisted wrist and hand strengthening exercises begin thereafter. Sport and heavy work tasks are allowed only after 3 months, according to the recovery of forearm muscle strength and endurance.

OUTCOMES

We examined 25 patients (12 women and 13 men), mean age 33 years (range, 13-69 years), who underwent an arthroscopically assisted foveal reattachment from 2006 to 2009. At a minimum follow-up of 6 months (mean 31 months; maximum 6 years), DRUJ stability was obtained in all but 5 patients. Pain at rest and under stress was reduced, reaching a statistical significance (P <.001). Flexion/extension wrist motion, pronosupination, and grip strength increased postoperatively. Overall objective wrist function was evaluated using the Mayo wrist score and results demonstrated a significant improvement (P <.001). Subjective hand function was assessed using both the DASH score and PRWE score. Both assessments demonstrated significant improvement (P <.001).

Wafer Resection

In the early stages of UCI, the central disc may show only partial thickness tear and attrition of the proximal surface against the prominent ulnar head, so that the distal surface as seen from the radiocarpal joint maintains a normal appearance and texture. In the typical case, however, the central disc is perforated. After debridement, the disc perforation is enlarged enough to provide good visualization and perform a wafer resection via the 3-4 and 6R portals. Forearm rotation facilitates the exposure of the ulnar head under the volar and dorsal margins of the TFCC to allow an adequate resection of the ulnar head. Conversely, in young subjects, when radiocarpal exploration reveals an intact TFCC, it is preferable to save the central disc and perform the wafer resection via DRUJ arthroscopy. The scope is introduced in the D-DRUJ portal providing good visualization of the shaver and burr inserted though the DF or volar portal (Fig. 32-17). Limited forearm rotation is usually required. The tear of the proximal disc is debrided and the ulnar head resected up to the foveal insertion of the TFCC, taking care not to damage the ligamentous fibers. The technique is moderately more difficult, due to the close proximity of scope and instruments. Care should be taken at the time of introduction of the burr, because its tip can be trapped in the soft tissues around the portals: use of a small cannula is advisable. Advantages of this procedure include reduced postoperative pain and the expected long-term benefit of a preserved load-bearing disc.[12,13]

OUTCOMES

From 2002 to 2011 we operated on 31 patients (18 males and 13 females) with a mean age of 40 years (range 17-63 years) with UCI. In 30 cases an ulna plus was present. In 4 cases it was due to wrist fracture; in 3 cases it was secondary to a resection of the radial head. In 3 cases a distal radius malunion coexisted. The arthroscopic wafer resection procedure gave good result in almost all the cases, improving the pronosupination, reducing pain, and increasing grip strength. Only 2 cases (6%) underwent an open surgical revision for persistent symptoms due to secondary synovitis. The cases due to distal radius malunion improved despite the fact that the ulnar head remained in the same preoperative position. No complications were seen.

Arthroscopic Sauvé-Kapandji Technique

The arthroscopic Sauvé-Kapandji (ASK) is an arthroscopic modification of the original open technique[14] that consists

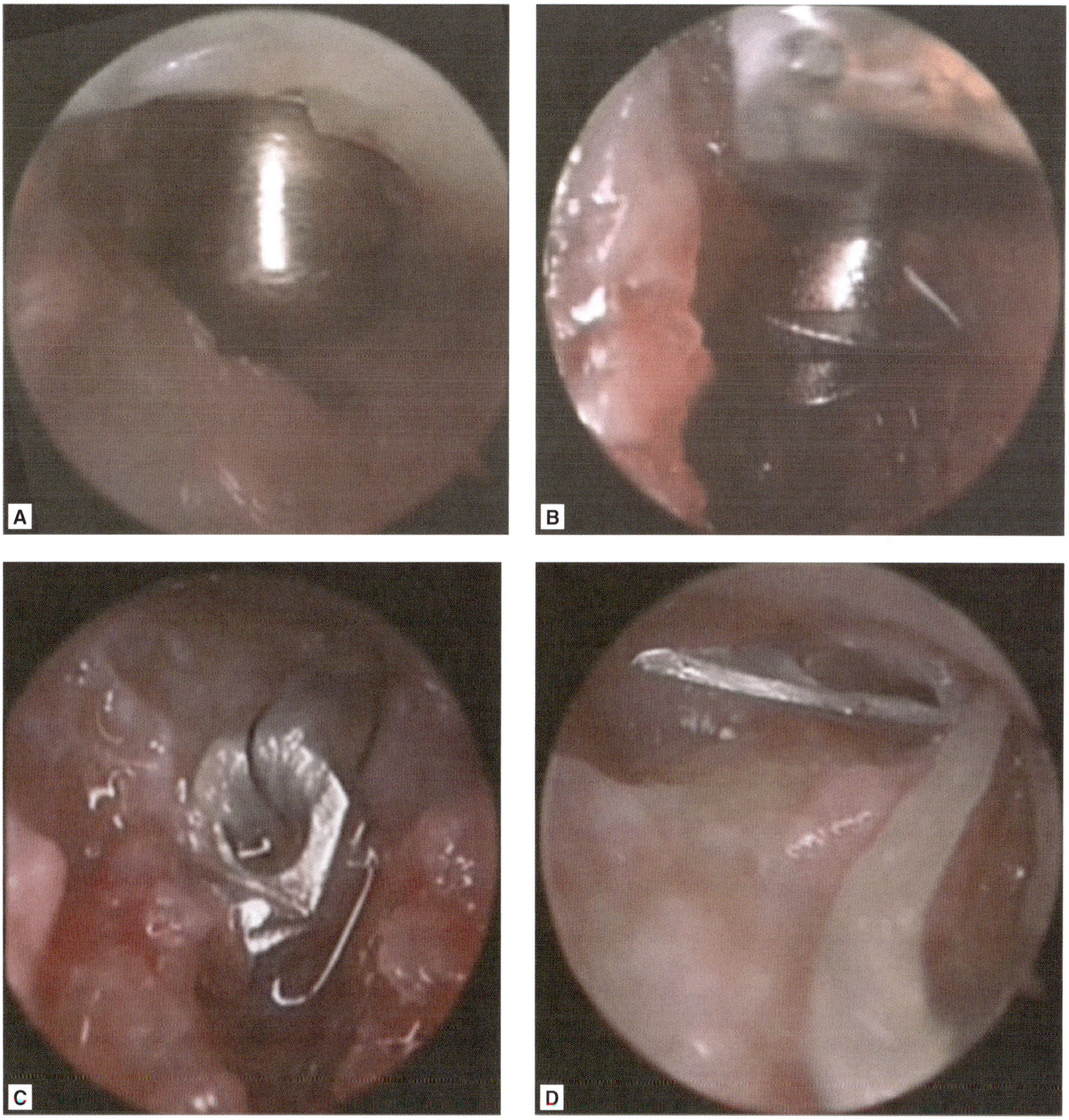

FIGURE 32-16 Arthroscopic reattachment of the TFCC through the DRUJ using a bone anchor. The scope is in the D-DRUJ portal and the DF portal is used for instrumentation (ie, the shaver to refresh the fovea) (**A**). The bone anchor is inserted into the fovea (**B**) and, at the end of the procedure, the sutures exit though the DF portal (**C**). Then the sutures are loaded on a needle that is introduced via the DF portal and pushed upward to pierce the TFCC and be retrieved from the radiocarpal joint (**D**).

of a DRUJ fusion and creation of an artificial pseudarthrosis of the ulnar neck. It requires a combination of arthroscopic access to the DRUJ and a mini-open approach to the distal ulna and ulnar neck. The technique can be successfully used for the treatment of primary or secondary DRUJ osteoarthritis and in rheumatoid patients. An unstable or arthritic DRUJ with or without UCI following a distal radius fracture is an ideal candidate for the ASK technique.[6] The first step of the procedure is radiocarpal arthroscopy, in which attention is focused to the UC joint, followed by DRUJ arthroscopy. The 3-4 portal is used for the scope and 6R for the probe. The UC arthroscopy is used to assess the condition of the TFCC and cartilage of both the lunate and the triquetrum, as they may be damaged by a coexisting UCI that should be treated during the same sitting. The ulnar head is exposed through the perforated TFCC and the DRUJ can be approached from the UC joint. In order to remove the cartilage on both the ulnar head and the sigmoid notch, a D-DRUJ portal is used to

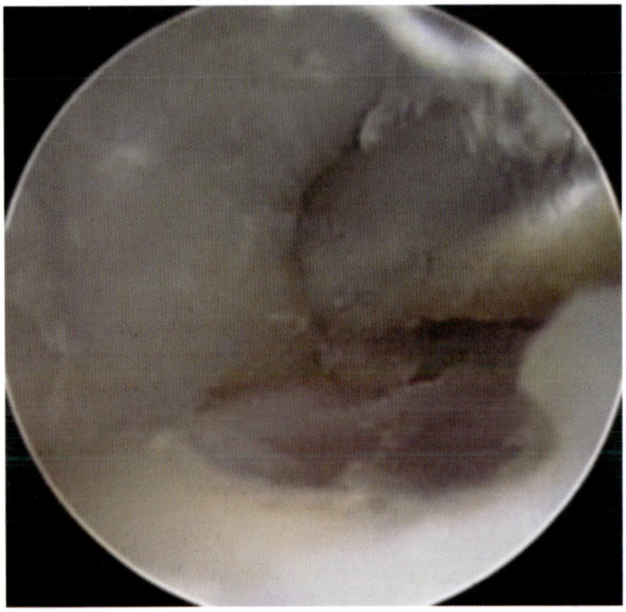

FIGURE 32-17 Arthroscopic image of wafer resection through the DRUJ. Scope in the D-DRUJ portal and burr in the DF portal.

introduce a motorized "burr" and/or radio-frequency device (Fig. 32-18A and B), while the scope is positioned in the 6R portal. Use of a 3.5-mm burr is recommended to speed up cartilage debridement and suction removal of the debris. The cartilage removal from the DRUJ should be done with the wrist in neutral pronosupination, because this is the site of joint contact, where the arthrodesis should be performed. Forearm rotation in pronation and anteroposterior translation of the ulnar head facilitate cartilage removal. When a sufficient area of subchondral bone is exposed on the opposing surfaces of both the ulnar head and the sigmoid notch, the forearm is positioned in neutral pronosupination to fix the DRUJ. Preliminary DRUJ fixation is achieved using a K-wire that is positioned anterior to the ECU tendon, under fluoroscopic control. Then a short vertical skin incision is made on the ulnar aspect of the wrist to allow cannulated drilling and introduction of a 2.5- to 3.0-mm cannulated screw across the DRUJ over the previous K-wire. At this time, forearm rotation is blocked in neutral pronosupination. Forearm rotation can be restored only after the ulnar osteotomy. Under fluoroscopic control, the correct level of the osteotomy, just proximal to the ulnar neck, is checked. The previous vertical skin incision is continued proximally to the level of the ulnar osteotomy, which is performed with an osteotome or oscillating saw. Usually, a bone block of 0.5 to 1 cm is resected from the ulnar neck. The screw across the DRUJ is then tightened to achieve optimal compression of the DRUJ. A 2.0-mm K-wire is drilled, parallel to the screw, to provide additional reinforcement to the screw fixation and avoid undue rotation of the distal ulna (Fig. 32-19). After the bone block is removed from the ulna, forearm rotation is checked and the stability of the ulnar stump is also assessed. At the end of the procedure, a final arthroscopic evaluation can be done, and with the probe, a good fixation and stability of the DRUJ can be appreciated. During all the arthroscopic surgery, the DRUJ is never surgically exposed. Postoperatively, an above-elbow cast is worn for 2 weeks with the forearm in neutral pronosupination and the elbow flexed at 90°. Rehabilitation and physical therapy is continued for 1 month after the removal of the cast.

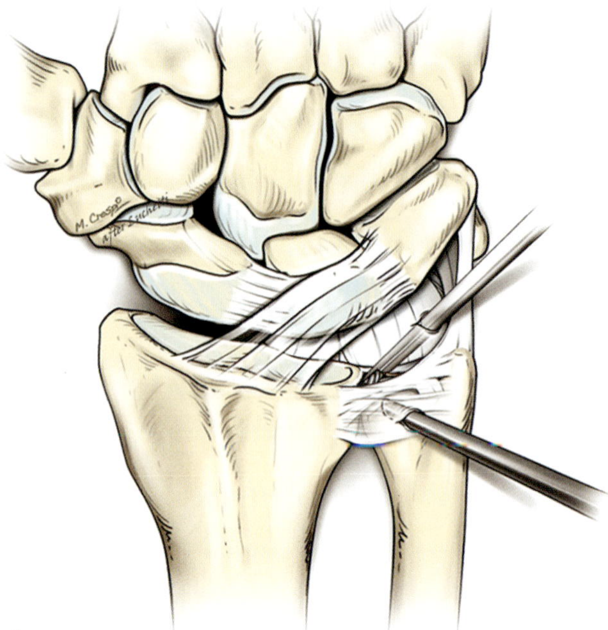

A

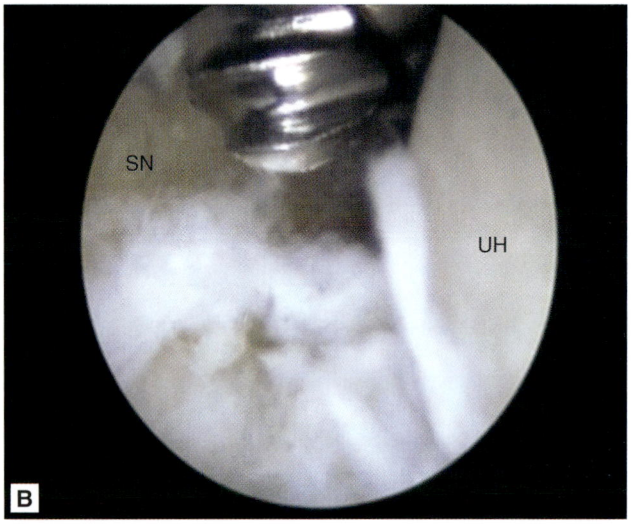

FIGURE 32-18 **A.** Drawing showing the technical procedure to resect the ulnar head articular surface. **B.** Arthroscopic images of the ulnar head (UH) articular surface resection. SN, sigmoid notch.

OUTCOMES

From 2003 to 2010, 4 patients (5 wrists) were operated on. The mean age was 54 years (range, 32-78). The male patient had a primary arthritis of the DRUJ without sign of articular

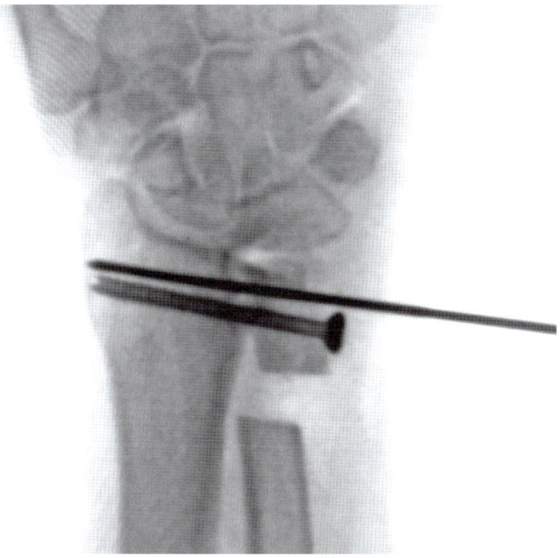

FIGURE 32-19 PA x-ray view of Sauvé-Kapandji procedure.

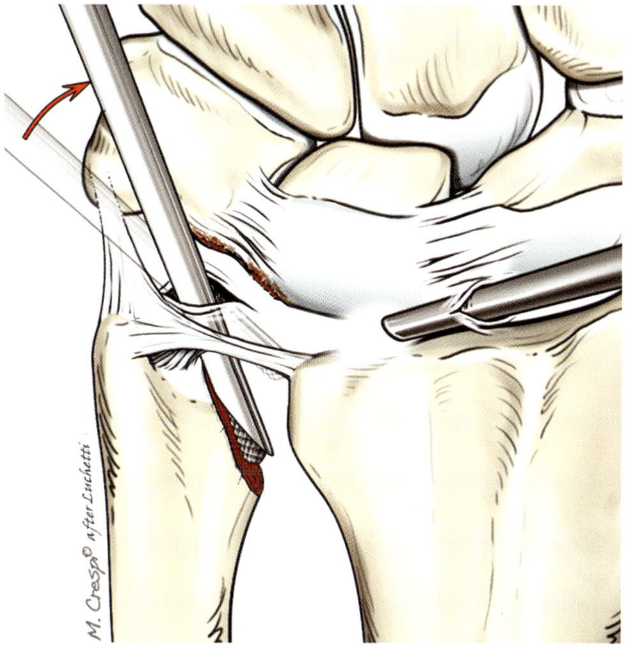

FIGURE 32-20 Technical procedure of arthroscopic Bowers procedure.

degeneration at the RC and MC joint. The youngest female had posttraumatic DRUJ and LT instability. She had 2 previous unsuccessful procedures for the DRUJ instability (arthroscopic and open surgery, respectively). At the last wrist (DRUJ) arthroscopy ulnar head chondromalacia was seen without radiological signs of DRUJ degeneration. The last 2 patients had DRUJ contracture due to posttraumatic arthritis with ulnar dorsal subluxation and UC abutment due to previous wrist fracture. In these cases an arthroscopic wafer resection was combined with an arthroscopic-assisted S-K procedure. At a mean follow-up of 52 months (range, 96-10 months) 4/5 patients went on to union. The mean VAS pain score improved from 7 to 0 at rest and from 9 to 2 after heavy work. The mean ROM (pronosupination) and grip strength increased consistently. The 1 patient in which the procedure failed was noncompliant with the rehabilitation and follow-up.

The patients who healed returned to their previous manual work. X-rays demonstrated complete fusion of the DRUJ in 4 cases, and a painless nonunion in the failed case.

Arthroscopic Ulnar Head Resection Technique (Arthroscopic Modified Bowers Technique)

Complete arthroscopic ulnar head resection[6] represents an extension of the technique of wafer resection. Thus, it creates a form of Bowers procedure,[15] in which the ulnar styloid and the foveal insertions of the RUL are preserved in continuity with the ulnar shaft (Fig. 32-20). An arthroscopic ulnar head resection is the simplest form of DRUJ arthroplasty to perform. It is indicated in low-demand patients with advanced DRUJ arthritis, in which the foveal fibers are still competent. The procedure starts with the resection of the dome of the ulnar head and continues proximally resecting the articulating portion of the ulnar head. The sigmoid notch must be left untouched. Dry arthroscopy can also be used.[7,8] A preliminary radiocarpal arthroscopic survey is performed, using the 3-4 portal for the scope and 6R for the probe and instruments. Often the TFFC shows a central perforation of the articular disc, which allows one to perform the resection through the tear. If the disc is preserved, the procedure requires use of the D-DRUJ and volar portals for the scope. An arthroscopic synovectomy is the first step of the procedure. Then a 2.9-mm burr is used to perform a wafer resection of the ulnar dome, in order to create space and to allow introduction of a 3.5-mm burr to speed up the proximal resection. The burr can be switched from the D-DRUJ and volar portals, with the scope in the opposite DRUJ portal or in the 6R portal if the disc is perforated. Particular attention is placed to preserve the volar and the dorsal limbs of the RUL and its foveal insertion and avoid secondary DRUJ instability. Careful management of the motorized burr should reduce the risk of damage to the flexor tendons and the ulnar neurovascular bundle or the EDM and ECU tendons around the D-DRUJ and volar portals, respectively. The ulnar stump is resected in a rounded fashion using slight forearm rotation as for a wafer resection. As the resection of the ulnar head proceeds, the range of pronosupination increases. The resection ends when the sigmoid notch is clearly visible, and sufficient pronosupination is restored, without impingement. Fluoroscopy could be useful to check the correct amount of ulnar head resection (Fig. 32-21). Postoperatively, an above-elbow cast is worn for 2 weeks with forearm in neutral rotation and the elbow flexed at 90°. Rehabilitation and physical therapy started after 2 weeks, and a Münster-type

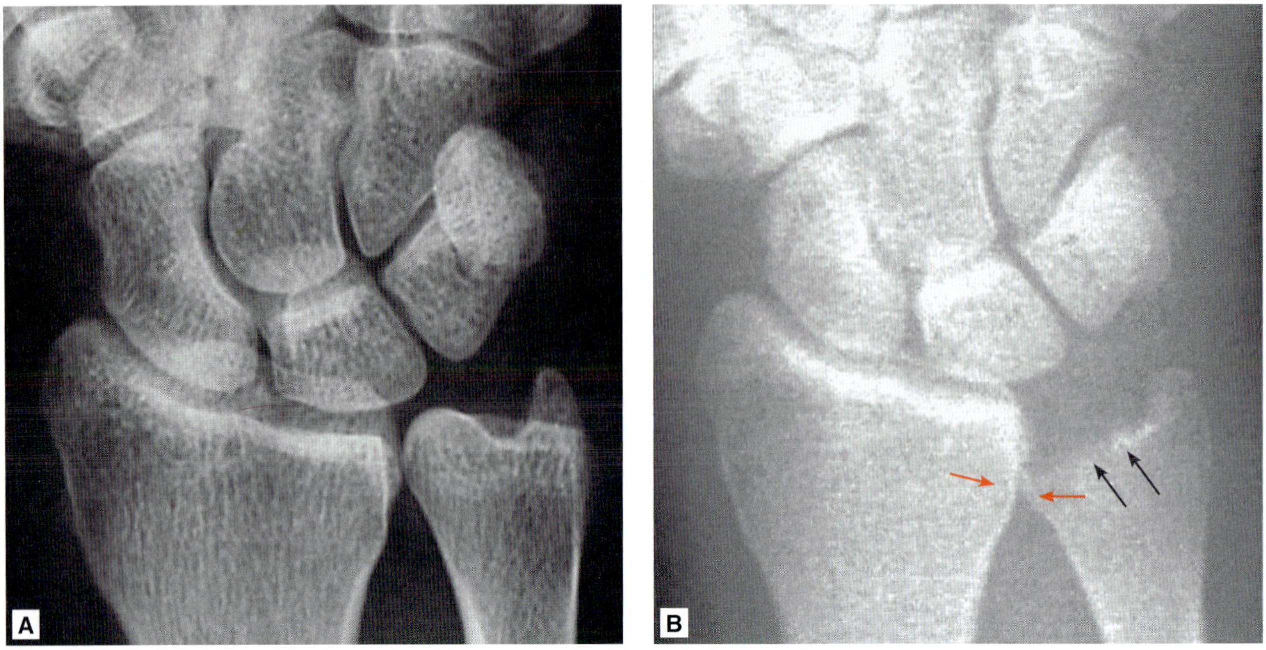

FIGURE 32-21 X-ray images of arthroscopic Bowers procedure (black arrows): preoperative (**A**) and postoperative (**B**). Note that part of the proximal ulnar head was maintained to protect the DRUJ from the ulnar impaction.

thermoplastic splint is worn between exercises for another 2 weeks. Progressive resisted wrist and hand strengthening exercises are started thereafter. The expected outcomes are usually good. However, such a procedure is not exempt from complications or unsatisfactory results as for the open surgery, even if it does not burn any bridges with regards to further open surgery.

COMPLICATIONS

The ulnar side of the wrist is anatomically complex with vessels and nerves that run in close proximity to the DRUJ. This condition is favorable for complications. In our experience, complete and partial lesions of the sensory nerves are rare.[16] One must be diligent to remember to use superficial skin incisions and perform the deeper dissection with blunt tipped instruments such as a mosquito forceps to enter into the DRUJ. We have no cases of infection. We have seen recurrence of DRUJ instability following a failed foveal repair, persistent pain in the UC joint after a wafer resection, and insufficient improvement in pronosupination following a DRUJ arthrolysis, and finally nonunion of the arthrodesis following an ASK procedure.

REFERENCES

1. Lawler EA, Adams BD. Arthroscopy of the distal radioulnar joint. In: Slutsky D, Nagle D, eds. *Techniques in Wrist and Hand Arthroscopy*. Philadelphia: Churchill Livingstone Elsevier; 2007:54–57.
2. Slutsky DJ. Arthroscopic evaluation of the foveal attachment of the triangular fibrocartilage. *Hand Clin*. 2011;27:255–261.
3. Slutsky DJ. Distal radioulnar joint arthroscopy and volar ulnar portal. *Tech Hand Up Extrem Surg*. 2007;11:38–44.
4. Whipple TL. Arthroscopy of the distal radioulnar joint. *Hand Clin*. 1994;10:589–592.
5. Atzei A. New trends in arthroscopic management of type 1-B TFCC injuries with DRUJ instability. *J Hand Surg Eur Vol*. 2009;34: 582–591.
6. Luchetti R. Arthroscopic ulnar head resection and Sauvé-Kapandji. In: del Piñal F, Mathoulin C, Nakamura T, eds. *Arthroscopic Management of Ulnar Pain*. Berlin: Springer-Verlag; 2012:315–334.
7. Atzei A, Luchetti R, Sgarbossa A, Carità E, Llusà M. Installation, voies d'abord et exploration normale en arthroscopie du poignet [Set-up, portals and normal exploration in wrist arthroscopy]. *Chir Main*. 2006;25:S131–S144.
8. del Piñal F, Garcia-Bernal FJ, Pisani D, Regalado J, Ayala H, Studer A. Dry arthroscopy of the wrist: surgical technique. *J Hand Surg Am*. 2007;32:119–123.
9. Atzei A, Rizzo A, Luchetti R, Fairplay T. Arthroscopic foveal repair of triangular fibrocartilage complex peripheral lesion with distal radioulnar joint instability. *Tech Hand Up Extrem Surg*. 2008;12: 226–235.
10. Snyder SJ. *Shoulder Arthroscopy*. New York: McGraw-Hill; 1994.
11. Luchetti R. The role of arthroscopy in post-traumatic stiffness. In: del Piñal F, Mathoulin C, Luchetti R, eds. *Arthroscopic Management of Distal Radius Fractures*. Berlin: Springer-Verlag; 2009:151–172.
12. Luchetti R, Atzei A, Borelli PP, Cozzolino R. Articolazione radioulnare distale: debridment della TFCC e wafer resection in plus dell'ulna. In: Adravanti P, Denti M, Mazzola C, Randelli P, Zorzi C, eds. *Artroscopia base ed avanzata*. Rome: CIC Edizioni Internazionali; 2012:733–744.
13. Mathoulin C. Ulnocarpal abutment: state of art and the role of arthroscopy. In: del Pinal F, Mathoulin C, Nakamura T, eds. *Arthroscopic Management of Ulnar Pain*. Berlin: Springer-Verlag; 2012:169–182.
14. Sauvé L, Kapandji M. Nouvelle technique de traitement chirurgical des luxation recidivantesisolees de l'extremiteeinferieure du cubitus. *J Chir*. 1936;47:589–594.
15. Bowers WH. Distal radioulnar joint arthroplasty: the hemiresection-interposition technique. *J Hand Surg Am*. 1985;10:169–178.
16. Luchetti R, Atzei A, Rocchi L. Fréquence et causes des mauvais résultats de l'arthroscopie du poignet. *Chir Main*. 2002;25:48–53.

33

Salvage Procedures of the DRUJ

Loukia K. Papatheodorou, MD
Dean G. Sotereanos, MD

INTRODUCTION

The distal radioulnar joint (DRUJ) is a complex articulation, between the sigmoid notch of the distal radius and the ulnar head, allowing significant rotational and translational motion. Degenerative changes of the DRUJ can be caused by posttraumatic arthritis (distal radius fracture, malunion), inflammatory arthritis (usually rheumatoid arthritis), osteoarthritis, or, rarely, long-standing DRUJ instability. Painful forearm rotation, increased pain with compression of the DRUJ, and decreased grip strength are the most common symptoms of DRUJ arthritis.

Stability of the DRUJ depends on bony and ligamentous structures including intrinsic stabilizers of the triangular fibrocartilage complex (TFCC) and extrinsic stabilizers of the distal forearm. Because of these interdependencies, treatment of the DRUJ is challenging since it is difficult to restore the original anatomy and function. Several surgical techniques have been developed for the treatment of DRUJ arthritis. The current salvage procedures not using a prosthetic implant include the Darrach procedure and its modifications, the hemiresection interposition technique (HIT), matched distal ulnar resection, and the Sauvé-Kapandji procedure.

DARRACH PROCEDURE

In 1912, Darrach described the resection of the entire ulnar head for the management of posttraumatic DRUJ dislocation.[1] Although distal ulnar resection had been previously reported, the procedure was popularized by Darrach and today it bears his name. The Darrach procedure has for many decades been considered the "gold standard" for management of chronic ulnocarpal or DRUJ arthritis.[2,3] However, numerous modifications of the Darrach procedure with soft tissue stabilization techniques have been proposed to reduce its major complications, radioulnar impingement and instability.[4–12]

Indications

The general indication for a distal ulnar resection is any condition that causes incongruity or arthritis of the DRUJ (inflammatory arthritis, posttraumatic arthritis, osteoarthritis), with resultant pain or stiffness.[13–15] The ideal candidate for the Darrach procedure is a patient with a relatively low-demand upper extremity without requirement of a load-bearing DRUJ.[3,15,16]

Contraindications

In patients with inflammatory arthropathy and coexisting ulnar translocation, an isolated Darrach procedure without radiocarpal stabilization is contraindicated to avoid exacerbating the ulnar translation. DRUJ instability in the patient without rheumatoid arthritis is considered a relative contraindication to the Darrach procedure.

Surgical Technique

The procedure is performed under general or regional anesthesia with the patient in supine position. The arm is supported on a standard table used for upper extremity and a tourniquet is used. An oblique dorsal approach over the fifth dorsal compartment is made.[1,9] An ulnar-based rectangle of retinaculum is raised for reinforcement after distal ulnar resection and careful attention is paid to avoid damaging the dorsal cutaneous branch of the ulnar nerve. Then a longitudinal capsulotomy is made deep to the fifth compartment beginning proximal to the dorsal radioulnar ligament and proceeding in a distal direction. Careful subperiosteal dissection allows elevation of a sleeve of periosteum along with the contiguous DRUJ capsule exposing the ulnar head.

Osteotomy of the distal ulna is performed just proximal to the sigmoid notch and the entire head is then removed along with the entire ulnar styloid. Care should be taken not to perform the osteotomy more proximal than the sigmoid notch. Next the edges of the distal ulna are trimmed and are smoothed with a small rasp. Closure is a critical element of the procedure and a secure multilayered closure is performed. The periosteum, DRUJ capsule, and retinaculum are repaired separately using nonabsorbable sutures and then routine skin closure follows. The wrist is maintained in a long arm splint with the elbow at 90° for 3 to 4 weeks. Active elbow and forearm exercises can begin at that time. Strengthening without the splint can begin at 6 to 8 weeks. Full activity is allowed at 3 months postoperatively.

The senior author (D.G.S.) described a modified Darrach procedure including distal ulnar resection combined with extensor carpi ulnaris (ECU) stabilization and a radial oblique osteotomy of the ulnar stump to prevent impingement.[17] The patient is positioned supine with the affected extremity fully pronated on a hand-table extension. The operation is performed under general or regional anesthesia and tourniquet control. A vertical dorsal incision is made from the ulnar head and is extended 4 cm proximally with care taken to avoid the dorsal cutaneous branch of the ulnar nerve. This approach provides excellent exposure of the distal ulna.

The extensor retinaculum is opened between the fifth and sixth compartments and the ECU tendon is exposed. Subperiosteal flaps, including the radioulnar joint capsule, are sharply elevated with a scalpel in a longitudinal fashion from the distal ulna. The TFCC is sharply elevated away from the ulnar styloid and then is debrided. The flaps are protected until final closure.

Osteotomy of the distal ulna for removal of the head is performed with a transverse osteotomy at the proximal extent of the sigmoid notch of the radius (Fig. 33-1). The radial border of the ulnar stump is then obliquely osteotomized and the sharp edges are smoothed with a small rasp (Fig. 33-2). The ECU tendon is then split longitudinally approximately 5 cm proximal to the resected end of the distal ulna. The radial half is harvested and the ulnar tendon strip remains intact. A 1/8-in bicortical drill hole is then made in the ulnar stump through a dorsal to volar direction (Fig. 33-3). Next the radial tendon strip is passed from volar to dorsal and is pulled taut with the wrist slightly ulnarly deviated (Fig. 33-4). The radial tendon strip then is sutured to itself, using a 2-0 nonabsorbable suture, while the ulna is held volar (Fig. 33-5). The forearm is pronated and supinated while the surgeon palpates between the bones to ensure that a smooth arc of motion is possible without impingement.

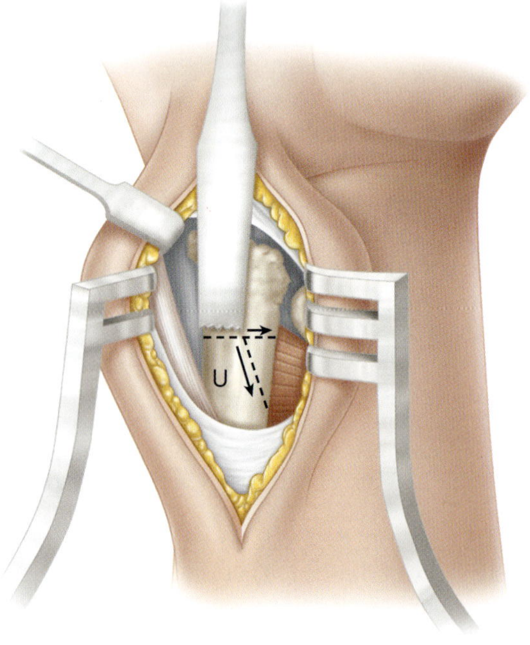

FIGURE 33-1 Schematic illustration of the proposed osteotomies, transverse osteotomy of the distal ulna and radial oblique osteotomy of the ulnar stump. U, ulna.

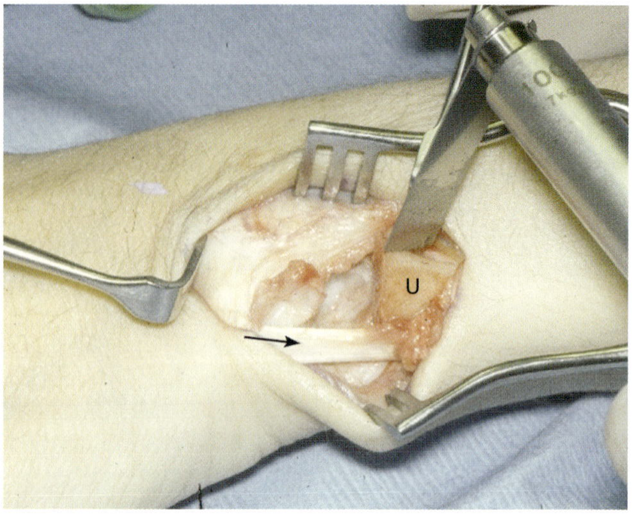

FIGURE 33-2 Intraoperative view of the radial oblique osteotomy of the ulnar stump after transverse osteotomy U, ulna; arrow, extensor carpi ulnaris tendon.

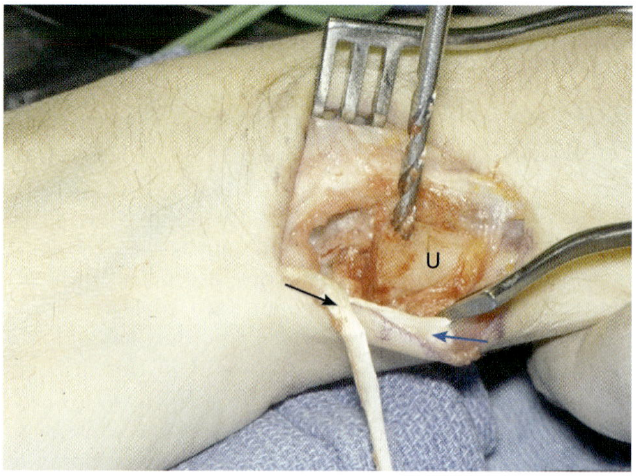

FIGURE 33-3 Intraoperative view of the bicortical drill hole in the ulnar stump through a dorsal to volar direction. U, ulna; black arrow, radial strip of the extensor carpi ulnaris tendon; blue arrow, ulnar strip of the extensor carpi ulnaris tendon.

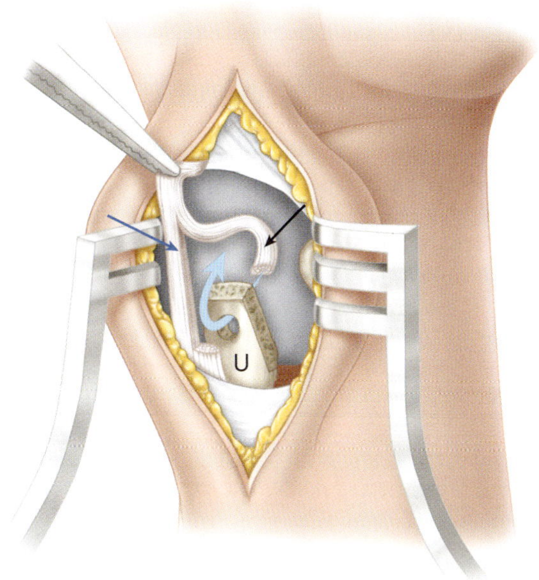

FIGURE 33-4 Schematic illustration, the radial strip of the extensor carpi ulnaris tendon is passed through the drill hole (black arrow). The ulnar strip of the extensor carpi ulnaris tendon remains intact (blue arrow).

Meticulous attention to closure is imperative. The subperiosteal flaps and capsule are snugly imbricated over the distal ulnar stump using an absorbable suture and then routine skin closure follows. The wrist is placed in a well-padded long arm splint in neutral pronation–supination and extension–flexion. At 6 weeks postoperatively the patient begins a rehabilitation program with active and active-assisted range of motion and progressive strengthening (Figs. 33-6 and 33-7).

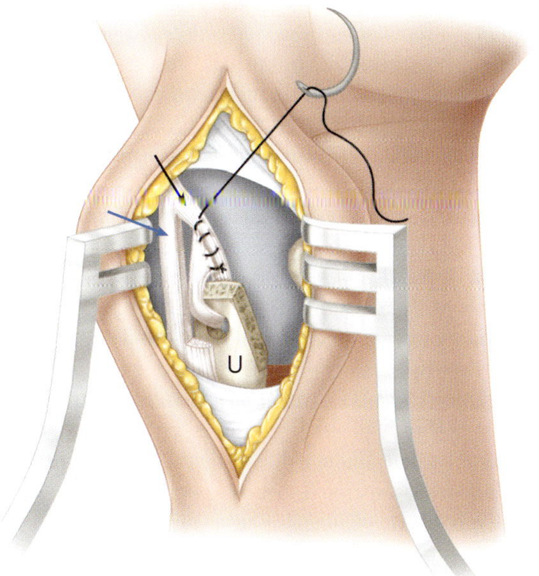

FIGURE 33-5 Schematic illustration, the radial strip of the extensor carpi ulnaris tendon is sutured to itself (black arrow). The ulnar strip of the extensor carpi ulnaris tendon remains intact (blue arrow).

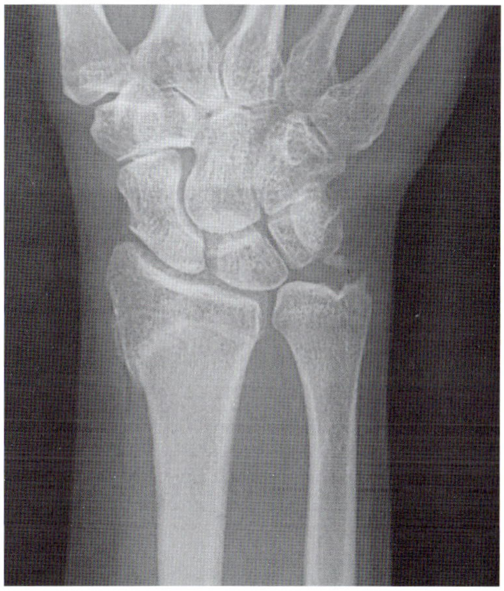

FIGURE 33-6 Preoperative PA view of a 38-year-old woman with post-traumatic DRUJ arthritis. Clinically, this patient was unable to pronate and supinate her wrist and had severe pain to ballottement of the ulna.

Complications

The distal ulnar Darrach resection has the inherent problem of loss of ulnar support of the carpus. Loss of linkage

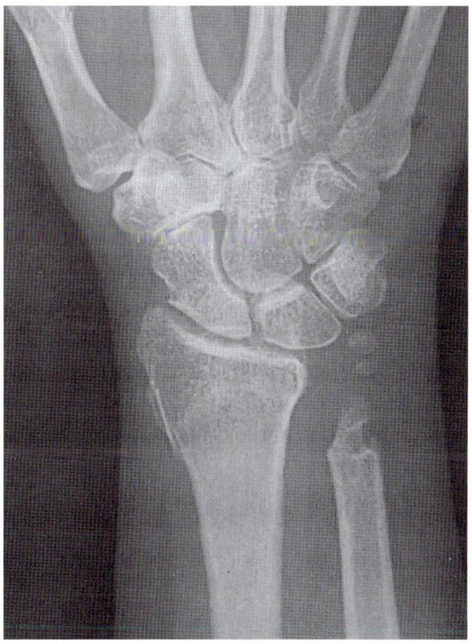

FIGURE 33-7 Postoperative PA view of the modified Darrach procedure with extensor carpi ulnaris stabilization. The patient was pain free 20 months postoperative.

between the radius and ulna results in radioulnar convergence, producing impingement of the ulnar stump against the radius usually accompanied by instability.[15,16,18-20] The distal radioulnar instability may manifest with crepitus, pain with forearm rotation, and grip weakness. Additional reported complications of the Darrach procedure include ulnar translocation of the carpus and attritional extensor tendon rupture by the ulnar stump.[8,19] The risk of damage to the dorsal cutaneous branch of the ulnar nerve can be lessened by careful dissection.

The modified Darrach procedure decreases the impingement using the combination of the distal ulnar resection with the oblique radial osteotomy of the ulnar stump. Additionally, the ECU stabilization prevents instability by augmenting a minimal subperiosteal distal ulnar resection and capsular repair.

Outcomes

It is difficult to compare the outcomes since there is a significant difference between rheumatoid patients and posttraumatic ulnar impaction. Most of the literature is more than 20 years old. The amount of instability and impingement is more common with increasing amounts of bony resection.[19] The resection should be limited to 2 cm or less. Rana and Taylor reported distal stump clicking if more than 3.5 cm was excised and no clicking if less than 2 cm was excised in patients with rheumatoid arthritis.[21] In patients with severe rheumatoid arthritis, especially those with active synovitis and lax ligaments, there is a risk of developing progressive ulnar translocation.[16,19] Gainor and Schaberg reported that excessive resection of more than 2 cm may contribute to ulnar translocation after reviewing their results in 25 patients (33 wrists) with rheumatoid arthritis at an average follow-up of 3.8 years.[22] Others feel the ulnar translocation is more a function of the rheumatoid arthritis than the Darrach resection. De Witte et al recently reviewed their experience in 15 women and 11 men with a mean age of 53 years (range, 24-80 years) who underwent a Darrach procedure for DRUJ stiffness, instability, nonunion, or substantial radioulnar length discrepancy after trauma.[23] At an average follow-up of 21 months (range, 4-60 months), the improvement in total arc of forearm rotation averaged 87° (range, 0°-160°), from an average of 49° to an average of 136° ($P < .001$). The proportion of patients with occasional or continuous pain after the Darrach procedure (7 after vs 16 prior; $P = .04$) was significantly reduced. Only 2 patients had reoperation related to the residual ulna.

Modification of the Darrach with ECU stabilization as the senior author's preference demonstrated good results with marked alleviation of pain and improvement in forearm rotation.[17] Fifteen patients (16 wrists) were reviewed at an average follow-up of 37 months. There was a marked alleviation in pain in 14/15 patients, with improved pain-free pronation/supination and increased grip strength.

HEMIRESECTION INTERPOSITION TECHNIQUE

In 1985, Bowers introduced the HIT of arthroplasty for preserving the functional elements of the ulnocarpal ligament complex eliminating the instability associated with the Darrach procedure.[24] The concept is to remove the articular surface of the ulnar head and retain the ulnar attachments of the TFCC (partial resection of ulnar head). The entire shaft and the ulnar styloid are left intact. An intact or reconstructable TFCC is a prerequisite to the success of the procedure.

Indications

The primary indication for the HIT is posttraumatic or degenerative arthritis of the DRUJ.[13,14,24] The HIT is useful in the early stages of rheumatoid arthritis.[25]

Contraindications

Patients with abutment or an ulnar positive variance are not suitable candidates unless a concomitant ulnar shortening procedure is performed. In patients with combined DRUJ arthritis and instability the HIT procedure can be performed along with a DRUJ stabilizing procedure; otherwise the instability will be exacerbated. Irreparable injury of the TFCC is a relative contraindication for the HIT since there is no advantage over the Darrach procedure.

Surgical Technique

The surgical approach for the HIT procedure as developed by Bowers is identical to the Darrach resection.[24] The difference lies in the amount of ulnar head resection and the soft tissue interposition after bone resection.

The DRUJ is approached dorsally through a longitudinal incision over the fifth extensor compartment. An ulnar-based flap of extensor retinaculum is elevated and an ulnar-based capsular flap is raised just proximal to the TFCC. Small rongeurs and a bur are used to resect the surface of the ulnar head. Instead of resecting the distal ulna at the proximal margin of the sigmoid notch (Darrach procedure), the seat and pole of the ulna are entirely resected and the medial cortex of the distal ulna is preserved from the diaphysis to the tip of the styloid. The integrity of the TFCC is left intact. The resected shaft should be round in cross-section and the ulna is tapered distally in a dowel shape. Great care is taken after resection to ensure full, unimpeded forearm rotation. Any osteophytes or prominent bone that may interfere with rotation must be removed.

If a preoperative or intraoperative diagnosis of ulnar abutment is rendered, an ulnar shortening is performed to avoid impingement between the triquetrum and the residual ulnar head or styloid. After the osteotomy, the ulnar-based capsular flap is interposed between the radius and the resected ulna. A free tendon graft (eg, palmaris longus) is used to increase the interposition bulk mitigating impingement of the resected ulna against the medial wall of the distal radius. In the modification technique, an ulnar-based retinacular flap is raised from the radial margin of the ECU sheath and interposed to avoid use of a free tendon graft.[14] The retinacular flap is interposed and sutured to the volar DRUJ to cover the resected surface. A routine skin closure follows. The extremity is immobilized in a long arm splint in neutral forearm rotation for 3 weeks. The postoperative rehabilitation depends on whether an ulnar shortening has been performed.

Complications

The ulna is vulnerable to fracture if excessive bone is resected or mechanical stresses exceed the biomechanical limitations of the arthroplasty.[24,26] Untreated ulnar positive variance may lead to stylocarpal impingement. Radioulnar impingement is also a known complication as reported with many Darrach modifications. Preexisting DRUJ instability may be exacerbated, but pain is usually reduced. Additional reported complications of HIT procedure include ECU tendonitis (when retinacular reconstruction of the ECU tendon sheath is performed) and neuroma of the ulnar dorsal sensory nerve.[24,26]

Outcomes

Bowers reported good results for pain relief and motion on 38 patients (27 of 38 had rheumatoid arthritis).[24,25] Patients with degenerative or posttraumatic arthritis had better results than patients with rheumatoid arthritis.[27] Failures were often related to residual ulnocarpal impaction. Many other authors have demonstrated generally favorable results using the HIT procedure with no pain in 76% and mild pain in 24% of patients.[27–30] The HIT procedure has additionally been reported to be effective in conjunction with a radial osteotomy for malunited distal radius fractures.[26] More recently, van Schoonhoven et al performed a retrospective study of 36 patients with a mean age of 53 years after an average follow-up of 34 months.[31] There was a statistically significant reduction in the visual analog pain score to 3.9 versus 7.8 preoperatively. The average DASH score measured 35. Pronation was largely unchanged from a mean of 74° to 76°, but supination significantly improved from 54° to 69°. The average grip strength increased from 40% to 64% as compared with the unaffected side. Using the modified Mayo wrist score, there were 6 excellent, 11 good, 10 satisfactory, and 4 poor results. Radioulnar impingement, however, was noted in 21 patients (painful in 14), requiring revision to an ulnar head implant in 5 patients. In 3 patients a secondary ulnar shortening had to be performed due to a remaining painful impaction of the distal ulna against the lunate and triquetrum.

MATCHED DISTAL ULNAR RESECTION

In this modification, described by Watson et al in 1986, the distal ulna is resected convexly at the DRUJ that matches the corresponding concave radius.[32] They suggest that if the procedure is done properly, there is no need to add interposition material between the distal radius and ulna.

Indications

Indications for matched distal ulnar resection include chronic subluxation, dislocation, incongruity, or other arthritic conditions of the DRUJ.[13,32]

Contraindications

Patients with ulnar positive variance and patients with preexisting or concomitant wrist pathology may not be suited for the procedure.

Surgical Technique

The surgical approach is identical to the approaches mentioned for prior procedures. The matched resection osteotomy is more proximal than the HIT osteotomy.[32,33] The distal ulna is resected in a long, sloping convex curve that matches the opposing concave radius. A 270° arc of the ulnar is resected to allow full pronation and supination. Any osteophytes or prominent bone that may interfere with rotation must be removed. An ulnar styloidectomy may be necessary to maximize radial and ulnar deviation.

Complications

The radius may exhibit a reverse slope along its medial border.[33] Any proximal protuberant portion of the radial sulcus at the sigmoid notch should be resected to prevent ulnar impingement. To avoid ulnocarpal abutment, the resected ulna should not be longer than the end of the adjacent radius.

Outcomes

Watson et al reported excellent results with improvement of symptoms in their series of 97 wrists over 21 years.[32,33] The results were better in patients who had isolated problems of the DRUJ, a preserved radiocarpal joint, and no other wrist instability. Few other reports described the results of the matched resection demonstrating good to excellent results in patients with posttraumatic DRUJ arthritis and rheumatoid arthritis.[30,34]

SAUVÉ-KAPANDJI PROCEDURE

In 1936, Sauvé and later Kapandji described an alternative technique to the resection of distal ulna.[35] This procedure consists of DRUJ fusion with creation of a pseudarthrosis of the ulna proximal to the fusion. The Sauvé-Kapandji procedure provides ulnar support of the wrist preserving the distal radioulnar and ulnocarpal ligaments.

Indications

Indications are similar to those for the Darrach procedure, including posttraumatic DRUJ arthritis, osteoarthritis, or rheumatoid arthritis.[13,14,35] The Sauvé-Kapandji procedure is especially useful for patients with rheumatoid arthritis since it provides bony support of the ulnar carpus and thus reduces the risk of ulnar translocation.[35,36] It is, also, particular useful for young, active, high-demand patients with posttraumatic or osteoarthritis of DRUJ, because retaining the ulnar head maintains the ulnocarpal buttress and the TFCC to allow a more physiological transmission of load from the hand to the forearm.[36,37]

Contraindications

Active infection or an unstable skin coverage is a contraindication to this procedure. Marked osteopenia and DRUJ instability are relative contraindications.

Surgical Technique

The patient is positioned supine with the upper extremity on a hand table. The operation is performed under general or regional anesthesia and tourniquet control. Although some modifications of the procedure have been described, the basic technique remains essentially unchanged since the procedure was first described.[35,38] A longitudinal dorsal incision, 6 to 8 cm long, is made along the ulnar border of the distal forearm. Care is taken to identify and protect the dorsal cutaneous branch of the ulnar nerve. The fifth extensor compartment is divided and the extensor digiti minimi is retracted radially. The extensor retinaculum and the DRUJ capsule are raised as an ulnar-based flap and the DRUJ is exposed using subperiosteal dissection. The ECU sheath should not be opened because it is an important DRUJ stabilizer.

The choice of fixation depends on the size and quality of the bone. If possible, a cannulated screw is utilized. Two parallel guide wires are inserted into the head just beneath the ECU sheath. Next the ulnar head is osteotomized using an oscillating saw just proximal to the flare of the head. A second cut proximal and parallel to the first is made removing a 10- to 15-mm segment of the ulna. The periosteum in the region of the gap is resected to prevent regrowth of ulna. If there is a positive ulnar variance, a longer segment of the ulna is removed. Then, a rongeur or osteotome is used to decorticate the articular surfaces of the ulnar head and sigmoid notch of the radius. With the forearm in neutral rotation, the ulnar head is held against the sigmoid notch so that ulnar neutral variance is obtained. The guide wires are driven into the radius and the proper position is confirmed fluoroscopically. Two cannulated compression screws are inserted or 1 screw and 1 of the guide wires are used for the fixation. The cancellous bone harvested from the resected ulnar segment can be placed at the fusion site. The fascia of the pronator quadratus is interposed at the pseudarthrosis site and is sutured to the volar aspect of the tendon sheath of the ECU to prevent regrowth and fusion of the cut bony ends. Closure in layers follows with repair of the retinacular compartments. ECU or flexor carpi ulnaris stabilization of the proximal ulnar stump can be used to gain additional stability of the proximal ulnar stump in young patients.[39,40] A long arm splint is used for 2 weeks followed by a short-arm cast until there is radiographic evidence of fusion. Regular activity is allowed once bony union has occurred.

Complications

Painful instability of the ulnar stump is a known complication of the Sauvé-Kapandji procedure.[37,41] Less common complications include fibrous or osseous union at the pseudarthrosis site and radioulnar nonunion or delayed union.[37,41] Hardware-related pain from screw heads can occur in necessarily removal. Injury to the dorsal cutaneous branch of the ulnar nerve is a potential complication and can be avoided with careful dissection.

Outcomes

In general, the results are reported to be good with elimination of pain, improvement of grip strength, and restoration of function in greater than 85% of patients.[38-40,42] Postoperative grip strength and return to work status are reportedly better than the Darrach procedure especially in younger active patients.[43] However, painful instability of the ulnar stump has been reported after the Sauvé-Kapandji procedure, although it developed less commonly than after the Darrach procedure.[37,41,44] Other studies have found instability of the ulnar stump to be more common, even though not always symptomatic.[36] De Smet and Van Ransbeeck surveyed 84 patients treated with the Sauvé-Kapandji procedure, 11 in combination with another wrist procedure.[45] There was significant pain decrease and high patient satisfaction (74%). The range of motion increased in the flexion/extension arc from 109° to 124° ($P = .006$) and, in those with limited forearm rotation, from 71° to 134° ($P = .006$). According to the Mayo Clinic wrist score, there were 20 excellent, 34 good, 18 fair, and 12 poor results. Minami et al compared 61 patients with painful DRUJ OA who were treated with a Darrach resection (20), a Sauvé-Kapandji procedure (25), or a HIT (16).[28] There were 36 men and 25 women with an average age of 59.8 years. There were 38 primary and 23 secondary osteoarthritis cases. At an average follow-up of 10 years (range, 5-14 years) the Darrach procedure was inferior to the Sauvé-Kapandji procedure and HIT, although this was not statistically significant. Forearm rotation improved in all of the groups and wrist flexion and extension and grip strength were better in the HIT and Sauvé-Kapandji patients.

FAILED DISTAL ULNAR RESECTION

Severe instability of the distal ulna after a resection can develop early or later most commonly after the Darrach procedure; however, it can also occur after HIT, Sauvé-Kapandji procedure, or any other modification. Despite modifications, the reported failure rate of the Darrach procedure remains between 7% and 50%.[2,3,16,20,46] The patient with a symptomatic failed distal ulnar resection experiences pain and upper extremity disuse, as a result of painful grinding and mechanical limitations to forearm rotation. Many techniques have been described for management of the failed distal ulnar resection with varying success to prevent recurrent impingement. The reported techniques include stabilization of the distal ulna using different local tendons, osteoplasties, soft tissue interposition, and combinations with more complex procedures.[6,7,10,14,47–49] Recently, distal ulnar replacement has become a popular option.[50–52] However, long-term survival of the implants has not been reported and there are concerns for implant longevity in the young, active patient. Problems such as loosening, bone resorption, dislocation, and implant instability are concerns for this patient population. In an effort to eliminate the symptoms of impingement by maintaining a wide distal radioulnar relationship and to avoid implant failure a technique using a biologically compatible allograft has been developed by the senior author (D.G.S.).[53,54] This technique relies on the interposition of an Achilles tendon allograft between the distal radius and the resected distal ulna.

Indications

This is primarily suited to the salvage of a failed distal ulnar implant arthroplasty, although it can be used for painful impingement between the distal ulnar stump and the radius from radioulnar convergence following a distal ulnar resection arthroplasty. The Achilles allograft interposition technique is an attractive alternative especially for the young, active patients, in whom an implant or alternative procedure may not be appropriate.

Contraindications

Marked stability of the proximal ulnar stump would preclude the use of this procedure.

Surgical Technique

The procedure is performed under general or regional anesthesia with tourniquet control.[53,54] The patient is positioned supine with the affected extremity on a hand-table extension. If possible, the previous surgical incisions are incorporated into the approach for the allograft interposition. A dorsal approach through the fifth dorsal compartment is preferred with care to preserve the dorsal cutaneous branch of the ulnar nerve. Subperiosteal exposure of the distal ulna is performed approximately 4 to 6 cm proximal to the distal stump. Frequently, the resected ulna develops reactive bone that may impinge on the distal radius or cause mechanical limitations to motion. The prominent bone is removed and a smooth surface of the ulnar stump is created. Then the medial cortex of the radius is exposed, by retracting the ulna volarly, and 3 or 4 unicortical suture anchors are placed into the medial cortex of the radius, proximal to the sigmoid notch where the impingement occurs. It is necessary to obtain a 2- to 3-cm area for fixation of the allograft to the medial radius to ensure that a large buffer is created between the 2 bones. Three or 4 drill holes are made in a medial-to-lateral direction in the distal ulna and then sutures are passed through each of the holes.

An Achilles tendon allograft is prepared for implantation by removing the calcaneal remnant. The allograft is then rolled onto itself to create a large interpositional "pillow" that will act as a soft tissue buffer between the radius and ulna. The allograft is then sutured between the radius and ulna (anchors to radius and drill holes to ulna) (Fig. 33-8). The size of the allograft pillow is determined by pronating and supinating the forearm with pressure applied to the ulnar aspect of the ulna to assess crepitus. If crepitus is noted, the allograft size is increased until no further crepitus occurs with passive ulnar displacement of the ulna toward the radius or with forearm rotation. With final allograft placement there should be significant padding between the radius and the ulna to prevent any palpable crepitus during forearm rotation under compression and to ensure that a smooth

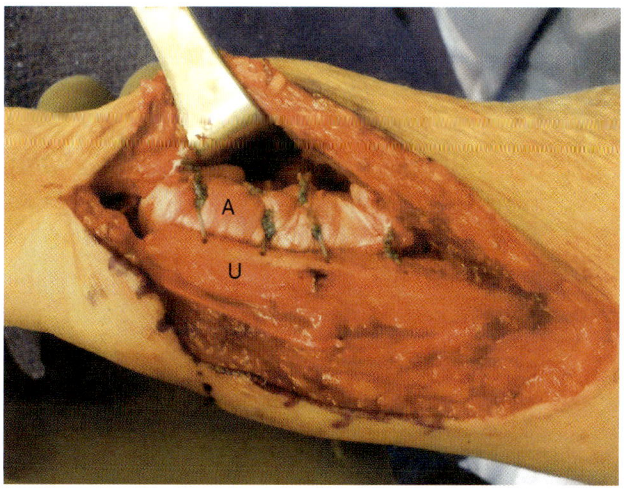

FIGURE 33-8 Intraoperative view of the final position of the allograft between distal radius and ulnar stump creating a pillow-shaped spacer. The allograft is sutured through anchors to radius and drill holes to ulna. A, allograft; U, ulna.

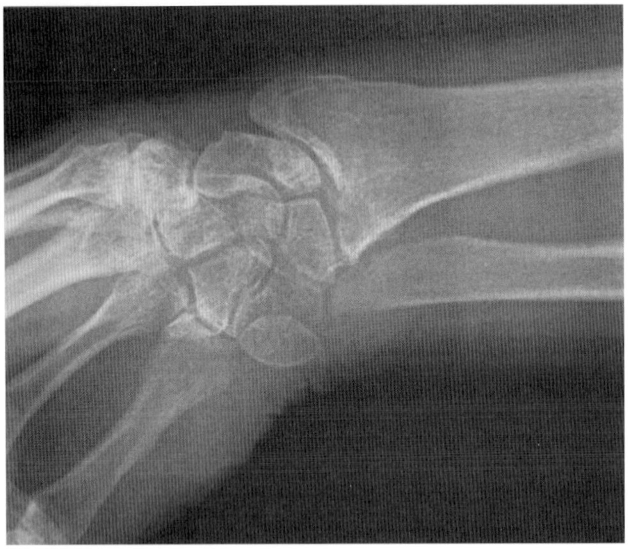

FIGURE 33-9 Preoperative gripping "weight-bearing," PA view, depicting contact between distal radius and ulnar stump after failed Darrach procedure.

arc of motion occurs without impingement (Figs. 33-9 and 33-10). No other tissues are used to stabilize the ulnar stump. Standard capsular and soft tissue closures are completed over the allograft and the retinaculum closed. After skin closure, a well-padded long arm splint is applied. The long arm splint is converted to a cast at the initial postoperative follow-up for 6 weeks. Protected range of motion and interval splintage is continued until 12 weeks postoperatively.

Complications

Great attention must be paid to the size of the allograft. When insufficient allograft bulk is used, the radioulnar space may not be maintained. The allograft should prevent the ulnar stump from contacting the radius during pronation and supination under compression. A possible complication is a radial shaft fracture, which is prevented by using micro-suture anchors for the graft fixation. We use the Micro FT Anchor (Arthrex) as a unicortical small anchor.

Asymptomatic ulnar shaft scalloping is also a potential complication. Cost, availability, and immunologic reaction are among disadvantages of all allografts. Despite these noted disadvantages of the allografts, they are currently widely used in orthopedic surgery. Immune reactions or infections with the Achilles allograft interpositional arthroplasty have not been reported, yet. The risk of damage to the dorsal cutaneous branch of the ulnar nerve can be lessened by careful dissection.

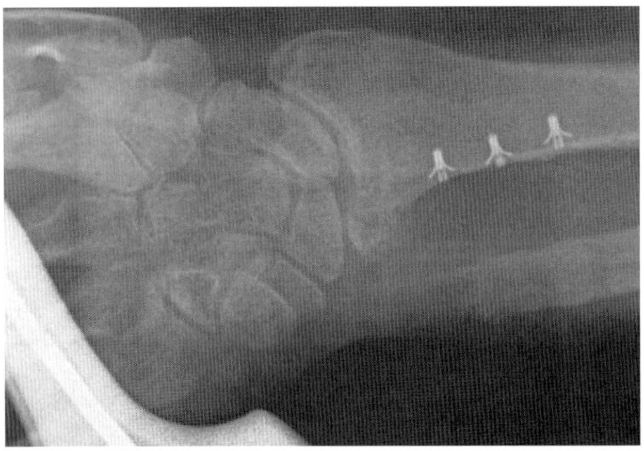

FIGURE 33-10 One-year postoperative gripping "weight-bearing," PA view. Note maintenance of the interosseous space, no impingement between both forearm bones.

Outcomes

The initial combined series includes 27 patients with failed distal ulnar resection with a mean age of 44 years (range 37-68 years). At a mean follow-up of 76 months, good (17/27 patients) to excellent (9/27 patients) results have been demonstrated with marked alleviation of pain and improvement in forearm rotation. Grip strength improved an average of 77% and the total arc of forearm rotation improved an average of 76°. Palpable crepitus was noted in 1 patient (worker compensation) whose result was graded as a failure and attributed to insufficient graft bulk. Radiographic evaluation revealed ulnar scalloping in 2 patients, 2 and 3 years postoperatively, respectively, although the patients remain asymptomatic. No graft-related complications were encountered. Although the Achilles allograft interposition does not restore normal biomechanics of the DRUJ, it can prevent impingement, crepitus, and painful convergence of the radius on the ulna especially in the position of neutral forearm rotation.

REFERENCES

1. Darrach W. Forward dislocation at the inferior radio-ulnar joint, with fracture of the lower third of the shaft of the radius. *Ann Surg.* 1912;56:801–802.
2. Dingman PV. Resection of the distal end of the ulna (Darrach operation); an end result study of twenty four cases. *J Bone Joint Surg Am.* 1952;34A:893–900.
3. Hartz CR, Beckenbaugh RD. Long-term results of resection of the distal ulna for post-traumatic conditions. *J Trauma.* 1979;19:219–226.
4. Spinner M, Kaplan EB. Extensor carpi ulnaris. Its relationship to the stability of the distal radio-ulnar joint. *Clin Orthop Relat Res.* 1970;68:124–129.
5. Webber JB, Maser SA. Stabilization of the distal ulna. *Hand Clin.* 1991;7:345–353.
6. Breen TF, Jupiter JB. Extensor carpi ulnaris and flexor carpi ulnaris tenodesis of the unstable distal ulna. *J Hand Surg Am.* 1989;14:612–617.
7. Tsai TM, Stilwell JH. Repair of chronic subluxation of the distal radio-ulnar joint (ulnar dorsal) using flexor carpi ulnaris tendon. *J Hand Surg Br.* 1984;9:289–294.
8. O'Donovan TM, Ruby LK. The distal radioulnar joint in rheumatoid arthritis. *Hand Clin.* 1989;5:249–256.
9. Nolan WB 3rd, Eaton RG. A Darrach procedure for distal ulnar pathology derangements. *Clin Orthop Relat Res.* 1992;275:85–89.
10. Leslie BM, Carlson G, Ruby LK. Results of extensor carpi ulnaris tenodesis in the rheumatoid wrist undergoing a distal ulnar excision. *J Hand Surg Am.* 1990;15:547–551.

11. Melone CP Jr, Taras JS. Distal ulna resection, extensor carpi ulnaris tenodesis, and dorsal synovectomy for the rheumatoid wrist. *Hand Clin.* 1991;7:335–343.
12. Fraser KE, Diao E, Peimer CA, Sherwin FS. Comparative results of resection of the distal ulna in rheumatoid arthritis and post-traumatic conditions. *J Hand Surg Br.* 1999;24:667–670.
13. Lichtman DM, Ganocy TK, Kim DC. The indications for and techniques and outcomes of ablative procedures of the distal ulna. The Darrach resection, hemiresection, matched resection, and Sauvé-Kapandji procedure. *Hand Clin.* 1988;14:265–277.
14. Adams BD. Distal radioulnar joint instability. In: Green DP, ed. *Green's Operative Hand Surgery*. 5th ed. Philadelphia: Churchill Livingstone; 2005:605–644.
15. Bell MJ, Hill RJ, McMurtry RY. Ulnar impingement syndrome. *J Bone Joint Surg Br.* 1985;67:126–129.
16. Bieber EJ, Linscheid RL, Dobyns JH, Beckenbaugh RD. Failed distal ulna resections. *J Hand Surg Am.* 1988;13:193–200.
17. Sotereanos DG, Leit ME. A modified Darrach procedure for treatment of the painful distal radioulnar joint. *Clin Orthop Relat Res.* 1996;325:140–147.
18. Kleinman WB, Graham TJ. Distal ulnar injury and dysfunction. In: Peimer CA, ed. *Surgery of the Hand and Upper Extremity*. New York: McGraw-Hill; 1996:667–709.
19. McKee MD, Richards RR. Dynamic radio-ulnar convergence after the Darrach procedure. *J Bone Joint Surg Br.* 1996;78:413–418.
20. Field J, Majkowski RJ, Leslie IJ. Poor results of Darrach's procedure after wrist injuries. *J Bone Joint Surg Br.* 1993;75:53–57.
21. Rana NA, Taylor AR. Excision of the distal end of the ulna in rheumatoid arthritis. *J Bone Joint Surg Br.* 1973;55:96–105.
22. Gainor BJ, Schaberg J. The rheumatoid wrist after resection of the distal ulna. *J Hand Surg Am.* 1985;10:837–844.
23. De Witte PB, Wijffels M, Jupiter JB, Ring D. The Darrach procedure for post-traumatic reconstruction. *Acta Orthop Belg.* 2009;75:316–322.
24. Bowers WH. Distal radioulnar joint arthroplasty: the hemiresection-interposition technique. *J Hand Surg Am.* 1985;10:169–178.
25. Bowers WH. Distal radioulnar joint arthroplasty. Current concepts. *Clin Orthop Relat Res.* 1992;275:104–109.
26. Fernandez DL. Radial osteotomy and Bowers arthroplasty for malunited fractures of the distal end of the radius. *J Bone Joint Surg Am.* 1988;70:1538–1551.
27. Imbriglia JE, Matthews D. Treatment of chronic post-traumatic dorsal subluxation of the distal ulna by hemiresection-interposition arthroplasty. *J Hand Surg Am.* 1993;18:899–907.
28. Minami A, Iwasaki N, Ishikawa J, Suenaga N, Yasuda K, Kato H. Treatments of osteoarthritis of the distal radioulnar joint: long-term results of three procedures. *Hand Surg.* 2005;10:243–248.
29. Glowacki KA. Hemiresection arthroplasty of the distal radioulnar joint. *Hand Clin.* 2005;21:591–601.
30. Bain GI, Pugh DM, MacDermid JC, Roth JH. Matched hemiresection interposition arthroplasty of the distal radioulnar joint. *J Hand Surg Am.* 1995;20:944–950.
31. van Schoonhoven J, Kall S, Schober F, Prommersberger KJ, Lanz U. The hemiresection-interposition arthroplasty as a salvage procedure for the arthrotically destroyed distal radioulnar joint. *Handchir Mikrochir Plast Chir.* 2003;35:175–180.
32. Watson HK, Ryu JY, Burgess RC. Matched distal ulnar resection. *J Hand Surg Am.* 1986;11:812–817.
33. Watson HK, Gabuzda GM. Matched distal ulna resection for post-traumatic disorders of the distal radioulnar joint. *J Hand Surg Am.* 1992;17:724–730.
34. Srikanth KN, Shahane SA, Stilwell JH. Modified matched ulnar resection for arthrosis of distal radioulnar joint in rheumatoid arthritis. *Hand Surg.* 2006;11:15–19.
35. Kapandji IA. The Kapandji-Sauve operation. Its techniques and indications in nonrheumatoid diseases. *Ann Chir Main.* 1986;5:181–193.
36. Vincent KA, Szabo RM, Agee JM. The Sauve-Kapandji procedure for reconstruction of the rheumatoid distal radioulnar joint. *J Hand Surg Am.* 1993;18:978–983.
37. Taleisnik J. The Sauve-Kapandji procedure. *Clin Orthop Relat Res.* 1992;275:110–123.
38. Millroy P, Coleman S, Ivers R. The Sauvé-Kapandji operation. Technique and results. *J Hand Surg Br.* 1992;17:411–414.
39. Lamey DM, Fernandez DL. Results of the modified Sauvé-Kapandji procedure in the treatment of chronic posttraumatic derangement of the distal radioulnar joint. *J Bone Joint Surg Am.* 1998;80:1758–1769.
40. Minami A, Kato H, Iwasaki N. Modification of the Sauvé-Kapandji procedure with extensor carpi ulnaris tenodesis. *J Hand Surg Am.* 2000;25:1080–1084.
41. Sanders RA, Frederick HA, Hontas RB. The Sauvé-Kapandji procedure: a salvage operation for the distal radioulnar joint. *J Hand Surg Am.* 1991;16:1125–1129.
42. De Smet LA, Van Ransbeeck H. The Sauvé-Kapandji procedure for posttraumatic wrist disorders: further experience. *Acta Orthop Belg.* 2000;66:251–254.
43. Minami A, Suzuki K, Suenaga N, Ishikawa J. The Sauvé-Kapandji procedure for osteoarthritis of the distal radioulnar joint. *J Hand Surg Am.* 1995;20:602–608.
44. Daecke W, Martini AK, Schneider S, Streich NA. Amount of ulnar resection is a predictive factor for ulnar instability problems after the Sauvé-Kapandji procedure: a retrospective study of 44 patients followed for 1-13 years. *Acta Orthop.* 2006;77:290–297.
45. De Smet LA, Van Ransbeeck H. The Sauve-Kapandji procedure for posttraumatic wrist disorders: further experience. *Acta Orthop Belg.* 2000;66:251–254.
46. Noble J, Arafa M. Stabilisation of distal ulna after excessive Darrach's procedure. *Hand.* 1983;15:70–72.
47. Kleinman WB, Greenberg JA. Salvage of the failed Darrach procedure. *J Hand Surg Am.* 1995;20:951–958.
48. Johnson RK. Stabilization of the distal ulna by transfer of the pronator quadratus origin. *Clin Orthop Relat Res.* 1992;275:130–132.
49. Wolfe SW, Mih AD, Hotchkiss RN, Culp RW, Kiefhaber TR, Nagle DJ. Wide excision of the distal ulna: a multicenter case study. *J Hand Surg Am.* 1998;23:222–228.
50. Fernandez DL, Joneschild ES, Abella DM. Treatment of failed Sauvé-Kapandji procedures with a spherical ulnar head prosthesis. *Clin Orthop Relat Res.* 2006;445:100–107.
51. Herbert TJ, van Schoonhoven J. Ulnar head replacement. *Tech Hand Up Extrem Surg.* 2007;11:98–108.
52. Willis AA, Berger RA, Cooney WP 3rd. Arthroplasty of the distal radioulnar joint using a new ulnar head endoprosthesis: preliminary report. *J Hand Surg Am.* 2007;32:177–189.
53. Sotereanos DG, Gobel F, Vardakas DG, Sarris I. An allograft salvage technique for failure of the Darrach procedure: a report of four cases. *J Hand Surg Br.* 2002;27:317–321.
54. Greenberg JA, Sotereanos D. Achilles allograft interposition for failed Darrach distal ulna resections. *Tech Hand Up Extrem Surg.* 2008;12:121–125.

34A

Partial Head Distal Radioulnar Joint Implants

Philippe Kopylov, MD, PhD
Magnus Tägil, MD, PhD

RATIONALE AND BASIC SCIENCE

Pronation/supination is extremely important for the function of the hand. We need both mobility to position the hand in space and stability through a full arc of rotation with loading during grip. The geometry of the forearm joint, consisting of the distal radioulnar joint (DRUJ) and the proximal radioulnar joint (PRUJ) together with the curvatures of the radius and ulna, determines the range of motion. The static and dynamic ligaments and muscles provide the stability.[1]

To be able to optimize the treatment to our patients when the DRUJ is injured or diseased, we need to understand the complexity of this joint. Primarily, we have to recognize the importance of the ulnar head and appreciate its various roles for the function of the DRUJ in unloaded and loaded forearm rotation. The rotational forces induced by simply holding a weight of any object in the hand are transferred from the hand, across the DRUJ and the interosseous membrane to the ulna and elbow joint. The ulnar head and the functional unit of the DRUJ form the keystone weight-bearing fundamental part of the hand and distal forearm. The ulnar head is important for maintaining adequate tension within the radioulnar ligaments and to keep the tension of the interosseous membrane. When removed, as in a Darrach procedure, the 2 forearm bones converge distally and the tensioning function of the ulnar head is lost. The stability of the pseudojoint that forms after a Darrach procedure differs during loading in pronation and supination as the contact area shifts anteriorly or dorsally, which often results in a painful clicking of the ulnar stump when performing a loaded rotation.

DRUJ Anatomy

The DRUJ is a trochoid joint as is the PRUJ. The sigmoid notch of the radius is concave and relatively shallow and the depth and inclination vary between subjects. The sigmoid notch is limited by 3 distinct margins. The distal margin with the radial insertion of the triangular fibrocartilage complex (TFCC) marks the separation between the radiocarpal joint and the DRUJ. Dorsally and palmarly, the margins are formed by the joint capsule. The ulnar head, on which the radius rotates, is an asymmetric semicylinder. The inclination of the articular surface varies between −15° and 20° and has an approximate 130° dorsopalmar arc. The articulation of the ulnar head with the sigmoid notch has a limited congruency since the radius of curvature is greater for the sigmoid notch than for the ulnar head and the stability is dependent on ligamentous and muscular constraints. Pronation and supination include rotation, distal/proximal sliding, and a volar/dorsal translation. In midpronation/supination, the sigmoid notch covers 60° to 80° of the ulnar head convexity, but at the extreme positions of rotation, less than 10% of the ulnar head is covered by the sigmoid notch. Hence, joint stability depends largely on the TFCC and the DRUJ ligaments. The ulnotriquetral ligaments and the radioulnar ligaments form a unique entity as they insert into the fovea and the proximal part of the ulnar styloid. They extend as 2 fans in perpendicular planes, in the coronal plane and transverse plane, respectively, which along with the dorsal radiocarpal ligament provide stable 3-dimensional static fixation of the radius and carpus to the ulnar head (Fig. 34A-1).

The Forearm Joint

In an anatomical study Hagert demonstrated how the PRUJ and DRUJ act together functionally as a bicondylar joint (Fig. 34A-2). The proximal "condyle," the radial head, rotates axially so that the radius rotates around the distal "condyle," the ulnar head.[2] The dorsal and palmar radioulnar ligaments consist of superficial components inserting directly onto the ulnar styloid, and deep components inserting into the fovea of the distal ulna. Hagert observed that in pronation, both the deep palmar fibers and the superficial dorsal fibers tighten, while in supination the deep dorsal fibers and the superficial palmar fibers tighten.[3] The deep fibers are aligned to provide a vector of force that resists sagittal plane motion of the radius and function as checkreins to translation of the radius on the ulna. In addition, the ulnolunate ligament, ulnotriquetral

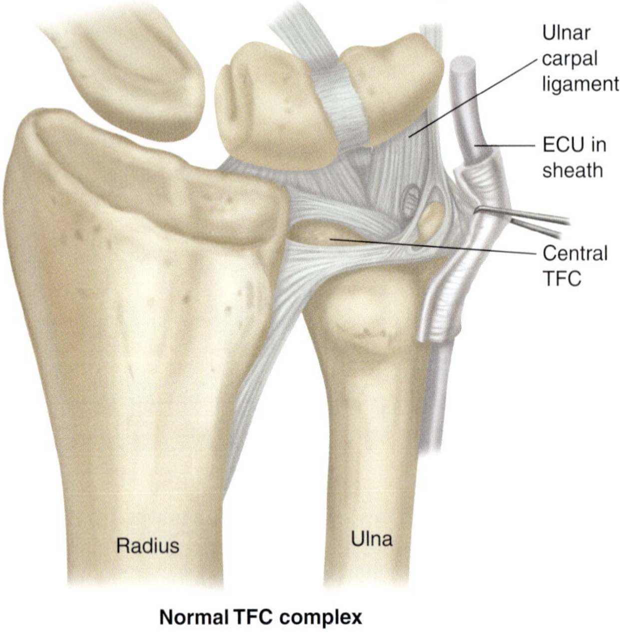

FIGURE 34A-1 The ulnotriquetral ligament and the palmar and dorsal radioulnar ligaments (DRUL, PRUL) extend as 2 fans in the coronal and transverse planes to provide static 3-dimensional fixation of the radius to the ulnar head.

ligament, interosseous membrane, and the deep portion of the ECU sheath act as secondary static stabilizers of the DRUJ. The ECU and pronator quadratus provide dynamic stability to the joint.[4] The ulnar head serves as a keystone that resists convergence of the radius and ulna and constitutes the weight-bearing part of the wrist. This provides the rationale for Hagert's fixed-point concept in which the ulnar head is the fixed point around which everything moves that is fundamental to ulnar head implants (Fig. 34A-3).

The Implant

The implant has to replicate the functions of the ulnar head. The forces across the DRUJ are related to both the forearm position in rotation and the muscle activity; therefore, the center of the rotational axis should be as close as possible to normal in order to allow existing ligaments to share the load and stabilize the implant all through the motion arc. The optimal rotational axis is reestablished when the interosseous membrane is rebalanced and tensed in every sector of the rotational motion arc. This is accomplished by reestablishing the offset of the DRUJ, spacing the joint, both in neutral, where most of the loaded activities of the daily life take place, and in the extremes of supination and pronation, where the contact area between the implant and the sigmoid notch is minimal and therefore the contact pressure will be the highest. Normally, resuture of the structures and ligaments should be enough to stabilize the joint, but reconstruction of the TFCC can also be performed with different techniques, using the palmaris longus tendon as a transplant. In all cases, the dorsal and volar stabilizing structures have to be appreciated, emphasizing the intact pronator quadratus on the volar side and an optimal positioning of the extensor carpi ulnaris and its tendon sheath on the dorsal side.

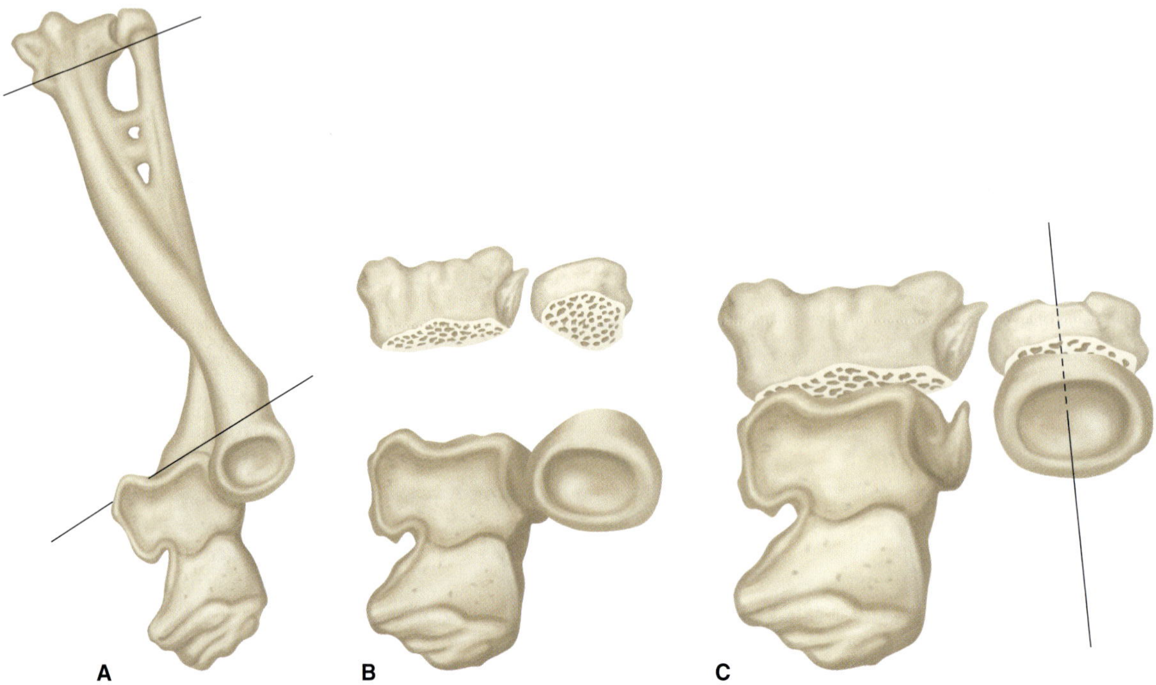

FIGURE 34A-2 The forearm joint as described by Hagert in 1992 with the proximal "condyle" the radial head and the distal "condyle" the ulnar head. DRUJ, distal radioulnar joint; PRUJ, proximal radioulnar joint.

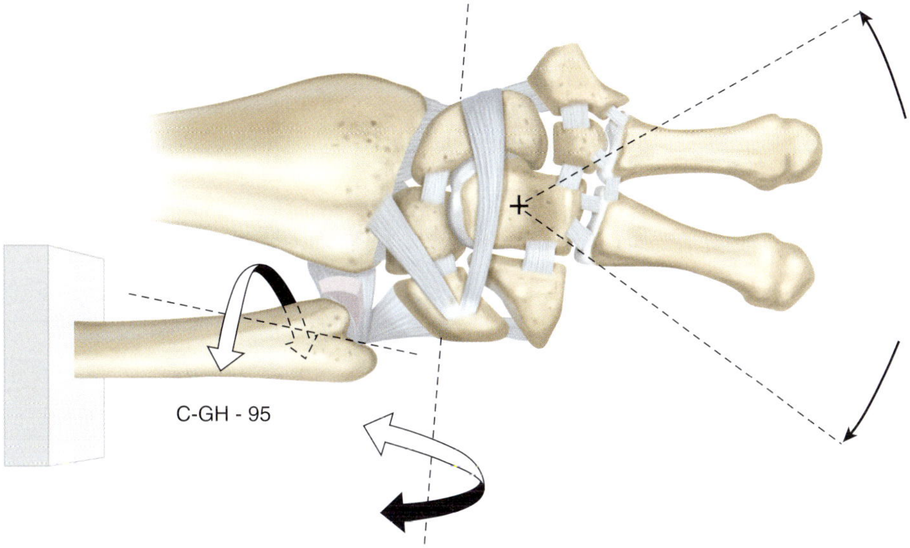

FIGURE 34A-3 This schematic drawing of the wrist shows the hand and carpus attached to the radius with possibility of flexion/extension and radial/ulnar deviation. The ulnar head is the load-bearing keystone of the DRUJ that allows pronation/supination in association with the PRUJ.

Replacement Prerequisites

The experience acquired and lessons learned from replacing other joints should preferably be used also for the DRU joint replacement. The basic technical principles and material choices are not different for this indication. The optimal implant should mimic, as closely as possible, the normal anatomical design and motion of the joint, respecting the configuration of the joint surfaces and the intrinsic and extrinsic stabilizing structures. The joint implant should be unconstrained in order to avoid abnormal loading on the interface surfaces and fixation structures and minimize the risk of material breakage or implant loosening. The implant can replace the joint partially or totally. In both cases, the friction between the different parts of the implant (total arthroplasty) or between the implant and the remaining anatomical surface (hemiarthroplasty) has to be considered in order to minimize the debris and the implant material or design chosen according to the prerequisites (cobalt chrome vs polyethylene and concavity vs convexity in total arthroplasties; pyrolytic carbon vs cartilaginous joint surface in hemiarthroplasties). In all cases the implant fixation to the bone remains a problem to be solved for which the experience in other types of joint arthroplasties can give important information (osseointegration, cement fixation, press fit, implant coating).

Salvage Procedures

When discussing joint arthroplasties, the reoperation options must be discussed, and acceptable salvage procedures such as fusion, resection, or interposition arthroplasties still be possible. This could for the DRU joint be a 1-bone forearm, which however is not a functional acceptable solution, or an ulnar head resection with known potential disabilities as discussed above. A single primary operation is always the best opportunity to succeed and secondary interventions will never reach the result they would have if used as the primary operation.

Indications

Some typical indications for implant arthroplasty include symptomatic arthrosis and posttraumatic osteoarthritis of the DRUJ following a distal radius and/or ulnar head fracture as well as replacement of the distal ulna in cases of advance rheumatoid arthritis. Other indications include an incongruous sigmoid notch following a distal radius osteotomy, and painful convergence of the ulnar head following a Darrach or hemiresection arthroplasty, Sauvé-Kapandji arthroplasty, or ulnar head excision for tumors. Preoperative considerations include determining whether the DRUJ joint surfaces are congruent and in need of a resurfacing or arthroplasty and whether the intrinsic and/or extrinsic ligament qualities are sufficient in strength to provide implant stability in all positions of pronation/supination. AP lateral and oblique x-ray views are performed as well as a CT or MRI to evaluate the status of the ulnar head and the sigmoid notch. Although the procedure can be performed at any time in skeletally mature patients, there is a higher failure rate in younger patients due to the higher functional demands. In inflammatory arthritis, the implant ideally should be performed earlier in the disease when the cartilage destruction is more prominent than the ligament destruction and the joint is still stable. Anatomical alignment of the radius and the ulna is a prerequisite for ulnar head replacement. Any malunion of the radial or ulnar shaft must be corrected either before or at the time of ulnar head replacement. Three questions have to be addressed before the decision is made to perform a DRUJ arthroplasty: Are the DRU joint surfaces congruent with the radius and ulnar bone geometry and in a physiologic relation to the forearm joint's 3 components—the PRUJ, radius curvature, and DRUJ? Are the intrinsic and/or extrinsic ligament quality sufficient in strength and structure to give stability to the implant in all positions of pronation/supination? Are the joint surfaces deteriorated and in need of a resurfacing or arthroplasty?

Contraindications

Contraindications for a nonconstrained total or partial ulnar head implant include DRUJ instability secondary to an unreconstructable TFCC or distal interosseous membrane, and following an Essex-Lopresti injury. A malunion of the distal radius would need a prior or simultaneous corrective osteotomy to provide correct alignment as would any ulnar shaft deformity. Advanced arthritis of the sigmoid fossa is relatively contraindicated unless a total joint replacement is performed. Previous infection, marked osteoporosis or cystic bone disease, and unstable soft tissue coverage are contraindications for all kind of implants constrained or nonconstrained.

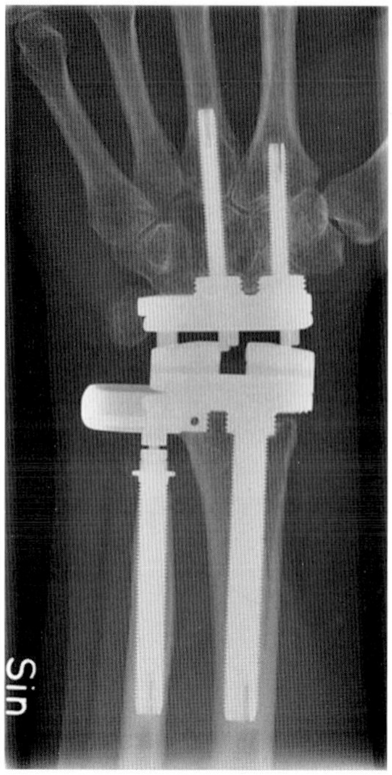

FIGURE 34A-4 Twelve-year follow-up of a combined radiocarpal and DRUJ wrist prosthesis. Note the osteointegration in radius, metacarpals, and ulna and the resorption of bone around the collar of the ulnar component. (Reproduced with permission from G. Lundborg.)

DRUJ IMPLANTS

Constrained Implants

In the beginning of the 1990s several groups presented, almost at the same time, relatively complicated mechanical systems in order to reconstruct the DRUJ. These constrained devices use multiple parts in order to restore the rotation and stability of the joint. Both Kapandji and Lundborg (Fig. 34A-4) reported anecdotal cases with custom-made implants, with or without concomitant radiocarpal replacement.[5] The concept of a constrained device has since been developed further by Scheker, who described and since 1997 uses an uncemented, semiconstrained modular prosthesis to replace the DRUJ (Fig. 34A-5). A polished peg fixed to the ulna end has freedom of movement within a polyethylene

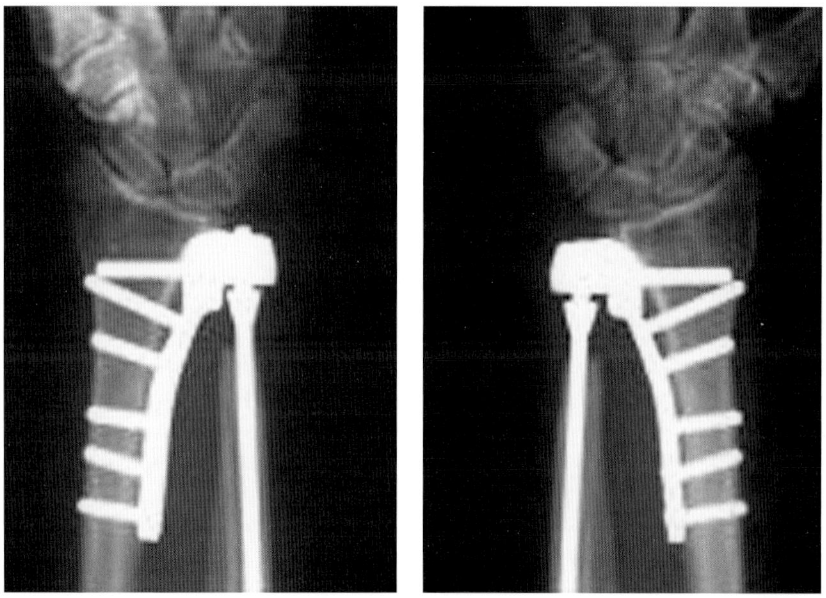

FIGURE 34A-5 Pictures in pronation and supination of an Aptis DRUJ implant.

ball secured to the radius ulnar border by a long plate. The system allows not only rotation but also freedom for an axial migration of the radius in relation to ulna. Good long-term results of this implant have been presented by several groups, all of which however report the surgical procedure to be complex and requiring a relatively important amount of reoperation for technical reasons.[6,7]

Nonconstrained Implants

THE SWANSON ULNAR HEAD PROSTHESIS

Alfred Swanson was one of the first in modern time who introduced the concept of replacement of the ulnar head as treatment of painful arthritis of the DRUJ. In 1973 he reported the use of a stemmed silicone implant acting as replacement of the resected ulnar head (Fig. 34A-6). His positive preliminary reports on pain were confirmed by others, but complications such as bone resorption, tilting or fracture of the implant, and synovitis were common and the prosthesis was abandoned.[8,9]

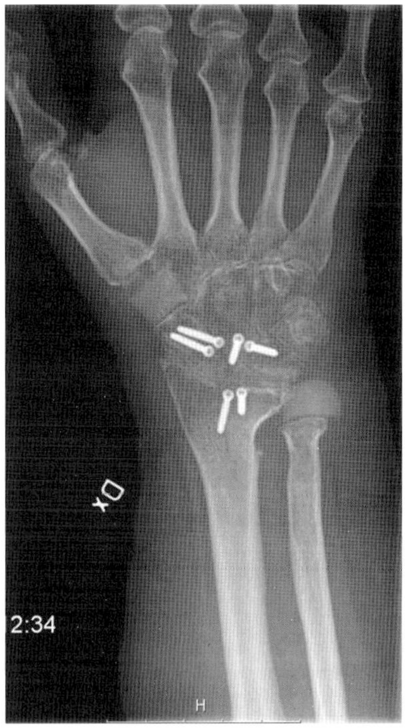

FIGURE 34A-6 Frontal radiographs of a rheumatoid patient wrist 15 years following a silicone ulnar head implant. The patient was symptom free following a wrist fusion and base of thumb silicone arthroplasty.

Total Head Implants

Primarily proposed as salvage procedure to treat symptomatic ulnar stump impingement syndrome, ulnar head implants are nowadays also used as primary treatment, avoiding the Darrach or Sauvé-Kapandji procedures and their potential complications (Fig. 34A-7A and B). The original ulnar head prosthesis, developed by Herbert and van Schoonhoven, was made in ceramic. Just as with steel, there is a discrepancy in the elastic modulus of ceramics compared with bone and a risk for radius erosion when used as a hemiprosthesis.[10,11] Other designs and material for ulnar head implant have since been presented without major improvements of the results. Most authors seem to agree on the results that can be obtained with a total ulnar

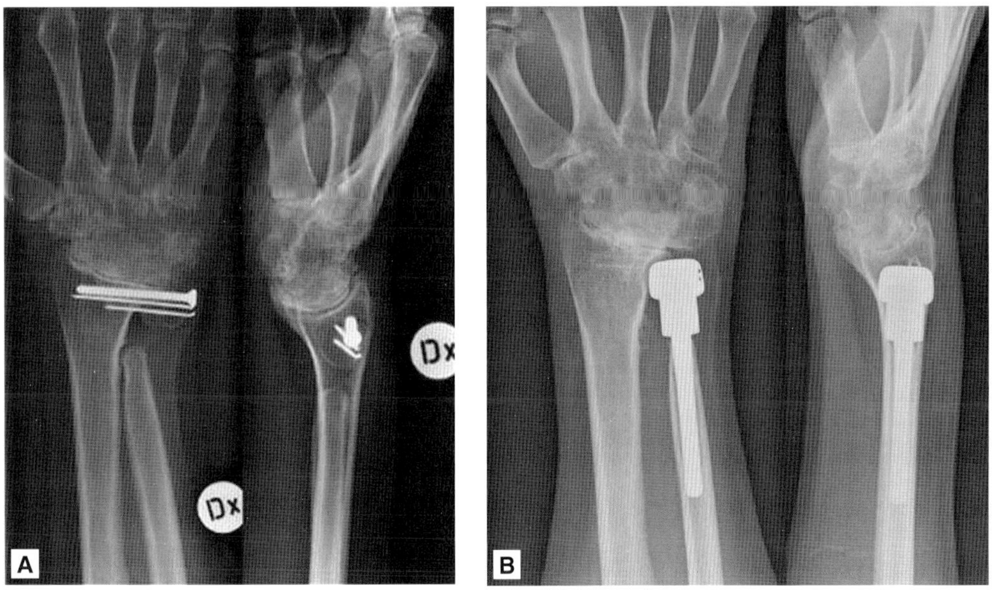

FIGURE 34A-7 **A.** A 42-year-old woman with juvenile rheumatoid arthritis 13 years following a Sauvé-Kapandji DRU joint resection arthroplasty presenting with complaints of painful DRUJ clicking and ulnar stump instability. **B.** The distal ulnar head fusion is excised and a total ulnar head implant is inserted restoring DRUJ stability with normal pain-free pronation/supination.

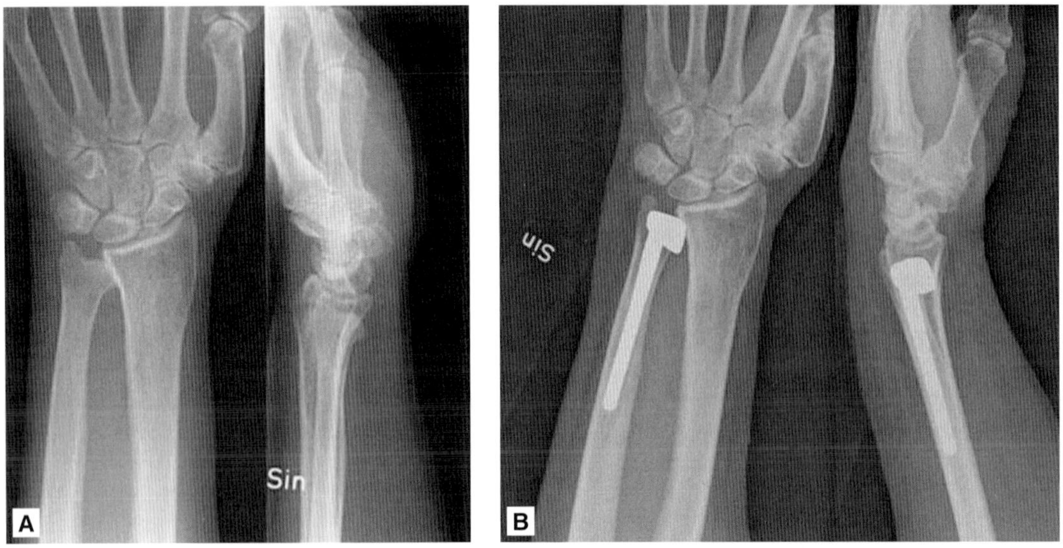

FIGURE 34A-8 **A.** AP and lateral view of a patient with primary DRUJ OA. **B.** Five years following insertion of a First Choice hemi-DRUJ prosthesis. The patient is pain free and has a full pronation/supination. Note the sigmoid notch erosion.

head implant, but concerns are raised mainly regarding the bone resorption appearing around the collar of the implant and the erosion of the radial sigmoid notch.[12] Various other procedures have been presented in order to stabilize these implants, reflecting the remaining problem of stability after deletion of the ulnar head using a technique that includes a destruction of the intrinsic stabilizers such as the TFCC and the ulnocarpal ligaments.

Partial Head Implants

In order to spare the intrinsic stabilizers and focus on the mere resurfacing of the joint, which may in fact be the core goal of any arthroplasty, partial ulnar head replacement has been proposed.[13-15] Only the articular portion of the injured or diseased ulnar head is substituted without resection or damage of the TFCC and the ulnocarpal ligaments and their insertions. The clinical results are promising with follow-ups now up to 5 years with pain-free pronation/supination, subjectively stable DRU joints giving a substantial improvement of the grip strength in the entire range of forearm rotation, and a reasonable revision rate (Figs. 34A-8A and B and 34A-9).

SURGICAL TECHNIQUE

The technique described below and especially the approach can be used for most of the implants.

Partial Ulnar Head Nonconstrained DRUJ Arthroplasty

The partial ulnar head nonconstrained hemi-DRUJ arthroplasty is the authors' first choice, combined with a distal radius osteotomy if necessary, since the system respects the TFCC and other soft tissue stabilizers. We avoid as long as possible the constrained implants and believe more in reconstruction or reinforcement of the ligaments than in mechanical solution to eventual instability. When primary stabilizers

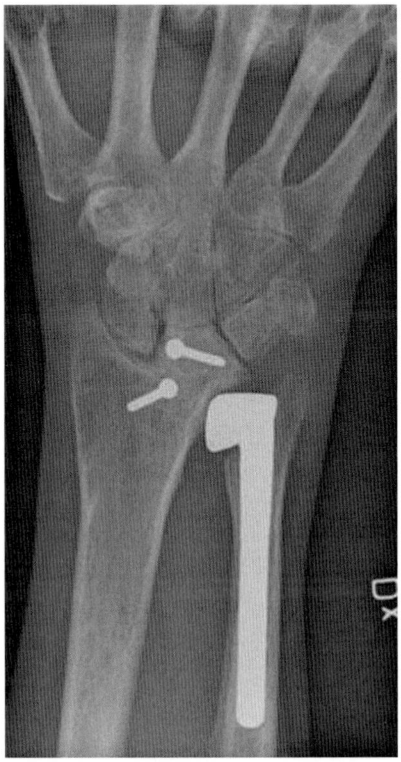

FIGURE 34A-9 Five-year follow-up of a First Choice hemi-DRUJ prosthesis in a patient with rheumatoid arthritis with a combined radiolunate fusion. Note the resorption of the distal ulna with a well-fixed stem.

are missing, as in rheumatoid arthritis, it seems possible to achieve stability through the secondary stabilizers and the reestablished joint congruency.

Preoperative Planning

A proper evaluation should be made of the status of the static and dynamic stabilizing structures. The anatomical prerequisites for postoperative stability have to be evaluated, such as the inclination of the DRUJ joint and the relative length of ulna, both of which affect the possibility of preserving the TFCC attachments during the preparation and cut. The size and position of the implant should be planned preoperatively using templates, both in the anteroposterior and in the lateral projections. The ulnar variance has to be measured on both wrists in order to plan the exact position of the ulnar head implant in relation to the radius.

Anatomical Approach

The patient is placed in the supine position under general anesthesia or axillary block. The shoulder is abducted to 90° and the elbow extended and the wrist in pronation. The approach is centered dorsally over the DRUJ preserving the dorsal ulnar veins and the dorsal branch of the ulnar nerve. The extensor digiti minimi (EDM) can be used as a landmark for localization of the DRUJ space and the fifth compartment is opened. The retinaculum is mobilized radially over the fourth compartment and ulnarly over the sixth compartment. The capsule overlaying the ulnar head is mobilized en bloc with the ECU tendon sheath and the tendon itself. In order to preserve the TFCC, the incision has to be made entirely proximal to this structure or the dissection should be made underneath it, in order to find the cleavage between the capsule and the dorsal part of the TFCC.[16] Once opened, the joint can be explored more easily, proximal and distal to the TFCC, using a Hohman retractor placed underneath the ulnar head. A gentle pronation of the radius facilitates delivery of the ulnar head into the operative field. A K-wire is placed at the distal ulnar border of the radius in order to indicate the radius length and make an easy positioning of the ulnar implant according to the measured and expected ulnar variance.

An awl is introduced radially into the fovea under fluoroscopic control, respecting the major ligament insertions, and then replaced by the reamer. The ulnar shaft is reamed to the desired implant stem length and size of the stem of the implant as planned preoperatively and the length is corrected as needed. The position is controlled in the fluoroscope. The saw guide for the hemi-DRUJ resurfacing implant is mounted on the reamer and the bone cut is made in 2 steps, with and without the intramedullary pointing device. The saw guide has to be parallel to the groove formed by the ECU tendon. At this step of surgery the procedure can be changed to a total ulnar head arthroplasty if necessary and for this purpose the saw guide appropriate to the procedure is used. In all cases the excised ulnar head is measured in order to choose the appropriate size of the implant. Some oversizing can be accepted to allow tensioning of the ligaments and the interosseous membrane, in order to increase the stability of the joint. The trial implant is inserted and checked fluoroscopically and clinically prior to insertion of the definitive implant. The capsule and the retinaculum, including the ECU tendon sheath, are repaired in anatomical position or along the border of the radius and dorsal margin of the sigmoid notch using transosseous stitches or bone anchors as necessary. The ECU has to be repositioned and centered dorsally, over the implant in pronation. Small sutures can be added to fixate the dorsal part of the TFCC to the capsule and retinaculum. The reconstruction of the fifth compartment is not mandatory since EDM has an adequate pulley more distally. After suture of the skin, a compressive dressing is applied for 2 weeks. In case of slight subluxation of the DRUJ, the reinsertion of the capsule on the dorsal margin of the sigmoid notch can be performed in pronation but tightened in supination, but is otherwise avoided since it carries the potential risk of decreased pronation. The remaining part of the ulnar head, including the styloid and the insertion of the main ligaments, allows for further stabilization procedures or reconstruction including free tendon transplants for TFCC reconstruction (Fig. 34A-10).

Postoperative Care

After wound closure a compressive dressing is applied for 2 weeks. The postoperative care has to be customized and depends on the patient, the intraoperative judgment of the stability of the device, and any concomitant procedures. As a general rule, pronation should be avoided for 2 to 3 weeks. The patient is immobilized in a splint in neutral position of pronation–supination and told to rotate the forearm from the neutral position to supination. After 2 to 3 weeks the plaster is changed to a removable splint. The patient starts active training of pronation and should reach full pronation–supination at 6 to 8 weeks.

PERSONAL OUTCOMES

Between November 2006 and October 2010, 15 patients (3 osteoarthritis and 12 rheumatoid arthritis patients), aged 61 years (range, 40-72 years), were operated for DRUJ reconstruction with the "First Choice" implant (Ascension Orthopedics). In the 12 rheumatoid patients, 10 had a concomitant partial or total wrist fusion. The patients were followed prospectively by independent observers, measuring range of motion, grip strength, VAS, and patient-administered outcome scores (DASH and COPM) as well as radiographically.

In the rheumatoid group, 1 patient was revised due to infection and 1 required reoperation due to stiffness. In

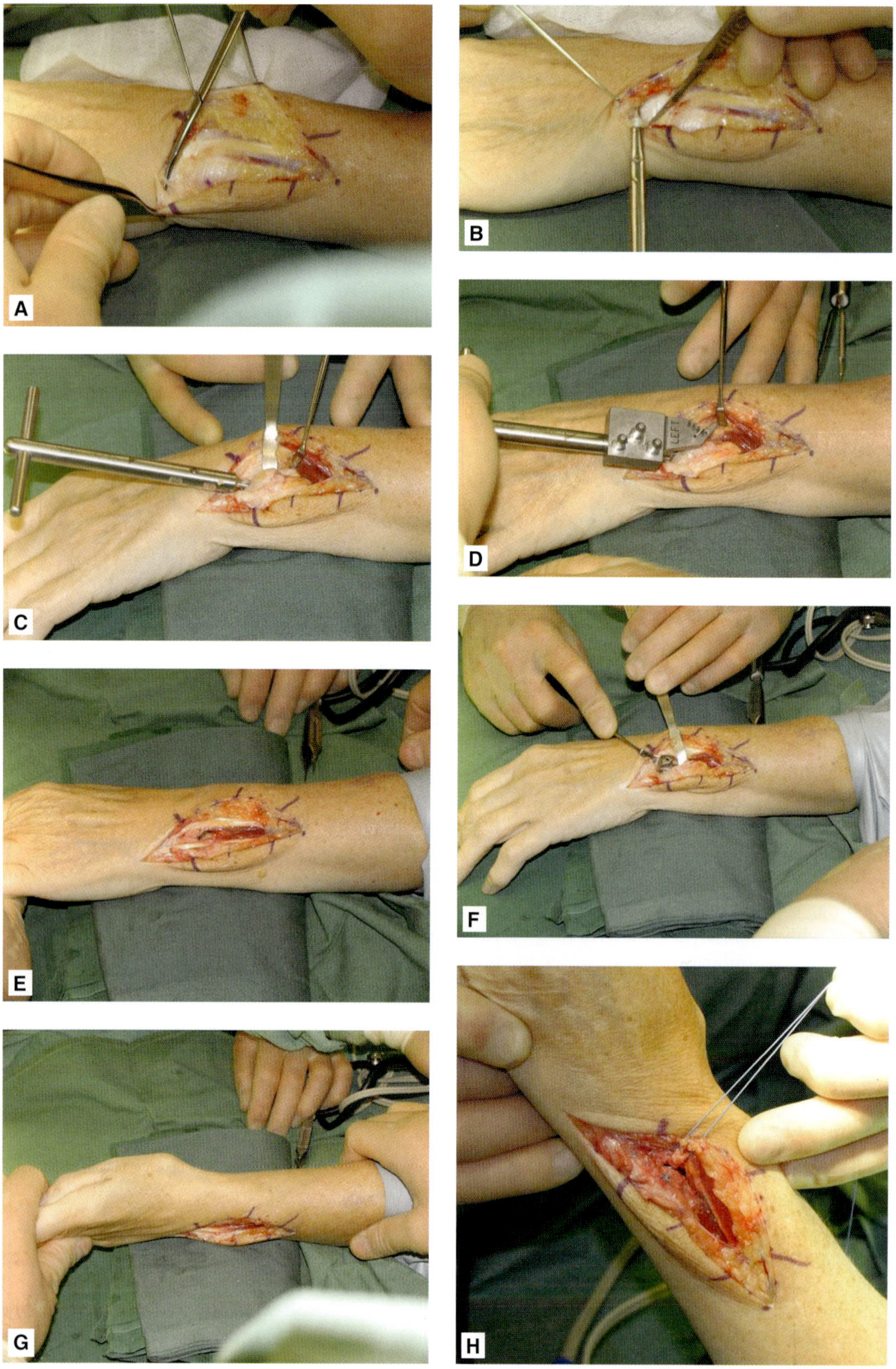

FIGURE 34A-10 **A-I.** Perioperative views of the implantation of a First Choice hemi-DRUJ prosthesis: the dorsal approach with preservation of the dorsal cutaneous branch of the ulnar nerve (**A**); the dorsal retinaculum is incised at the level of the EDM just above the DRU joint and dissected ulnarly (**B**); the ulnar head is exteriorized and the reamer can be introduced in the ulnar shaft with preservation of the TFCC and the ulnotriquetral ligament (**C**); the saw guide in place (**D**) allows a precise resection of the ulnar head with preservation of the styloid and ligament attachments (**E**). The prosthesis is introduced in the reamed ulnar shaft (**F**). The testing of the pronation–supination shows good stability of the joint (**G**); if necessary, the extensor retinaculum is sutured directly to the dorsal border of the sigmoid notch in order to increase stability (**H**). After suture and restoration of the anatomy the prosthesis is stable and does not protrude in pronation (**I**).

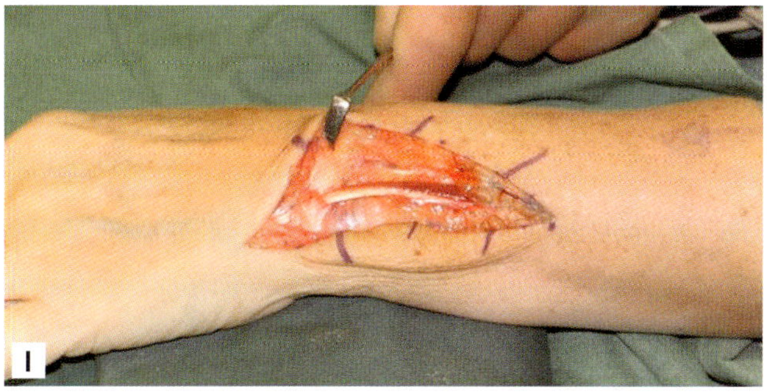

FIGURE 34A-10 (*Continued*).

the osteoarthritic group 1 patient had a painful clicking on forearm rotation and was reoperated on for dorsal capsular reattachment. The pronation was 67° preoperatively and 74° (40°-90°) after 1 year. Supination was 66° preoperatively and 60° (0°-90°) after 1 year. The mean grip strength of the operated hand increased from 85% to 153% of the contralateral at 1 year (P = .16). The DASH score remained unchanged between preoperative levels of 50 (32-69) and after 1 year at 44 (14-83). Subjective function as measured with the functional evaluation test of activities canadian occupational performance measure (COPM)[17] improved from 3.59 to 5.44 regarding performance and from 2.95 to 5.6 regarding satisfaction. The VAS (0-100) pain at rest decreased from 37 to 11 and VAS pain at activity from 50 to 29.

CONCLUSION

Only a full understanding of the role of the ulna and the ulnar head in the anatomy of the DRUJ and the forearm makes it possible to use an arthroplasty for this joint. It is mandatory to differentiate between the function in relation with the wrist joint and the forearm joint. The restitution of a pain-free pronation/supination/rotation of the forearm is best performed without deterioration of the stability of the DRUJ and for this purpose when necessary the use of an implant has to be discussed. The resection of the ulnar head today seems avoidable and in all cases the preservation of the anatomy and the stabilizing structures of the DRUJ should be recommended.

REFERENCES

1. Dahlquist J. *Biomechanical Study of Human Forearm* [master's thesis]. Lund: Lund Technical University; 2003.
2. Hagert CG. The distal radio ulnar joint in relation to the whole arm. *Clin Orthop*. 1992;275:56-64.
3. Hagert CG. Distal radius fracture and the distal radioulnar joint anatomical considerations. *Handchir Mikrochir Plast Chir*. 1994;26(1):22-26.
4. Gordon KD, Kedgley AF, Ferreira LM, King GJ, Johnson JA. Effect of simulated muscle activity on distal radioulnar joint loading in vitro. *J Orthop Res*. 2006;24(7):1395-1404.
5. Kapandji AI. Distal radioulnar prosthesis. *Ann Chir Main Memb Super*. 1992;11(4):320-332.
6. Ganser J. The Scheker-Aptis prosthesis for the distal radio ulnar joint. In: Røkkum M, ed. *Wrist and Joint Replacements*. FESSH Instructional Course. Oslo: FESSH; 2011.
7. Scheker LR. Implant arthroplasty for the distal radioulnar joint. *J Hand Surg Am*. 2008;33(9):1639-1644.
8. Sagerman SD, Seiler JG, Fleming LL, Lockerman E. Silicone rubber distal ulnar replacement arthroplasty. *J Hand Surg Br*. 1992;17(6):689-693.
9. Stanley D, Herbert TJ. The Swanson ulnar head prosthesis for post traumatic disorders of the distal radio ulnar joint. *J Hand Surg Br*. 1992;17(6):682-688.
10. Herbert TH, van Schoonhoven J. Ulnar head replacement. *Tech Hand Up Extrem Surg*. 2007;11(1):98-108.
11. van Schoonhoven J, Fernandez DL, Bowers WH, Herbert TJ. Salvage of failed resection arthroplasties of the distal radio ulnar joint using a new ulnar head prosthesis. *J Hand Surg Am*. 2000;25(3):438-446.
12. Herzberg G. Periprosthetic bone resorption and sigmoid notch erosion around ulnar head implants a concern? *Hand Clin*. 2010;26(4):573-577.
13. Conaway DA, Kuhl TL, Adams BD. Comparison of the native ulnar head and a partial head resurfacing implant. *J Hand Surg Am*. 2009;34(6):1056-1062.
14. Garcia-Elias M. Eclypse. Partial ulnar head replacement for the isolated radioulnar joint arthrosis. *Tech Hand Up Extrem Surg*. 2007;11(1):121-128.
15. Kopylov P, Tägil M. Distal radioulnar joint replacement. *Tech Hand Up Extrem Surg*. 2007;11(1):109-114.
16. Garcia-Elias M, Smith DE, Llusa M. Surgical approach of the triangular fibro cartilage complex. *Tech Hand Up Extrem Surg*. 2003;7(4):134-140.
17. Case-Smith J. Outcomes in hand rehabilitation using occupational therapy services. *Am J Occup Ther*. 2003;57(5):499-506.

Distal Radioulnar Joint Implants

34B

David J. Slutsky, MD

Distal ulnar implant arthroplasties can be divided into constrained and unconstrained prostheses. The unconstrained prosthesis consists of an anatomic distal ulnar replacement with or without soft tissue reconstruction. The options include a distal ulnar arthroplasty (ulnar head replacement) alone or distal ulnar replacement and resurfacing of the sigmoid fossa. There are a number of hemiarthroplasties that have been used as distal ulnar head replacements. These include the Herbert-Martin prosthesis (KLS Martin, Tuttinger, Germany), the uHead® cobalt chrome prosthesis with titanium-coated stem (Small Bone Innovations, Morrisville, Pennsylvania), the partial or complete pyrolytic carbon prosthesis (Ascension Orthopedics), and the Eclypse® (Tornier, Inc, Cedex, France) pyrocarbon partial head implant.

INDICATIONS

A primary indication for an ulnar head implant arthroplasty is symptomatic distal radioulnar joint (DRUJ) arthrosis. Another common indication is posttraumatic DRUJ osteoarthritis (OA) following a distal radius and/or ulnar head fracture or an irreducible fracture dislocation. An ulnar head replacement is indicated in advanced rheumatoid arthritis and for painful convergence of the ulnar stump following a Darrach or hemiresection arthroplasty, Sauvé-Kapandji procedure, or ulnar head excision for tumors.

CONTRAINDICATIONS

Contraindications for a nonconstrained or partial ulnar head implant include DRUJ instability secondary to an unreconstructable triangular fibrocartilage complex (TFCC) or distal interosseous membrane, previous infection, marked osteoporosis or cystic bone disease, unstable soft tissue coverage, and persistent DRUJ instability following an Essex-Lopresti injury. Inadequate soft tissue for the flap repair may result in instability of the prosthesis and may be contraindicated in patients with severe ligamentous laxity, scarring, or destructive rheumatoid arthritis. A malunion of the distal radius would need a prior or simultaneous corrective osteotomy to provide correct alignment as would any ulnar shaft deformity. Advanced arthritis of the sigmoid fossa is relatively contraindicated unless a total joint replacement is performed. Prior wrist fusion has been associated with an increased risk of prosthetic loosening; hence, cement fixation of the distal ulnar implant is recommended in the face of a prior total wrist fusion.

uHead® ENDOPROSTHESIS

The uHead® endoprosthesis is a modular endoprosthesis that consists of a metal stem with a shaft that can be press-fit or cemented into the intramedullary canal of the distal ulna. A metal semispheric ulnar head of cobalt–chrome alloy is connected to an intramedullary stem of cobalt–chrome alloy with a titanium-sprayed finish through a tight-fit Morse-taper junction. There are 2 stem-neck designs: an extended collar for revision of previous distal ulnar complete resection and a normal collar for primary procedures calling for ulnar head excision and for revision of failed distal ulnar head resection procedures. The head has a provision for suture fixation of the TFCC and extensor carpi ulnaris (ECU) subsheath to the device for the initial soft tissue stabilization. To ensure adequate length correction after previous surgery, differently sized ulnar head components and extended collars are available to compensate for shortening of the ulna after ulnar head resection (Fig. 34B-1A-F).

SURGICAL TECHNIQUE

The DRUJ is approached through a dorsal ulnar incision.[1] The extensor retinaculum is reflected and the dorsal cutaneous branch of the ulnar nerve is identified and protected. The DRUJ capsule is divided and retracted along with ECU subsheath. The triangular fibrocartilage (TFC) is either reflected and suture tagged or left attached to the ulnar styloid that is released (divided) from the ulnar head. The uHead® has 2 resection guides for a normal length and extended collar

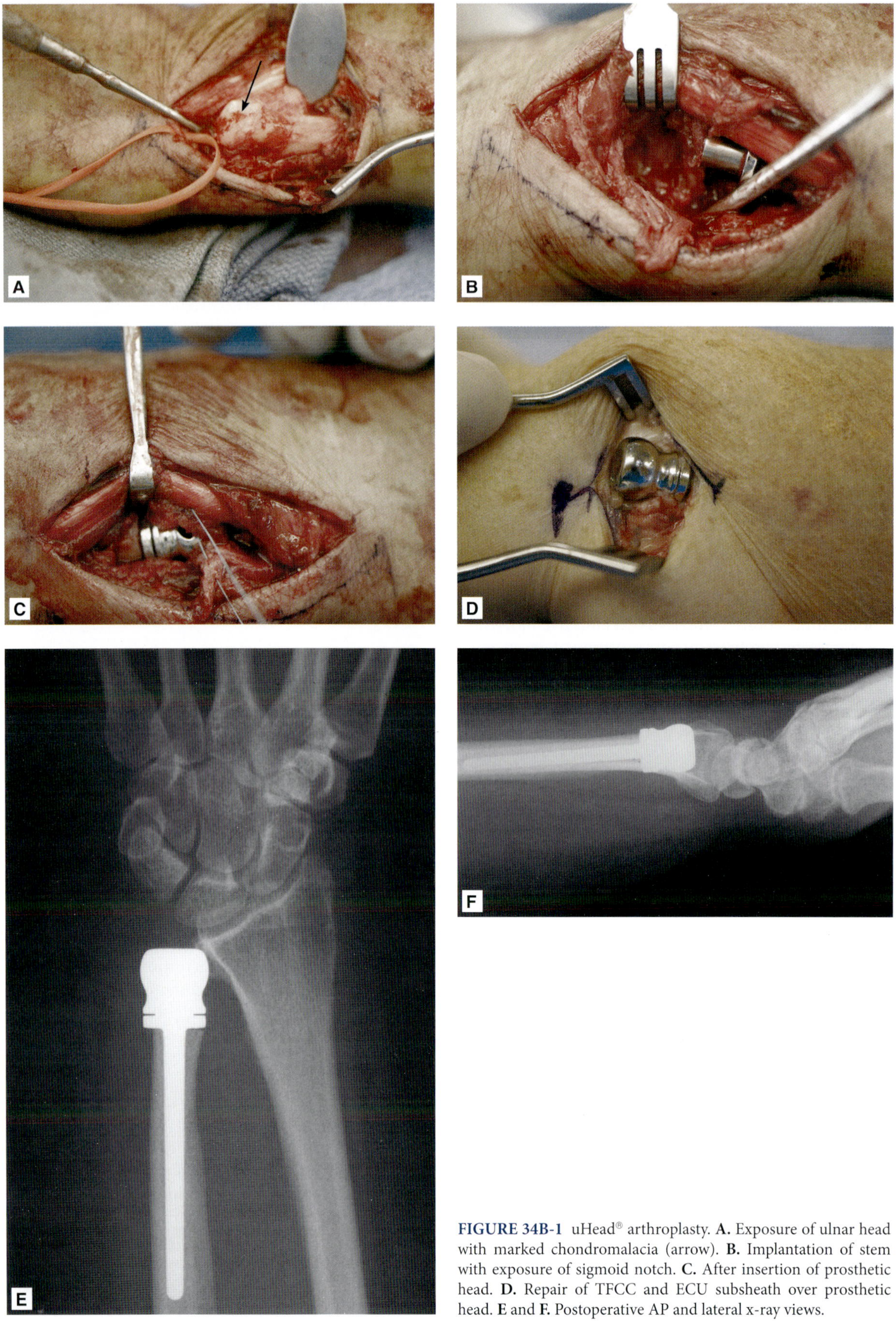

FIGURE 34B-1 uHead® arthroplasty. **A.** Exposure of ulnar head with marked chondromalacia (arrow). **B.** Implantation of stem with exposure of sigmoid notch. **C.** After insertion of prosthetic head. **D.** Repair of TFCC and ECU subsheath over prosthetic head. **E** and **F.** Postoperative AP and lateral x-ray views.

designs for early and late prosthesis replacement. After ulnar head resection, the intramedullary canal of the distal ulna is broached to match the expected stem size of the ulnar implant. The ulnar head size is also templated either directly from x-ray of the planned resected ulna or from the opposite distal ulna. The trial of the ulnar head and prosthesis are inserted and are tested clinically for stability, length, and position. The ulnar head should be neutral or negative ulnar variance. The ulnar head should be stable during testing of forearm rotation and not be too loose or unstable or overstuffed. The ulnar head should match or be smaller than the normal ulnar head size.

Prior to ulnar head linkage with the intramedullary stem component the TFC and ECU subsheath are attached by nonabsorbable 2 0 or 3 0 suture through the drill holes in the ulnar head. After prosthetic insertion, the soft tissues about the DRUJ are tightened in neutral rotation. The extensor retinaculum is repaired and the skin closed. A long arm splint is applied for 8 weeks to allow for bone ingrowth to the sintered titanium stem and soft tissue healing followed by strengthening exercises.

OUTCOMES

Kakar et al reviewed the results of 47 patients with an average age of 48 years (range 19-74 years) who received a unilateral DRUJ implant at a mean follow-up of 56 months (range, 16-126 months).[2] The indications for surgery included DRUJ injury due to a distal radius fracture in 22 wrists, repetitive overuse in 7, inflammatory disease in 7, DRUJ dislocation in 5, and other causes in 6. Forty patients had a total of 52 previous procedures related to the distal ulna. Cement fixation was used in 5 patients. The postoperative pain score decreased from 5 to 2 ± 2. The mean Mayo wrist score improved from 41 ± 9 to 69 ± 12 points after surgery, a mean improvement of 29 ± 12 points. There was an increase in postoperative grip and key pinch strength as well as wrist motion, but these changes did not reach statistical significance. At the final radiographic follow-up of 4.1 years (range, 13 months to 11.5 years), 37% of implants had greater than 2 mm of lucency around the stem and 40% had pedestal formation at the tip. A total of 16 implants (34%) had evidence of greater than 5 mm dorsal instability on the lateral radiograph. In addition, 57% demonstrated radiographic evidence of ulnar head erosion or osteolysis of the sigmoid notch. There were 8 implants that failed during a 6-year follow-up, giving an implant survival of 83%. Five were for aseptic loosening necessitating implant exchange, 1 was revised with the addition of a sigmoid notch replacement, and 2 were converted to a total DRUJ prosthesis (APTIS Medical, Louisville, Kentucky) because of persistent pain and instability despite attempts at soft tissue stabilization.

COMPLICATIONS

Four patients had complications, 1 early and 3 late. There was 1 intraoperative nondisplaced fracture of the ulna, 1 patient with a painful neuroma of the dorsal cutaneous branch of the ulnar nerve, and 1 patient with symptomatic instability of the ulnar head prosthesis, which was restored at revision surgery with a distally based strip of flexor carpi ulnaris (FCU) tendon (Linscheid-Hui procedure). Two patients had intramedullary stem loosening that was revised with bone cement at 14 to 16 months.

SIGMOID NOTCH PROSTHESIS

The STABILITY prosthesis (Small Bone Innovations) is part of a modular system consisting of the uHead® ulnar head prosthesis and a polyethylene sigmoid notch resurfacing implant. The sigmoid notch implant comes in 2 sizes and consists of a cobalt chrome radial plate with a titanium coating and fixation screws and an ultra-high-molecular-weight polyethylene insert. The insert slides onto the plate following plate fixation and is secured via a peripheral and ramp lock snap fit. The implants are designed so that any size sigmoid notch can accommodate any size head.

Indications

There is a high incidence of sigmoid notch erosion following ulnar head replacement, which is the main indication for surgery. While erosion alone has not been linked directly to pain, there is some concern regarding the overall impact on clinical symptomatology and on long-term implant survival.

Contraindications

This implant cannot be used with poor radial bone stock, active infection, or ulnar head implant instability. It has not been used as a stand-alone implant.

Surgical Technique

The DRUJ approach is the same as described for the ulnar head implant. The sigmoid notch component is placed after preparation of the ulnar shaft for ulnar head replacement. A trial head and saddle tool is placed onto the ulnar stem prior to placement of the final ulnar head prosthesis. This trial head and saddle tool is cannulated allowing the surgeon to drill a guidewire into the sigmoid notch. The position of the guidewire is then verified with posterior–anterior and lateral fluoroscopy. Once the position has been confirmed, the trial head is then removed and a cannulated drill is passed over the guidewire to create a pilot hole for the sigmoid implant. The implant is then pressed into position and a cancellous bone screw is then placed into the sigmoid component firmly fixing it to the distal radius. The polyethylene insert is then placed onto the sigmoid component. The final ulnar head stem and prosthesis are then inserted into the ulnar shaft. The joint is reduced and the capsule is closed (Fig. 34B-2A-H). A sugar tong splint is used for 2 weeks

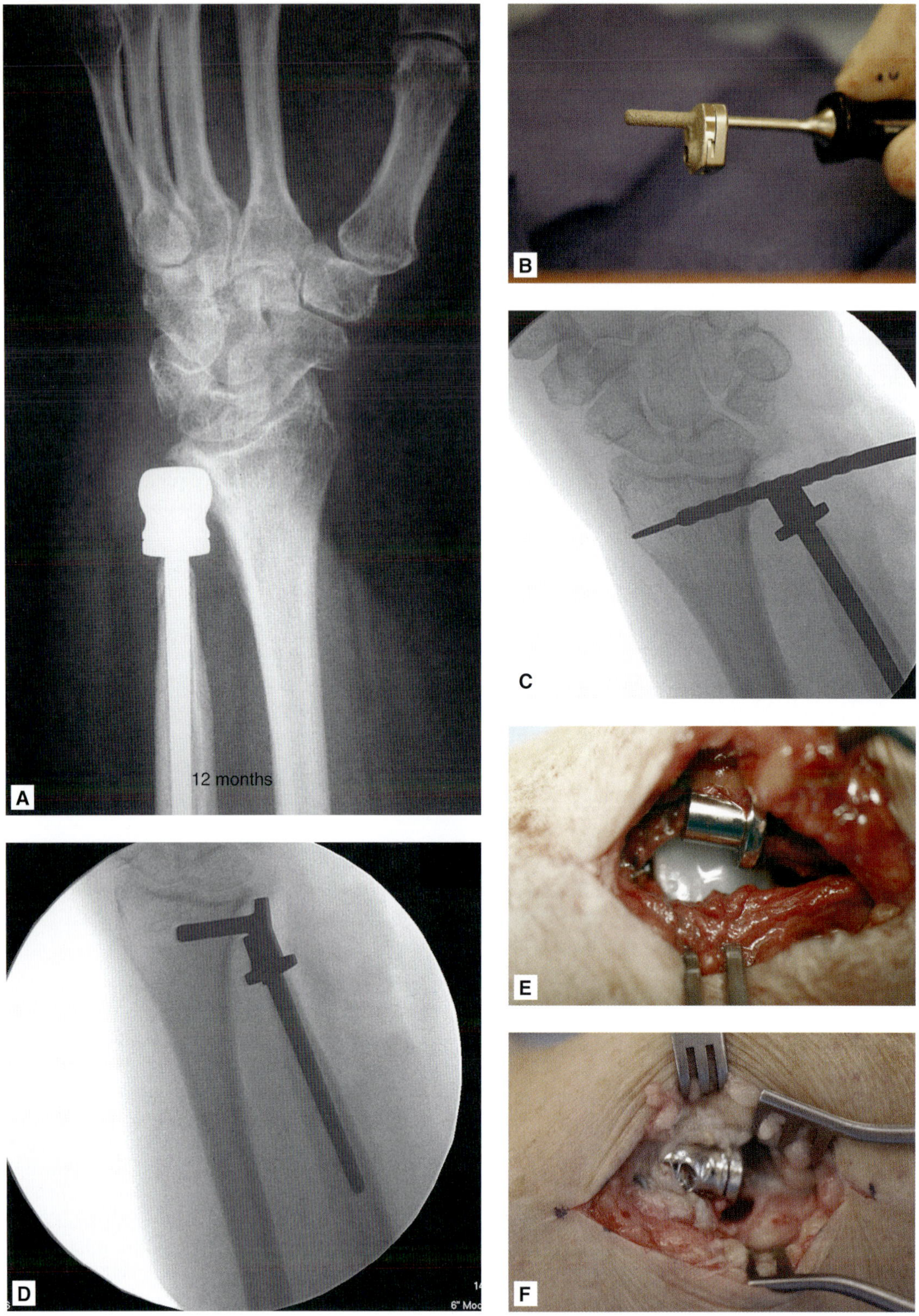

FIGURE 34B-2 STABILITY Sigmoid Notch replacement. **A.** Painful sigmoid notch erosion in a 50-year-old female at 1 year following a uHead® arthroplasty. **B.** Photo of porous-coated sigmoid notch insert. **C.** Intraoperative photo illustrating the sigmoid notch implant with the polyethelene insert. **D.** Drill hole for STABILITY plate implantation. **E.** X-ray following STABILITY implant insertion. **F.** Clinical photo of polyethylene lining.

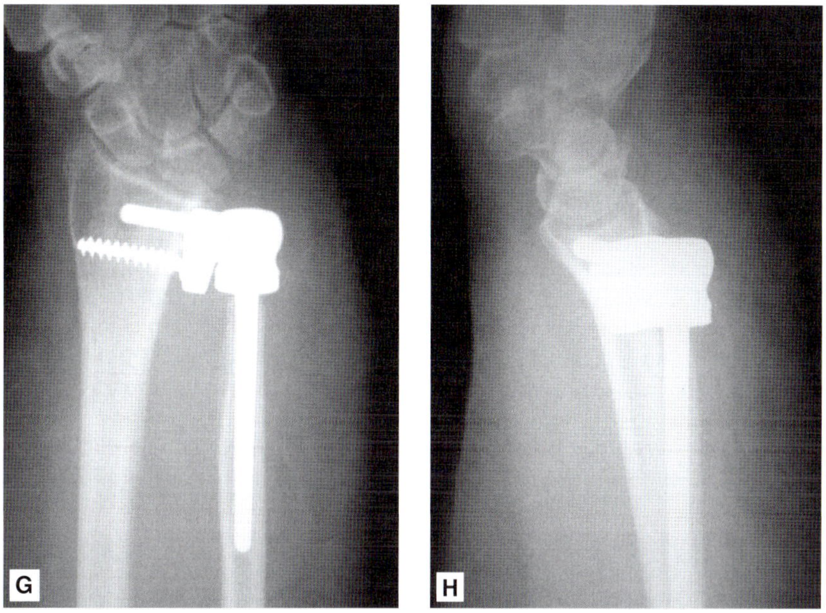

FIGURE 34B-2 (*Continued*) **G.** Soft tissue reconstruction following insertion of the uHead®. **H.** Postoperative x-ray.

followed by a Muenster cast or long arm cast in full forearm supination for 4 additional weeks, followed by range of motion exercises at 6 weeks. The patients are allowed to return to regular activities at 12 weeks.

Outcomes

Moran and coworkers performed a retrospective review of 4 patients with a mean age of 42.5 years (range 35-51 years) who had undergone placement of the STABILITY Sigmoid Notch Total DRUJ System.[3] The mean follow-up was 46 months (range 36-66 months). All patients had an average of 4 (range 2-7) prior operative procedures before receiving a total DRUJ replacement. Successful implant of the total DRUJ was achieved in each patient. Subluxation was defined by drawing a longitudinal line through the center of the radius and the ulnar head and the distance between the 2 lines at the distalmost aspect of the sigmoid notch was measured. A difference of 5 mm was defined as a sign of dorsal implant instability while a negative measurement greater than 5 mm indicated volar instability. The implants were evaluated for loosening, which was defined as greater than 2 mm of lucency around the ulnar prosthetic stem or greater than 2 mm of lucency around the screws of the sigmoid implant. Radiographs were also evaluated for osteolysis under the ulnar head and collar pedestal formation at the tip of the stem. The average preoperative visual analog pain scale (VAS) score (scale 1-10) was 8 and averaged 2.5 at the final follow-up. The preoperative grip strength averaged 7.5 kg (range 4-12 kg) and improved postoperatively to an average of 25.5 kg (range 10-32 kg). The forearm rotation remained stable or improved in all patients with a mean final pronation of 80° (range 60°-90°) and mean supination of 64° (range 45°-90°). There was no clinical evidence of instability noted in any of the forearms. Patient satisfaction was 100% with all patients stating they would have the operation again. There were no secondary procedures performed with implant survival of 100% at an average of 46 months. There was no evidence of ulnar stem or sigmoid notch loosening and no evidence of dorsal or volar instability. There was also no evidence for polyethylene wear or particular synovitis. All ulnar shafts showed evidence of tapering and 2 of the 4 had evidence of pedestal formation.

SALVAGE

In late cases of distal ulnar resection associated with DRUJ instability reconstruction of the ligament support of the DRUJ may be necessary. Options for the later include use of the FCU, brachioradialis (BR), or palmaris longus (PL) tendons. Gupta has described the BR wrap procedure that consists of rerouting the insertion of the BR from radial to ulna dorsally or volarly to reconstruct the dorsal and volar DRUJ capsule.[4]

Indication/Contraindication

The BR wrap can be used for an unstable DRUJ with a preserved ulnar head as well as following an ulnar head implant arthroplasty. Active infection is a main contraindication. A previous release of the BR tendon during internal fixation of the distal radius precludes the use of this procedure. Inadequate soft tissue coverage should be managed with pedicled or free tissue transfer prior to performing the BR wrap.

Surgical Technique

The BR is first identified through a 4-cm radial incision proximal to the first extensor compartment.[4] A second 4-cm incision is made more proximally at the musculotendinous junction. The superficial radial nerve is identified and gently retracted. The muscle is gently teased off the tendon to increase the graft length. The BR tendon is released and pulled into the wrist incision. The DRUJ is exposed through a midlateral incision between the ECU and FCU, protecting the DCBUN. The pronator quadratus (PQ) muscle is identified on the palmar aspect of the radius. A channel is dissected by subperiosteally elevating a strip of the PQ from the radial to the ulnar incision. The free proximal end of the BR tendon is now passed in this channel from the radial to the ulnar side, leaving the BR attached at its radial styloid insertion and retrieved in the ulnar incision. Suture anchors are inserted on the palmar and dorsal rim of the sigmoid notch, and used to prevent any palmar or dorsal into which the ulnar head may sublux. Prosthetic replacement of the sigmoid notch and/or the ulnar head is now carried out. The flat BR tendon is draped over the ulnar head replacement and while holding the ulnar head reduced in the sigmoid notch, the BR is sutured tightly to the dorsal rim of the sigmoid notch using the suture anchor. The remaining BR tendon is then passed palmar to the extensor tendons, so that it lies on the dorsal cortex of the radius. It is delivered into the radial incision, where it is sutured to the intact portion of the BR tendon with nonabsorbable sutures proximal to the first extensor compartment. This holds the replaced ulnar head well reduced relative to the radius in all planes while at the same time allowing the ulnar head to rotate in the sigmoid notch. The ulnar part of the TFCC and other remaining ulnar soft tissue stabilizers may be sutured to the distal part of the BR as it wraps around the ulnar head, thus forming a soft tissue hood around the replaced ulnar head. If the ulnar head subluxation is primarily on the dorsal side, the BR tendon is routed from the dorsal to palmar side (Fig. 34B-3A-F). The patient is immobilized in a sugar tong splint for 2 weeks, followed by gentle active and passive range of motion exercises.

HERBERT-MARTIN CERAMIC ULNAR HEAD IMPLANT

Herbert started using a Swanson silicone ulnar head implant in 1981 for patients with symptomatic posttraumatic arthritis of the DRUJ, but because of the poor midterm outcomes he developed a modular ulnar head prosthesis with assistance from the Department of Biomechanical Engineering, University of New South Wales.[5] They chose ceramic (zirconium oxide) as the material most suitable for articulation with joint cartilage. They decided to use a noncemented stem made of porous-coated titanium because of its known biocompatibility and a modulus of elasticity (100,000 N/mm^2) that is very similar to that of bone. The Herbert ulnar head prosthesis (Martin Medizintechnik) first became available early in 1995, and the first 5 cases were carried out at that time, with encouraging short-term results. A multicenter clinical trial was initiated later that year, and the prosthesis was released for general use in 1998. The indications and contraindications are as described above.

Surgical Technique

A dorsal approach is performed between the fifth and sixth extensor compartments raising an ulnar-based capsular-retinacular flap.[5] A resection guide is hooked over the distal end of the radius, and the appropriate resection level as determined from the preoperative x-rays is marked. An oscillating saw is used for the osteotomy and the ulnar head is removed, while preserving the TFCC. Any TFCC tears are repaired or patched using a flap of retinaculum. The ulnar shaft is hand reamed to the appropriate diameter with progressively larger reamers. The sigmoid fossa is debrided of any loose osteophytes, debris, or scar tissue. Two holes are drilled through the dorsal rim of the sigmoid for later flap reattachment. A trial prosthesis is inserted to check the length ensuring that the flap does not impinge on the TFCC in full pronation; otherwise more bone is resected. If the resection is too proximal, a stem with a longer collar is used. The ulnar flap is manually advanced over the prosthesis and held down onto the dorsal rim of the sigmoid to assess the range of motion as well as the implant stability.

Any necessary adjustments are made such as changing the head size, tightening, or releasing the flap and/or adjacent soft tissues to ensure a stable reduction with a full range of rotation. The position is checked under fluoroscopy prior to inserting the definitive prosthesis. The stem is press-fit without cement, using the impactor to ensure that the collar sits flush on the distal end of the ulna. The head is impacted on the distal cone of the stem to ensure a good interference fit between the 2 components. The flap is reattached with sutures through the sigmoid drill holes prior to implant reduction, and then sutured to the dorsal rim of the TFCC.

In patients with painful instability following a Sauvé-Kapandji procedure a resection of the fusion mass and insertion of the prosthesis is preferred if either the fusion has not healed completely or the original fusion has been performed in an ulna-plus situation leading to additional symptoms of ulnar impaction syndrome. If this is not an option, Fernandez et al have described using a specially designed spherical head to articulate within the previously fused ulnar head following reaming of a socket into the proximal fusion mass.[6]

Outcomes

Van Schoonhoven and Lanz reviewed the results of ulnar head replacement using the Herbert ceramic ulnar head implant for painful instability following a resection arthroplasty of the DRUJ in 76 patients with a mean follow-up of 95 (61-124) months.[7] The VAS was reduced from a mean

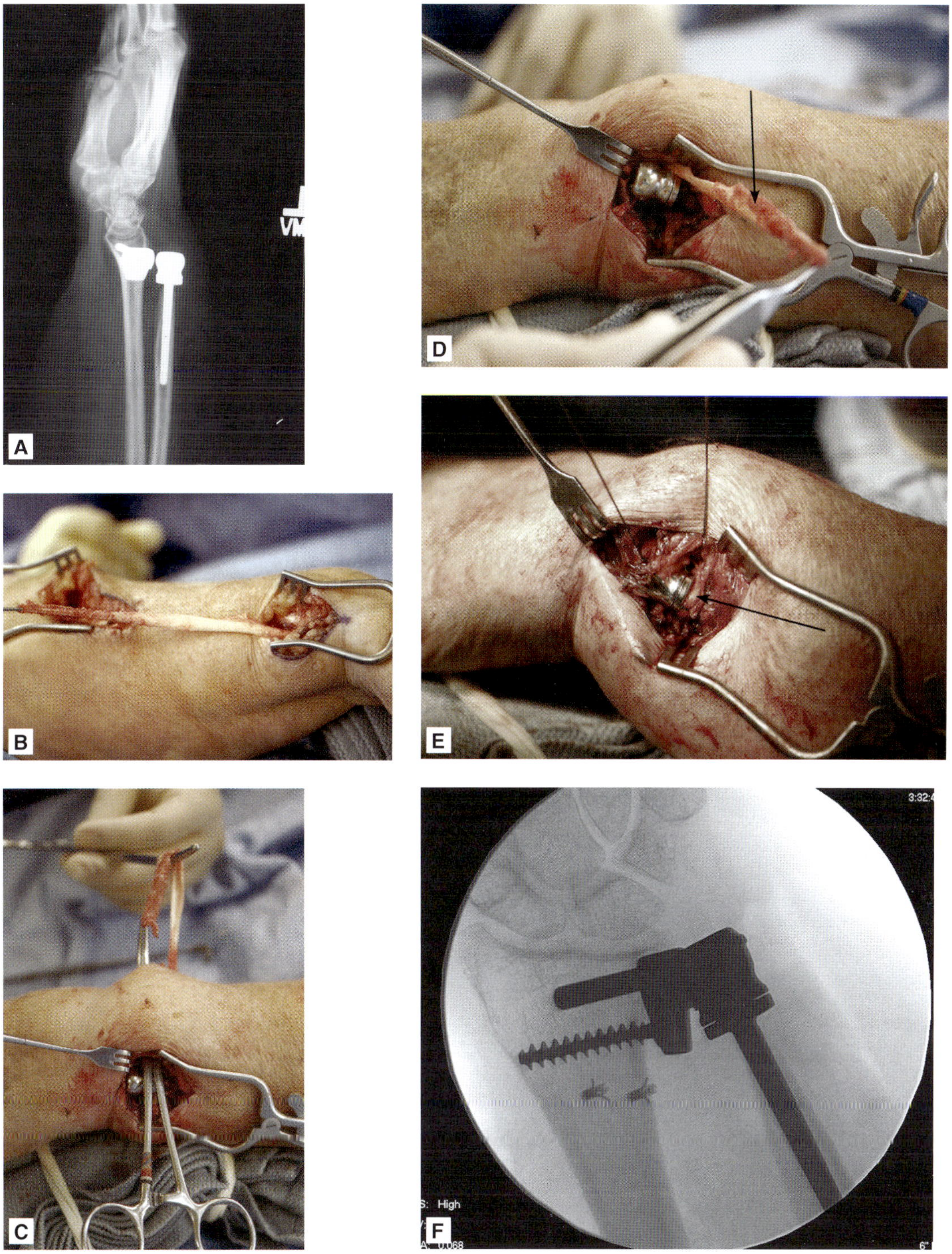

FIGURE 34B-3 Brachioradialis wrap. **A.** Unstable uHead® prosthesis. **B.** Harvesting of brachioradialis tendon. **C.** Rerouting BR tendon palmar to the pronator quadratus. **D.** BR tendon wrapped around uHead®. **E.** Soft tissue repair. **F.** Intraoperative x-ray showing a congruent reduction of the prosthesis.

of 8.7 preoperatively to 2.0. Preoperative grip strength averaged 42% compared with the contralateral side and increased to a mean of 74%. Forearm rotation improved from a mean of 126° to 144°. The overall satisfaction was found to be very high with a mean of 8.4 on a visual scale from 0 to 10. Radiographically, early bone resorption at the distal end of the ulna under the collar of the prosthesis was seen in 6 patients and averaged 2 mm. It was common to find some reactive bone remodeling at the sigmoid fossa, which was seen in 5 patients. These bone reactions were felt to be harmless and resolved after 12 to 18 months. There were no signs of late loosening of the stem on long-term follow-up.

PYROCARBON PARTIAL HEAD IMPLANT

Indications

A pyrocarbon partial head implant (Eclypse®) is indicated in all those conditions where one would consider performing a hemiresection-interposition arthroplasty (Bowers procedure).[8] These include isolated OA of the DRUJ, posttraumatic deformity of the articular surface of the ulnar head with preservation of the sigmoid notch, and ulnar head degeneration secondary to chronic inflammatory disease such as chondrocalcinosis or rheumatoid arthritis, provided there is no major DRUJ instability.

Contraindications

Eclypse® is not indicated in the presence of DRUJ instability owing to rupture or insufficiency of both the distal radioulnar and ulnocarpal ligaments. If only the radioulnar ligaments are disrupted but the ulnocarpal ligaments still maintain some level of stability, the implant may be used. Other contraindications are when the sigmoid is not concave and congruent, or if the radius exhibits substantial malalignment, which would require a corrective osteotomy prior to implantation. If there is a noncorrectable radial deformity that makes it impossible for the implant to articulate with the radius or if the ulnar head has been excised to a level where no contact can be reestablished between the Eclypse® and the sigmoid notch, this implant should not be utilized. In the latter cases, a total ulnar head implant or a total DRUJ prosthesis would be indicated.

Surgical Technique

A dorsoulnar skin incision centered on the ulnar head is made, identifying and protecting the DCBUN. The fifth extensor compartment is released longitudinally, and an ulnar-based retinacular flap is elevated taking care not to enter the DRUJ joint. If the ECU tendon is unstable and subluxes toward the palmar corner of the wrist in supination and ulnar deviation, an ECU sling is reconstructed using a portion of extensor retinaculum. An ulnar-based capsular flap is developed and detached off the medial edge of the radius by dividing the peripheral fibers that attach to the dorsal radioulnar ligament. The forearm is then fully pronated and the ulnar head is dorsally subluxed into the wound. Two osteotomy cuts are performed using a specialized guide, including a transverse osteotomy of about half the diameter of the ulnar head, perpendicular to the longitudinal axis of the ulna, and a longitudinal osteotomy along the sagittal plane at the level of the fovea and adjacent to the styloid process. This second cut is perpendicular to the plane of flexion–extension of the elbow to create a flat surface parallel to the sigmoid notch of the radius. The implant rests on the top of this horizontal surface, so that the radius rotates around its center, during supination to pronation. An awl is introduced at the center of the basistyloid fovea parallel to the ulnar diaphysis. A drill is used to create a 40-mm long vertical tunnel in the metaphysis. If the drill abuts the cortical bone, the small, 3.5-mm diameter stem is used, whereas a 4.5- or 5.5-mm drill is used with larger canals and a medium-size stem is press-fit. The 4 legs of the stem are rectangular shaped and are compressed with a specially designed clamp during insertion to facilitate stem impaction and allow proper orientation. The stem has a semicircular horizontal plate with a flat edge and a central peg for the ulnar head insertion. The flat edge of this plate is inset parallel to the sagittal osteotomy. Once fully inserted, the proximal tips of the 4 legs expand, which maximizes the stability of the implant while allowing bone formation among the vertical slits formed by the 4 legs. The DRUJ stability is assessed throughout the entire range of forearm rotation. The ulnar head should move easily around the central peg, continuously adjusting its position to match the changing space between radius and ulna. The titanium stem usually undergoes bony incorporation in about 6 weeks; hence, the patient is protected from passive hyperpronation or supination during that period. A loose ulnar head is not problematic, as long as the central stem prevents any possibility of implant dislocation since the implant serves mostly as a spacer that maintains proper separation of the 2 bones. The capsule is repaired in layers.

Outcomes

Garcia-Elias initially reported 3 cases (47, 56, and 60 years old). At a 10-month follow-up the mean pronation was 75°, supination 80°, and lifting averaged 4 kg.[8] He later reviewed 13 patients following an arthroplasty.[9] At an average follow-up of 12 months (range 7-25), the patients had minimal discomfort at the extremes of motion, with a mean pronation of 75° and supination of 65°. In another series 14 patients who were treated with the Eclypse® implant were evaluated.[10] The mean DASH score at the latest follow-up was 31 (range 0-63). Thirteen patients had no pain at rest while 3 had slight pain, 8 had no pain with light activity while 6 had slight pain, and 2 had moderate pain. During heavy activity 5 had no pain, 2 had slight pain, 6 had moderate pain, and 3 had severe pain. The average pronation was 86° (100% of the opposite side) and the average supination was 69° (93% of the opposite side).

SEMICONSTRAINED DRUJ PROSTHESIS

Absence of an intact DRUJ, as occurs following an ulnar head resection, causes the distal ulnar stump to impinge on the radius metaphysis when loading the DRUJ such as when lifting a drinking glass. This impingement may not be evident on regular posteroanterior x-rays since the forearm is not loaded in this position.[11] A cross-table lateral obtained when the person is holding a weight against gravity with the forearm in the neutral position demonstrates the impingement. Scheker has designed a semiconstrained DRUJ implant that can be used in cases of DRUJ instability (APTIS® distal radioulnar joint total replacement prosthesis, APTIS Medical). The DRUJ prosthesis is a semiconstrained ball-and-socket joint comprising a radial component and an ulnar component. The radial component is shaped in the form of a plate with a hemisocket on the distal end. The body of the plate, with its 5 screw holes, is contoured to fit against the distal 6 to 7 cm of the interosseous crest, in the area of the sigmoid notch. The plate is fixed to the radius by a peg that is driven into the distal radius in an ulnoradial direction, in addition to screw fixation of the plate with 3.5-mm cortical screws. The hemisocket, which is part of the plate, is directed ulnarward and is designed to receive the ultra-high-molecular-weight polyethylene ball of the ulnar component. The other half of the socket consists of a cover that encloses the ultra-high-molecular-weight polyethylene ball and is fixed to its counterpart on the plate by means of 2 screws. The radial component is available in 2 sizes, small (size 20) and large (size 30), which fit with the corresponding sizes of the ulnar component. The ulnar component consists of an 11 cm long plasma-coated fluted stem. The most distal end of the stem bears a highly polished peg that fits into the hole of an ultra-high-molecular-weight polyethylene ball. The stems are provided in 2 diameters, 4.5 and 5.0 mm, and have correspondingly sized ultra-high-molecular-weight polyethylene balls. Each size couples with the small and large radial components, respectively.

Indications

This implant is ideally used in patients who have a nonreconstructable painful instability of the ulnar head with erosive changes in the DRUJ. It can also be used after a failed ulnar head resection or following failed ulnar head arthroplasty.

Contraindications

Severe osteoporosis, unresolved osteomyelitis, and systemic disease contraindicate the use of the prosthesis. The implant is bulkier than an ulnar head prosthesis; hence, inadequate soft tissue coverage precludes the use of this implant.

Surgical Technique

The forearm is placed in full pronation and a 7- to 8-cm hockey stick incision is made above the dorsal lateral aspect of the distal ulna, turning radially just distal to the head of the ulna.[12] The incision is deepened through the interval between the extensor digiti quinti minimi and ECU sheath, which is released from the ulna, taking care to protect the DCBUN. A fascial flap can be created to later provide a barrier between the prosthesis and tendons. If present, the head of the ulna is then excised at the neck level while preserving the radial attachment of the TFCC. Excising the ulnar head facilitates the exposure of the radius by allowing the ulnar shaft to be retracted palmarward. Any DRUJ osteophytes are excised and the interosseous membrane is elevated 8 to 9 cm proximally. The radial plate trial is then placed over the interosseous surface of the radius and held with K-wires. The distal end of the trial should be 3 mm proximal to the radiocarpal joint in the area of the sigmoid notch to prevent radiocarpal impingement, with the palmar edge of the plate aligned with the volar edge of the radius. A 2.5-mm drill bit is used to drill a transverse hole through the sliding guide hole of the trial followed by a tap and 3.5-mm screw. Once the final position is confirmed, the distal K-wires are removed and the radial peg drill bit is passed through the center distal guide hole of the trial. The trial component is removed and replaced with the radial plate component that is held by screws. A short 18-mm distal screw is used to prevent impingement against the transverse peg.

With the forearm fully pronated, a specially designed measuring device is inserted along the ulna and into the hemisocket of the radial component. With the measuring device in place, the proximal edge of the metal lip below the ball indicates the appropriate level of resection to provide 1 mm of tolerance. An extended stem with a lengthened collar can be used when too much bone has been lost due to injury or previous surgery. A 0.062-in guidewire is inserted into the medullary canal followed by a cannulated drill bit. The canal is reamed to a depth of 11 cm until the shoulder of the medullary reamer comes into contact with the distal end of the ulnar shaft. The ulnar stem component is introduced using a plastic impactor. The ulnar component is completed by placing the ultra-high-molecular-weight polyethylene ball over the distal peg of the ulnar stem. This combination replaces the function of the ulnar head. Finally, the cover is positioned over the radial socket and secured with 2 screws to encapsulate the ultra-high-molecular-weight polyethylene ball, which recreates the stabilizing effects of an intact TFCC and completes the prosthesis (Fig. 34B-4A-J). The wound is closed and a bulky splint is applied, followed by wrist motion and forearm rotation at 2 weeks.

Outcomes

Scheker's group interviewed/examined 31 patients who had received the prosthesis, at a mean follow-up of 5.9 years (range, 4-9 years). The forearm pronation increased from a mean of 65° (range, 5°-90°) to 74° (range, 20°-90°) and the supination increased from 53° (range, 5°-90°) to 70° (range, 20°-90°). The grip strength increased from a mean of 10 to 24 kg. Weight bearing was restored or increased in 29 of 31 patients, while greatly diminishing and/or eliminating DRUJ pain.

Fox et al presented the outcomes of 10 patients with a mean age of 47 years who received the APTIS® prosthesis at a mean follow-up of 3.3 years (2.2-4.0 years) and after a mean of 4 prior wrist surgeries.[13] One patient required revision of a loose ulnar stem at 7 months. Five patients were treated with secondary procedures for either extensor tendon irritation or prominent radial-sided screw tips. The average forearm rotation remained unchanged versus the preoperative status. In a similar study Axelsson reviewed 9 patients treated with the APTIS® prosthesis after a mean of 3.4 prior surgeries (range 1-7) and a mean follow-up of 35 months (range 12-62 months).[14] The median VAS decreased from 6 preoperatively to 0.5. The median DASH score improved from 43 to 29. The median grip increased from 17 to 21 kg. There were no radiographic signs of loosening.

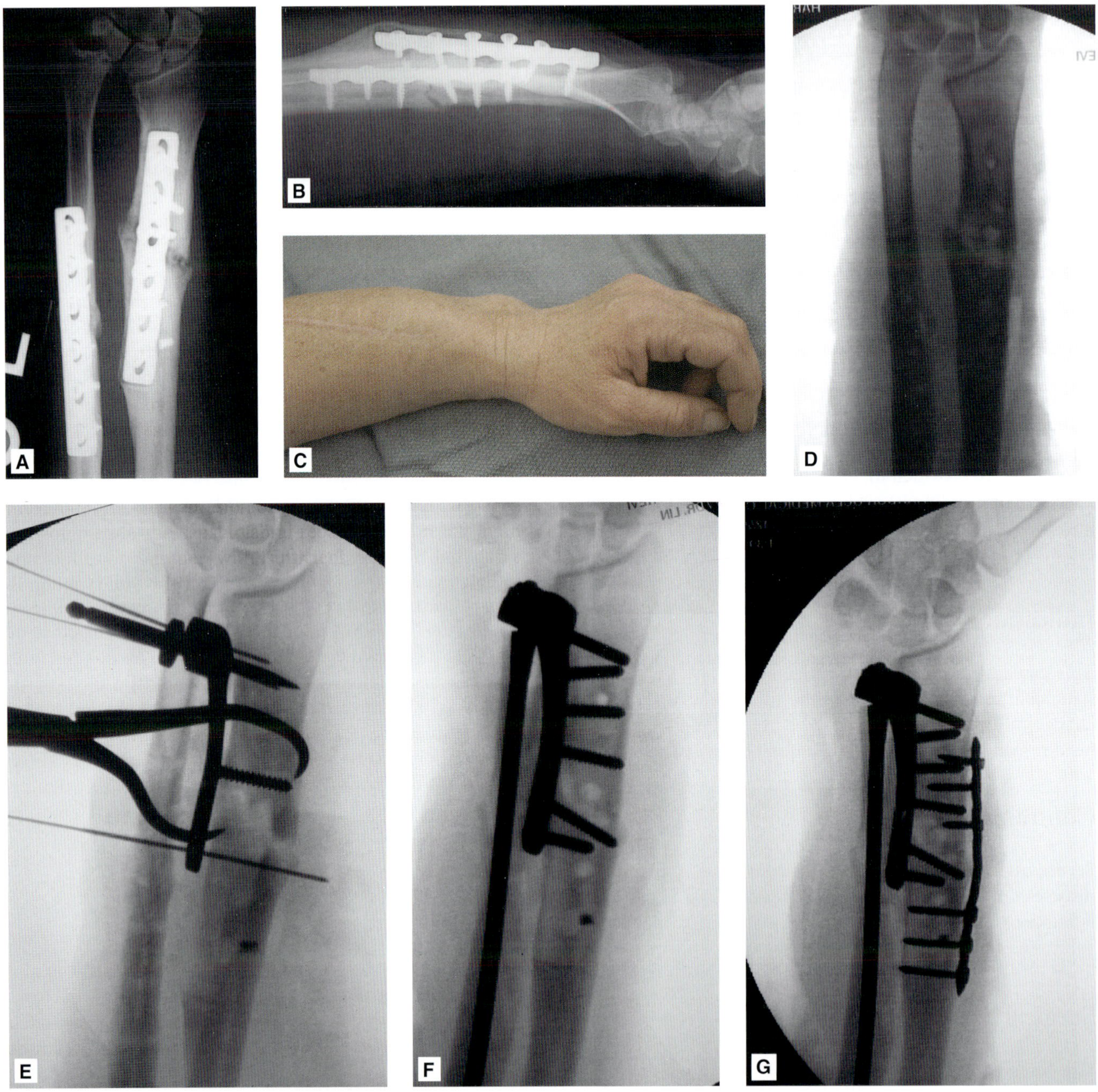

FIGURE 34B-4 APTIS® distal radioulnar joint prosthesis. **A** and **B.** AP and lateral views of a nonunion of the radius and ulnar with a marked ulnar variance and DRUJ disruption. **C.** Clinical appearance of the forearm. **D.** Intraoperative x-ray following plate removal showing the marked radioulnar height discrepancy. **E.** Provisional stabilization of the radius nonunion with the radial plate. **F.** Intraoperative x-ray following insertion of the prosthesis. **G.** Additional plating of the nonunion of the radius.

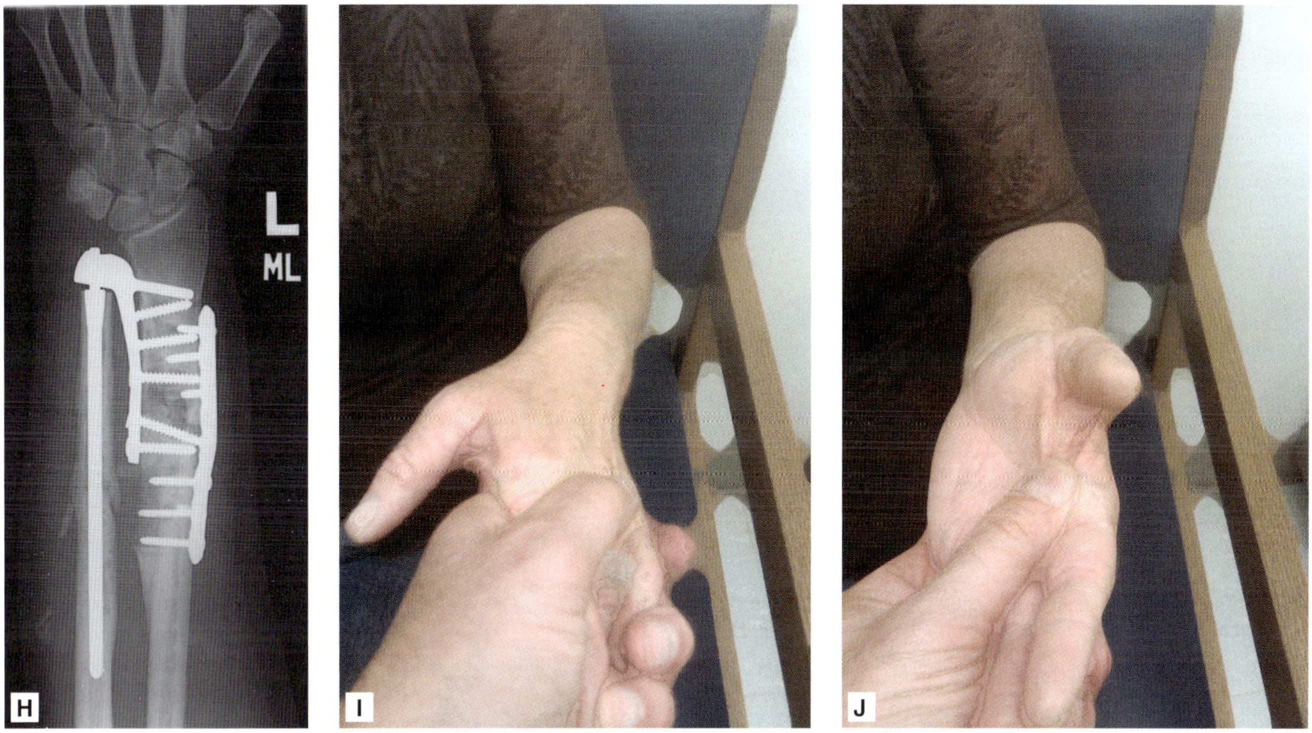

FIGURE 34B-4 (*Continued*) **H.** X-ray appearance at 2 years. **I** and **J.** Limited but stable arc of pronation and supination.

REFERENCES

1. Berger RA, Cooney WP 3rd. Use of an ulnar head endoprosthesis for treatment of an unstable distal ulnar resection: review of mechanics, indications, and surgical technique. *Hand Clin.* 2005;21:603–620, vii.
2. Kakar S, Swann RP, Perry KI, Wood-Wentz CM, Shin AY, Moran SL. Functional and radiographic outcomes following distal ulna implant arthroplasty. *J Hand Surg Am.* 2012;37:1364–1371.
3. Ewald T, Skeete K, Moran S. Total wrist and sigmoid notch replacement. *J Wrist Surg.* 2012;1:23–30.
4. Gupta A. Brachioradialis wrap: a new method of stabilizing the distal radioulnar joint. In: Slutsky DJ, ed. *Principles and Practice of Wrist Surgery.* Philadelphia: Elsevier Inc; 2012.
5. Herbert TJ, van Schoonhoven J. Ulnar head replacement. *Tech Hand Up Extrem Surg.* 2007;11:98–108.
6. Fernandez DL, Joneschild ES, Abella DM. Treatment of failed Sauve-Kapandji procedures with a spherical ulnar head prosthesis. *Clin Orthop Relat Res.* 2006;445:100–107.
7. Van Schoonhoven J, Lanz U. Salvage operations and their differential indication for the distal radioulnar joint. *Orthopade.* 2004;33:704–714.
8. Garcia-Elias M. Eclypse: partial ulnar head replacement for the isolated distal radio-ulnar joint arthrosis. *Tech Hand Up Extrem Surg.* 2007;11:121–128.
9. Garcia-Elias M. Partial ulnar head (eclypse) replacement. In: Slutsky DJ, ed. *The Principles and Practice of Wrist Surgery.* Philadelphia: Elsevier Inc; 2012.
10. Gilham N. *IWIW Meeting*; 2011; Las Vegas, NV.
11. Shaaban H, Giakas G, Bolton M, et al. The load-bearing characteristics of the forearm: pattern of axial and bending force transmitted through ulna and radius. *J Hand Surg Br.* 2006;31:274–279.
12. Scheker LR. Implant arthroplasty for the distal radioulnar joint. *J Hand Surg Am.* 2008;33:1639–1644.
13. Fox T, Wagner E, Berger RA, Kakar S. Linked distal radioulnar joint arthroplasty: short-term outcome of the APTIS® prosthesis. *J Hand Surg.* 2012;37:29–30.
14. Axelsson P. Good early outcomes of total joint implant arthroplasty as a secondary procedure at the distal radioulnar joint. *J Hand Surg.* 2012;37:30–31.

V

FOREARM

35

Forearm Fractures

John Kadzielski, MD
David C. Ring, MD, PhD

INTRODUCTION

Diaphyseal fractures of the forearm are usually relatively high-energy injuries in active patients with good bone quality. It is important to evaluate the proximal radioulnar joint (PRUJ) and distal radioulnar joint (DRUJ), particularly if only 1 of the forearm bones is fractured. The advent of plates and screws of adequate length, thickness, and metallurgy transformed the care of these injuries and remains the treatment of choice for all but the most contaminated or devitalized fractures. The forearm is a joint as well as a strut, so anatomic alignment and early mobilization are important. Angulation of more than 10° or loss of the normal bow of the radius is associated with decreased forearm rotation and—on occasion—DRUJ instability or arthrosis.[1,2] Nonunions are associated with the degree of injury complexity, infection, and a plate that is too short or too thin.[13,16]

RATIONALE AND BASIC SCIENCE

The forearm is a both a strut that helps place the hand in space and an articulation that helps position the hand for better manipulation of objects. The diaphyseal ulna is fairly straight with a gentle apex posterior bow proximally, which is best appreciated on the lateral x-ray. It is triangular in its cross-section and becomes more cylindrical distally (Fig. 35-1). The radius is angulated in both the anteroposterior and lateral planes. The bow of the radius allows it to rotate over the ulna without impingement. The annular, quadrate, and interosseous ligaments contribute to the stability of the PRUJ. The dorsal and volar radioulnar ligaments, the ligamentum subcruentum, the ulnar collateral ligament, and the subsheath of the extensor carpi ulnaris combine to form a structure known as the triangular fibrocartilage complex and confer stability to the DRUJ. The articular disc component of the triangular fibrocartilage complex may help cushion the articulation of the distal ulna with the carpus. Methods of fixation strive to recreate these anatomic relationships, restore soft tissue integrity and balance, and provide sufficient stability to allow for immediate use of the arm for light functional activities and active self-assisted stretching exercises.

INDICATIONS

All diaphyseal fractures of both forearm bones in adults are treated with plate and screw fixation. Skeletally mature girls older than 10 and boys older than 12 are treated like adults because there is limited remodeling of diaphyseal fractures near the end of growth. Cast treatment may be considered if near-anatomic reduction is achieved in older skeletally immature patients.

The indications for operative treatment of an isolated diaphyseal ulnar fracture are debated. Nonunion is uncommon with nonoperative treatment, even when the arm is not immobilized. The patients and the treating surgeon should be aware that isolated diaphyseal ulnar fractures can remain painful and limiting for up to 3 months even if the fractures are secondary to low-energy trauma. Fractures with greater than 50% loss of bony apposition or greater than 10° of angulation are considered for surgery.

Isolated diaphyseal radius fractures with or without dislocation of the DRUJ (ie, Galeazzi fractures[11]) and isolated ulnar fractures with disruption of the PRUJ (ie, Monteggia fractures[19]) are treated with plate and screw fixation in adults.

The timing for surgical repair is dictated by the associated injuries and additional factors that may be associated with the trauma including an acute-onset carpal tunnel syndrome or a compartment syndrome. Diaphyseal forearm fractures can be difficult to reduce; therefore, it is expedient to operate within a week of injury. Most patients with this injury are admitted and have an operation within 1 to 2 days.

CONTRAINDICATIONS

Contraindications to operative management of these fractures include fractures in skeletally immature patients who have substantial remodeling potential. In patients with

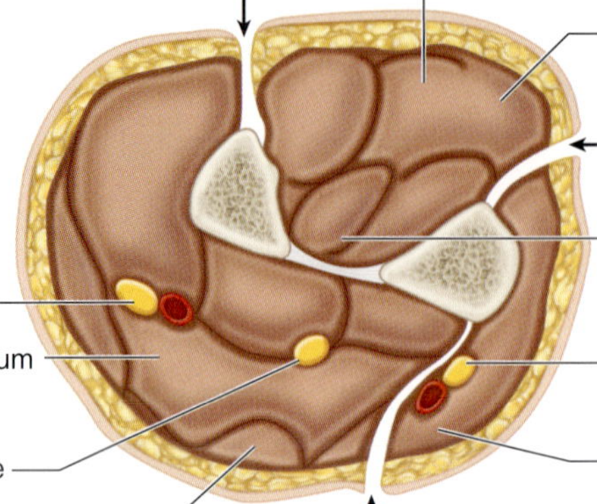

FIGURE 35-1 Cross-sectional view of the distal third of the forearm.

life-threatening injuries, forearm fracture care is of a lower priority with the exception of open fractures, and fractures with vascular injury or any compartment syndrome. A very severe contaminated or devitalized open fracture might be initially debrided and stabilized with an external fixator prior to definitive plate and screw fixation.

SURGICAL TECHNIQUES

Isolated Ulnar Fracture

Isolated ulnar fractures (Fig. 35-2A and B) can be plated under tourniquet control and general or regional anesthesia with the patient positioned supine with the arm on a hand table or in the lateral decubitus position with the arm over a pillow bolster or an arm holder. An incision centered at the fracture site is made directly over the subcutaneous border of the ulna. The internervous plane is between the extensor carpi ulnaris innervated by the radial nerve and the flexor carpi ulnaris that is innervated by the ulnar nerve (Fig. 35-1). Once the fracture is exposed, the incision can be extended proximally and distally to facilitate the reduction and plate application.

An extraperiosteal dissection is performed on the volar aspect of the ulna to preserve the muscular and periosteal arterial perforators and to keep the dissection away from the interosseous space to diminish the risk of synostosis.

A 3.5-mm dynamic compression plate or the equivalent should be used (Fig. 35-3A and B). In the case of a transverse fracture the plate is prebent to compress at the opposite cortex of the fracture site first. For oblique fractures, interfragmentary compression is applied using a lag screw at 90° to the fracture plane either through the plate or separate from it. The reduction is checked fluoroscopically.

Both-bone Forearm Fracture

With a both-bone forearm fracture our preference is to position the patient in the supine position with the arm extended on a hand table under tourniquet control and general anesthesia rather than a regional block in order to monitor for a compartment syndrome postoperatively.

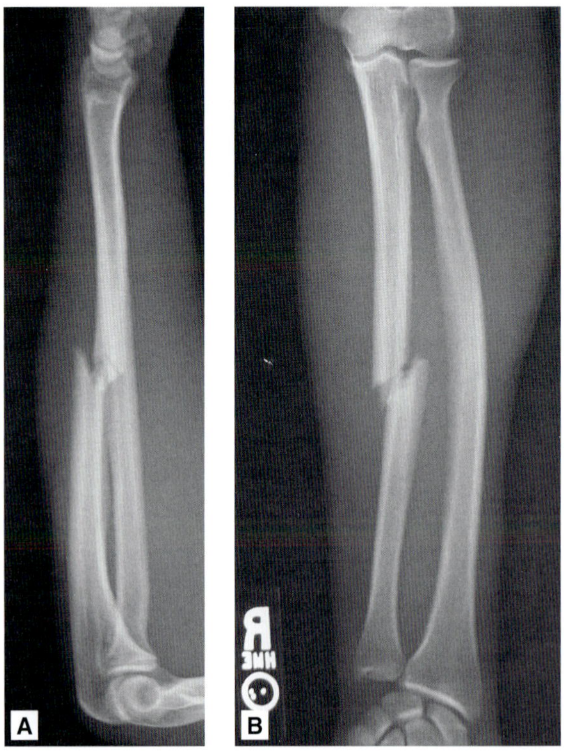

FIGURE 35-2 Lateral (A) and AP (B) x-rays of the forearm showing a diaphyseal ulnar fracture.

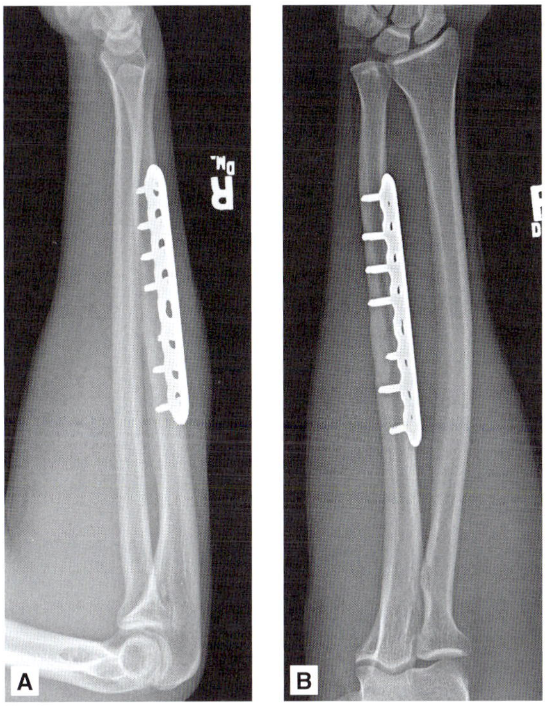

FIGURE 35-3 Lateral (**A**) and AP (**B**) x-rays of the forearm showing 3.5-mm plate fixation of the diaphyseal ulnar fracture.

We suggest addressing the least comminuted bone first, because it is easier to ensure a correct alignment if the fracture lines lock into place. Diaphyseal fractures can be difficult to reduce, especially in heavily muscled individuals. Indirect reduction techniques such as using a push–pull screw or a temporary external fixator can facilitate this step (Fig. 35-4A-C). Alignment and provisional fixation of the less comminuted fracture with a plate and at least 2 screws on each side of the fracture helps restore the anatomic relationships and tissue balance, facilitating the reduction and fixation of the more complex fracture.

The ulna is plated as described above. An anterior (Henry) exposure is used for exposing the radius because it is extensile and there is less risk of a posterior interosseous nerve proximally (Fig. 35-5). A longitudinal incision is made centered over the fracture site on a line that is drawn between the scaphoid tuberosity and the radial aspect of the biceps tendon.

The deep fascia is released ulnar to the brachioradialis (Fig. 35-6A-C). An internervous plane is developed between the brachioradialis (radial nerve) and flexor carpi radialis (median nerve). The radial artery is retracted medially with the flexor pronator muscles, ligating the radial branches. The superficial branch of the radial nerve is identified and retracted radially with the brachioradialis.

For proximal third fractures, keeping the forearm in supination helps protect the posterior interosseous nerve by sweeping it laterally. If the anatomy is distorted and proximal edge of the supinator is ill-defined, the posterior interosseous nerve is identified within the supinator muscle and

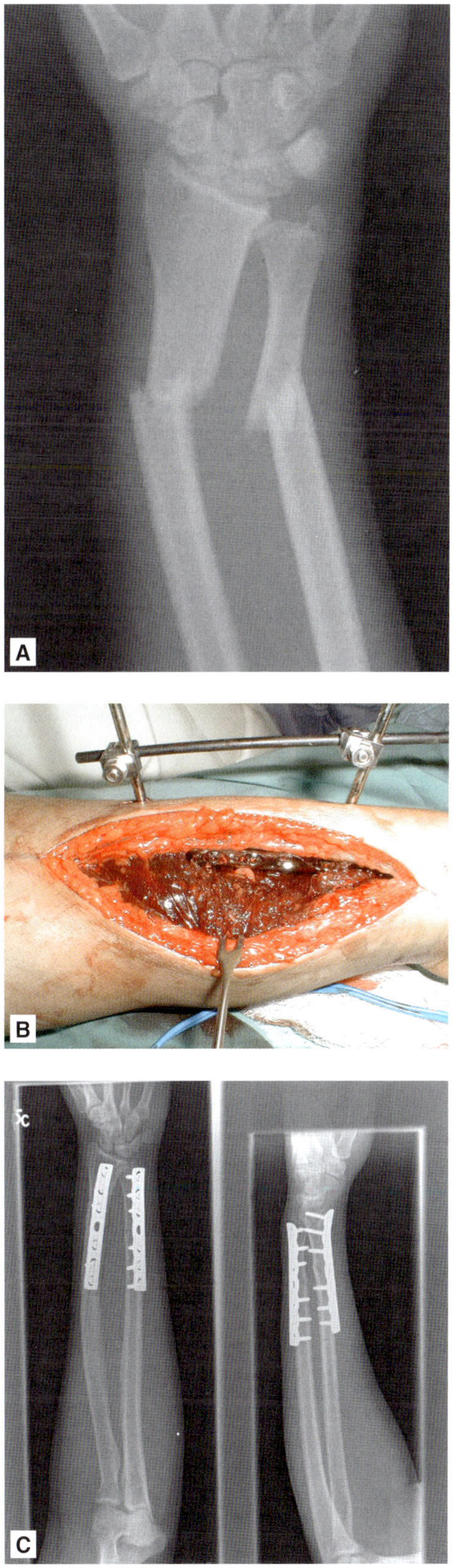

FIGURE 35-4 External fixator applied for provisional fixation to facilitation open reduction and internal fixation of both-bone forearm fracture (**A-C**).

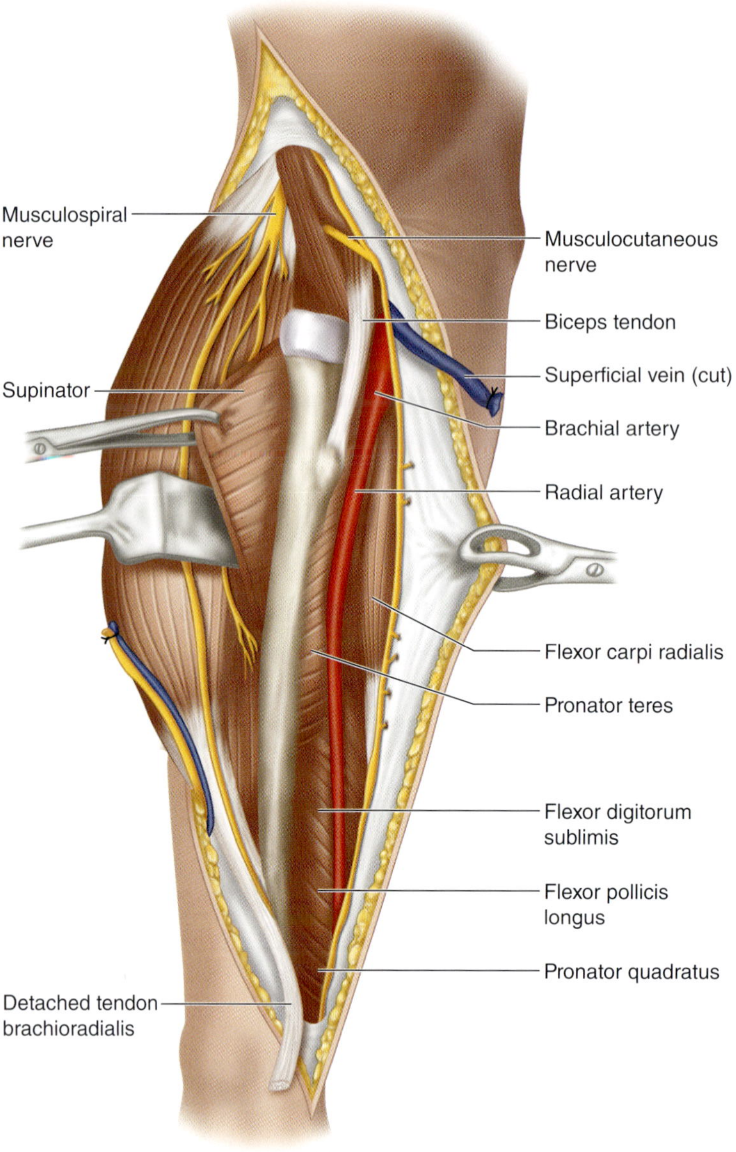

FIGURE 35-5 Anterior Henry approach to the radius.

protected. The plate can be applied over the flat tendinous insertion of the pronator teres if necessary. In the distal half of the radius, the flexor pollicis longus and the pronator quadratus are elevated extraperiosteally and retracted for plate application on the volar surface of the radius, which is flat and aids fracture realignment. Use of a long straight plate can decrease the natural bow of the radius, which can limit forearm rotation. Commercially available precontoured plates can mitigate this. An alternative is to apply the plate radially that limits the need for muscle stripping and allows the surgeon to contour the plate to restore the radial bow.

The original recommendation of Anderson et al[3] to bone graft regions of comminution involving more than one-third of the diameter of the bone is no longer applicable. With the use of more modern 3.5-mm limited contact plates, indirect reduction techniques, and limited soft tissue elevation. We reviewed 41 patients with diaphyseal fractures of both forearm bones who were treated with plating.[4] Five patients (12%) had a nonunion of 1 or both bones (12%). No single factor was associated with nonunion. In particular, the use of bone graft was not associated with a higher rate of union.

Passive forearm rotation and DRUJ stability are evaluated after provisional plate fixation (Fig. 35-7A). The image intensifier is used to assess the implant position, the PRUJ and DRUJ, pronation and supination, and the fracture reduction. Remember that an AP and lateral view of the radius can be obtained by simply rotating the forearm, whereas a cross-table view is required to obtain a lateral view of the ulna.

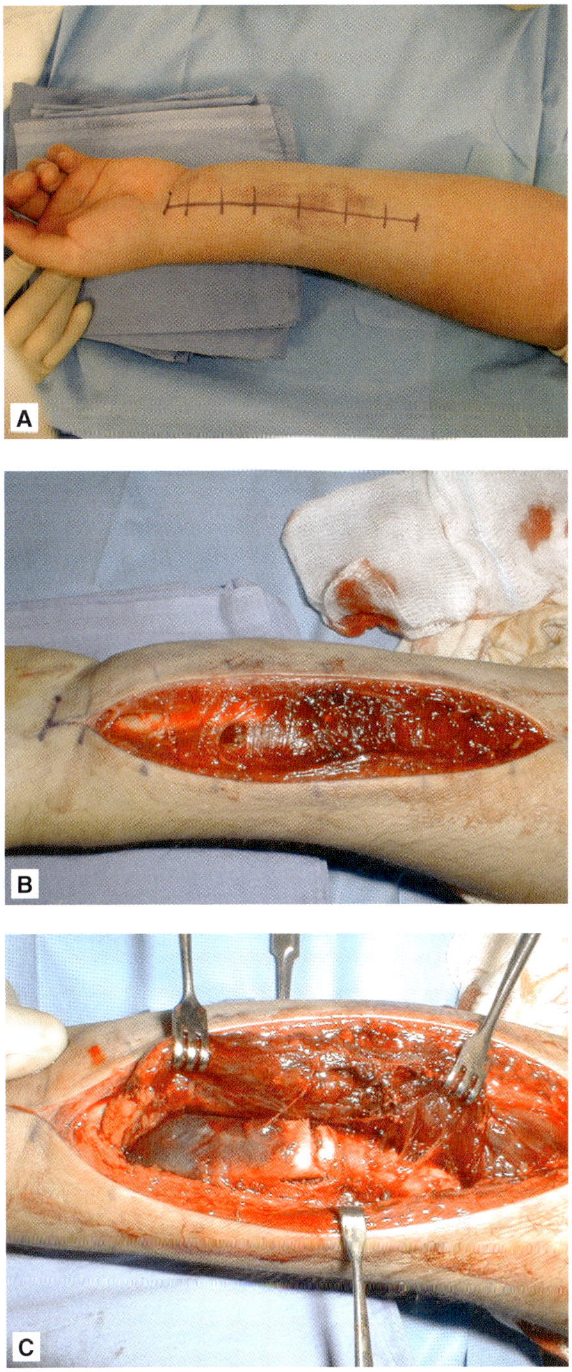

FIGURE 35-6 An anterior Henry approach (**A**-**C**) with an internervous plane following the radial after between the brachial radialis (radial nerve) and the flexor carpi radialis (median nerve).

It is our preference to fill most of the holes in the plate with screws rather than using minimal screw plate fixation[5,6] (Fig. 35-7B). A splint is included in the postoperative dressing for comfort. It can immobilize the wrist, forearm, and elbow, or only the wrist for distal fractures or isolated fractures of the elbow. Active-assisted use and stretching of the arm can be initiated as soon as patients feel comfortable,

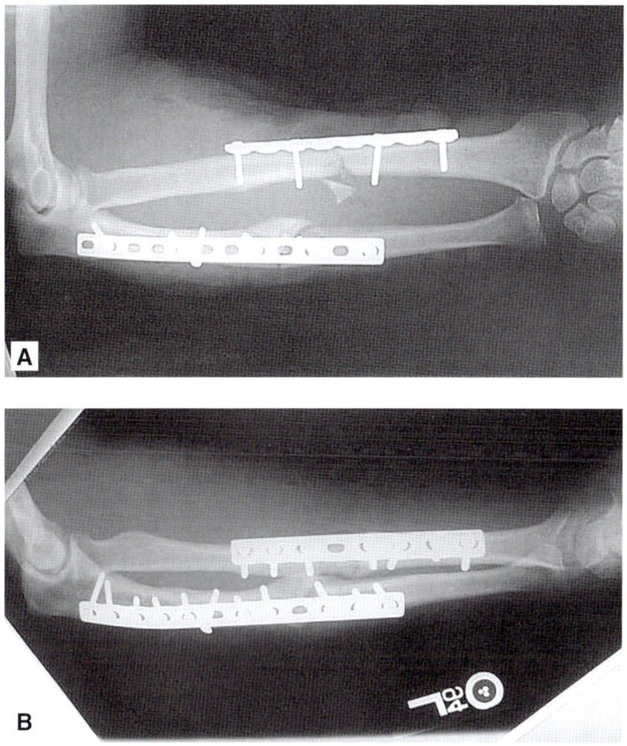

FIGURE 35-7 Intraoperative x-rays showing provisional (**A**) and definitive (**B**) fixation of a diaphyseal both-bone forearm fracture.

usually within a few days of surgery. Strengthening is instituted at 2 months if there are signs of early bony union and full activities can be resumed after 4 months. The plates are not removed routinely. If there is a problem due to hardware irritation implant, we prefer to delay removal for 18 months.

DIAPHYSEAL RADIUS FRACTURES WITH AND WITHOUT DRUJ DISLOCATION

A Galeazzi fracture–dislocation is defined as a fracture of the middle to distal one-third of the radial diaphysis with simultaneous dislocation of the DRUJ. When there is a fracture of the base of the ulnar styloid, fixation of that fracture in addition to the radius will restore DRUJ stability. In the absence of an ulnar styloid base fracture, the question is whether or not to cross-pin the ulna or repair the TFCC. This is only an issue when there is radial shortening of more than 5 mm on radiographs made prior to fixation of the radius (Fig. 35-8A-C). Even then, it is not clear that any specific treatment of the DRUJ is needed.[7,8]

Early studies demonstrated uniformly poor results with nonoperative management. Mikic reported an 80% failure rate with conservative management in 86 adults with Galeazzi fracture–dislocations due to both inability to control progressive displacement of the radius fracture and

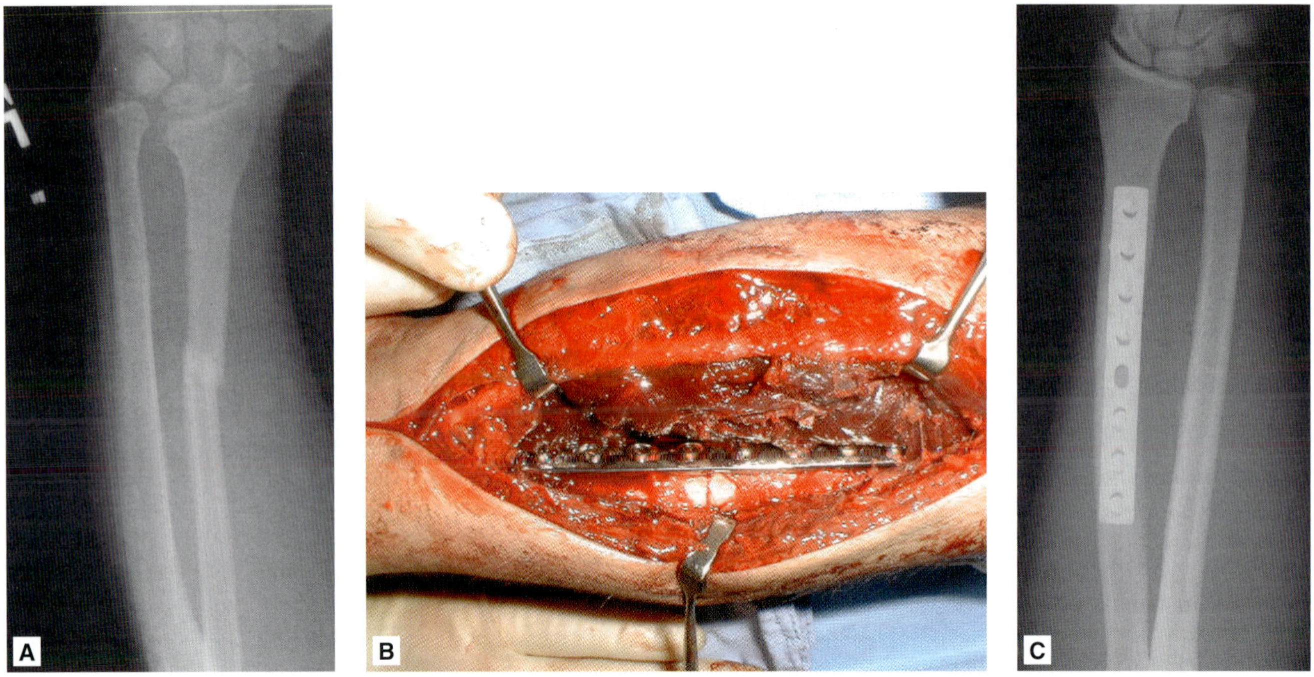

FIGURE 35-8 X-ray of forearm showing a Galeazzi fracture (**A**) open reduction and internal fixation through an anterior Henry approach (**B**) with postoperative x-ray (**C**).

recurrent subluxation or dislocation of the DRUJ despite cast immobilization.[9] Open reduction and plate and screw fixation is now standard.

Bony congruity between the ulnar head and sigmoid notch of the radius only contributes approximately 20% of total DRUJ stability. The TFCC is considered the primary stabilizer of the DRUJ, and the interosseous membrane (IOM) a secondary restraint. The IOM is organized into a central band (also called the interosseous ligament), 1 to 5 accessory bands, a dorsal proximal interosseous band, and an inconstant distal band. In a biomechanical study Watanabe et al[10] showed that it is a specific injury to the distal portion of the IOM that results in the increased dorsal–volar instability at the DRUJ throughout a range of forearm rotation when the TFCC and distal radioulnar ligaments are incompetent. When the midportion of the IOM (including the central band) is sectioned together with the distal IOM, the DRUJ becomes unconstrained.

Rettig and Raskin[11] found that 12 of 22 patients with fractures occurring within 7.5 cm of the midarticular surface of the distal radius had persistent DRUJ instability following ORIF of the radial shaft fracture treated with Kirschner-wire fixation of the ulna to the radius. Three of 12 patients also underwent a concomitant open repair of the triangular fibrocartilage complex as the DRUJ was irreducible. In contrast, only 1 of 18 patients with a fracture of radial shaft more than 7.5 cm from the midarticular surface had percutaneous fixation of an unstable DRUJ.

In a retrospective review of 36 patients with radial shaft fractures treated with plate and screw fixation, Ring et al observed a similar, but not as strict, trend toward DRUJ stability with proximal and middle third fractures. In their series 5 out of 8 distal third fractures were associated with DRUJ instability, while only 4 out of 28 proximal/middle third radius fractures had DRUJ involvement.[7]

Surgical Technique

The volar approach to the radial shaft fracture has been described above. A 3.5-mm AO dynamic compression plate or equivalent is used and locking plates are considered only if bone quality is poor. Interfragmentary compression with 3.5-mm cortical lag screws is used for oblique fracture lines.

After plate fixation of the radius, the DRUJ is then evaluated. We have found it unnecessary to treat the DRUJ if it is unstable, but some authors recommend forearm immobilization in supination or cross-pinning.

On rare occasion, an open reduction of the DRUJ is necessary due to interposition of extensor retinaculum, DRUJ capsule, extensor carpi ulnaris, or a digital extensor tendon. A dorsal approach to the DRUJ is performed between the fifth and sixth extensor compartments protecting the dorsal sensory branch of the ulnar nerve. The extensor retinaculum is elevated and an L-shaped capsulotomy is performed, although the ulnar head may be buttonholed through the dorsal capsule with dorsal DRUJ dislocations. The DRUJ is inspected for loose bodies and traumatic chondromalacia, and then debrided. If the deep fibers of the TFCC are avulsed from the fovea, they can be reattached through drill holes or using suture anchors.

Displaced ulnar styloid base fractures are repaired with a 24- or 26-gauge stainless steel figure-of-8 tension band construct with or without K-wires. Fixation of a large ulnar styloid fracture stabilizes the DRUJ allowing mobilization of the forearm and wrist as comfort allows.

MONTEGGIA FRACTURES

The diagnosis of Monteggia fracture, which is a fracture of the ulna that is associated with a radial head dislocation, should be ruled out in every patient with an isolated ulnar shaft fracture, especially with proximal ulnar fractures. The PRUJ is disrupted if the axis of the radius fails to intersect the center of the sphere of the capitellum on all views, but the ulnohumeral joint is aligned.

Monteggia fractures with the radial head displaced either anteriorly or laterally usually reduce with anatomic reduction and stabilization of the ulna with 3.5-mm dynamic compression plates or the equivalent. Persistent subluxation of the radial head is nearly always a result of persistent malalignment of the ulna and exploration of the radiocapitellar joint to address the annular ligament is rarely necessary (Fig. 35-9). Posterior radial head dislocation is usually part of the posterior Monteggia lesion or posterior olecranon fracture–dislocation and is best considered in the context of traumatic elbow instability. We recommend against temporary fixation of the radiocapitellar joint.

ESSEX-LOPRESTI FRACTURES

An Essex-Lopresti lesion is a radial head fracture that is associated with a disruption of the interosseous ligament and TFCC resulting in longitudinal radioulnar dissociation. Some radioulnar dissociation injuries also involve a diaphyseal fracture of the radius and/or ulna. Key concepts to keep in mind when treating these fractures are (1) restoration of alignment through the anatomic reduction of all fractures; (2) restoration of radiocapitellar alignment with repair or replacement of the fractured radial head; and (3) addressing the soft tissue injury with direct tissue repair, immobilization, or pinning of the forearm.

As the forearm is loaded axially in compression, the IOL is loaded in tension. Tears of the IOL appear to occur in the midsubstance of the tendon; however, there are some reports of injury to the ulnar insertion. Longitudinal stability can be assessed intraoperatively by applying an axial load to the radius resulting in a dynamic positive ulnar variance.[12]

There is debate regarding repair of the soft tissue injuries (including the IOL in addition to the TFCC) or immobilization with either a long arm cast or two 0.062-in Kirschner wires between the radius and the ulna with the forearm in mid-supination.

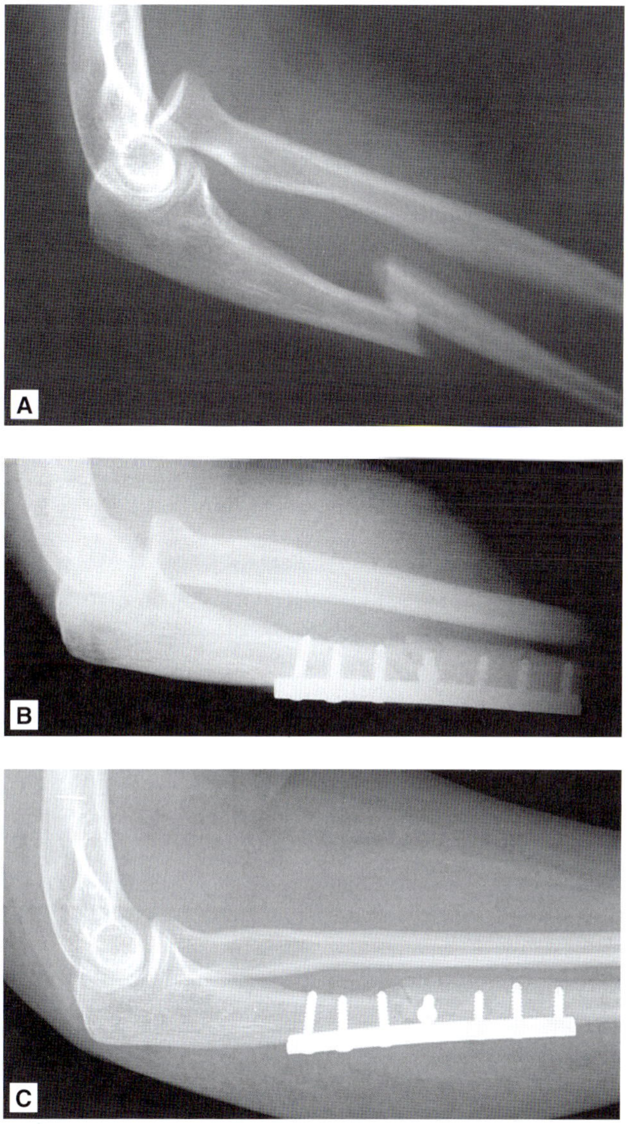

FIGURE 35-9 X-rays of the forearm show a Monteggia fracture (**A**) treated with open reduction and plate fixation (**B**). If the reduction of the ulnar is near anatomic, the reduction of the radiocapitellar joint (**C**) is usually stable.

Complications

Common adverse events include infection, compartment syndrome, malunion, nonunion, and refracture. Infection rates are around 3% in open fractures and lower in closed injuries.[13]

In general, the incisions used to reduce and plate forearm fractures are adequate to release the forearm compartments, but unexpected postoperative pain out of proportion and pain with passive finger extension, particularly with progressive numbness, should lead to return to the operating room for a more extensive fasciotomy.

If the patient has altered mental status or fails to offer a reliable examination, intracompartmental pressure monitoring is indicated. Cutoff pressure values for compartmental release in the forearm are controversial. Pressures above 30 mm Hg are considered elevated. Surgeons should strongly consider releasing when pressures are above 45 mm Hg or within 30 mm Hg of the diastolic blood pressure. Fractures in the proximal one-third of the forearm where there is more muscle may have a higher propensity to develop compartment syndromes than distal fractures.

Nonunion rates have been reported to be 5% when adequate technique is used in compliant patients.[13] Nonunions are related to the use of mechanically inadequate plates, for example, semitubular plates, malreduction, and injury severity.[18,21] Nonunions are usually atrophic and can be satisfactorily managed with autogenous cancellous graft, restoration of mechanical alignment, and plate fixation (Fig. 35-10). For bony defects we have used cancellous autograft alone,[18,21] while other authors advocate a structural corticocancellous graft.[17]

Plate removal after initial fracture healing was initially recommended by the AO/ASIF, but given that refractures both through the original fracture site and through screw holes as well as posterior interosseous nerve injury have been observed during removal, many surgeons remove a plate only if it causes irritation, which is rare. Factors associated with refracture include initial comminution or lack of absolute stability, stress shielding with larger implants, for example, 4.5-mm plates, radiolucency under the implant, insufficient protection following plate removal, and implant removal less than 12 months after fixation.

Outcomes

Historically, Anderson et al reported >96% union rate with the use of iliac crest bone graft when needed in their series of 137 fractures using compression plates.[3] Similarly, Chapman et al reported 98% union rates with 3.5-mm dynamic compression plates in 129 fractures.[13] Since these studies, alternative strategies have been employed to enhance results without substantial improvement. Two randomized prospective trials comparing all-locked constructs, for example, the point contact fixator versus dynamic compression plating and locked compression plating versus dynamic compression plating, failed to show any statistical benefit.[14,15] A more recent body of literature has emerged embracing a more minimalistic concept of fixation leaving some screw holes empty to increase the working distance of the plate, but we still recommend filling all of the holes when possible.[6,16] There are retrospective data that suggest good results from newer more rigid anatomic intramedullary devices, but these devices have not proved superior to dynamic compression plating that is still the reference standard.

We reviewed 71 adult and pediatric patients at an average of 21 years after diaphyseal fractures of both the radius

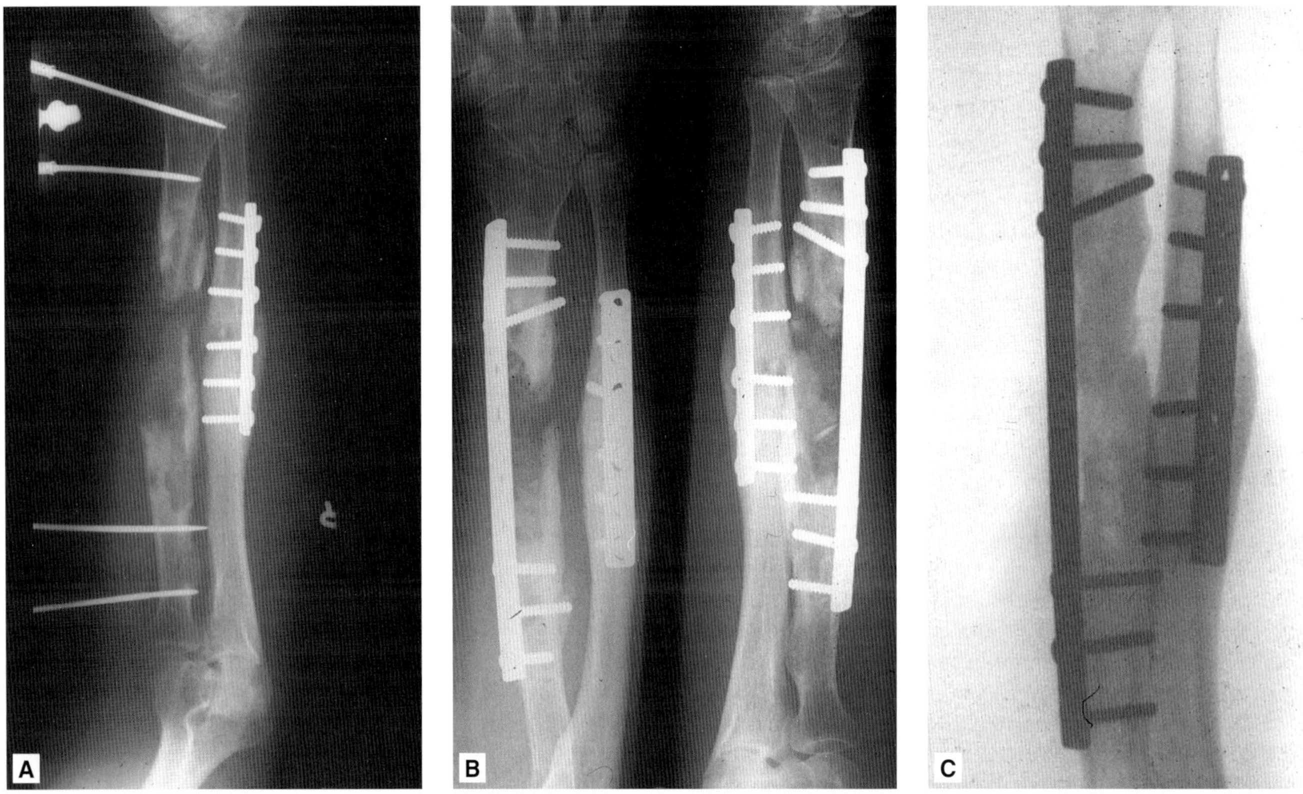

FIGURE 35-10 X-rays of the forearm showing a nonunion of the radius (**A**) treated with autologous cancellous bone graft with interval healing 3 months (**B**) and 6 months (**C**).

and the ulna.[17] Twenty-five of the 35 patients who were skeletally immature at the time of injury were treated nonoperatively, and 31 of the 36 skeletally mature patients were treated operatively. The average DASH score was 8 points (range, 0-54); 97% of patients had excellent or satisfactory results according to the criteria of Anderson et al, and 72% reported no pain. Both the forearm rotation and the wrist flexion/extension arc were 91% of the uninjured side; grip strength was 94%. There were small but significant differences in rotation (151° vs 169°; $P = .004$) and wrist flexion–extension (123° vs 142°; $P = .002$) compared with the results in the uninjured arm. There was no difference in disability between patients who were skeletally mature and those who were skeletally immature at the time of injury. Pain, pain catastrophizing (misinterpretation of nociception), and grip strength were the most important predictors of disability.

With the current techniques of plate and screw fixation, diaphyseal nonunions of the radius and ulna are unusual.[18] We reviewed the records of 35 patients with an atrophic ununited diaphyseal fracture of the forearm who were treated with 3.5-mm plate and screw fixation and autogenous cancellous bone grafting. A segmental osseous defect with an average size of 2.2 cm (range, 1-6 cm) was present in each patient. The atrophic nonunion was associated with an open fracture in 20 patients, suboptimal fixation in 22, a fracture–dislocation of the forearm in 9, and infection in 11. All fractures healed without additional intervention within 6 months. Two patients had a subsequent Darrach resection of the distal part of the ulna for the treatment of arthrosis of the DRUJ. After an average duration of follow-up of 43 months, the final arc of motion averaged 121° in the forearm, 131° at the elbow, and 137° at the wrist, with an average grip strength of 83% compared with that of the contralateral limb. According to the system of Anderson and colleagues, 5 patients had an excellent result, 18 had a satisfactory result, 11 had an unsatisfactory result (because of elbow stiffness related to associated elbow injuries in 3 and because of wrist stiffness in 8), and 1 had a poor result (because of malunion).

Forty-eight patients with Monteggia fractures were followed for an average of 6.5 years (range, 2-14 years).[19] There were 25 women and 23 men, and the average age was 52 years (range, 18-88 years). According to the Bado classification, there were 7 type I, 38 type II (26 with a fractured radial head, 10 with a fracture coronoid), 1 type III, and 2 type IV injuries. The ulna was fixed with a tension band wire construct supplemented with screws in 3 patients (all of whom had a Bado type II fracture). An ulnar diaphyseal fracture was fixed with an intramedullary Steinmann pin in 1 patient. The remaining patients had fixation with a plate and screws. The fracture of the radial head was treated with either complete or partial excision of the fragments in 12 patients (with replacement with a silicone prosthesis in 2), open reduction and internal fixation in 10 patients, and no intervention in 4 patients. Nine patients, all of whom had a Bado type II fracture, needed a reoperation within 3 months after the initial operation; 5 had revision of a loose ulnar fixation device, 3 had resection of the radial head, and 1 had removal of a wire that had migrated from the radial head into the elbow articulation. Other important complications included proximal radioulnar synostosis in 3 patients, ulnar malunion in 3, posterolateral rotatory instability of the ulnohumeral joint in 1, and instability of the DRUJ in 1. The average score according to the system of Broberg and Morrey was 86 points (range, 15-100 points). The result was excellent for 18 patients, good for 22, fair for 2, and poor for 6. Six of the 8 patients who had an unsatisfactory (fair or poor) result had had a Bado type II fracture with a concomitant fracture of the radial head. These unsatisfactory results were related to a malunited fracture of the coronoid process in 2 patients, a proximal radioulnar synostosis in 1, a malunited fracture of the coronoid process and a proximal radioulnar synostosis in 1, a malunion of the ulna in 1, and painfully restricted rotation of the forearm after operative fixation of a comminuted fracture of the radial head in 1. The other 2 unsatisfactory results were in a patient who had had a Bado type I fracture and in 1 who had had a Bado type IV fracture.

We evaluated 11 adult patients who had surgical treatment of an anterior (Bado type I) Monteggia fracture at a median follow-up of 20 years (range, 7-34 years).[20] Two patients had subsequent surgery to address a nonunion and 3 elbows had radiographic signs of arthrosis. The mean arc of elbow flexion increased from 110° (range, 35°-140°) at early follow-up to 120° (range, 40°-150°) at late follow-up. The mean arc of forearm rotation increased from 145° (range, 90°-180°) to 149° (range, 90°-180°). The mean Broberg and Morrey score increased from 89 points (range, 62-100 points) to 94 points (range, 76-100 points). The median DASH score was 7 points (range, 0-34 points) at long-term follow-up. There was no statistical difference between early and late range of motion or Broberg and Morrey score.

We examined 17 patients with persistent malalignment following surgical treatment of a posterior Monteggia fracture who were treated with realignment of the ulna and fixation with a contoured dorsal plate.[21] Fifteen patients had loose fixation and 12 patients had subluxation or dislocation of the ulnohumeral joint. Sixteen patients had fracture of the radial head and 9 patients had fracture of the coronoid process. Nine patients had ancillary procedures on the radial head, 4 had ancillary procedures on the coronoid, 5 had hinged external fixation, and 1 had fascial arthroplasty. Seven patients had another surgery before the final evaluation related to a complication in 6 patients and a subsequent injury in 1 patient. At the final evaluation at an average of 59 months the fracture was healed and the ulnohumeral joint was reduced concentrically in all 17 patients. The average arc of elbow flexion was 108° and the average arc of forearm rotation was 134°. The average American Shoulder and Elbow Surgeons Elbow Evaluation Score was 88. According to the system of Broberg and Morrey, the final result was rated excellent for 5 patients, good for 9, fair for 2, and poor for 1. One patient had fascial arthroplasty as part of the index procedure and 9 patients had radiographic signs of ulnohumeral arthrosis.

Rettig and Raskin reported excellent results in 38/40 patients following surgery. Two patients with a type I fracture–dislocation had a poor result and subsequently required DRUJ reconstruction at an average of 9 months following the initial injury due to pain and limited supination. We evaluated 17 patients with an isolated diaphyseal fracture of the radius (7 with DRUJ disruption) at an average of 19 years after surgery (range, 13-33 years).[8] There were no significant differences between patients with and without DRUJ dislocation. No patient had greater laxity of the DRUJ than the opposite uninjured side. The average modified Mayo wrist score was 96 (range, 85-100), the average Mayo Elbow Performance Index was 95 (range, 80-100), and the average DASH score was 5 (range, 0-33).

REFERENCES

1. Richards RR. Chronic disorders of the forearm. *J Bone Joint Surg Am.* 1996;78:916–930.
2. Schemitsch EH, Richards RR. The effect of malunion on functional outcome after plate fixation of fractures of both bones of the forearm in adults. *J Bone Joint Surg Am.* 1992;74:1068–1078.
3. Anderson LD, Sisk TD, Tooms RE, Park WI. Compression-plate fixation in acute diaphyseal fractures of the radius and ulna. *J Bone Joint Surg Am.* 1975;57:287–297.
4. Ring D, Rhim R, Carpenter C, Jupiter JB. Comminuted diaphyseal fractures of the radius and ulna: does bone grafting affect nonunion rate? *J Trauma.* 2005;59:438–441 [discussion 42].
5. Lindvall EM, Sagi HC. Selective screw placement in forearm compression plating: results of 75 consecutive fractures stabilized with 4 cortices of screw fixation on either side of the fracture. *J Orthop Trauma.* 2006;20:157–162 [discussion 62–63].
6. Bradley CD, Mundis G, Angen JO. Clinical results of minimal screw plate fixation of forearm fractures. *Am J Orthop.* 2011;36:477–480.
7. Ring D, Rhim R, Carpenter C, Jupiter JB. Isolated radial shaft fractures are more common than Galeazzi fractures. *J Hand Surg Am.* 2006;31:17–21.
8. van Duijvenbode DC, Guitton TG, Raaymakers EL, Kloen P, Ring D. Long-term outcome of isolated diaphyseal radius fractures with and without dislocation of the distal radioulnar joint. *J Hand Surg Am.* 2012;37:523–527.
9. Mikic ZD. Galeazzi fracture–dislocations. *J Bone Joint Surg Am.* 1975;57:1071–1080.
10. Watanabe H, Berger RA, Berglund LJ, Zobitz ME, An KN. Contribution of the interosseous membrane to distal radioulnar joint constraint. *J Hand Surg Am.* 2005;30:1164–1171.
11. Rettig ME, Raskin KB. Galeazzi fracture–dislocation: a new treatment-oriented classification. *J Hand Surg Am.* 2001;26:228–235.
12. Smith AM, Urbanosky LR, Castle JA, Rushing JT, Ruch DS. Radius pull test: predictor of longitudinal forearm instability. *J Bone Joint Surg Am.* 2002;84-A:1970–1976.
13. Chapman MW, Gordon JE, Zissimos AG. Compression plate fixation of acute fractures of the diaphysis of the radius and ulna. *J Bone Joint Surg Am.* 1989;71:159–169.
14. Saikia K, Bhuyan S, Bhattacharya T, Borgohain M, Jitesh P, Ahmed F. Internal fixation of fractures of both bones forearm: Comparison of locked compression and limited contact dynamic compression plate. *Indian J Orthop.* 2011;45:417–421.
15. Leung F, Chow SP. A prospective, randomized trial comparing the limited contact dynamic compression plate with the point contact fixator for forearm fractures. *J Bone Joint Surg Am.* 2003;85-A:2343–2348.
16. Sterns P, Drury WJ. Complications of plate fixation of forearm fractures. *Clin Orthop Relat Res.* 1983;175:25–29.
17. Bot AG, Doornberg JN, Lindenhovius AL, Ring D, Goslings JC, van Dijk CN. Long-term outcomes of fractures of both bones of the forearm. *J Bone Joint Surg Am.* 2011;93:527–532.
18. Ring D, Allende C, Jafarnia K, Allende BT, Jupiter JB. Ununited diaphyseal forearm fractures with segmental defects: plate fixation and autogenous cancellous bone-grafting. *J Bone Joint Surg Am.* 2004;86:2440–2445.
19. Ring D, Jupiter JB, Simpson NS. Monteggia fractures in adults. *J Bone Joint Surg Am.* 1998;80:1733–1744.
20. Guitton TG, Ring D, Kloen P. Long-term evaluation of surgically treated anterior Monteggia fractures in skeletally mature patients. *J Hand Surg Am.* 2009;34:1618–1624.
21. Ring D, Tavakolian J, Kloen P, Helfet D, Jupiter JB. Loss of alignment after surgical treatment of posterior Monteggia fractures: salvage with dorsal contoured plating. *J Hand Surg Am.* 2004;29:694–702.

VI

ELBOW

36

Fractures of the Elbow

Michael R. Hausman, MD
Shawn M. Kutnik, MD

Fractures about the elbow remain challenging, having justifiably earned monikers such as "terrible triad." Relatively recent advances in understanding the pathoanatomy and a belated appreciation of the importance of concomitant soft tissue injuries have informed treatment and led to changes in management.

BASIC PRINCIPLES OF ARTHROSCOPIC FRACTURE FIXATION

Arthroscopy is, in essence, a surgical approach. As such, it should afford optimal exposure and visualization of the operative site with minimal collateral damage to adjacent tissues. If it does not achieve these goals, another approach should be selected.

While elbow arthroscopy can be performed from the prone, lateral decubitus, or supine position, our preference is the supine position with use of an elbow positioner to access the anterior and posterior compartments (Fig. 36-1). This allows the arm to be moved intraoperatively and affords easy conversion to an open procedure as well as use of the image intensifier. The timing of intervention is also important. If possible, a delay of about 2 days is beneficial to allow for some clot formation on the fracture surfaces. Otherwise, higher inflow pressures (>30 mm Hg) are required to control bone bleeding and swelling results in decreased working time.[1] In the 25 to 30 mm Hg pressure range, prolonged working times are possible with minimal swelling and, thus, conversion to an open procedure would not be problematic.

The joint capsule is usually thin and pliant having been distended by the fracture hematoma. As such, entering the joint of an elbow with an intra-articular fracture is usually quite easy. Specialized instruments such as cannulated screws, small Freer elevators with a hole drilled in the end, 28-gauge stainless steel wire for suture shuttling, and a modified skin hook for holding fragments and passing sutures are helpful.

DISTAL HUMERUS FRACTURES

Distal humerus fractures have an incidence of 5.7 per 100,000 people per year.[2] They account for some of the most challenging injuries to manage, particularly when intra-articular and comminuted. The loss of elbow function that results from improperly treated fractures imparts a major functional impairment with an inability to reach the head and peroneal area.[3] Strict adherence to the principles of open reduction and internal fixation using more advanced implant designs has greatly improved the results of operative intervention.[4] Elbow arthroscopy holds further promise for decreasing soft tissue trauma required for exposure.

Indications

The role of nonoperative management of distal humerus fractures is quite limited as the historical "bag of bones" treatment resulted in a high incidence of poor outcomes.[5] The advent of modern implants and improved understanding of the methods of stable fixation make most fractures reconstructable. Nonoperative management is now reserved only for patients unable to tolerate anesthesia or with chronic, irreversible conditions that limited preinjury function and independence.[4]

The 90/90 method of plating, recommended by the AO/ASIF group, is still currently used by many surgeons.[6] Certain fracture patterns may be amenable to 90/90 plating, but when there is a comminuted, crushing injury of the lateral column, the posterior lateral column plate only provides for a limited number of unicortical screws so as not to penetrate the articular surface. These posterior to anterior screws frequently achieve only marginal distal fixation of the articular fragments, particularly in osteopenic patients.[7] The biomechanical and clinical evidence now supports a parallel plate construct for such challenging fractures.[7,8] However, recognize that the very distal, intra-articular fracture with comminution of the lateral column and trochlea may not be

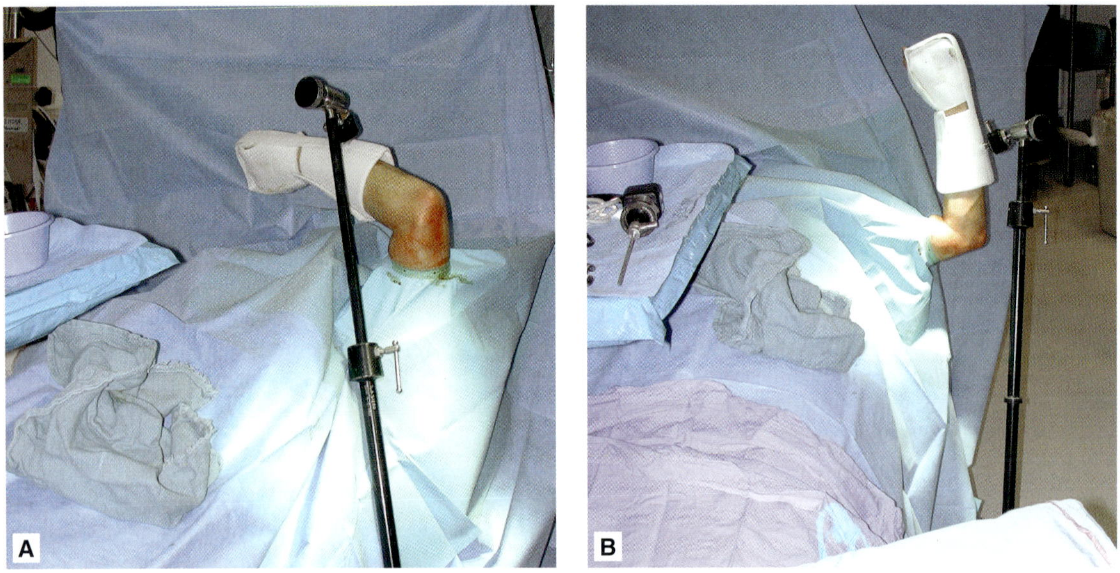

FIGURE 36-1 The authors' preferred patient positioning for elbow arthroscopy: supine with a McConnell arm positioner. **A.** Position for access to the posterior compartment. **B.** Position for anterior elbow access.

reparable in the geriatric patient and preparation for a total elbow arthroplasty (TEA) or hemiarthroplasty is advised.

McKee et al cited failure of ORIF as a rationale for TEA.[9] While there are some encouraging short-term results, the lifetime limitations on activities and difficult salvage of TEA failures merit caution and reserve. In addition, their conclusions may no longer be valid since the patients in the internal fixation group underwent 90/90 rather than parallel plating, which may have negatively impacted the outcomes.

Given these risks and limitations we will make every effort to fix the fracture. Contoured plates are placed in a parallel fashion along the medial and lateral columns. This optimizes the distal fixation as well as the supracondylar stability provided that treatment protocols are followed as outlined below.[10] Bone loss is effectively managed with tricortical grafts to replace comminuted segments of the medial and lateral columns and augment stability. While 2 cm of shortening at the supracondylar level to increase bony contact is advocated by some, this may compromise motion because of impingement in the coronoid and olecranon fossae. Finally, recognizing that both open and arthroscopic contracture release are effective in restoring functional motion, bony union is now prioritized over motion. If the fixation is anything less than stable and rigid, longer periods of immobilization to achieve union with a subsequent, staged contracture release is preferred to early motion and loss of fixation.

Surgical Technique of Open Reduction Internal Fixation

From the supine position the elbow is flexed over the patient's chest and held in place with an elbow positioner (Fig. 36-2). A sterile tourniquet is applied to allow for proximal extension of the exposure as necessary. Well-described approaches to the distal humerus include the paratricipital, triceps-reflecting, triceps-reflecting anconeus pedicle, triceps-splitting, and olecranon osteotomy. Complete exposure and visualization of all of the fracture fragments is a prerequisite for successful reconstruction and the choice of approach is ultimately at the surgeon's discretion. An olecranon osteotomy has been shown to provide maximal exposure of distal humerus intra-articular fractures[4] and facilitate achieving an anatomic reduction of the articular surface. Furthermore, a TEA can still be performed even if an olecranon osteotomy has been done.

A straight posterior incision is made directly over the olecranon. Curving the incision around the olecranon is not recommended as the cutaneous blood supply of the skin directly over the olecranon is precarious. The dissection is carried out down to the level of the triceps fascia. Full-thickness skin flaps are elevated laterally to the level of the intermuscular septum and medially until the ulnar nerve is visualized. The ulnar nerve is carefully mobilized by releasing the arcade of Struthers, Osborne ligament, and the fibrous aponeurosis between the 2 heads of the flexor carpi ulnaris (FCU). While many advocate subcutaneous transposition at the end of the procedure,[4] our preference is to leave it in situ and avoid circumferential dissection unless absolutely necessary. There is no conclusive evidence on the best approach for managing the ulnar nerve and leaving it in situ simplifies revision surgery or contracture release should it be necessary. This is supported by a recent study by Wiggers et al of 17/107 patients who developed an ulnar neuropathy following internal fixation of a distal humerus fracture.[11] There was a higher incidence of ulnar neuropathy in columnar fractures, which they attributed to the additional handling of the ulnar nerve that occurred with the reduction of a columnar fracture and

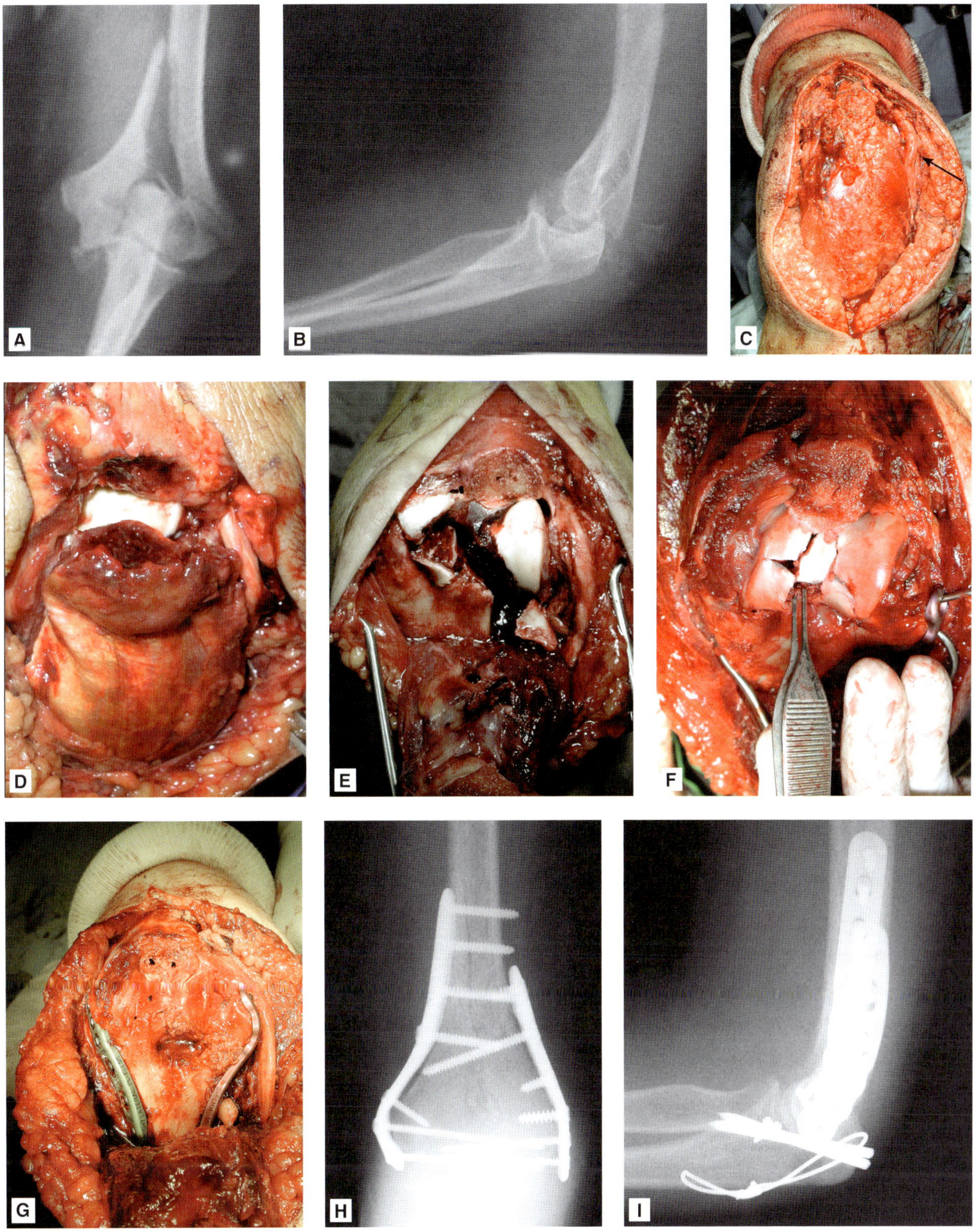

FIGURE 36-2 ORIF of the distal humerus. **A** and **B.** AP and lateral radiographs of a comminuted, intra-articular distal humerus fracture. **C.** Full-thickness skin flaps elevated through a posterior incision. The ulnar nerve has been freed and mobilized to protect it through the remainder of the case. **D.** The olecranon osteotomy is reflected proximally exposing the underlying distal humerus. **E.** Exposure of the articular surface demonstrates the degree of comminution. **F.** The joint is carefully pieced together with every effort made to minimize stripping of any remaining periosteal attachments. **G.** Application of precontoured parallel plates to the medial and lateral columns of the distal humerus with strict adherence to O'Driscoll's principles will maximize the stability of the construct. **H** and **I.** Postoperative x-rays show reduction of the fracture and support of the articular surface. The osteotomy has been secured with a tension band construct. Arrow, ulnar nerve.

application of a medial plate rather than the nerve transposition per se.[11]

With the nerve protected and olecranon exposed, preparations are made for an olecranon osteotomy. Our current practice is to use a 1-piece, low-profile fixation system (TriMed Olecranon Sled™), but acceptable options include tension band fixation, plating, or a cancellous lag screw as described in the section "Olecranon Fractures." A Chevron osteotomy is made with use of an osteotome and finished by cracking the anterior cortex to create precisely interdigitating surfaces without a saw blade or osteotome kerf to ensure an accurate reduction. The triceps and attached olecranon are elevated off the posterior aspect of the humerus at the medial and lateral intermuscular septae. Note that the radial nerve will be found 8 to 10 cm proximal to the lateral epicondyle as it passes around the posterior surface of the humerus and care should be taken to find and protect it if proximal exposure is required.

Exposure of the distal humerus now allows for reduction of the articular surface. Every effort should be made to minimize stripping of any remaining periosteal attachments by using a small dental pick, skin hook, or K-wires as joysticks to manipulate the fragments into a reduced position. The anterior aspect of the distal humerus is the most critical for a functional joint and the medial trochlea is essential in maintaining articular stability. Reconstruction therefore best proceeds in a systematic fashion by first addressing the anterior trochlea and capitellum, then the medial trochlea, and finally the posterior fragments.[7] Bone defects in these regions may require prolonged immobilization to allow for complete bony fusion. Provisional stabilization of these pieces with wires is useful, but no screws are placed in the distal fragments prior to plate application.

With the articular surface aligned and temporarily held in place, fixation of the major distal fragment (articular surface) to the shaft proceeds with precontoured plates applied to the medial and lateral columns running parallel along their respective supracondylar ridges. Plates of appropriate length should be selected to engage at least 8 cortices proximal to the fracture and provisionally held with K-wires. Reliable union of the distal fragment to the shaft is maximized by executing 7 technical objectives that each contribute to the stability of the construct as outlined by O'Driscoll[10]: (1) every screw in the distal fragment should pass through a plate; (2) every screw in the distal fragment should be anchored in a fragment on the opposite side that is also fixed by a plate; (3) as many screws as possible should be placed in the distal fragments (minimum 4-5 screws); (4) every screw in the distal fragment should be as long as possible; (5) every screw in the distal fragment should engage as many articular fragments as possible; (6) screws in the distal fragment should lock together by interdigitation to create a fixed-angle structure; (7) plates should be applied with compression at the supracondylar level (unless comminution of the column makes this impossible).

Temporary wires are removed and the elbow is taken through the full range of passive motion under fluoroscopy. Stability of the construct now dictates whether early motion is possible or if prolonged casting is necessary. The olecranon osteotomy is reduced and fixed with the chosen fixation method. The ulnar nerve is repositioned into the epicondylar groove and the overlying skin flaps are closed over a drain. The patient is placed in a long arm posterior splint to support the fixation.

Arthroscopic-assisted Fixation of Unicondylar Distal Humerus Fractures

As discussed above, the major challenge in distal humerus fixation is adequate visualization of the articular surface. In standard open techniques, a large exposure and arthrotomy is necessary to achieve what is readily visible through small arthroscopic portals. Paratricipital approaches afford limited visualization of the articular surface unless the capsule and collateral ligaments are released to allow for subluxation or dislocation of the elbow, which is undesirable. Arthroscopy allows direct assessment of the articular reduction in cases of simpler, unicondylar, intra-articular fractures (Fig. 36-3).

With the joint surface under direct arthroscopic visualization from either the standard anteromedial or anterolateral portal, a thick Steinmann pin (1/8 in) is used to manipulate the larger fragment with attached muscle origins into position. The fracture is temporarily fixed in place with a transcondylar wire or a stout Steinmann pin. The reduction is confirmed arthroscopically and radiographically. A medial- or lateral-sided incision, as dictated by the fracture, is then made through the skin and subcutaneous tissue directly over the appropriate column without need for additional arthrotomy or muscular dissection. For the medial column, this incision should precede the initial pin placement in order to avoid iatrogenic injury to the ulnar nerve, which must be identified by opening the cubital tunnel. For the lateral column, care should be taken to avoid past pointing of pins through the medial trochlea that can injure the ulnar nerve. The precontoured plate is then applied over the stabilizing pin and provisionally fixed with an additional transcondylar screw through the plate. The initial pin can be removed and replaced with a screw through the plate to conform to O'Driscoll's principles. Remaining screws are inserted in the same fashion as described above.

Total Elbow Arthroplasty in the Acute Setting

The increased use of semiconstrained total joint replacements for acute fractures of the distal humerus has been described.[9] Although its proponents emphasize better functional scores in otherwise unsalvageable joints, these studies are short term. In our view, the strict weight-bearing demands combined with questionable longevity of the implants relegate this treatment to the very select group of elderly patients who are older than 65 years of age with low physical demands. It is our belief that adherence to the above fixation principles, liberal use of tricortical autograft to manage bone loss, and prolonged immobilization with a staged contracture release yield improved outcomes in even osteoporotic fractures.[3]

Rehabilitation

Postoperative treatment needs to be individualized to the stability of the final construct. Early postoperative motion is used only with stable fixation; otherwise it is better to immobilize the elbow until the fracture has adequately healed and then proceed with an elbow release if necessary. Elbow motion without adequate bony stability risks a loss of alignment and predisposes to a delayed or nonunion or avascular necrosis of the articular fragments.

Complications

One study reported a 35% complication rate including stiffness, malunion, nonunion, fixation failure, heterotopic ossification, and ulnar neuropathy.[9]

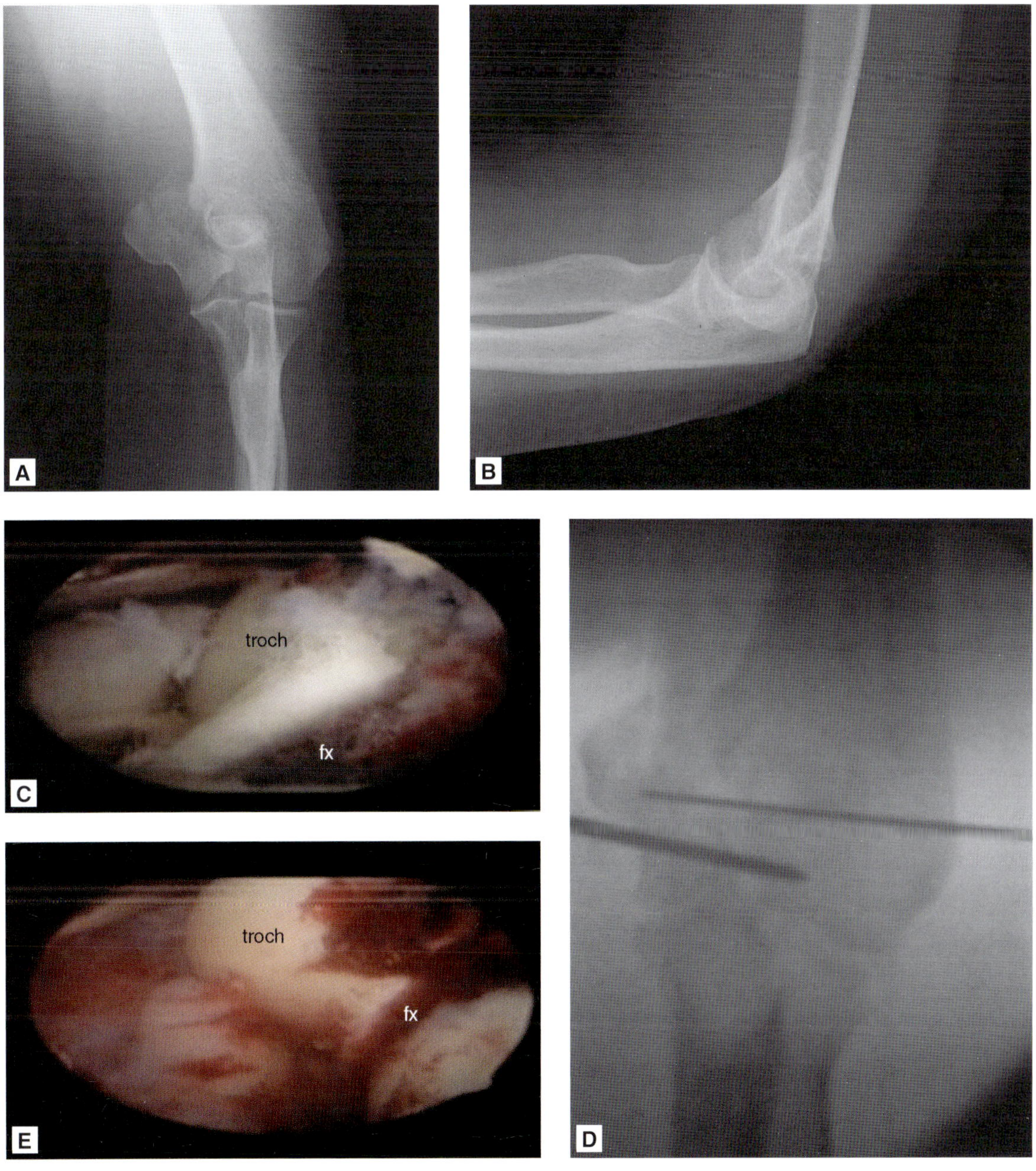

FIGURE 36-3 Arthroscopic fixation of the distal humerus. **A** and **B.** A comminuted medial condyle fracture as seen on x-ray. **C.** Arthroscopically, the trochlear articular fragment is seen. **D** and **E.** A limited medial approach is made to protect the ulnar nerve so that a heavy Steinmann pin can be inserted as a joystick to manipulate the fragment into a reduction. K-wires placed from lateral to medial temporarily stabilize the reduction while a transcondylar screw is inserted (in a lag fashion, if necessary) to achieve an anatomic reduction.

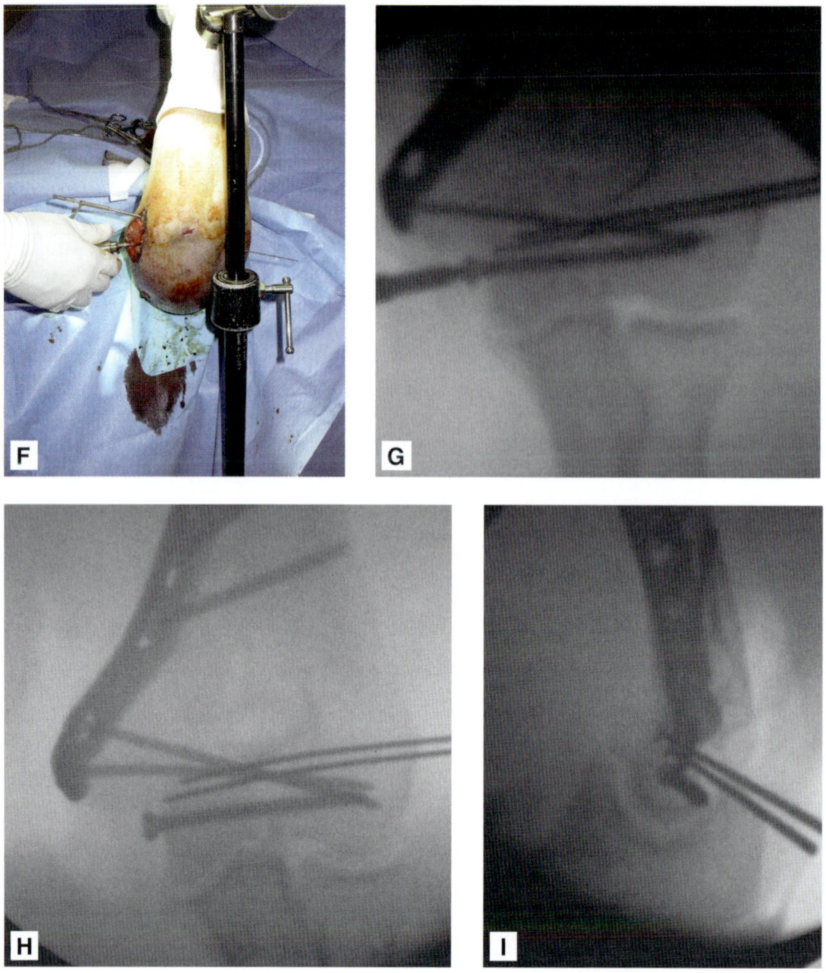

FIGURE 36-3 (*Continued*) **F** and **G.** A medial plate is applied without disturbing the flexor-pronator origin. The intact lateral condyle allows an exemption from the usual "4-5" distal screw rule since the intact lateral column acts as a "plate," thus achieving 4 distal screws that secure the articular surface to the shaft. **H** and **I.** Reduction of a lateral column fracture involves similar steps from the lateral side. fx, fracture line; troch, medial trochlea.

Postoperative ulnar nerve problems are one of the most common complications and there is conflicting evidence in the literature regarding the optimum treatment. While the nerve should routinely be identified and, if necessary, mobilized during exposure for its protection, some studies have suggested further benefit by transposing it anteriorly.[4] As our goal is to achieve bony union even at the expense of postoperative stiffness, we prefer to leave the nerve in situ and close the underlying fascia to protect it from the hardware. This keeps it in a known location so a planned contracture release can be done with less concern for iatrogenic injury.

The incidence of heterotopic ossification without the use of routine prophylaxis varies in the literature from 0% to 21%.[4] We have found it rare enough that we do not routinely use prophylaxis. One prospective randomized trial comparing postoperative prophylactic radiation with a control group in posttraumatic elbow fixation demonstrated a significant and unexpectedly high nonunion rate in the radiation group leading to premature termination of the study.[12] When it does occur, the standard treatment of heterotopic ossification is excision of the heterotopic bone after 3 months to restore elbow motion. In the absence of a progressive loss of elbow motion, erythema, and swelling that is suggestive of ongoing bone formation, earlier resection is possible.

Modern fixation techniques have improved the results of treatment, but 20% to 25% of patients still may go on to a nonunion or malunion. This usually can be successfully addressed with a revision of the internal fixation with the use of bone graft and prolonged immobilization, which often requires a contracture release at a second stage. The plates and screws are not removed during this procedure unless they specifically impede motion so as not to weaken the bone and predispose to stress refracture. A TEA may be used for salvage, but the failure rate is substantial.

RADIAL HEAD FRACTURES

Fractures of the radial head represent the most common fracture about the elbow.[13] The majority of fractures that are treated nonoperatively heal without a functional deficit.[14] Those fractures that require surgery are treated with internal fixation, radial head replacement, or resection depending on the fracture pattern and associated injuries.

The routine workup of radial head fractures includes a careful assessment of the areas of tenderness or swelling since at least 50% of these fractures have associated injuries.[15] Specific attention should be directed to pain about the forearm or wrist that may be indicative of an Essex-Lopresti lesion. Epicondylar tenderness is potentially indicative of a ligamentous disruption. Stress testing of the collateral ligaments without anesthesia is notoriously difficult and unreliable. The elbow motion should be assessed for any mechanical block that could be suggestive of fragment impingement. If pain is a limiting factor, it is helpful to aspirate the fracture hematoma and inject local anesthetic into the joint through the soft spot on the lateral aspect of the elbow between the radial head and the lateral upper condyle. Standard x-rays include an AP, oblique, and lateral with the elbow extended. If there is a highly comminuted radial head fracture or if there is a suspicion of other bony injury, a CT scan of the elbow in extension is invaluable in surgical planning and may demonstrate posterolateral or posteromedial instability.

Classification

The Mason classification is the most common one in use today. It was modified by Hotchkiss to quantify the extent of head and neck involvement.[16] Type I fractures have less than 2 mm of displacement of the head or neck with no mechanical limitation to forearm rotation (pronation/supination). Type II fractures demonstrate displacement of more than 2 mm without severe comminution and may be excised or internally fixed assuming adequate bone quality. Type III fractures are severely comminuted and may not be reconstructable, requiring excision or replacement to restore elbow motion.

Indications

Type I fractures are best treated nonoperatively and emphasize early motion to prevent stiffness with protected weight bearing until healing is evident. Type II fractures are best treated with internal fixation in the form of screws, plates, or bioabsorbable pins and type III fractures are treated with either resection or a radial head arthroplasty.

Functionally, the radial head acts as a secondary stabilizer to valgus restraint in the normal elbow.[17] It maintains the congruity of the radiocapitellar joint and contributes to varus stability by tensioning the lateral collateral ligament (LCL) complex. In the ligament deficit elbow its role as a stabilizer becomes critical and precludes excision. Likewise, the presence of an injury to the interosseous membrane or DRUJ (Essex-Lopresti) requires fixation or replacement of the head to restore appropriate length to the lateral forearm and prevent proximal migration of the radius. This migration dramatically alters the biomechanics of the wrist and few reliable alternatives exist once it has occurred.[16]

The decision of replacement or fixation is then dictated by the fracture pattern. All efforts should be made to maintain the native radial head if possible but not at the expense of tenuous fixation. Ring et al showed markedly decreased functional results with internal fixation when more than 3 articular fragments are present and therefore recommend an arthroplasty.[18]

Surgical Technique of Open Reduction and Internal Fixation

The patient is positioned supine over an arm board with a tourniquet. The arm is kept in the pronated position throughout to minimize risk of injury to the posterior interosseous nerve (PIN). In the setting of an injury to the LCL that is combined with a radial head fracture, one can use the posterolateral Kocher approach between the anconeus and the extensor carpi ulnaris (ECU) to expose the radial head and repair the LCL through the same incision. Our preferred approach for these fractures is through a standard Kaplan approach to facilitate the anterior exposure needed for an ORIF while decreasing the risk of iatrogenic injury. A straight lateral incision is made directly over the lateral epicondyle and extended distally along the radiocapitellar joint. Keeping this approach anterior to the anconeus avoids the LCL complex arising from the posterior aspect of the lateral epicondyle. The fibers of the extensor digitorum communis are split in line with the skin incision, exposing the underlying capsule that is then sharply incised directly over the radiocapitellar joint. The exposure can be extended by elevating the capsule directly off the humerus while staying anterior to the LCL. Distally, the dissection continues over the radial head, but it should not extend to the neck to avoid injury to the PIN. If exposure of the neck is needed due to the fracture pattern or the need for a plate, the obliquely oriented fibers of the supinator muscle should be identified. This muscle is elevated off the proximal radius starting at its most posterior aspect.[16] If further exposure is required, the PIN should be identified to ensure it is not inadvertently injured by retractors or hardware placement.

With the fractured head exposed, the wound is irrigated and the hematoma evacuated. An assessment of the injury is done after rotating the forearm into full pronation and supination. If a small fragment is identified that is impeding motion, it can be excised, but ORIF is preferred.[19] Displaced fragments are reduced with direct manipulation or with a dental pick. Small K-wires may be used as joysticks to manipulate larger fragments into position. A priority is given to reconstruction of the articular surface with temporary stabilization with K-wires, followed by definitive fixation with mini-fragment screws (1.5 or 2.0 mm), headless miniscrews, minicondylar plates (2.0 or 2.4 mm), and bioabsorbable pins depending on the fracture pattern (Fig. 36-4). The radial head fragments may be excised and reconstructed on the back table prior to replacing them and fixing them to the shaft. All hardware should be placed in the "safe zone" that consists of a 100° arc in which

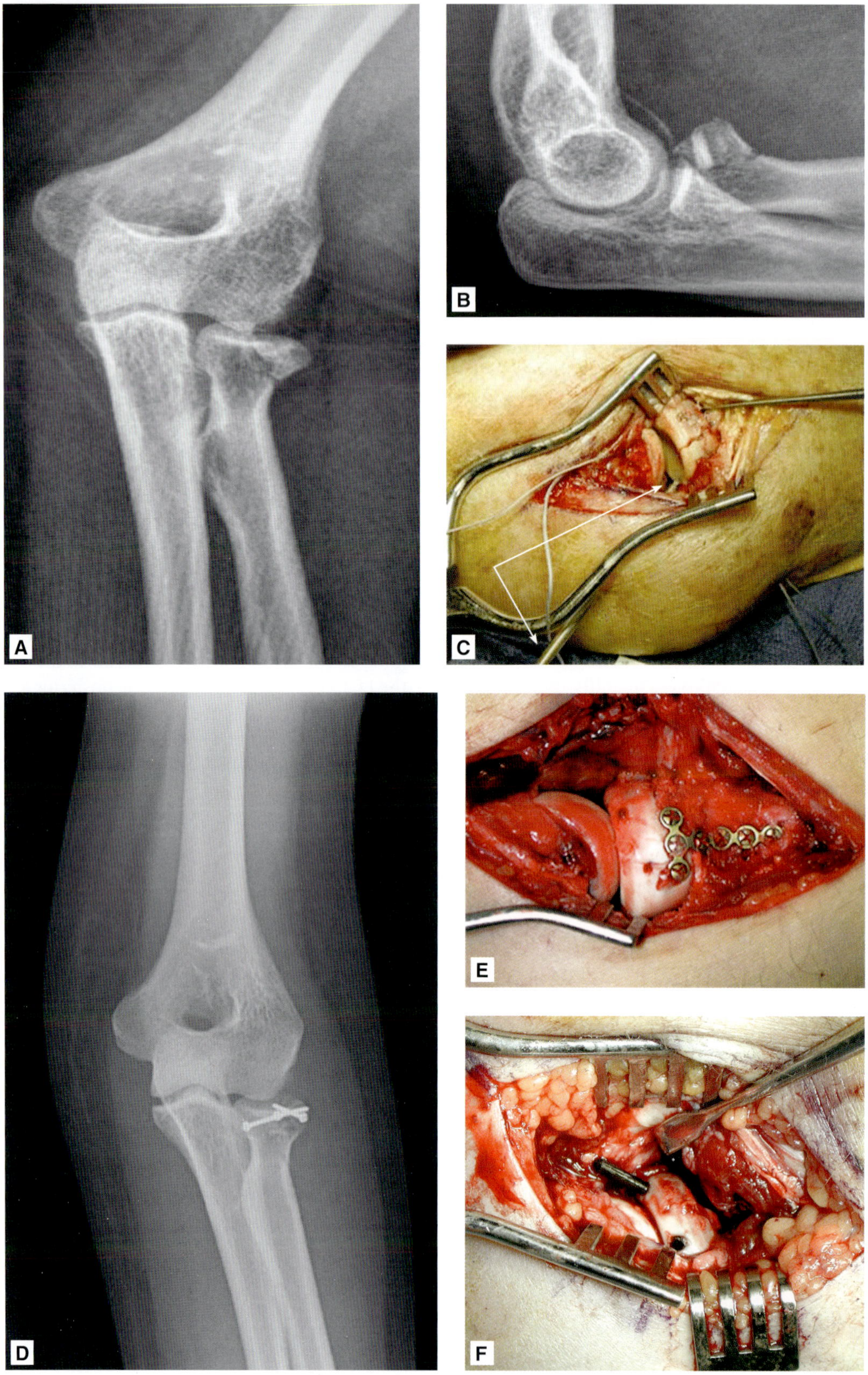

FIGURE 36-4 Methods of radial head fixation. **A** and **B.** AP and lateral x-rays demonstrating a type II radial head fracture amenable to ORIF. **C** and **D.** Screw fixation of the fracture in the "safe zone." A bioabsorbable pin has been inserted through a posterior percutaneous incision in order to secure the radial head to the shaft. **E.** Buttress plating to secure the radial head to the shaft. **F.** Insertion of bioabsorbable pins. Arrow, percutaneous drilling for bioabsorbable pin insertion.

any hardware will not impinge on the proximal radioulnar articulation through full supination and pronation. This zone is the angle defined between the palpable landmarks of the radial styloid and Lister's tubercle.[20] Screws may be countersunk below the chondral surface. The elbow is taken through full motion to assess for hardware impingement. The muscular intervals are closed with absorbable sutures. A tear of the LCL should be reattached at this point with bone anchors to restore lateral stability.

Hardware irritation remains a concern if the fixation extends to the neck.[21] Some available methods are at least 2 obliquely oriented, countersunk screws, bioabsorbable pins, or K-wires in opposing planes to increase the rigidity of the fixation.[21] This avoids the need for increased exposure and the necessary soft tissue stripping required for plate placement. If head–neck fixation is necessary, our preference is bioabsorbable pins placed intramedullarly down the shaft. Concerns regarding seroma formation and synovitis have not been borne out in our experience.

Arthroscopic-assisted reduction and fixation of radial head fractures has been reported, but we prefer a small lateral or anterolateral approach due to the limited arthroscopic visualization of the radial head fragments.[22]

Surgical Technique of Radial Head Arthroplasty

Various implants have been used to replace the native radial head including monopolar, bipolar, cemented, and press fit varieties. None has been conclusively shown to be superior. However, much attention has been directed at poor outcomes with silastic implants in regards to mechanical failure, inflammatory arthritis, and reactive synovitis.[23] We however have reported good long-term results with silastic implants, but they are not suitable in an unstable elbow or Essex-Lopresti injury.[24] There has been a trend toward the use of metal prostheses, but potential complications include loosening,[25] capitellar erosion, and osteopenia.[26]

The procedure is performed with the patient in the supine position but with the arm kept in pronation during the procedure to minimize risk of injury to the PIN (Fig. 36-5). If the

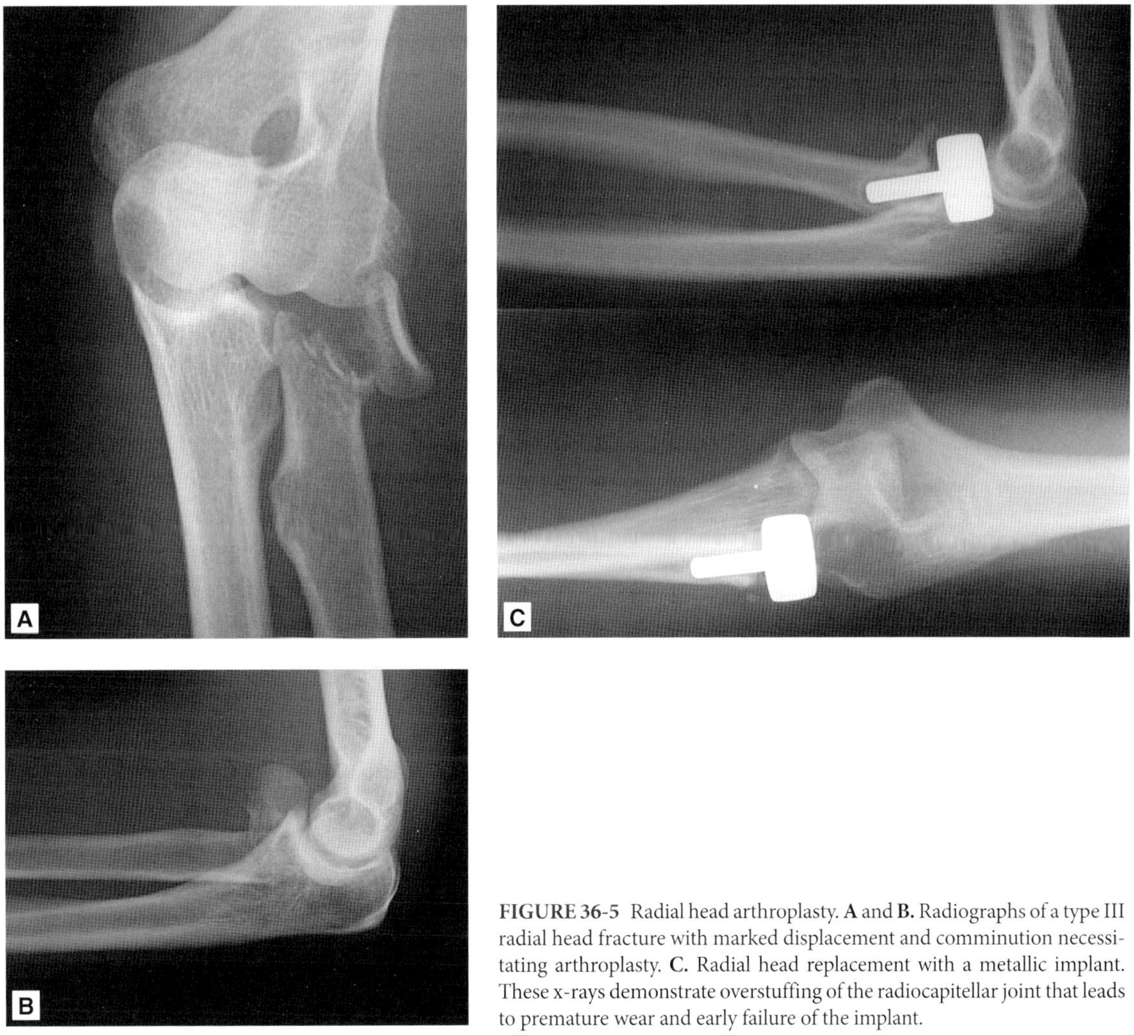

FIGURE 36-5 Radial head arthroplasty. **A** and **B.** Radiographs of a type III radial head fracture with marked displacement and comminution necessitating arthroplasty. **C.** Radial head replacement with a metallic implant. These x-rays demonstrate overstuffing of the radiocapitellar joint that leads to premature wear and early failure of the implant.

lateral ulnar collateral ligament (LUCL) is torn, the Kocher approach provides excellent exposure of the entire head. With an intact ligament, staying anterior with splitting of the EDC will avoid inadvertent injury and iatrogenic instability. The capsule is incised over the radiocapitellar joint, but not infrequently there is a traumatic rent that can be enlarged to complete the exposure.

An osteotome or sagittal saw is used at the head–neck junction to remove any remaining attached bone. Every effort should be made to retrieve all of the radial head fragments for reconstruction on the back table to aid in the sizing of the implant. A common error is to overstuff the joint especially in the face of a LUCL injury. For this reason, it is recommended that the final diameter and thickness of the implant be slightly undersized in comparison to the patient's native head.[27] Two methods are available for reliably determining the correct thickness of the radial head implant intraoperatively. In the van Riet method, the implant should rest flush with the proximal edge of the lesser sigmoid notch when viewed from a lateral perspective. If it is too thick, the implant will sit proud and extend beyond this point. Alternatively, any gapping of the lateral ulnohumeral joint when viewed from an extended lateral approach or with use of an angled dental mirror is indicative of overstuffing.[27]

Planars are available if desired to prepare the neck and optimize the seating of the implant. The cancellous bone of the radial neck is removed with increasing size reamers until some cortical chatter is appreciated. As with implant sizing, it is preferable to choose a stem that is 1 size smaller than the final reamer. After insertion of a trial implant, the radial head prosthesis is inserted. If difficulty is encountered in obtaining the necessary angle for implant insertion, particularly in the ligamentously stable elbow, it is helpful to pull the radial neck into view with a posteriorly placed retractor. In unusual circumstances, it may be necessary to perform a partial LUCL takedown from its origin off the lateral epicondyle. Fluoroscopy is used to confirm a concentric reduction, but bear in mind that it is difficult to evaluate correct implant sizing intraoperatively. Joint stability should be restored by ligament repair or reconstruction, not by overstuffing the radiocapitellar joint. Closure is done in layers with reapproximation of the capsule and muscular interval.

Rehabilitation

Postoperatively, patients are splinted for 3 to 5 days. They are then started on supervised and self-administered overhead ROM exercises while avoiding valgus stress. Strengthening begins at 10 weeks.

Complications

Regardless of treatment, the most common complication is postoperative elbow stiffness. Other complications include hardware irritation, nonunion or malunion, arthritis, and osteonecrosis.[13] Prominent hardware may be removed if necessary after 4 to 6 months. Nonunion is best addressed with a delayed excision of the radial head as repeat attempts at fixation are often unsuccessful.[28]

CAPITELLAR FRACTURES

Coronal plane fractures of the distal humerus involving the capitellum and trochlea represent less than 1% of humerus fractures.[29] Recent studies have shown that routine radiographic studies often underestimate their complexity. Frequently the lateral aspect of the trochlea and lateral column are involved in addition to a high incidence of other associated injuries.[30] Therefore, treatment requires visualization of the anterior articular surface as well as the posterior cortex of the lateral column that may have suffered fracture or plastic deformation.

Classification

The Bryan and Morrey classification is based on AP, lateral, and oblique x-ray views. Type I (Hans-Steinhal) is a capitellar shear fracture. Type II (Kocher-Lorenz) is an osteochondral flake. Type III is a comminuted fracture of the capitellum. The McKee modification adds a type IV capitellar fracture indicating extension to the trochlea.[31] While this classification system is useful as a descriptor, it does not lend itself well to treatment recommendations. Therefore, Dubberley et al proposed a classification scheme based on a retrospective review designed to direct treatment options.[32] In their system, a type 1 fracture primarily involves the capitellum with or without the lateral trochlear ridge (Bryan-Morrey type I equivalent). Type 2 fractures extend to the trochlear groove but remain as 1 fragment (similar to the McKee type IV). And type 3 fractures represent separate trochlear and capitellar fragments. These types were then subdivided to denote absence (A) or presence (B) of posterior comminution.

Indications

The result of nonoperative management of capitellar fractures is unpredictable with a high incidence of posttraumatic arthritis, contractures, and instability.[31] The current standard is therefore operative fixation and stabilization.[33] While plain radiographs may show large, displaced fragments, a CT scan is recommended due to the high incidence of extension to the lateral trochlea and posterior column with associated comminution that may be underappreciated on the standard views.[34] This will help the surgeon determine the full extent of necessary exposure to adequately stabilize all injured areas. Associated elbow instability should be carefully investigated as well.

With the rare exception of completely nondisplaced stable fractures, capitellar fractures should be fixed operatively. The literature has included descriptions of fixation with screws, plates, tension band wiring, and suture stabilization. Arthroscopic fixation of capitellar fractures has also been described.[2] Regardless of the method chosen, the goal is to achieve stable fixation while avoiding the main blood supply to the capitellar fragments that comes from perforating vessels that pass through the posterior aspect of the condyles.

Surgical Technique for Open Reduction Internal Fixation

Appropriate positioning of the patient is based on the intended surgical approach (Fig. 36-6). In the case of capitellar fractures, preoperative imaging determines to what extent exposure of the articular surface will be necessary for adequate visualization and fixation. In fractures that do not extend to the trochlear groove (Dubberley type 1), the exposure is through an extensile lateral approach centered proximally over the lateral epicondyle and distally over the radiocapitellar joint.[33] The wrist extensors and anterior capsule are elevated off the lateral supracondylar ridge. The forearm is kept in pronation to protect the radial nerve and retractors are placed deep to the brachialis. Posterior exposure of the lateral column is facilitated by elevation of the lateral triceps from the posterior distal humerus and proximal ulna. Further visualization may be obtained by release of the LUCL, but this should be avoided if at all possible. If not, the ligament should be released from the origin at the lateral epicondyle and then reattached rather than sectioned midsubstance. If the expectation for full articular exposure is anticipated (Dubberley type 2 or 3), our preference is an olecranon osteotomy to preserve the LCL and completely visualize the involved surfaces.

With complete exposure, reduction of the articular fragments is best done with a dental pick, small bone tenaculum, or a large skin hook. Care should be taken to avoid stripping the remaining periosteum to minimize the risk of AVN. In instances of plastic deformation, bone graft should

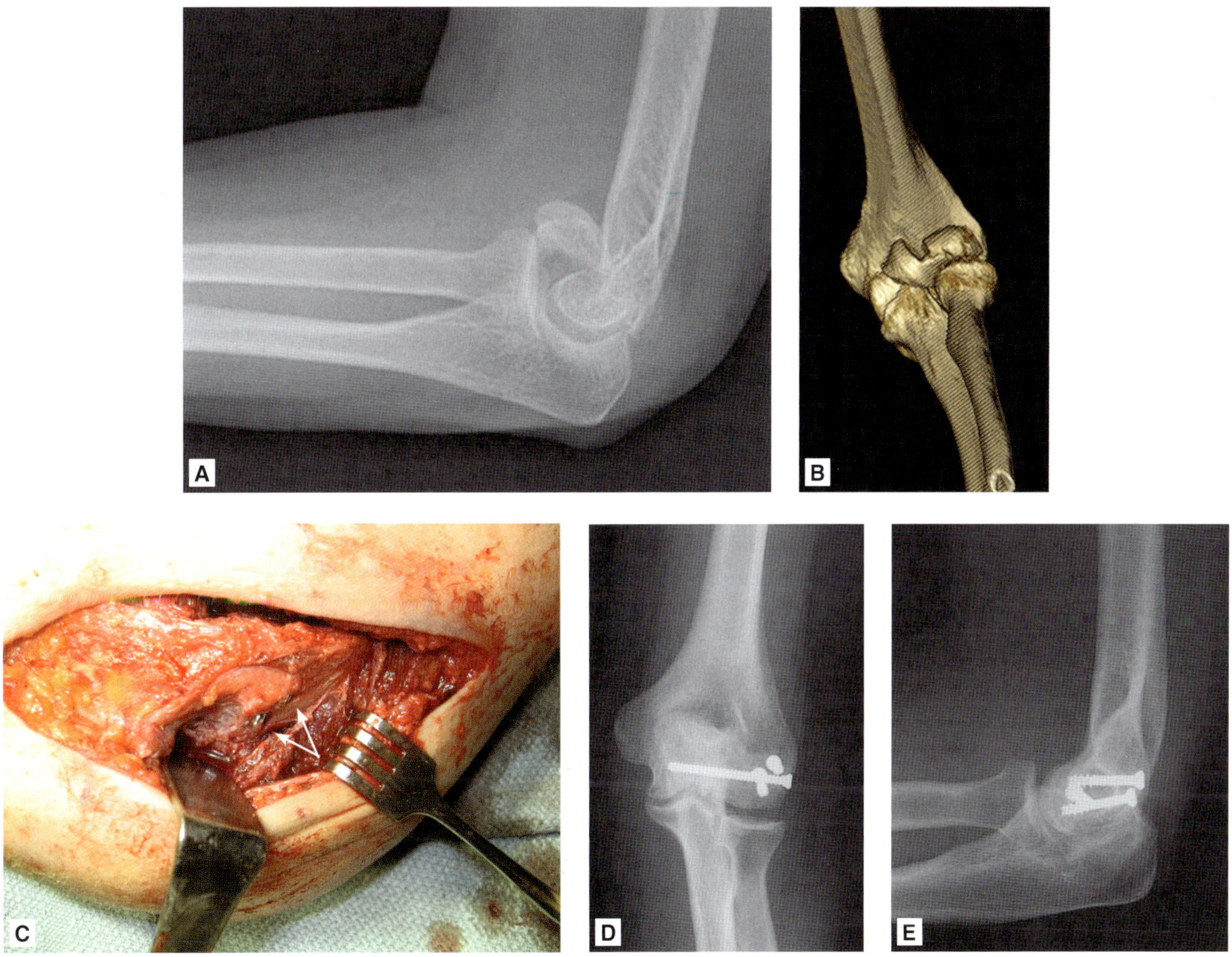

FIGURE 36-6 Capitellum ORIF. **A.** Lateral x-ray and (**B**) 3D recon CT of a Dubberley type 2 capitellar fracture. **C.** Intraoperatively, 2 screws are placed in a divergent fashion from posterior to anterior. **D** and **E.** Placement of a third, transcondylar screw increases the strength of the fixation. Arrows, posterior to anterior screws.

be prepared to fill the void once the fragments are disimpacted. Small K-wires may be used for provisional fixation but should be placed away from the planned definitive fixation. The goal is stable, anatomic restoration of the joint surface. Screws can be placed anterior to posterior or posterior to anterior depending on the size of the fragment. Small capitellar fragments are preferably stabilized with headless compression screws placed in an anterior to posterior direction and buried beneath the subchondral surface. These have been shown in biomechanical studies to have superior fixation over posteroanterior cancellous screws.[35] Anterior placement also avoids further disruption of the main blood supply to the capitellar fragments from the posterior condylar vessels. Typically 2 screws are placed in a divergent fashion to avoid rotational malalignment, but supplemental fixation in the form of additional screws, threaded K-wires, bioabsorbable pins, or lateral column plates may be required depending on the extent of injury.[33] Osteochondral "flakes" cannot be adequately fixed with screws. Therefore, suture fixation is recommended.

Arthroscopic Screw Fixation of the Capitellum

The patient is positioned for an anterior approach to the elbow (Fig. 36-7). The proximal anteromedial portal is established and fracture hematoma is evacuated. Elbow extension will typically reduce the fracture, but it tends to redisplace with flexion as the radial head comes in contact with the fragment. In this case, a trocar placed through the proximal anterolateral portal will provide stabilization of the fragment as the elbow is flexed to help the radial head "ride over" the capitellum. A trocar placed through the proximal anterolateral portal can then reduce the fragment allowing the radiocapitellar joint to function as a shoehorn preventing

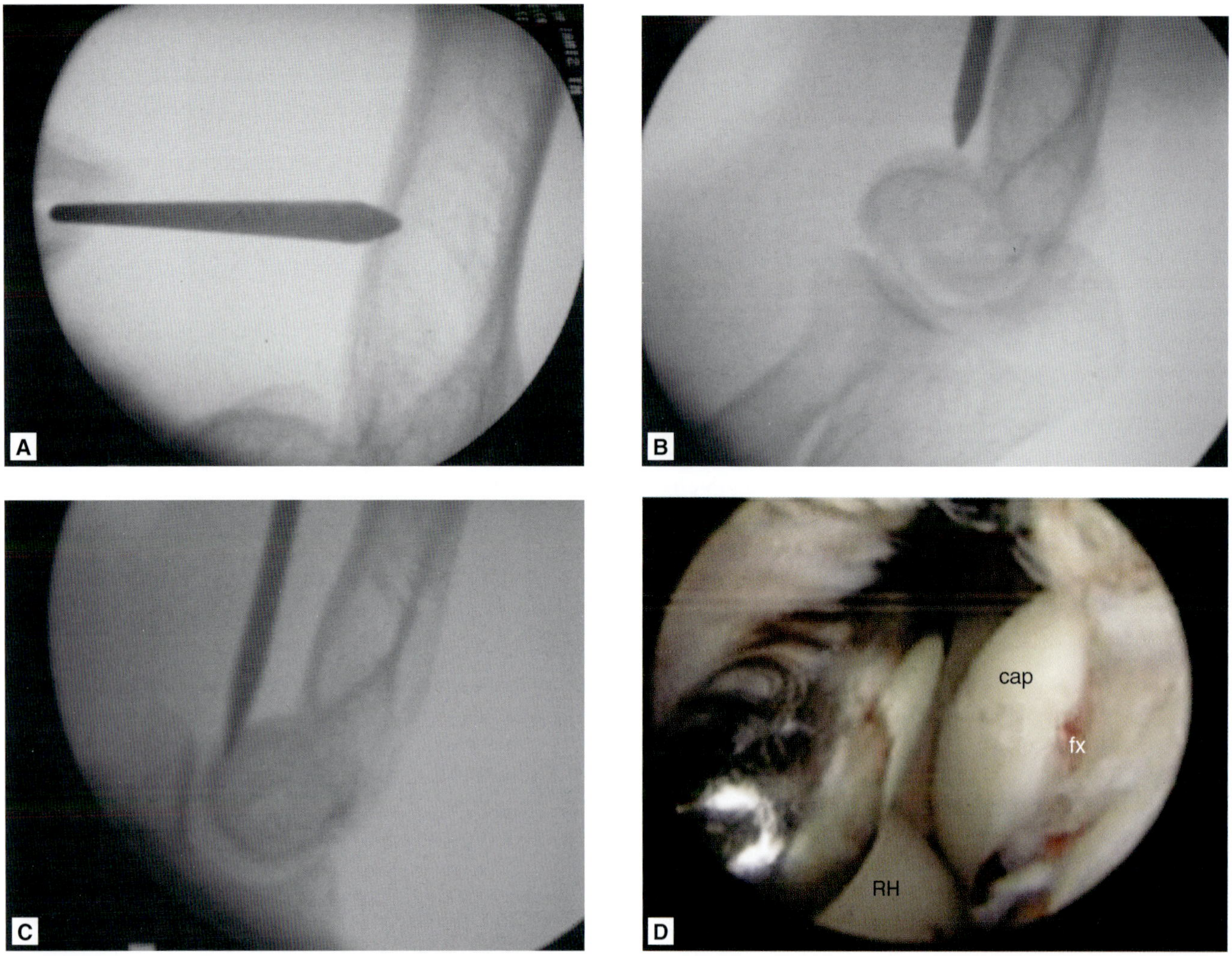

FIGURE 36-7 Arthroscopic fixation of a type 2 capitellar fracture. **A.** A "high" proximal anterolateral portal is marked out under radiologic guidance and created proximal to the fracture. **B** and **C.** Extension frequently will reduce the fracture, but in this case a complete reduction does not occur. Therefore, the trocar is used to push the fragment into an anatomic reduction. **D.** This is confirmed with the arthroscopic view from the anterolateral portal.

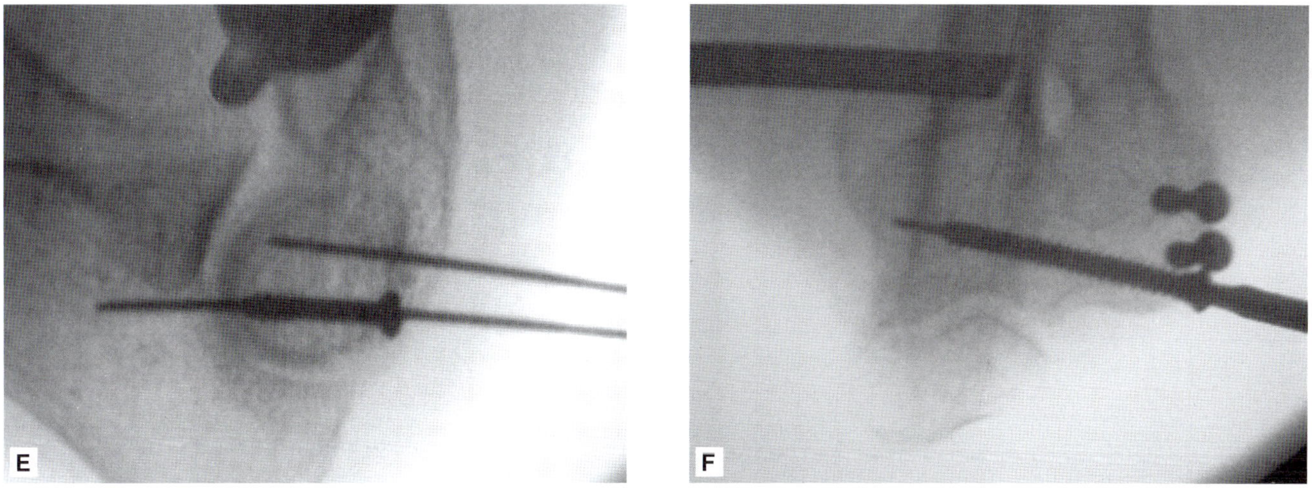

FIGURE 36-7 (*Continued*) **E.** Fixation is achieved with cannulated screws, again using the arthroscope to confirm optimal placement and length. **F.** Note the use of a transcondylar screw to reinforce the fixation, permitting early use and therapy; cap, capitellum; fx, fracture line; olec, olecranon; RH, radial head.

redisplacement by the radial head with the elbow in more than 90° of flexion. The reduction is confirmed by fluoroscopy with the above steps repeated as necessary to align the shear fragment appropriately. Alternatively, the trocar may be placed through an anteromedial or accessory anterolateral portal to obtain a reduction.

Given the high incidence of posterior comminution and plastic deformation, the reduction should be assessed posteriorly. The transtriceps or distal posterolateral portal allows access to the posterior aspect of the lateral column by passing down the lateral gutter. It may be necessary to use a "soft spot" posterior radiocapitellar portal for a 3.5-mm shaver to remove debris in this area and improve visualization.

Once an accurate reduction is confirmed, small posterior incisions are made to insert guidewires for at least 2 cannulated screws. Under direct visualization of the articular surface from an anterior portal or from the lateral gutter, the trajectory of the guidewires is confirmed by advancing them until they are visible just beneath the cartilage to calculate screw length. A cannulated 3.5-mm screw 2 to 4 mm shorter than the measured length is selected. This ensures that the longest possible screw is being used to avoid undersizing. If anterior to posterior placement is desired, the guidewires are further advanced until they can be extracted through a more distal "soft spot" portal and screws are inserted from this trajectory. If the fracture pattern allows, a transcondylar screw placed from lateral to medial will substantially increase the strength of the fixation. Care should be taken to assess the reduction of the trochlear ridge if the fracture extends medially.

Arthroscopic Suture Fixation of Capitellar Fragments

The above techniques are appropriate for fragments large enough for screw fixation. Small fragments and osteochondral flakes present a challenge due to the inadequate purchase with standard screws. To address this we use a novel technique of suture fixation of these fragments. Its utility is best served in Kocher-Lorenz fragments, but the indications may be expanded to include fixation of osteochondritis dissecans (OCD) lesions in the pediatric population.

A standard arthroscopic setup for access to the posterior compartment is performed (Fig. 36-8). The arthroscope is placed in the distal posterolateral portal and moved to the lateral gutter. It is carefully advanced over the top of the distal humerus just lateral to the olecranon to reach the posterior radiocapitellar joint. From this view a 3.5-mm shaver is inserted through the "soft spot" portal to debride the area and improve the visualization. A probe is inserted to check for instability of the fragment and outline its dimensions. A second accessory portal is established just distal to the soft spot with insertion of a guidewire into the joint. This is placed in the center of the lesion and aimed to exit out the posterior lateral column of the distal humerus. Fluoroscopy will confirm the trajectory. The guidewire is advanced through the bone and out the skin posteriorly. A longitudinal incision directly over this guidewire down to the bone of the posterior lateral column will assist with the remainder of the case. If the fragment is too proximal to place the guidewire from anterior to posterior in the capitellum, the wire may be inserted from the posterior aspect of the lateral column while observing the fragment with the arthroscope to assure it is centered intra-articularly.

An arthroscopic grasper is inserted through the soft spot portal to grab the end of the wire in the joint. This is used to stabilize and compress the fragment during drilling and to prevent the wire from advancing. A tunnel is drilled through the humerus to just under the subchondral bone using a cannulated drill, sequentially increasing the size from 2.5 to 3.0-3.5 mm in diameter. The wire is removed and an 18-gauge spinal needle inserted through the tunnel until it is visualized in the joint space. A 0-PDS suture is passed through the needle and retrieved out the

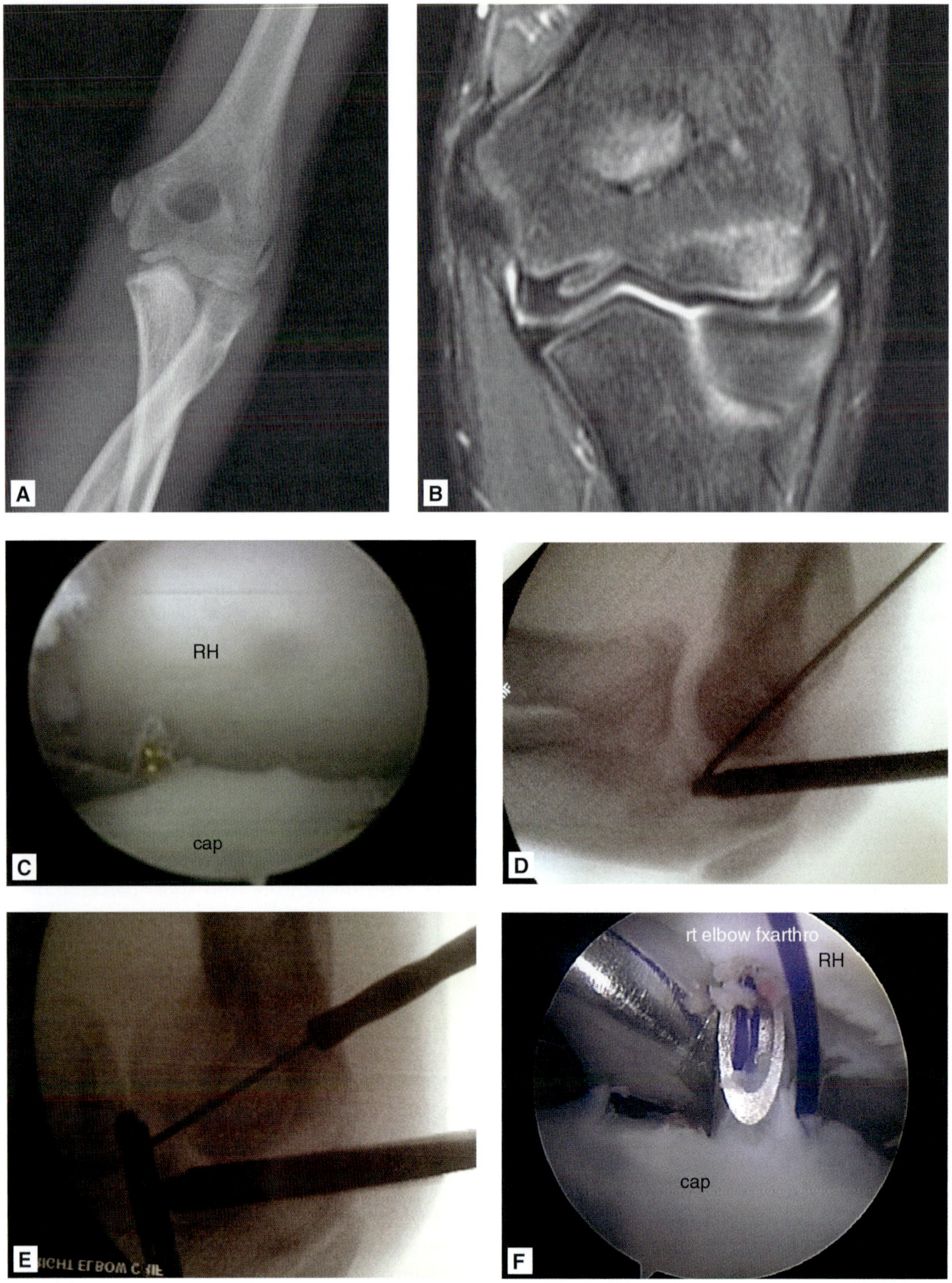

FIGURE 36-8 Arthroscopic suture fixation of a capitellar fracture. **A** and **B.** AP x-ray and MRI demonstrate a large osteochondral fragment. **C.** Viewing from the posterior radiocapitellar portal, a guidewire is advanced through the center of the fragment until it is just visible inside the joint. **D.** Its trajectory is confirmed fluoroscopically. **E.** An arthroscopic grasper secures the guidewire and underlying fragment as the tunnel is reamed from posterior to anterior. **F.** A spinal needle is passed into the joint and used to shuttle 0-PDS fixation sutures out an accessory portal.

soft spot portal with an arthroscopic grasper. This process is repeated as necessary depending on the number of desired fixation sutures. Then, from the same posterolateral incision, another guidewire is drilled through the humerus and aimed to exit just medial to the defect. The spinal needle is used to pass a 3-0 Prolene suture into the joint and is again retrieved. This is used to shuttle one of the original PDS sutures to the posterolateral column incision (adjacent to where the PDS sutures enter the bone). Additional fixation points are possible around the defect in a similar manner,

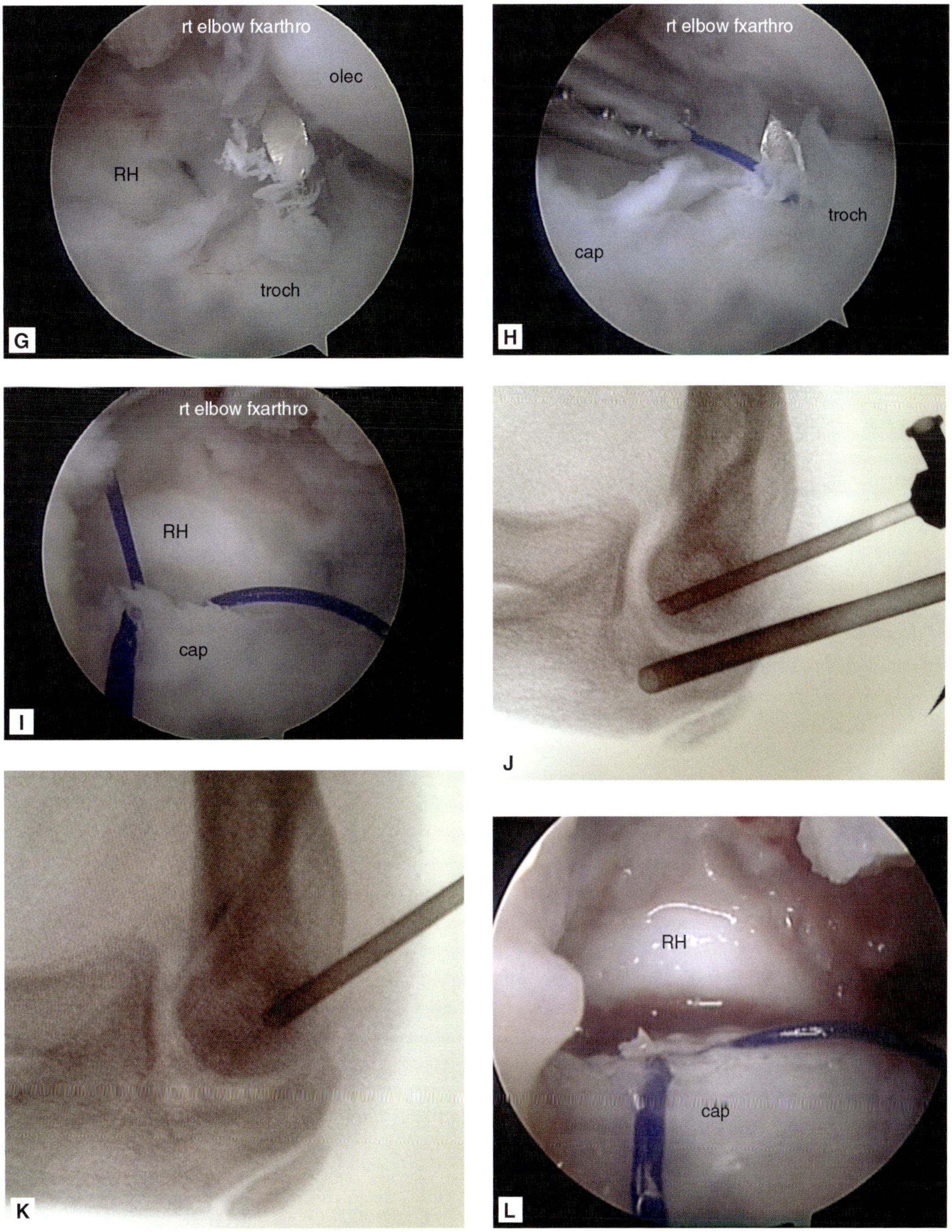

FIGURE 36-8 (*Continued*) **G.** A second point of fixation is made medial to the defect with (**H**) a Prolene suture used to shuttle the fixation suture out posteriorly. **I.** Multiple fixation points are chosen to adequately secure the fragment. **J.** Drilling of the tunnel to just under the subchondral bone allows insertion of the cannula. **K.** Bone graft is packed into the defect to support the fixation and sutures are tied using arthroscopic sliding knots posteriorly. **L.** Final dry views demonstrate fixation of the fragment.

taking care to stay deep to the LUCL and proximal to the fragment itself.

In the case of an OCD lesion, a cannula is inserted through the posterior tunnel to just under the fragment. Autologous bone graft harvested from the iliac crest is packed through this cannula to support the fragment and promote healing. As the process continues the cannula is slowly removed in order to fill as much of the tunnel as possible. Grafting is not necessary for an acute type II (Kocher-Lorenz) capitellar fragment. Finally, each fixation suture is tied individually using an arthroscopic sliding knot along the posterior aspect of the humerus. Final views of the joint should demonstrate stable fixation of the fragment. For OCD cases, this examination is performed dry so as not to wash out the impacted graft. Due to the difficulty of achieving rigid, stable fixation with these fragments, healing is prioritized over motion and the elbow is immobilized until evidence of healing is seen on MRI, usually at 3 months.

Rehabilitation

If stable fixation is achieved, early motion is instituted. If any question about stability exists or if significant comminution is present, the elbow should be immobilized to prioritize healing over motion.

Complications

The most commonly described complications from this fracture are AVN, degenerative arthritis, and heterotopic ossification. Not surprisingly, these occur more commonly in more extensive injuries with greater comminution.[32] Minimizing dissection and achieving an anatomic reduction limit the incidence of these serious complications. The development of heterotopic ossification in capitellum fractures is relatively unusual and routine prophylaxis is not indicated.

OLECRANON FRACTURES

Fractures of the proximal ulna and olecranon account for 10% of fractures about the elbow.[36] The pattern of injury spans from simple transverse fractures to complex, comminuted fractures and those associated with elbow instability. Depending on the type of fracture, success has been reported with nonoperative management, fragment excision with triceps advancement, and internal fixation with tension band, intramedullary fixation, or plates.[36] The prognosis depends on the severity of the injury and associated soft tissue trauma.

Classification

The Mayo classification of olecranon fractures categorizes them based on displacement, stability, and comminution. Mayo type I fractures are minimally displaced and stable with less than 2 mm of displacement and no change in position with increasing elbow flexion to 90°. These are often treated nonoperatively whether A (noncomminuted) or B (comminuted). Type II fractures maintain elbow stability through intact collateral ligaments but are otherwise displaced and are best treated operatively. Type III fractures are classified in the setting of associated elbow instability and multiple studies have documented a poorer outcome with all methods of fixation in this type.[37]

Indications

The current standard is to fix displaced fractures of the olecranon operatively. Conversion of the distraction force of the triceps across the fracture site with tension band fixation is appropriate for displaced, transverse fracture patterns. Comminuted and oblique fractures are better served with plate fixation as tension bands will lead to further displacement or shortening of the olecranon articular surface and incongruity with the distal humerus. Limited contact-dynamic compression (LC-DC) plates provide excellent fixation strength, but precontoured plates have seen increasing popularity due to ease of placement and an increased number of fixation points in the proximal fragment. It is very important to examine the elbow under anesthesia to be certain that there is no instability, as tension band fixation is not adequate for a Monteggia-type fracture.

Surgical Technique for Tension Band Fixation

The exposure is achieved through a posterior, extensile longitudinal incision directly over the ulna (Fig. 36-9). Full-thickness flaps are elevated medially and laterally directly off the bone to expose the fracture site. Reduction is readily achieved with direct manipulation of the fracture fragments and may be temporarily held with the bone tenaculum or K-wires. A characteristic "bare area" devoid of articular cartilage is present at the junction of the anterior third to posterior two-thirds of the articulation and must be recognized and restored to avoid narrowing the trochlear fossa and obtaining an incongruous radius of curvature.[38] Fluoroscopic views should demonstrate a concentric reduction of the ulnohumeral joint. Two-millimeter K-wires have been described for tension band fixation, but our preference is to use larger intramedullary 3-mm Steinmann pins since smaller wires are subject to bending loads with flexion and extension of the elbow.[3] The pins are inserted through the olecranon tip under fluoroscopic control to engage the anterior cortex. Penetrating the anterior cortex increases the pullout strength, but care must be taken to avoid overpenetration and injury of the anterior interosseous nerve (AIN) or impingement on the proximal radius that would impair forearm rotation.[39] Pins with a threaded tip also prevent backing out. The pins are backed out slightly after penetrating the far cortex, bent or cut, and impacted against the bone. A drill hole is then made through the ulna distally at a point equidistant from the olecranon tip to the fracture. An 18-gauge wire is passed through this hole and around the pins in a figure-of-8 fashion deep to the triceps muscle and tendon. The loops should be tightened with knots on both the radial and ulnar sides of the bone as this construct is more stable than a single knot.[40] Hardware irritation is a concern that often requires hardware removal following fracture healing.[38]

Surgical Technique for Intramedullary Fixation

Simple fixation with a single 6.5-mm cannulated cancellous screw with a washer passed intramedullary down the ulna

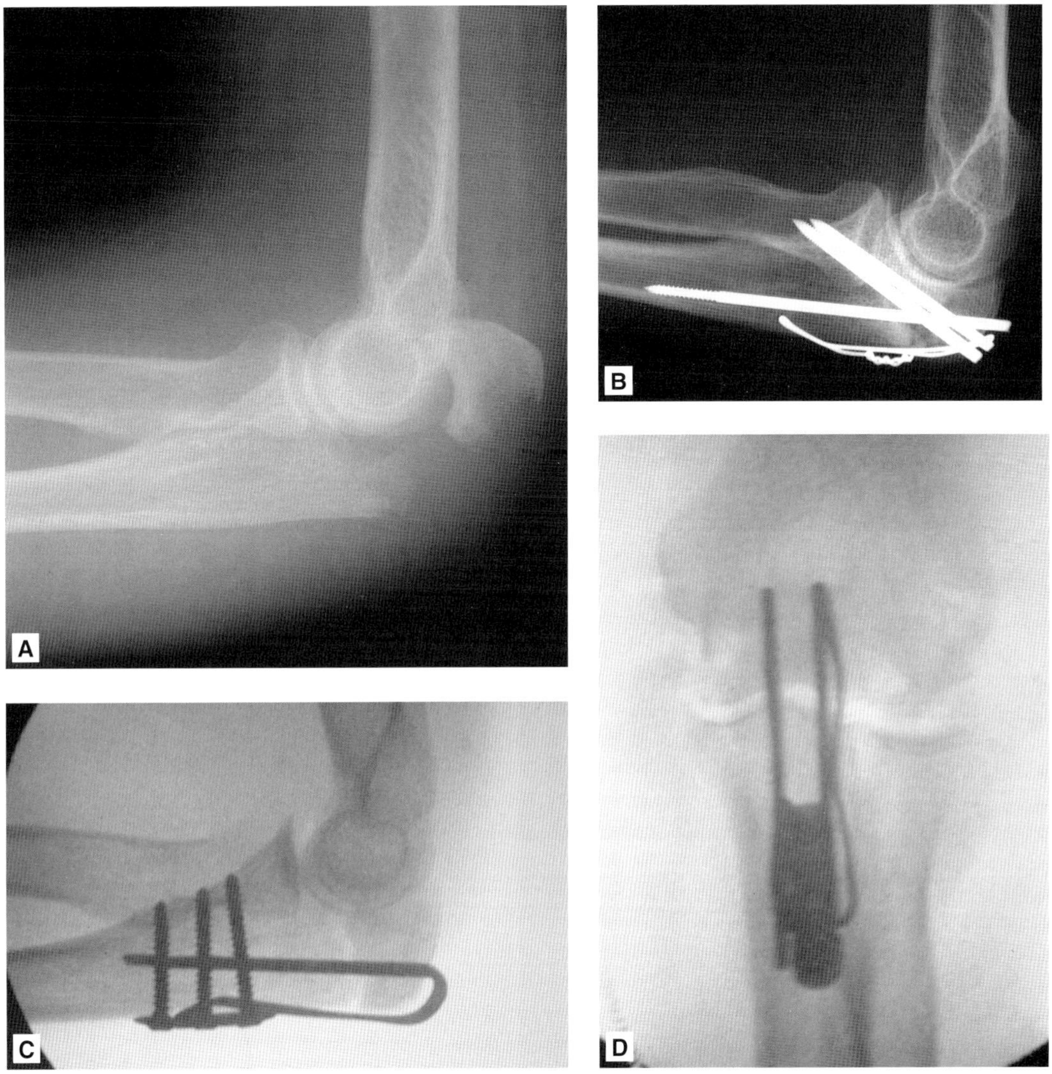

FIGURE 36-9 **A.** Proximal ulnar fracture amenable to (**B**) tension band fixation. **C** and **D.** Use of the Trimed Olecranon Sled™ to fix a transverse fracture of the proximal ulna.

over a guidewire has been described.[36] While this is conceptually easy to do through a small percutaneous incision posteriorly along the olecranon border, its application is limited. The biomechanical strength is less than other described techniques and inadequate for comminuted, oblique, or osteoporotic fractures. Its use is reserved for transverse fractures in bone of adequate density. The Trimed Olecranon Sled™ is a combination of tension band and intramedullary fixation and may also be used for simpler, noncomminuted fractures. Other intramedullary devices, such as the multiscrew OlecraNail™ (Mylad Orthopedic Solutions), are also available.

Surgical Technique for Plate Fixation

Plating affords the highest biomechanical strength of all the constructs.[41] LC-DC plates provide excellent fixation of all types of ulnar fractures and may be used for any Mayo classification, although they are certainly advised for more distal fractures and Monteggia variants. The disadvantage of simpler plate systems is the limited number of screws in the proximal fragment. The construct may be strengthened by applying the plate along the lateral, rather than the posterior, surface of the proximal ulna so that bicortical fixation can be achieved by screws passing lateral to medial in the fragment (taking appropriate precautions for the ulnar nerve). Precontoured plates have a lower profile and more screws can be placed through the proximal fragment.[38] These plates should always be applied directly along the dorsal aspect of the ulna and under compression when the fracture pattern allows. Comminution is readily accommodated by static plate fixation augmented by bone graft as necessary.

The exposure is the same as previously described along the subcutaneous border of the posterior ulna (Fig. 36-10). The plate length should be chosen to accommodate at least 3 screws with 6 cortices on each side of the fracture. The plate should sit directly against bone proximally by splitting the

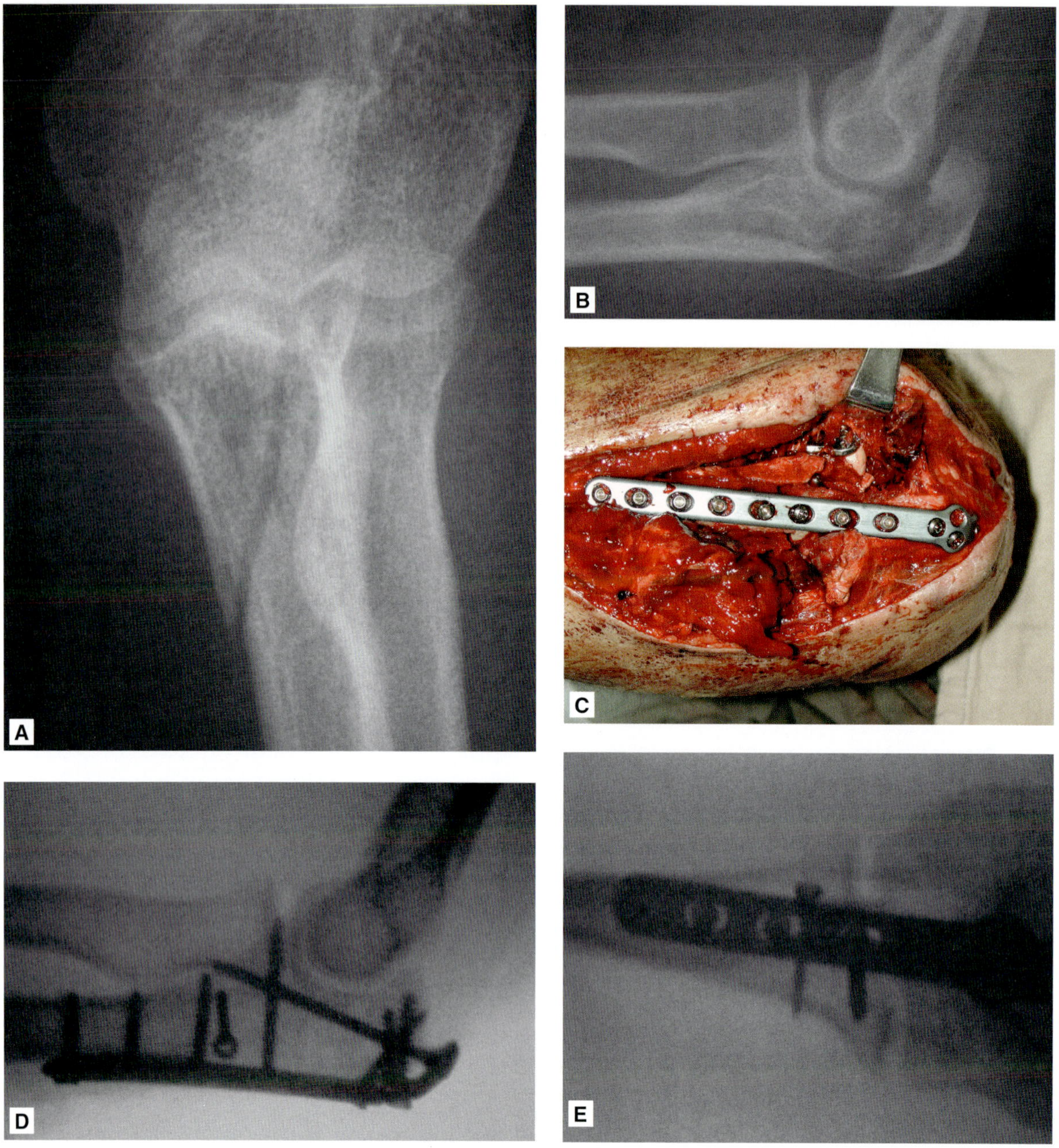

FIGURE 36-10 **A** and **B.** AP and lateral radiographs of a proximal ulnar fracture requiring plate fixation. **C.** Precontoured plate application posteriorly along the ulna and (**D** and **E**) fixation with multiple screws.

triceps fascia. Precontoured plates are easily positioned and may be temporary held with K-wires. 3.5-mm LC-DC plates should be bent to accommodate the curve of the proximal ulna. While site-specific plates are generally strong enough to provide adequate stabilization, the construct may be reinforced by a 90/90 construct with a low-profile plate applied to the lateral surface of the proximal ulna. A lateral plate (which provides good fixation from the coronoid level distally) may also be combined with a tension band construct proximally if fracture-specific precontoured plates are not available.

Surgical Technique for Triceps Advancement

Severely osteoporotic bone may not accommodate adequate fixation to allow early motion. In these elderly patients, function is more readily restored with fragment excision and triceps advancement. Contraindications to this technique include instability, incompetence of the medial ulnar collateral ligament (MUCL), interosseous membrane or DRUJ disruption, and associated coronoid fracture.[41] Up to 50% of the olecranon can be removed without compromising function.

Further resection beyond this level has been shown to have a linear reduction in elbow stability.[36] The triceps is reattached with a nonabsorbable Krakow stitch passed through drill holes in the remaining ulna. The goal is to recreate a congruent transition from triceps tendon to articular surface. This provides greater elbow stability but comes at the expense of a decreased moment arm and weaker extension,[38] although this is well tolerated in the elderly patient population. Resistance exercises are avoided until 12 weeks postoperatively.

Rehabilitation

The patients are initially splinted for 5 to 7 days following fixation and early motion is allowed if fixation is stable. Longer periods of immobilization are recommended if any concern of stability exists. Strengthening is avoided until evidence of healing is seen on radiographs.

Complications

Hardware irritation, more common after tension band fixation, occurs in up to 80% of cases. Its incidence is less with use of plate fixation, but some studies have shown up to 20% of patients still requiring removal after healing.[38]

The incidence of postoperative stiffness is also quite common and should be viewed as less a complication than a consequence of the elbow trauma. The area of pathology is usually quite focal and resection of the posteromedial capsule and posterior MUCL alone will frequently restore full motion.

Nonunion and malunion are uncommon in these injuries with the reported incidence of 1% to 5%. If they do occur, options include fragment excision, revision fixation with compression plating and bone graft, and arthroplasty in select cases of an elderly patient with an unreconstructable injury.[36]

Posttraumatic arthrosis is more likely in proximal ulnar fractures with other associated injuries such as elbow instability, coronoid, or radial head fractures.

MONTEGGIA FRACTURES

Monteggia fractures are defined as traumatic ulnar fractures with dislocation of the radiohumeroulnar joint. This requires disruption of the annular and quadrate ligaments to allow a dissociation of the proximal radioulnar joint. Intact portions of the interosseous membrane and TFCC maintain the alignment of the distal forearm. Reduction of the ulna restores the congruity of the proximal radioulnar joint and, therefore, the radiocapitellar articulation. The outcomes tend to mirror the fracture complexity.[42]

Classification

Despite its limitations, the Bado classification is widely used today. As originally described, Bado type I fractures represent an anterior dislocation of the radial head with any fracture of the ulnar diaphysis at any level. These injuries are more common in children and rare in adults. Bado type II injuries are distinguished by the presence of an anterior ulnar cortical fragment leading to posterior angulation of the ulnar fracture and an associated posterolateral dislocation of the radial head. Bado type III fractures are ulnar metaphyseal fractures with a lateral or anterolateral radial head dislocation and are also more common in children. Finally, a type IV is a fracture of the radius and ulna at the same level proximally with an anterior dislocation of the radial head.

Indications

An anatomic reduction of the ulnar fracture is critical for establishing a stable, congruent articulation of the radioulnar and radiocapitellar joints.[42] Although useful for proximal ulnar fractures, tension band fixation and intramedullary screws are not sufficient to restore adequate stability in Monteggia injuries.[42] Stabilization is best achieved with 3.5-mm LC-DC plates or fracture-specific precontoured plates. These provide a uniform stiffness and flexibility while resisting fatigue failure at extreme bending stresses. The plates should be applied along the lateral or dorsal border of the ulna, with 90/90 fixation reserved for cases that are especially unstable. Theoretically, 90/90 fixation offers the advantage of extra, bicortical fixation in the proximal fragment but, again, requires protection of the ulnar nerve.

Surgical Technique for Internal Fixation

Monteggia fractures are best approached directly along the subcutaneous border of the ulna at the site of injury as described previously. Full-thickness flaps are elevated directly off the bony surface for complete exposure. It is desirable to have at least 3 screws or 6 cortices on each side of the fracture and the plate length should be selected as such. Provisional reduction is readily achieved with reduction clamps as the plate is positioned and held temporarily with K-wires. If the fracture pattern allows, the plate should be applied with compression across the fracture. In comminuted fractures, autogenous corticocancellous bone graft is used to fill any gaps created by comminution.

In the unusual instance of residual incongruity of the radiocapitellar joint, the ulnar fixation should be carefully scrutinized to ensure an appropriate reduction of the fracture and restoration of length. If it is deemed adequate, disruption of the LCL is suspected. An open reduction of the radiocapitellar joint from a lateral approach allows for ligament repair and direct approximation of the radiocapitellar joint.

Associated fractures of the radial head or proximal radius should be approached through a separate lateral, midaxial incision. While it is tempting to treat this through the same posterior incision used to access the ulna, this approach is thought to increase the incidence of proximal radioulnar synostosis.

Rehabilitation

The postoperative management is consistent with that of other fractures about the elbow. An assessment of stability is made intraoperatively and follow-up radiographs are done to confirm the maintenance of a concentric reduction. Bony healing is prioritized over motion and prolonged immobilization may be necessary. No strengthening is started until evidence of healing is evident on x-rays. Loss of pronation and supination is more common than a function-limiting loss of flexion/extension.

CORONOID FRACTURES

The last decade has seen dramatic changes in the treatment of coronoid fractures. Even though they were initially thought to be of little functional importance, the results of nonoperative management have been disappointing.[43] Biomechanical studies have since revealed that even small and apparently insignificant coronoid fractures may be associated with significant elbow instability. The treatment of these injuries has evolved toward operative fixation.[43]

Classification

The earliest adopted classification of coronoid fractures by Regan and Morrey utilized a lateral x-ray of the elbow to classify these fractures based on morphology. Type I fractures represent a small fleck of bone off the tip of the coronoid. Type II fractures involve less than 50% of the coronoid process while type III are coronoid base fractures involving more than 50%. Due to its simplicity, this system is still widely used but fails to incorporate oblique fracture patterns such as the anteromedial or anterolateral facet fractures that often require operative treatment.[44] Furthermore, the treatment recommendations derived from this study may not always apply because it was performed in elbows with intact ligaments. This is rarely the case in a true, clinical coronoid fracture and the incidence of instability may be underestimated.

Indications

The coronoid is critical for elbow stability. In conjunction with the radial head, it acts as an anterior buttress to prevent posterior dislocation of the elbow.[45] The only other structure restraining anterior displacement of the humerus on the ulna is the posterior MUCL and the posteromedial capsule, which are frequently ruptured in elbow fracture dislocations. Even small tip fractures (type I) are shearing or avulsion fractures that, in the adult, imply some degree of ulnohumeral or radiocapitellar instability with an associated ligament injury. Attempts to quantify the percentage of coronoid involvement that requires fixation to restore stability have been conflicting and it is likely that the ligamentous

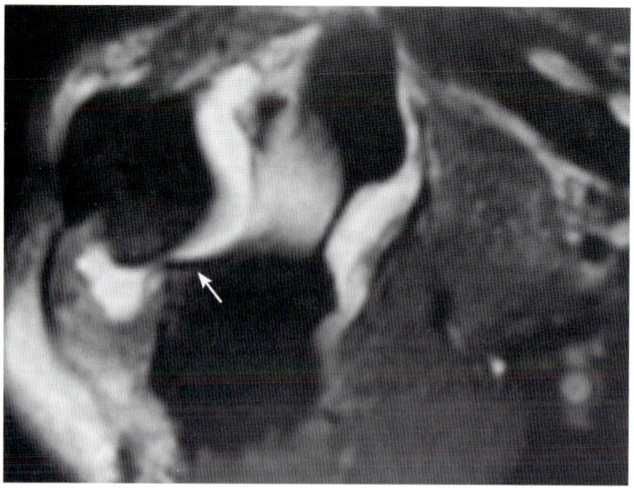

FIGURE 36-11 A "sag sign" seen in cross-sectional tomographic images indicates posteromedial (seen here) or posterolateral rotatory instability, depending upon whether the abnormal joint opening is medial or lateral.

disruption in the setting of a type I or II fracture is the more critical determinant.[46] These injuries should be approached cautiously and careful clinical and radiographic examination for any ulnohumeral instability is mandatory. The surgeon should also determine the direction of instability, for example, posterolateral or posteromedial. This can frequently be gleaned from the axial cuts of a CT scan looking for a "sag sign" in the olecranon fossa (Fig. 36-11) to determine the direction of displacement.

Type II and III fractures should be assumed unstable until proven otherwise and treated surgically. Fractures of the anteromedial facet are indicative of varus posteromedial instability. They require fixation with a buttress plate as the only other stabilizers against posteromedial rotatory subluxation are the posterior MUCL and posteromedial capsule.[44]

The surgical approach is dependent on not only the size and location of the coronoid fragment but also the choice of fixation and need for exposure. A preoperative CT scan is invaluable in evaluating the extent of injury and surgical planning.

Surgical Technique for Open Reduction Internal Fixation of Coronoid Fractures

The patient is positioned supine with the elbow flexed over the body and held with a positioner (Fig. 36-12). A single midline posterior or separate medial and lateral incisions may be used as described above. The ulnar nerve is exposed and decompressed. It may be transposed at the conclusion of case depending on the surgeon's preference. The origin of the flexor-pronator mass is exposed at the medial epicondyle and carefully elevated off the ulna in a distal to proximal direction to expose the sublime tubercle, coronoid process,

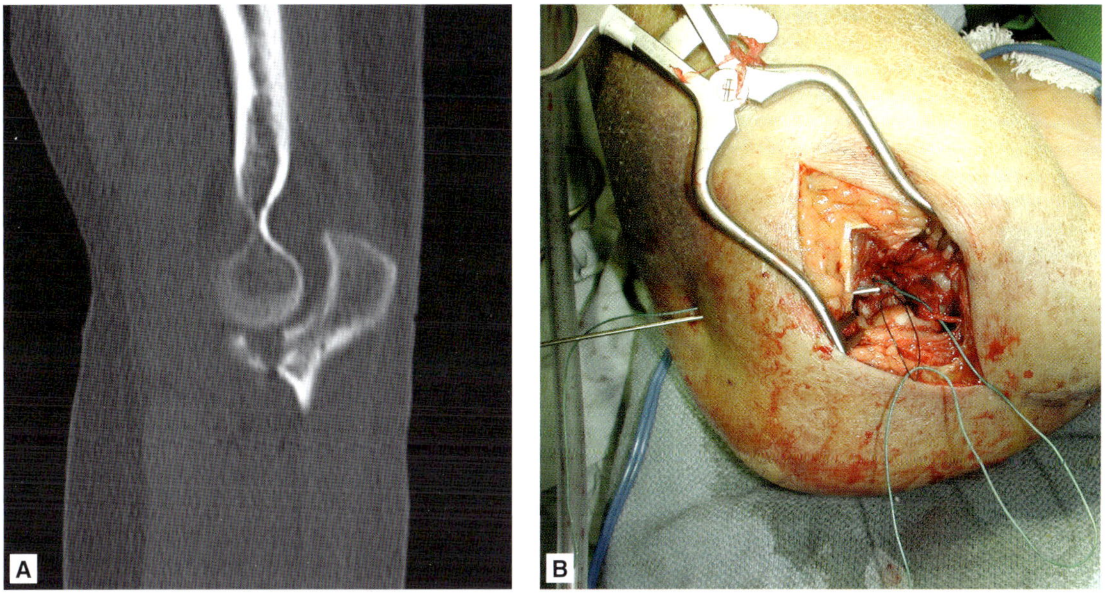

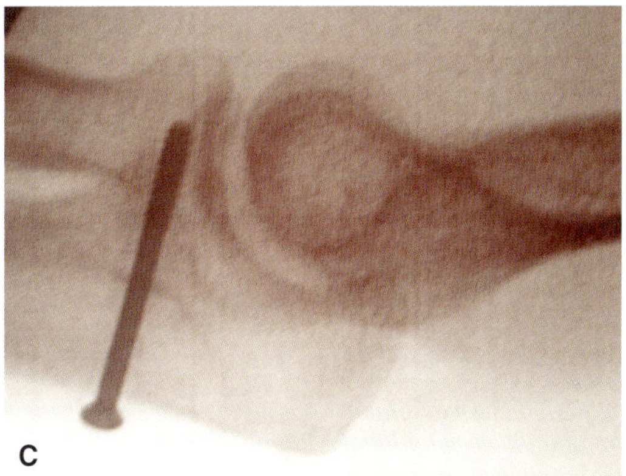

FIGURE 36-12 Coronoid fracture fixation. **A.** CT of coronoid fx demonstrates posterior subluxation of the joint. **B.** Suture lasso fixation of a coronoid fracture. The Hewson suture passer is used to shuttle the sutures posteriorly. They are tied over arthroscopic sliding knots to secure the fragment under compression. **C.** In larger fragments, screws may be inserted through the same approach over guidewires.

and the medial collateral ligament. Dissecting from distal to proximal simplifies the procedure as there is a clear transition from the distal muscle portion to the fibrous MUCL insertion on the sublime tubercle.[47] Provisional stabilization is accomplished with reduction clamps or K-wires. This approach allows for placement of a buttress plate directly against the posteromedial facet or screw fixation. If the fragment is large enough, partially threaded cannulated screws are placed over guidewires through the posterior ulna. An ACL guide will assist with aligning the guidewires to penetrate the posterior ulnar cortex into the center of the fragment while reduction is held. These wires should angle slightly from distal posterior to proximal anterior in the coronoid so that distally directed forces on the coronoid from the trochlea tend to compress, rather than distract, across the fracture site. Two screws are preferred if the fragment size allows (3.0 or 3.5 mm). Fluoroscopy should be used to confirm guidewire and screw placement and concentric reduction. The LCL is repaired to its origin from the anteroinferior aspect of the lateral epicondyle at its isometric point using a braided, Kevlar-reinforced suture. The MUCL should be reconstructed rather than repaired if torn, but this will not protect against posteromedial rotatory instability that, if present, is an indication for supplemental static external fixation to ensure a stable, concentric reduction.

Surgical Technique for Suture Lasso

This is the preferred technique if the fragment is severely comminuted or too small to accommodate screw fixation or buttress plating (Fig. 36-12). The exposure is done as above or through the classic medial over-the-top approach or the proximally extended lateral approach, depending on the configuration of the fracture and the need to treat associated injuries, such as a radial head fracture. A Kevlar-reinforced suture is passed over the top of the coronoid fragment and through its attached anterior capsule. A free needle is then used to pass each limb of the suture through the base of the fracture and out the posterior cortex of the ulna.[47] These sutures are tied along the subcutaneous border of the posterior ulna to secure the fragment.

Surgical Technique for Anterolateral or Anteromedial Coronoid Fractures

Anterolateral fragments may be accessible from an extended anterolateral exposure, particularly if the radial head is removed for replacement (Fig. 36-13). The lateral midaxial incision is extended proximally and the ECRB and, if necessary, a portion of the brachioradialis is reflected from the humerus being mindful of the radial nerve. Fixation by lag screws or a circlage suture may then be performed. Hardware should always be angled slightly in a distal to proximal direction to permit maximal coronoid fragment purchase and to

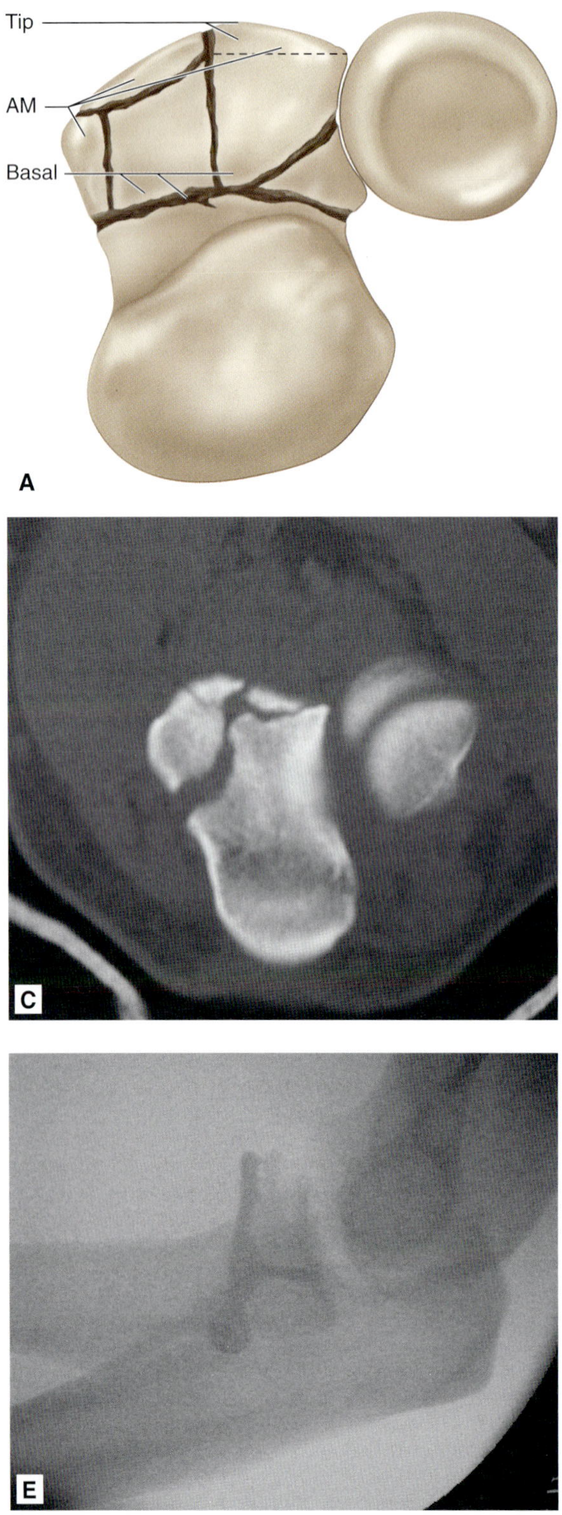

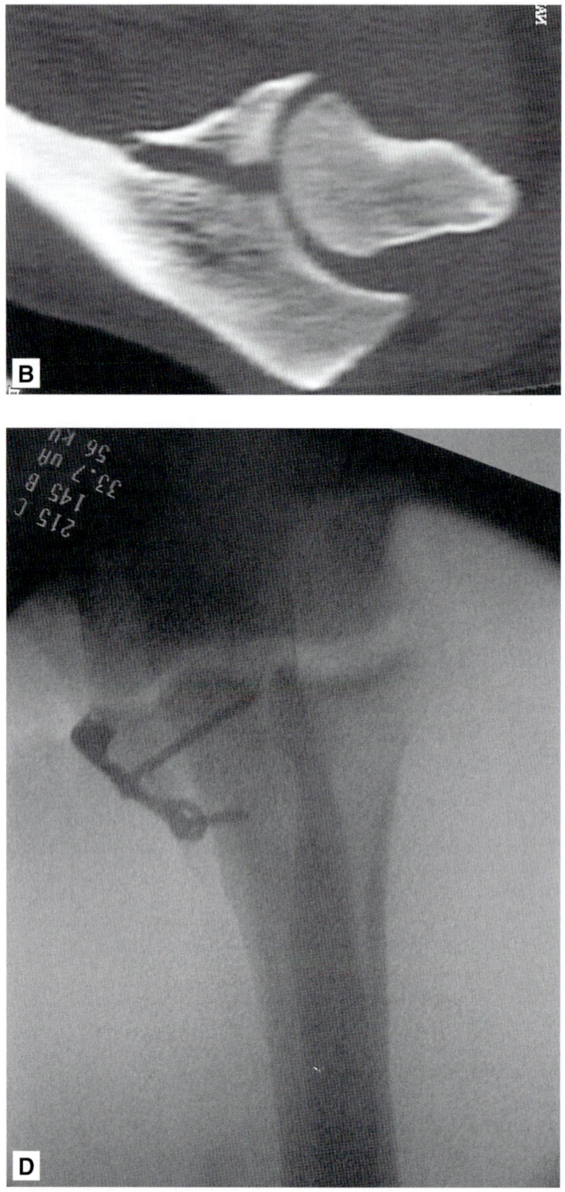

FIGURE 36-13 Oblique coronoid fractures. **A.** Additional fracture patterns are easily missed on plain x-rays, (Reproduced with permission from O'Driscoll SW, Jupiter J, Cohen MS, Ring D, McKee MD. Difficult elbow fractures: pearls and pitfalls. In: Ferlic DC, ed. *Instructional Course Lectures*, Vol 52. Rosemont, IL: American Academy of Orthopaedic Surgeons; 2003.) but (**B** and **C**) CT scan clearly demonstrates the oblique pattern of injury. **D** and **E.** Fixation with a buttress plate supports the fracture and stabilizes against posteromedial rotatory instability.

"trap" the coronoid fragment between the anterior surface of the proximal ulna and the screw, thus providing a buttress against distal displacement.

Anteromedial facet fragments must be approached through the medial side and are fixed with a buttress plate. The interval depends on the size of the fragment, but access to the entire medial border of the proximal ulna may be needed. This can be done by splitting the flexor-pronator mass and reflecting anterior and posterior muscles groups, or by reflecting the entire flexor-pronator mass from the humerus and proximal ulna anteriorly with the ulnar nerve included in the musculotendinous bundle. In some circumstances, the surgeon may also take advantage of concomitant fractures of the radial head or proximal ulna to use as viewing portals through which to treat the coronoid.

However it is approached and fixed, the overarching goal is stable restoration of the ulnohumeral joint. Fixation of the coronoid alone is often not enough in the presence of other injured structures. Ligament repair or reconstruction, radial head fixation or replacement, and proximal ulnar fixation may all be necessary along with supplemental static external fixation.

Arthroscopic Fixation of the Coronoid

Transverse fractures of the coronoid tip and anterolateral fractures are amenable to arthroscopic fixation (Fig. 36-14). This imparts additional stability to the elbow with minimal surgical trauma.

The standard anteromedial and anterolateral portals are established. Evacuation of the hematoma with a 3.5-mm shaver in the anteromedial portal will generally permit adequate visualization of the coronoid. Debridement of significant synovitis along the anterior capsule may also be necessary. This is most often the difficult portion of the procedure, particularly with soft tissue swelling and capsular avulsion. A few extra minutes spent debriding this area to achieve good visualization is invaluable, as is the use of retractors. Low inflow pressures (<30 mm Hg) will minimize swelling and prolong working time. A small, modified skin hook is then introduced through the anteromedial portal to grab and reduce the coronoid fragment. It should be remembered that the coronoid will fit intimately against the trochlea when properly reduced. Fluoroscopy is used to determine the optimal entrance site for the cannulated screw guidewires along the posterior cortex of the proximal ulna aiming to pass into the coronoid. These wires should angle slightly from distal posterior to proximal anterior in the coronoid. A drill guide, if available, is also helpful.

If the fragment is of sufficient size to pass 2 partially threaded cannulated screws (3.0 or 3.5 mm), this is the preferred fixation. It should be further reinforced with a circlage loop of suture passed through the screws to achieve a mattress suture effect, much like an umbrella embracing the tip of the fragment. Most fractures, however, will not accept 2 screws. Therefore, a single screw should be placed to target the center of the largest fragment dimension. The correct position of the wires is confirmed with fluoroscopy and direct visualization through the arthroscope. The guidewire is then grasped with a locking arthroscopic forceps as the cannulated drill bores a tunnel through the bone. This will prevent inadvertent extraction as well as stabilize and compress the fragment to the coronoid base. A partially threaded cannulated screw is selected and should be slightly undersized to maintain 1 mm of bone between the cortex of the coronoid and the screw. This will avoid abrasion of the sutures against the screw.

The fixation is then reinforced with the circlage sutures passed through the cannulated screws into the joint. Depending on the orientation of the fracture, these sutures will be passed down the border of the coronoid medially or laterally. If there are 2 screws, passage of the suture is straightforward and a #2 Kevlar-reinforced suture may be shuttled through the screws. If the size of the fragment does not permit the use of 2 screws, the suture is passed through the screw and is then shuttled either laterally, using an 18-gauge spinal needle passed through the proximal radioulnar joint, or medially, deep to the flexor-pronator mass and ulnar nerve. Great care must be taken in passing the medial circlage suture due to the proximity of the nerve. A small Freer elevator with a hole drilled in it is preloaded with the 28-gauge wire. It is passed exactly along the medial bone of the proximal ulna ensuring it is deep to the ulnar nerve. The wire is then used to shuttle out the circlage suture. Sliding knots are used to cinch the sutures tightly along the posterior border of the ulna. No adverse effects have been noted from an intra-articular suture of this type, although the knot on the posterior border of the proximal ulna can be irritating. If this is the case, the sutures are easily removed once the fracture has healed.

ELBOW INSTABILITY AND ASSOCIATED FRACTURES ("TERRIBLE TRIAD")

As outlined above, coronoid fractures are frequently associated with elbow instability. Any fixation of the coronoid should therefore include an evaluation and repair of a torn LCL. Depending on the fracture pattern, disruption of the posterior medial collateral ligament may be involved as well. In the event of persistent instability despite adequate fixation and repair, a static external fixator is applied to stabilize the ulnohumeral joint. Note that the anterior band of the MUCL is the primary stabilizer against valgus forces, but cannot prevent posteromedial rotatory instability. Hence, even MUCL reconstruction would not prevent this problem. Under no circumstances is it acceptable to leave the operating room with a subluxed joint.

The combination of an elbow dislocation, radial head fracture, and coronoid fracture is commonly referred to as the "terrible triad" in light of its notoriously poor outcome. Posttraumatic arthritis, recurrent instability, chronic pain, and functional deficits are common long term. Although its

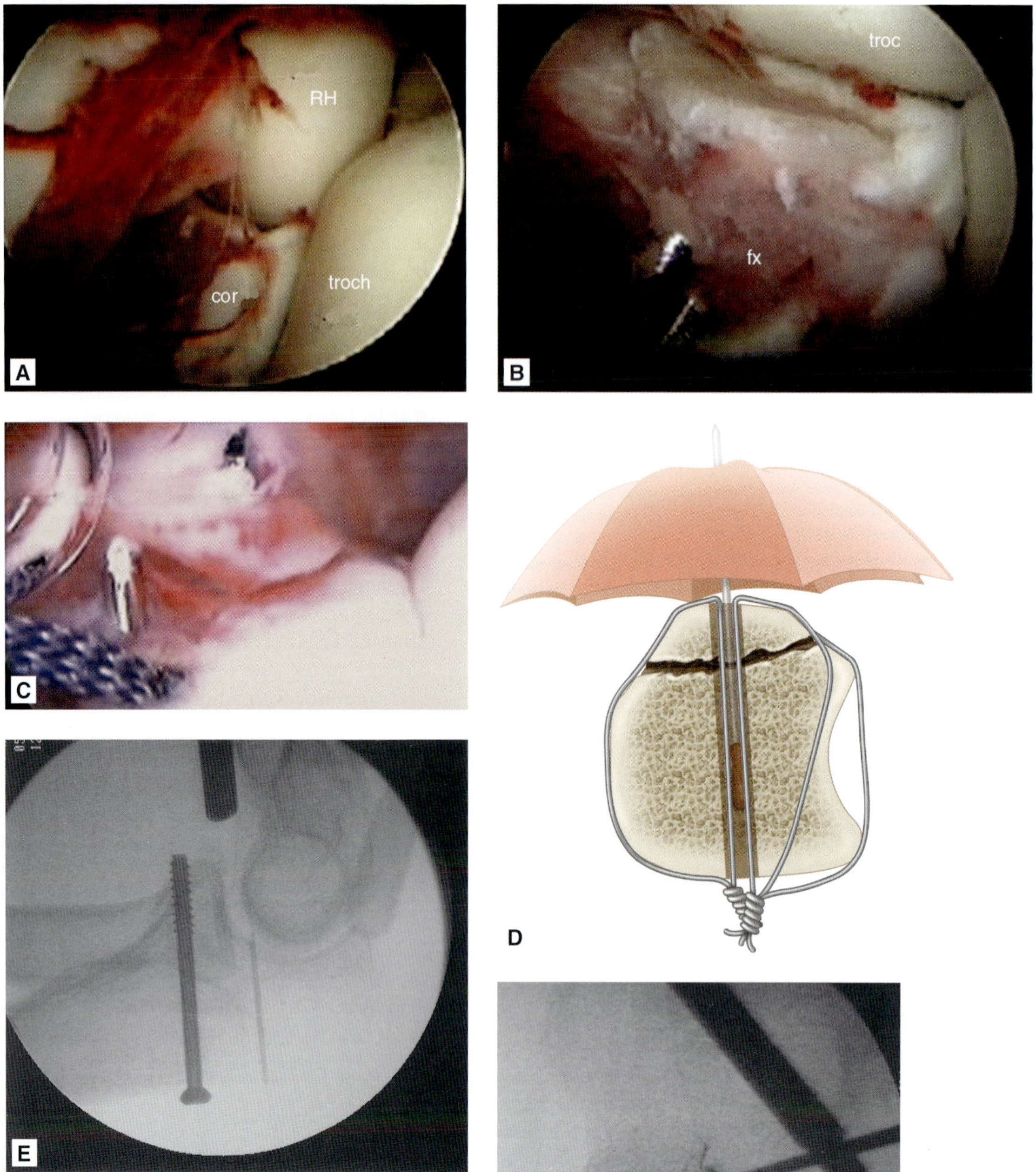

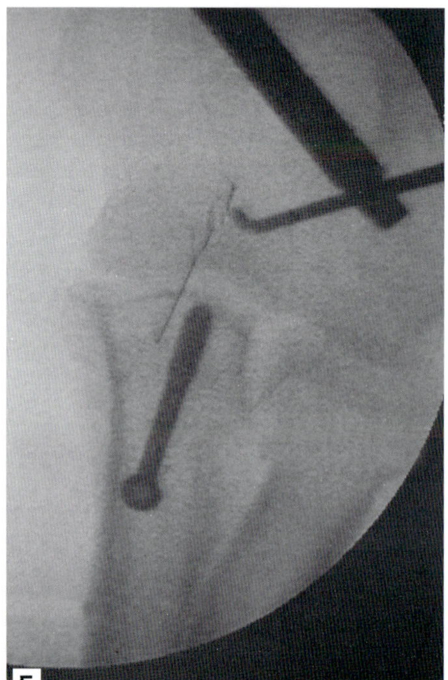

FIGURE 36-14 Arthroscopic coronoid fixation. **A.** The coronoid fracture is visualized and (**B**) guidewires are directed from the posterior proximal ulna to the base of the coronoid. The tip of the coronoid is then reduced and, under arthroscopic visualization, a guidewire and cannulated screw are placed in the coronoid from the subcutaneous border of the proximal ulna. Fluoroscopy helps determine the approximate entrance point. A second, medial hole is drilled over another guidewire for passage of a circlage suture using a suture retriever or 28-gauge wire. **C** and **D.** A Kevlar-reinforced suture is passed through the cannulated screw and through the second hole, and then exiting to the posterior border of the ulna. **E** and **F.** The coronoid circlage suture is tied after ORIF of the radial head using an arthroscopic sliding knot. The radial head fracture is then fixed through a small, lateral approach. cor, coronoid; fx, fracture line; RH, radial head; troch, trochlea.

complexity can be daunting, a systematic approach to treatment simplifies this and provides a more dependable and reproducible method of appropriate fixation. McKee et al described a standard protocol to approaching these injuries. It includes initial fixation or replacement of the radial head, fixation of the coronoid fracture, repair of the LCL complex, and, for residual instability, reconstruction of the medial collateral ligament and/or application of an external fixator[48] (Fig. 36-15). Persistent posteromedial instability or marginal fixation of the anteromedial coronoid fragment is an indication for static external fixation in order to achieve the primary goal of a stable, reduced elbow.[44] Motion can

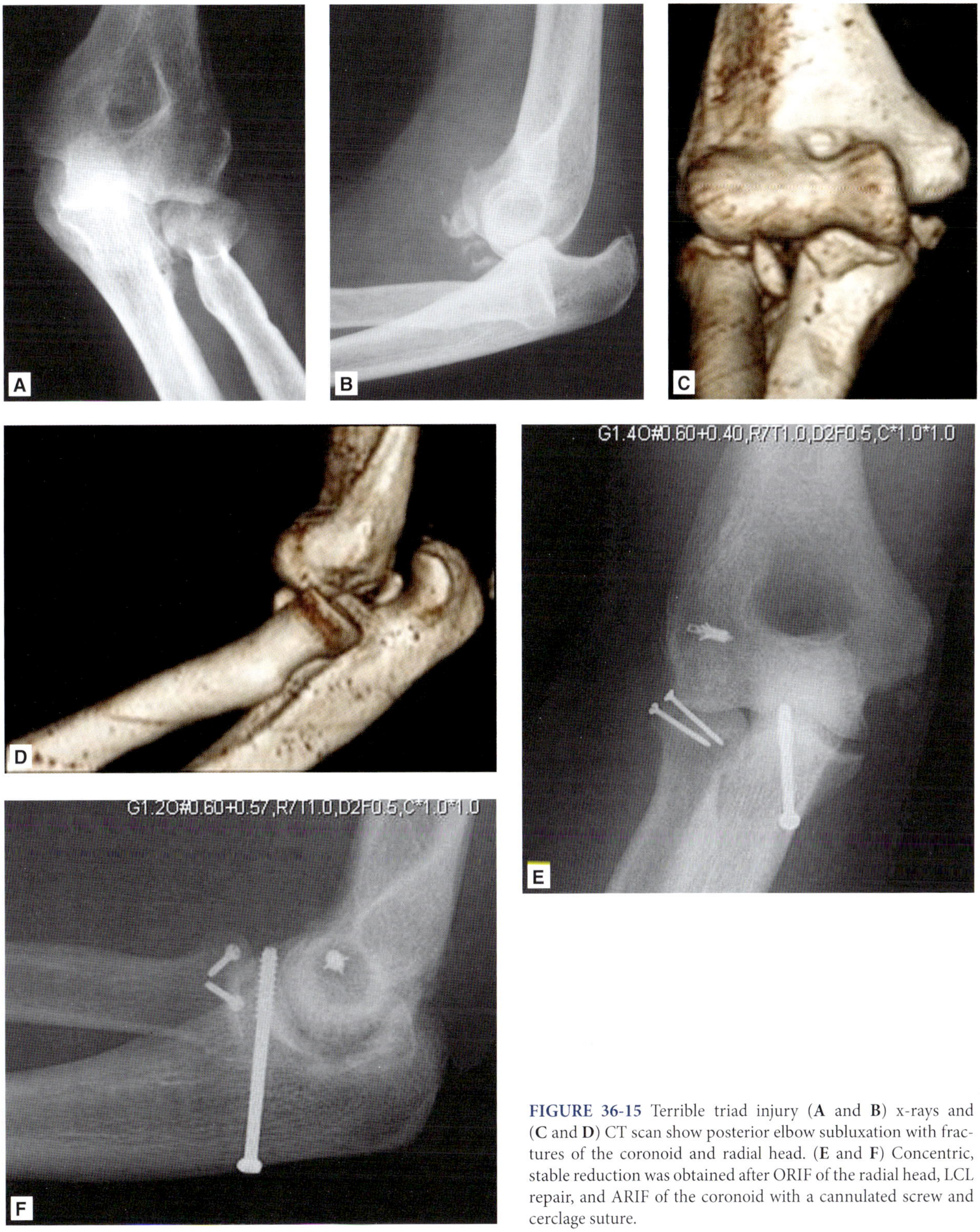

FIGURE 36-15 Terrible triad injury (**A** and **B**) x-rays and (**C** and **D**) CT scan show posterior elbow subluxation with fractures of the coronoid and radial head. (**E** and **F**) Concentric, stable reduction was obtained after ORIF of the radial head, LCL repair, and ARIF of the coronoid with a cannulated screw and cerclage suture.

be reliably restored by means of subsequent arthroscopic or open release if necessary, but an unstable elbow is an intractable problem.

If an external fixator is needed, many authors advocate dynamic external fixation to allow for some postoperative motion and the technique is well described.[49] While conceptually attractive, this requires perfect placement of the central pin through the axis of rotation, something far easier to describe than perform. Any deviation from this axis will unevenly distribute the load across the joint creating abnormal stress at a focal region or hinging the joint into a subluxed position and compromising fixation. As we discussed in the treatment of distal humerus fractures, our preference is to prioritize stability over motion and it is our practice to apply a static external fixator, if needed, and plan on staged contracture release once injured structures have healed.

Complications

As with the other fractures, common complications include ulnar nerve palsy, heterotopic ossification, stiffness, and posttraumatic arthrosis. While some element of posttraumatic arthrosis is probably inevitable, stable well-aligned joints have been shown to degenerate to a lesser degree.[45] Stiffness, likewise, is common but less problematic with the current success of contracture release. Recurrent subluxation is a feared complication but preventable with careful attention to each aspect of fixation.

CONCLUSION

A changing paradigm for treatment of elbow fractures and fracture/dislocations, combined with improved instrumentation, implants, and surgical technique, has improved the results of these challenging injuries.[4,10,13,42–44,48] Prioritizing healing and a stable, congruent reduction over early motion may require a staged contracture release, but helps avoid nonunion, avascular necrosis, or stiffness with instability, for which there are no good solutions.

REFERENCES

1. Hsu JW, Gould JL, Fonseca-Sabune H, Hausman MR. The emerging role of elbow arthroscopy in chronic use injuries and fracture care. *Hand Clin.* 2009;25:305–321.
2. Robinson CM, Hill RM, Jacobs N, Dall G, Court-Brown CM. Adult distal humeral metaphyseal fractures: epidemiology and results of treatment. *J Orthop Trauma.* 2003;17:38–47.
3. Hausman MR, Panozzo A. Treatment of distal humerus fractures in the elderly. *Clin Orthop Relat Res.* 2004;425:55–63.
4. Nauth A, McKee MD, Ristevski B, Hall J, Schemitsch EH. Distal humeral fractures in adults. *J Bone Joint Surg Am.* 2011;93:686–700.
5. Zagorski JB, Jennings JJ, Burkhalter WE, Uribe JW. Comminuted intraarticular fractures of the distal humeral condyles: surgical vs. nonsurgical treatment. *Clin Orthop Relat Res.* 1986;202:197–204.
6. Helfet DL, Hotchkiss RN. Internal fixation of the distal humerus: a biomechanical comparison of methods. *J Orthop Trauma.* 1990;4:260–264.
7. Sanchez-Sotelo J, Tochia ME, O'Driscoll SW. Principle-based internal fixation of distal humerus fractures. *Tech Hand Up Extrem Surg.* 2001;5:179–187.
8. Zalavras CG, Vercillo MT, Jun B, Otarodifard K, Itamura JM, Lee TQ. Biomechanical evaluation of parallel versus orthogonal plate fixation of intra-articular distal humerus fractures. *J Shoulder Elbow Surg.* 2011;20:12–20.
9. McKee MD, Veillette CJ, Hall JA, et al. A multicenter, prospective, randomized, controlled trial of open reduction-internal fixation versus total elbow arthroplasty for displaced intra-articular distal humeral fractures in elderly patients. *J Shoulder Elbow Surg.* 2009;18:3–12.
10. O'Driscoll SW. Optimizing stability in distal humeral fracture fixation. *J Shoulder Elbow Surg.* 2005;14(1 suppl S):186S–194S.
11. Wiggers JK, Brouwer KM, Helmerhorst GT, Ring D. Predictors of diagnosis of ulnar neuropathy after surgically treated distal humerus fractures. *J Hand Surg Am.* 2012;37:1168–1172.
12. Hamid N, Ashraf N, Bosse MJ, et al. Radiation therapy for heterotopic ossification prophylaxis acutely after elbow trauma: a prospective randomized study. *J Bone Joint Surg Am.* 2010;92:2032–2038.
13. Pike JM, Athwal GS, Faber KJ, King GJW. Radial head fractures—an update. *J Hand Surg Am.* 2009;34:557–565.
14. Herbertsson P, Josefsson PO, Hasserius R, Karlsson C, Besjakov J, Karlsson MK. Displaced Mason type I fractures of the radial head and neck in adults: a fifteen- to thirty-three-year follow-up study. *J Shoulder Elbow Surg.* 2005;14:73–77.
15. van Riet RP, Morrey BF. Documentation of associated injuries occurring with radial head fracture. *Clin Orthop Relat Res.* 2008;466:130–134.
16. Hotchkiss RN. Displaced fractures of the radial head: internal fixation or excision? *J Am Acad Orthop Surg.* 1997;5:1–10.
17. Morrey BF, Tanaka S, An KN. Valgus stability of the elbow. A definition of primary and secondary constraints. *Clin Orthop Relat Res.* 1991;265:187–195.
18. Ring D, Quintero J, Jupiter JB. Open reduction and internal fixation of fractures of the radial head. *J Bone Joint Surg Am.* 2002;84:1811–1815.
19. Beingessner DM, Dunning CE, Gordon KD, Johnson JA, King GJ. The effect of radial head fracture size on elbow kinematics and stability. *J Orthop Relat Res.* 2005;23:210–217.
20. Caputo AE, Mazzocca AD, Santoro VM. The nonarticulating portion of the radial head: anatomic and clinical correlations for internal fixation. *J Hand Surg Am.* 1998;23:1082–1090.
21. Smith AM, Morrey BF, Steinmann SP. Low profile fixation of radial head and neck fractures: surgical technique and clinical experience. *J Orthop Trauma.* 2007;21:718–724.
22. Michels F, Pouliart N, Handelberg F. Arthroscopic management of Mason type 2 radial head fractures. *Knee Surg Sports Traumatol Arthrosc.* 2007;15:1244–1250.
23. Vanderwilde RS, Morrey BF, Melberg MW, Vinh TN. Inflammatory arthritis after failure of silicone rubber replacement of the radial head. *J Bone Joint Surg Br.* 1994;76:78–81.
24. Maghen Y, Leo AJ, Hsu JW, Hausman MR. Is a silastic radial head still a reasonable option? *Clin Orthop Relat Res.* 2011;469:1061–1070.
25. Popovic N, Lemaire R, Georis P, Gillet P. Midterm results with a bipolar radial head prosthesis: radiographic evidence of loosening at the bone–cement interface. *J Bone Joint Surg Am.* 2007;89:2469–2476.
26. Van Riet RP, Van Glabbeek F, Verborgt O, Gielen J. Capitellar erosion caused by a metal radial head prosthesis: a case report. *J Bone Joint Surg Am.* 2004;86:1061–1064.
27. Athwal GS, Frank SG, Grewal R, Faber KJ, Johnson J, King GJW. Determination of correct implant size in radial head arthroplasty to avoid overlengthening: surgical technique. *J Bone Joint Surg Am.* 2010;92(suppl 1) (part 2):250–257.
28. Herbertsson P, Josefsson PO, Hasserius R, Besjakov J, Nyqvist F, Karlsson MK. Fractures of the radial head and neck treated with radial head excision. *J Bone Joint Surg Am.* 2004;86:1925–1930.
29. Hardy P, Menguy F, Guillot S. Arthroscopic treatment of capitellum fracture of the humerus. *Arthroscopy.* 2002;18:422–426.
30. Guitton TG, Doornberg JN, Raaymakers EL, Ring D, Kloen P. Fractures of the capitellum and trochlea. *J Bone Joint Surg Am.* 2009;91:390–397.
31. McKee MD, Jupiter JB, Bamberger HB. Coronal shear fractures of the distal end of the humerus. *J Bone Joint Surg Am.* 1996;78:49–54.
32. Dubberley JH, Faber KJ, MacDermid JC, Patterson SD, King GJ. Outcome after open reduction and internal fixation of capitellar and trochlear fractures. *J Bone Joint Surg Am.* 2006;88:46–54.

33. Ruchelsman DE, Tejwani NC, Kwon YW, Egol KA. Coronal plane partial articular fractures of the distal humerus: current concepts in management. *J Am Acad Orthop Surg*. 2008;16:716–728.
34. Brouwer KM, Bolmers A, Ring D. Quantitative 3-dimensional computed tomography measurement of distal humerus fractures. *J Shoulder Elbow Surg*. 2012;21:977–982 [Epub ahead of print].
35. Elkowitz SJ, Polatsch DB, Egol KA, Kummer FJ, Koval KJ. Capitellum fractures: a biomechanical evaluation of three fixation methods. *J Orthop Trauma*. 2002;16(7):503–506.
36. Newman SD, Mauffrey C, Krikler S. Olecranon fractures. *Injury*. 2009;40:575–581.
37. Morrey BF. Current concepts in the treatment of fractures of the radial head, the olecranon, and the coronoid. *Instr Course Lect*. 1995;44:175–185.
38. Veillette CJ, Steinmann SP. Olecranon fractures. *Orthop Clin North Am*. 2008;39:229–236.
39. Parker JR, Conroy J, Campbell DA. Anterior interosseous nerve injury following tension band wiring of the olecranon. *Injury*. 2005;36:1252–1253.
40. Fyfe IS, Mossad MM, Holdsworth BJ. Methods of fixation of olecranon fractures. An experimental mechanical study. *J Bone Joint Surg Br*. 1985;67:367–372.
41. Hak DJ, Golladay GJ. Olecranon fractures: treatment options. *J Am Acad Orthop Surg*. 2000;8:266–275.
42. Eathiraju S, Mudgal CS, Jupiter JB. Monteggia fracture–dislocations. *Hand Clin*. 2007;23:165–177.
43. Doornberg JN, Ring DC. Fracture of the anteromedial facet of the coronoid process. *J Bone Joint Surg Am*. 2006;88:2216–2224.
44. O'Driscoll SW, Jupiter JB, Cohen MS, Ring D, McKee MD. Difficult elbow fractures: pearls and pitfalls. *Instr Course Lect*. 2003;52: 113–134.
45. Ring D. Fractures of the coronoid process of the ulna. *J Hand Surg Am*. 2006;31:1679–1689.
46. Schneeberger AG, Sadowski MM, Jacob HA. Coronoid process and radial head as posterolateral rotatory stabilizers of the elbow. *J Bone Joint Surg Am*. 2004;86:975–982.
47. Steinmann SP. Coronoid process fracture. *J Am Acad Orthop Surg*. 2008;16:519–529.
48. McKee MD, Pugh DM, Wild LM, Schemitsh EH, King GJ. Standard surgical protocol to treat elbow dislocations with radial head and coronoid fractures. *J Bone Joint Surg Am*. 2004;86:1122–1130.
49. Pennig D, Gausepohl T, Mader K. Transarticular fixation with the capacity for motion in fracture dislocations of the elbow. *Injury*. 2000;31(suppl 1):35–44.

37

Simple Elbow Dislocations—A Practical Guide

Michael A.C. Lapner, MD, FRCSC
George S. Athwal, MD, FRCSC

RATIONALE AND BASIC SCIENCE

The elbow is a trochoginglymoid joint with motion occurring in flexion–extension and pronation–supination arcs.[1] Stability is conferred by the unique osteology of 3 articulations: the distal humerus and proximal ulna, proximal radius and ulna, and radiocapitellar joints. Soft tissues play an important role in stability through ligaments, joint capsule, common extensor origin, and flexor pronator mass (Fig. 37-1).[1–5] The medial collateral ligament has 3 bundles: anterior, posterior, and transverse. The anterior bundle, a primary elbow stabilizer, is important in resisting valgus stresses.[1,6–8] The lateral collateral ligament comprises the lateral ulnar collateral (LUCL), radial collateral ligament (RCL), and annular ligament. The LUCL, another primary stabilizer, imparts stabilization during varus stress and in the setting of posterolateral rotatory instability.[5] The RCL stabilizes the ulnohumeral and radiocapitellar joints while the annular ligament stabilizes the proximal radioulnar joint (PRUJ). The common extensor origin and flexor pronator mass are dynamic secondary stabilizers.[5]

Simple elbow dislocations are soft tissue injuries lacking fractures. A dislocation is still considered simple if small coronoid tip fractures or fleck avulsions of the collateral ligaments are present.[9]

EPIDEMIOLOGY AND MECHANISM OF INJURY

The elbow is the second most commonly dislocated joint and 10% to 25% of all elbow injuries include dislocation.[1,10–12] Simple dislocations comprise 51% to 74% of all dislocations.[1,10] In a recent study the incidence of simple dislocations was 5 per 100,000 person years, with the highest risk at ages 10 to 19. There was an almost equal risk of dislocation in all other age brackets. Posterior or posterolateral dislocations are most common,[1,13] while anterior are rare, and divergent even less common.[1,13] Associated injuries are not uncommon and include proximal humerus, distal radius and ulna, perilunate, and scaphoid fractures.[3]

Classification is based on the direction of the dislocation and commonly includes posterior, lateral, medial, anterior, and divergent. Dislocations can also be classified as acute, subacute (2-6 weeks), and chronic (>6 weeks).[9]

The mechanism of injury is typically a fall on an outstretched hand.[1] An axial force is applied through the flexed, valgus joint with the forearm in supination. It is theorized that a progressive soft tissue failure occurs from lateral to medial: first the LCL is disrupted followed by the anterior capsule, and lastly the MCL.[5,11] The Horii ring of elbow instability includes 3 stages. Stage 1 involves disruption of the ulnar component of the LCL with a posterolateral subluxation and reduction is spontaneous. Stage 2 occurs with progressive disruption both anteriorly and posteriorly with an incomplete posterolateral dislocation, termed perched. Stage 3 is divided into 3a (anterior bundle of MCL intact) and 3b, all soft tissues disrupted. Dislocation is the final sequence of the stages.[5]

Postreduction radiographs must be scrutinized for fractures including those of the radial head, capitellum, or coronoid. The congruence of the joint must be assessed. The drop sign may be the only radiographic indication of a reduced dislocation (Fig. 37-2). The drop sign measures the distance from the trochlear sulcus to the olecranon articular surface and increased values are suggestive of instability.[14] Radiographs may also reveal a subtle impaction injury called the Osborne-Cotterill lesion.[15] This osseous defect occurs on the posterolateral aspect of capitellum, caused by the dislocated radial head.[16]

The management of an elbow dislocation begins with a history, physical examination, and plain radiograph evaluation. Computed tomography may be utilized if further osseous assessment is required. Reduction of the dislocation is generally performed under conscious sedation; however, local anesthetic, general anesthesia, or regional anesthesia may also be used. Fluoroscopy is beneficial in determining postreduction stability and for the reduction maneuver. Various methods of reduction have been described. For the

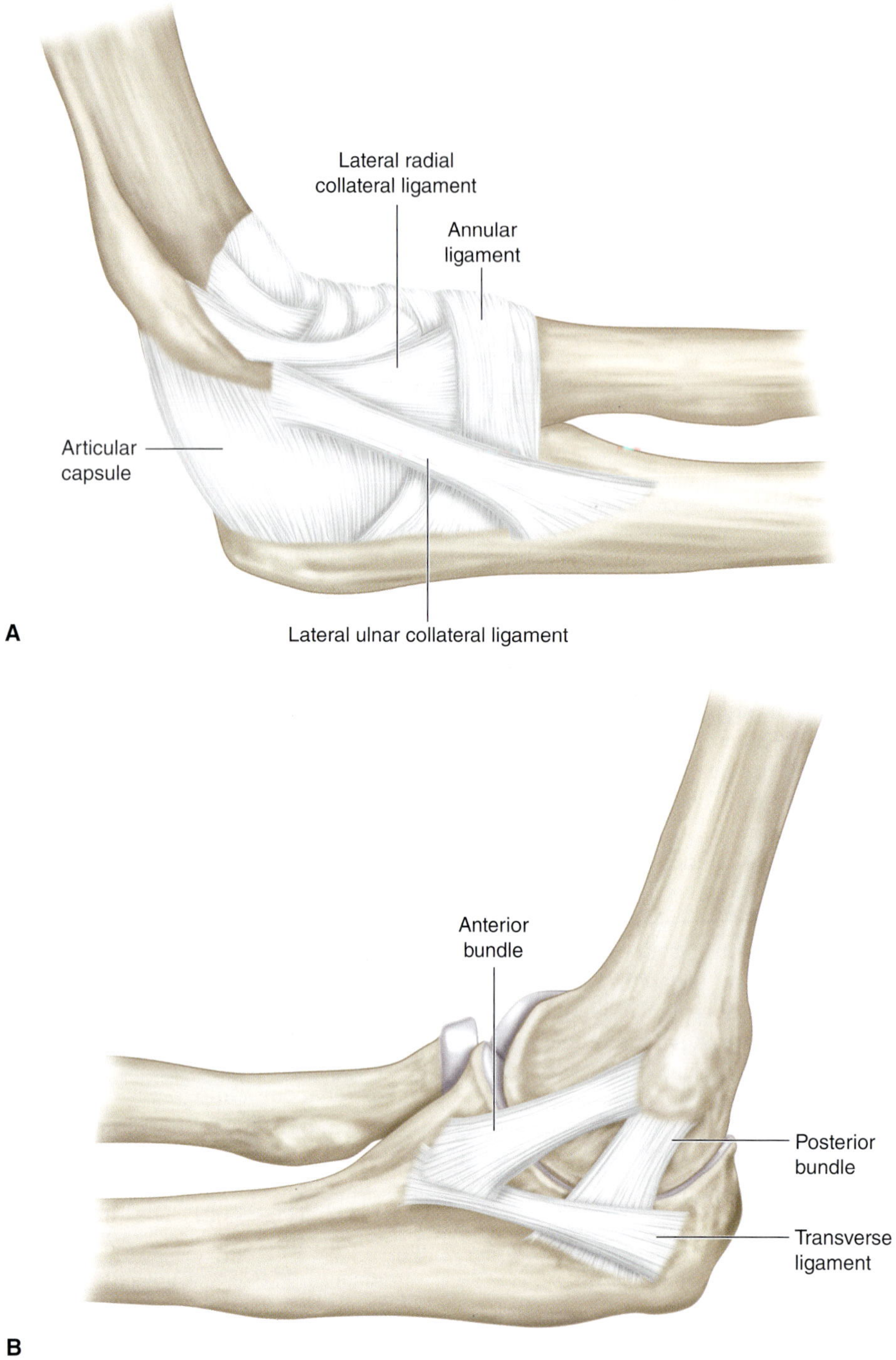

FIGURE 37-1 Anatomy of the lateral (**A**) and medial (**B**) collateral ligaments. (Adapted with permission from Bain GI, Mehta JA. Anatomy of the elbow joint and surgical approaches. In: Baker CL Jr, Plancher KD, eds. *Operative Treatment of Elbow Injuries*. New York: Springer-Verlag; 2001:1–27.)

typical posterolateral dislocation the patient is positioned supine with slight elbow flexion. The coronoid must be disengaged from distal humerus in order to prevent shearing and resultant osteochondral damage. This is accomplished by having the physician apply longitudinal traction to forearm while an assistant applies countertraction on the arm. Medial or lateral displacement is first corrected followed by a gentle force on the olecranon with elbow flexion to reduce the joint. A postreduction examination is then performed. The elbow is tested for stability in both pronation and supination and documented.[1,5,9,11,17–19] The patient is placed in a sling if the elbow is stable, or in a posterior splint at 90° of flexion if unstable, and seen within 3 to 7 days for clinical and radiographic follow-up examination. Anterior dislocations

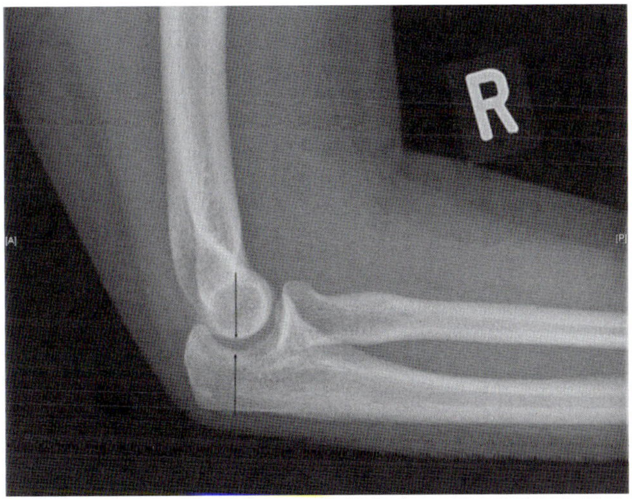

FIGURE 37-2 The drop sign.

are less common and may be caused by higher-energy mechanisms. Reduction is performed by positioning the elbow in slight flexion and applying traction to the forearm; some authors suggest performing the reduction in the operating room.[1] Divergent dislocations are extremely rare and various methods have been described to reduce the elbow including reducing the radius to ulna and then the forearm to humerus or reducing the radius to humerus and then the ulna to the humerus. Neurovascular assessment is required prior to and after any reduction.

Indications

In general, most simple elbow dislocations are managed effectively with nonoperative techniques. The indications for nonoperative management include a stable, concentrically reduced elbow including those with a drop sign.[20] Radiographs are taken in the clinic at the first follow-up visit and active range of motion exercises initiated. The timing of activation of range of motion is controversial, but there is agreement that it should commence within 1 to 2 weeks of injury. Stability is defined as a flexion–extension arc from 60° to full flexion. Range of motion through this stable arc may be initiated at the first follow-up visit with an extension-block splint or a hinged brace.

The indications for operative treatment include an irreducible joint, inability to maintain reduction, or an open dislocation.[21] The failure to maintain reduction at 60° of flexion despite positioning the elbow in pronation or supination typically requires surgical intervention.[11,22,23] Elbows with open injuries, vascular compromise, or compartment syndrome are also indications for surgery.[11] Controversy exists in the surgical management of simple elbow dislocations; options include repair of the LCL alone (commonly), or repair of the LCL and MCL.[24] Generally, if the elbow is stable after LCL repair, the MCL may be left unrepaired if the patient's vocation or activities do not risk positions of varus stress. Other surgical options include external fixation and transarticular pinning.

Contraindications

Contraindications to surgery include a stable elbow. Relative contraindication includes a medical history that precludes the patient from undergoing an operation.

Surgical Technique

Surgical options for simple elbow dislocations include repair of the LCL, LCL and MCL repair, static or dynamic external fixation, ligament repair and external fixation, or transarticular pinning.

The ligament(s) can be repaired with a transosseous technique or using suture anchors. The transosseous technique, our preferred method, requires high-strength #2 braided suture, a suture passer or shuttle, drills, fluoroscopy, and possibly a cortical button to augment the repair in osteopenic bone.

The patient should be positioned supine or semilateral. A sterile or nonsterile tourniquet may be applied depending on arm and cuff size, leaving room for proximal dissection if required. A regional block or general anesthetic may be used. One of 2 incisions may be selected—posterior or lateral. The posterior incision is fashioned in the midline with full-thickness fasciocutaneous flaps. The advantages of the posterior incision are that fewer cutaneous nerves cross the incision[25] and that deep medial and lateral approaches can be conducted through the same skin incision. A lateral incision may be beneficial in obese or vasculopathic patients where larger flaps may be at risk of healing issues. If a medial repair is planned when using a posterior incision, the ulnar nerve is identified and may be transposed to an anterior subcutaneous location.

The common extensor origin is often avulsion off the lateral epicondyle allowing for easy access to the lateral elbow.[26] If intact, the interval between the anconeus and extensor carpi ulnaris is used to access the radial head and ruptured LCL. Inspecting a bare area on the epicondyle can help identify the LCL origin. The isometric origin of the LCL on the lateral epicondyle is selected as the center point of a circle created by the radius of curvature of the capitellum. This can be confirmed by observing ligament/suture tension by taking the elbow through a flexion and extension arc with the ligament origin centered on the capitellum.[27,28] As mentioned above, options for repair of the collateral ligaments include a transosseous bone tunnel technique, suture anchors, or interference screws with each sharing the same underlying principle of anatomic repair.[29] The common extensor origin is often repaired with the LCL or can be repaired as a second superficial layer to the lateral supracondylar ridge. Following LCL repair, the elbow is tested for stability in both pronation and supination in varying degrees of flexion with fluoroscopic imaging assistance. If the elbow is stable, the wound may be closed in layers. If still unstable, a medial dissection is carried out. The MCL is exposed after mobilizing or splitting the flexor pronator tendon. At times, the flexor pronator mass is avulsed from the humerus facilitating dissection.[26] The anterior bundle of the MCL must be repaired to its anatomic footprint on the sublime tubercle (insertion) or the medial epicondyle (origin). Reconstruction of the MCL or LCL is rarely required in the acute circumstance. After MCL repair, the flexor pronator mass is repaired with drill holes through the supracondylar ridge. Following repair, range of motion and stability are again tested in neutral, pronation, and supination.

If still unstable or in an obese patient with a very heavy arm, consideration should be given to an external fixator to further protect the repairs.[30] Both static and hinged external fixators are commercially available. Static fixators, our preferred method, have the benefit of ease of application and lower complication rates, but risk stiffness.[31] When using hinged external fixators, one must ensure the axis pin is inserted in the isometric point.[32] Transarticular pinning, although historic, may still be considered when external fixation is unavailable.

Rehabilitation

The postreduction management of simple elbow dislocations involves early active range of motion, as several studies have reported the detrimental effects of prolonged immobilization.[9,33–36] Flexion contracture, pain, and time away from work increase if motion is not initiated within the first 7 to 10 days. If stable after reduction, then full active motion is initiated. A sling may be used for 2 to 3 weeks for comfort.

A controlled motion program with an extension-block splint may be used for unstable elbows. The forearm is positioned in maximal stability (typically pronation) and progressively extended until full motion is achieved (Fig. 37-3).

The overhead rehabilitation protocol may be considered in unstable elbows to limit the effect of gravitational forces that may contribute to ulnohumeral separation (Fig. 37-4).[37] Overhead exercises with active elbow flexion and extension are comfortably performed with the patient supine, shoulder flexed 90°, and neutral rotation, with the forearm in a position of stability (pronation or supination). This technique may assist with flexion contractures by activating the triceps. Exercises are performed every 2 to 4 hours during the day.

If a dynamic external fixator is utilized, active range of motion is typically allowed and the fixator is removed at 4 to 6 weeks. With a static fixator, removal usually occurs at 3 to 4 weeks followed by a fluoroscopic assessment of stability.

Complications

Complications of simple elbow dislocations include heterotopic ossification, stiffness, neurovascular injuries, persistent instability, or chronic dislocations.[38,39]

Prevention of stiffness occurs with early range of motion protocols.[34–36] If there is failure of progressive motion or range of motion is less than 30° to 130°, static progressive splinting may be initiated 4 to 8 weeks after injury.[3] Flexion contractures may be treated with an extension volar orthosis and adjusted until full extension is achieved. Restricted flexion may be managed with adjustable flexion cuffs. Aggressive stretching should be avoided.[3] If there is a failure of progression, or failure with static splinting, a turnbuckle orthosis may also be applied.[36] Generally, these are initiated after 6 weeks as sufficient bony and soft healing has taken place at this point. If there is less than 10° of progression over 3 to 4 months, surgical release can be considered if there is interference with patient function.

Indomethacin use for heterotopic ossification prevention is controversial and largely based on the orthopedic hip literature.[40] Radiation may be used in those patients with head injuries (700 cGy single dose). Neurovascular injury has been reported.[3,35,40] Ulnar neuropathy is the most common nerve injury with persistent symptoms occurring in less than 10% of patients. Brachial artery injury is rare. Chronic instability is uncommon if adequate treatment is performed early.[3,20,35,41] For the small proportion of patients who remain unstable, operative intervention may be considered. Chronic dislocations are infrequently seen and treatment depends on the patient's functional demands with options including observation, open reconstruction, arthroplasty, or fusion.[9,42]

Outcomes

For the simple elbow dislocation treated closed, the literature supports an early range of motion protocol.[18,33–36,41,43] Superior results are observed with minimal, less than 1 week of immobilization, followed by progressive active mobilization and strengthening. Final range of motion, return to full activity, and return to work are improved in those with early motion protocols.[33–35] In a retrospective study comparing reduction followed by plaster splint for 2 weeks with reduction and sling, both groups had excellent outcomes; however, the sling group had significantly better QuickDASH and Mayo Elbow Performance Index scores.[33] Slight postreduction subluxation, referred to as the drop sign, may be managed similarly with active elbow exercises and avoidance of varus stress.[14,20] Patients treated operatively may report higher rates of pain with activity, weather-related symptoms, weakness, and pain at rest compared with a nonsurgically treated cohort.[26]

In a comparative trial of 26 patients treated with 3 weeks of casting versus 24 patients treated with immediate functional treatment (three 10-minute sessions per day with initial progressive ROM starting at 50° to 100°, and a sling at rest), Rafai et al showed that functional treatment had better outcomes with 96% normal extension versus 81% in the casted group. There was no difference in pain, instability, or heterotopic ossification.[44]

Josefsson et al, in a randomized controlled trial comparing closed versus open treatment with ligament repair, reported

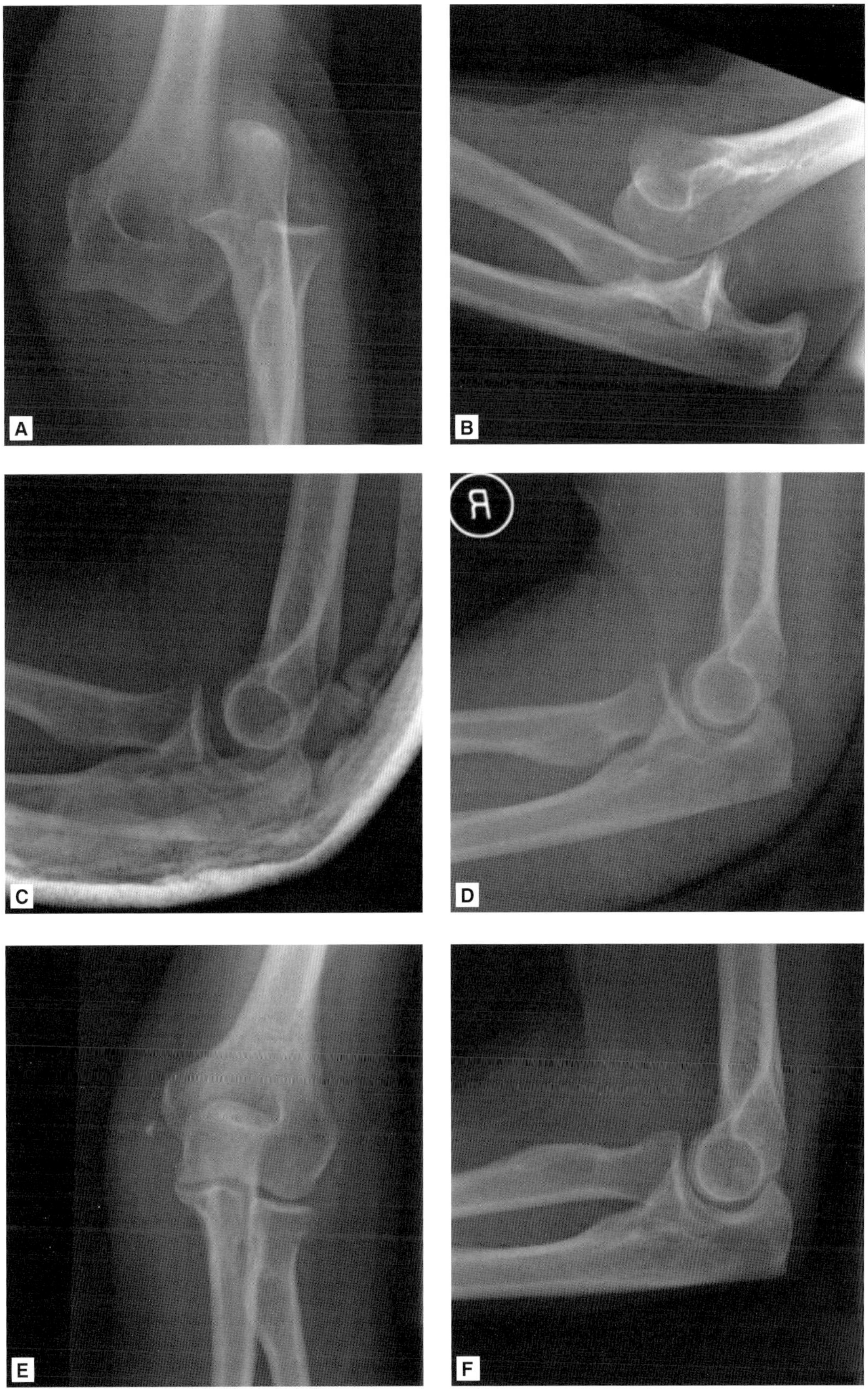

FIGURE 37-3 Anteroposterior (**A**) and lateral (**B**) radiographs demonstrating a simple posterolateral elbow dislocation. A postreduction lateral view with the forearm in neutral rotation (**C**) reveals an incongruent ulnohumeral joint and posterolateral rotatory instability. Elbow reduction by position forearm in full pronation (**D**). The 3-month follow-up anteroposterior (**E**) and lateral (**F**) images demonstrate a concentrically reduced joint.

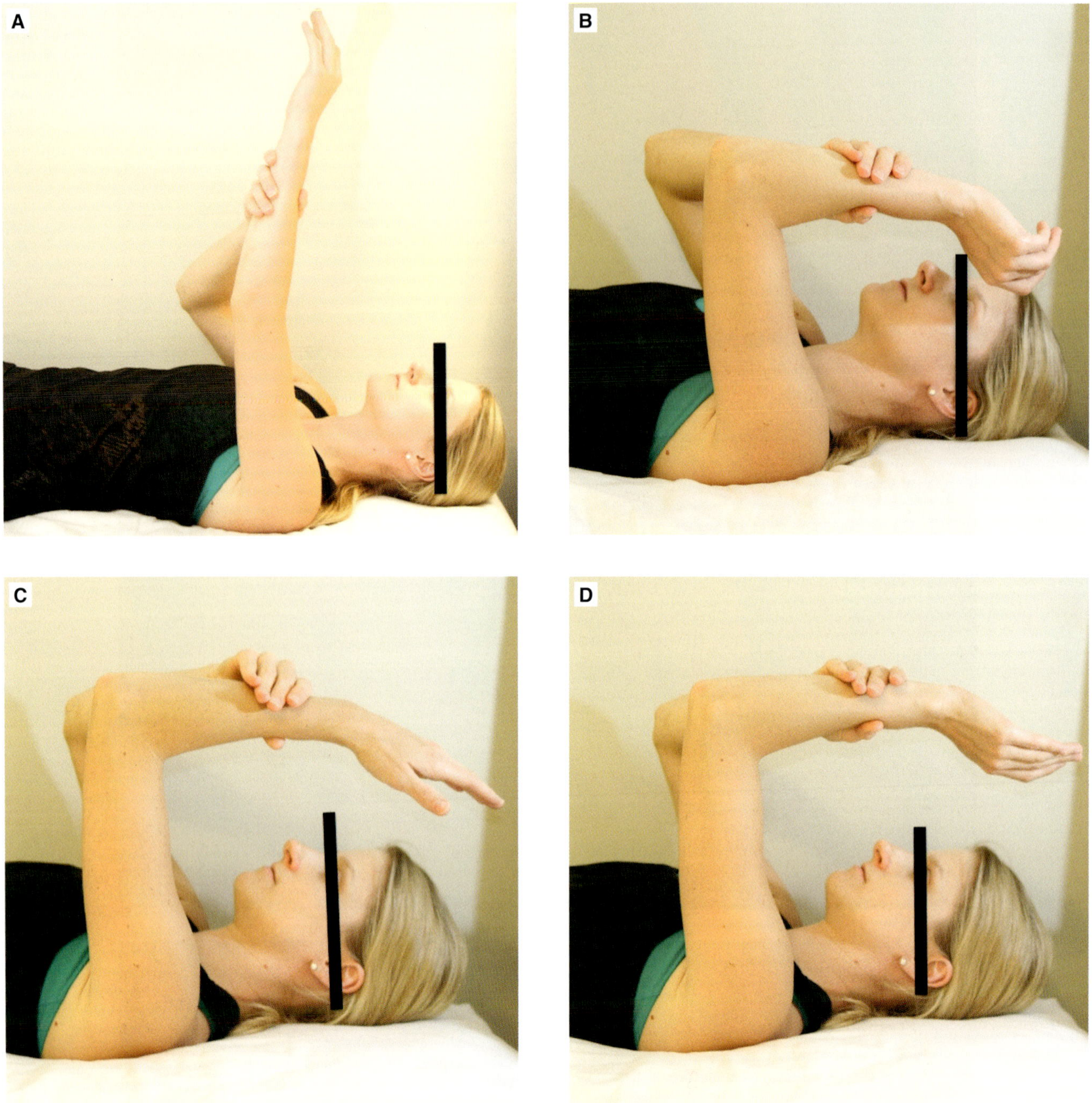

FIGURE 37-4 Overhead rehabilitation protocol for LCL deficiency. Images **A** and **B** demonstrate active elbow extension and flexion with forearm pronated, respectively. Images **C** and **D** demonstrate active supination and pronation of forearm with elbow at 90°, respectively.

better final range of motion in the closed cohort, although it did not achieve statistical significance.[26] A subgroup analysis revealed that even unstable elbows performed similarly in both groups (grip, pain, instability). Additionally, no cases of recurrent dislocation were reported.

For longer-term follow-up, a retrospective comparative study between closed and open treatment for simple elbow dislocations demonstrated no difference in final outcomes at 3- to 7-year follow-up.[41] Duckworth et al, in a series of 23 patients with slight residual subluxation after a simple dislocation, reported that with avoidance of varus stress and active range of motion exercises, patients had stable elbows with normal radiographic parameters at 2-year follow-up.[20]

Micic et al reported on 20 patients with simple elbow dislocations with postreduction instability treated with anatomic ligament repair. At the time of surgery, the authors observed LCL avulsions in 80%, MCL avulsions in 55%, common extensor injuries in 80%, and flexor pronator injuries

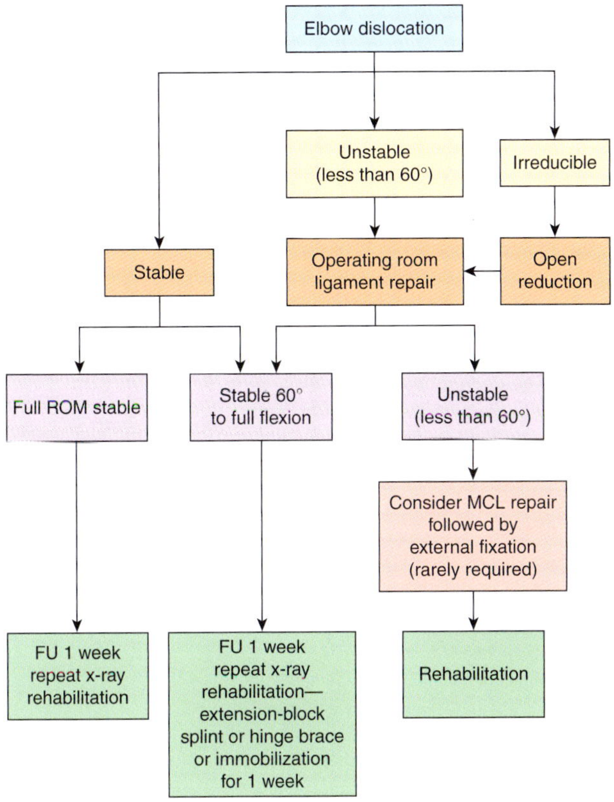

FIGURE 37-5 Algorithm of simple elbow dislocation management.

in 60%. At a mean 2-year follow-up, the mean Mayo Elbow Performance Index was 93/100 and extension loss averaged 14°. Fourteen patients developed heterotopic ossification, but none required further surgery.[22]

Long-term follow-up studies on simple elbow dislocations have demonstrated that patients generally have satisfactory outcomes.[45] However, the injury may not be completely benign as Anakwe et al reported, in a series of 110 patients, an 8% rate of subjective instability without recurrent dislocations and minor limitations in range of motion on the injured side. The results obtained, including the subjective instability (8%), stiffness (56%), and pain (62%), could have been a reflection of the categorical questionnaires used in the study.[46] In another long-term study by de Haan et al, 86 patients were identified with simple and complex dislocations and 42 were reviewed at follow-up. The authors concluded that good results were obtained with early functional range of motion in most patients.[47]

In summary, the vast majority of simple elbow dislocations can be treated nonoperatively with an early active range of motion rehabilitation protocol. A treatment algorithm is demonstrated in Figure 37-5. Patients with a stable reduction between 60° and full flexion can be rehabilitated with an extension-blocking orthosis. Instability in greater degrees of flexion may require operative repair. Typically the LCL is repaired first and stability is usually obtained. However, in case of persistent instability, MCL repair and possibly an external fixator may be required.

REFERENCES

1. Hildebrand KA, Patterson SD, King GJ. Acute elbow dislocations: simple and complex. *Orthop Clin North Am*. 1999;30(1):63–79.
2. Bryce CD, Armstrong AD. Anatomy and biomechanics of the elbow. *Orthop Clin North Am*. 2008;39(2):141–154, v.
3. Linscheid RL, Wheeler DK. Elbow dislocations. *JAMA*. 1965;194(11):1171–1176.
4. McKee MD, Schemitsch EH, Sala MJ, O'Driscoll W. The pathoanatomy of lateral ligamentous disruption in complex elbow instability. *J Shoulder Elbow Surg*. 2003;12(4):391–396.
5. O'Driscoll SW, Morrey BF, Korinek S, An KN. Elbow subluxation and dislocation. A spectrum of instability. *Clin Orthop Relat Res*. 1992;(280):186–197.
6. Hotchkiss RN, Weiland AJ. Valgus stability of the elbow. *J Orthop Res*. 1987;5(3):372–377.
7. King GJ, Glauser SJ, Westreich A, Morrey BF, An KN. In vitro stability of an unconstrained total elbow prosthesis. Influence of axial loading and joint flexion angle. *J Arthroplasty*. 1993;8(3):291–298.
8. Sojbjerg JO, Ovesen J, Gundorf CE. The stability of the elbow following excision of the radial head and transection of the annular ligament. An experimental study. *Arch Orthop Trauma Surg*. 1987;106(4):248–250.
9. Sheps DM, Hildebrand KA, Boorman RS. Simple dislocations of the elbow: evaluation and treatment. *Hand Clin*. 2004;20(4):389–404.
10. Josefsson PO, Nilsson BE. Incidence of elbow dislocation. *Acta Orthop Scand*. 1986;57(6):537–538.
11. Kuhn MA, Ross G. Acute elbow dislocations. *Orthop Clin North Am*. 2008;39(2):155–161, v.
12. Stoneback JW, Owens BD, Sykes J, Athwal GS, Pointer L, Wolf JM. Incidence of elbow dislocations in the United States population. *J Bone Joint Surg Am*. 2012;94(3):240–245.
13. Conn JJ, Wade PA. Injuries of the elbow: a ten year review. *J Trauma*. 1961;1(3):248–268.
14. Coonrad RW, Roush TF, Major NM, Basamania CJ. The drop sign, a radiographic warning sign of elbow instability. *J Shoulder Elbow Surg*. 2005;14(3):312–317.
15. Osborne G, Cotterill P. Recurrent dislocation of the elbow. *J Bone Joint Surg Br*. 1966;48(2):340–346.
16. Jeon IH, Micic ID, Yamamoto N, Morrey BF. Osborne-Cotterill lesion: an osseous defect of the capitellum associated with instability of the elbow. *AJR Am J Roentgenol*. 2008;191(3):727–729.
17. Cohen MS, Hastings H 2nd. Acute elbow dislocation: evaluation and management. *J Am Acad Orthop Surg*. 1998;6(1):15–23.
18. Duckworth AD, Ring D, Kulijdian A, McKee MD. Unstable elbow dislocations. *J Shoulder Elbow Surg*. 2008;17(2):281–286.
19. Ross G, McDevitt ER, Chronister R, Ove PN. Treatment of simple elbow dislocation using an immediate motion protocol. *Am J Sports Med*. 1999;27(3):308–311.
20. Duckworth AD, Kulijdian A, McKee MD, Ring D. Residual subluxation of the elbow after dislocation or fracture–dislocation: treatment with active elbow exercises and avoidance of varus stress. *J Shoulder Elbow Surg*. 2008;17(2):276–280.
21. Hobgood ER, Khan SO, Field LD. Acute dislocations of the adult elbow. *Hand Clin*. 2008;24(1):1–7.
22. Micic I, Kim SY, Park IH, Kim PT, Jeon IH. Surgical management of unstable elbow dislocation without intra-articular fracture. *Int Orthop*. 2009;33(4):1141–1147.
23. O'Driscoll SW, Jupiter JB, King GJ, Hotchkiss RN, Morrey BF. The unstable elbow. *Instr Course Lect*. 2001;50:89–102.
24. McKee MD, Pugh DM, Wild LM, Schemitsch EH, King GJ. Standard surgical protocol to treat elbow dislocations with radial head and coronoid fractures. Surgical technique. *J Bone Joint Surg Am*. 2005;87(suppl 1, pt 1):22–32.
25. Dowdy PA, Bain GI, King GJ, Patterson SD. The midline posterior elbow incision. An anatomical appraisal. *J Bone Joint Surg Br*. 1995;77(5):696–699.
26. Josefsson PO, Gentz CF, Johnell O, Wendeberg B. Surgical versus nonsurgical treatment of ligamentous injuries following dislocation of the elbow joint. A prospective randomized study. *J Bone Joint Surg Am*. 1987;69(4):605–608.
27. Cheung EV. Chronic lateral elbow instability. *Orthop Clin North Am*. 2008;39(2):221–228, vi–vii.

28. Nestor BJ, O'Driscoll SW, Morrey BF. Ligamentous reconstruction for posterolateral rotatory instability of the elbow. *J Bone Joint Surg Am.* 1992;74(8):1235–1241.
29. Langer P, Fadale P, Hulstyn M. Evolution of the treatment options of ulnar collateral ligament injuries of the elbow. *Br J Sports Med.* 2006;40(6):499–506.
30. Jupiter JB, Ring D. Treatment of unreduced elbow dislocations with hinged external fixation. *J Bone Joint Surg Am.* 2002;84-A(9): 1630–1635.
31. Tashjian RZ, Katarincic JA. Complex elbow instability. *J Am Acad Orthop Surg.* 2006;14(5):278–286.
32. Tan V, Daluiski A, Capo J, Hotchkiss R. Hinged elbow external fixators: indications and uses. *J Am Acad Orthop Surg.* 2005;13(8): 503–514.
33. Maripuri SN, Debnath UK, Rao P, Mohanty K. Simple elbow dislocation among adults: a comparative study of two different methods of treatment. *Injury.* 2007;38(11):1254–1258.
34. Mehlhoff TL, Noble PC, Bennett JB, Tullos HS. Simple dislocation of the elbow in the adult. Results after closed treatment. *J Bone Joint Surg Am.* 1988;70(2):244–249.
35. Protzman RR. Dislocation of the elbow joint. *J Bone Joint Surg Am.* 1978;60(4):539–541.
36. Royle SG. Posterior dislocation of the elbow. *Clin Orthop Relat Res.* 1991;(269):201–204.
37. Pipicelli JG, Chinchalkar SJ, Grewal R, Athwal GS. Rehabilitation considerations in the management of terrible triad injury to the elbow. *Tech Hand Up Extrem Surg.* 2011;15(4):198–208.
38. McKee MD, Bowden SH, King GJ, et al. Management of recurrent, complex instability of the elbow with a hinged external fixator. *J Bone Joint Surg Br.* 1998;80(6):1031–1036.
39. Cheng SL, Morrey BF. Treatment of the mobile, painful arthritic elbow by distraction interposition arthroplasty. *J Bone Joint Surg Br.* 2000;82(2):233–238.
40. Martin BD, Johansen JA, Edwards SG. Complications related to simple dislocations of the elbow. *Hand Clin.* 2008;24(1):9–25.
41. Josefsson PO, Johnell O, Gentz CF. Long-term sequelae of simple dislocation of the elbow. *J Bone Joint Surg Am.* 1984;66(6):927–930.
42. Chloros GD, Wiesler ER, Stabile KJ, Papadonikolakis A, Ruch DS, Kuzma GR. Reconstruction of Essex-Lopresti injury of the forearm: technical note. *J Hand Surg Am.* 2008;33(1):124–130.
43. van der Ley J, van Niekerk JL, Binnendijk B. Conservative treatment of elbow dislocations in adults. *Neth J Surg.* 1987;39(6):167–169.
44. Rafai M, Largab A, Cohen D, Trafeh M. Pure posterior luxation of the elbow in adults: immobilization or early mobilization. A randomized prospective study of 50 cases. *Chir Main.* 1999;18(4):272–278.
45. Schippinger G, Seibert FJ, Steinböck J, Kucharczyk M. Management of simple elbow dislocations. Does the period of immobilization affect the eventual results? *Langenbecks Arch Surg.* 1999;384(3):294–297.
46. Anakwe RE, Middleton SD, Jenkins PJ, McQueen MM, Court-Brown CM. Patient-reported outcomes after simple dislocation of the elbow. *J Bone Joint Surg Am.* 2011;93(13):1220–1226.
47. de Haan J, Schep NW, Zengerink I, van Buijtenen J, Tuinebreijer WE, den Hartog D. Dislocation of the elbow: a retrospective multicentre study of 86 patients. *Open Orthop J.* 2010;4:76–79.

38

Elbow Arthroscopy

Julie E. Adams, MD
Scott P. Steinmann, MD

RATIONALE AND BASIC SCIENCE PERTINENT TO THE PROCEDURE

Elbow arthroscopy is an emerging technique for treatment of a variety of conditions about the elbow. Previously, elbow arthroscopy was abandoned as it was deemed to be inherently unsafe.[1] However, in recent years, an increased understanding of the anatomy about the elbow and techniques to make arthroscopy less risky have emerged. In addition, recent interest in "minimally invasive" techniques to accelerate rehabilitation has expanded interest in arthroscopy of the elbow.

INDICATIONS

The ideal indication for elbow arthroscopy is loose body extraction. Other indications include debridement for septic elbow arthritis, synovectomy for rheumatoid arthritis or hemophilic arthritis, debridement for osteoarthritis, contracture release, treatment of osteochondral defects, tennis elbow release, and for diagnostic purposes. In addition, there is an emerging role of elbow arthroscopy for treatment of selected fractures about the elbow as well as for instability of the elbow in some cases.[2–24]

CONTRAINDICATIONS

Contraindications to elbow arthroscopy include lack of surgeon experience with the procedure and available arthroscopic equipment and setup; in addition, prior submuscular or intramuscular ulnar nerve transposition is generally considered a contraindication. Prior subcutaneous nerve transposition is not necessarily a contraindication to arthroscopy; however, the path of the nerve should be conclusively identified prior to surgery, by intraoperative ultrasound, palpation, or via an incision and direct exposure.[25] Caution should be exercised in the setting of prior surgery in general, as especially an anterolateral incision may have resulted in scarring and possible tethering of the radial nerve. In addition, prior surgery may have distorted the normal anatomy making surgery more risky. Need for an open incision, such as for removal of hardware, reconstruction of ligaments, placement of prostheses, or transposition of the ulnar nerve, may make arthroscopy an extra step in the procedure and less desirable. In addition, for arthritic elbows, pain experienced throughout the arc of motion rather than just at end arc of motion may indicate that elbow arthroscopy and simple debridement will be less effective than alternative open reconstructive procedures (such as arthroplasty) for relief of pain.[16,17]

SURGICAL TECHNIQUE

General anesthesia is preferred, as the patient's neurovascular status may be evaluated in the recovery room shortly after the procedure. Either a nonsterile tourniquet may be applied high on the arm and the arm prepped and draped distal to the tourniquet or a sterile tourniquet may be applied after the arm has been prepped and draped from the fingertips to the axilla.

Patient positioning may be supine, prone, or in the lateral decubitus position. We prefer a lateral position, in which the patient is positioned with the aid of an inflatable bean bag. The arm is secured with a dedicated arm holder. Commercially available arm holders may be used; alternatively, modifications of a knee holder or custom-made holders may be used.

The arm is placed such that the elbow is higher than the shoulder (Fig. 38-1). Care is taken to avoid pressure on the antecubital fossa, and that the support of the arm holder is sufficiently proximal (Fig. 38-2).

The arm is draped and positioned such that the elbow can be freely flexed and extended and that full access to the elbow can be maintained (Fig. 38-3).

Arthroscopic equipment is the standard knee arthroscopy equipment with a 30°, 4.5-mm arthroscope. Cannulas that lack trephinations are especially useful for elbow arthroscopy. Cannulas with trephinations can allow escape

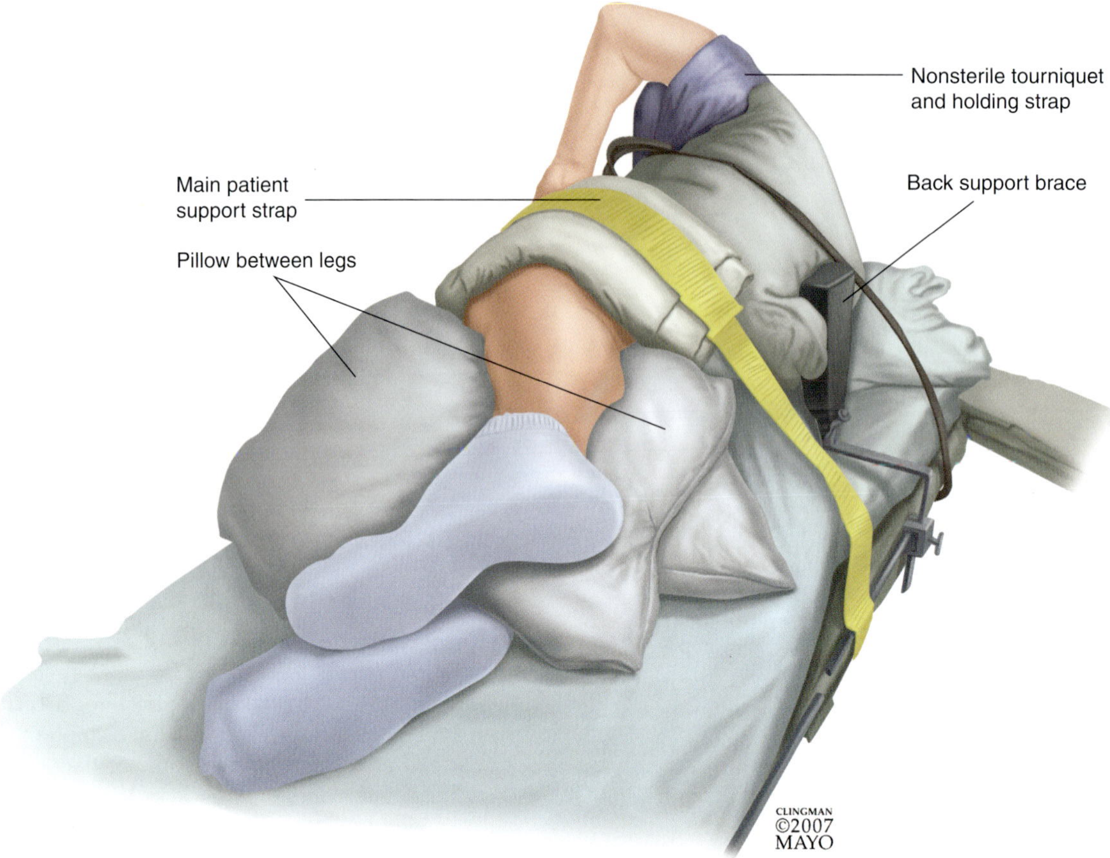

FIGURE 38-1 Operative setup demonstrating the patient in the lateral decubitus position. (With permission of Mayo Foundation for Medical Education and Research. All rights reserved.)

of fluid out into the soft tissues, worsening swelling and limiting the working time of the procedure. A radiofrequency ablator is useful to control bleeding and debride synovitis. A variety of standard arthroscopic biters and graspers are helpful, as are burrs and shavers. The shaver importantly is not hooked up to suction, as there may be a tendency to suck in soft tissue during shaving. In the elbow, given the proximity of the neurovascular structures, the margin of safety may be slight and avoidance of shaver suction may help prevent inadvertent injury to named structures. Rather, the shaver is allowed to drain freely to the floor. A variety of commercially available purpose-made retractor devices are available. In addition, one might use Howarth retractors, Freer elevators, blunt trocars, and other such devices for the same purpose.

Portal Placement

In general, standard portals include the anterolateral, anteromedial, posteromedial, and direct posterior portals. Accessory portals include the soft spot portal (direct lateral portal), distal ulnar portal, and accessory retraction portals in the anterior joint laterally and medially.

It is most helpful to mark out bony and soft tissue landmarks and the intended portal sites prior to any work being done on the elbow; doing so helps make the markings more accurate than attempting to mark landmarks that may be altered or obscured by fluid extravasation after work has commenced. In particular, the path of the ulnar nerve is marked and the elbow is examined to exclude or note presence of a subluxating ulnar nerve. In addition, the radiocapitellar joint, lateral and medial epicondyles, olecranon, and intramuscular septum are marked, as are the intended portal sites.

The tourniquet is inflated to 200 or 250 mm Hg after elevation of the arm. Regardless of the portal placement, the procedure starts with insufflation of the joint with saline through the direct lateral portal or at the first portal site placed. Typically, 25 to 30 cm^3 of saline is insufflated into the joint via an 18-gauge needle and syringe. Appropriate placement into the joint is confirmed by slight extension of the elbow as fluid is placed and the joint is distended. Following insufflation of the joint, portals may be placed. Order of portal placement depends in part on the preference and experience of the surgeon, and the pathology to be addressed. In most cases the authors prefer initial portal placement anterolaterally, and then creation of an anteromedial portal. The anterolateral portal is the portal that in most cases has the

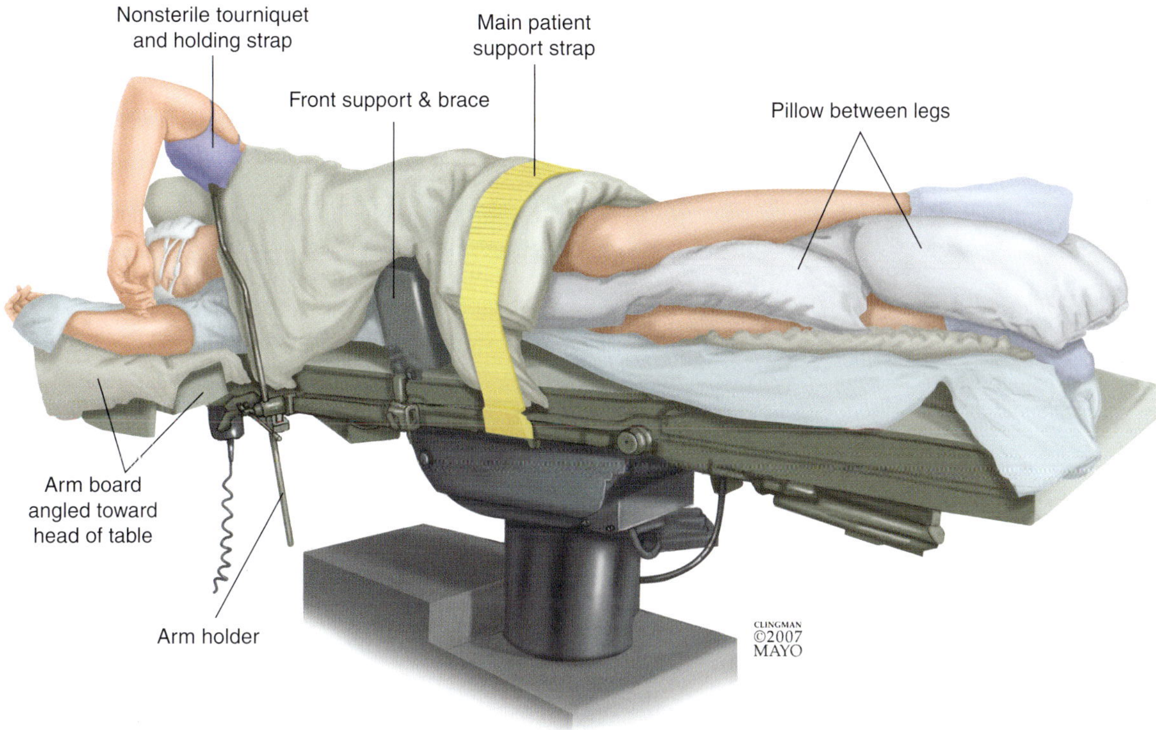

FIGURE 38-2 Operative setup demonstrating the patient in the lateral decubitus position. The arm is draped free such that the elbow is higher than the shoulder. (With permission of Mayo Foundation for Medical Education and Research. All rights reserved.)

least margin of safety and is closest to an important named neurovascular structure; we prefer creating this portal first before fluid extravasation and distension alters palpable landmarks. Nevertheless, many surgeons prefer starting anteromedially, which is perfectly acceptable.

ANTEROLATERAL PORTAL

This portal is placed just anterior to the radiocapitellar joint. Care is taken to err somewhat proximally (increasing the margin of safety) rather than more distally (closer to the PIN). A finger is placed on the radial head and radiocapitellar joint, and position is confirmed by forearm rotation (Fig. 38-4). A spinal needle or 18-gauge needle and syringe are used to localize the joint. It is important to have a 3D visualization and sense of the joint position; the needle is aimed proximally and centrally toward the elbow joint. The intra-articular location is confirmed by tactile feel; aspiration and injection of saline should elicit an easy egress of fluid and slight passive extension of the elbow with joint distension.

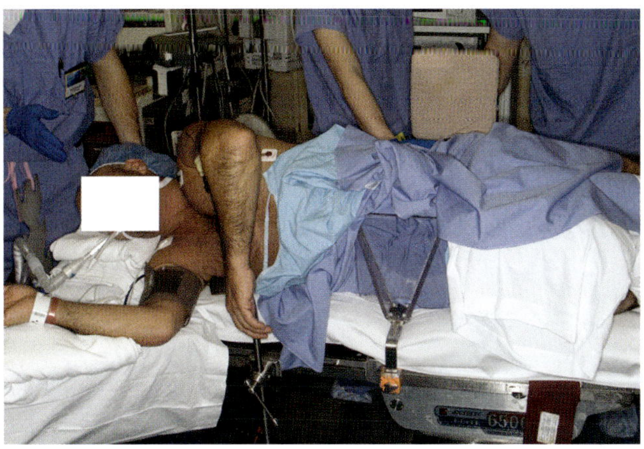

FIGURE 38-3 The operative setup is demonstrated in this photograph documenting free access to the elbow.

Portals are created in the usual fashion, with skin incised only with a #15 blade, and then blunt dissection down to the capsule with a hemostat to decrease risk of injury to cutaneous nerves. When the capsule is breached, a sudden egress of fluid confirms appropriate positioning at the joint. A blunt trocar and arthroscopy sheath is then placed at the portal site.

ANTEROMEDIAL PORTAL

This portal is approximately 1 to 2 cm distal and 1 to 2 cm anterior to the medial epicondyle. It goes through the flexor pronator mass and has a high margin of safety from neurovascular structures. Typically we make this portal after visualizing from the anterolateral portal and palpating while viewing to choose the appropriate portal site. The portal may be made from an inside-out technique, by exchanging the

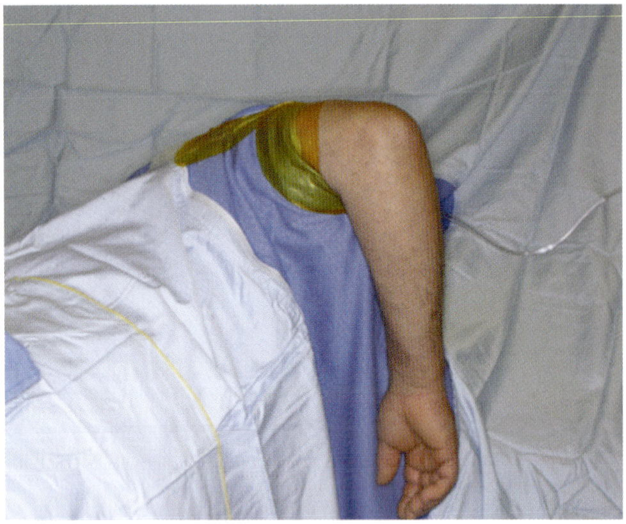

FIGURE 38-4 Intraoperative positioning of the patient such that full access to the elbow is demonstrated.

camera for a blunt trocar and advancing it toward the medial skin (Fig. 38-5). A second sheath can then be introduced from medial, allowing for this working portal to be used. A Wissenger switching stick is often useful as well as visualization is swapped from lateral to medial.

ACCESSORY ANTERIOR PORTALS

Accessory portals may be placed anteriorly for retraction.

Anteromedially, an accessory portal may be placed just anterior to the supracondylar ridge and intramuscular septum, 2 cm superior to the medial epicondyle.

The anterolateral accessory portal may be placed 2 cm superior to the lateral epicondyle, and just anterior to the supracondylar ridge.

DIRECT LATERAL OR "SOFT SPOT" PORTAL

This portal is useful to see and treat osteochondral defects. It is created through the center of a triangle made between the tip of the olecranon, lateral epicondyle, and radial head. This palpable "soft spot" is covered by the anconeus, through which the trocar must traverse.

DISTAL ULNAR PORTAL

This portal is also particularly useful to visualize the posterior capitellum, commonly affected by osteochondral defects. It is created by sliding along the lateral border of the ulna toward the elbow joint from a starting point 3 to 4 cm distal to the radiocapitellar joint[7] (Figs. 38-6 and 38-7).

POSTERIOR PORTALS

Direct Posterior Portal. This portal is made 2 to 3 cm above the proximal edge of the olecranon. It traverses the thick triceps and thus requires incision through the skin and triceps with the knife blade. A blunt trocar is helpful to abrade the posterior humerus and thereby remove posterior olecranon fat to help create a visualization space. This is really a potential space; thus, it is useful to place the shaver and blindly shave at the olecranon fossa to remove tissue and create a working and visualization space. This portal is relatively safe provided the position of the ulnar nerve is kept in mind. After creation of a working space, this portal is used most for visualization.

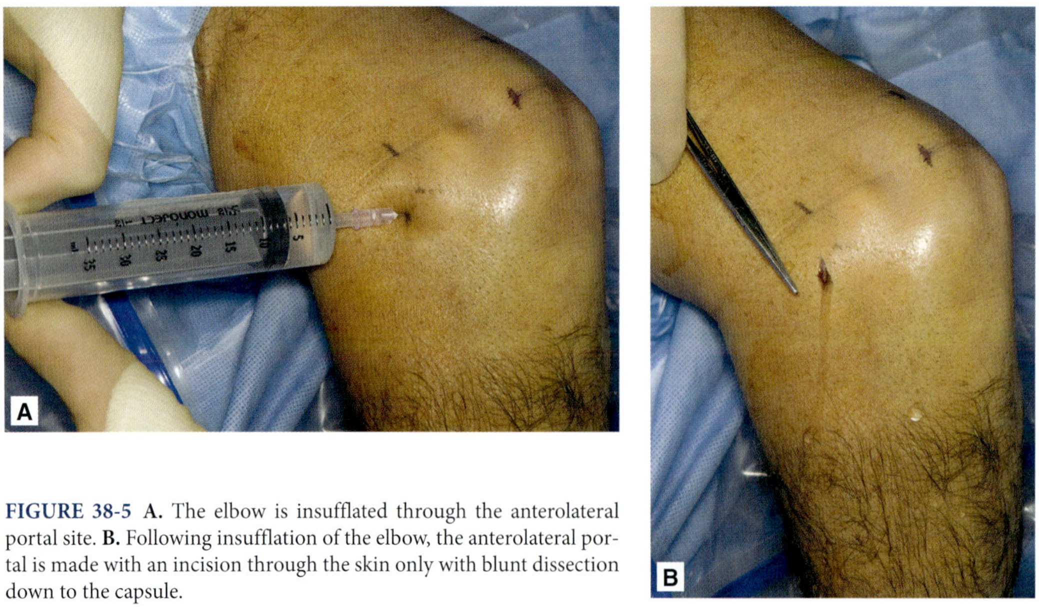

FIGURE 38-5 **A.** The elbow is insufflated through the anterolateral portal site. **B.** Following insufflation of the elbow, the anterolateral portal is made with an incision through the skin only with blunt dissection down to the capsule.

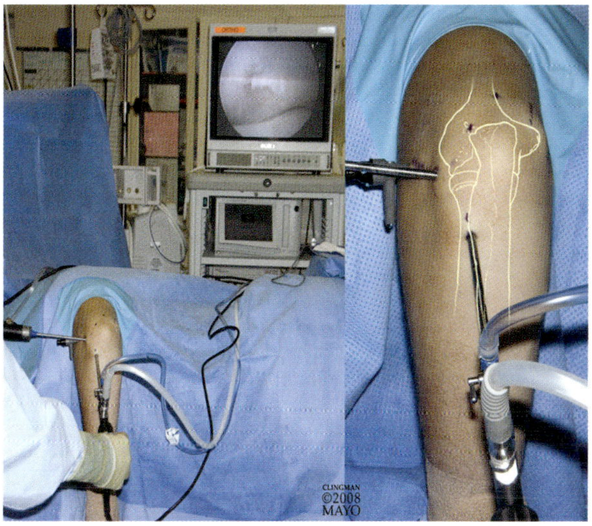

FIGURE 38-6 The distal ulnar portal allows enhanced visualization of the capitellum to address osteochondral lesions. (With permission of Mayo Foundation for Medical Education and Research. All rights reserved.)

Posterolateral Portal. This portal is made near level with the proximal edge of the olecranon on the posterolateral surface. It is predominantly a working portal, and again has a high margin of safety away from named neurovascular structures.

COMPLICATIONS

Published reports document injury to all major peripheral nerves about the elbow. In 1 series of 473 elbow arthroscopies, the ulnar nerve was most commonly involved, followed by the superficial radial nerve, and then the PIN, AIN, and medial antebrachial cutaneous nerve. Fortunately, in this series, all nerve injuries were transient; however, in other reports, nerve injury has been permanent.[17,26,38]

Nerve injury is more common in the setting of rheumatoid arthritis, in which the capsule is thinned or absent; profound preoperative contractures; and the setting of distorted anatomy. It is likely that neurovascular injuries about the elbow are underreported. Certainly, even following

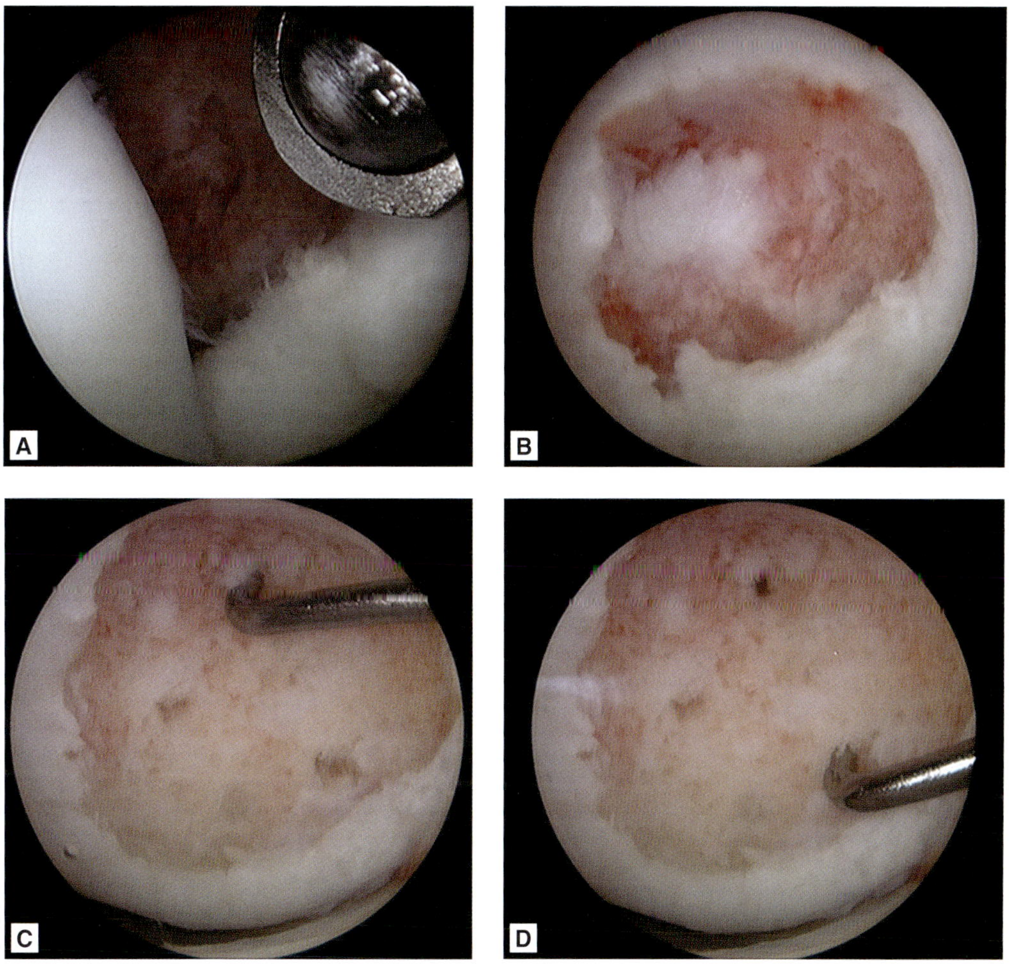

FIGURE 38-7 These images from intraoperative arthroscopy demonstrate an osteochondral lesion (**A**). The distal ulnar portal has been used to visualize the lesion and a shaver or burr used to remove the lesion (**B**). Microfracture techniques (**C** and **D**) are performed to promote fibrocartilage development.

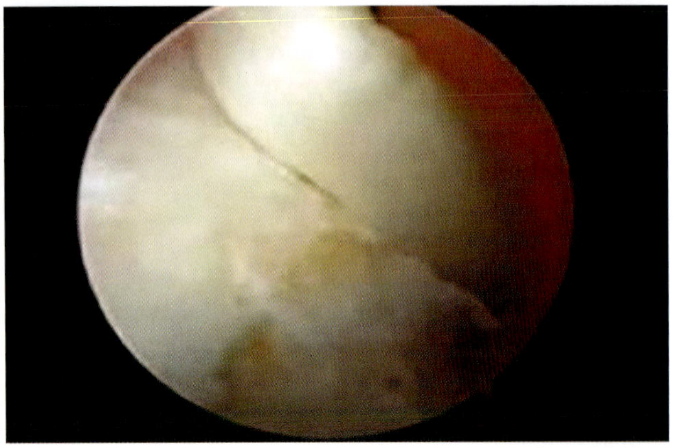

FIGURE 38-8 The ulnar nerve may be decompressed arthroscopically, as seen in this image.

careful precautions, the risk of neurovascular injury in conjunction with elbow arthroscopy cannot be entirely eliminated.[17]

One controversy is the role of and need for ulnar nerve decompression in the setting of contracture release. Certainly, many patients with stiff or arthritic elbows have concomitant ulnar neuritis. Some suggest need for ulnar nerve decompression even in asymptomatic elbows if there is an anticipated large restoration of motion or with a certain preoperative threshold loss of motion. Little information exists regarding the need for ulnar nerve decompression. Currently, the authors release the nerve if there are preoperative symptoms; 1 of us (J. E. A.) has a very low threshold for ulnar nerve release, performing an open decompression if there is to be a substantial improvement in motion; the other (S. P. S.) often decompresses the nerve arthroscopically if needed but has a more wait-and-see approach (Fig. 38-8). Future research is likely to provide more than level V expert opinion evidence regarding the need for ulnar nerve decompression.

Heterotopic ossification is believed to be less common following elbow arthroscopy than open procedures; however, this complication does occur in conjunction with elbow arthroscopy. The role of, duration, and compliance with heterotopic ossification prophylaxis are uncertain; however, we often prescribe indomethacin SR 75 mg daily for 6 weeks.[16,39–41]

Joint space infection is unusual following elbow arthroscopy; however, persistent drainage from the joint or development of fistulae has been more common.[29]

OUTCOMES

Outcomes following elbow arthroscopy have been reported in the literature for a variety of conditions. However, no series to date documents that this procedure is superior to open procedures. Rather, elbow arthroscopy should be considered as yet another tool to be used for treatment of various pathologies. We have personal experience with elbow arthroscopy for treatment of hemophilic arthropathy, rheumatoid arthritis and osteoarthritis, loose body excision, osteochondral defects, contracture release, elbow instability, tennis elbow release, and fractures. Our experience suggests an acceptable complication rate and satisfactory outcomes. Our largest experience has been in the setting of osteoarthritis of the elbow.[16] In this series, we described the outcomes following arthroscopic debridement in 41 patients (42 elbows) with primary osteoarthritis of the elbow (Fig. 38-9). Similar to others, we have documented an increase in range of motion and patient satisfaction.[13,42–45] At an average follow-up of 176.3 weeks, significant improvements occurred in mean flexion, from 117.3° preoperatively to 131.6° ($P < .0001$); extension, from 21.4° to 8.4° ($P < .0001$); supination, from 70.7° to 78.6° ($P = .0056$); and Mayo Elbow Performance Index scores ($P < .0001$), with 81% good to excellent results. Pain decreased significantly ($P < .0001$). Complications were rare ($n = 2$) and included heterotopic ossification and ulnar dysesthesias. Similarly, we recently evaluated our experience with the outcomes of arthroscopic ulnar nerve decompression at the elbow in a series of patients with associated osteoarthritis.[46] Thirteen patients (15 elbows) with an average age of 51 years (range, 20–75 years) underwent an arthroscopic ulnar nerve decompression, osteophyte resection, and capsulectomy during the same procedure. At an average follow-up of 47 months there were 7 excellent, 5 good, 1 fair, and 2 poor results using the Dellon classification. Three patients with severe compression preoperatively underwent reoperation because of persistent or recurrent symptoms. Elbow arthroscopy has an emerging role in acute trauma. We assessed 7 patients who underwent an arthroscopic-assisted treatment of a coronoid fracture with an average age of 37 years and an average follow-up of 31.8 months.[18] The Regan-Morrey fracture types were II ($n = 4$) and III ($n = 3$), which were treated with an arthroscopic reduction and plate fixation (1), screws (2), and threaded Steinmann pins (2); 2 fractures were debrided. Three patients had immediate (2) or delayed (1) lateral ulnar collateral ligament repair. The range of motion averaged 9° to 133° in flexion–extension and 87°/79° in pronosupination. The Mayo Elbow Performance scores were 100 in 5 of 6 patients (1 unavailable). There was 1 case of heterotopic ossification and 1 delayed ulnar neuropathy.

Reddy et al did a chart review of 172 patients (184 arthroscopies) at an average follow-up of 42.3 months (range, 7-115 months).[47] Ninety-six patients had posterior impingement (51%), 72 had loose bodies, and 32 had degenerative joint disease. There were 51 patients (56%) with an excellent surgical result, 37 patients (36%) with a good result, 12 patients (11%) with a fair result, and 4 patients (4%) with a poor result.

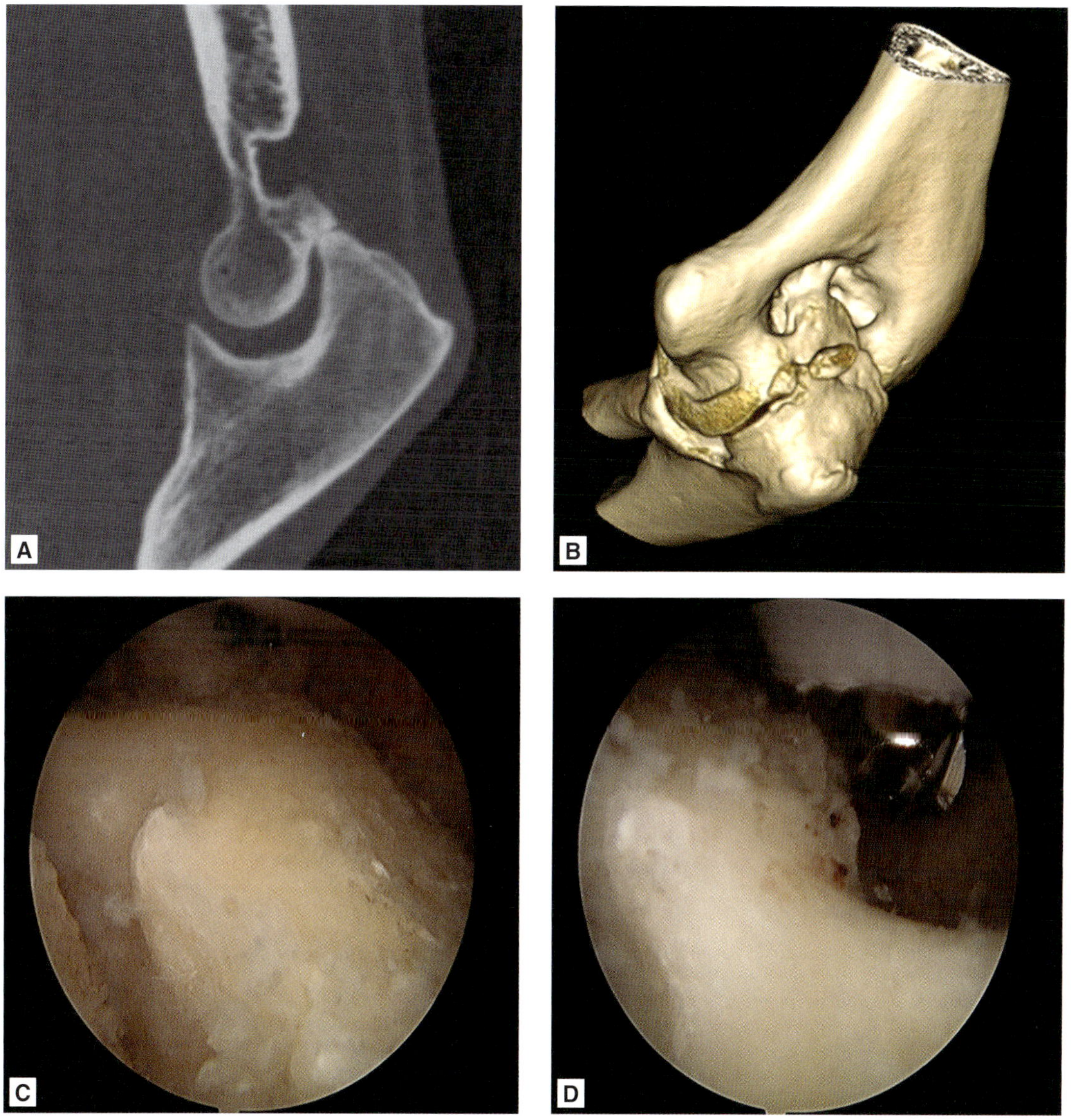

FIGURE 38-9 Preoperative (**A** and **B**) CT scans of a 38-year-old man demonstrate osteoarthrosis in this elbow. Intraoperative (**C** and **D**) visualization of the removal of the impinging bone in the olecranon fossa.

REFERENCES

1. Burman MS. Arthroscopy of the elbow joint. A cadaver study. *J Bone Joint Surg Am*. 1932;14:349–350.
2. Adams JE, Reding MT. Hemophilic arthropathy of the elbow. *Hand Clin*. 2011;27:151–163, v.
3. Yeoh KM, King GJ, Faber KJ, Glazebrook MA, Athwal GS. Evidence-based indications for elbow arthroscopy. *Arthroscopy*. 2012;28:272–282.
4. Miyake J, Masatomi T. Arthroscopic debridement of the humeral capitellum for osteochondritis dissecans: radiographic and clinical outcomes. *J Hand Surg Am*. 2011;36:1333–1338.
5. Cefo I, Eygendaal D. Arthroscopic arthrolysis for posttraumatic elbow stiffness. *J Shoulder Elbow Surg*. 2011;20:434–439.
6. Tucker SA, Savoie FH 3rd, O'Brien MJ. Arthroscopic management of the post-traumatic stiff elbow. *J Shoulder Elbow Surg*. 2011;20:S83–S89.
7. van den Ende KI, McIntosh AL, Adams JE, Steinmann SP. Osteochondritis dissecans of the capitellum: a review of the literature and a distal ulnar portal. *Arthroscopy*. 2011;27:122–128.
8. Savoie FH 3rd, O'Brien MJ, Field LD, Gurley DJ. Arthroscopic and open radial ulnohumeral ligament reconstruction for posterolateral rotatory instability of the elbow. *Clin Sports Med*. 2010;29:611–618.
9. Kang HJ, Park MJ, Ahn JH, Lee SH. Arthroscopic synovectomy for the rheumatoid elbow. *Arthroscopy*. 2010;26:1195–1202.
10. Savoie FH 3rd, VanSice W, O'Brien MJ. Arthroscopic tennis elbow release. *J Shoulder Elbow Surg*. 2010;19:31–36.
11. Savoie FH 3rd, Field LD, Gurley DJ. Arthroscopic and open radial ulnohumeral ligament reconstruction for posterolateral rotatory instability of the elbow. *Hand Clin*. 2009;25:323–329.
12. Savoie FH 3rd. Guidelines to becoming an expert elbow arthroscopist. *Arthroscopy*. 2007;23:1237–1240.
13. Krishnan SG, Harkins DC, Pennington SD, Harrison DK, Burkhead WZ. Arthroscopic ulnohumeral arthroplasty for degenerative arthritis

of the elbow in patients under fifty years of age. *J Shoulder Elbow Surg.* 2007;16:443–448.
14. Steinmann SP, King GJ, Savoie FH 3rd. Arthroscopic treatment of the arthritic elbow. *J Bone Joint Surg Am.* 2005;87:2114–2121.
15. Savoie FH 3rd, Nunley PD, Field LD. Arthroscopic management of the arthritic elbow: indications, technique, and results. *J Shoulder Elbow Surg.* 1999;8:214–219.
16. Adams JE, Wolff LH 3rd, Merten SM, Steinmann SP. Osteoarthritis of the elbow: results of arthroscopic osteophyte resection and capsulectomy. *J Shoulder Elbow Surg.* 2008;17:126–131.
17. Steinmann SP. Elbow arthroscopy: where are we now? *Arthroscopy.* 2007;23:1231–1236.
18. Adams JE, Merten SM, Steinmann SP. Arthroscopic-assisted treatment of coronoid fractures. *Arthroscopy.* 2007;23:1060–1065.
19. Hausman MR, Klug RA, Qureshi S, Goldstein R, Parsons BO. Arthroscopically assisted coronoid fracture fixation: a preliminary report. *Clin Orthop Relat Res.* 2008;466:3147–3152.
20. Hausman MR, Qureshi S, Goldstein R, et al. Arthroscopically-assisted treatment of pediatric lateral humeral condyle fractures. *J Pediatr Orthop.* 2007;27:739–742.
21. Hsu JW, Gould JL, Fonseca-Sabune H, Hausman MH. The emerging role of elbow arthroscopy in chronic use injuries and fracture care. *Hand Clin.* 2009;25:305–321.
22. Cohen MS, Romeo AA, Hennigan SP, Gordon M. Lateral epicondylitis: anatomic relationships of the extensor tendon origins and implications for arthroscopic treatment. *J Shoulder Elbow Surg.* 2008;17: 954–960.
23. Lattermann C, Romeo AA, Anbari A, et al. Arthroscopic debridement of the extensor carpi radialis brevis for recalcitrant lateral epicondylitis. *J Shoulder Elbow Surg.* 2010;19:651–656.
24. van den Ende KI, Steinmann SP. Arthroscopic treatment of septic arthritis of the elbow. *J Shoulder Elbow Surg.* 2012;21:1001–1005.
25. Sahajpal DT, Blonna D, O'Driscoll SW. Anteromedial elbow arthroscopy portals in patients with prior ulnar nerve transposition or subluxation. *Arthroscopy.* 2010;26:1045–1052.
26. Gay DM, Raphael BS, Weiland AJ. Revision arthroscopic contracture release in the elbow resulting in an ulnar nerve transection: a case report. *J Bone Joint Surg Am.* 2010;92:1246–1249.
27. Adams JE, Steinmann SP. Nerve injuries about the elbow. *J Hand Surg Am.* 2006;31:303–313.
28. Haapaniemi T, Berggren M, Adolfsson L. Complete transection of the median and radial nerves during arthroscopic release of post-traumatic elbow contracture. *Arthroscopy.* 1999;15:784–787.
29. Kelly EW, Morrey BF, O'Driscoll SW. Complications of elbow arthroscopy. *J Bone Joint Surg Am.* 2001;83-A:25–34.
30. Lynch GJ, Meyers JF, Whipple TL, Caspari RB. Neurovascular anatomy and elbow arthroscopy: inherent risks. *Arthroscopy.* 1986;2:190–197.
31. Marshall PD, Fairclough JA, Johnson SR, Evans EJ. Avoiding nerve damage during elbow arthroscopy. *J Bone Joint Surg Br.* 1993;75:129–131.
32. Miller CD, Jobe CM, Wright MH. Neuroanatomy in elbow arthroscopy. *J Shoulder Elbow Surg.* 1995;4:168–174.
33. O'Driscoll SW, Morrey BF. Arthroscopy of the elbow. Diagnostic and therapeutic benefits and hazards. *J Bone Joint Surg Am.* 1992;74:84–94.
34. Papilion JD, Neff RS, Shall LM. Compression neuropathy of the radial nerve as a complication of elbow arthroscopy: a case report and review of the literature. *Arthroscopy.* 1988;4:284–286.
35. Park JY, Cho CH, Choi JH, Lee ST, Kang CH. Radial nerve palsy after arthroscopic anterior capsular release for degenerative elbow contracture. *Arthroscopy.* 2007;23:1360 e1361–e1363.
36. Ruch DS, Poehling GG. Anterior interosseus nerve injury following elbow arthroscopy. *Arthroscopy.* 1997;13:756–758.
37. Thomas MA, Fast A, Shapiro D. Radial nerve damage as a complication of elbow arthroscopy. *Clin Orthop Relat Res.* 1987:130–131.
38. Verhaar J, van Mameren H, Brandsma A. Risks of neurovascular injury in elbow arthroscopy: starting anteromedially or anterolaterally? *Arthroscopy.* 1991;7:287–290.
39. Gofton WT, King GJ. Heterotopic ossification following elbow arthroscopy. *Arthroscopy.* 2001;17:E2.
40. Sodha S, Nagda SH, Sennett BJ. Heterotopic ossification in a throwing athlete after elbow arthroscopy. *Arthroscopy.* 2006;22:802 e801–e803.
41. Hughes SC, Hildebrand KA. Heterotopic ossification—a complication of elbow arthroscopy: a case report. *J Shoulder Elbow Surg.* 2010;19:e1–e5.
42. DeGreef I, Samorjai N, De Smet L. The Outerbridge-Kashiwaghi procedure in elbow arthroscopy. *Acta Orthop Belg.* 2010;76:468–471.
43. Cohen AP, Redden JF, Stanley D. Treatment of osteoarthritis of the elbow: a comparison of open and arthroscopic debridement. *Arthroscopy.* 2000;16:701–706.
44. Redden JF, Stanley D. Arthroscopic fenestration of the olecranon fossa in the treatment of osteoarthritis of the elbow. *Arthroscopy.* 1993;9:14–16.
45. McLaughlin RE 2nd, Savoie FH 3rd, Field LD, Ramsey JR. Arthroscopic treatment of the arthritic elbow due to primary radiocapitellar arthritis. *Arthroscopy.* 2006;22:63–69.
46. Kovachevich R, Steinmann SP. Arthroscopic ulnar nerve decompression in the setting of elbow osteoarthritis. *J Hand Surg Am.* 2012;37:663–668.
47. Reddy AS, Kvitne RS, Yocum LA, Elattrache NS, Glousman RE, Jobe FW. Arthroscopy of the elbow: a long-term clinical review. *Arthroscopy.* 2000;16:588–594.

39

Arthroscopic and Open Management of Instability of the Elbow

Felix H. Savoie, III, MD
Michael J. O'Brien, MD

RATIONALE AND BASIC SCIENCE PERTINENT TO THE PROCEDURE

History

There has been a growing interest in the management of instability of the elbow, driven primarily by the high demand of patients to resume normal activity after injury. Since the landmark reports by Jobe et al[1] on reconstruction of the medial ulnar collateral ligament (MUCL) in baseball players and by O'Driscoll et al[2] on posterolateral rotatory instability (PLRI), the management of ligament injuries of the elbow has advanced dramatically.

Reconstruction of the MUCL in athletes was defined by the initial report by Jobe et al,[1] which changed a career-ending injury into one where the majority of players are able to resume their career. Their technique has been modified over the years by Altchek, Conway, ElAttrache, and Andrews, along with many others.[3] The so-called Tommy John surgery has caught the public imagination with its high-profile success stories. More recently, Smith et al[4] and Richard et al[5] have reported successful results of repair of the ligament in younger athletes who are performing at a high level but who do not yet have the more severe panligamentous damage noted in professional athletes.

Basic Science

In general, the ligaments of the elbow are extracapsular, with an abundant blood supply and an excellent healing environment. Stability of the elbow is afforded by a combination of these ligaments, the bony anatomy, and dynamic muscle contraction.[6]

MUCL

The anatomy of the MUCL, specifically the origin from the distal, lateral aspect of the epicondyle, was first accurately described by Callaway et al.[7] Prior to that description it was thought to originate more medially, near the tip. This led Richard et al[5] and Smith et al[4] to design successful repair techniques that more accurately replicated the normal anatomy.

The medial collateral ligament consists of an anterior and a posterior bundle with a transverse ligament in between.[8] The anterior bundle is the primary restraint to valgus stress. It originates on the central two-thirds of the anteroinferior aspect of the medial humeral epicondyle. The humeral attachment is spread around the base of the medial epicondyle across its distal and posterior-distal aspects, thus spanning across the site of the flexion–extension axis that emerges from the center of the circular medial end-face of the trochlea at the distal edge of the epicondyle. The anterior bundle inserts at the base of the coronoid, on average 18 mm posterior from the tip. The width of its origin averages about 10 mm and involves 67% of the epicondyle in the coronal plane. The mean length of the anterior bundle is about 27 mm, with a width of 4 to 5 mm. Some studies have also shown that the anterior medial collateral ligament can be subdivided into anterior and posterior bands. These bands demonstrate a different tension in various positions of the elbow, due to a cam effect. A central portion that remains isometric throughout elbow movement has also been suggested, and can be used as a guide for ligament reconstruction. This deep bundle runs from 5 mm anterior to the distal tip of the medial epicondyle to the most prominent part of the sublime tubercle on the ulna. The posterior bundle of the medial collateral ligament inserts slightly posterior to the anterior medial collateral ligament and fans out along the base of the greater sigmoid notch. It has an average width of 8 mm and a thickness of 4 to 8 mm. The function of this ligament is to restrain valgus stress, especially during flexion.

The mechanical properties of the collateral ligaments were measured by Regan et al.[9] They found that the anterior band of the MCL was the strongest, with a tensile strength of 261 ± 71 N, while the posterior band had a tensile strength of 159 ± 40 N. The lateral collateral ligament had a tensile strength of 233 ± 116 N. By comparison, the palmaris longus tendon strength was 358 ± 88 N and its stiffness was more than 6 times greater than the ligaments.

Morrey and An at the Mayo clinic did multiple studies on the function of the MUCL.[10] The most anterior fibers of the anterior band of the MUCL are close to being isometric and, therefore, tight throughout the range of elbow flexion–extension. Moving posteriorly across the width of the MUCL complex, there is an increasing tendency for the ligament fibers to slacken as the elbow is extended; hence, the posterior band of the MUCL is only tightened completely when it becomes wrapped around the distal aspect of the epicondyle beyond 90° of elbow flexion. Morrey and An found that the MUCL resisted approximately one-third of the valgus stress applied to the elbow when it was extended. In addition, they noted that because the anterior joint capsule was tight in this position, it also took one-third of the load, with the articular surfaces taking the remainder. As the elbow flexed, the MUCL took a larger proportion of the load, reaching 54% at 90° flexion. Thus, they felt that the MCL was the primary restraint to valgus laxity. Cutting the anterior band of the MCL led to 14° of valgus laxity at 70° of elbow flexion. At this point, the posterior band became tight; if this was also cut, the elbow became unstable, with up to 31° of valgus deformity.

Pronation, axial load, and varus stress are thought to cause a fracture of the anteromedial coronoid, with avulsion of the lateral collateral ligament at its origin and disruption of the posterior bundle of the medial collateral ligament. This injury pattern results in posteromedial rotatory instability (PMRI). This instability pattern typically occurs after a fall on the outstretched hand where the forearm is pronated, axially loaded, and undergoes a varus stress. The anteromedial coronoid fails as the trochlea rotates and displaces anteriorly, while the lateral collateral ligament fails under tension at the lateral epicondyle. The posterior bundle of the MCL also tears due to ulnar rotation. Baseball pitchers and other high-velocity overhead athletes may develop acute or chronic valgus instability due to rupture or attenuation of the anterior bundle of the MCL.

Radioulnohumeral Ligament (RUHL)

Four distinct bundles comprise the lateral collateral ligament complex: the lateral ulnar collateral ligament, the radial collateral ligament, the annular ligament, and the accessory lateral collateral ligament. It is a key stabilizer for varus stress and posterolateral stability.

The most important part of the lateral collateral ligament complex is the lateral ulnar collateral ligament, which is responsible for the prevention of posterolateral elbow instability. The origin is situated on the center of the lateral epicondyle of the humerus, blends with the annular ligament, and inserts onto the tubercle of the supinator crest. The radial collateral ligament, which originates at the center of the lateral epicondyle, extends to the annular ligament. This ligament provides an additional origin for the supinator muscle. The radial collateral ligament has an average length of 20 mm and a width of 8 mm.

The annular ligament inserts on the anterior and posterior margins of the radial notch and encircles the radial head, binding it to the lesser sigmoid notch of the ulna to prevent inferior or lateral subluxation. The collective function of the annular ligament and the radial collateral ligament is to maintain stability during varus stress and posterolateral directed forces on the elbow. The annular ligament, together with the quadrate ligament, also stabilizes the proximal radioulnar joint. Various components of the lateral collateral ligament play a different role in maintaining stability during varus stress. The anterior and posterior parts of the radial collateral ligament are taut in extension and flexion, respectively, while the middle part is taut in midrange. The lateral ulnar collateral ligament is taut in extreme elbow flexion and is tightened further with additional varus stress. The interosseous membrane between the ulna and the radius prevents divergence of the radius or ulna and regulates the forces acting on these 2 bones. Together with the distal radioulnar joint it is a key component in forearm rotation and stability. In general, the lateral collateral ligament structures are less important for elbow stability than the medial collateral ligament complex. Morrey and An found that the trochlea was more important than the lateral ligaments for resisting varus stresses, contributing 75% at 90° of flexion. As the elbow reached full extension, the tightening of the anterior capsule caused the soft tissues to become more dominant, with the lateral collateral ligaments contributing 14% and the anterior capsule 32%.

The principal clinical problem associated with disruption of the lateral ligaments is PLRI. This is associated with the radial head subluxing posterior to the capitellum as a result of translation and rotation of the forearm.

PLRI has been described as an instability pattern of the elbow that results from an incompetent radial ulnohumeral ligament complex (RUHLC).[2] O'Driscoll et al found that for PLRI to occur the ulna had to supinate 41° out of its articulation with the trochlea, carrying the head of the radius posteriorly while pivoting on the intact medial collateral ligament, which resulted in 15° of valgus from the elbow's normal carrying angle. Supination, axial load, and valgus stress typically result in injury to the lateral collateral ligament with or without associated radial head and coronoid fractures. Dunning et al[11] stated that both the RUHL and the radial collateral ligament must be sectioned to achieve PLRI. They also stated that they could not visually differentiate the 2 ligaments at their humeral origin. They could only differentiate the RUHL from the RCL by identifying the distal extent of the RUHL at the supinator crest of the ulna. Seki et al[12] were able to show that sectioning just the anterior band of the lateral collateral complex induced instability. This suggests that an intact RUHL alone cannot stabilize the elbow. These data demonstrate that the entity of PLRI is, in fact, a spectrum of injury. Although originally described as a sequelae of an elbow dislocation, these anatomic studies and the report by Kalainov and Cohen,[13] and more recently by Savoie et al,[14] support that there is a continuum of injury between PLRI and frank elbow dislocation.

Examination

Medial instability is best demonstrated by the moving valgus extension overload (VEO) test described by O'Driscoll, who reported it as both sensitive (100% in 17 patients) and specific (75% in 4 patients). The patient is positioned such that the arm is abducted to 90° and is in maximum external rotation. The test is begun with the elbow in maximum flexion. The examiner grasps the patient's wrist with 1 hand and places the other hand to pivot on the lateral aspect of the elbow. While applying a valgus stress to the elbow, the elbow is moved from full flexion to full extension. Pain on the medial side of the elbow between 70° and 120° of elbow flexion denotes a positive test for MUCL pathology. Pain with the elbow at 45° is more indicative of a capitellar osteochondral defect, while pain at terminal extension may indicate a trochlear chondral defect. It is important to evaluate areas of tenderness and range of motion, and also compare the elbow side to side for valgus laxity, milk test, and VEO test in addition to the moving VEO test.

VALGUS EXTENSION OVERLOAD TEST

Some overhead-throwing athletes with physiological MUCL laxity or chronic MUCL insufficiency will develop osteophytes at the posteromedial olecranon, with pain at terminal extension. To test for VEO syndrome, the elbow is gently forced into full extension with a valgus stress. Pain with this test or tenderness to palpation over the posteromedial aspect of the olecranon denotes a positive test and may indicate symptomatic abutment of osteophytes on the olecranon or in the olecranon fossa.

VALGUS STRESS TEST

The patient is seated with the shoulder in maximal external rotation to lock the humerus in position, and the elbow is placed in 25° to 30° of flexion to unlock the olecranon from the olecranon fossa and to relax the anterior capsule. The examiner then braces the patient's hand and wrist between their own arm and chest wall and applies a valgus stress to the elbow while palpating the medial ulnohumeral joint for increased opening with no definitive end point. A soft end point may also indicate an attenuated or incompetent ligament. The degree of instability is measured in millimeters of ulnohumeral opening and is considered positive when greater than 3 mm.

MILKING MANEUVER

This test derives from a common stretching maneuver done by baseball pitchers during warm-ups. The patient begins by placing the affected elbow on the antecubital fossa of the contralateral arm and then grasps the thumb of the affected extremity with the unaffected extremity. Pulling downward on the thumb, with the elbow flexed greater than 90°, creates a valgus stress, thus loading the MUCL. Pain elicited at the medial elbow, with or without apprehension, denotes a positive test for MCL injury. If the patient is not flexible enough to perform this unaided, the examiner may re-create the same effect by forward elevating and maximally externally rotating the arm of the patient and then applying a valgus stress to the flexed elbow. A positive test elicits pain at the medial elbow.

HYPERPRONATION TEST

The elbow is placed in 90° of flexion and the examiner maximally pronates the patient's forearm while palpating the medial ulnohumeral joint for gapping. This test is best performed under anesthesia and can be best appreciated with fluoroscopic imaging.

PMRI pattern typically occurs after a fall on the outstretched hand where the forearm is pronated, axially loaded, and incurs a varus stress. The anteromedial coronoid fails as the trochlea rotates and displaces anteriorly, while the lateral collateral ligament fails under tension at the lateral epicondyle. The posterior bundle of the MCL also tears due to ulnar rotation. Tests for this type of instability include the varus stress and the reverse pivot shift test.

LATERAL PIVOT SHIFT TEST

Lateral instability is best demonstrated clinically with the pivot shift test of the elbow. This test, as first described by O'Driscoll et al, in the supine position may elicit gross instability, pain, and apprehension[2] and is difficult to perform in the awake patient due to apprehension and guarding. The patient is positioned supine on the examination table with the shoulder placed in full forward elevation and in full external rotation. The examiner stands at the head of the table, grasps the patient's wrist with 1 hand, and braces the lateral aspect of the patient's elbow with the other hand. Beginning with the elbow extended, the examiner fully supinates the patient's forearm, applies an axial load with simultaneous valgus stress, and brings the elbow from extension to flexion. A positive test occurs when a palpable clunk is generated as the radial head reduces from the posteriorly subluxated or dislocated position to become reduced on the capitellum. Reduction usually occurs as the elbow approaches 40° of flexion. Taking the elbow from a flexed to an extended position causes the radial head to subluxate or dislocate posterior to the capitellum. A posterolateral skin dimple may be seen while the radial head is dislocated. O'Driscoll subsequently modified this test to one in which a positive test is denoted by apprehension of this maneuver. This is more easily elicited in the awake patient and is one of the most sensitive special tests for PLRI.

REVERSE PIVOT SHIFT TEST

This reduction test is performed in an analogous fashion to the lateral pivot shift test. The patient is supine, with the affected shoulder in full forward elevation. With the elbow in extension, the forearm is pronated and a varus and axial load is applied to subluxate the elbow. As the elbow is gradually flexed the joint will reduce with an audible clunk or grinding sensation from the associated coronoid fracture.

In throwers, one should also evaluate the shoulder and trunk stability along with hip strength by the 1 leg squat test. Radiographs are usually negative, while ultrasound (US) and MR arthrograms (MRA) are more definitive in the evaluation of the ligament. In young athletes (age <20), it is important to determine the structural status of the ligament to see if they are a candidate for repair versus reconstruction.

Two other clinical tests, described by Regan et al,[9] include pushing up from an arm chair with the palms facing inward and having the patient push up from a prone or wall leaning position—first with the forearms maximally pronated and then repeating the test with the forearms supinated—to reproduce the pain and instability the patient is feeling. We prefer to examine the elbow with the patient in the prone position and use the table as a base to stabilize the humerus. We begin by manually trying to rotate the forearm from the humerus in 90° of flexion, and then use the wrist to supinate and rotate the forearm to reproduce the radial column subluxation away from the humerus. The radial head movement on the capitellum is more easily seen and felt in this position, and the elbow can be flexed and extended while maintaining the subluxation force.

POSTEROLATERAL DRAWER TEST

The patient lies supine with the shoulder extended and externally rotated. The elbow is flexed to 90° and the examiner grasps the proximal forearm while applying a posteriorly directed force. Subluxation of the radial head and ulna denotes a positive test as these rotate away from the humerus and pivot on the MUCL.

HYPERSUPINATION TEST

This is easier to perform on the awake patient than the lateral pivot shift and posterolateral drawer tests. Unlike the lateral pivot shift test, which is a reduction maneuver, this test re-creates instability. The patient is positioned with the elbow at 90° of flexion. The examiner grasps the patient's wrist with 1 hand and places the thumb of the other hand on the posterolateral aspect of the radiocapitellar joint. With hypersupination of the patient's forearm, the examiner palpates for radial head glide, subluxation, or dislocation with respect to the capitellum. If instability is noted, pronation of the forearm will reduce the radial head. A dimple may be seen with subluxation of the radial head and, in addition, rotation of the ulna away from the lateral epicondyle may occur. The test should be repeated at about 45° of elbow flexion if it is equivocal or negative at 90°. Performing this test under fluoroscopy will demonstrate the instability with posterolateral subluxation of the radial head on the capitellum and associated rotation of the ulna away from the trochlea.

Imaging

Imaging studies for PLRI can be helpful. Radiographs may reveal an avulsion fragment from the posterior humeral lateral epicondyle in acute cases. However, often radiographs are normal. A stress radiograph or fluoroscopy while performing the pivot shift test may show the radial head and proximal ulna moving together in a subluxed and posterolaterally rotated position. Magnetic resonance imaging (MRI) of the elbow has been described to identify a lesion in the RUHL.[15] It has been our experience that MRIs are most helpful when contrast is added. This can be either a formal arthrogram or, in the case of in-office MRI, an injection of 20 to 30 cc^3 of sterile normal saline just before the scan that can greatly enhance the effectiveness of the test.

Indications for Surgery

MEDIAL

The primary indication for surgery in medial instability is the injury to the ligament in an athlete involved in a throwing sport who wishes to continue in that sport. Thus, the ideal patient is a young athlete, usually age 12 to 20 for repair and 17 to 35 for reconstruction. This ligament is not involved in most day-to-day activities, and repair or reconstruction is usually not indicated in nonathletic patients. The main decision in these patients is that of repair versus reconstruction. In young patients with proximal or distal avulsion and a normal-appearing ligament, repair is preferable over reconstruction. In most professional athletes, the ligament is usually more diffusely damaged and reconstruction with either autograft or allograft is preferable.

LATERAL

The primary indication for lateral repair is functional impairment of activities of daily living and a failure of nonoperative treatment. The ideal patient would be one who sustained a traumatic dislocation, was properly treated, and regained motion but is left with shifting of the elbow on supination extension maneuvers without damage to lateral musculature. The usual problem in lateral instability is making the proper diagnosis. The more subtle findings include a lateral shift/click of the radial head in 90° of flexion. Lateral radiographs may show a subtle posterior shift of the radial head on the capitellum. MRA may be of use, but requires careful inspection of the ligaments in chronic situation.

Contraindications

The main contraindications for surgery for instability are those commonly noted for any surgical procedure: failure to meet appropriate indications, ongoing infections, and a lack of training to do the proper operation.

Surgical Technique

INSTRUMENTATION

The main equipment for all 4 surgeries that will be discussed below includes a standard arthroscopy system, with a bridge on the arthroscope to allow easy switching between portals, 18-gauge spinal needles, PDS suture for shuttling, retrograde suture graspers (we favor the 30° Ideal™ suture retriever [DePuy Mitek, Raynham, Massachusetts]), anchors, drill bits, and small reamers and small interference screws for supplemental fixation. A Hewson™ suture retriever (Smith & Nephew, Andover, Massachusetts) and small curettes are quite useful in most cases. A pump for the arthroscope is usually not used but, if used, should be on a very low pressure setting in order to minimize swelling and thereby potentially complicate the open surgery.

MUCL Repair

TULANE TECHNIQUE

The patient is positioned prone with the arm elevated on a small bump. The arthroscope is introduced via a proximal anteromedial or proximal anterolateral portal and a diagnostic arthroscopy performed with careful attention for capsular damage, associated lateral laxity, and loose bodies. The inflow is left anterior and the arthroscope placed posterior central to evaluate the olecranon fossa and posteromedial olecranon tip for impingement and chondromalacia. Once completed, the shoulder is internally rotated and the hand placed on the arm board, allowing easy access to the medial elbow. A 3-cm incision is made from the tip of the medial epicondyle distally, approximately 1 cm anterior to the path of the ulnar nerve in the forearm (Fig. 39-1). The medial antebrachial cutaneous nerve is protected by retracting it anteriorly. The flexor pronator fascia is incised just posterior to the medial conjoined tendon septum and the interval in the muscle posterior to this vertical band is developed down to the MUCL. The ligament is carefully inspected to determine its areas of damage (Fig. 39-2).

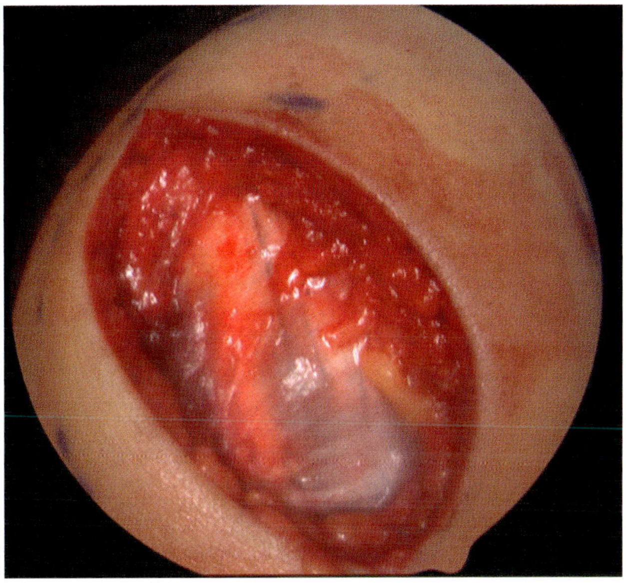

FIGURE 39-1 The incision for the medial approach begins at the tip of the medial epicondyle and extends distally toward the wrist, paralleling the fibers of the flexor pronator muscle and 1 cm anterior to the course of the ulnar nerve in the forearm.

An incision is made along its anterior edge to allow evaluation of the underside of the ligament (Fig. 39-2B). Once it has been confirmed that it is normal except for the area of tearing, a double-loaded, absorbable anchor is inserted into the base of the medial epicondyle at the junction of the trochlea and the distal medial epicondyle. The first set of sutures is passed in horizontal mattress fashion through the ligament just outside the tear site and the second 5 to 8 mm distal to the first (Fig. 39-3). The ulnar nerve is quite close to the posterior aspect of the ligament, so it should be carefully protected during suture passage. The sutures are tied in sequence and the elbow cycled to confirm an anatomic repair. The flexor pronator muscle is allowed to fall back into its normal position and the fascia closed with absorbable suture, as is the skin.

The patient is splinted for the first week and then placed into a hinged elbow brace full time for the next 6 weeks. Rehabilitation of the scapula is started immediately and progressed to shoulder, core, and lower extremity during the first 8 weeks in the brace. A return to throw and hit program is initiated in the brace near the 8-week mark, depending on shoulder and scapular strength. If there is no pain over the medial elbow, the brace is removed at 12 weeks and the patient is progressed back into play under PT and ATC supervision.

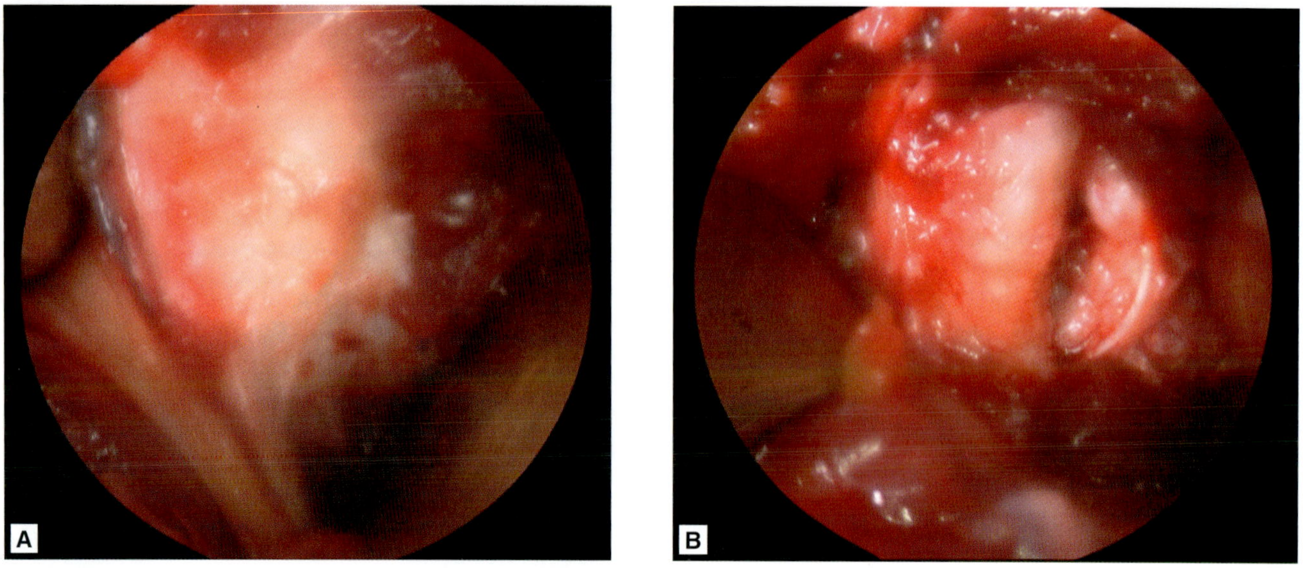

FIGURE 39-2 **A.** The view of the MUCL via a flexor pronator split. **B.** The underside of the ligament.

MUCL Reconstruction

The approach used by Smith et al[16] for MUCL repair is also used for the reconstruction, but extended slightly both proximally and distally (Fig. 39-4). The fascial sheath over the ulnar nerve is identified and split to allow direct visualization of the nerve. Once the ligament is visualized, it is carefully examined. The sublime tubercle of the ulna is evaluated for the quality and shape of the bone. Either converging drill holes anterior and posterior to the tubercle or a single tunnel directly centered on the tubercle is made. If the converging tunnels are used (classic Jobe technique), we usually make 4-mm tunnels. If a single tunnel is made (Conway's DANE technique), then it is a single 5-mm tunnel directly through the tubercle, tapped to allow a 5.5- or 6-mm screw (Fig. 39-5). The middle of the graft is then placed into the tunnels and fixated with an absorbable interference screw. A single 5- or 6-mm tunnel is then drilled into the medial epicondyle at the anatomic origin site of the MUCL (Fig. 39-6). Connecting drill holes are then made from posterior inferior and posterior superior to connect to the more posterior aspect of the single tunnel. The graft is pulled through the center tunnel, 1 limb out the top drill hole and 1 out the bottom. The graft limbs are then crossed and sutured to each other (Fig. 39-7). The residual ligament is repaired to the graft and the flexor pronator fascia repaired as well.

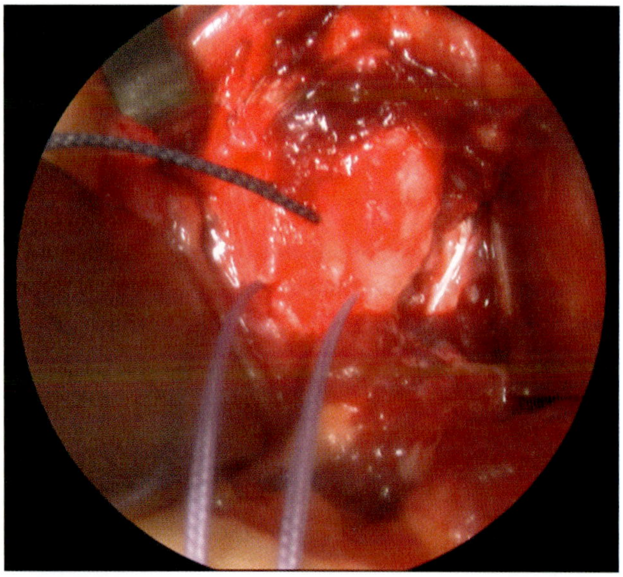

FIGURE 39-3 Passing of the dual mattress sutures through the proximal end of the MUCL tear.

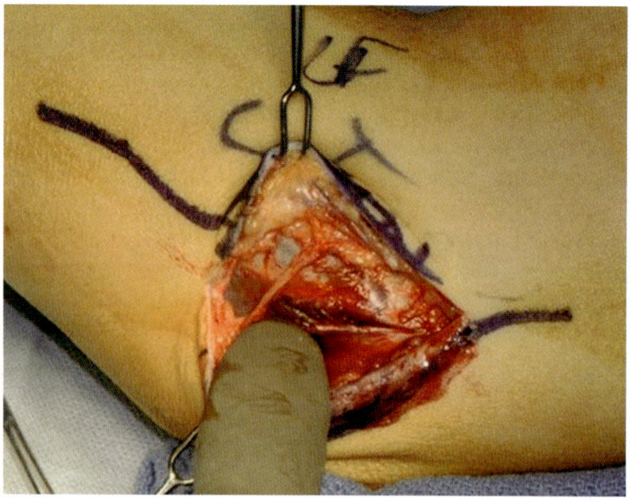

FIGURE 39-4 The flexor pronator approach of Smith and Altchek to the MUCL.

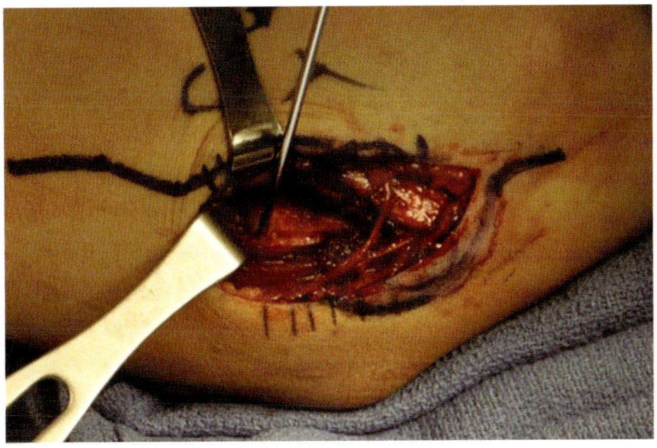

FIGURE 39-5 The ulnar tunnels are drilled and the graft passed.

Rehabilitation for the reconstructed elbow is similar to that described for the repair, just much slower due to the need for graft incorporation. However, as an extra-articular ligament with abundant blood supply, one should expect graft incorporation to occur at a rapid rate. Our patients are splinted for the first week, and then placed in a hinged elbow brace set at 30° to 120° for the next 4 weeks and at full ROM for the following 16 weeks. Scapular, core, and leg exercises are initiated the first week and progressed with a focus on correct scapular positioning during all activities. Rotator cuff exercises are added at week 3 and pain-free elbow stretching and exercises at week 4. Usually around week 12, throwing and hitting are added while keeping the brace on if all the rest of the body has returned to normal. Most athletes return in 6 months.

ARTHROSCOPIC LATERAL AND POSTEROLATERAL REPAIR

In the elbow with an acute or chronic avulsion of the RULC, arthroscopic repair can be quite effective. The procedure

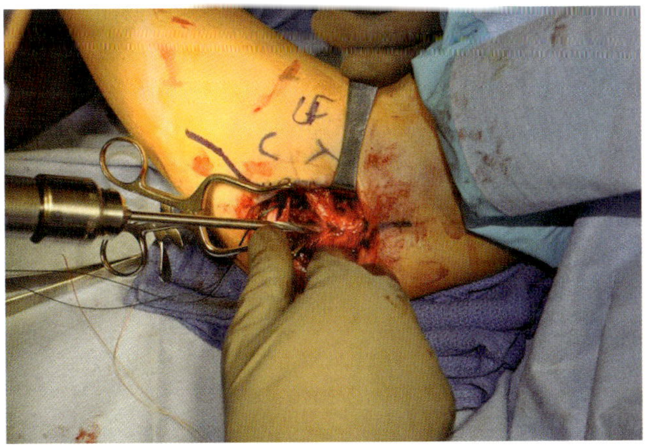

FIGURE 39-6 The humeral tunnel is drilled into the condyle and then converging tunnels made and the graft passed through the tunnels.

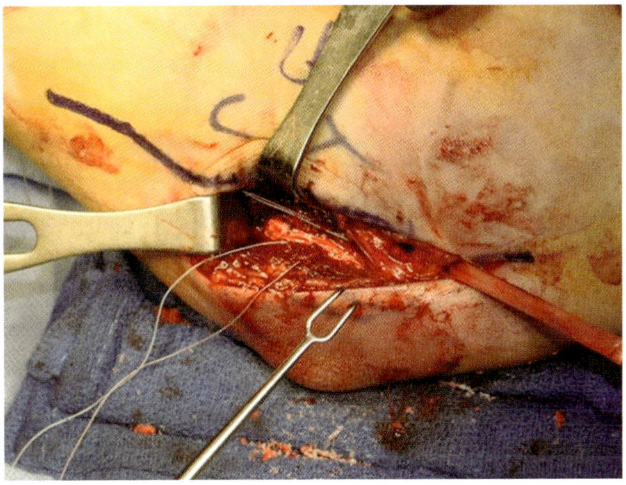

FIGURE 39-7 The graft in place for MUCL reconstruction.

begins with the establishment of a proximal anterior medial portal and a diagnostic anterior compartment arthroscopy. In the acute setting, it may be necessary to establish a lateral portal to clean out the associated hematoma (Fig. 39-8). The tearing of the anterior capsule is readily apparent acutely, and most often one can also see the damage to the brachialis muscle visible through the torn capsule. The main area of interest here is to view the annular ligament for damage and place a suture in it if necessary. One can also view "around the corner" of the proximal capitellum for damage to the collateral ligament part of the RULC (Fig. 39-9). The arthroscope is then placed into the posterior central portal and the hematoma in the back of the elbow compartment evacuated via a proximal posterior lateral portal. Both of these portals need to be relatively proximal to allow for the later repair of the ligament, usually at least 3 cm above the olecranon tip. A view of the medial gutter will show hemorrhage and sometimes tearing of the capsule near the posterior aspect

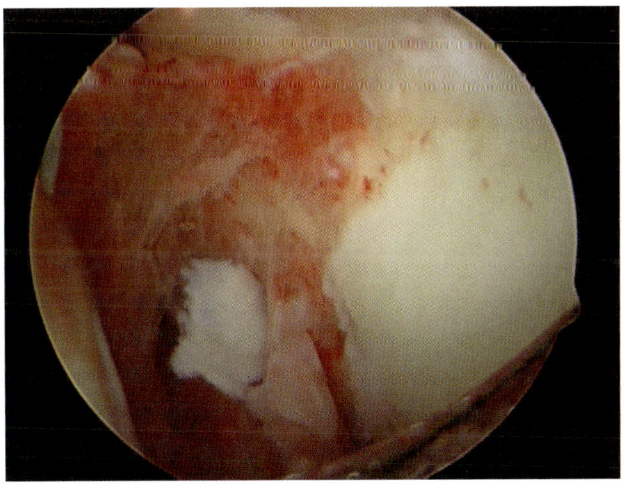

FIGURE 39-8 Hematoma and tearing of the anterior capsule.

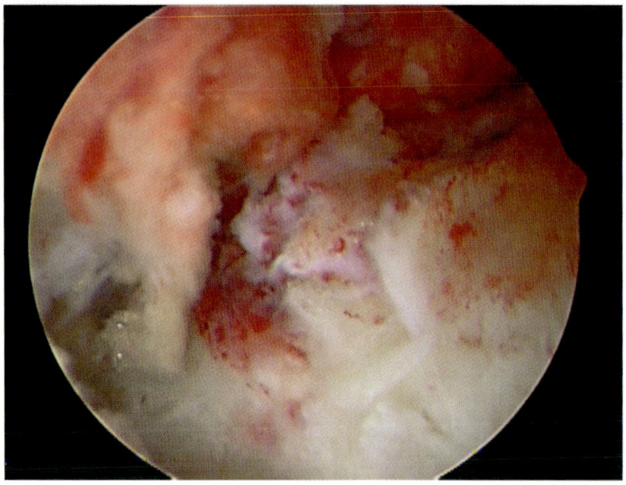

FIGURE 39-9 Damage to the lateral capsule from dislocation of the elbow.

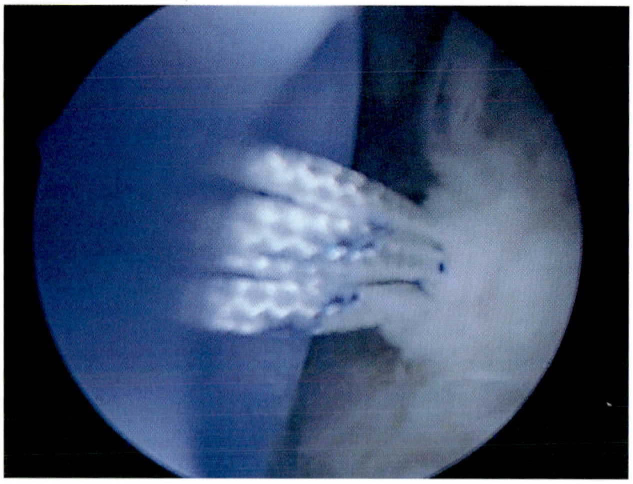

FIGURE 39-11 Anchor placement into the posterior aspect of the distal lateral epicondyle.

of the medial epicondyle. The lateral gutter and capsule is then evaluated. It is very important to stay close to the ulna as the lateral gutter is evaluated and the hematoma debrided as the avulsed ligament and bone fragments are displaced distally and may inadvertently be removed by the shaver (Fig. 39-10). The lateral aspect of the posterior humerus should also be lightly debrided and the site of avulsion localized. It is usually directly lateral and slightly inferior to the center of the olecranon fossa. Once the area of damage has been defined an arthroscopic anchor may be placed into the humerus at the site of origin of the RUHL (Fig. 39-11). The limbs of the suture are then retrieved to place 2 horizontal mattress sutures through the uninjured part of the ligament. In the case of a bony avulsion, we place 1 set of sutures around the bone fragment and the other distal to the fragment (Fig. 39-12A and B). The sutures are tensioned while

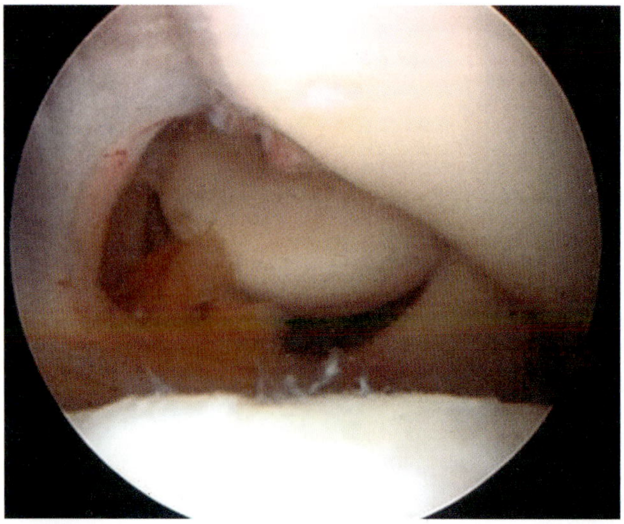

FIGURE 39-10 Damage to the lateral and posterior lateral capsule, which is allowing the elbow to gap open.

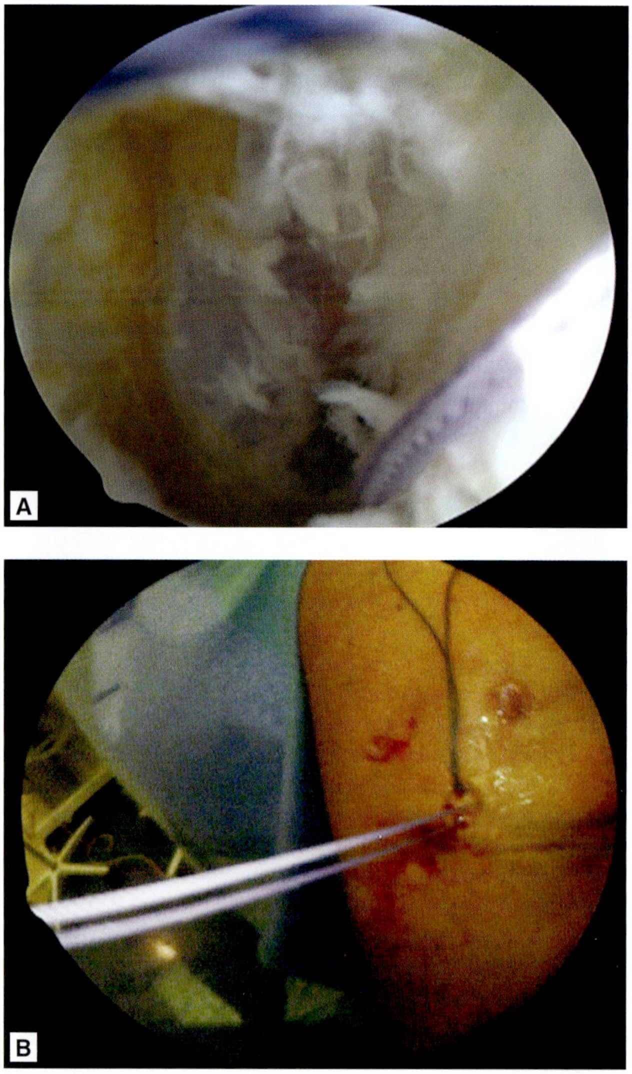

FIGURE 39-12 Sutures through the RUHL prior to tightening: (**A**) arthroscopic view; (**B**) open view.

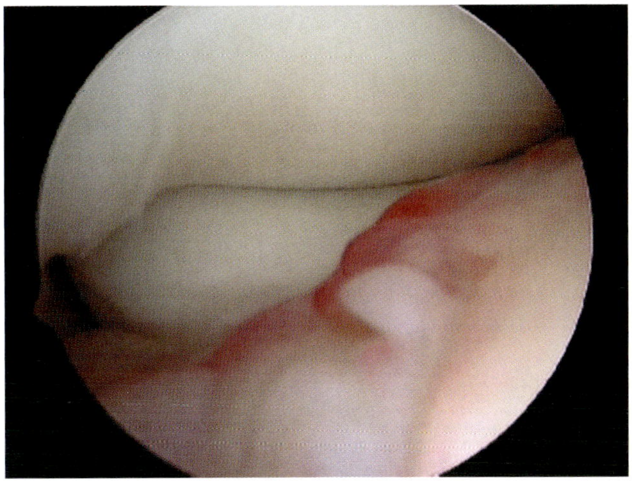

FIGURE 39-13 Anterior view after RUHL repair showing the properly restored tension to the annular ligament.

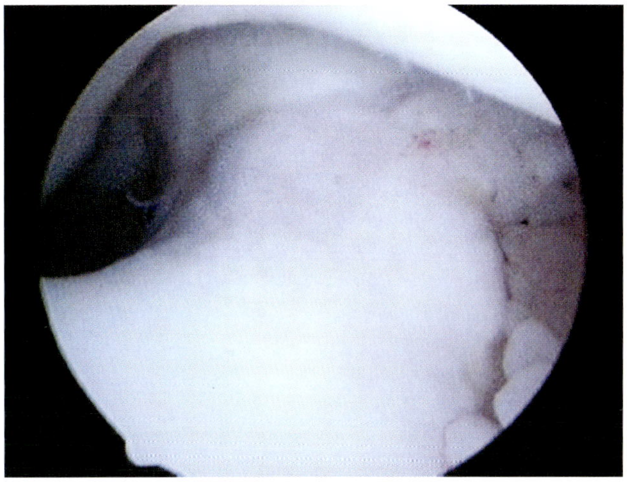

FIGURE 39-14 The drive-through sign of the elbow, pathognomonic of PLRI.

viewing with the arthroscope, which should have the effect of pushing it (the arthroscope) out of the lateral gutter. The elbow is then extended and the sutures are tied beneath the anconeus muscle, tightening the ligament. Motion and stability is then evaluated with the arthroscope back in the anterior compartment (Fig. 39-13).

ARTHROSCOPIC PLICATION

The development of an arthroscopic technique for the treatment of chronic PLRI was described by Smith et al in 2001.[4] Chronic posterolateral instability is more readily seen during examination under anesthesia and on arthroscopic evaluation. While viewing from the proximal anterior medial portal, the ulnar and radial head can be seen to subluxate posterolaterally during the performance of a pivot shift test. In most cases the annular ligament is intact as the entire proximal radioulnar joint shifts on the humerus. One common finding is the ability to move an arthroscope, placed down the posterolateral gutter from the posterior central portal, straight across the ulnohumeral articulation into the medial gutter. This maneuver is not possible in a stable elbow, and is termed the "drive-through sign of the elbow" and is somewhat analogous to the "drive-through sign" in shoulder instability (Fig. 39-14). The elimination of the laxity that allows this maneuver is one of the key aspects of confirming an adequate arthroscopic reconstruction in patients with PLRI.

The arthroscopic technique for chronic instability has 2 key features: plication of the 2 major components of the complex and then repair of the complex to the humerus. We believe both components can be managed via arthroscopic techniques if there is enough ligamentous and capsular tissue. This assessment is in part determined by the preoperative evaluation, including palpation of the structures in the area to be reconstructed, the amount of prior surgery, and the tissue present on MRA findings. If adequate tissue is present, the tissue in the posterolateral gutter is assessed arthroscopically and prepared with a shaver or rasp. Four to 7 absorbable sutures are then placed in oblique fashion beginning at the most distal extent of the RUHL complex attachment to the ulna. The sutures are placed into the lateral gutter via an 18-gauge spinal needle that slides along the radial border of the ulna. The first suture is delivered into the joint through the midportion of the annular ligament (Fig. 39-15). Subsequent sutures are brought into the joint in a progressively more proximal position. Each suture is immediately retrieved with a retrograde suture retriever that passes into the joint from the posterior lateral aspect of the lateral epicondyle (Fig. 39-16). It is quite important that the retrograde retriever comes under the entire RUHL near its proximal attachment to the humerus. The suture should

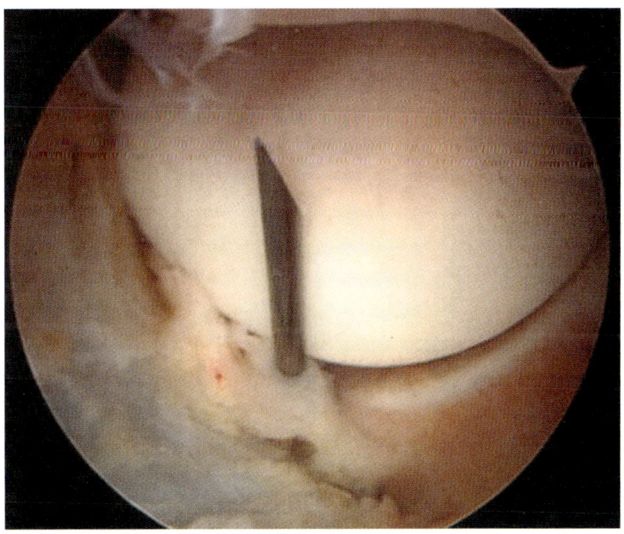

FIGURE 39-15 Placement of the spinal needle along the ulna and under the annular ligament for suture delivery.

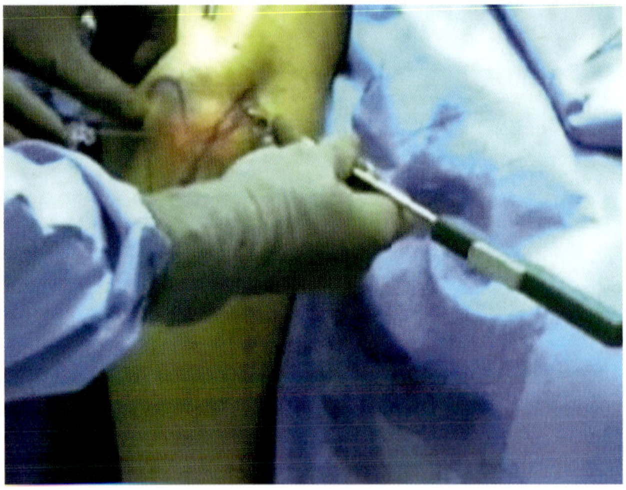

FIGURE 39-16 Outside view of retrograde retriever being placed into the joint posterior to lateral epicondyle at site of origin of the RUHL.

span the capsule from the ulna to the humerus (Fig. 39-17). Once all the sutures have been placed, they are retrieved 1 at a time percutaneously through the existing skin portals under, or in some cases over, the anconeus muscle and pulled to tension the sutures and evaluate the plication. If the reconstruction has been properly performed and the tissue is adequate for plication, the arthroscope is driven out of the lateral gutter as this tensioning occurs. The arthroscope is then removed, the elbow extended, and the sutures are then tied individually from distal to proximal. The examination under anesthesia is repeated and the arthroscope placed into the posterior central and proximal anterior medial portals to evaluate adequacy of the reconstruction. If there is laxity or subluxation still present after the sutures are pretensioned, an anchor can be placed at the isometric point of the lateral epicondyle as in the acute repairs and 1 limb of suture can pass under all of the loops of the plication sutures to a retriever and then retrieved over the plicated sutures to pull the entire plicated complex back to the humerus. This is usually noted as part of the preoperative planning and is accomplished before the plication sutures are tied.

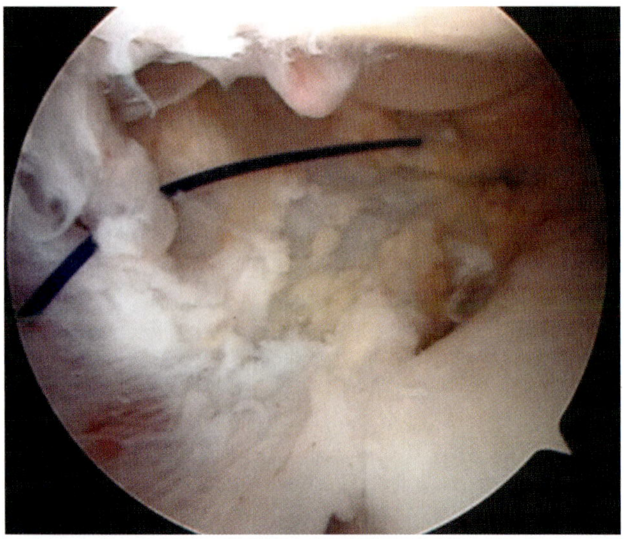

FIGURE 39-17 First suture spanning the entire RUHL complex.

REHABILITATION AFTER LATERAL REPAIRS

In both the acute and chronic cases, the patients are placed in a splint or brace with the elbow in approximately −30° of extension to relax tension on the repair. Fluoroscopy or radiographs should be used to check the reduction after the splint is applied, as additional flexion may be necessary to tighten the reconstruction and keep the joint reduced. The first postoperative visit is usually scheduled within 3 to 5 days of the surgery and the patient placed into a hinged elbow brace that allows comfortable movement, usually 30° to 45°. Shoulder, periscapular, wrist, and hand exercises are initiated and allowed as long as they do not produce pain in the elbow. The patient is seen at 2-week intervals and the motion slowly increased as pain and swelling allows. Once the repair begins to mature, usually between 5 and 8 weeks, physical therapy is increased to include more aggressive upper extremity and core exercises with the elbow brace in place. We expect normal motion of the elbow by 8 weeks postoperatively, if not earlier in the postoperative phase. Depending on individual progression, patients are allowed to start strengthening exercises out of brace at 10 to 12 weeks. They must be able to perform all strengthening exercises pain free in the brace prior to progression out of the brace.

OPEN LATERAL RECONSTRUCTION TECHNIQUE

The open technique for plication and repair is similar to that described by O'Driscoll et al.[2] After a diagnostic arthroscopy confirms the instability and the absence of associated pathology an extensile posterolateral approach is used and the anconeus muscle split or retracted anteriorly to access the RUHL complex. The ligaments are plicated and then repaired to the humerus as described in the section "Arthroscopic Lateral and Posterolateral Repair" if adequate tissue is found to allow repair. In revision surgery or in patients with inadequate tissue for repair, a palmaris autograft or gracilis allograft may be used to reconstruct the joint. The supinator crest of the ulna just posterior to the radial neck is dissected free and the insertion site identified. A 4- to 6-mm tunnel is created in this spot. A Beath pin is drilled from this point out the ulnar side of the ulna and used to pull a passing suture out this side of the arm. The midportion of the graft is then pulled into the ulna and fixed using an interference screw technique. The 2 free limbs are then brought superiorly, pulling 1 under the annular ligament and 1 over the ligament and attached to the isometric point on the posterior aspect of the lateral epicondyle. The graft should be slightly lax in extension and tighten with flexion (Fig. 39-18).

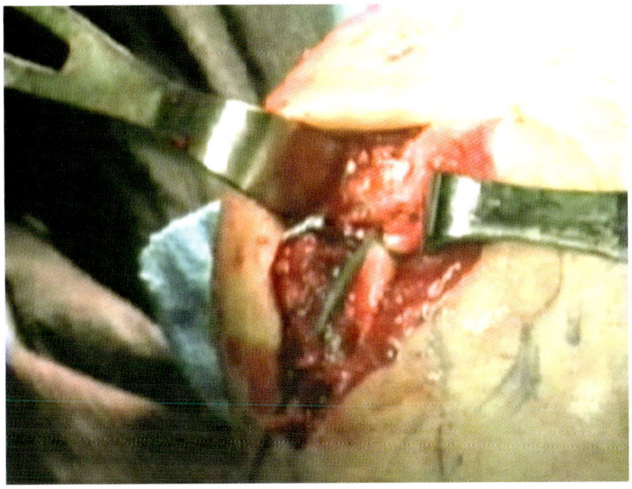

FIGURE 39-18 Graft being positioned for placement into the humerus.

Results

MUCL: Savoie et al[17] reported on the results of repair in a series of 60 athletes. Fifty-eight were able to return to sport at the same or higher level of play. Cain et al,[18] in the largest series to date of over 1200 MUCL reconstructions, had an 85% return to the same or higher level of play.

LUCL: In a series of arthroscopic lateral reconstructions, Savoie et al[14] performed a PLRI repair, plication, or graft. Forty-one patients (20 arthroscopic and 21 open) had a combined plication and repair, 10 patients (6 open and 4 arthroscopic) had acute or subacute repairs for recurrent elbow instability, and 3 patients (all open) were reconstructed with a free tendon graft. Ten of the 20 arthroscopically treated plication/repair patients and 11 of 21 open plication/repair patients had the addition of an anchor to supplement the arthroscopic suture plication.

The average follow-up was 41 months (range 12-103 months). Overall Andrews-Carson scores for all repairs improved from 145 to 180 (P <.0001).[19] Subjective scores improved from 57 to 85 (P <.0001) and objective scores improved from 88 to 95 (P = .008). Subdividing the technique yielded these overall results: arthroscopic repairs improved from 146 to 176 (P = .0001) and open repairs 144 to 182 (P <.001). Acute repairs seemed to perform the best, with 9 of 10 returning to normal activities and 1 to near normal. There was no statistical difference between the results of open versus arthroscopic repair.

Conclusions

MUCL: Both repair and reconstruction have shown to provide successful results in throwing athletes. Repair should be reserved for avulsion-type injuries in relatively younger patients with an otherwise normal ligament. Reconstruction, while technically more demanding, has been shown to allow a successful return to play at the highest levels in a majority of patients.

RUHL: Both arthroscopic and open treatments have been shown to provide satisfactory results. The key in either technique is an understanding of the anatomy and the location of the damage.

REFERENCES

1. Jobe FW, Stark H, Lombardo SJ. Reconstruction of the ulnar collateral ligament in athletes. *J Bone Joint Surg Am*. 1986;68(8):1158–1163.
2. O'Driscoll SW, Bell DF, Morrey BF. Posterolateral rotatory instability of the elbow. *J Bone Joint Surg Am*. 1991;73(3):440–446.
3. Azar FM, Andrews JR, Dugas JR, et al. Operative treatment of ulnar collateral ligament injuries of the elbow in athletes. *Am J Sports Med*. 2000;28(1):16–23.
4. Smith JP, Savoie FH, Field LD. Posterolateral rotatory instability of the elbow. *Clin Sports Med*. 2001;20(1):47–58.
5. Richard MJ, Aldridge JM 3rd, Wiesler ER, Ruch DS. Traumatic valgus instability of the elbow: pathoanatomy and results of direct repair: surgical technique. *J Bone Joint Surg Am*. 2009;91(suppl 2):191–199.
6. Miyake J, Moritomo H, Masatomi T, et al. In vivo and 3-dimensional functional anatomy of the anterior bundle of the medial collateral ligament of the elbow. *J Shoulder Elbow Surg*. 2012;21(8):1006–1012.
7. Callaway GH, Field LD, Deng XH, et al. Biomechanical evaluation of the medical collateral ligament of the elbow. *J Bone Joint Surg Am*. 1997;79(8):1223–1231.
8. O'Driscoll SW, Jaloszynski R, Morrey BF, et al. Origin of the medial ulnar collateral ligament. *J Hand Surg Am*. 1992;17:164–168.
9. Regan WD, Korinek SL, Morrey BF. Biomechanical study of ligaments around the elbow joint. *Clin Orthop*. 1991;271:170–179.
10. Morrey BF, An KN. Functional anatomy of the ligaments of the elbow. *Clin Orthop Relat Res*. 1985;201:84–90.
11. Dunning CE, Zarzour ZD, Patterson SD, Johnson JA, King GJ. Ligamentous stabilizers against posterolateral rotator instability of the elbow. *J Bone Joint Surg Am*. 2001;83-A(12):1823–1828.
12. Seki A, Olsen BS, Jensen SL, Eygendaal D, Sojbjerg JO. Functional anatomy of the lateral collateral ligament complex of the elbow: configuration of Y and its role. *J Shoulder Elbow Surg*. 2002;11(1):53–59.
13. Kalainov DM, Cohen MS. Posterolateral rotatory instability of the elbow in association with lateral epicondylitis. A report of three cases. *J Bone Joint Surg Am*. 2005;87(5):1120–1125.
14. Savoie FH III, Field LD, Gurley DJ. Arthroscopic and open radial ulnohumeral ligament reconstruction for posterolateral rotatory instability of the elbow. *Hand Clin*. 2009;25:323–329. doi:10.1016/j.hcl.2009.05.010.
15. Potter HG, Weiland AJ, Schatz JA, Paletta GA, Hotchkiss RN. Posterolateral rotator instability of the elbow: usefulness of MR imaging in diagnosis. *Radiology*. 1997;204:185–189.
16. Smith GR, Altcheck DW, Pagnani MJ, Keeley JR. A muscle-splitting approach to the ulnar collateral ligament of the elbow: neuroanatomy and operative technique. *Am J Sports Med*. 1996;24(5):575–580.
17. Savoie FH III, Trenhaile SW, John Roberts J, Field LD, Ramsey JR. Primary repair of ulnar collateral ligament injuries of the elbow in young athletes: a case series of injuries to the proximal and distal ends of the ligament. *Am J Sports Med*. 2008;36(6):1066–1072. doi:10.1177/0363546508315201.
18. Cain EL Jr, Andrews JR, Dugas JR, et al. Outcome of ulnar collateral ligament reconstruction of the elbow in 281 athletes: results in 743 athletes with minimum 2-year follow-up. *Am J Sports Med*. 2010;38:2426–2434.
19. Andrews JR, Carson WG. Arthroscopy of the elbow. *Arthroscopy*. 1985;1(2):97–107.

40

Elbow Arthroplasty

Graham JW King, MD, MSc, FRCSC

Elbow arthroplasty is being increasingly utilized for the management of arthritis, fractures, nonunions, osteonecrosis, tumors, and instability. With an aging population and improvements in the medical management of rheumatoid arthritis, traumatic and posttraumatic conditions are now the most frequent indications for elbow arthroplasty. Radial head arthroplasty, distal humeral hemiarthroplasty, and total elbow arthroplasty are most commonly performed. Recently, unicompartmental radiocapitellar arthroplasty systems have become available; however, the indications and efficacy of these devices have not yet been well elucidated.

RADIAL HEAD ARTHROPLASTY

Rationale and Basic Science

The radial head is important for both load transfer and stability of the elbow and forearm. Forces across the elbow joint may exceed 4 times body weight for certain strenuous activities.[1] Up to 60% of elbow loads pass across the radiocapitellar joint.[2] Excision of the radial head results in not only a loss of load transfer across this articulation but also an increase in tension in the medial collateral ligament and a concentration of forces on the lateral aspect of the ulnohumeral joint.[3] Forces across the ulnohumeral joint have been estimated to reach 9 times body weight after radial head excision. In the setting of a medial collateral ligament injury the radial head is an important secondary valgus stabilizer of the elbow. The radial head also resists posterolateral rotatory instability of the elbow by virtue of the concavity of the articulating dish of the radial head resisting translation off the more spherical capitellum.[4] The radial head tensions the lateral collateral ligament that passes across it. The radial head serves as an important axial stabilizer, particularly in the setting of a disrupted interosseous membrane.[5]

Metallic radial head arthroplasty has been shown to restore the axial and valgus stability of the forearm and elbow.[4] Bipolar radial head arthroplasties are less effective at maintaining elbow stability than monopolar implants in the setting of concomitant ligament injuries.[6] The tilting action of the bipolar head increases the tendency for radiocapitellar joint subluxation relative to that of a monopolar implant or the native elbow because of the reduced concavity-compression effect of this type of articulation.[7] Metallic radial head arthroplasty decreases the joint contact surface area on the capitellum and increases the articular cartilage contact pressures.[8] These biomechanical alterations may result in the development of degenerative arthritic changes of the capitellum over the longer term. Recently a pyrolytic carbon radial head has become available. Its lower stiffness relative to a metallic implant has theoretical advantages; however, initial experience with this device resulted in some catastrophic failures due to dissociation of the coupling mechanism between the head and stem.[9] Further studies with this device are needed.

The optimal fixation method of radial head arthroplasty continues to be controversial with some systems employing a smooth stem that permits toggling in the canal and others attempting to achieve rigid fixation using cement or osteointegration of a porous surface. Recent in vitro biomechanical studies have shown that larger press-fit stems provide sufficient stability to permit osteointegration; however, the insertion of these larger stems has resulted in problems such as fractures and stress shielding of the radial neck.[7] Loose rough stems seem to have a higher incidence of symptoms than smooth stem devices.[10] Comparative clinical studies are needed.

The anatomy of the native radial head and neck is complex and variable (Fig. 40-1). The radial head has an elliptical shape that is variably offset from the axis of the radial neck.[11] The articulating concave dish is also somewhat elliptical and has a larger radius of curvature than the capitellum, making this articulation only moderately constrained. About two-thirds of the margin of the radial head articulates with the lesser sigmoid notch of the proximal ulna. This portion is flattened while the nonarticular portion is more rounded and devoid of articular cartilage. The radial head is surrounded by the annular ligament that blends with the radial collateral and lateral ulnar collateral ligaments to form the

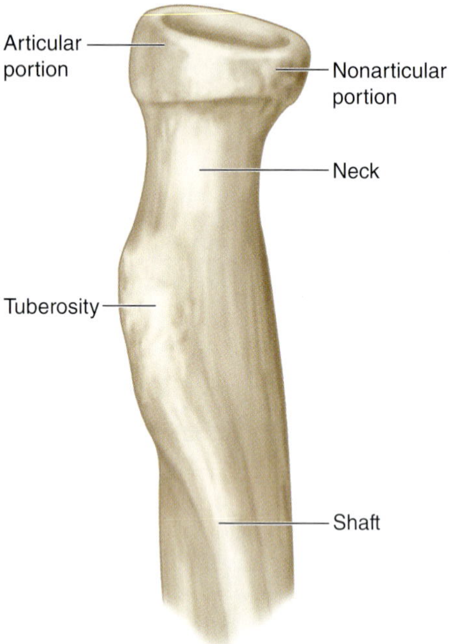

FIGURE 40-1 The radial head is variably eccentric and is offset from the radial neck. The articulating margin is flattened while the portion that does not articulate with the radial head is more rounded and often nearly devoid of articular cartilage. (Reproduced with permission from King GJW. Fractures of the head of the radius. In: Wolfe SW, Hotchkiss RN, Pederson WC, Kozin SH, eds. *Green's Operative Hand Surgery*. 6th ed. Philadelphia: Elsevier, Churchill Livingstone; 2011:788 [chapter 21, Fig. 21.7]. Copyright Elsevier.)

lateral collateral ligament, the major varus and posterolateral rotatory stabilizer of the elbow (Fig. 40-2). The blood supply of the radial head is provided by both intraosseous and extraosseous sources. Fractures of the radial neck disrupt the interosseous blood supply and often the extraosseous supply that perforates through the periosteum at the head and neck junction.[12] This results in a propensity for avascular necrosis and nonunion of fractures of the radial neck after open reduction and internal fixation.

Indications

Radial head arthroplasty is indicated for the management of displaced, unrepairable, comminuted fractures of the radial head and neck. Radial head arthroplasty is also employed for the management of nonunions and malunions or to manage elbow or forearm instability following a previous radial head resection. Acute radial head excision can be considered for comminuted radial head fractures with or without an associated ligamentous or osseous injury, but it is mandatory in the face of an Essex-Lopresti injury. The adverse biomechanical consequences of radial head excision, the frequency of occult concomitant ligament injuries, and the high incidence of posttraumatic arthritis in long-term outcome studies have resulted in an increased use of primary radial head arthroplasty for the management of comminuted unrepairable fractures.[13,14] Since the incidence of concomitant injuries to the collateral ligaments of

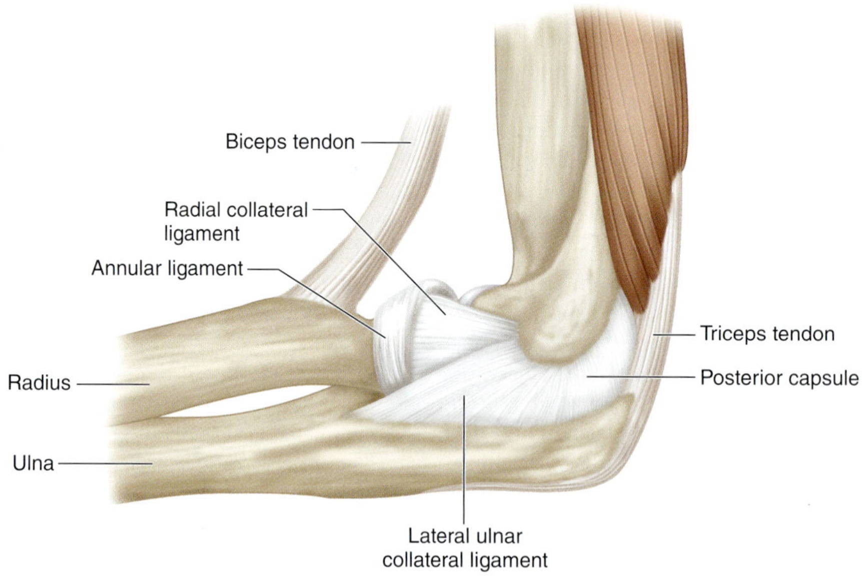

FIGURE 40-2 The lateral collateral ligament has 3 components: the annular ligament, the radial collateral ligament, and the lateral ulnar collateral ligament. The radial head is surrounded by the annular ligament that stabilizes the radial head within the sigmoid notch. The radial collateral ligament arises from the lateral epicondyle and blends with the annular ligament. The lateral ulnar collateral ligament arises from the lateral epicondyle and inserts on the crista supinatoris of the proximal ulna. (Reproduced with permission from King GJW. Fractures of the head of the radius. In: Wolfe SW, Hotchkiss RN, Pederson WC, Kozin SH, eds. *Green's Operative Hand Surgery*. 6th ed. Philadelphia: Elsevier, Churchill Livingstone; 2011:789 [chapter 21, Fig. 21.9]. Copyright Elsevier.)

the elbow or interosseous membrane has exceeded 75% in most studies of comminuted radial head fractures, many surgeons routinely replace the radial head in all acute, displaced fractures that cannot be reliably fixed with open reduction and internal fixation.

The prerequisites for secondary radial head replacement are the presence of capitellar bone and cartilage that is suitable to articulate with a prosthesis and a proximal radius that aligns or can be made to align with the native capitellum. In the setting where the capitellum is too damaged to be suitable for placement of a metallic prosthesis, however, an implant is required to manage elbow or forearm instability; a unicompartmental radiocapitellar joint arthroplasty may be considered. The effectiveness and reliability of these new devices remain unknown at this time.[15]

Radial head implants can be used at any age, although there is a clear tendency to aggressively preserve the radial head in younger patients and to replace the radial head in the elderly where osteoporosis and compromised vascularity make the success of radial head reconstruction less likely. The decision as to which radial head fracture requires operative management is difficult to make on the basis of preoperative imaging; some patients who are expected to do well with conservative care do not. During surgery the decision between open reduction and internal fixation versus excision with arthroplasty is often challenging as problems with fracture healing and fixation failure are not always possible to anticipate. Primary radial head excision can be considered; however, concomitant ligament injures may be subtle and the late salvage of elbow or forearm instability has been less successful than primary repair and radial head arthroplasty. The optimal design and material of a radial head implant has not been determined. The variability in size and shape of a proximal radius makes it difficult for "off-the-shelf" implant to precisely replicate the kinematics and contact mechanics of the native radial head. Erosion of the capitellum and lesser sigmoid notch may occur when using well-fixed monoblock implants that do not optimally align with the capitellum. This has resulted in designs that favor adaption of the implant to ensure optimal articular contact and kinematics of the radial head with the capitellum. This is currently achieved using a smooth, polished implant with a slightly undersized stem that can move within the radial neck or the use of a bipolar implant that accommodates by mobility within the polyethylene articulation.[16,17] Modular prostheses are popular as they address the mismatch between the size of the medullary canal of the radial neck and the radial head and allow the surgeon the versatility of choosing the thickness and diameter of the implant independently. Eccentric prostheses attempt to approximate the anatomic shape of the proximal radius. These implants rely on accurate positioning and rigid fixation of the stem into the proximal radius to avoid articular maltracking. Unfortunately, obtaining routine osteointegration of uncemented radial stems has been problematic clinically.[10] There are no reported randomized clinical trials comparing radial implant design concepts.

Contraindications

The presence of active infection is an absolute contraindication to the use of a radial head implant. A capitellum that does not have a spherical shape is also an absolute contraindication to using a radial head arthroplasty without capitellar reconstruction. Relative contraindications include the presence of an open growth plate and patients where the radial neck cannot be made to align with the capitellum; a bipolar radial head implant might be possible to use in this situation if the malalignment is not too severe. The lack of articular cartilage on the capitellum is a relative contraindication, although underlengthening of the radial head or a concomitant interposition arthroplasty to resurface the capitellum can be considered while still proceeding with a radial head arthroplasty.

Surgical Technique

Radial head replacement can be performed with the patient supine and the arm placed across the chest with the surgeon standing or on a hand table with the surgeon sitting. General or regional anesthesia is employed as is routine administration of prophylactic antibiotics. A sterile tourniquet is applied and inflated.

A posterior midline or lateral skin incision can be used. The posterior midline incision is extensile allowing the surgeon to access the medial side of the elbow if required to manage concomitant fractures of the coronoid or medial collateral ligament. A posterior incision is longer but has a reduced chance of injuring cutaneous nerves.[18] A direct lateral incision is shorter and decreases the risk of seromas or hematomas relative to a posterior incision (Fig. 40-3).

The deep surgical approach depends on the presence of concomitant ligamentous injuries. In the setting of a lateral collateral ligament injury with concomitant varus and posterolateral rotatory instability a Kocher approach between the anconeus and extensor carpi ulnaris is preferred. Typically a humeral avulsion of the lateral collateral ligament and extensor muscles allows for adequate exposure of the radial head for replacement. The annular ligament should be divided to adequately visualize the radial head and neck. If the lateral collateral ligament is intact, a common extensor tendon splitting approach is performed (Fig. 40-4). An incision is made extending from the lateral epicondyle through the common extensor tendon and annular ligament at the midaxis of the radial head. The forearm is maintained in pronation during lateral surgical approaches to the proximal radius to reduce the proximity of the posterior interosseous nerve.[19] This incision is turned up the lateral supracondylar ridge to detach the radial collateral ligament and extensor carpi radialis brevis and longus to allow adequate exposure of the radial head. Posterior dissection should be avoided to preserve the attachment of the lateral ulnar collateral ligament on the lateral epicondyle and hence prevent the development of varus and posterolateral rotatory instability.

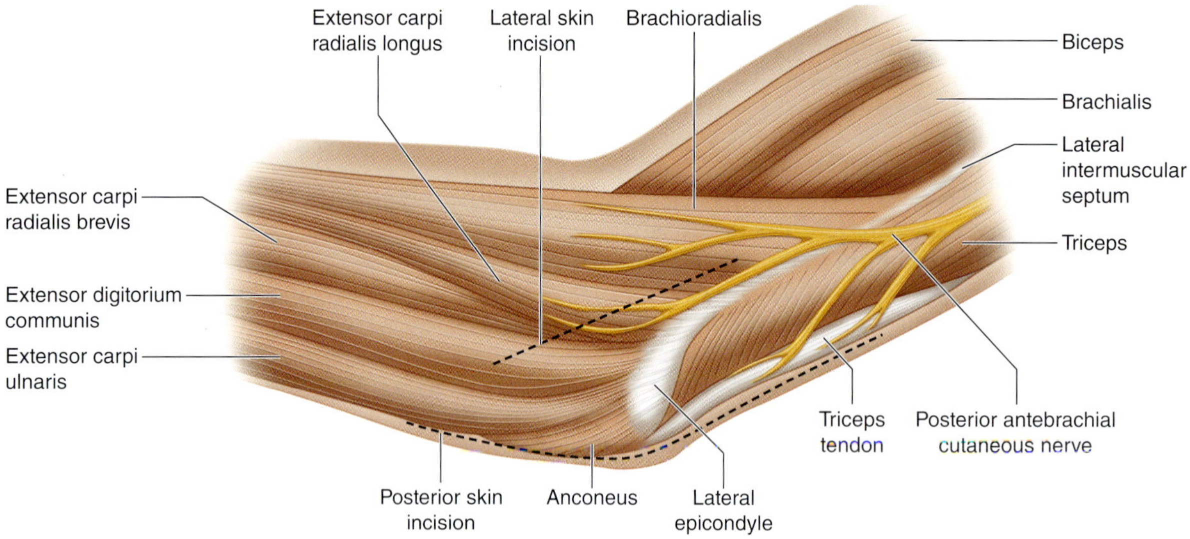

FIGURE 40-3 A posterior or lateral skin incision can be used to approach the radial head. A common extensor tendon splitting approach is preferred if the lateral collateral ligament is intact, while the anconeus/extensor carpi ulnaris interval is preferred if the radial head is intact. (Illustration reproduced with permission from Wright Medical Technology, Inc.)

The precise surgical technique for radial head replacement depends on the prosthesis system employed. Fragments of the radial head are removed and the radial neck is divided at the level of the head–neck junction or at the level of the fracture. The diameter and thickness of the radial head are selected based on the size of the reconstructed excised radial head. The minor diameter of the elliptical radial head is chosen as the correct diameter of an axisymmetric radial head. The thickness of the prosthesis is decided using the height of the excised and reconstructed radial head (Fig. 40-5). Since overlengthening of the radius has been shown to result in capitellar wear and pain, the placement of a radial head implant that is too thick should be avoided.[20] The lateral ligaments are often incompetent in patients with a radial head fracture; therefore, the space between the radial head and capitellum should not be used to choose the correct thickness of the prosthesis. The radial head implant should articulate at the proximal aspect of

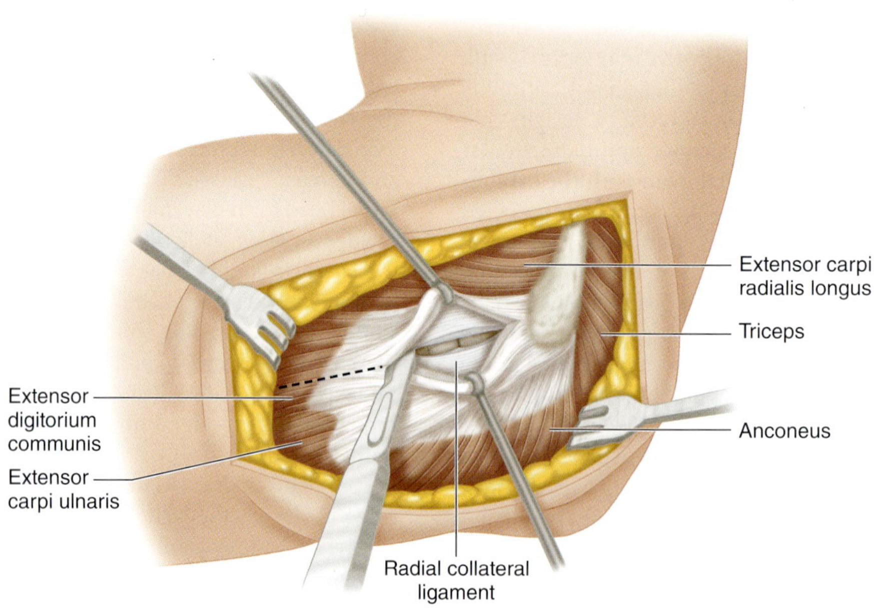

FIGURE 40-4 If the lateral collateral ligament is intact, a common extensor tendon splitting approach is used. The forearm is maintained in pronation while dividing the annular and radial collateral ligaments to protect the posterior interosseous nerve. (Illustration reproduced with permission from Wright Medical Technology, Inc.)

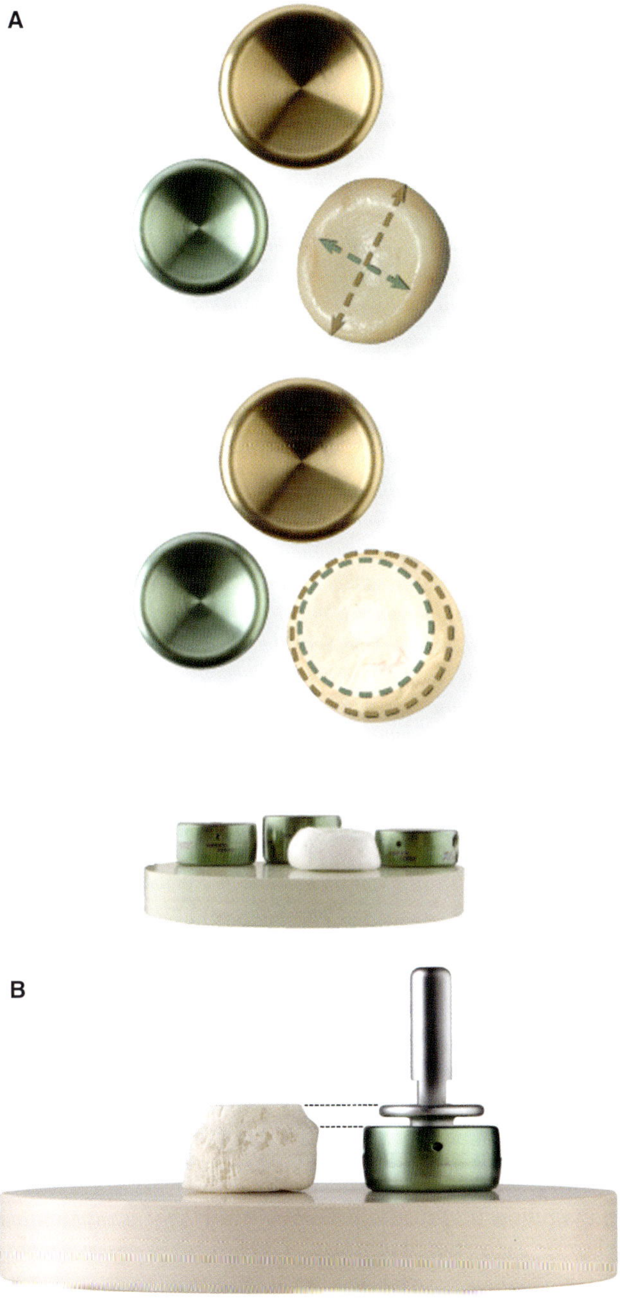

FIGURE 40-5 A. The radial head fragments are assembled on the back table. The minor diameter is selected for the optimal implant size as this closely replicates the size of the articular dish. **B.** The thickness of the implant is selected based on the height of articular portion of the radial head and any involvement of the neck is added to the stem length of the implant. (Images reproduced with permission from Wright Medical Technology, Inc.)

the lesser sigmoid notch of the ulna that is about 2 mm distal to the tip of the coronoid.[21] A fluoroscopic evaluation of the elbow should be performed after insertion of the trial prosthesis. The medial ulnohumeral joint space should be parallel and the ulnar variance equal to that of the opposite wrist.[22] The lateral ulnohumeral joint space may be wider

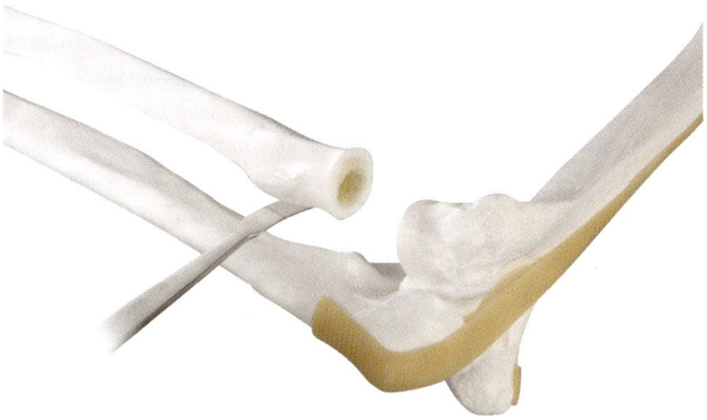

FIGURE 40-6 A homan retractor is placed behind the radial neck and the proximal radius is delivered laterally to facilitate preparation of the radial neck and insertion of the prosthesis. (Image reproduced with permission from Wright Medical Technology, Inc.)

as a normal variant and should not be used to evaluate the correct length of the prosthesis. A contralateral elbow radiograph can be useful in deciding whether previously placed radial head prosthesis is overlengthened.[23,24] In the setting where a radial head is not available as it has previously been excised, contralateral templating of the normal elbow should be performed preoperatively.

In order to facilitate preparation of the radial neck and insertion of an assembled modular prosthesis, the radial neck is retracted laterally. A homan retractor is placed around the posterior aspect of the radial neck and the radius is pulled laterally by prying the retractor against the proximal ulna (Fig. 40-6). Anteriorly based homan retractors should not be used due to risk of compression of the posterior interosseous nerve. The medullary canal should be prepared using the reamers for the system to be employed. In the setting where a smooth stem uncemented implant is used, a stem 1 mm smaller than the final reamer is typically selected to achieve a nontight fit of the stem. Using trial components the congruity of the radial capitellar joint and alignment of the elbow and forearm are checked both visually and fluoroscopically. Repair of the annular ligament is critical to ensure optimal articular tracking of a smooth stem monopolar radial head implant as well as for a bipolar radial head implant.

If a common extensor tendon splitting approach was utilized, a side-to-side closure of the annular ligament and common extensor tendon is performed (Fig. 40-7). The extensor carpi radialis longus and brevis and radial collateral ligament are reattached to the lateral epicondyle and supracondylar ridge. If the lateral collateral ligament is deficient, locking Krackow sutures are placed in the lateral ulnar collateral, radial collateral, and annular ligaments as well as in the common extensor fascia. These sutures are then passed through a drill hole placed at the center of the axis of motion of the elbow that can be approximated as the center of a circle defined by the curvature of the capitellum. Two drill holes are placed posterior to the supracondylar ridge and the sutures are tied over the posterior bone bridge after

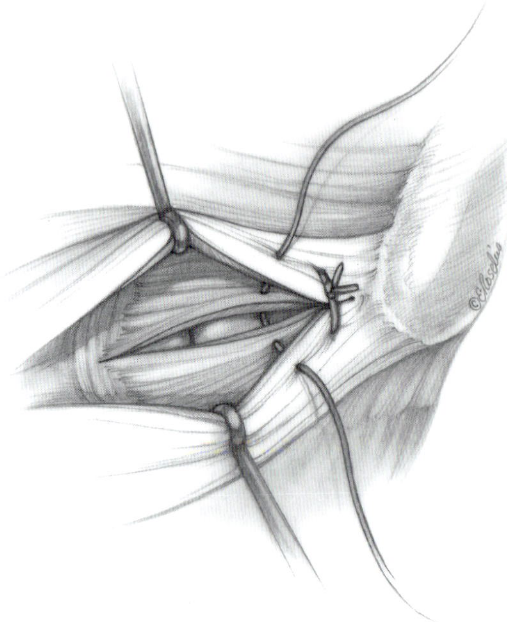

FIGURE 40-7 The annular ligament and common extensor tendon are repaired to maintain optimal articular tracking of the radial head. If the lateral collateral ligament was detached or injured, it should be repaired using transosseous bone tunnels to restore elbow stability. (Illustration reproduced with permission from Wright Medical Technology, Inc.)

appropriate tensioning of the lateral soft tissues. If the posterior bone is soft, a drill hole should be placed anterior and posterior to the supracondylar ridge allowing the sutures to be tied over strong cortical bone, thereby avoiding fixation failure. The lateral collateral ligament should be tensioned carefully when there is a concomitant medial ligament injury as the elbow can be pulled into excessive valgus.[25]

When performing a radial head arthroplasty, management of concomitant elbow injuries is critical (Fig. 40-8). In the setting of a coronoid fracture access to the coronoid can be facilitated by radial head excision such that internal fixation with sutures or screws can be achieved from a lateral surgical approach. Fractures of the proximal ulna should also be stably fixed such as transolecranon or Monteggia fracture–dislocations (Fig. 40-9). If a comminuted coronoid fracture cannot be fixed through the radial head excision, a medial approach should be performed and coronoid repair achieved with suture, screw, and/or plate fixation. A medial approach should also be performed to repair the medial collateral ligament in the unlikely event that the elbow is still unstable after repairing the coronoid, radial head, and lateral collateral ligament.[26]

Complications

Complications are frequent in patients undergoing radial head arthroplasty; however, given the high incidence of associated ligamentous and osseous injuries in patients with comminuted radial head fractures, a causal relationship to the prosthesis is often unclear. The most common complications of radial head arthroplasty are stiffness, osteoarthritis, capitellar erosions, loosening, elbow instability, and heterotopic ossification.[16,17,27] Damage to the posterior interosseous nerve can occur with zealous retraction anterior to the radial neck or if the dissection is carried too distally. Radial neck fractures can occur with the insertion of press-fit prostheses; fixation with cerclage wires may be required.

Radiolucency around smooth stem implants is common; however, its presence does not correlate with patient's symptoms.[16,28] Stem lucencies are expected given that the stem toggles within the radial neck. Loosening of press-fit stems has been reported and seems to be more commonly associated with patient's symptoms and may lead to revision or removal of these implants[10] (Fig. 40-10). Placement of an overlengthened radial head prosthesis can occur if the gap between the capitellum and implant is used to guide the thickness of the radial head prosthesis due to the high incidence of concomitant lateral collateral ligament injuries in patients requiring a radial head arthroplasty. Overlengthening of the radial head prosthesis has been reported to cause capitellar erosion and decreased flexion; revision is required.[20] Osteoarthritis of the ulnohumeral joint has been common in follow-up studies with a higher incidence in patients in whom a radial head implant is used to treat chronic posttraumatic elbow disorders.[29]

Outcomes

The results of metallic radial head implants have been good to excellent in the majority of patients in multiple clinical studies. While stiffness is common and pain relief often incomplete, the majority of patients undergoing radial head implants have multiple associated injuries making it difficult to determine the outcome of the prosthesis in isolation from that of the associated injuries. The average Mayo Elbow Performance Index (MEPI) scores range from 80 to 90 in the majority of published reports (out of a total of 100 points).

Grewal et al prospectively followed 27 patients treated with a modular smooth stem radial head implant.[16] Functional recovery was achieved by 6 months. The average MEPI was 83. Twenty-two patients had a good or excellent result. Mild osteoarthritis was noted in 19% of patients. Fifty percent of their patients had lucencies around the stem, but these were nonprogressive and did not correlate with residual patient symptoms. Doornberg et al reviewed 27 patients at a mean of 3.5 years following smooth stem modular radial head replacement.[30] Twenty-two patients had a good or excellent result; the mean MEPI was 85. The average range of motion was from 20° to 131° of flexion, 73° of pronation, and 57° of supination. Seventeen patients had lucencies around the neck of the prosthesis, but these were not associated with pain.

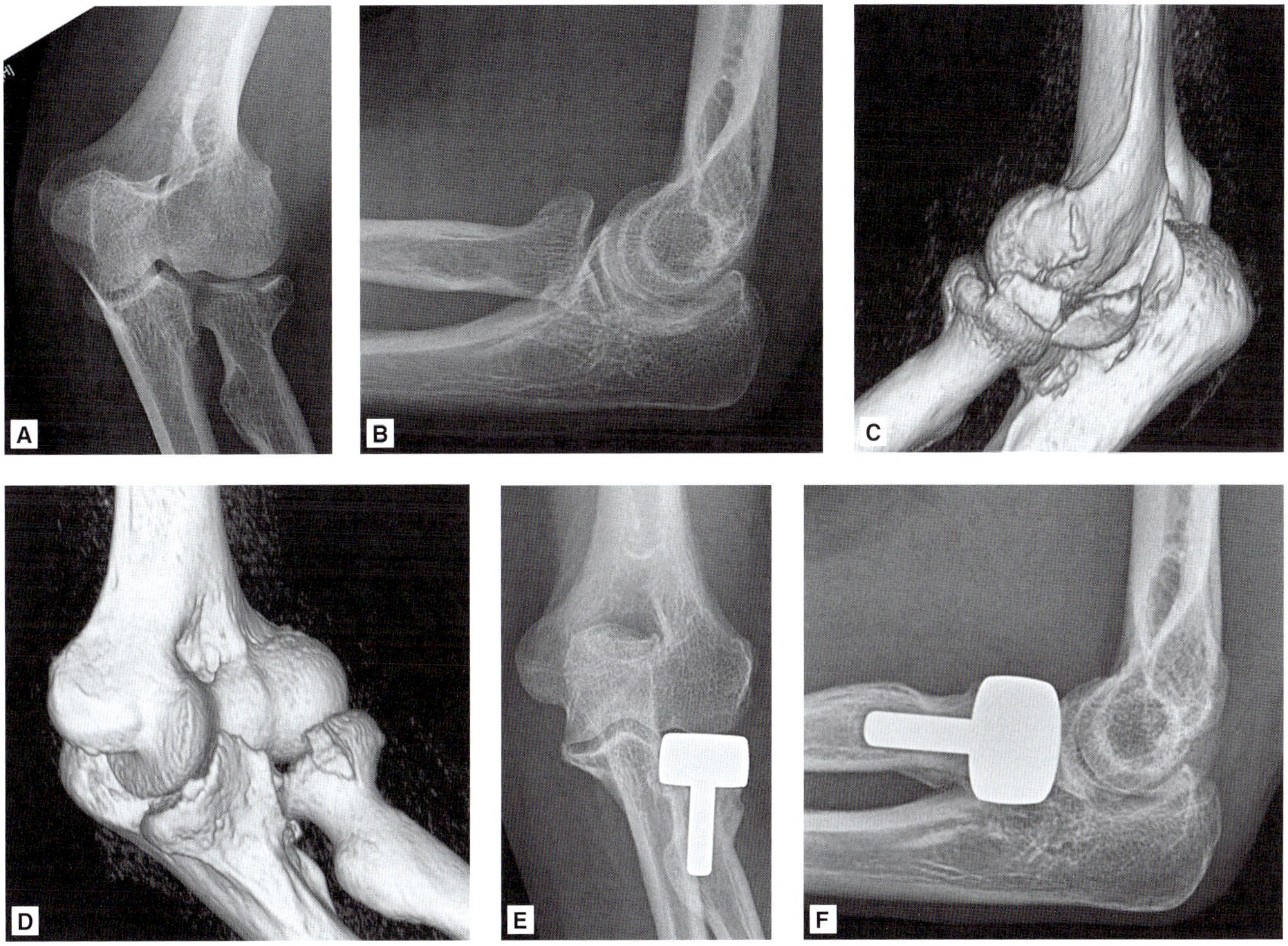

FIGURE 40-8 **A** and **B.** A 54-year-old man with a block to forearm rotation following a fall off a bike. Anteroposterior and lateral radiographs demonstrate an elbow effusion with an elevated anterior fat pad with a subtle displaced radial head fracture. **C** and **D.** CT images demonstrate a comminuted radial head fracture with significant displacement. **E** and **F.** Two-year postoperative radiographs following radial head replacement and repair of a lateral collateral ligament injury diagnosed at surgery. The patient had no pain, full rotation, and a 10° flexion contracture.

The clinical results of delayed radial head arthroplasty for the treatment of radial head nonunions, malunions, failed open reduction, and internal fixation, and for the management of chronic instability have been similar to that of an acute radial head arthroplasty; however, the incidence of osteoarthritis is higher. At a mean 8-year follow-up, Shore et al reviewed 32 patients treated with a metallic radial head arthroplasty for chronic reconstruction.[29] The average MEPI was 83; 21 patients had a good or excellent result. Posttraumatic arthritis was noted in 74%. None of the implants required revision. Given the differences in patient profile and concomitant injuries in patients undergoing acute and chronic radial head reconstruction, it is difficult to critically compare the outcome of acute versus delayed surgery.

At a mean 8-year follow-up of 51 patients with a cemented bipolar radial head replacement, Popovic et al reported that 39 had a good or excellent clinical outcome.[31] However, osteolysis was seen in 37 patients and there were 10 complications. Zunkiewicz et al reported a mean MEPI of 92 at an average of 3 years following a smooth stem bipolar implant.[17] Osteolysis was not noted as an issue with this device at this early follow-up. Flinkkila et al reviewed 37 patients who had metallic press-fit prostheses at an average of 4 years.[10] Early stem loosening occurred in 12 patients and of these 9 required removal due to pain and progressive osteolysis. The average MEPI was 86. Comparative clinical trials are needed to compare the outcome of the different prosthesis design concepts.

TOTAL ELBOW ARTHROPLASTY

Rationale and Basic Science

The first total elbow arthroplasty was reported by Dee in 1972.[32] This was a cemented, fully constrained linked prosthesis that excised the distal humerus condyles. Unfortunately, the good early results of these constrained implants were not sustained due to a high incidence of aseptic loosening.[33]

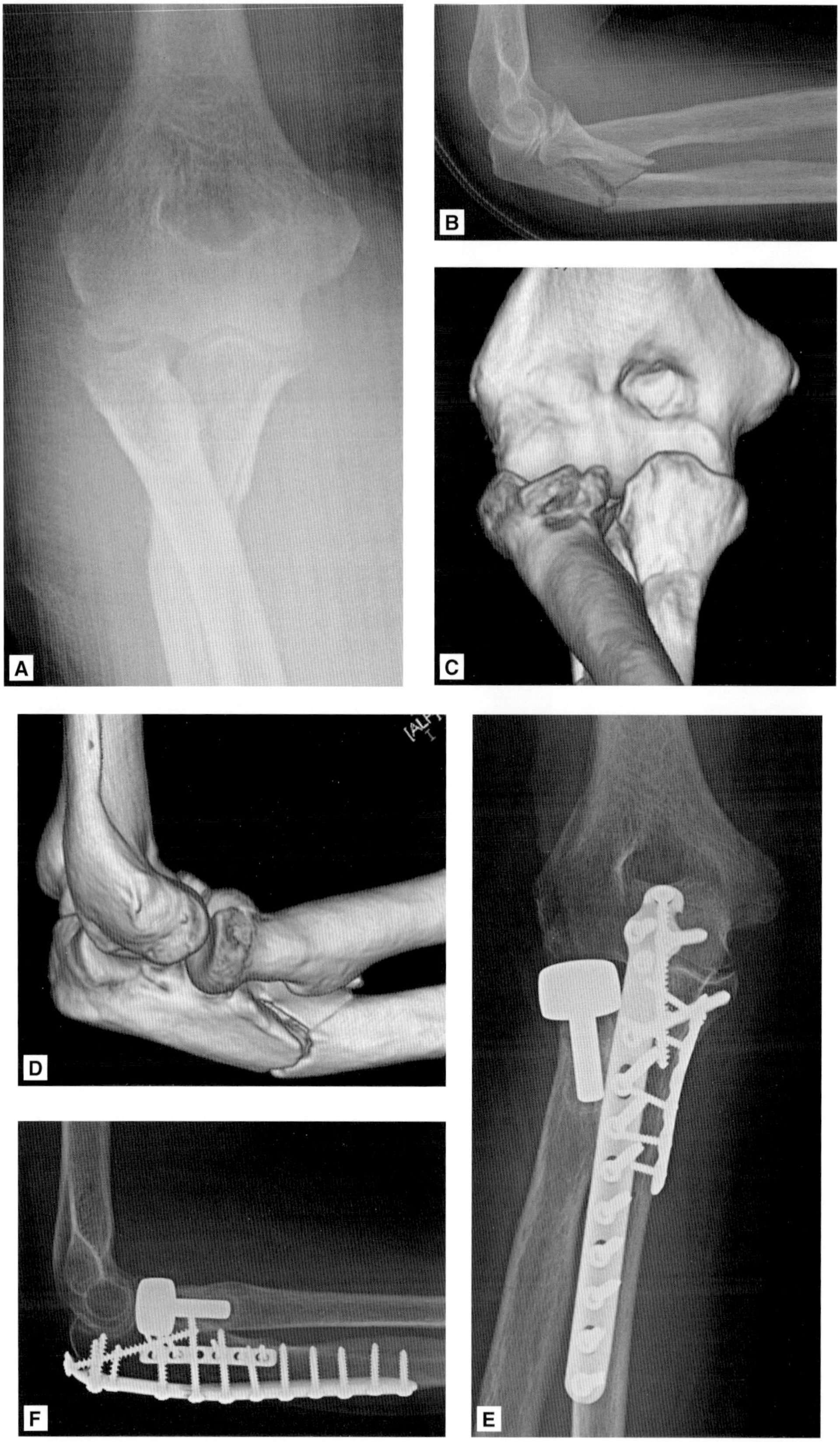

FIGURE 40-9 **A** and **B.** A 64-year-old woman with a posterior Monteggia fracture–dislocation following a slip and fall. Anteroposterior and lateral radiographs demonstrate radial head and proximal ulnar fractures. **C** and **D.** CT images demonstrate a comminuted partial articular radial head and proximal ulnar fracture. **E** and **F.** One-year postoperative radiographs following radial head replacement and open reduction and internal fixation of the ulnar shaft. The patient achieved a functional range of motion; however, the ulnar plate was symptomatic and required removal.

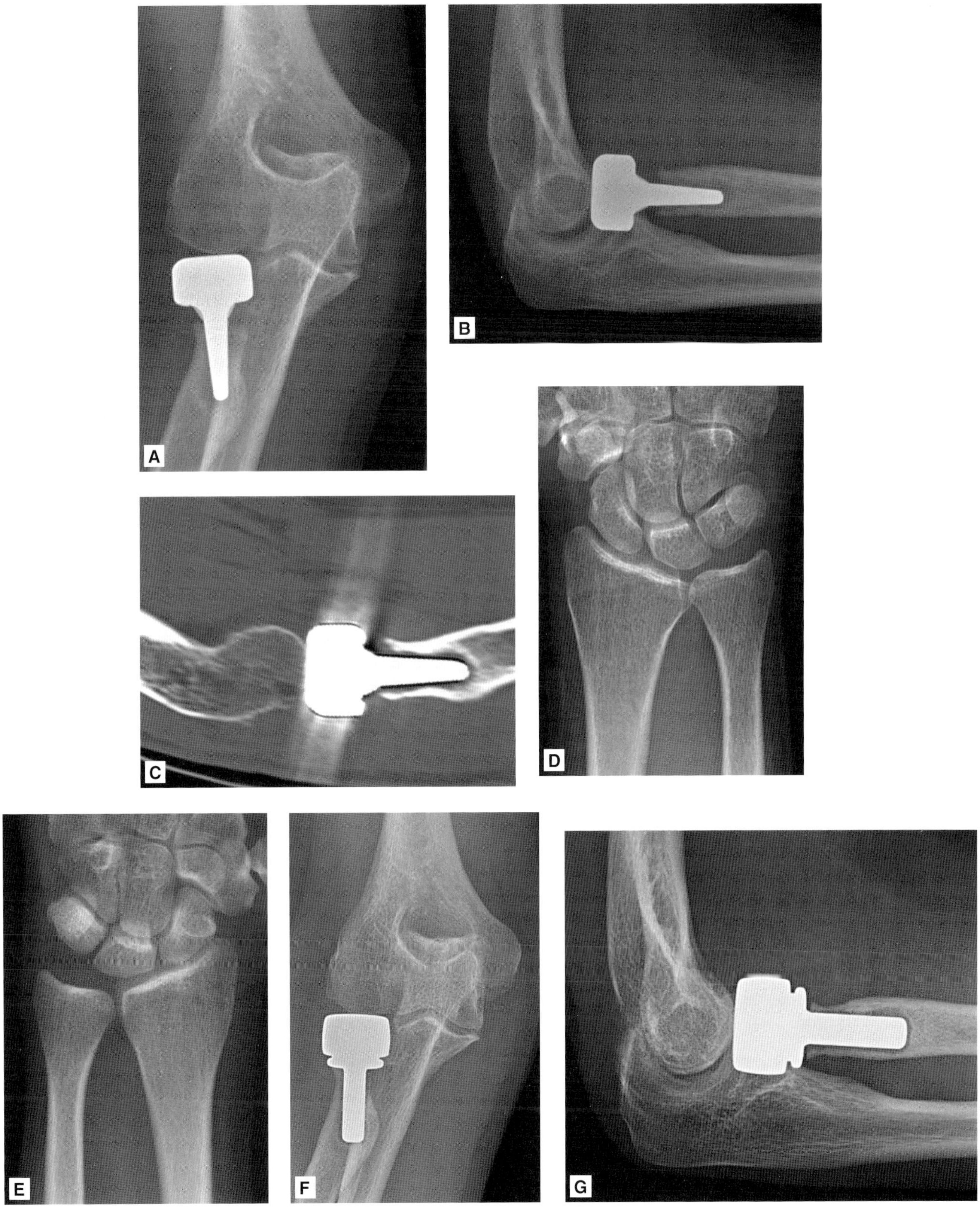

FIGURE 40-10 **A** and **B.** A 24-year-old woman 2 years following a radial head replacement for a comminuted radial head fracture. The patient complained of both wrist and elbow pain. Anteroposterior and lateral radiographs demonstrate an underlengthened radial head arthroplasty with a gap between the implant and radial neck. **C.** CT confirmed a loose radial stem. **D** and **E.** Anteroposterior wrist radiographs demonstrate radial shortening of the affected forearm. **F** and **G.** Two-year postoperative revision arthroplasty with a smooth stem radial head implant; the patient's wrist and elbow pain were minimal.

Biomechanical studies subsequently demonstrated that the elbow does not have a fixed axis of rotation, but rather it behaves as a loose hinge whereby the axis normally moves during elbow flexion and extension.[34]

A better understanding of the kinematics and stability of the normal elbow resulted in the parallel development of unlinked resurfacing-type arthroplasties and loose hinge linked devices. Unlinked devices allow load sharing between the prosthesis and the surrounding joint capsule, ligaments, and muscles; however, these implants have an increased risk of instability relative to that of a linked articulation.[35] The loose hinge linked implants theoretically dissipate stresses across the articulation during elbow motion through the soft tissues rather than applying these to the mechanical articulation or stem fixation.[36]

More recently convertible types of elbow arthroplasties have been developed that allow the surgeon to choose between an unlinked and a linked prosthesis depending on the integrity of the surrounding osseous and ligament structures of the elbow. Some implants allow for the incorporation of a radial head prosthesis that may be important in the setting of an unlinked implant to improve stability.[37] Early attempts to achieve stable prosthesis fixation without a humeral or ulnar stem failed and all commercially available devices now are stemmed. Most implants rely on cement fixation; however, 1 uncemented humeral component design has reliably achieved osteointegration.[38] Smooth stem cemented implants have a higher incidence of loosening than rough stems, possibly due to distraction forces that occur across the elbow with certain activities.[39,40] Correct alignment and position of the axis of motion is important with respect to restoring normal motion pathways and humeral stem loading in biomechanical studies; however, the importance of prosthesis positioning has yet to be confirmed clinically.[41]

Indications

The most common indications for a total elbow arthroplasty are rheumatoid arthritis, osteoarthritis, comminuted distal humeral fractures, distal humeral nonunions, dysfunctional instability, osteonecrosis, hemophilic arthropathy, and periarticular elbow tumors. The ideal candidates are low-demand elderly patients with either rheumatoid arthritis or an acute distal humeral fracture. Total elbow arthroplasty has been less successful in the management of younger patients with posttraumatic arthritis.

Contraindications

Active infection is an absolute contraindication for a total elbow arthroplasty. Patients who are unwilling to be compliant with the postoperative long-term restrictions of an elbow arthroplasty should be managed with alternative options. A history of prior infection, a suboptimal soft tissue envelope, and a nonfunctional hand are relative contraindications.

Surgical Technique

The surgical technique will depend on the elbow arthroplasty system to be employed. Elbow arthroplasty is performed in the supine or lateral decubitus position. Patients should receive standard prophylactic intravenous antibiotics. A sterile tourniquet should be employed. A posterior midline incision is placed medial to the tip of the olecranon to prevent injury to longitudinally running cutaneous nerves.[18] To reduce the incidence of flap necrosis, full-thickness flaps are elevated on the deep fascia to optimize skin perfusion. The ulnar nerve should be identified and transposed.

The deep surgical approach to the elbow is at the surgeon's discretion. In the setting of distal humeral bone loss a paratricipital approach should be employed as it avoids detachment of the triceps from the olecranon preserving triceps strength.[42] This is particularly useful in patients with comminuted distal humeral fractures where adequate access to the proximal ulna can be achieved and elbow stiffness is not a problem. The paratricipital approach follows the medial–lateral margins of the triceps. In the setting of elbow stiffness and where distal humeral bone stock is preserved, detachment of the triceps from the olecranon facilitates exposure for preparation and insertion of a total elbow arthroplasty. The triceps can be elevated from the olecranon in a medial–lateral direction (Byan-Morrey) or from the lateral to medial direction (extended Kocher).[43,44] Alternatively, a triceps splitting approach can be employed where the triceps is split centrally and elevated both medially and laterally off the tip of the olecranon (Fig. 40-11). Some surgeons prefer the use of a triceps tongue approach where a portion of the triceps is left attached to the olecranon to facilitate later repair.[45] The lateral and medial collateral ligaments are sectioned from the humeral epicondyles and the posterior capsule and fat pad are excised. The elbow is dislocated by hyperflexion allowing the olecranon to move away from the humerus. The anterior capsule is elevated off the anterior aspect of the distal humerus to facilitate exposure and allow for placement of a bone graft behind the anterior flange of the humeral component that is typical of most implant systems.

An appropriate sized implant is selected depending on the system employed. Using the supplied instrumentation bony cuts on the distal humerus, proximal ulna, and proximal radius (if applicable) are made and trial prostheses are inserted. The radial head may be retained in the setting of acute fractures or when arthritic involvement is not extensive. A trial reduction is critical to ensure that the implants are tracking correctly. If an unlinked implant is planned and articular tracking is suboptimal, the implant needs to be repositioned. The prerequisites to the use of an unlinked implant include the presence of a good triceps and elbow flexor mechanism, adequate collateral ligaments, absence of significant preexisting deformity, and restoration of the lateral joint reactive forces by either retaining or replacing the radial head. When these prerequisites are not met or the trial implants are maltracking, a linked implant should

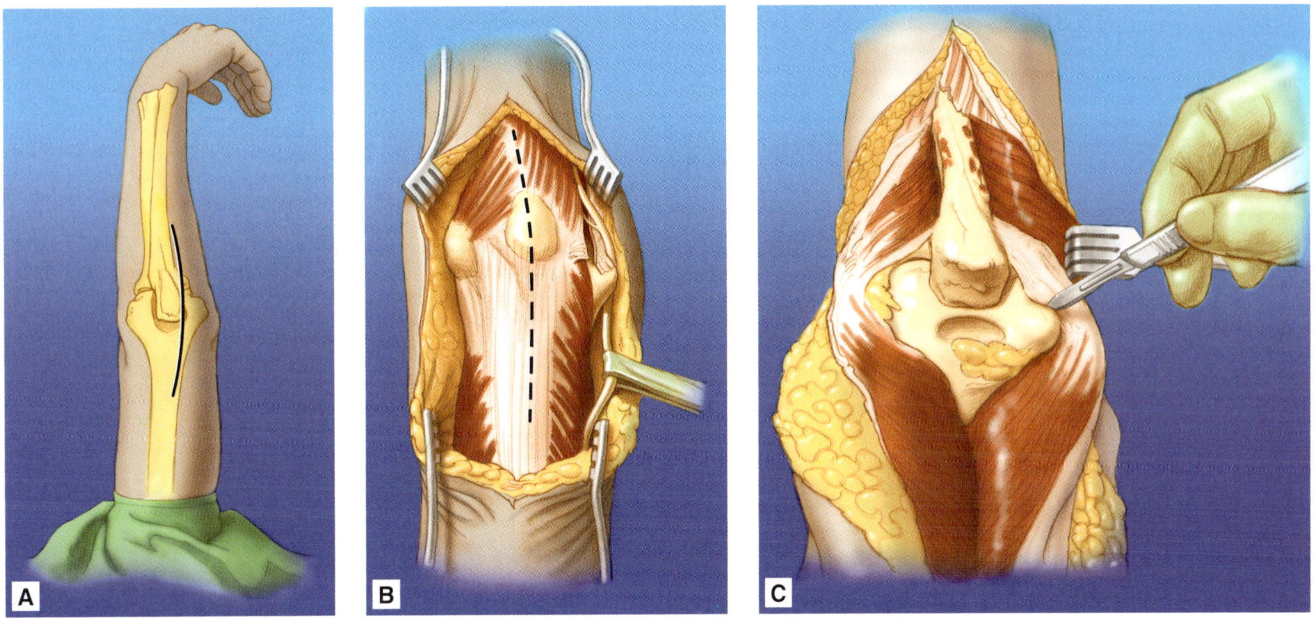

FIGURE 40-11 **A-C.** Triceps splitting approach to the proximal ulna. The skin incision is placed medial to the olecranon tip and an ulnar nerve transposition is completed. The triceps is split centrally and elevated medially and laterally off the olecranon. The collateral ligaments are released from the medial and lateral epicondyles to allow the elbow to subluxate to access the articulation. (Illustrations reproduced with permission from Tornier, Inc.)

be performed. If the radial head is to be replaced, it should track congruously with the capitellum throughout motion; if it cannot be made to articulate congruously, a radial head component should not be employed. Linked implants are used routinely in elderly low-demand patients because wear and loosening are less of a concern.

If the trial reduction of the implant is adequate, cement restrictors are placed within the humeral, ulnar, and, if applicable, proximal radial canal. The medullary canals are lavaged and dried and antibiotic-containing cement is injected retrograde using a cement gun with a narrow nozzle. The implant components are then inserted in the appropriate position and orientation. Excess cement is removed from around the arthroplasty prior to the cement setting. The joint is reduced and held still as the cement sets. A cancellous bone graft is placed behind the anterior flange of the humeral component where indicated and possible. The linkage mechanism is placed if a linked arthroplasty is to be performed. A secure repair of the collateral ligaments back to the epicondyles and implant is required if an unlinked arthroplasty is employed. If the triceps was detached, it should be repaired back to the olecranon through drill holes using locking nonabsorbable Krackow sutures (Fig. 40-12). The ulnar nerve is secured in the anterior subcutaneous transposed location and the wound is closed in layers over a hemovac drain.

Postoperative management depends on the type of arthroplasty performed. If the arthroplasty is linked, the elbow is immobilized in near full extension using a bulky dressing with an anterior splint. If an unlinked arthroplasty is performed, the elbow is immobilized in 70° of flexion using an anterior splint to avoid posterior wound pressure. Drains are removed 1 day postoperatively and antibiotics are administered for 24 hours. After 10 to 14 days depending on the patient age, comorbidities, and quality of their skin, the splint is removed and range of motion exercises are commenced if soft tissue healing is secure.[46]

Rehabilitation depends on whether a linked or unlinked arthroplasty has been performed and also on in the integrity of the triceps mechanism. In the setting with an unlinked implant where the collateral ligaments have been reattached, a collar and cuff is employed for 6 weeks to protect the collateral ligament repair. Elbow extension should initially be limited to 40° and gradually increased until full extension of the elbow is achieved by 6 weeks postoperatively. If a linked arthroplasty is performed, and no specific precautions are required, unrestricted active motion can be initiated following removal of the initial splint. If the triceps was detached, gravity-assisted extension is performed and full postoperative flexion is avoided for 6 weeks until triceps healing is secure. A nighttime extension splint can be useful in patients having difficulty gaining full extension. Patients are advised not to lift more than 2 to 5 kg following a total elbow arthroplasty.[46]

Complications

Complications are common following total elbow arthroplasty. Fortunately, as surgeons' experience improves and with advances in implant and instrument designs, the incidence of these complications seems to be decreasing over time. Intraoperative complications include cortical

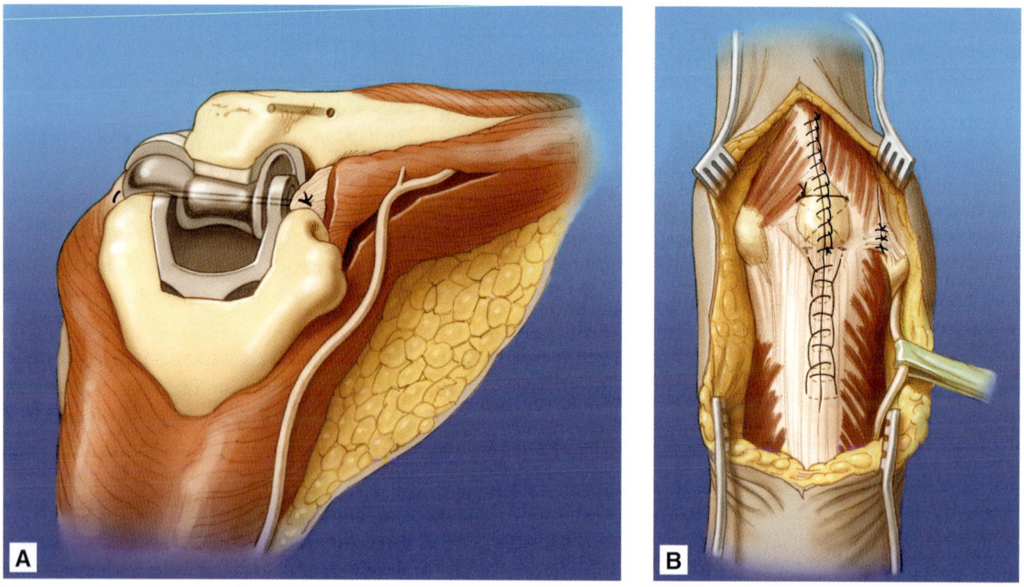

FIGURE 40-12 **A.** The collateral ligaments must be securely repaired back to the medial and lateral epicondyles when an unlinked elbow arthroplasty is performed to restore elbow stability. **B.** The triceps is reattached to the olecranon using transosseous sutures. (Illustrations reproduced with permission from Tornier, Inc.)

perforations, fractures, and nerve injuries. Common early postoperative complications include delayed wound healing, flap necrosis, infection, and triceps insufficiency. If an unlinked arthroplasty is performed, acute or subacute instability can also occur. Long-term complications include infection, aseptic loosening, polyethylene wear, stem fractures, linkage failure, and periprosthetic fractures.[47,48]

Outcomes

Over 90% of patients following a linked or unlinked total elbow arthroplasty achieve significant pain relief, joint stability, and functional motion. The outcome of linked and unlinked arthroplasties tends to be similar in the literature. There are no good comparative clinical trials demonstrating whether the theoretical benefit of an unlinked arthroplasty has any clinical advantage over a linked device. Patients undergoing an unlinked device tend to have greater problems with postoperative stiffness perhaps due to less bone shortening, less soft tissue release, and a tendency for more protective postoperative mobilization programs.

The results of unlinked arthroplasty have been more variable than linked arthroplasty (Fig. 40-13). Ewald et al reported excellent outcomes in 202 patients at an average of 6-year follow-up following a capitellocondylar total elbow arthroplasty.[49] They had a 1.5% incidence of revision for postoperative instability and a 1.5% incidence of revision for aseptic loosening. Seven percent of their patients had a wound complication. Other authors have reported up to a 20% incidence of instability when using this same unlinked device suggesting that careful patient selection and surgical technique are essential to achieve a good outcome.[50] The Souter-Strathclyde unlinked total elbow arthroplasty is more constrained and has had a lower incidence of problems with instability; however, humeral loosening, particularly the short stem humeral component, has been more problematic.[51] Excellent long-term outcomes have been reported for the Kudo unlinked total elbow arthroplasty. Tanaka et al reported a 100% survivorship of the metal-backed ulnar components and a 72% survivorship of elbows with an all-polyethylene ulnar component at an average of 13 years.[38]

The results of linked total elbow arthroplasty in patients with rheumatoid arthritis have been excellent with Gill and Morrey reporting 92% survivorship at an average of 10-year follow-up[52] (Fig. 40-14). Bushing wear was noted in 15% of patients. Similar results have been reported in patients following the management of acute distal humeral fractures; however, mechanical failure has been more common in patients treated for posttraumatic conditions (Fig. 40-15). Schneeberger et al reported 11 major complications in 39 patients treated with a total elbow arthroplasty for posttraumatic arthritis at an average of 5 years postoperatively.[53] Five of their patients had ulnar stem fractures and 2 patients had problems with major polyethylene bushing wear (Fig. 40-16).

There are limited results available with convertible total elbow devices. Bassi et al reported on the short-term results of the Acclaim prosthesis.[54] At 3-year follow-up clinical loosening was not observed; however, 20% had some evidence of loosening radiographically and 2 patients had clinical instability that required conversion to a linked prosthesis.

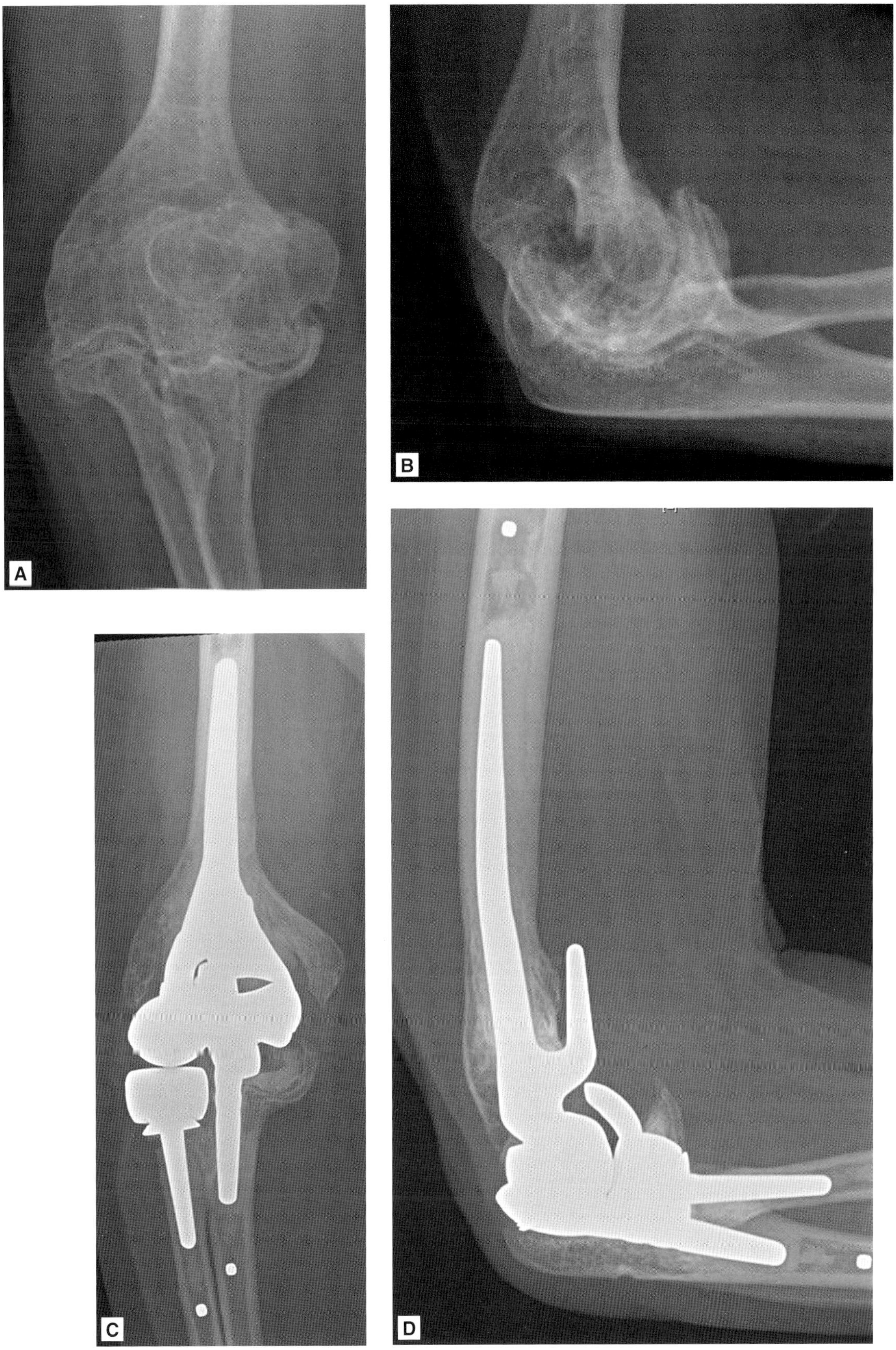

FIGURE 40-13 **A** and **B.** Anteroposterior and lateral radiographs of a 60-year-old woman with juvenile rheumatoid arthritis. She presented with disabling stiffness and pain. **C** and **D.** Two years following an unlinked total elbow arthroplasty her elbow was stable and pain free and she regained a functional range of motion. Note the need to contour the humeral component during surgery due to the small size of her medullary canals.

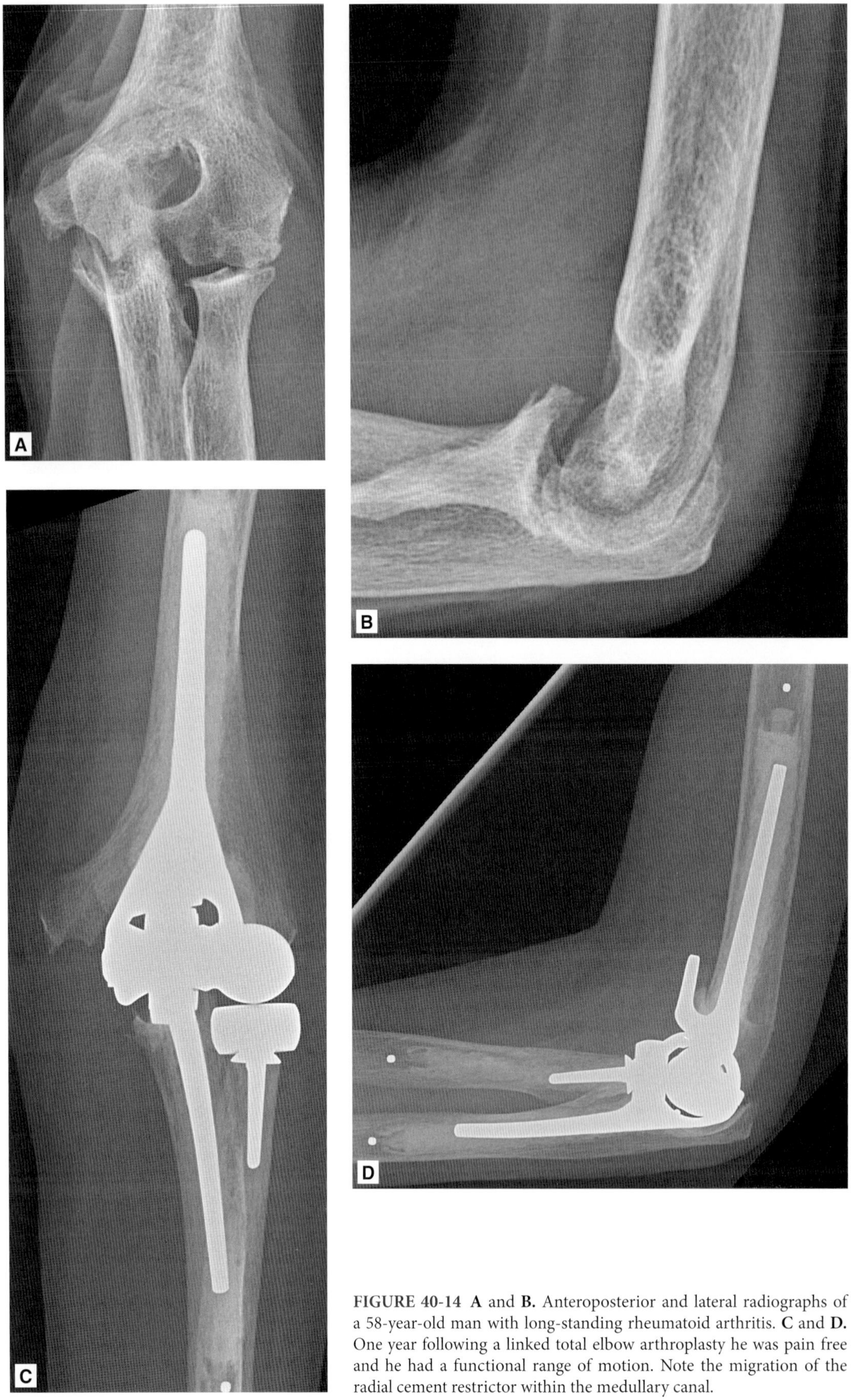

FIGURE 40-14 **A** and **B.** Anteroposterior and lateral radiographs of a 58-year-old man with long-standing rheumatoid arthritis. **C** and **D.** One year following a linked total elbow arthroplasty he was pain free and he had a functional range of motion. Note the migration of the radial cement restrictor within the medullary canal.

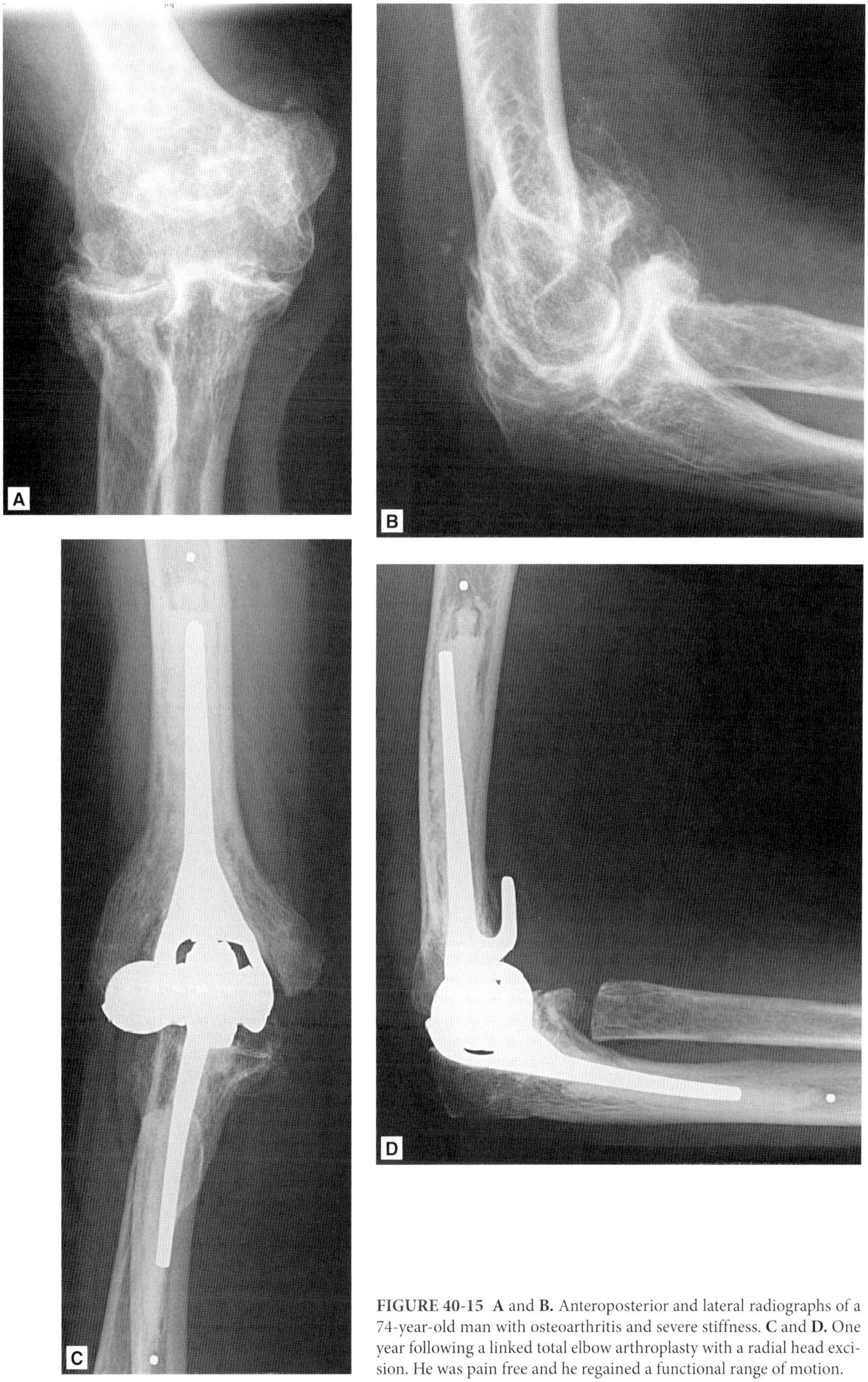

FIGURE 40-15 **A** and **B.** Anteroposterior and lateral radiographs of a 74-year-old man with osteoarthritis and severe stiffness. **C** and **D.** One year following a linked total elbow arthroplasty with a radial head excision. He was pain free and he regained a functional range of motion.

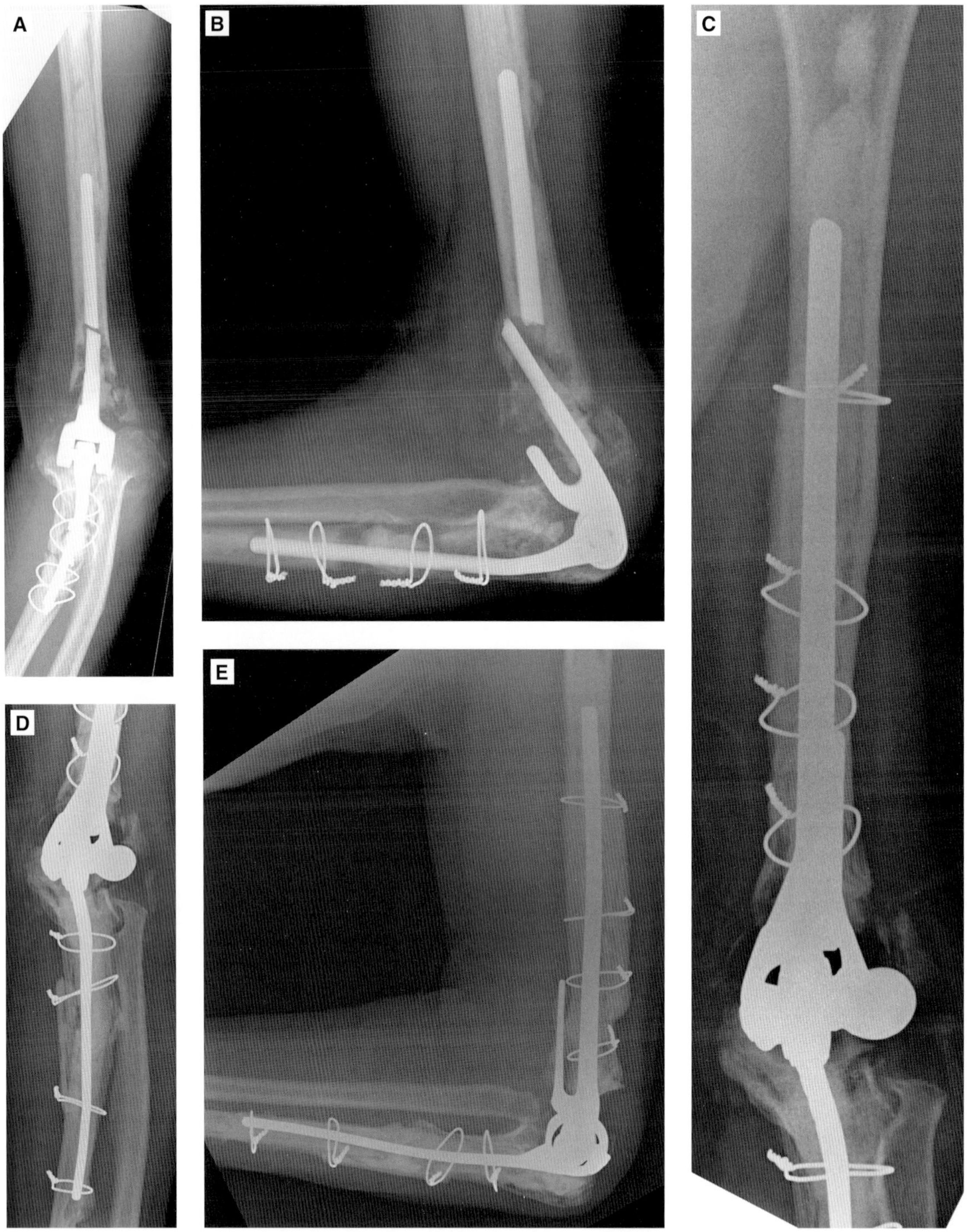

FIGURE 40-16 **A** and **B.** Anteroposterior and lateral radiographs of a 65-year-old man with bearing wear and a fractured humeral stem after a fourth revision elbow arthroplasty. Note the cement migration without the use of cement restrictors. **C** to **E.** Two years following allograft reconstruction and a linked total elbow arthroplasty. He had mild pain and a functional range of motion.

DISTAL HUMERAL HEMIARTHROPLASTY

Rationale and Basic Science

Distal humeral hemiarthroplasty avoids the need for replacement of the ulna and therefore the need to use polyethylene. While hemiarthroplasty of the distal humerus was performed as early as 1927, it has only recently become more commonly used as devices specifically designed for this indication have become available.

While the concern about polyethylene wear is avoided, the articulation of metal on cartilage raises the possibility of degenerative cartilage changes and possible erosion of the underlying ulna and radial bones. Theoretically, patients undergoing a distal humeral hemiarthroplasty could have reduced restrictions on their postoperative activity relative to the typical 2 to 5 kg that has been recommended for patients undergoing total elbow arthroplasty. There is no literature evaluating the biomechanical effects of distal humeral hemiarthroplasty to date and there are limited anthropometric studies of the distal humerus.[55]

Indications

The ideal candidate for distal humeral hemiarthroplasty has not been defined. The most common indication would be a distal humeral fracture, nonunion or avascular necrosis. Comminuted coronal shear fractures of the distal humerus with preserved epicondyles are a good indication as condylar reconstruction is not required as is typically the case for patients with supracondylar fractures. Patients being considered for distal humeral hemiarthroplasty are typically younger and more active than patients who would be candidates for a total elbow arthroplasty.

Contraindications

Given the limited data on the effectiveness of distal humeral hemiarthroplasty, this procedure is contraindicated in patients who are elderly or low demand where a total elbow arthroplasty would be expected to have a good result. Active infection is an absolute contraindication. Other absolute contraindications would be the lack of condylar bone stock and collateral ligaments to allow effective restoration of elbow stability following replacement of the distal humeral articulation. Relative contraindications are preexisting elbow arthritis and patients who are unable or unwilling to live within the restrictions of a distal humeral hemiarthroplasty. Distal humeral hemiarthroplasty is relatively contraindicated in patients who do not have an intact radial column. In this setting a radial head prosthesis should be considered to stabilize the elbow and assist in load transfer.

Surgical Technique

The surgical technique is at the discretion of the operating surgeon and the type of hemiarthroplasty to be performed. There is currently no hemiarthroplasty implant that is FDA approved in the United States; however, these implants are widely available worldwide. Patient preparation and positioning is similar to that described previously for total elbow arthroplasty. It is important to preserve the integrity of the condyles to restore stability after placement of the hemiarthroplasty. In most distal humeral fractures the condyles and epicondyles are fractured in which case the distal humeral arthroplasty is inserted using a paratricipital approach. The width of the articulation of the ulna and radial head determines the size of implant to be used. Depth of insertion is judged by reassembling one of the condyles if possible. The proximal aspect of the olecranon fossa is also a useful landmark as this is at the same location as the anterior flange of the humeral component. A trial reduction should be performed to evaluate soft tissue tension and condylar length prior to cementing the definitive implant. The flat posterior portion of the distal humerus is a useful guide for the rotational positioning of the prosthesis in the setting of fractures of the distal humeral condyles; the implant should be internally rotated 14° relative to the posterior humeral cortex.[56] A cement restrictor is placed in the medullary canal and the canal is lavaged and dried. Antibiotic cement is injected retrograde using a cement gun and the prosthesis is inserted and held in the appropriate position and orientation until the cement has set. A bone graft is placed behind the anterior flange of the implant. After insertion of the prosthesis the epicondyles and condyles are reconstructed using tension band wiring or plate fixation. Unicortical or bicortical screws placed anterior or posterior to the implant stem facilitate secure fixation of supracondylar plates. If the collateral ligaments and condyles are intact such as in the setting of coronal shear fractures, nonunions, or avascular necrosis, an olecranon osteotomy can be used to allow insertion of the implant while maintaining the stability of the elbow. Standard techniques for olecranon osteotomy fixation are performed, either tension band wiring or plate fixation. Accurate positioning of the distal humeral hemiarthroplasty is critical to avoid malarticulation and early implant failure. Implant sizing is critical to ensure congruous tracking of the implant with the ulna and radial head. If stable condylar reconstruction and ligament stability is not achievable, conversion to a linked total elbow arthroplasty is advisable.

Outcomes

There are little data available on the outcomes of distal humeral hemiarthroplasty. The majority of the studies have small patient numbers and short-term follow-up. They often include a mixture of clinical indications. The majority of patients achieve a functional outcome; however, similar to total elbow arthroplasty, complications are not infrequent,

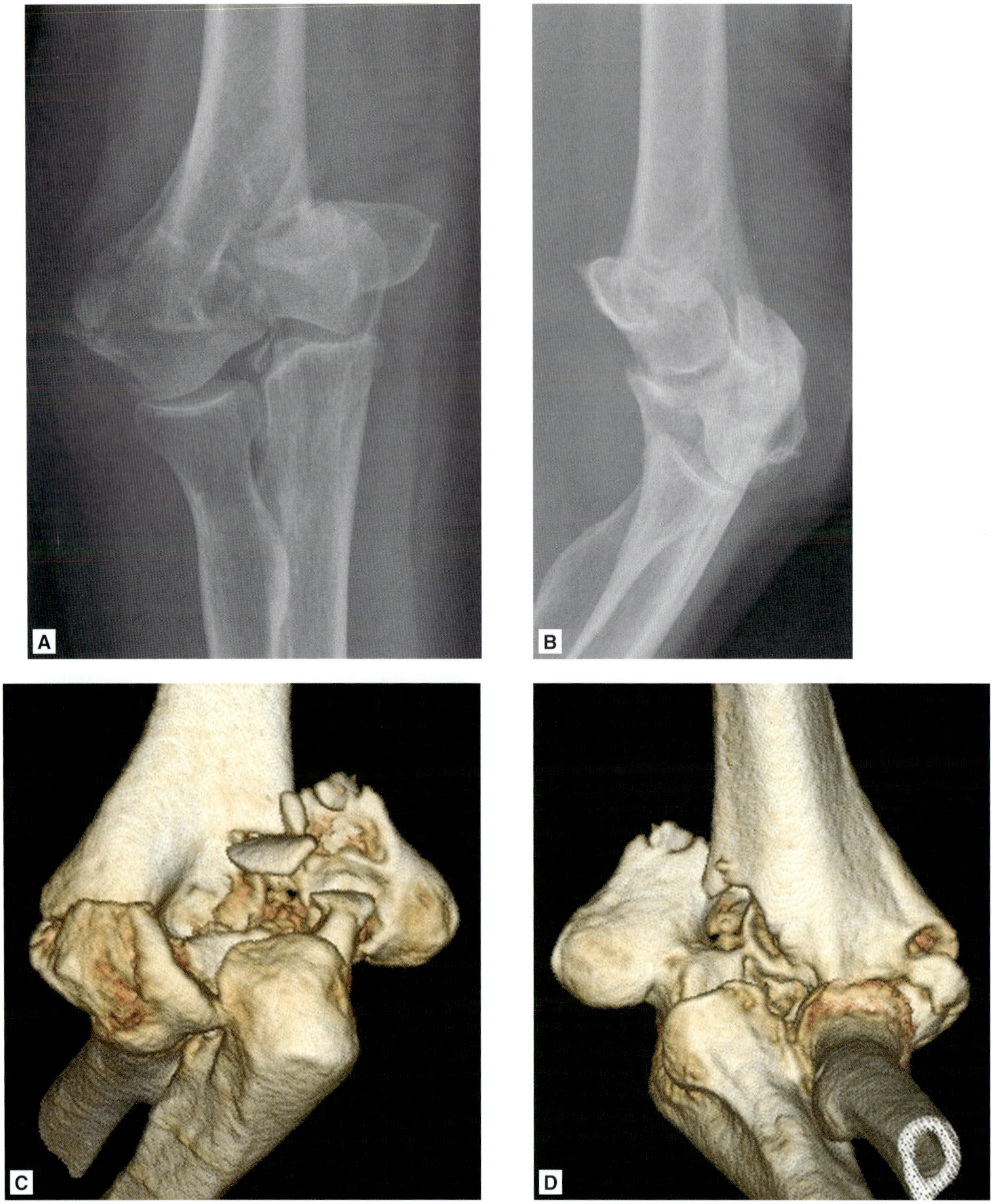

FIGURE 40-17 **A** and **B.** Anteroposterior and lateral radiographs of a distal humerus fracture in a 69-year-old woman after a low-energy fall. **C** and **D.** CT shows comminution of the articulation.

although most are treatable and allow retention of the arthroplasty. Street and Stevens developed an anatomically shaped metallic distal humerus hemiarthroplasty and reported their initial experience with this device in 10 patients.[57] Their best results were in patients with posttraumatic conditions. The implant was unreliable in patients with rheumatoid and hemophilic arthritis. Swoboda and Scott reported that the capitellocondylar humeral component, which is not anatomically shaped, could provide reasonable short-term benefit in young patients with rheumatoid arthritis, but the results were not as reliable as a total elbow arthroplasty.[58] Adolfsson and Nestorson reviewed 8 patients at an average of 4 years

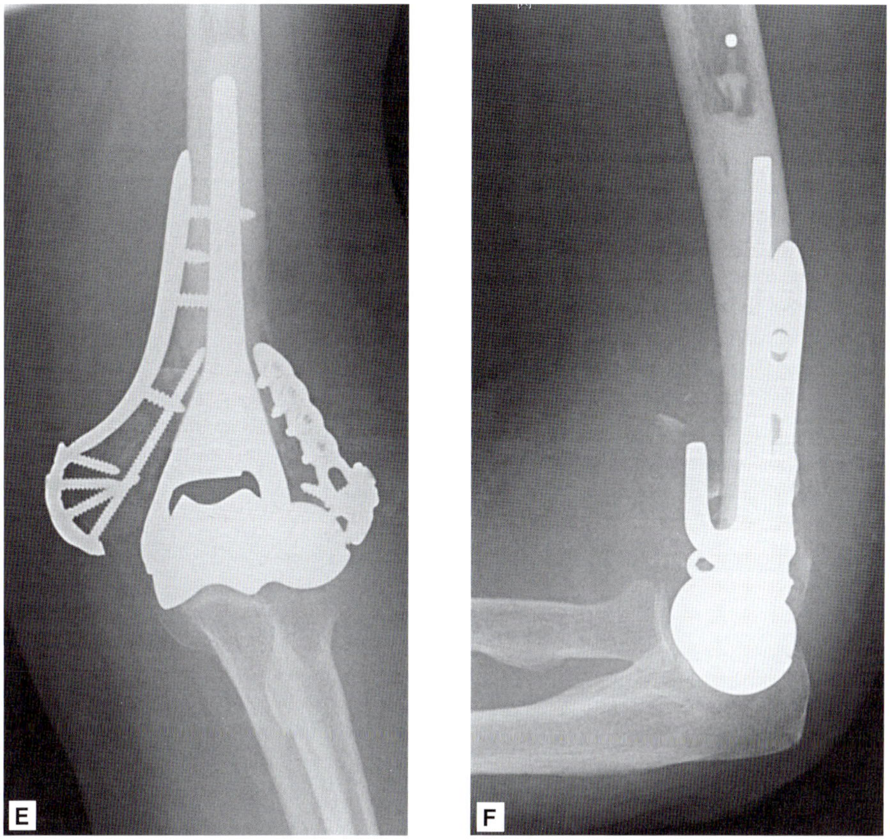

FIGURE 40-17 (*Continued*) **E** and **F.** Radiographs 2 months postoperative distal humeral hemiarthroplasty with condylar fixation.

following distal humeral hemiarthroplasty using the Kudo humeral component.[59] The clinical outcomes were good or excellent; however, erosion of the ulna and radius was noted, perhaps because the articulation of the implant does not closely replicate the shape of the native distal humerus. Burkhart et al reported their experience in 8 patients with an acute distal humeral fracture and 2 patients with a non-union at an average of 1 year postoperatively.[60,61] They used an anatomically shaped latitude humeral hemiarthroplasty (Fig. 40-17). Nine of the patients had a good or excellent result. Long term follow-up studies are required to evaluate the durability of these more anatomically shaped devices that are designed to closely replicate the shape of the distal humerus articulation. Degenerative cartilage changes and osseous erosions remain a concern in the longer term.

REFERENCES

1. Amis AA, Dowson D, Wright V. Elbow joint force predictions for some strenuous isometric actions. *J Biomech.* 1980;13(9):765–775.
2. Halls AA, Travill A. Transmission of pressures across the elbow joint. *Anat Rec.* 1964;150:243–248.
3. Morrey BF, An KN. Articular and ligamentous contributions to the stability of the elbow joint. *Am J Sports Med.* 1983;11(5):315–319.
4. Beingessner DM, Dunning CE, Gordon KD, Johnson JA, King GJ. The effect of radial head excision and arthroplasty on elbow kinematics and stability. *J Bone Joint Surg Am.* 2004;86A(8):1730–1739.
5. Sellman DC, Seitz WH Jr, Postak PD, Greenwald AS. Reconstructive strategies for radioulnar dissociation: a biomechanical study. *J Orthop Trauma.* 1995;9(6):516–522.
6. Schneeberger A, Sadowski MM, Jacob HAC. Coronoid process and radial head as posterolateral rotatory stabilizers of the elbow. *J Bone Joint Surg Am.* 2004;86A(5):975–982.
7. Chanlalit C, Shukla DR, Fitzsimmons JS, An KN, O'Driscoll SW. The biomechanical effect of prosthetic design on radiocapitellar stability in a terrible triad model. *J Orthop Trauma.* 2012;26:539–544.
8. Liew VS, Cooper IC, Ferreira LM, Johnson JA, King GJ. The effect of metallic radial head arthroplasty on radiocapitellar joint contact area. *Clin Biomech (Bristol, Avon).* 2003;18(2):115–118.
9. Sarris IK, Kyrkos MJ, Galanis NN, Papavasiliou KA, Sayegh FE, Kapetanos GA. Radial head replacement with the MoPyC pyrocarbon prosthesis. *J Shoulder Elbow Surg.* 2012;21:1222–1228.
10. Flinkkila T, Kaisto T, Sirnio K, Hyvonen P, Leppilahti J. Short- to mid-term results of metallic press-fit radial head arthroplasty in unstable injuries of the elbow. *J Bone Joint Surg Br.* 2012;94(6):805–810.
11. King GJ, Zarzour ZD, Patterson SD, Johnson JA. An anthropometric study of the radial head: implications in the design of a prosthesis. *J Arthroplasty.* 2001;16(1):112–116.
12. Koslowsky TC, Schliwa S, Koebke J. Presentation of the microscopic vascular architecture of the radial head using a sequential plastination technique. *Clin Anat.* 2011;24(6):721–732.
13. van Riet RP, Morrey BF, O'Driscoll SW, Van Glabbeek F. Associated injuries complicating radial head fractures: a demographic study. *Clin Orthop Relat Res.* 2005;441:351–355.
14. Davidson PA, Moseley JB Jr, Tullos HS. Radial head fracture. A potentially complex injury. *Clin Orthop Relat Res.* 1993;(297):224–230.
15. Giannicola G, Angeloni R, Mantovani A, et al. Open debridement and radiocapitellar replacement in primary and post-traumatic arthritis of the elbow: a multicenter study. *J Shoulder Elbow Surg.* 2012;21(4):456–463.

16. Grewal R, MacDermid JC, Faber KJ, Drosdowech DS, King GJ. Comminuted radial head fractures treated with a modular metallic radial head arthroplasty. Study of outcomes. *J Bone Joint Surg Am.* 2006;88(10):2192–2200.
17. Zunkiewicz MR, Clemente JS, Miller MC, Baratz ME, Gray R, Cohen MS. Radial head replacement with a bipolar system: a minimum 2-year follow-up. *J Shoulder Elbow Surg.* 2012;21:98–104.
18. Dowdy PA, Bain GI, King GJ, Patterson SD. The midline posterior elbow incision. An anatomical appraisal. *J Bone Joint Surg Br.* 1995;77(5):696–699.
19. Diliberti T, Botte MJ, Abrams RA. Anatomical considerations regarding the posterior interosseous nerve during posterolateral approaches to the proximal part of the radius. *J Bone Joint Surg Am.* 2000;82(6):809–813.
20. Birkedal JP, Deal DN, Ruch DS. Loss of flexion after radial head replacement. *J Shoulder Elbow Surg.* 2004;13(2):208–213.
21. Doornberg JN, Linzel DS, Zurakowski D, Ring D. Reference points for radial head prosthesis size. *J Hand Surg Am.* 2006;31(1):53–57.
22. Rowland AS, Athwal GS, MacDermid JC, King GJ. Lateral ulnohumeral joint space widening is not diagnostic of radial head arthroplasty overstuffing. *J Hand Surg Am.* 2007;32(5):637–641.
23. Athwal GS, Frank SG, Grewal R, Faber KJ, Johnson J, King GJ. Determination of correct implant size in radial head arthroplasty to avoid overlengthening: surgical technique. *J Bone Joint Surg Am.* 2010;92(suppl 1, Pt 2):250–257.
24. Athwal GS, Rouleau DM, MacDermid JC, King GJ. Contralateral elbow radiographs can reliably diagnose radial head implant overlengthening. *J Bone Joint Surg Am.* 2011;93(14):1339–1346.
25. Fraser GS, Pichora JE, Ferreira LM, Brownhill JR, Johnson JA, King GJ. Lateral collateral ligament repair restores the initial varus stability of the elbow: an in vitro biomechanical study. *J Orthop Trauma.* 2008;22(9):615–623.
26. Mathew PK, Athwal GS, King GJ. Terrible triad injury of the elbow: current concepts. *J Am Acad Orthop Surg.* 2009;17(3):137–151.
27. Moro JK, Werier J, MacDermid JC, Patterson SD, King GJ. Arthroplasty with a metal radial head for unreconstructible fractures of the radial head. *J Bone Joint Surg Am.* 2001;83-A(8):1201–1211.
28. Fehringer EV, Burns EM, Knierim A, Sun J, Apker KA, Berg RE. Radiolucencies surrounding a smooth-stemmed radial head component may not correlate with forearm pain or poor elbow function. *J Shoulder Elbow Surg.* 2009;18(2):275–278.
29. Shore BJ, Mozzon JB, MacDermid JC, Faber KJ, King GJ. Chronic posttraumatic elbow disorders treated with metallic radial head arthroplasty. *J Bone Joint Surg Am.* 2008;90(2):271–280.
30. Doornberg JN, Parisien R, van Duijn PJ, Ring D. Radial head arthroplasty with a modular metal spacer to treat acute traumatic elbow instability. *J Bone Joint Surg Am.* 2007;89(5):1075–1080.
31. Popovic N, Lemaire R, Georis P, Gillet P. Midterm results with a bipolar radial head prosthesis: radiographic evidence of loosening at the bone–cement interface. *J Bone Joint Surg Am.* 2007;89(11): 2469–2476.
32. Dee R. Total replacement arthroplasty of the elbow for rheumatoid arthritis. *J Bone Joint Surg Br.* 1972;54(1):88–95.
33. Garrett JC, Ewald FC, Thomas WH, Sledge CB. Loosening associated with G.S.B. hinge total elbow replacement in patients with rheumatoid arthritis. *Clin Orthop Relat Res.* 1977;66(127):170–174.
34. Morrey BF, Chao EY. Passive motion of the elbow joint. *J Bone Joint Surg Am.* 1976;58(4):501–508.
35. King GJ, Itoi E, Niebur GL, Morrey BF, An KN. Motion and laxity of the capitellocondylar total elbow prosthesis. *J Bone Joint Surg Am.* 1994;76(7):1000–1008.
36. O'Driscoll SW, An KN, Korinek S, Morrey BF. Kinematics of semi-constrained total elbow arthroplasty. *J Bone Joint Surg Br.* 1992;74(2):297–299.
37. Gramstad GD, King GJ, O'Driscoll SW, Yamaguchi K. Elbow arthroplasty using a convertible implant. *Tech Hand Up Extrem Surg.* 2005;9(3):153–163.
38. Tanaka N, Kudo H, Iwano K, Sakahashi H, Sato E, Ishii S. Kudo total elbow arthroplasty in patients with rheumatoid arthritis: a long-term follow-up study. *J Bone Joint Surg Am.* 2001;83-A(10):1506–1513.
39. Jeon IH, Morrey BF, Sanchez-Sotelo J. Ulnar component surface finish influenced the outcome of primary Coonrad-Morrey total elbow arthroplasty. *J Shoulder Elbow Surg.* 2012;21(9):1229–1235.
40. Cheung EV, O'Driscoll SW. Total elbow prosthesis loosening caused by ulnar component pistoning. *J Bone Joint Surg Am.* 2007;89(6): 1269–1274.
41. Brownhill JR, Pollock JW, Ferreira LM, Johnson JA, King GJ. The effect of implant malalignment on joint loading in total elbow arthroplasty: an in vitro study. *J Shoulder Elbow Surg.* 2012;21(8):1032–1038.
42. Alonso-Llames M. Bilaterotricipital approach to the elbow. Its application in the osteosynthesis of supracondylar fractures of the humerus in children. *Acta Orthop Scand.* 1972;43(6):479–490.
43. Bryan RS, Morrey BF. Extensive posterior exposure of the elbow. A triceps-sparing approach. *Clin Orthop Relat Res.* 1982;(166):188–192.
44. Kocher T. *Textbook of Operative Surgery.* 3rd ed. London: Adam and Charles Black; 1911.
45. Mehta JA, Bain GI. Surgical approaches to the elbow. *Hand Clin.* 2004;20(4):375–387.
46. Szekeres M, King GJ. Total elbow arthroplasty. *J Hand Ther.* 2006;19(2):245–253.
47. Gay DM, Lyman S, Do H, Hotchkiss RN, Marx RG, Daluiski A. Indications and reoperation rates for total elbow arthroplasty: an analysis of trends in New York State. *J Bone Joint Surg Am.* 2012;94(2):110–117.
48. King GJ, Adams RA, Morrey BF. Total elbow arthroplasty: revision with use of a non-custom semiconstrained prosthesis. *J Bone Joint Surg Am.* 1997;79(3):394–400.
49. Ewald FC, Simmons ED Jr, Sullivan JA, et al. Capitellocondylar total elbow replacement in rheumatoid arthritis. Long-term results. *J Bone Joint Surg Am.* 1993;75(4):498–507.
50. Davis RF, Weiland AJ, Hungerford DS, Moore JR, Volenec-Dowling S. Nonconstrained total elbow arthroplasty. *Clin Orthop Relat Res.* 1982;(171):156–160.
51. Trail LA, Nuttall D, Stanley JK. Comparison of survivorship between standard and long-stem Souter-Strathclyde total elbow arthroplasty. *J Shoulder Elbow Surg.* 2002;11(4):373–376.
52. Gill DR, Morrey BF. The Coonrad-Morrey total elbow arthroplasty in patients who have rheumatoid arthritis. A ten to fifteen-year follow-up study. *J Bone Joint Surg Am.* 1998;80(9):1327–1335.
53. Schneeberger AG, Adams R, Morrey BF. Semiconstrained total elbow replacement for the treatment of post-traumatic osteoarthrosis. *J Bone Joint Surg Am.* 1997;79(8):1211–1222.
54. Bassi RS, Simmons D, Ali F, et al. Early results of the Acclaim elbow replacement. *J Bone Joint Surg Br.* 2007;89(4):486–489.
55. Shiba R, Sorbie C, Siu DW, Bryant JT, Cooke TD, Wevers HW. Geometry of the humeroulnar joint. *J Orthop Res.* 1988;6(6):897–906.
56. Sabo MT, Athwal GS, King GJ. Landmarks for rotational alignment of the humeral component during elbow arthroplasty. *J Bone Joint Surg Am.* 2012;94(19):1794–1800.
57. Street DM, Stevens PS. A humeral replacement prosthesis for the elbow: results in ten elbows. *J Bone Joint Surg Am.* 1974;56(6):1147–1158.
58. Swoboda B, Scott RD. Humeral hemiarthroplasty of the elbow joint in young patients with rheumatoid arthritis: a report on 7 arthroplasties. *J Arthroplasty.* 1999;14(5):553–559.
59. Adolfsson L, Nestorson J. The Kudo humeral component as primary hemiarthroplasty in distal humeral fractures. *J Shoulder Elbow Surg.* 2012;21(4):451–455.
60. Burkhart KJ, Muller LP, Schwarz C, Mattyasovszky SG, Rommens PM. Treatment of the complex intraarticular fracture of the distal humerus with the latitude elbow prosthesis. *Oper Orthop Traumatol.* 2010;22(3):279–298.
61. Burkhart KJ, Nijs S, Mattyasovszky SG, et al. Distal humerus hemiarthroplasty of the elbow for comminuted distal humeral fractures in the elderly patient. *J Trauma.* 2011;71(3):635–642.

41A

Tendon Repairs About the Elbow—Part A: Distal Biceps Tendon Ruptures

Kevin Eng, MBBS, FRACS
Gregory I. Bain, MBBS, FRACS, FA(Ortho) A, PhD

INTRODUCTION

Distal biceps rupture usually affects male patients between 30 and 60, although it can extend from the second to eighth decade.[1] The most common presentation involves an explosive eccentric contracture against resistance. It is a rare injury making up 3% to 12% of all biceps injuries,[2] with an incidence of 1.2 per 100,000 people.[3] Risk factors include male gender, smoking,[3] anabolic steroid use,[4] and weight lifting.[2]

BACKGROUND/ETIOLOGY

Anatomy

The biceps has 2 bellies. The long head and short head of the biceps have a defined footprint.[5] The long head passes radial to the short head and inserts onto the proximal part of the radial tuberosity. The short head inserts distal to this in a fan-like pattern. In some patients the tendons of the short and long head are independent, but this is rare.[6] Both tendons are ensheathed by the biceps aponeurosis (lacertus fibrosus) that consists of 3 layers (Fig. 41A-1). It comes off the medial aspect of the biceps tendon to insert into the subcutaneous border of the ulna via the deep fascia of the forearm.

Siebenlist et al found that the native strength of the cadaveric tendon was 379 N, and presumably the load must be higher than this to rupture.[7]

The biceps footprint measures a mean length of 21 mm and a width of 7 mm and has footprint of 108 mm^2.[6] The tendon attaches to this posterior rim, and the bursa attaches to the remainder of the tuberosity. The apex of the radial tuberosity is 65° (range 15°–120°) posterior to the ulnar side of the fully supinated radius[8] (Figs. 41A-2 to 41A-4).

Pathophysiology

The pathophysiology of distal biceps tendon ruptures is unclear. Hypertrophic lipping on the radial tuberosity, radial bursitis, and a watershed area of poor arterial supply resulting in local weakness may predispose to tears.[9–11]

Bilateral cases have been reported at a rate of 8%, a mean of 4.6 years apart. This is much higher than the background incidence, and may suggest an underlying predisposition.[12]

The tendon most commonly tears at its insertion. Tears within the length of the tendon and at the musculotendinous junction are rare.[13] Partial-thickness tears are also possible.[14] The tendon is more likely to retract if the bicipital aponeurosis is also torn.

Regardless of the predisposing factors, the most common mechanism is rapid eccentric loading of the arm in flexion.

Natural History of Tendon Rupture

An unrepaired rupture leads to a deficit of 27% in supination strength and 47% loss of supination endurance compared with the normal contralateral arm. Flexion strength and endurance is decreased by 21%.[15] More recently, Freeman et al found a mean 25% reduction in supination strength but only a 7% loss of flexion when compared with the normal contralateral arm. The loss of flexion strength was not statistically significant.[16]

PRESENTATION, INVESTIGATION, AND TREATMENT OPTIONS

History

There is usually a history of a sudden and sharp extension load to an elbow flexed at 90° with the biceps in a contracted state. This is followed by sharp pain, typically in the antecubital fossa, but sometimes felt in the posterolateral elbow. There may be an audible "pop."[1]

Examination

For several days post injury, there may be an ecchymosis over the antecubital fossa. There is a palpable gap in the biceps

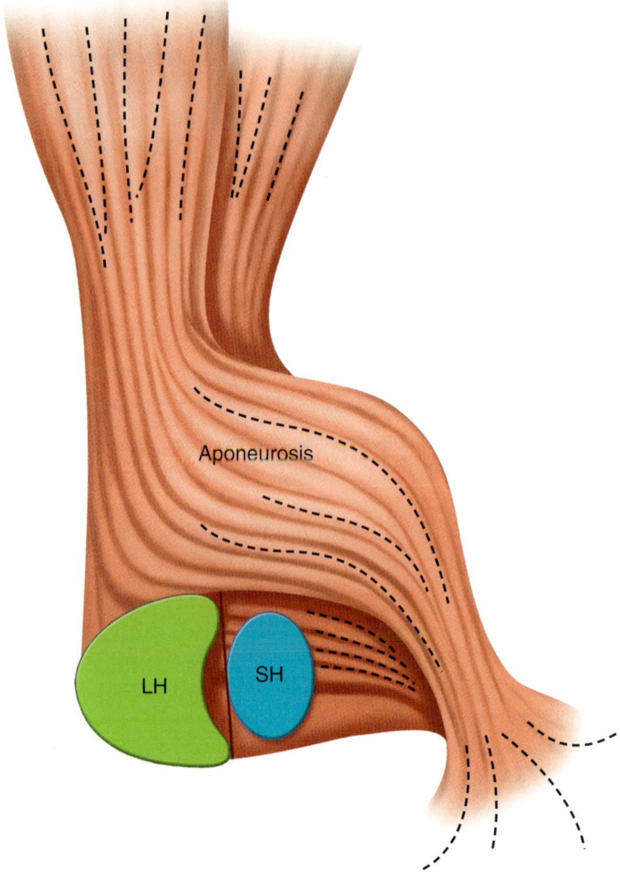

FIGURE 41A-1 Distal biceps tendon anatomy. LH, long head; SH, short head. (Reproduced with permission from Eames et al.[5])

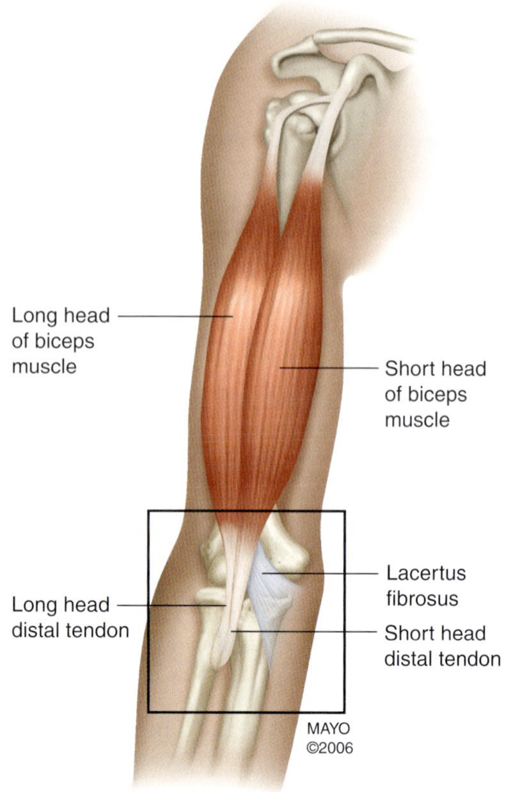

FIGURE 41A-2 Distal biceps tendon insertional anatomy. (Reproduced with permission from Athwal et al.[6] Copyright © 2007 by the American Society for Surgery of the Hand.)

tendon. Tenderness may be elicited over the radial tuberosity. There is weakness of supination against resistance. Weakness of flexion is less marked as the brachialis compensates.

The signs of a partial rupture are more subtle. There may be crepitus or grinding on passive rotation of the forearm[14] and weakness of resisted supination. A direct tuberosity compression test has been described for aiding the diagnosis of partial tears. The examiner palpates the lateral aspect of the fully supinated radius 2.5 cm distal to the radiocapitellar joint. The patient then rotates the forearm. If this elicits more pain than the normal contralateral side, the test is positive.[17]

Several clinical tests have been described to aid the diagnosis of complete rupture. The senior author's preference is to simply perform passive rotation of the patient's forearm with the elbow flexed to 90° and observe the biceps muscle belly compared with the opposite side. If there is no movement, a complete rupture is likely. Ruland et al described a "squeeze test."[18] The patient is seated with the elbow flexed to 60° and the forearm in slight pronation. The surgeon squeezes the muscle belly of biceps with both hands. Forearm supination should be observed if the distal biceps is intact. O'Driscoll et al described the hook sign. The patient is asked to actively supinate and flex the elbow to 90°. The examiner is then able to hook their finger under the distal biceps tendon from the lateral aspect of the elbow. In the case of a complete rupture of the distal biceps tendon, the examiner is unable to satisfactorily hook their finger under the tendon.[19]

Imaging

Plain radiographs are not particularly helpful in the diagnosis of distal biceps tendon ruptures. The only finding on an x-ray may be irregular changes in the radial tuberosity that may predispose to a rupture.[20]

Ultrasound has been used to diagnose distal biceps tears. A newer technique involving a medial approach through the pronator window has resulted in more complete visualization of the ulnarly facing radial tuberosity and distal biceps insertion.[21] Dynamic imaging may be helpful in revealing partial tears.[22] However, it is less reliable than magnetic resonance imaging (MRI).

MRI can depict the level of the tear and whether the injury is a partial-thickness tear. A recent study showed a 100% specificity, but 59.1% sensitivity in detecting partial tears. The missed partial tears were reported as having "tendinopathy" and were all low grade (<50%).[23]

Giuffre and Moss[22] described an MRI view that allows a longitudinal view of the tendon to be obtained in 1 slice allowing easier recognition of pathology, the FABS view

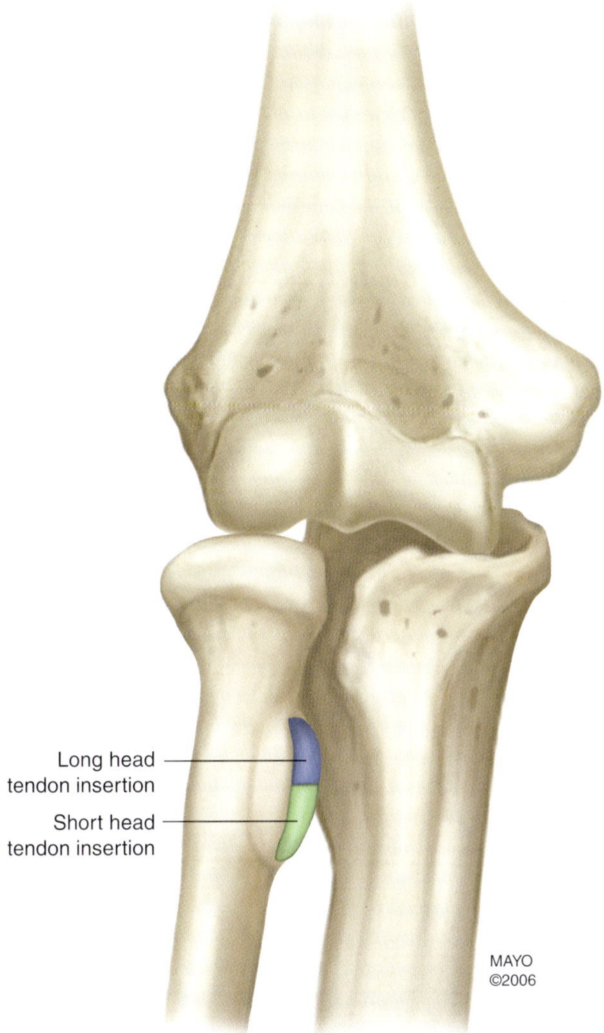

FIGURE 41A-3 Anatomy of the biceps footprint. (Reproduced with permission from Athwal et al.[6] Copyright © 2007 by the American Society for Surgery of the Hand.)

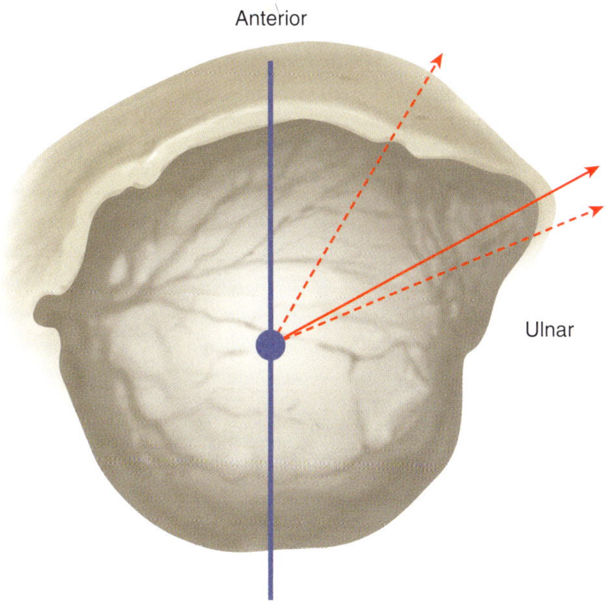

FIGURE 41A-4 A Faxitron image of a proximal radius demonstrates the angular orientation of the bicipital tuberosity (solid red line) and the leading and trailing edges of the biceps brachii tendon insertion (dashed red lines). The anterior posterior reference (blue) is established by a line passing through the center of the radius and a posterior cortical trough marking the midsagittal plane of the radius. (Reproduced with permission from Forthman et al.[8])

(flexed, abducted, and supinated view). The patient lies prone with the shoulder abducted to 180°, the elbow flexed, and the forearm supinated (Fig. 41A-5).

Biceps tendon endoscopy enables the surgeon to directly examine the biceps insertion and is most useful in investigation of partial tears.[24] A longitudinal 2.5-cm incision is made over the palpable biceps tendon about 2 cm distal to the elbow crease. The lateral cutaneous nerve of the forearm is identified and protected. The surgeon uses a digit to palpate the tendon and the bursa. The bursa is then insufflated with normal saline under gravity feed. A small entry point is made on the radial side of the bursa to allow access of the arthroscope. The tendon can then be visualized to its insertion as well as associated synovitis and bursitis. Dynamic assessment of the tendon can be made by pronating and supinating the forearm. A hook probe can assist in assessment of the insertion.

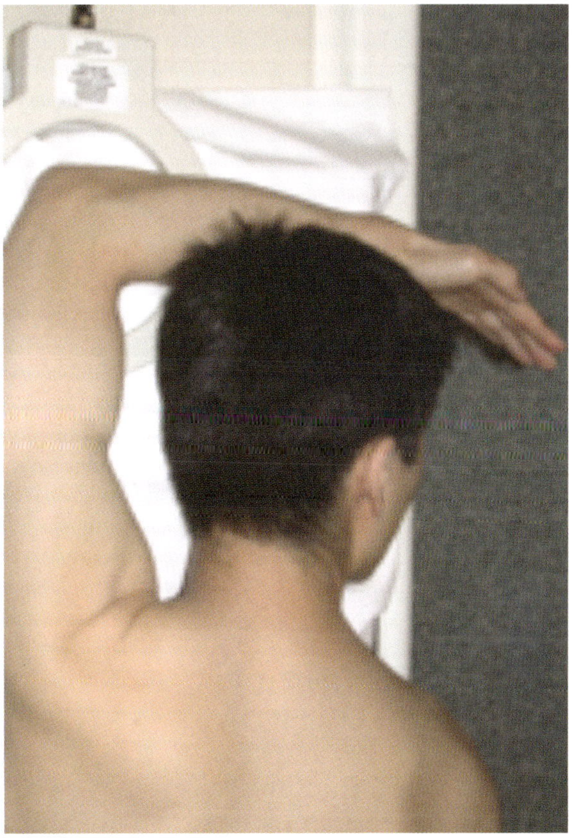

FIGURE 41A-5 FABS view. (Reproduced with permission from Giuffre and Moss.[22])

TABLE 41A-1: Classification of Insertional (Zone 3) Distal Biceps Tendon Ruptures

Grade	Injury	Signs		Treatment
Grade 0	Distal biceps tendinosis	Pain on resisted supination and flexion	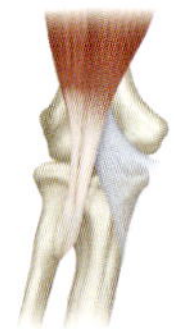	Nonoperative
Grade 1	Distal biceps tendon partial tear	Pain and weakness on resisted supination and flexion	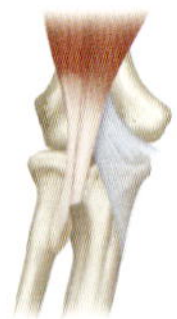	Biceps endoscopy
Grade 2	Combined short and long head avulsion, lacertus intact, minimal muscle retraction	Marked weakness of resisted supination and flexion. Positive Hook test	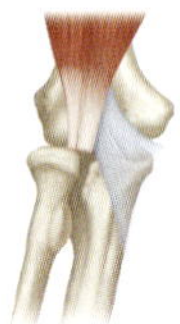	Biceps tendon repair
Grade 3	Complete tendon rupture with torn lacertus fibrosus and muscle retraction	Marked weakness of resisted supination and flexion. Positive Hook test. "Empty" cubital fossa	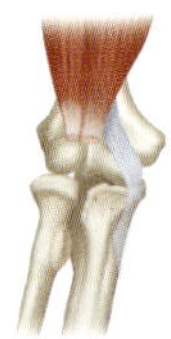	Biceps tendon repair ± lacertus repair
Grade 4	Delayed presentation	Persistent weakness of resisted supination and flexion. Positive Hook test. Proximal retraction of muscle belly	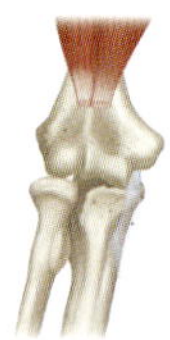	Autograft or allograft reconstruction procedure

Classification

Distal biceps injury can be classified according to degree (partial or complete), temporally (acute or chronic), or anatomically where zone 1 is preaponeurotic (musculotendinous junction), zone 2 is aponeurotic, and zone 3 is postaponeurotic (tendon–bone interface). Most injuries occur in zone 3, and we have devised a classification for these injuries (Table 41A-1).

An acute rupture presents within 4 weeks of injury. Within 4 weeks a direct repair of the tendon is usually possible. A reconstructive procedure may be indicated in chronic biceps tears (greater than 4 weeks old).

SURGICAL TECHNIQUES AND REHABILITATION

Partial-thickness Ruptures

Partial-thickness ruptures of the distal biceps tendon have a variable prognosis. The patient is advised to avoid heavy activity, followed by graduated stretching and strengthening exercises. This treatment is more effective in tears of less than 50% of the tendon, and in patients with lower demands.[1]

Debridement of the distal biceps tendon has limited success.[25] If this fails, the surgeon may consider completing the tear, and reattaching the tendon (see the sections "Operative Techniques—2 Incision," "Operative Techniques—Single Anterior Incision," and "Operative Techniques—Chronic Biceps Tendon Rupture").[26,27]

Acute Full-thickness Ruptures

Acute complete ruptures of the distal biceps tendon usually require operative repair. Nonoperative management may be considered if the patient has low demands or if there is a high surgical risk.

Operative Techniques—2 Incision

The 2-incision technique of distal biceps tenodesis was initially described by Boyd and Anderson. This was modified by Morrey and became popular due to lower rates of heterotopic ossification and synostosis.

The anterior approach is through a 3- to 4-cm transverse incision over the antecubital fossa. The tendon is secured with a grasping stitch. The forearm is then fully supinated and a blunt artery forceps is passed abutting the medial border of the radius through to the dorsolateral aspect of the forearm until it visibly tents the skin. It is of utmost importance that the tip of the forceps passes along the radius only and does not breach the periosteum of the ulna to minimize the risk of radioulnar synostosis. An incision is made on the dorsolateral aspect of the forearm over the tip of the forceps and blunt dissection is performed down to the radius.

The forearm is pronated, placing the posterior interosseous nerve (PIN) away from the operative field, and bringing the radial tuberosity into view. The surface of the tuberosity is burred and drill holes made through the tuberosity. Using forceps, the sutures attached to the proximal portion of the tendon are passed through radius to the dorsolateral wound and tied over bone. Aggressive use of lavage may minimize the risk of heterotopic ossification and synostosis.[28]

Operative Techniques—Single Anterior Incision

SURGICAL APPROACH

Multiple tenodesis techniques exist through a single anterior approach with limited dissection required. Tenodesis of the distal biceps tendon using suture anchors,[29,30] Endobuttons,[31,32] and Biotenodesis interference screws[33] has been described.

Combinations of cortical button and interference screw fixation have good results.[34] Intramedullary Endobuttons have been utilized, aiming to minimize injury to the PIN[35] by not breaching the posterior cortex of the radius.

Endoscopically assisted procedures with anchors[36] as well as the Endobutton technique have been published.[37]

SENIOR AUTHOR'S SURGICAL TECHNIQUE

The senior author developed the Endobutton technique in 1994 and has since performed over 150 cases. The greater majority returned to full activities. However, we have had complications including hematoma, infection, PIN palsy, and fracture through the burr holes in the proximal radial neck. The PIN recovered spontaneously and the radial neck fracture healed with internal fixation and bone graft. We have seen cases of heterotopic bone, but these are insignificant. We have not had any major cases of heterotopic ossification and no cases of radioulnar synostosis.

Based on a number of concepts we have made some changes to our technique to optimize the anatomic restoration of the biceps footprint, and therefore flexion and supination mechanics, in a safe and reliable manner.

While the short head of the biceps tendon is a stronger supinator in most positions,[38] the long head may have a larger contribution to supination force in the fully supinated forearm.[39] We believe that this strength is important particularly in the power position required for heavy lifting; with the elbow at 90° of flexion and full supination. In this position the lacertus is tense that passively tightens the biceps tendon[5] and increases its strength. It is less important in the "precision" position with the hand and forearm in pronation when writing, for example. *The normal position of the footprint is a mean of 65° (range 15°–120° from the anterior apex of the radius) to the ulnar side.*[8] *Placing the repair anterior to the footprint does not restore the supination strength.*[40]

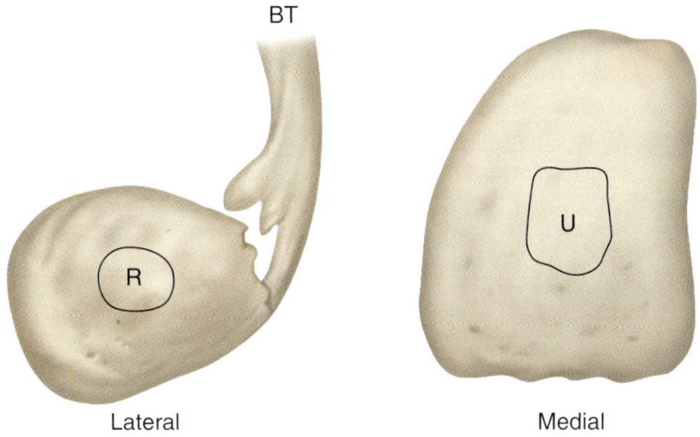

FIGURE 41A-6 Axial view of the left forearm with the arm in full supination. Note the ulnar position of the biceps tuberosity, making access with a drill difficult.

A single longitudinal anterior incision is made distal to the antecubital fossa. The dissection is continued through the deep fascia and the proximal portion of the torn tendon is retrieved. Two braided number 2 nonabsorbable sutures are anchored to the distal biceps tendon using a Bunnell stitch. This leaves 4 "trailing" sutures exiting the distal end of the tendon.

The radial tuberosity is exposed with blunt digital dissection using the tract of the biceps tendon, which is still obvious in the acute setting. The forearm is fully supinated and right angle retractors used to aid exposure.

To restore the biceps anatomically the tendon should not be attached to the radius from anterior to posterior, but more medial to lateral (as the radial tuberosity lies ulnar with the arm in full supination) (Fig. 41A-6).

However, it is technically difficult to access the ulna/posterior aspect of the radial tuberosity from a single anterior incision.

The author currently pronates the arm approximately 70° to place 2 drill holes from the radial cortex starting immediately *opposite* the tuberosity, and drilling toward and through the radial tuberosity. The drill is therefore aimed from anterolateral to posteromedial (Fig. 41A-7).

The sutures from the distal biceps tendon are passed through the holes in an anterograde fashion from tuberosity to opposite cortex using a suture passer. They are then threaded through the Endobutton, tensioned, and tied so that the button lies against the opposite cortex (Fig. 41A-8).

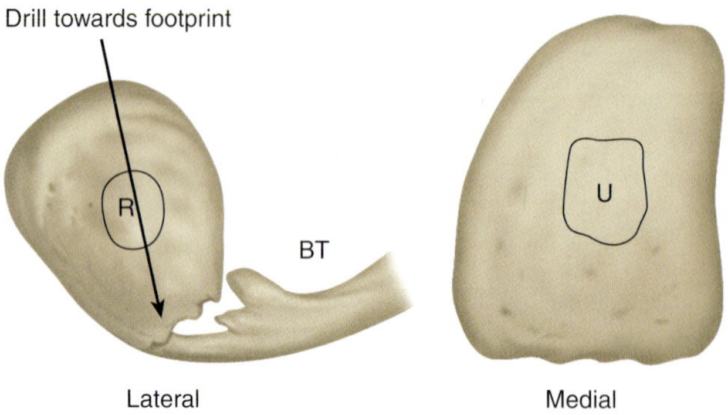

FIGURE 41A-7 Pronation of the arm 70° allows "retrograde" drilling toward the biceps insertion.

Postoperative rehabilitation consists of immediate range of motion with no resisted supination of flexion for 6 weeks.

This technique utilizes a single anterior incision and provides an anatomic footprint repair that is aimed to improve both supination and flexion strength. The drill is aimed away from the PIN[31] and the Endobutton is placed under direct vision, preventing entrapment of the PIN under the button (Fig. 41A-9). It minimizes the risk of synostosis and proximal radius fracture associated with the large burr holes.

Multiple studies have been performed assessing the biomechanical properties of these various repair techniques. Pullout strength of distal biceps tendon repairs using bone tunnels, suture anchors, Biotenodesis screws, and Endobuttons was evaluated.[41] The authors found an ultimate load of 232 N for suture anchors and up to 440 N for Endobuttons. None of the Endobuttons failed in cyclic testing. A systematic review assessing the biomechanical pullout strength and complication rates of distal biceps tendon repairs showed that the Endobutton technique had a superior pullout strength, and that the 2-incision technique for repair led to increased loss of forearm rotation compared with single anterior incision techniques.[42] The Endobutton withstood 2000 cycles at a mean of 166 N before failure.[43] Rose suggested immediate rehabilitation could be done with a maximum of 900-g weights.

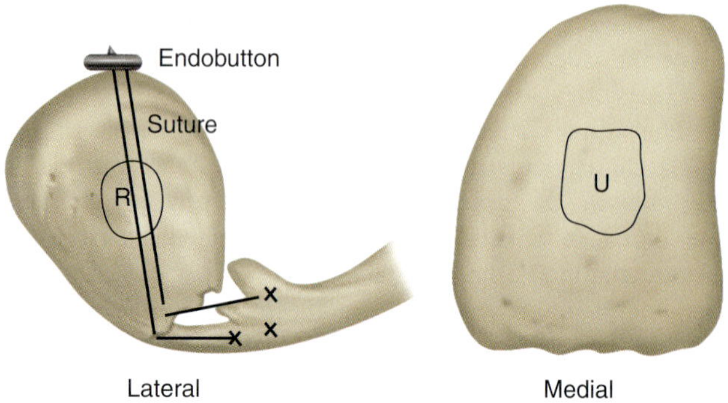

FIGURE 41A-8 Suture from distal biceps (Bunnell type) passed from radial tuberosity to opposite cortex and tied over Endobutton.

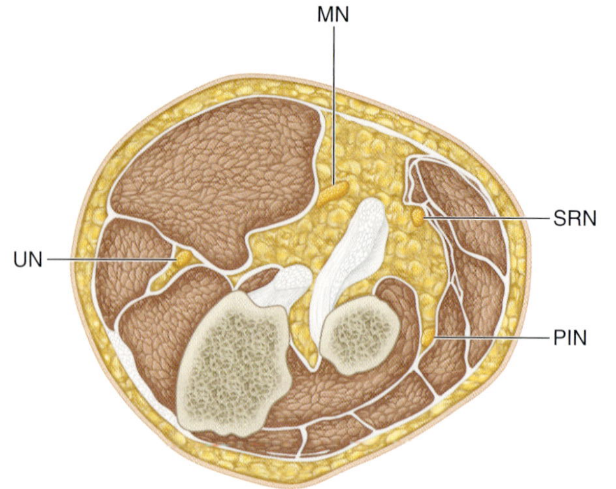

FIGURE 41A-9 Diagram showing the position of the major nerves in relation to the radial tuberosity. MN, median nerve; PIN, posterior interosseous nerve; SRN, superficial radial nerve; UN, ulnar nerve.

Operative Techniques—Chronic Biceps Tendon Rupture

The management of the chronic distal biceps tendon tear is an interesting problem. If the patient has a low demand or if there is a high surgical risk, nonoperative treatment should be offered (see Table 41A-2).

Surgery requires a more extensive approach and the surgeon needs to be competent in the exposure of the major neurovascular structures in the cubital fossa. The bursa to radial tuberosity will still be patent, even after some years, although the dissection is more difficult.

The retraction and mobility of the tendon will be quite variable. If the lacertus fibrosis is still intact, the tendon can usually be directly repaired, although it will be tight and there will be a fixed flexion deformity. The senior author releases the lacertus from the tendon, repairs the tendon to the tuberosity, and lastly repairs the lacertus. This ensures it does not deform the line of the tendon, and does not compress the median nerve and the brachial artery beneath the lacertus. It is our experience that even a 70° flexion deformity repaired with an Endobutton will correct over the period of about 1 month, with gentle active mobilization.

TABLE 41A-2: Treatment Options for Chronic Biceps Rupture

Treatment	Comment
Nonoperative	Persistent weakness and fatigue pain
Primary repair	Tendon mobilization and repair
Autograft reconstruction	Hamstring,[44] FCR,[45] donor-site morbidity
Allograft reconstruction	Achilles tendon,[49] fascia lata,[48] infection risk

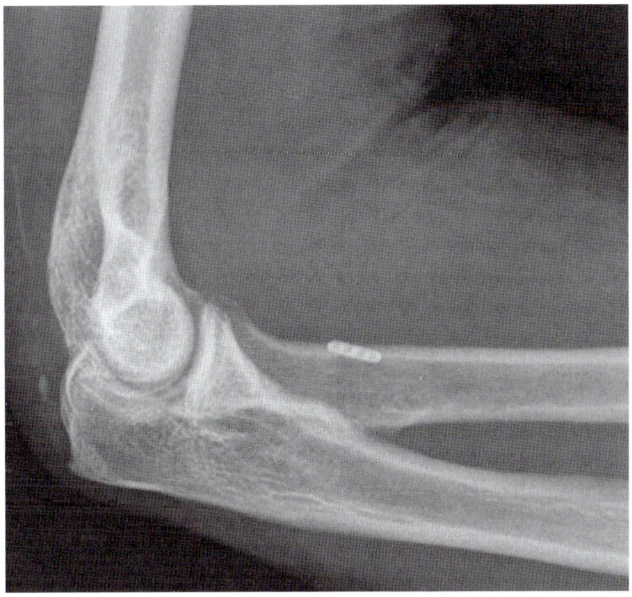

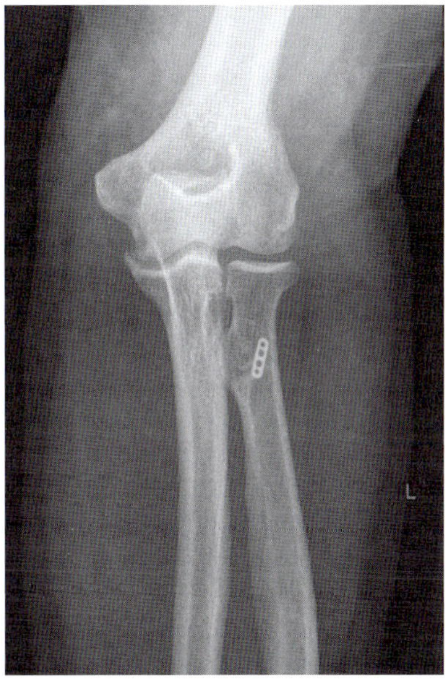

FIGURES 41A-10 and **41A-11** Postoperative radiographs of biceps repair. Note the Endobutton lies *opposite* the radial tuberosity.

If the lacertus is torn and the tendon retracts, primary repair may not be possible and a tendon graft may be required. The muscle is mobilized, using blunt dissection. The tendon is teased from the adjacent tissues, which can include unraveling the concertinaed tendon, releasing the tendon from a bursal cocoon, or releasing an invaginated tendon into the muscle substance. Factors that will direct us to a tendon graft include tendon retracted into the arm, a delay greater than 6 months since injury, a muscle tendon unit that cannot be delivered to the elbow skin crease, a tendon that is shorter than 5 cm, and failed previous surgery.

Tendon autograft such as from flexor carpi radialis[45] or semitendinosus[46] can be interwoven into the distal part of the retracted biceps muscle and distal tendon, and using any 1 of the aforementioned fixation techniques to repair it to the radial tuberosity (Figs. 41A-10 and 41A-11). The author's preferred technique is to use a hamstring tendon autograft with an Endobutton (Fig. 41A-12).

Allograft tendon has also been utilized with success.[47-49]

OUTCOMES

The outcome of surgical repair for distal biceps tendon rupture is good. The largest reported series of distal biceps tendon repairs using a single incision technique found that 96% were satisfied or very satisfied with the outcome of surgical repair at an average of 29 months after surgery.[30] The mean DASH score was no different from healthy controls, and the range of movement and strength of supination and flexion were comparable to the contralateral limb. Positive workers' compensation status adversely affected the DASH scores of the patients. In a series of 27 patients Dillon et al found the Endobutton gave return of 101% of flexion strength and 99% supination strength with no loss of motion. This group included patients with a chronic tear that was primarily repaired without tendon augmentation.[50] Peeters et al[51] reviewed 26 patients who had a mean of 16-month follow-up. There was a mean flexion strength of 80% and a supination strength of 91%.

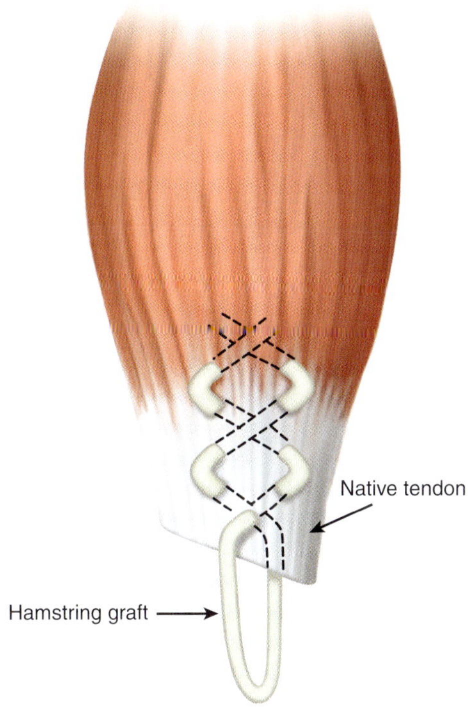

FIGURE 41A-12 Hamstring autograft woven through the distal biceps. (Reproduced with permission from Hallam and Bain.[44])

COMPLICATIONS

Reported complications include failure of repair, heterotopic ossification, radioulnar synostosis, nerve palsies, loss of motion, weakness, and arterial injury. Complication rates are higher for chronic injuries and revisions. The Boyd-Anderson approach had the highest rate of synostosis.

Nerve palsies are usually transient, and involve the lateral cutaneous nerve of the forearm, superficial branch of the radial nerve, and PIN. Rarely, the median nerve is involved.[36] Aggressive retraction can contribute.

Rarer complications include osteolysis in bioabsorbable screw fixation,[52] chronic regional pain syndrome, cold intolerance, and cramping.[50] In the series of Peeters et al, 3 had Endobuttons that did not abut the cortex. One had to be removed. They did not use x-rays intraoperatively.[51] We use this routinely and recommend it to check the position of the Endobutton.

REFERENCES

1. Ramsey ML. Distal biceps tendon injuries: diagnosis and management. *J Am Acad Orthop Surg.* 1999;7(3):199–207.
2. D'Alessandro DF, Shields CL Jr, Tibone JE, Chandler RW. Repair of distal biceps tendon ruptures in athletes. *Am J Sports Med.* 1993;21(1):114–119.
3. Safran MR, Graham SM. Distal biceps tendon ruptures: incidence, demographics, and the effect of smoking. *Clin Orthop Relat Res.* 2002;(404):275–283.
4. Visuri T, Lindholm H. Bilateral distal biceps tendon avulsions with use of anabolic steroids. *Med Sci Sports Exerc.* 1994;26(8):941–944.
5. Eames MH, Bain GI, Fogg QA, van Riet RP. Distal biceps tendon anatomy: a cadaveric study. *J Bone Joint Surg Am.* 2007;89(5):1044–1049.
6. Athwal GS, Steinmann SP, Rispoli DM. The distal biceps tendon: footprint and relevant clinical anatomy. *J Hand Surg Am.* 2007;32(8):1225–1229.
7. Siebenlist S, Lenich A, Buccholz A, et al. Biomechanical in vitro validation of intramedullary cortical button fixation for distal biceps tendon repair. *Am J Sports Med.* 2011;39(8):1762–1768.
8. Forthman CL, Zimmerman RM, Sullivan MJ, Gabel GT. Cross-sectional anatomy of the bicipital tuberosity and biceps brachii tendon insertion: relevance to anatomic tendon repair. *J Shoulder Elbow Surg.* 2008;17(3):522–526.
9. Davis WM, Yassine Z. An etiological factor in tear of the distal tendon of the biceps brachii; report of two cases. *J Bone Joint Surg Am.* 1956;38-A(6):1365–1368.
10. Morrey BF. Injury of the flexors of the elbow: biceps in tendon injury. In: Morrey BF, ed. *The Elbow and Its Disorders.* Philadelphia: WB Saunders; 2000:468–478.
11. Seiler JG 3rd, Parker LM, Chamberland PD, Sherbourne GM, Carpenter WA. The distal biceps tendon. Two potential mechanisms involved in its rupture: arterial supply and mechanical impingement. *J Shoulder Elbow Surg.* 1995;4(3):149–156.
12. Green JB, Skaife TL, Leslie BM. Bilateral distal biceps tendon ruptures. *J Hand Surg Am.* 2012;37(1):120–123.
13. Schamblin ML, Safran MR. Injury of the distal biceps at the musculotendinous junction. *J Shoulder Elbow Surg.* 2007;16(2):208–212.
14. Dellaero DT, Mallon WJ. Surgical treatment of partial biceps tendon ruptures at the elbow. *J Shoulder Elbow Surg.* 2006;15(2):215–217.
15. Baker BE, Bierwagen D. Rupture of the distal tendon of the biceps brachii. Operative versus non-operative treatment *J Bone Joint Surg Am.* 1985;67(414):7.
16. Freeman CR, McCormick KR, Mahoney D, Baratz M, Lubahn JD. Nonoperative treatment of distal biceps tendon ruptures compared with a historical control group. *J Bone Joint Surg Am.* 2009;91(10):2329–2334.
17. Abboud JA, Ricchetti ET, Tjoumakaris FP, Bartolozzi AR, Hsu JE. The direct radial tuberosity compression test: a sensitive method for diagnosing partial distal biceps tendon ruptures. *Curr Orthop Pract.* 2011;22(1):76.
18. Ruland RT, Dunbar RP, Bowen JD. The biceps squeeze test for diagnosis of distal biceps tendon ruptures. *Clin Orthop Relat Res.* 2005;(437):128–131.
19. O'Driscoll SW, Goncalves LB, Dietz P. The hook test for distal biceps tendon avulsion. *Am J Sports Med.* 2007;35(11):1865–1869.
20. Chew ML, Giuffre BM. Disorders of the distal biceps brachii tendon. *Radiographics.* 2005;25(5):1227–1237.
21. Smith J, Finnoff JT, O'Driscoll SW, Lai JK. Sonographic evaluation of the distal biceps tendon using a medial approach. *J Ultrasound Med.* 2010;29(5):861–865.
22. Giuffre BM, Moss MJ. Optimal positioning for MRI of the distal biceps brachii tendon: flexed abducted supinated view. *AJR Am J Roentgenol.* 2004;182(4):944–946.
23. Festa A, Mulieri PJ, Newman JS, Spitz DJ, Leslie BM. Effectiveness of magnetic resonance imaging in detecting partial and complete distal biceps tendon rupture. *J Hand Surg Am.* 2010;35(1):77–83.
24. Eames MH, Bain GI. Distal biceps tendon endoscopy and anterior elbow arthroscopy portal. *Tech Shoulder Elbow Surg.* 2006;7(3):139–142.
25. Durr HR, Stabler A, Pfahler M, Matzko M, Refior HJ. Partial rupture of the distal biceps tendon. *Clin Orthop Relat Res.* 2000;(374):195–200.
26. Bourne MH, Morrey BF. Partial rupture of the distal biceps tendon. *Clin Orthop Relat Res.* 1991;(271):143–148.
27. Vardakas DG, Musgrave DS, Varitimidis SE, Goebel F, Sotereanos DG. Partial rupture of the distal biceps tendon. *J Shoulder Elbow Surg.* 2001;10(4):377–379.
28. Mazzocca AD, Spang JT, Arciero RA. Distal biceps rupture. *Orthop Clin North Am.* 2008;39(2):237–249, vii.
29. Barnes S, Coleman S, Gilpin D. Repair of avulsed insertion of biceps. A new technique in four cases. *J Bone Joint Surg Br.* 1993;75-B(6):938–939.
30. McKee MD, Hirji R, Schemitsch EH, Wild LM, Waddell JP. Patient-oriented functional outcome after repair of distal biceps tendon ruptures using a single-incision technique. *J Shoulder Elbow Surg.* 2005;14(3):302–306.
31. Bain GI, Prem H, Heptinstall RJ, Verhellen R, Paix D. Repair of distal biceps tendon rupture: a new technique using the Endobutton. *J Shoulder Elbow Surg.* 2000;9(2):120–126.
32. Greenberg JA. Endobutton repair of distal biceps tendon ruptures. *J Hand Surg Am.* 2009;34(8):1541–1548.
33. John CK, Field LD, Weiss KS, Savoie FH 3rd. Single-incision repair of acute distal biceps ruptures by use of suture anchors. *J Shoulder Elbow Surg.* 2007;16(1):78–83.
34. Heinzelmann AD, Savoie FH, Ramsay JR, Field LD, Mazzocca AD. A combined technique for distal biceps repair using a soft tissue button and biotenodesis interference screw. *Am J Sports Med.* 2009;37(5):989–994.
35. Arbuthnot JE, Deans VM, Morgan D, Colville J, Sloan R, Selvey DM. The intramedullary Endobutton® technique: the outcome of repair of acute distal biceps rupture. *Eur J Orthop Surg Traumatol.* 2009;19(3):155–157.
36. Grégory T, Roure P, Fontès D. Repair of distal biceps tendon rupture using a suture anchor. *Am J Sports Med.* 2009;37(3):506–511.
37. Sharma S, MacKay G. Endoscopic repair of distal biceps tendon using an endobutton. *Arthroscopy.* 2005;21(7):897.e891–897.e894.
38. Jarrett CD, Weir DM, Stuffmann ES, Jain S, Miller MC, Schmidt CC. Anatomic and biomechanical analysis of the short and long head components of the distal biceps tendon. *J Shoulder Elbow Surg.* 2012;21:942–948.
39. Prud'homme-Foster M, Louati H, Parai M, Dervin G. *Evaluation of the Long and Short Heads of the Distal Biceps Contribution to Elbow Flexion Strength and Forearm Supination Strength.* AHSS. 2011.
40. Schmidt CC, Weir DM, Wong AS, Howard M, Miller MC. The effect of biceps reattachment site. *J Shoulder Elbow Surg.* 2010;19(8):1157–1165.
41. Mazzocca AD, Burton KJ, Romeo AA, Santangelo S, Adams DA, Arciero RA. Biomechanical evaluation of 4 techniques of distal biceps brachii tendon repair. *Am J Sports Med.* 2007;35(2):252–258.
42. Chavan PR, Duquin TR, Bisson LJ. Repair of the ruptured distal biceps tendon: a systematic review. *Am J Sports Med.* 2008;36(8):1618–1624.
43. Rose DM, Archibald JD, Sutter EG, Belkoff SM, Wilckens JH. Biomechanical analysis suggests early rehabilitation is possible after single-incision EndoButton distal biceps repair with FiberWire. *Knee Surg Sports Traumatol Arthrosc.* 2011;19:1019–1022.

44. Hallam P, Bain GI. Repair of chronic distal biceps tendon ruptures using autologous hamstring graft and the Endobutton. *J Shoulder Elbow Surg*. 2004;13(6):648–651.
45. Levy HJ, Mashoof AA, Morgan D. Repair of chronic ruptures of the distal biceps tendon using flexor carpi radialis tendon graft. *Am J Sports Med*. 2000;28(4):538–540.
46. Wiley WB, Noble JS, Dulaney TD, Bell RH, Noble DD. Late reconstruction of chronic distal biceps tendon ruptures with a semitendinosus autograft technique. *J Shoulder Elbow Surg*. 2006;15(4):440–444.
47. Darlis NA, Sotereanos DG. Distal biceps tendon reconstruction in chronic ruptures. *J Shoulder Elbow Surg*. 2006;15(5):614–619.
48. Kaplan FTD, Rokito AS, Birdzell MG, Zuckerman JD. Reconstruction of chronic distal biceps tendon rupture with use of fascia lata combined with a ligament augmentation device: a report of 3 cases. *J Shoulder Elbow Surg*. 2002;11(6):633–636.
49. Sanchez-Sotelo J, Morrey BF, Adams RA, O'Driscoll SW. Reconstruction of chronic ruptures of the distal biceps tendon with use of an Achilles tendon allograft. *J Bone Joint Surg Am*. 2002;84-A(6):999–1005.
50. Dillon MT, Bollier MJ, King JC. Repair of acute and chronic distal biceps tendon ruptures using the EndoButton. *Hand (N Y)*. 2011;6(1): 39–46.
51. Peeters T, Ching-Soon NG, Jansen N, Sneyers C, Declerg G, Verstreken F. Functional outcome after repair of distal biceps tendon ruptures using the endobutton technique. *J Shoulder Elbow Surg*. 2009;18(2): 283–287.
52. Potapov A, Laflamme YG, Gagnon S, Canet F, Rouleau DM. Progressive osteolysis of the radius after distal biceps tendon repair with the bioabsorbable screw. *J Shoulder Elbow Surg*. 2011;20(5):819–826.

41B

Tendon Repairs About the Elbow—Part B: Triceps Tendon Rupture

Morne Scheepers, MD
Kevin Eng, MBBS, FRACS
Gregory I. Bain, MBBS, FRACS, FA(Ortho) A, PhD

RATIONALE AND BASIC SCIENCE

Introduction

Distal triceps tendon ruptures are rare. They account for less than 1% of all tendon injuries.[1] Due to the low incidence few clinical trials have been published, and the literature consists largely of case series.

Distal triceps tendon ruptures have a more even prevalence between genders when compared with biceps ruptures; however, males are still more commonly affected with a ratio of 3:2. The mean age is 33 years (range from 7 to 80 years).[2] Three major etiological groups have been reported: acute traumatic failure of a normal tendon due to excessive loads such as those encountered in body building[3] and American Football[4]; second, a pathological group where the tendon-bone interface is weakened; lastly, an iatrogenic group, largely after elbow arthroplasty.

Background/Etiology

ANATOMY

The triceps has 3 heads. The long head arises from the infraglenoid tubercle. The lateral head arises from the posterior surface of the humerus from a linear origin extending from the surgical neck to the deltoid origin, and lies lateral to the long head. These 2 heads converge distally to form a fused flat tendon that inserts into the posterior part of the proximal end of the olecranon. The medial head originates medial to the radial groove and the lateral head. The origin then widens to include the posterior surface of the humerus as it runs distally, including each intermuscular septum. It lies *deep* to the long and lateral heads. A fourth head of the triceps muscle has also been described in rare cases.[5]

The long and lateral heads give rise to a conjoined superficial tendon that inserts onto the olecranon. The superficial fibers continue as the triceps expand and insert into the posterior crest of the ulna medially and the fascia of the extensor carpi ulnaris laterally. The deeper medial head remains muscular more distally until close to the insertion where it gives rise to a deep separate tendon that inserts in part to the olecranon, in part to the flattened fused tendon of the long and lateral heads, and in part to the posterior aspect of the elbow joint capsule, preventing impingement of the capsule on extension of the elbow. The mean tendon width is 30.56 mm.[6]

The bony footprint on the olecranon has a flat distal insertion, whereas the proximal aspect is dome shaped (Fig. 41B-1). It is 20.9 mm wide and 13.4 mm long and the proximal border is 14.8 mm from the olecranon tip.[7]

PATHOPHYSIOLOGY

The most common site of triceps tears is at the insertion of the tendon with or without a bony avulsion (Fig. 41B-2). It is rare for the tendon to tear at the musculotendinous junction[9] or within the muscle belly.[10] The patient may also have associated fractures of the radial head[11] or distal radius.[12]

Distal triceps tendon ruptures can be categorized into 3 etiological groups. The *acute* traumatic group incorporates healthy individuals (typically athletes) with normal tissues in whom the cause is a single episode of trauma. This typically occurs during a large eccentric contraction. The sudden deceleration causes the triceps muscle to avulse its distal attachment from the olecranon of the ulna, occasionally taking a small piece of bone with it.[13]

The second *pathological* group has preexisting pathology weakening the tendon or the bone. The tendon can commonly be damaged following local steroid injection,[14] anabolic steroids,[15] or infection. The bone may be weakened by hyperparathyroidism,[16] renal osteodystrophy,[17] or osteogenesis imperfecta.[18] In these patients the forces causing rupture may be within normal physiological limits.

The third is the *iatrogenic* group in whom the triceps tendon has failed following surgical mobilization. This has

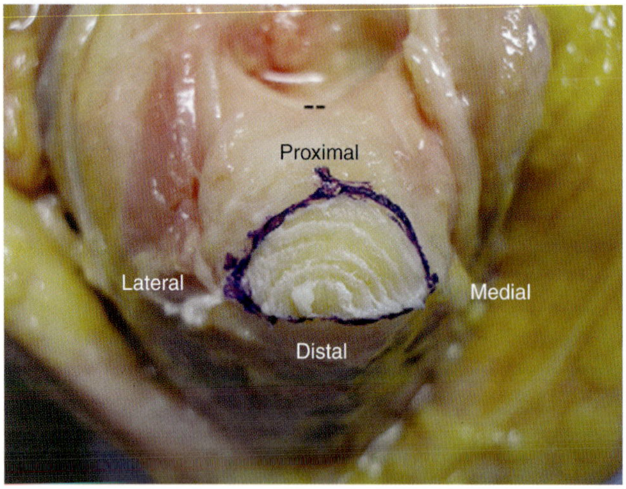

FIGURE 41B-1 Footprint of the triceps tendon insertion on a cadaveric olecranon. The border of the triceps tendon insertion has been highlighted showing the dome-shaped appearance. (Reproduced with permission from Keener et al.[7] Copyright Elsevier.)

been reported in 2% to 11% of cases following total elbow arthroplasty.[19–21]

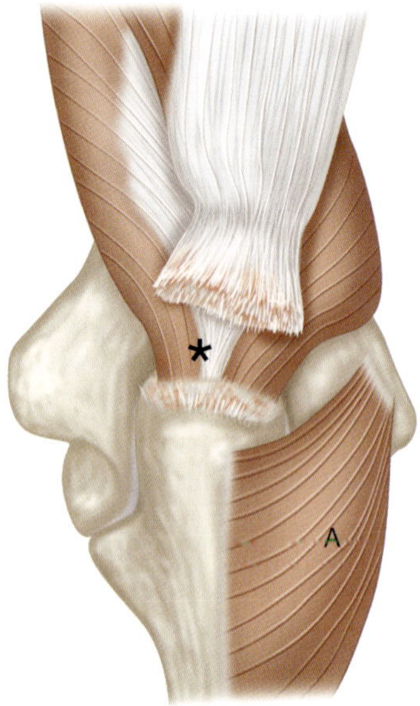

FIGURE 41B-2 3D reconstruction of the posterior aspect of the elbow demonstrating a complete tear of the conjoined long and lateral part of the tendon that is retracted to reveal an intact medial head insertion (*). The anconeus (A) is also demonstrated. (Courtesy Dr. Michael Stadnick.)

Presentation, Investigation, and Treatment Options

Since rupture may be partial or complete and may coexist with other injuries, its diagnosis is frequently missed.[22]

HISTORY

For acute injuries the typical history is of a fall onto an outstretched hand, often during sports. The patient may describe an extending elbow that has been forced into flexion during the fall. The patient will complain of pain and swelling at the insertion site of the triceps. Direct trauma to the extensor surface of the arm has also been reported, although this is much less common.

In the pathological group the patient is likely to have had prodromal symptoms of elbow pain and may have sought treatment for this prior to tendon rupture. The mechanism is low energy.

The iatrogenic group will present following a procedure that required mobilization of the extensor mechanism and will not typically report an acute trauma. These patients may not be aware of their triceps weakness in the postoperative period because they utilize gravity-assisted extension.

All groups will have functional limitations such as altered ability to push up from a chair or transfer from bed. Overhead activities may also be affected.

EXAMINATION

Examination will reveal swelling and tenderness over the triceps insertion. A palpable defect may be felt. The patient will exhibit weakness of elbow extension; however, in some patients there can be a functional strength due to an intact triceps expansion. It is important to assess extension by the examiner holding the arm extended overhead, and release it and ask the patient to actively extend their elbow against gravity and then against the examiner's power. It should then be compared with the opposite limb. In chronic distal triceps rupture extensor lag of up to 30° may be present.

IMAGING

Plain radiographs should be performed to exclude avulsion fracture of the olecranon that is suggestive of a tendon rupture. While ultrasound can identify partial and complete ruptures,[23] magnetic resonance imaging (MRI) is the authors' preferred investigation. It can distinguish between partial- and full-thickness tears and demonstrate retraction (Fig. 41B-3), which may aid operative planning.[24]

Natural History of Triceps Tendon Rupture

Full-thickness ruptures will perform poorly with nonoperative management.[25] The triceps muscle is the major elbow extensor (anconeus provides only minimal extension), and loss may lead to extension weakness.[26]

INDICATIONS FOR SURGERY

The main indication for surgery is a full-thickness tear with weakness that adversely affects the patient's functional level. The authors recommend surgery unless there is high risk

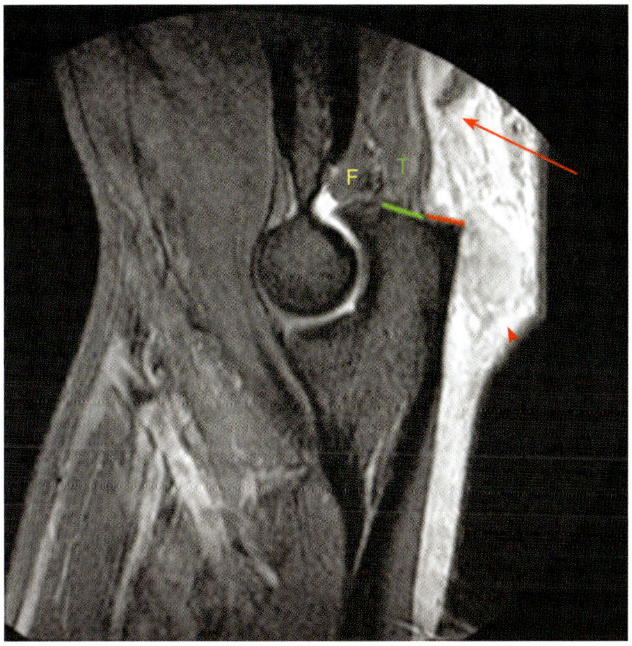

FIGURE 41B-3 MRI scan of posterior component of the distal triceps tendon that is completely avulsed and retracted (red arrow). The anterior or deep component of the distal triceps remains intact (T). Note the exposed surface of the olecranon from which the posterior component has been avulsed (red line) and the remaining intact attachment of the primarily muscular anterior component (green line). The posterior fat pad (F) is also identified (red arrowhead) and is found posterior to the olecranon. (Reproduced with permission from Bodor.[8])

of complications or low demand for functional triceps use. It is important to assess the stage of injury when deciding what type of surgical intervention is indicated (Table 41B-1). Acute ruptures are classified as injuries that occurred *less than 3 weeks prior*. Early surgical repair constantly provides good functional outcomes.[22]

Partial tears of the distal triceps tendon may be treated nonoperatively. A study of National Football League players reported good outcomes in 6 patients treated nonoperatively for partial tendon rupture.[4] These authors recommend nonoperative treatment if the tear involves up to 75% of the triceps tendon.

TABLE 41B-1: Overview of Management for Triceps Tendon Ruptures

Type of Tear	Recommended Management
Full-thickness tear	
Acute	Surgical repair
Chronic	Surgical repair or reconstruction
Iatrogenic	Surgical repair or reconstruction
Pathological	Surgical reconstruction
Partial-thickness tear	
Acute	Conservative management
Chronic	Conservative management

SURGICAL TECHNIQUE

Surgical Techniques—Acute Full-thickness Ruptures (Repair)

The patient is placed in a lateral position with the affected arm placed over a bolster. A midline incision and direct posterior approach is used to dissect down to the triceps muscle. The tendon and footprint are debrided. The tendon may be found to be retracted into the muscle belly. The tendon is extracted and a heavy nonabsorbable suture such as 5 Ethibond or FiberWire is passed through the proximal portion of the tendon with a grasping suture (eg, a Krakow suture). Two transverse holes are drilled in the olecranon, and the suture is passed through and tied pulling the end of the tendon down and affixing it to the olecranon (Fig. 41B-4). The senior author uses tensionable rotator cuff anchors. These allow solid fixation with correct tensioning. Others have utilized “transosseus-equivalent” double-row constructs that accurately restore the triceps “footprint” and have reported good biomechanical results[6] (see Fig. 41B-5).

If there is an avulsion fracture attached to the tendon, it may be possible to augment the repair with internal fixation of the avulsion fracture with a screw and washer. This repair technique is effective if the injury is treated early (within 3 weeks).[25]

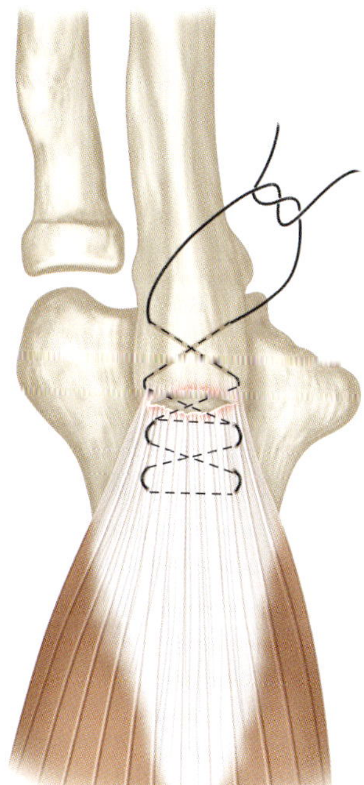

FIGURE 41B-4 Demonstration of triceps tendon fixation to the olecranon via a suture passed through 2 transverse holes drilled in the olecranon. (Reproduced with permission from van Riet et al.[25])

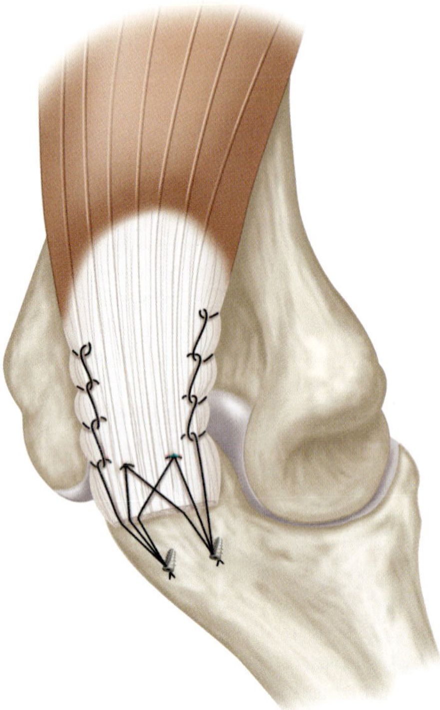

FIGURE 41B-5 Illustration of triceps repair using double-row constructs. (Reproduced with permission from Yeh et al.[6] Copyright Sage Publications.)

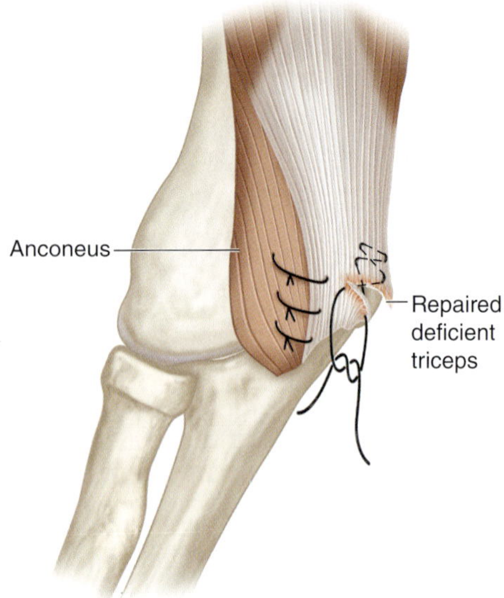

FIGURE 41B-6 Chronic full-thickness tear repair involving suture of the retracted triceps tendon to the anconeus muscle.

Surgical Techniques—Chronic Full-thickness Tears (Reconstruction)

If operative treatment is delayed, retraction of the tendon into the muscle belly and subsequent scarring can make this a difficult entity to treat operatively. The same posterior approach is used, and the extent of retraction is assessed. The ruptured tendon is mobilized distally. If primary repair can be performed, this is preferable.

If the retraction is moderate, an anconeus slide may be performed. The distal portion of the anconeus is detached and reattached to the olecranon. The retracted triceps tendon is sutured to the medial border of the proximal portion of anconeus, effectively using anconeus as an augmentation to bridge the deficient length of triceps (Fig. 41B-6).

More severe deficiencies of the triceps tendon may not be easily augmented with an anconeus slide. Tendon augmentation is used in this situation and is interwoven through the proximal portion of the ruptured triceps tendon (Fig. 41B-7). This is fixed to the olecranon, bridging the gap between the torn tendon and the olecranon. The senior author's preference is to use a gracilis tendon autograft weaved in a Bunnell-type pattern and fixed through oblique drill holes in the ulna.

An alternative technique is to use an Achilles tendon allograft, with a small piece of calcaneum still attached. The piece of calcaneum is trimmed and internally fixed to the proximal tip of the olecranon with a screw. The elbow is flexed to 20° to 30° and the triceps muscle is mobilized distally as far as possible. The Achilles tendon is then sutured to the triceps tendon, augmenting it for the deficient length. The strength of this repair can be further improved by pulling the Achilles fascia proximally and suturing it to the medial and lateral margins of the triceps muscle belly.[27]

Arthroscopic Repair

An arthroscopic technique for repair of isolated avulsions of the medial head of the triceps tendon has been described by Athwal et al.[28] For this procedure the patient is placed in the lateral decubitus position with the elbow flexed over a bolster. A posterior central portal is made to visualize the olecranon fossa. The arthroscope is then placed through a proximal posterolateral port with the resector inserted via a posterocentral port (Fig. 41B-8). The posterior capsular insertion on the olecranon is excised that allows the medial head of the triceps tendon to be identified superiorly. The free head of the tendon is mobilized and debrided, and a ratcheted grasper placed through a distal posterolateral working port and used to grasp the free tendon head and assess mobility with a trial reduction. Two double-loaded 5-mm metallic suture anchors are placed into the insertional footprint on the olecranon (Figs. 41B-9 and 41B-10). A suture shuttle is then passed percutaneously through an 18-gauge spinal needle to pass the sutures through the intact portion of the triceps and the reduced medial head of tendon. This step is repeated to pass all limbs of the double-loaded anchors, creating a horizontal mattress stitch on the subcutaneous border of the triceps. Finally the sutures are tied to reduce the tear to its footprint (Fig. 41B-11).

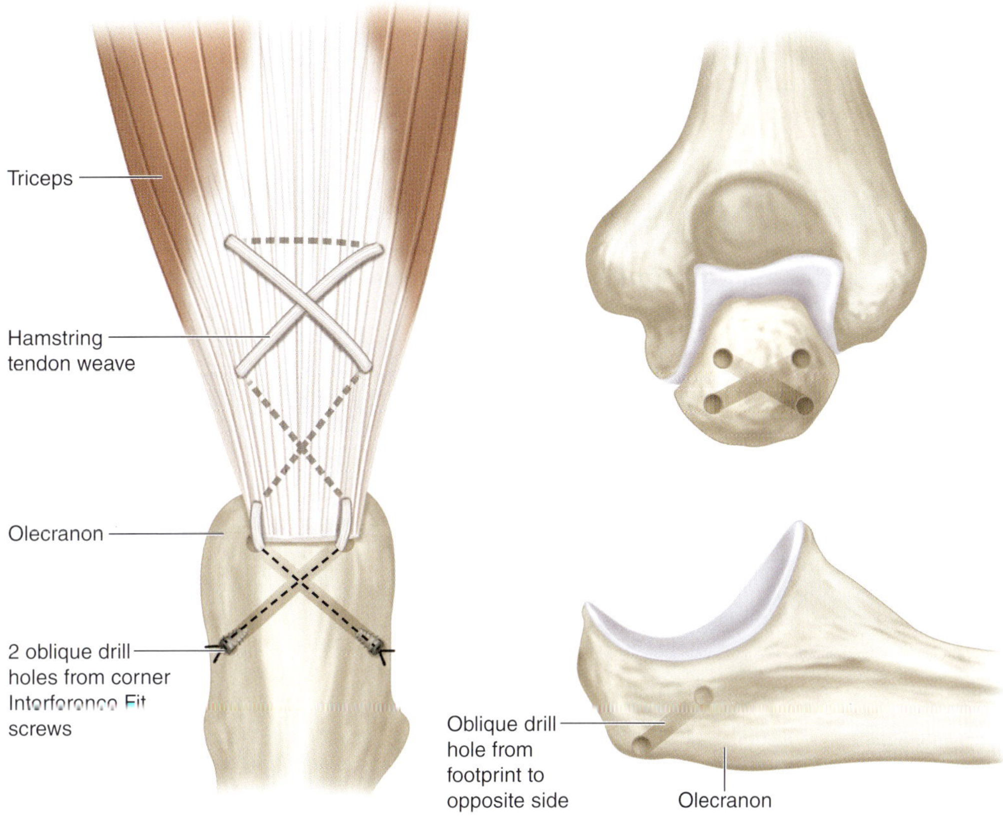

FIGURE 41B-7 Hamstring tendon augmentation for chronic triceps tendon repair.

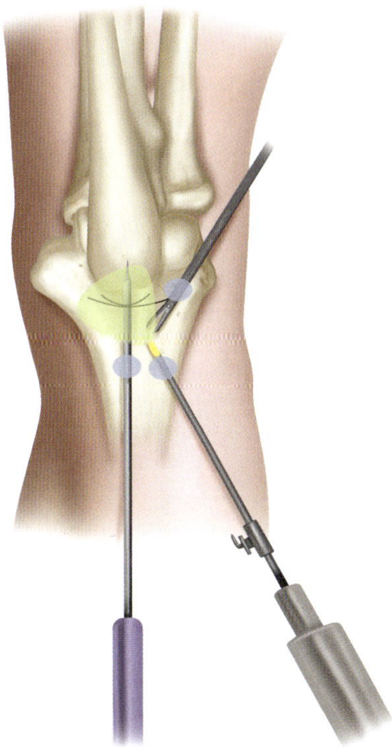

FIGURE 41B-8 Illustration of port placement for arthroscopic repair of ruptured triceps tendon. (Reproduced with permission from Athwal et al.[28] Copyright Elsevier.)

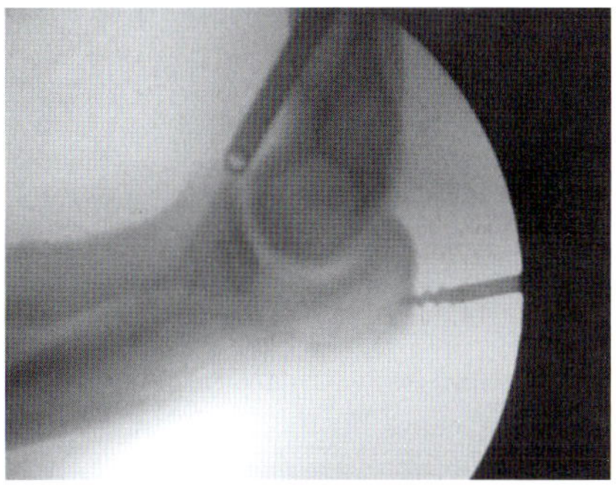

FIGURE 41B-9 Image intensifier showing the anchor placement. (Reproduced with permission from Athwal et al.[28] Copyright Elsevier.)

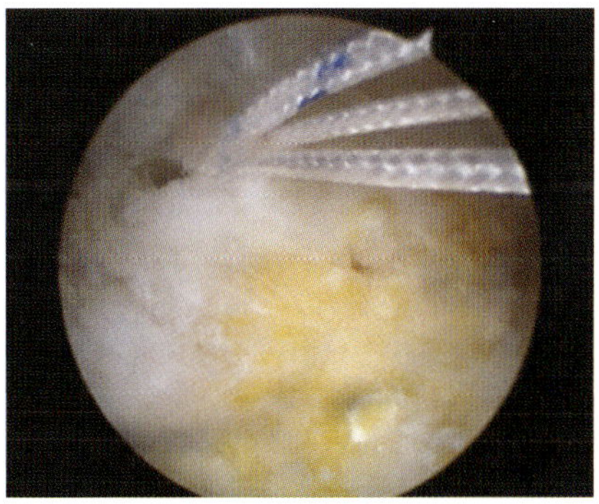

FIGURE 41B-10 The debrided footprint and anchor. (Reproduced with permission from Athwal et al.[28] Copyright Elsevier.)

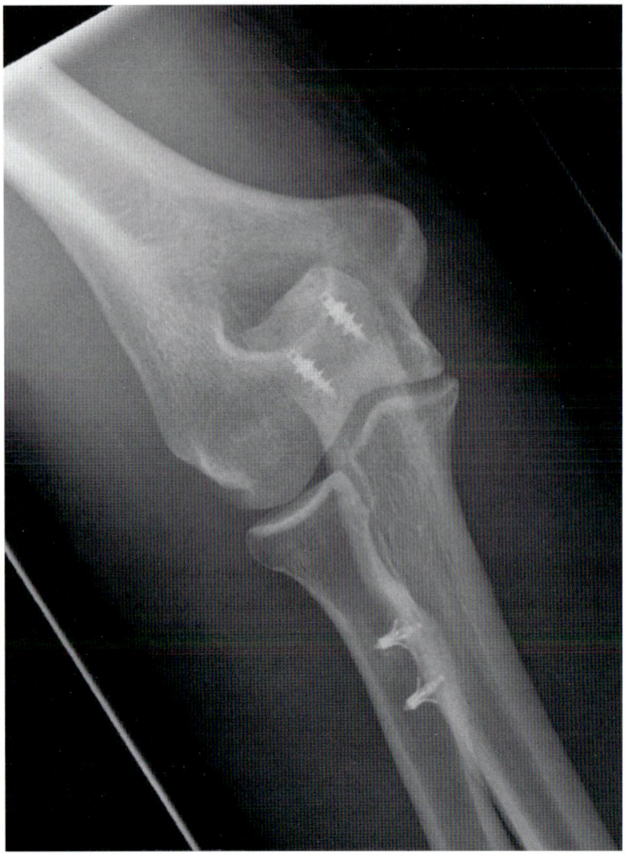

FIGURE 41B-11 X-ray showing the final anchor position in a patient who also had a bicep tendon repair. (Reproduced with permission from Athwal et al.[28] Copyright Elsevier.)

REHABILITATION AND OUTCOMES

There is no clear consensus on rehabilitation following operative treatment of distal triceps repair or reconstruction. Comparison of early mobilization, cast immobilization, and mobilization in a hinged brace found no significant effect of the rehabilitation regime on retear rates.[25] The quality of tendon and bone, and the strength of the repair and reconstruction are factors to consider. The authors favor immobilization in extension for 4 weeks with resisted extension introduced after 3 months.

There are few large studies on triceps tendon repairs. The outcome of surgical intervention depends on the etiology. Acute traumatic injuries have a favorable outcome. Mair et al identified 21 partial and complete triceps tendon ruptures in 19 professional football players in the United States.[4] Seven players had prodromal symptoms prior to injury, and 5 had received a cortisone injection. Eleven players with complete tears underwent surgical repair. Of the 10 players with partial tears, 6 healed without surgery. One patient completed the tear and required surgery. Three had residual pain and weakness and underwent surgical repair in the post season. Except for 1 patient, all of the players were able to return to play. van Riet et al reviewed the results of 23 tendon repairs. Thirteen patients returned for examination and 6 responded to a phone questionnaire.[25] Eight patients had a complete rupture, whereas 15 were partial tears. There were 14 primary repairs (with 3 reruptures) and 9 reconstructive procedures. At an average follow-up of 93 months (range, 7-264 months), elbow motion averaged 10° to 136°. Triceps strength was noted to be 4/5 or 5/5 in the 13 patients who were examined. Isokinetic testing of 10 patients showed that average peak strength was 82% of that of the untreated extremity. The results after repair and reconstruction were comparable, but the patients' recovery was slower after reconstruction. Bava et al reviewed 5 patients with a mean age of 47 years (range, 35-54 years) who underwent a suture anchor repair following a traumatic tendon rupture.[29] At a mean follow-up of 32 months the mean DASH score was 1.4, the mean American Shoulder and Elbow Surgeons elbow score was 99.2, the mean Mayo Elbow Performance Index was 95.8, the mean Oxford Elbow Score for pain was 98.8, the mean Oxford Elbow Score for function was 100, and the mean Oxford Elbow Score for the social domain was 96.2.

Celli et al reviewed the charts of 14 patients (16 elbow arthroplasties) with a mean age of 54 years, who required reconstruction for a triceps tendon insufficiency following a total elbow arthroplasty.[21] The procedures included direct suture in 7 elbows, anconeus rotation in 4, and an Achilles tendon allograft in 4. At a mean follow-up of 67 months, 15/16 could extend against gravity. Eleven patients had an excellent outcome, 3 had a good outcome, and 2 were classified as failures using the Mayo Elbow Performance Score.

SNAPPING TRICEPS SYNDROME

Rationale and Basic Science

INTRODUCTION

Another relatively rare condition that can affect the elbow is snapping triceps syndrome. This is a dynamic condition where the distal tendon of the triceps muscle dislocates (or "snaps") over the medial epicondyle of the elbow during flexion, or extension from a flexed position.

Individuals with snapping triceps experience localized tenderness and a snapping sensation over the medial aspect of the elbow. The condition usually coexists with ulnar nerve instability. The patient will often present with cubital tunnel syndrome in addition to the localized elbow symptoms.

ANATOMY AND PREDISPOSING FACTORS

In snapping triceps the position of the musculotendinous junction of the medial triceps head is of particular interest. The more distal the musculotendinous transition, the smaller the distance between the medial epicondyle and the medial edge of the triceps tendon, meaning the tendon can more easily pass over the medial epicondyle and dislocate.[30]

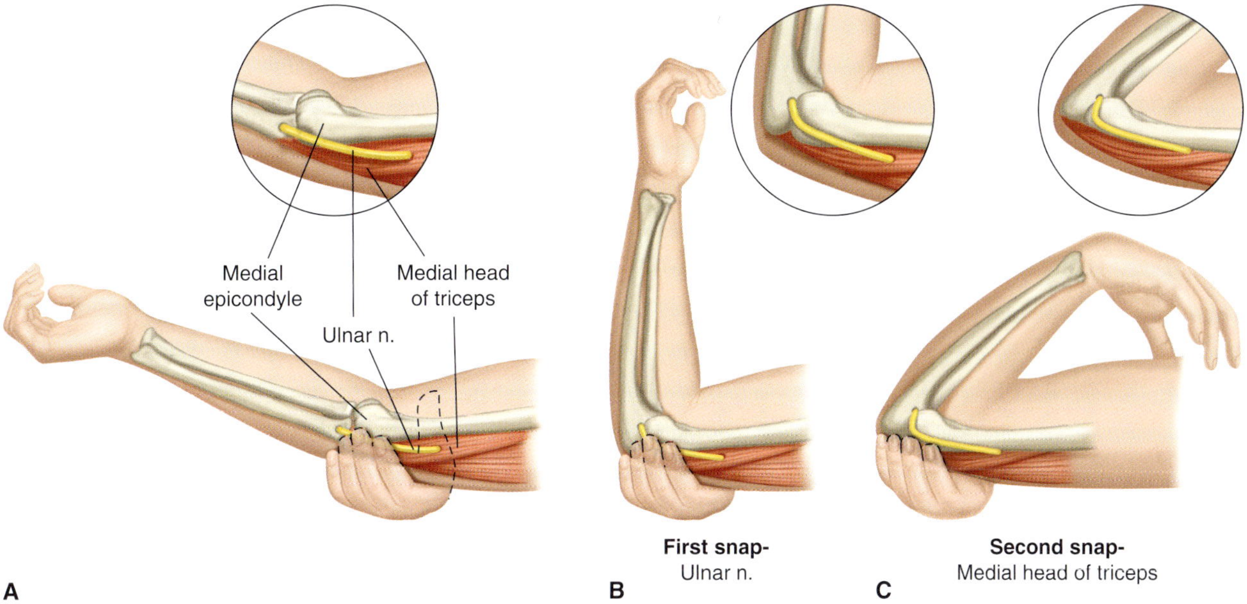

FIGURE 41B-12 **A.** Ulnar nerve and medial triceps head posterior to the medial epicondyle with the arm fully extended. **B.** At 70° to 90° the ulnar nerve dislocates. **C.** At approximately 115° the medial head dislocates. (Reproduced with permission from Spinner and Goldner.[33] Copyright Wolters Kluwer Health.)

A distal musculotendinous junction along with other structural features such as varus malalignment of the humerus,[31] hypoplasia of the medial epicondyle, and hypertrophy of the distal triceps muscle belly has also been implicated as a causative factor for snapping triceps.[32]

When the elbow is flexed, the distal triceps tendon is compressed against distal humerus that causes the tendon to flatten out.[30] Instead of the tendon sliding lateral to the epicondyle, this flattening out combined with the predisposing factors described previously allows the tendon to dislocate over the medial epicondyle.

PRESENTATION AND INVESTIGATION

Patients have pain over the medial aspect of the elbow that is accompanied by snapping and ulnar nerve paresthesia. Because snapping triceps usually coexists with ulnar nerve dislocation, patients may experience 2 separate palpable and audible snaps. The ulnar nerve is the first to dislocate at approximately 70° to 90° of elbow flexion followed by snapping of the triceps tendon at approximately 115° (Fig. 41B-12).[33] The symptoms are exacerbated during activities such as push-ups that require resisted elbow flexion or extension from a flexed position.

Examination may reveal 2 distinct snaps as described earlier with pain over medial elbow on palpation.[33] A case series publication of 17 patients (22 elbows) with snapping triceps found that snapping triceps and concurrent ulnar nerve dislocation were present in all 22 elbows.[34]

When the condition is suspected clinically, MRI performed with the elbow fully extended and fully flexed or dynamic ultrasonography may show the snapping structures.[35] The authors recommend using an experienced sonographer as the condition is rare.

Management and Indications for Surgery

The initial step in addressing this syndrome is conservative management that includes advice to avoid aggravating activities in addition to the use of nonsteroidal anti-inflammatory medications, physiotherapy, and splinting of the elbow.[30] If symptoms persist after a 3- to 6-month trial of nonoperative therapy, surgical intervention is indicated.

Surgical Treatment

Surgical intervention gives the opportunity to address the related problems of snapping triceps and ulnar nerve dislocation. The snapping triceps can be addressed via 2 methods. The most common method is to resect the portion of the triceps tendon that dislocates over the epicondyle. If the offending area is too large and will compromise the triceps, the medial tendon is partially detached from its insertion on the olecranon and transposed laterally to the central tendon.[33] The ulnar nerve can also be transposed anteriorly if clinically indicated.

Outcomes

There are only isolated case reports on the surgical treatment of this condition; hence, no meaningful conclusions can be made.

REFERENCES

1. Anzel SH, Covey KW, Weiner AD, Lipscomb PR. Disruption of muscles and tendons; an analysis of 1, 014 cases. *Surgery*. 1959;45(3):406–414.
2. Viegas SF. Avulsion of the triceps tendon. *Orthop Rev*. 1990;19(6):533–536.
3. Sherman OH, Snyder SJ, Fox JM. Triceps tendon avulsion in a professional body builder. A case report. *Am J Sports Med*. 1984;12(4):328–329.
4. Mair SD, Isbell WM, Gill TJ, Schlegel TF, Hawkins RJ. Triceps tendon ruptures in professional football players. *Am J Sports Med*. 2004;32(2):431–434.
5. Tubbs RS, Salter EG, Oakes WJ. Triceps brachii muscle demonstrating a fourth head. *Clin Anat*. 2006;19(7):657–660.
6. Yeh PC, Stephens KT, Solovyova O, et al. The distal triceps tendon footprint and a biomechanical analysis of 3 repair techniques. *Am J Sports Med*. 2010;38(5):1025.
7. Keener JD, Chafik D, Kim HM, Galatz LM, Yamaguchi K. Insertional anatomy of the triceps brachii tendon. *J Shoulder Elbow Surg*. 2010;19(3):399–405.
8. Bodor D. Distal triceps injuries. <www.radsource.us>. MRI Web Clinic; March 2010.
9. Bach BR Jr, Warren RF, Wickiewicz TL. Triceps rupture. A case report and literature review. *Am J Sports Med*. 1987;15(3):285–289.
10. Aso K, Torisu T. Muscle belly tear of the triceps. *Am J Sports Med*. 1984;12(6):485–487.
11. Levy M, Goldberg I, Meir I. Fracture of the head of the radius with a tear or avulsion of the triceps tendon. A new syndrome? *J Bone Joint Surg Br*. 1982;64(1):70–72.
12. Lee ML. Rupture of the triceps tendon. *Br Med J*. 1960;2(5193):197.
13. Sollender JL, Rayan GM, Barden GA. Triceps tendon rupture in weight lifters. *J Shoulder Elbow Surg*. 1998;7(2):151–153.
14. Stannard JP, Bucknell AL. Rupture of the triceps tendon associated with steroid injections. *Am J Sports Med*. 1993;21(3):482–485.
15. Lambert MI, St Clair Gibson A, Noakes TD. Rupture of the triceps tendon associated with steroid injections. *Am J Sports Med*. 1995;23(6):778.
16. Preston FS, Adicoff A. Hyperparathyroidism with avulsion of three major tendons. Report of a case. *N Engl J Med*. 1962;266:968–971.
17. Mankin HJ. Rickets, osteomalacia, and renal osteodystrophy. Part II. *J Bone Joint Surg Am*. 1974;56(2):352–386.
18. Match RM, Corrylos EV. Bilateral avulsion fracture of the triceps tendon insertion from skiing with osteogenesis imperfecta. A case report. *Am J Sports Med*. 1983;11(2):99–102.
19. Hildebrand KA, Patterson SD, Regan WD, MacDermid JC, King GJ. Functional outcome of semiconstrained total elbow arthroplasty. *J Bone Joint Surg Am*. 2000;82(10):1379–1386.
20. Kelly EW, Coghlan J, Bell S. Five- to thirteen-year follow-up of the GSB III total elbow arthroplasty. *J Shoulder Elbow Surg*. 2004;13(4):434–440.
21. Celli A, Arash A, Adams RA, Morrey BF. Triceps insufficiency following total elbow arthroplasty. *J Bone Joint Surg Am*. 2005;87(9):1957–1964.
22. Chamseddine AH, Jawish RM, Alasiry AA, Zein HK. Ruptures and avulsions of the distal tendon of triceps brachii. *Eur J Orthop Surg Traumatol*. 2011;22(3):175–185.
23. Tagliafico A, Gandolfo N, Michaud J, Perez MM, Palmieri F, Martinoli C. Ultrasound demonstration of distal triceps tendon tears. *Eur J Radiol*. 2012;81:1207–1210.
24. Kijowski R, Tuite M, Sanford M. Magnetic resonance imaging of the elbow. Part II: abnormalities of the ligaments, tendons, and nerves. *Skeletal Radiol*. 2005;34(1):1–18.
25. van Riet RP, Morrey BF, Ho E, O'Driscoll RW. Surgical treatment of distal triceps ruptures. *J Bone Joint Surg Am*. 2003;85-A(10):1961–1967.
26. Blackmore SM, Jander RM, Culp RW. Management of distal biceps and triceps ruptures. *J Hand Ther*. 2006;19:154–169.
27. Morrey BF. Radial head fractures. In: Morrey BF, ed. *The Elbow and Its Disorders*. Philadelphia: WB Saunders Company; 2000.
28. Athwal GS, McGill RJ, Rispoli DM. Isolated avulsion of the medical head of the triceps tendon: an anatomic study and arthroscopic repair in 2 cases. *Arthroscopy*. 2009;25(9):983–988.
29. Bava ED, Barber FA, Lund ER. Clinical outcome after suture anchor repair for complete traumatic rupture of the distal triceps tendon. *Arthroscopy*. 2012;28:1058–1063.
30. Vanhees MKD, Geurts GFAE, Van Riet RP. Snapping triceps syndrome: a review of the literature. *Shoulder Elbow*. 2010;2(1):30–33.
31. Spinner RJ, O'Driscoll SW, Davids JR, Goldner RD. Cubitus varus associated with dislocation of both the medial portion of the distal triceps and ulnar nerve. *J Hand Surg Am*. 1999;24(4):718–726.
32. Spinner RJ, An KN, Kim KJ, Goldner RD, O'Driscoll SW. Medial or lateral dislocation (snapping) of a portion of the distal triceps: a biomechanical, anatomic explanation. *J Shoulder Elbow Surg*. 2001;10(6).561–567.
33. Spinner RJ, Goldner RD. Snapping of the medial head of the triceps: diagnosis and treatment. *Tech Hand Up Extrem Surg*. 2002;6(2):91–97.
34. Spinner RJ, Goldner RD. Snapping of the medial head of the triceps and recurrent dislocation of the ulnar nerve. Anatomical and dynamic factors. *J Bone Joint Surg Am*. 1998;80(2):239–247.
35. Spinner RJ, Hayden FR Jr, Hipps CT, Goldner RD. Imaging the snapping triceps. *AJR AM J Roentgenol*. 1996;167(6):1550–1551.

Soft Tissue Coverage of the Elbow

42A

Frances Sharpe, MD
Milan Stevanovic, MD

Injuries or surgical procedures about the elbow that result in exposed bone, joint, nerves, tendons, or implants require durable soft tissue reconstruction. The goals in treating soft tissue defects are to provide wound closure, decrease the risk of infection, decrease tissue edema, and allow early mobilization and rehabilitation of the elbow. Since local tissue may be involved in the zone of injury, it is useful to be familiar with several options for treating soft tissue loss about the elbow. The type of coverage should be appropriate for the size and etiology of the defect as well as the general health and needs of the patient. This chapter addresses the treatment of large soft tissue defects, which cannot be addressed by skin grafts or local random fasciocutaneous flaps.

In addition to providing soft tissue coverage, we recommend the use of durable soft tissue coverage over areas of scarred unstable tissue as a prophylactic treatment. This is particularly important in the multiply operated elbow and in the setting of a poor soft tissue envelope where arthroplasty is planned.

TYPES OF COVERAGE

Primary Closure

Primary closure or delayed primary closure is useful for small soft tissue defects, where there is no immediately underlying bone, joint, dead space, or implant. Primary closure is limited by the size of the defect and the extensibility and vascularity of the surrounding skin.

Healing by Secondary Intention

Wound healing by secondary intention can be considered when structural integrity is preserved and there is no exposed joint, bone, neurovascular structure, or tendon without paratenon. This can be achieved with serial wet-to-moist dressing changes or with a wound closure system such as the wound VAC™. This is a closed-system vacuum device that reduces the risk of secondary infection and uses a vacuum system to contract the wound size and reduce swelling.

Skin Grafting

Split-thickness or full-thickness skin grafting is appropriate for any size defect that has a tissue bed that will accept a graft. Skin graft will reliably provide coverage over exposed subcutaneous tissue, muscle, tendon with paratenon, or bone with periosteum. The latter 2 conditions may be undesirable as recipient tissue bed because skin graft directly overlying tendon or bone can result in an unstable scar susceptible to breakdown. At the dorsal surface of the elbow, split-thickness skin graft should be used with caution since this does not provide durable coverage and must be able to withstand repeated flexion and extension of the elbow.

Local Random Flaps

Local random flaps are not based on any vascular pattern or pedicle, but are perfused through dermal and subdermal plexus. Local skin flaps can be used to close small defects when primary closure creates excessive tension on tissue margins, or where a small defect is not amenable to skin grafting, for example, an area over a bony prominence, or over an exposed tendon. Although these flaps have the advantage of providing wound closure with similar-texture skin, they have limited applicability in the upper extremity due to the relatively poor vascularity and limited tissue mobility.

Axial Fasciocutaneous Flaps

Axial fasciocutaneous flaps are based on recognized arteriovenous systems, which supply a defined territory of skin and subcutaneous tissue. These can be harvested as wide-based peninsular flaps, or as island flaps, where the pedicle is fully mobilized. Peninsular flaps do not require isolation of the pedicle and are usually used as transposition flaps

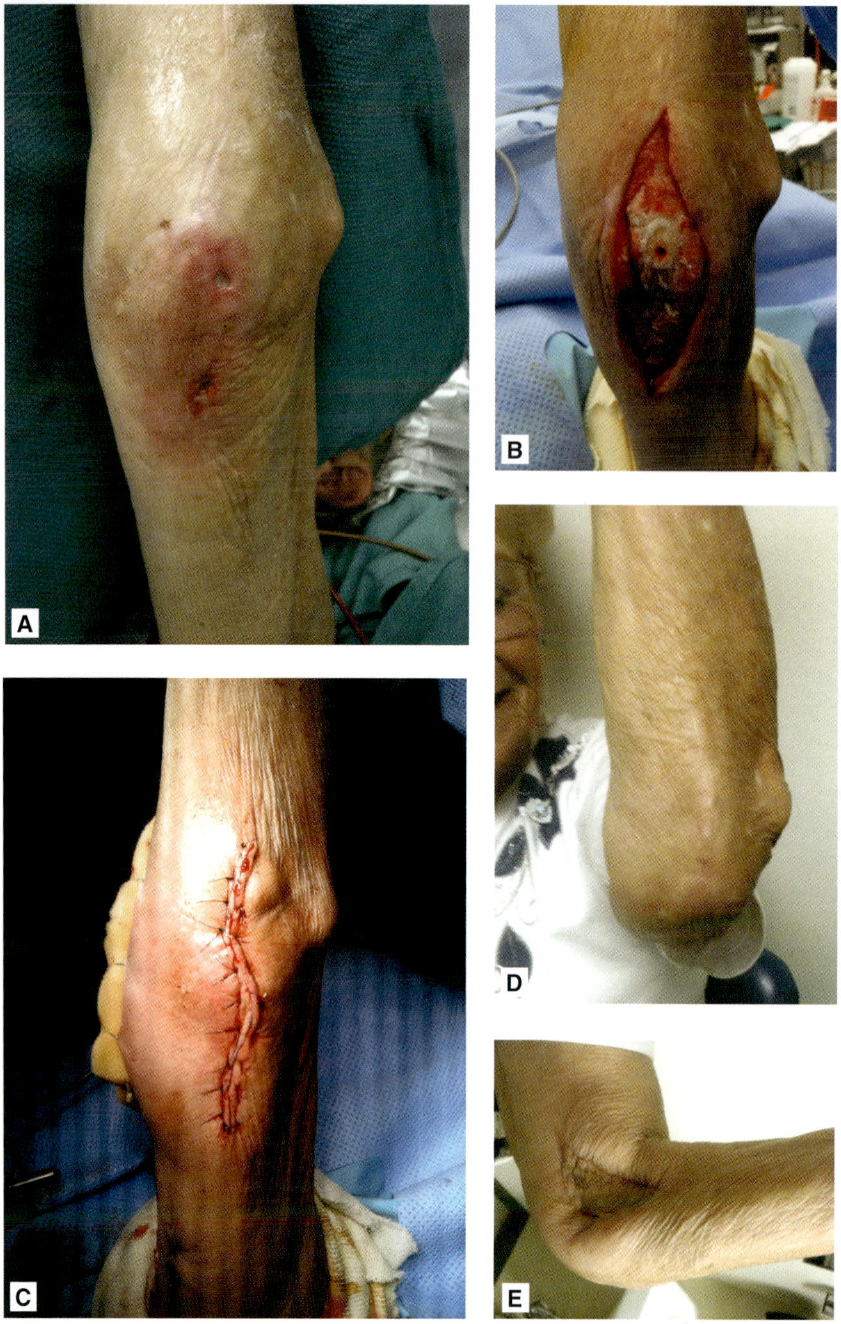

FIGURE 42A-1 This 78-year-old woman was 10 years out from a total elbow arthroplasty. At her initial surgery, she had delayed wound healing. At the time of her revision surgery, she underwent a rhomboid rotational flap to improve soft tissue coverage at the elbow. She did not heal her wound despite prolonged splinting. At 6 weeks post revision TEA, she underwent a fascial transposition flap. The wound was healed by 3 weeks. **A.** Six weeks postoperative revision total elbow arthroplasty. **B.** Intraoperative debridement with bone track created by suture used for triceps repair. **C.** Fasciocutaneous transposition with tissue mobilized from the medial elbow. **D.** Wound healing at 5 weeks—dorsal view. **E.** Wound healing at 5 weeks—medial view. (Copyright © Milan Stevanovic, MD and Frances Sharpe, MD.)

(Fig. 42A-1). Island flaps are similar to the peninsular flap; however, the vascular pedicle is isolated and mobilized. This allows greater versatility in coverage because of the increased arc of rotation. Most of these flaps also can be taken as free flaps. Examples in the arm and forearm include the lateral arm flap, the posterior interosseous flap, the ulnar artery flap, and the radial forearm flap.[1-16]

Distant Pedicle Flaps: 2-stage Flaps (Temporary Pedicle Flaps)

Distant pedicled flaps are one of the most reliable means of achieving coverage of large soft tissue defects, when recipient vessels are not available, or when the patient is a poor candidate for other types of reconstruction.[17-20] These flaps rely on the vascularity of the recipient tissue bed, and do not bring a permanent independent blood supply to the defect. They have been reported to cover defects as large as 22 cm in length.[17] Although seldom used, they remain an important reconstructive option in select patients. The main limitations of these flaps are related to the prolonged immobilization required for 2-stage procedures. This prolonged immobilization can significantly compromise functional recovery. Increased difficulties are encountered not only with stiffness and contracture at the elbow and shoulder but also with edema and stiffness of the hand and fingers.

Additional surgical requirements for flap division and subsequent flap contouring are another source of morbidity. At the time of flap division, if there is any suspicion of compromised circulation to the flap, a 7- to 10-day delay in final insetting at the recipient site will reduce the risk of flap necrosis. Donor-site cosmesis is of greater concern when the donor site cannot be closed primarily. These flaps also have been critiqued for their bulk and need for secondary surgeries for contouring.

Local Muscle Pedicle Flaps

Local muscle rotational flaps can be used to cover small defects about the elbow where there is exposed nerve, vessel, tendon, bone, or implant. Their arc of rotation generally allows for coverage of anterior and posterior wounds. Several local muscle rotational flaps have been described in small series, often only as case reports. These include the brachioradialis (Fig. 42A-2A), the extensor carpi radialis longus, the anconeus, and the flexor carpi ulnaris (FCU) (Fig. 42A-2B).[21–30] These muscles often lie within the zone of injury, limiting their use in these situations.

Distant Muscle Pedicle Flaps: 1 Stage

The latissimus dorsi (LD) rotational flap is the only distant pedicled muscle rotational flap that provides coverage of moderate to large soft tissue defects about the elbow. The muscle and its neurovascular pedicle lie well away from the

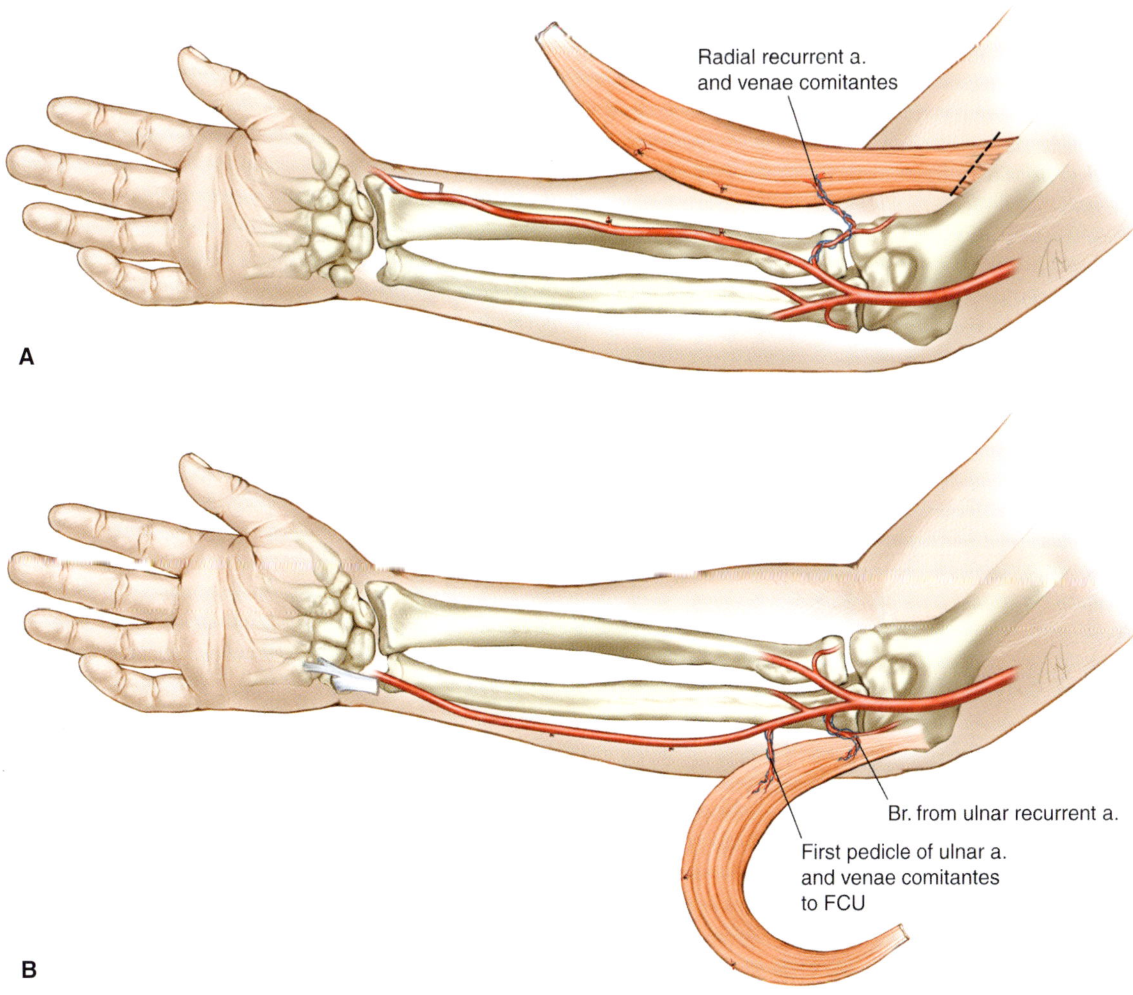

FIGURE 42A-2 **A.** Schematic drawing of brachioradialis flap. **B.** Schematic drawing of flexor carpi ulnaris flap. (Copyright © Milan Stevanovic, MD and Frances Sharpe, MD.)

elbow and are generally outside of the zone of injury. Because this is a 1-stage procedure, rehabilitation can be started within the first week of reconstruction.

Free-tissue Transfer

When local rotational flaps or distant 1-stage pedicle flaps are not suitable for soft tissue reconstruction, free-tissue transfer should be considered. Free-tissue transfer may provide the best functional and cosmetic outcome, and can be performed as a single-stage reconstruction, allowing early rehabilitation of the elbow.

Selection of the donor site depends on several factors. These include the size and location of the defect, any underlying structural or functional deficit, the presence of exposed or prominent implants, and the general health status of the patient. For example, functional morbidity at the donor site is more critical in the polytrauma patient, who is already functionally compromised. Many options for free-tissue transfer exist; these include fascial, fasciocutaneous, muscle, musculocutaneous, and osteocutaneous flaps.

Fascial free flaps can be used for defects that do not require the filling of a dead space. More commonly used fascial flaps include the temporoparietal fascia, radial forearm fascia, and parascapular fascia. They are particularly useful in the hand, where they provide thin pliable coverage, and allow tendon gliding.

The lateral arm and radial and ulnar forearm flaps can be taken as sensory flaps, which can be important in providing protective sensation over areas subject to pressure breakdown. Despite this advantage, these flaps have some donor-site morbidity with complaints of chronic aching, dysesthesias, and poor cosmetic appearance.

SURGICAL PROCEDURES

The procedures we use most frequently are described below. Although we sometimes use other techniques, we find these procedures to be reliable and durable with consistent anatomy. They require no microsurgical techniques and can be performed relatively quickly.

Local Muscle Rotational Flap: Anconeus

ANATOMY

The anconeus is a small triangular muscle crossing the lateral elbow. Its origin lies on the posterior surface of the lateral epicondyle of the humerus and it inserts on the lateral proximal olecranon. The muscle is supplied through 2 constant arterial pedicles, the medial collateral artery and the recurrent posterior interosseous artery, which anastomose within the muscle belly. The medial collateral artery is a terminal branch of the profunda brachii. It always travels with the radial nerve branch to the anconeus and enters the muscle on its proximal deep surface. From an arterial standpoint, the anconeus can be mobilized on either its proximal or distal pedicle. However, mobilization on the distal pedicle (recurrent posterior interosseous artery) requires sacrifice of the nerve leading to atrophy and scarring of the flap. The anconeus is innervated by branches of the radial nerve. The muscle measures approximately 2.5 cm in width and 7 cm in length. It functions as a minor elbow extensor and may play a role in augmenting lateral stability of the elbow.

INDICATIONS

The anconeus is very useful and available for small defects on the posterior and lateral elbow. Schmidt et al described 3 areas of coverage that include the lateral radiocapitellar joint, the distal triceps tendon at its insertion, and the olecranon.[27,28] The anconeus can be expected to reliably cover a 5- to 7-cm^2 defect. It can be harvested without measurable functional deficit.

CONTRAINDICATIONS

There are no specific contraindications other than defect size and local involvement in the zone of injury. Lateral-sided elbow instability is a relative contraindication. However, collateral ligament reconstruction can be performed in conjunction with soft tissue coverage.

SURGICAL TECHNIQUE

General hand surgery instrumentation is typically adequate for the surgical dissection. Loupe magnification is not necessary, but preferred. The procedure can be performed with the patient in a supine, lateral, or prone position, depending on other procedures being performed. When soft tissue coverage alone is performed, we prefer a supine position. The elbow and forearm are supported on towels as needed. The donor site for harvesting split-thickness skin graft should be considered in the surgical site preparation. A sterile tourniquet is used during the muscle dissection, but is released once the muscle has been mobilized. General anesthesia or regional anesthesia may be used based on patient and anesthesiologist preference.

The skin incision is centered over the lateral epicondyle and extends obliquely to the lateral border of the olecranon, near the distal insertion of the anconeus. The antebrachial fascia is exposed and the interval between anconeus and extensor carpi ulnaris is opened. The dissection of the anconeus must be carried to its distal-most insertion, which lies approximately 10 cm from the lateral epicondyle. The interval between the anconeus and the extensor carpi ulnaris is more easily identified distally.

The tip of the anconeus is elevated from its insertion. Supraperiosteal dissection is carried out along the inferior border of the ulna. The radiocapitellar joint capsule is protected. The recurrent posterior interosseous arterial pedicle is ligated, and the muscle is mobilized to its origin. The

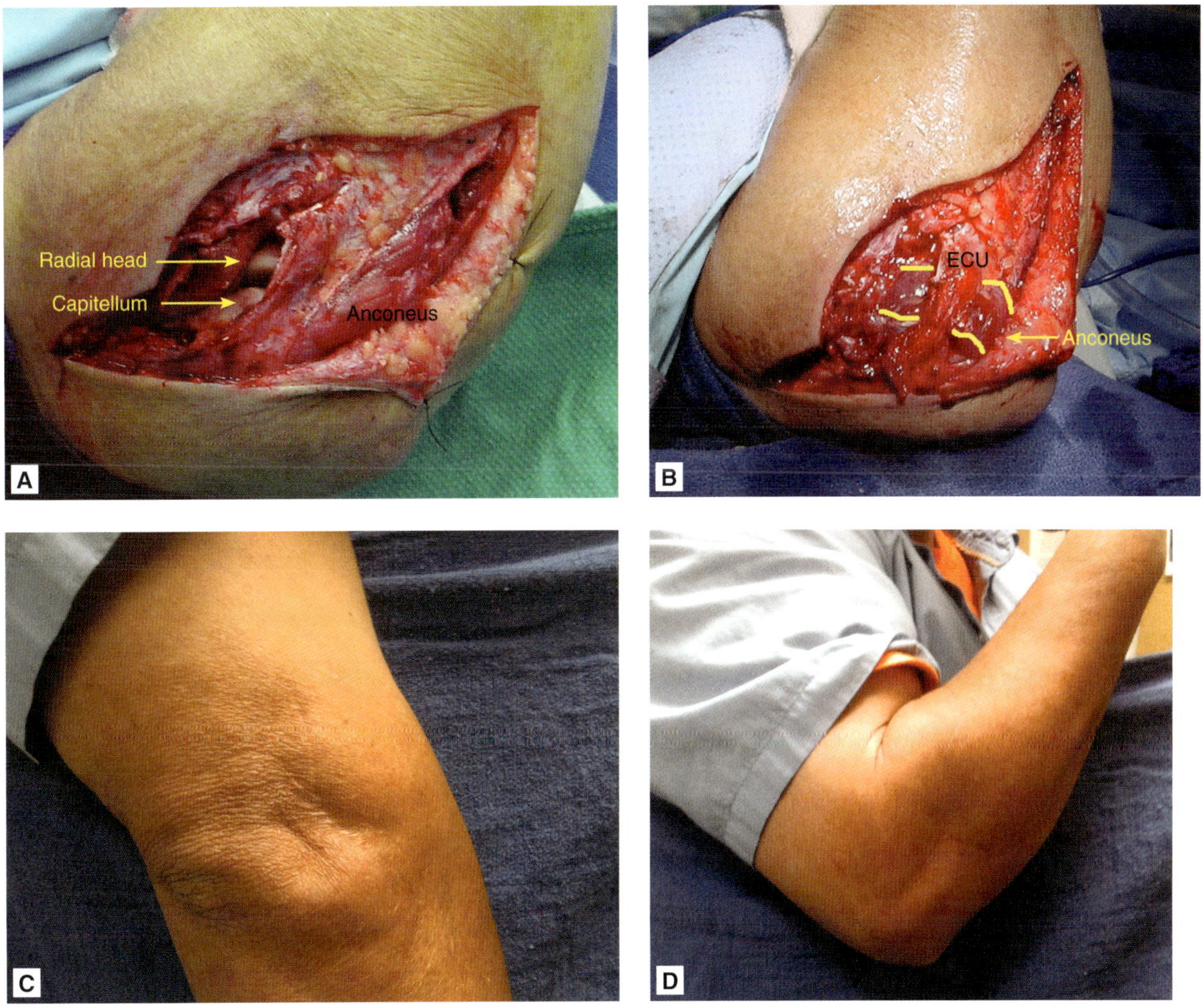

FIGURE 42A-3 This 53-year-old brick layer was surgically treated for lateral epicondylitis. He presented with a draining wound and was treated for presumed infection with multiple debridements. He failed to heal and was referred to our department. He was felt to have a chronic synoviocutaneous fistula. Lateral ulnar collateral ligament and capsular reconstruction was performed with tissue allograft. An anconeus muscle flap was used to cover the reconstruction. Primary wound closure was possible. **A.** Status post wound debridement showing lateral capsular deficiency and anconeus muscle. **B.** Anconeus muscle rotated below the extensor carpi ulnaris muscle and covering the lateral joint. **C.** Five years postoperative wound healing showing full extension. **D.** Five years postoperative flexion. (Copyright © Milan Stevanovic, MD and Frances Sharpe, MD.)

origin can also be released to increase the arc of rotation on its proximal pedicle from the medial collateral artery. If the muscle origin off the lateral epicondyle is released, the proximal pedicle (medial collateral artery) should be identified and protected. A split-thickness skin graft is used to cover any exposed muscle (Fig. 42A-3).

An overzealous dissection of the proximal anconeus and proximal release of the muscle origin can place the proximal pedicle and nerve at risk for injury. An underestimation of the defect size may make the anconeus unsuitable or inadequate to provide coverage. Debridement of the wound should be performed prior to committing to the use of the anconeus for coverage. Alternative coverage options should be considered prior to the time of surgery if the defect size is intraoperatively determined to be too large or distant.

Local Muscle Rotational Flap: Flexor Carpi Ulnaris

ANATOMY

The FCU is the ulnar-most superficial flexor of the forearm. It has 2 heads of origin: 1 from the medial epicondyle of the distal humerus and the other from the proximal ulna. The dominant pedicle is from the ulnar artery or the ulnar recurrent artery (a branch of the ulnar artery). The FCU muscle is usually supplied by several pedicles along the length of the muscle, but is well perfused by the proximal 1 to 2 pedicles. These pedicles are small 1- to 2-mm vessels (Fig. 42A-4A). The muscle is innervated by the ulnar nerve, which enters the proximal muscle just distal to the medial epicondyle. The

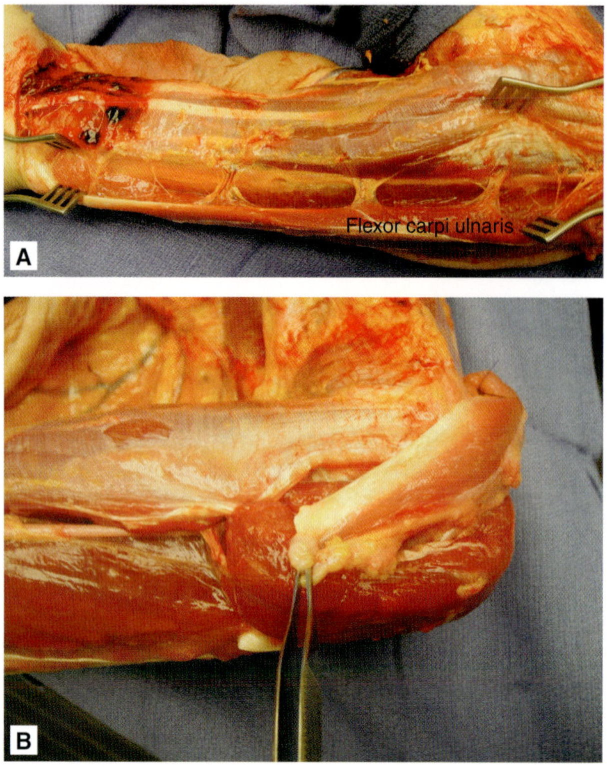

FIGURE 42A-4 **A.** Vascular anatomy of the flexor carpi ulnaris. **B.** Fan-folding of the flexor carpi ulnaris showing wider area of posterior elbow coverage. (Copyright © Milan Stevanovic, MD and Frances Sharpe, MD.)

average muscle belly measures 5 cm in width and 20 cm in length. The muscle belly extends to the wrist flexion crease in most specimens.

INDICATIONS

As with most local rotational muscle flaps for the elbow, the size and arc of rotation limits the use of these flaps for small- to medium-sized defects on the anterior, posterior, or medial elbow. The largest defect we have covered on the posterior elbow is 6 × 8 cm. The FCU can also be used to cover neurovascular structures, arteriovenous shunts, and vascular prosthetic grafts.[23,29,30]

CONTRAINDICATIONS

The FCU muscle should not be sacrificed when other coverage options with a lower morbidity are available. For patients who are anticipated to return to their previous level of function and require a strong wrist flexor, alternatives to the use of the FCU should be explored.[31] Specific contraindications to the use of the FCU are an absent ulnar artery, absent innervation to the FCU, and inclusion of the FCU in the zone of injury. The biggest controversy over the use of the FCU flap for soft tissue coverage is the potential donor-site morbidity associated with using the dominant flexor and ulnar deviator of the wrist.

SURGICAL TECHNIQUE

General hand surgery instrumentation is typically adequate for the surgical dissection. Microvascular ligaclips and bulldog clamps for 1- to 2-mm vessel size should be available. Bipolar cautery can help with hemostasis around neurovascular structures. Loupe magnification is useful in identifying the perforating branches from the ulnar artery.

The procedure is preferably done in the supine position. The donor site for harvesting split-thickness skin graft should be considered in the surgical site preparation. A sterile tourniquet is used for the dissection of the FCU. The tourniquet is released prior to ligation of the second most distal perforating pedicle, so that muscle perfusion can be assessed. General anesthesia is preferred, but the surgery can be performed under a regional block if the patient has a contraindication to general anesthesia. An Allen test is performed to assess the patency of both radial and ulnar arteries to rule out an absent ulnar artery with atypical vascular pedicles to the FCU.

A longitudinal incision is made along the ulnar border of the FCU muscle from the wrist flexion crease to the medial epicondyle. The incision is tailored proximally to the area of defect by a medial incision. The acuity of the angle of the skin flaps should be 60° or greater.

The distal end of the musculotendinous junction is identified and transected. The muscle is mobilized from the surrounding fascia and from the ulna. There are typically between 5 and 7 pedicles to the FCU from the ulnar artery. A relatively distal proximal pedicle can limit the arc of rotation of the flap. If the proximal pedicles lie very distally, it is possible that the flap is supplied closer to its insertion by a branch from the recurrent ulnar artery. The proximal pedicles should be evaluated before ligating the distal pedicles. With the tourniquet released, the perfusion of the muscle is assessed. The more distal pedicles are clamped with a bulldog clamp. If perfusion remains unchanged, the most distal perforators are ligated, leaving the proximal 2 pedicles intact. The flap is generally well perfused by the proximal 2 perforators. If necessary, the second of the most proximal perforators can also be sacrificed to allow a greater arc of rotation of the flap. The muscle belly is completely freed from surrounding tissue and fascia and rotated on its proximal pedicle(s). It is then brought over the posterior elbow and sutured to the recipient site with 3-0 absorbable suture. Torsion of the pedicle during rotation of the flap can result in vascular compromise. Good perfusion of muscle flap should be confirmed before skin closure. Tension-free closure is important to prevent compression of the pedicles. The posterior elbow defect is covered with a split-thickness skin graft (Fig. 42A-5). In order to maximize the surface area that can be covered by this flap, the muscle should be transected at the wrist level. Longitudinal incisions along the muscle fascia allow the muscle to be spread out to cover a wider surface area. In addition, *fan-folding* of the muscle increases the width of coverage (Fig. 42A-4B). Also, the tendinous portion of the FCU can be used for a vascularized ligament reconstruction of the collateral ligaments of the elbow.

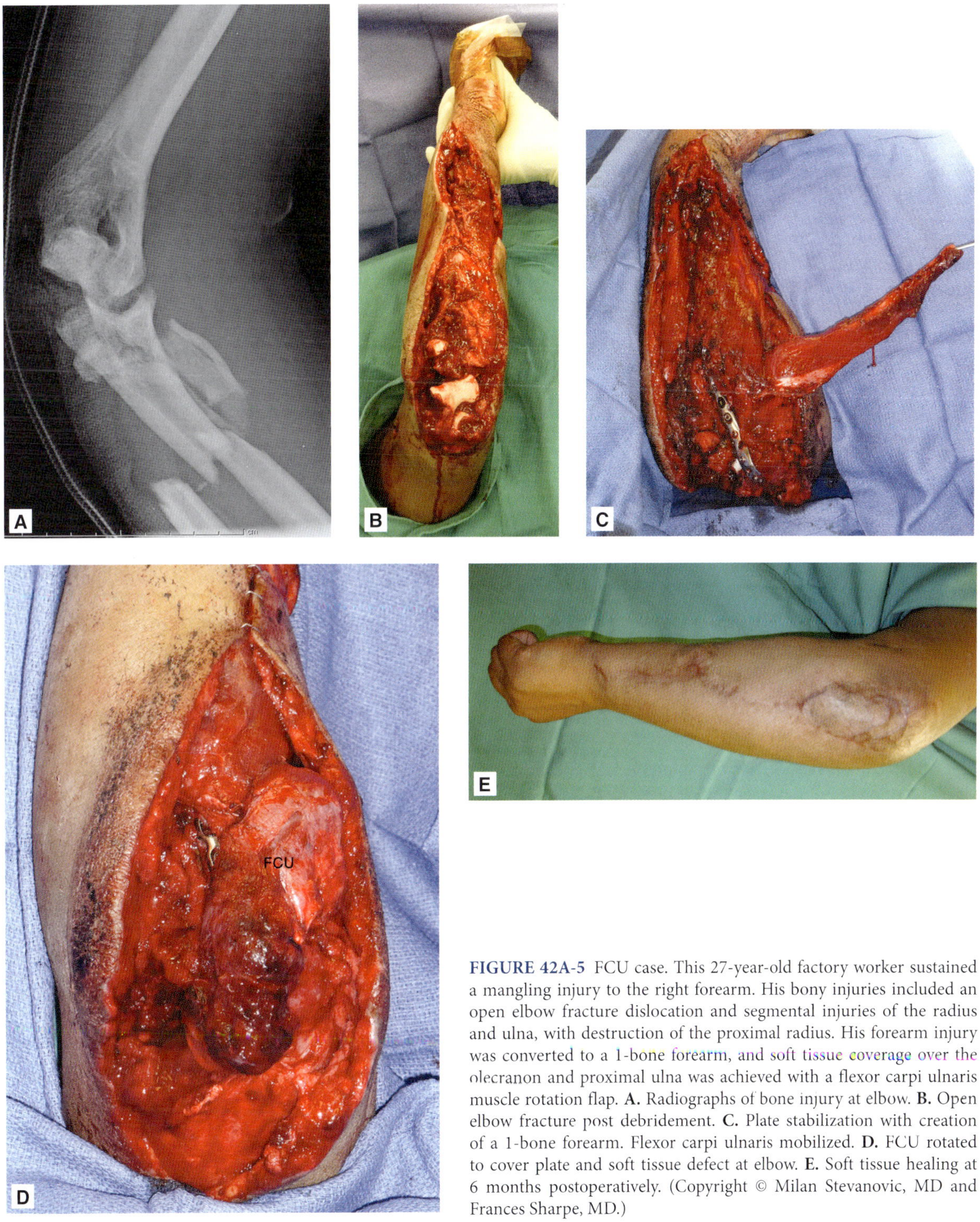

FIGURE 42A-5 FCU case. This 27-year-old factory worker sustained a mangling injury to the right forearm. His bony injuries included an open elbow fracture dislocation and segmental injuries of the radius and ulna, with destruction of the proximal radius. His forearm injury was converted to a 1-bone forearm, and soft tissue coverage over the olecranon and proximal ulna was achieved with a flexor carpi ulnaris muscle rotation flap. **A.** Radiographs of bone injury at elbow. **B.** Open elbow fracture post debridement. **C.** Plate stabilization with creation of a 1-bone forearm. Flexor carpi ulnaris mobilized. **D.** FCU rotated to cover plate and soft tissue defect at elbow. **E.** Soft tissue healing at 6 months postoperatively. (Copyright © Milan Stevanovic, MD and Frances Sharpe, MD.)

For optimizing the durability of the final outcome, the innervation to the FCU should be left intact. If it is not, the rotated muscle flap becomes very scarred and atrophic. Although a thicker soft tissue envelope can be achieved by harvesting the FCU with an overlying skin paddle, this can result in poor donor-site cosmesis.

Radial Forearm Flap

ANATOMY

The radial forearm flap is located on the volar surface of the forearm. The position of the donor site on the forearm is determined by the size of the defect and the length of the pedicle required to rotate the flap to the defect. The flap is supplied by the radial artery and its fascial perforators. The radial artery supply to the hand is sacrificed with this flap. In the proximal forearm, the radial artery lies proximally between the brachioradialis muscle and the pronator teres. Distally, the artery lies between the tendons of the brachioradialis and the flexor carpi radialis. Along the course of the radial artery numerous branches are present to supply the radial muscles of the forearm. There are also branches present that perforate the fascia, supplying the antebrachial fascia and its overlying subcutaneous tissue and skin. The radial forearm flap is based on these perforating branches and they must be protected throughout the dissection. In the distal forearm, there are numerous perforating branches. In the proximal forearm there are fewer branches and inadvertent injury to these perforators can result in loss of the proximal portion of this flap. The venous outflow for the flap is provided by the venae comitantes of the radial artery. The cephalic vein can sometimes be included in the flap, but it is not critical for flap outflow.[32] The main concern with the use of this flap relates to the cosmetic appearance at the donor site. This is reported to be a significant source of patient dissatisfaction, particularly in women. There are conflicting data regarding functional outcome related to grip and pinch strength and loss of dorsiflexion at the wrist.[33–35]

INDICATIONS

The radial forearm flap is perhaps the most versatile and reliable rotational flap for hand and elbow soft tissue reconstruction.[6,15,35–37] The flap provides thin durable coverage. When used for elbow coverage, the incorporation of the medial or lateral antebrachial cutaneous nerve can make this a sensate flap and provide sensory protection for large areas of reconstructed soft tissue about the elbow. A large skin flap can be harvested alone or with vascularized tendon and/or bone graft. Alternately, vascularized fascia alone can be taken as free or rotational tissue.[38] The long pedicle provides a wide arc of rotation, allowing for easy circumferential coverage of the elbow. Thus, the indications for this flap are for small to large soft tissue defects about the elbow. Since vascularized bone and tendon can be harvested with this flap, the radial forearm flap is uniquely capable of providing the elements for reconstruction of small bone defects and/or collateral ligaments in conjunction with soft tissue coverage.

CONTRAINDICATIONS

The absolute contraindication for a radial forearm flap is incomplete or inadequate perfusion of the hand through the ulnar artery or previous injury of the radial artery. Before using the radial forearm flap, a careful preoperative assessment is necessary to evaluate the blood supply to the hand. An Allen test and Doppler examination of the radial and ulnar arteries should be performed. An incomplete superficial arch or an absent ulnar artery is an absolute contraindication for use of this flap.

Relative contraindications include previous history of surgery on the volar forearm, patients with history of peripheral vascular disease or other vascular disorders, and patients for whom the cosmetic appearance of the donor site would affect the patient's profession or self-image. Patients should be counseled about the donor-site appearance, the potential for cold intolerance, and the remote risk of vascular compromise to the hand. They should also be aware of sensory deficits associated with harvesting a sensate flap.

SURGICAL TECHNIQUE

General hand surgery instrumentation is typically adequate for the surgical dissection. Microvascular ligaclips (small and medium) and bulldog clamps for 2- to 4-mm vessel size should be available. A sterile Doppler is not usually necessary, as the radial artery is easily palpated. Loupe magnification is useful and preferred. The procedure is performed in the supine position.

A sterile tourniquet is used for the dissection. Gravity elevation or light Esmarch exsanguination is used in order to allow better visualization of the septocutaneous perforating branches. General anesthesia is preferred, but the surgery can be performed under a regional block.

The flap is designed on the volar aspect of the forearm. The flap size and design depend on the size and shape of the defect to be covered (Fig. 42A-6). The position of the skin island on forearm depends on location of the defect. It should be positioned sufficiently distal to allow the skin island to be rotated to the area needing coverage. After outlining the flap, the incision follows the course of the radial artery. Proximally it is tailored toward the defect, following the anticipated arc of the flap. We do not recommend tunneling of the flap below the skin.

The course of the radial artery is approximated along a line drawn from the biceps tendon to the radial side of the flexor carpi radialis tendon at the proximal wrist crease. The skin island is marked. The incision is started distally, identifying the cephalic vein and the radial artery that lies between the tendons of the brachioradialis and flexor carpi radialis. The skin paddle is incised down to the antebrachial fascia. The fascia is sharply divided in line with the skin incision. The fascia is tacked to the subdermal layer with a 4-0 absorbable suture to prevent shearing injuries to the fascial perforators. The dissection is then continued in the subfascial plane starting on the ulnar side of the flap. The flap is elevated to the radial artery. It is critical to stay above the paratenon throughout the dissection. As the dissection approaches the radial artery the intermuscular septum must be included in the dissection to preserve the septocutaneous perforators that supply the skin paddle. The flap is then elevated from radial side in the same fashion. Retraction of the brachioradialis and eversion of its ulnar border allow better visualization of the radial artery and its pedicles. Prior to ligating the radial artery, the artery is provisionally clamped with a microvascular clamp, and the tourniquet is released. The perfusion of the hand is checked. If it is satisfactory, the

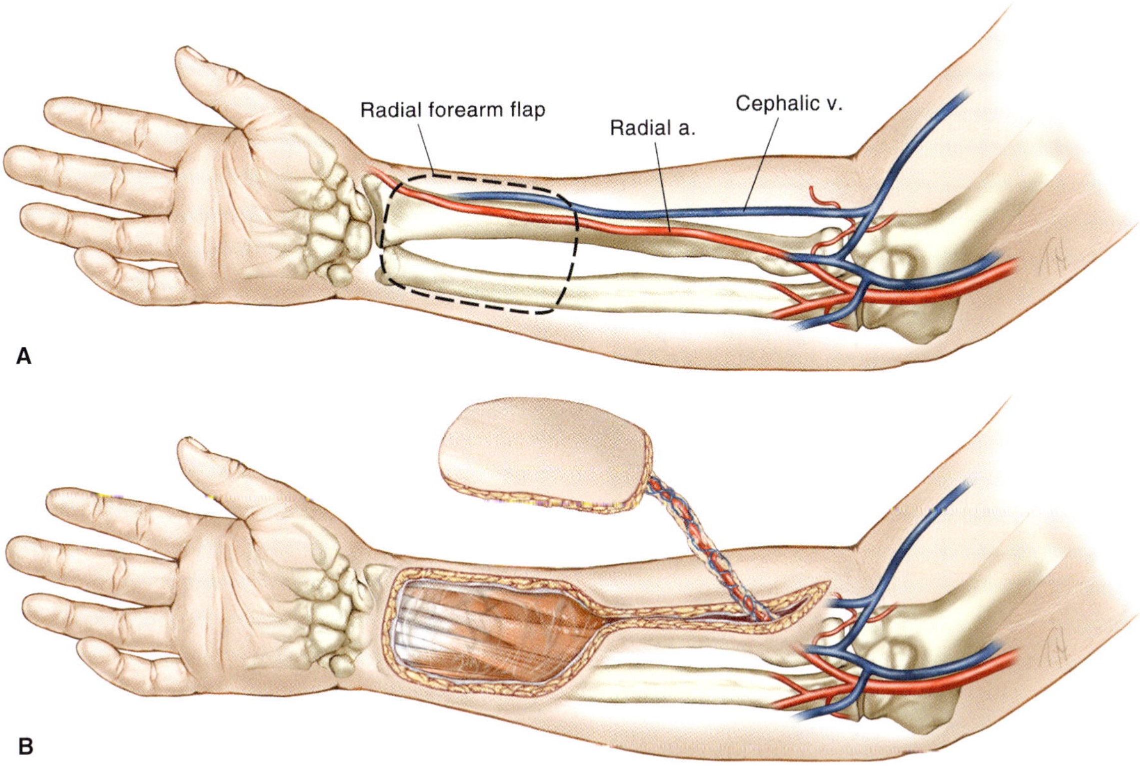

FIGURE 42A-6 Radial forearm flap. **A.** Outline of the flap on the forearm. **B.** Flap raised on its radial artery pedicle. (Copyright © Milan Stevanovic, MD and Frances Sharpe, MD.)

arm is re-exsanguinated and the tourniquet is reinflated. The radial artery and cephalic vein are ligated in the distal incision site, and the remainder of the flap is elevated together with the radial artery and cephalic vein. Depending on the distance to the defect, the radial artery and its venae comitantes can be traced proximally as far as the bifurcation of the brachial artery to allow a greater arc of rotation. The flap is inset into the defect in a standard manner (Fig. 42A-7). Kinking of the proximal pedicle during rotation of the flap can lead to flap congestion and failure.

A composite vascularized flap can also be harvested, as a tendinocutaneous graft or osteotendinocutaneous flap. The brachioradialis, flexor carpi radialis, and palmaris longus can be utilized either alone or in combination for triceps tendon reconstruction or augmentation or for a vascularized medial or lateral ligament reconstruction.

The donor site can rarely be closed primarily and requires split-thickness skin grafting. Use of nonmeshed skin graft provides a more cosmetic donor-site scar. The skin edges should be sutured to the adjacent epimysium to prevent further spreading of the skin edges. Preservation of the paratenon is important to prevent failure of the skin graft over the donor site. If the paratenon has been harvested with the flap, an attempt should be made to provide muscular coverage over the tendon(s). When this is not possible, consider resection of noncritical portions of tendon. After covering the donor site with a split-thickness skin graft, a bolster dressing is placed over the graft for 3 to 4 weeks. This prolonged period of maintaining the dressing has reduced the incidence of tendon adhesions in our experience. The forearm is splinted to prevent muscle shearing forces across the skin graft for the first 3 weeks.

Donor site morbidity may be decreased by a suprafascial dissection of the flap as injection studies have shown that the dominant subcutaneous vessels and their anastomosing vessels lie superficial to the fascia.[39]

Distant Muscle Rotational Flap: Latissimus Dorsi

ANATOMY

The LD is a broad thin muscle originating from the thoracodorsal fascia and inserting on the proximal medial humerus between the insertions of pectoralis major and teres major. It is a strong fan-shaped muscle supplied by the thoracodorsal artery and innervated by the thoracodorsal nerve, which arises as a terminal branch from the posterior cord. The proximal location of the neurovascular pedicle provides a wide arc of rotation for rotational coverage of the head, neck shoulder, arm, and elbow.

INDICATIONS

The LD is a versatile flap that can be harvested as a muscle or musculocutaneous flap. Due to its size and arc of rotation, this muscle or musculocutaneous flap can be used to cover large soft tissue defects of the upper extremity. In

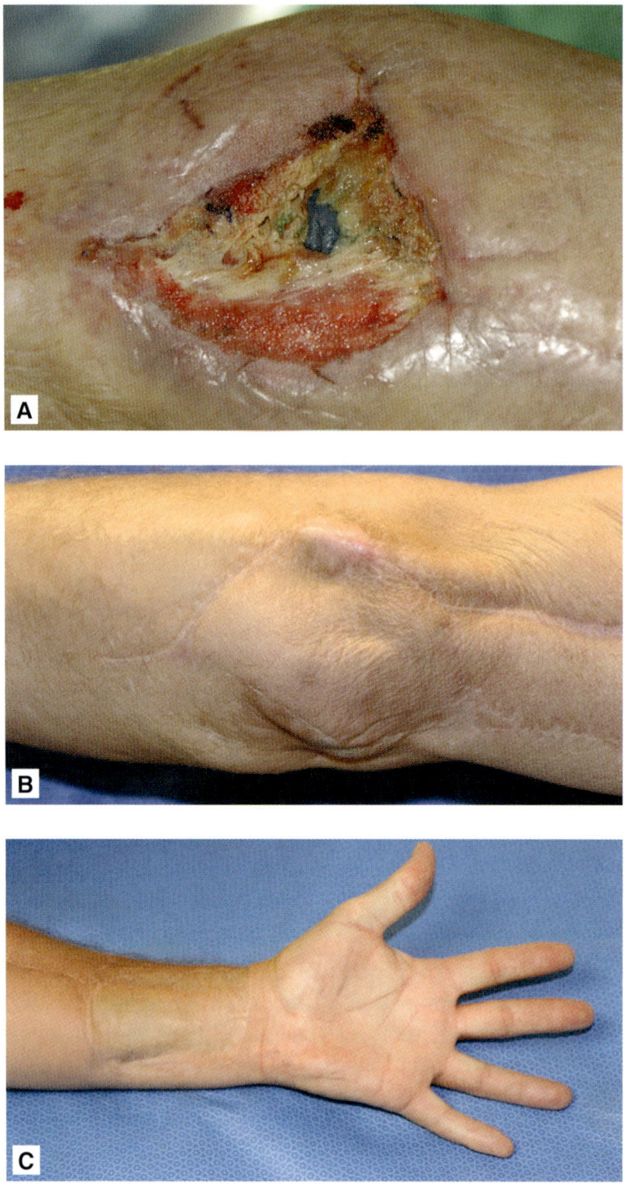

FIGURE 42A-7 This 40-year-old patient had sustained an open supracondylar humerus fracture. Wound healing was complicated by soft tissue necrosis and failure of the skin graft. Bone and suture were exposed. Following debridement of the wound, there was also exposed hardware. A radial forearm rotational flap was used to cover the defect. **A.** Chronic posterior elbow wound. **B.** Healed radial forearm flap at 2 years. **C.** Donor site at 2-year follow-up. (Copyright © Milan Stevanovic, MD and Frances Sharpe, MD.)

anatomic and clinical studies, it has been shown to reach 6 to 8 cm distal to the olecranon as a rotational flap.[40,41] The LD is particularly useful when the patient's zone of injury prevents the use of local tissue for soft tissue coverage as well as for large soft tissue defects. The neurovascular supply to this muscle allows the latissimus to also be rotated as a functional muscle transfer. At the elbow this can be used for reconstruction of elbow flexion or extension and can be done in combination with coverage of soft tissue defects.[40–51]

CONTRAINDICATIONS

Absolute contraindications for this flap are patient conditions that require use of crutches or a wheelchair, such as paraplegia or severe lower extremity injuries. Ipsilateral shoulder girdle weakness, previous surgeries about the shoulder girdle, previous trauma affecting the subclavian or axillary artery, tumor resection, and lymph node dissection in the area of the thoracodorsal artery and nerve are further contraindications. Relative contraindications include patients with family history of breast cancer that might need future reconstruction.

SURGICAL TECHNIQUE

General hand surgery instrumentation is typically adequate for the surgical dissection. Microvascular ligaclips (small and medium) and bulldog clamps for 2- to 4-mm vessel size should be available. A sterile Doppler is used to assess the distal flap circulation. Bipolar cautery is important for dissection around the pedicle. Long lighted retractors can be helpful if providing exposure through more limited skin incisions.

The patient is positioned in the lateral decubitus position. The entire lateral side from the ilium to the shoulder girdle and including the affected arm is included in the prep. Dorsally this should extend to the spinous processes and ventrally to the midumbilical line. The operative arm can be supported on a sterile Mayo stand. Prolonged abduction of the arm can cause a traction neurapraxia to the brachial plexus and periodic repositioning of the arm should be performed. Donor site for harvesting split-thickness skin graft should be considered in the surgical site preparation and is most conveniently done from the ipsilateral lateral thigh. The contralateral side should be well padded. An axillary roll should be placed to prevent compression of the brachial plexus and to prevent circulatory compromise to the upper extremity. A sterile tourniquet may be used for debridement of the defect site or for additional procedures that need to be performed at the elbow. General anesthesia is necessary for this procedure.

The skin incision follows the course of the latissimus along its midline axis. The incision extends from the axilla to approximately 4 fingerbreadths cephalad to the posterior iliac crest (Fig. 42A-8). In general, we prefer to transfer the latissimus as a muscle transfer rather than a musculocutaneous transfer. Indications for inclusion of a skin paddle for elbow coverage are limited. Our principal indication would be a massive soft tissue defect or if the muscle is to be used as a functional transfer. Inclusion of a skin paddle in this scenario is to prevent muscle adhesion and improve gliding. If a skin paddle is to be used, it is designed to fit the skin defect at the elbow. It is important to measure the size of the defect at the completion of the debridement of the traumatic wound.

During the dissection of the skin paddle, the incision is beveled away from the skin incision. The incision is carried down to the muscle fascia. Skin flaps are elevated in the suprafascial plane first toward the anterior margin of the latissimus and then toward the posterior margin. The anterior margin

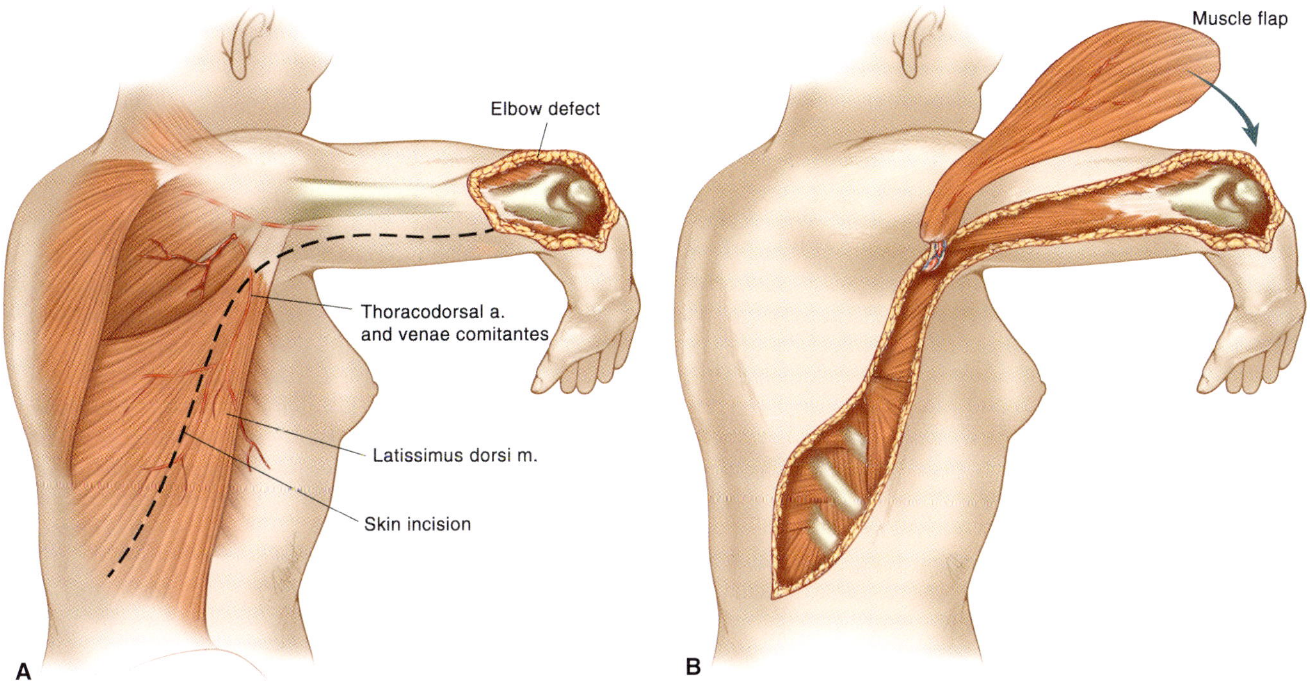

FIGURE 42A-8 Latissimus dorsi rotational flap. **A.** Skin incision for the latissimus dorsi. **B.** Flap elevated and rotated on the thoracodorsal pedicle. (Copyright © Milan Stevanovic, MD and Frances Sharpe, MD.)

of the latissimus is most easily identified and separated from adjacent muscles in the midpoint of the muscle. The anterior margin is mobilized and traced toward its caudal origin. As the iliac crest is approached, the fibrous origin of the latissimus must be tediously dissected from the fibers of the abdominal oblique muscles at the thoracodorsal fascia.

The fibrous origin of the latissimus is released from the thoracodorsal fascia and the muscle is elevated along its deep surface from caudad to cephalad. Deep perforating branches should be identified and cauterized or ligated. As the dissection continues cephalad, care should be taken to identify and protect the distal slips of the serratus anterior and the teres major muscle. The latissimus may be tightly adherent to the chest wall origin of the serratus anterior and to the scapular origin of the teres major, making it difficult to distinguish between the muscle planes. Electrical stimulation of the muscle fibers of the latissimus can help distinguish between the fibers of the latissimus and adjacent muscles.

During the dissection toward the axilla, the branch of the thoracodorsal artery that supplies the distal slips of the serratus anterior should be identified. The branch origin is variable in location. If the distal slips of serratus are not to be included in the rotational flap, the branch is ligated close to its takeoff from the thoracodorsal artery. We recommend the use of a 2-0 suture ligature rather than hemoclips. Hemoclips may loosen or dislodge and lead to significant bleeding. Small perforating branches of the thoracodorsal artery are also ligated. The thoracodorsal artery must be protected from stretching or twisting during the remainder of the dissection.

Attention is then directed cephalad to the insertion of the latissimus on the proximal humerus. Release of the humeral insertion of the latissimus allows greater mobilization of the muscle. We release 80% of the insertion regardless since this changes the muscle resting length and reduces muscle contraction that might disrupt the muscle after it is inset. The remaining intact 20% of the insertion helps prevent traction injury to the pedicle.

The tendinous portion of the latissimus is identified and dissected along its anterior surface toward its insertion on the humerus. Since the tendinous insertion of the LD and teres major are often conjoined, special attention is necessary to release only the insertion of the LD. It is important to remember that the axillary nerve lies just superior and medial to the latissimus insertion. Careful dissection in this area is necessary to avoid injury to the nerve. If the latissimus is to be used as a functional transfer, the release of the insertion is performed close to the bony insertion of the latissimus on the humerus.

The thoracodorsal pedicle is mobilized. We do not separately identify the thoracodorsal nerve. Although some surgeons do sacrifice the nerve when not performing a functional transfer, we spare the nerve in order to preserve some of the muscle thickness and elasticity and limit some of the fibrotic changes that occur in denervated flaps. The neurovascular pedicle is mobilized, and the surrounding fascia is completely released to prevent kinking of the pedicle over tight fascial bands. Ligating the vascular branch to the serratus anterior and more proximal perforating branches will improve length and mobility of the vascular pedicle.

The muscle can now be rotated on its pedicle to cover defects on any surface of the elbow. The pedicle should not be twisted, and there should be no tension on the pedicle at the time of insetting. During transposition, we do not recommend tunneling of the latissimus below a subcutaneous bridge. This can compress the muscle and/or pedicle, leading to myonecrosis.

The latissimus is inset below the subcutaneous tissue. The muscle fascia is tacked to the subcutaneous tissue layer beginning proximally to prevent traction on the pedicle. Periodically during insetting, the color of the vena comitantes is monitored. Any change or darkening of the venous return suggests possible venous obstruction proximally. This may be caused by kinking of the pedicle at the axilla. After the muscle is completely inset, a Doppler probe is used to check the patency of the vessel in full elbow extension and at 90° of elbow flexion. If the pulse is completely obliterated at 90° of flexion, the muscle is stretched too far distally and should be reinset. Failure to recognize these potential areas of vascular compromise can lead to partial or complete flap necrosis. When the entire latissimus muscle is used, the flap closest to the origin may not be adequately supplied on the proximal pedicle. This portion of the flap should be carefully checked once the muscle is rotated. If perfusion is questionable, this portion of the muscle flap should be resected. Exposed muscle is covered with a split-thickness skin graft. After application of the dressing, the arm is placed in 30° to 40° of shoulder abduction and 40° to 60° of elbow flexion. In this position, swelling about the axilla will be less likely to cause compression of the vascular pedicle. Gentle passive range of motion may be initiated at 1 week.

If the latissimus is to be used for simultaneous soft tissue coverage and functional reconstruction, the resting length of the muscle must be marked. This is done by placing the arm in full flexion. Marking sutures are sewn into the muscle belly at 5-cm intervals, starting from the muscle insertion and measuring toward the origin. When the muscle is inset for functional reconstruction, the resting length must be restored. This is done by insetting the muscle such that the marking sutures placed at the time of harvesting the muscle are restored to 5-cm intervals. Any excess muscle is resected. It is better to harvest a skin paddle with the latissimus to cover a functional muscle transfer. This tissue provides a better gliding surface for the muscle than a split-thickness skin graft. The skin paddle is inset. Any remaining exposed muscle is covered with split-thickness skin graft. For reconstruction of elbow flexion, the latissimus is inserted into the residual stump of the biceps. The resting length is set with the elbow in full extension, and the elbow is immobilized in approximately 90° of elbow flexion. When a reconstruction is done for elbow extension, the muscle resting length is set with the elbow in maximum flexion. Postoperatively, the elbow is immobilized in maximum extension. The period of immobilization for a functional reconstruction must be for a minimum of 8 weeks, followed by a gentle program of remobilization (Fig. 42A-9).

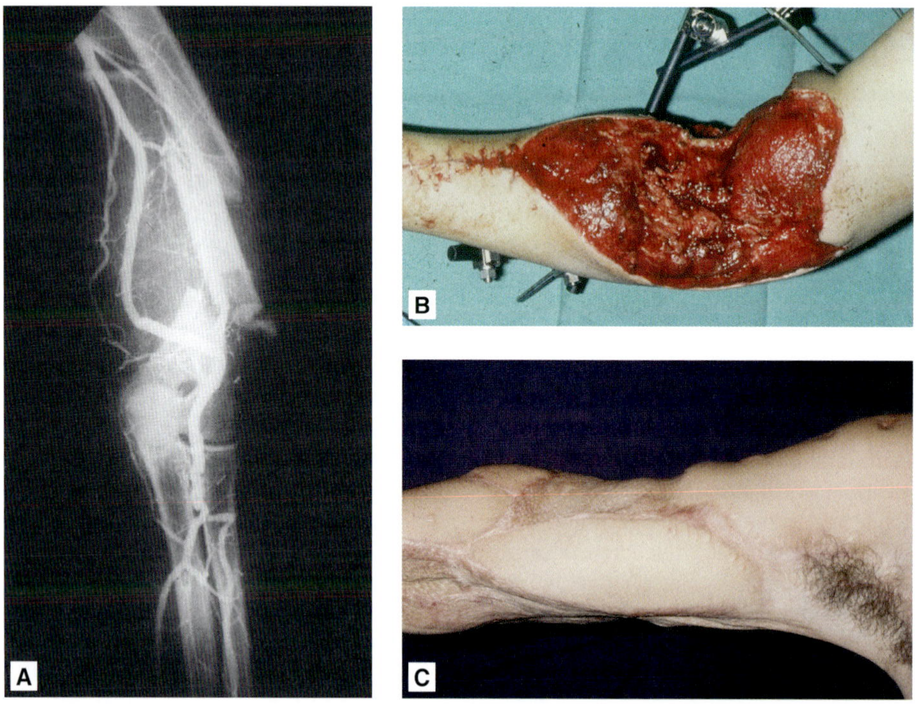

FIGURE 42A-9 A 23-year-old patient who sustained a crush injury of the arm and elbow. A vascular repair without bone stabilization was performed at an outside institution. An external fixator was used for stabilization due to the vascular repair that was performed in a shortened position. A rotational myocutaneous latissimus flap was used to cover the soft tissue defect on the arm and circumferentially around the elbow. **A.** Angiogram showing bone and vascular repair. **B.** Soft tissue defect following external fixation and debridement. **C.** Healed latissimus flap at 1 year. (Copyright © Milan Stevanovic, MD and Frances Sharpe, MD.)

COMPLICATIONS

The most serious complication following soft tissue coverage of the elbow is partial or complete loss of the flap. In the early stages this results from arterial inflow or venous outflow problems. In later stages of recovery, this can be related to infection. Careful attention to debridement of necrotic and poorly vascularized tissue, appropriate treatment of infected or contaminated wounds prior to soft tissue coverage, and adequate antibiotic therapy can reduce the risks of infection. Large donor sites can be prone to seroma formation. Specific cosmetic and functional losses related to the specific donor tissue should be considered and the procedure that allows the best coverage with the least deficit should be selected.

OUTCOMES

It is difficult to provide outcome data for soft tissue coverage procedures. Many of the techniques described are presented as small series or case reports. Functional outcomes are often more related to the underlying pathology rather than the specific coverage procedure. In larger series, the coverage procedures were performed for a variety of underlying pathologies. Elhassan et al reviewed 20 patients who underwent anconeus rotational flaps. The anconeus reliably covered defects with an average size of 4 × 3 cm. The most common diagnosis was a chronic draining olecranon bursitis. The average time to wound healing was 3 weeks. There were 2 wound dehiscences, which healed with local wound care.[52]

The FCU outcomes have been reported in a few small series.[23,30,53,54] In a cadaveric study by Wysocki et al, the FCU was found to reliably cover a defect width of 2 to 4 cm at the olecranon. They were able to correlate width of coverage with forearm circumference. In our experience of clinical and cadaveric dissections, we were able to cover defects between 2 and 5 cm in width. Fan-folding of the FCU provides a greater width of coverage. Without fan-folding, the FCU can reach 8 to 9 cm proximal to the olecranon tip with the elbow flexed at 90°.

Jutte et al performed cadaveric dissections to evaluate the distal extent of a rotational LD flap for elbow coverage. They found that the latissimus consistently reached the olecranon and frequently was able to provide coverage to the proximal forearm. They did not recommend coverage more than 6 cm from the tip of the olecranon on the posterior elbow.[40] Our clinical experience paralleled that of Jutte's. In our reported series, we had complications in 2 of 9 latissimus flaps, the first related to hematoma that formed from loss of a ligaclip on a branch to the serratus. The other complication was a partial flap necrosis at the distal flap when coverage past 8 cm distal to the olecranon tip was attempted.[55]

The most comprehensive paper on this subject was performed by Choudry et al. Ninety-nine flaps were reviewed. Pedicled flaps accounted for 65% of the coverage procedures. The most common of these was the radial forearm flap followed by LD. The overall complication rate was 31%, 30 minor complications that did not require additional reconstructive procedures. There were 12 major complications that did require additional coverage procedures. The highest complication rate was seen in the LD rotational flaps when used to cover defects distal to the olecranon tip.[56]

Any of the above procedures when appropriately sized to the soft tissue defect and performed with careful technique can provide durable soft tissue coverage and facilitate early range of motion of the elbow. As noted above, complications can and do occur. The risks of complications can be reduced through appropriate flap selection, careful attention to pedicle positioning, and vigilant postoperative monitoring.

REFERENCES

1. Akpuaka F. The radial recurrent fasciocutaneous flap for coverage of posterior elbow defects. *Injury*. 1991;22(4):332–334.
2. Bunkis J, Ryu R, Walton R, Epstein L, Vasconez L. Fasciocutaneous flap coverage for periolecranon defects. *Ann Plast Surg*. 1985;14(4):361–370.
3. Coessens B, Vico P, DeMey A. Clinical experience with the reverse lateral arm flap in soft-tissue coverage of the elbow. *Plast Reconstr Surg*. 1993;92(6):1133–1136.
4. Cormack G, Lamberty B. Fasciocutaneous vessels in the upper arm: application to the design of new fasciocutaneous flaps. *Plast Reconstr Surg*. 1984;74(2):244–249.
5. Culbertson J, Mutimer K. The reverse lateral upper arm flap for elbow coverage. *Ann Plast Surg*. 1987;18(1):62–69.
6. Hentz V, Pearl R, Grossman J, Wood M, Cooney W. The radial forearm flap: a versatile source of composite tissue. *Ann Plast Surg*. 1987;19(6):485–498.
7. Lanzetta M, Bernier M. The lateral forearm flap: an anatomic study. *Plast Reconstr Surg*. 1997;99(2):460–464.
8. Lazarou SA, Kaplan I. The lateral arm flap for elbow coverage. *Plast Reconstr Surg*. 1993;91:1349–1354.
9. Lovie M, Duncan G, Glasson D. The ulnar artery forearm free flap. *Br J Plast Surg*. 1984;37:486–492.
10. Orgill D, Pribaz J, Morris D. Local fasciocutaneous flaps for olecranon coverage. *Ann Plast Surg*. 1994;32(1):27–31.
11. Parry S, Ward J, Mathes S. Vascular anatomy of the upper extremity muscles. *Plast Reconstr Surg*. 1988;81(3):358–363.
12. Penteado C, Masquelet A, Chevrel J. The anatomic basis of the fascio-cutaneous flap of the posterior interosseous artery. *Surg Radiol Anat*. 1996;8:209–215.
13. Tan B-K, Lim B-H. The lateral forearm flap as a modification of the lateral arm flap: vascular anatomy and clinical implications. *Plast Reconstr Surg*. 2000;105(7):2400–2404.
14. Timmons M, Missotten F, Pode M, Davies D. Complications of radial forearm donor sites. *Br J Plast Surg*. 1986;39:176–178.
15. Tizian C, Sanner F, Berger A. The proximally pedicled arteria radialis forearm flap in the treatment of soft tissue defects of the dorsal elbow. *Ann Plast Surg*. 1991;26(1):40–44.
16. Pranti L, Schreml S, Schwarze H, et al. A safe and simple technique using the distal pedicled reversed upper arm flap to cover large elbow defects. *J Plast Reconstr Aesthet Surg*. 2008;61(5):546–551.
17. Burstein F, Salomon J, Stahl R. Elbow joint salvage with the transverse rectus island flap: a new application. *Plast Reconstr Surg*. 1989;79(9):492–497.
18. Davis W, McGraw J, Carraway J. Use of a direct, transverse, thoracoabdominal flap to close difficult wounds of the thorax and upper extremity. *Plast Reconstr Surg*. 1977;67(10):526–532.
19. Fisher J. External oblique fasciocutaneous flap for elbow coverage. *Plast Reconstr Surg*. 1985;75(1):51–59.
20. Sbitany U, Wray R. Use of the rectus abdominis muscle flap to reconstruct an elbow defect. *Plast Reconstr Surg*. 1986;77(6):988–989.
21. Janevicius R, Greager J. The extensor carpi radialis longus muscle flap for anterior elbow coverage. *J Hand Surg Am*. 1992;17A(1):102–106.

22. Lalikos J, Fudem GM. Brachioradialis musculocutaneous flap closure of the elbow utilizing a distal skin island. *Ann Plast Surg.* 1997;39(2):201–204.
23. Meals R. The use of a flexor carpi ulnaris muscle flap in the treatment of an infected nonunion of the proximal ulna. *Clin Orthop.* 1989;240:168–172.
24. Ohtsuka H, Imagawa S. Reconstruction of a posterior defect of the elbow joint using a extensor carpi radialis longus myocutaneous flap: case report. *Br J Plast Surg.* 1985;38:238–240.
25. Rohrich R, Ingram A. Brachioradialis muscle flap: clinical anatomy and use in soft-tissue reconstruction of the elbow. *Ann Plast Surg.* 1995;35(1):70–76.
26. Sanger J, Ye Z, Yousif N, Matloub H. The brachioradialis forearm flap: anatomy and clinical application. *Plast Reconstr Surg.* 1994;94(5):667–674.
27. Schmidt C, Kohut G, Greenberg J, Kann S, Idler R, Kiefhaber T. The anconeus muscle flap: its anatomy and clinical application. *J Hand Surg Am.* 1999;24A(2):359–368.
28. Fleager K, Cheung E. The "anconeus slide" rotation flap for management of posterior wound complications about the elbow. *J Shoulder Elbow Surg.* 2011;20(8):1310–1316.
29. Wysocki R, Gray R, Fernandez J, Cohen M. Posterior elbow coverage using whole and split flexor carpi ulnaris flaps: a cadaveric study. *J Hand Surg Am.* 2008;33(10):1807–1812.
30. Lingaraj K, Lim A, Puhaindran M, Kumar P. Case report: the split flexor carpi ulnaris as a local muscle flap. *Clin Orthop Relat Res.* 2007;455:262–266.
31. Raskin K, Wilgis E. Flexor carpi ulnaris transfer for radial nerve palsy: functional testing of long-term results. *J Hand Surg Am.* 1995;20A:737–743.
32. Lin CS, Lai CS, Chiu CC. Venous drainage in the reverse forearm flap. *Plast Reconstr Surg.* 1984;74(4):508–512.
33. Meland N, Core G, Hoverman V. The radial forearm flap donor site: should we vein graft the artery? A comparative study. *Plast Reconstr Surg.* 1993;91(5):865–869.
34. Richardson D, Fisher S, Vaughan E, Brown J. Radial forearm flap donor-site complications and morbidity: a prospective study. *Plast Reconstr Surg.* 1997;99:109–115.
35. Jones N, Jarrahy R, Kaufmann M. Pedicled and free radial forearm flaps for reconstruction of the elbow, wrist, and hand. *Plast Reconstr Surg.* 2008;121:887–898.
36. Govila A, Sharma D. The radial forearm flap for reconstruction of the upper extremity. *Plast Reconstr Surg.* 1990;86:920.
37. Song R, Gao Y, Song Y, Yu Y, Song Y. The forearm flap. *Clin Plast Surg.* 1982;9(1):21–26.
38. Ismail T. The free fascial forearm flap. *Microsurgery.* 1989;10:155.
39. Schaverien M, Saint-Cyr M. Suprafascial compared with subfascial harvest of the radial forearm flap: an anatomic study. *J Hand Surg Am.* 2008;33(1):97–101.
40. Jutte D, Rees R, Nanney L, Bueno R, Lynch J. Latissimus dorsi flap: a valuable tool in lower arm reconstruction. *South Med J.* 1987;80(1):37–40.
41. Stevanovic M, Sharpe F, Thommen V, Itamura J, Schnall S. Use of the pedicled latissimus dorsi rotational flap for coverage of soft tissue defects at the elbow. *J Shoulder Elbow Surg.* 1999;8(6):634–643.
42. Chang L, Goldberg N, Chang B, Spence R. Elbow defect coverage with a one-staged tunneled latissimus flap. *Ann Plast Surg.* 1994;32(5):496–502.
43. Harvey E, Aponte R, Levin L. Application of the island pedicle latissimus dorsi flap for soft tissue coverage of the elbow. *Can J Plast Surg.* 1999;7(1):23–26.
44. Minami A, Ogino T, Ohnishi N, Itoga H. The latissimus dorsi musculocutaneous flap for extremity reconstruction in orthopedic surgery. *Clin Orthop.* 1990;260:201–206.
45. Mordick T, Britton E, Brantigan C. Pedicled latissimus dorsi transfer for immediate soft tissue coverage and elbow flexion. *Plast Reconstr Surg.* 1996;99(6):1742–1744.
46. Park C, Shin K. Functioning free latissimus dorsi muscle transplantation: anterogradely positioned usage in reconstruction of extensive forearm defect. *Ann Plast Surg.* 1991;27(1):87–91.
47. Pruzansky M, Kelly M, Weinberg H. Latissimus dorsi musculocutaneous flap for elbow extension. *J Surg Oncol.* 1991;47:62–66.
48. Sadove R, Vasconez H, Arthur K, Draud J, Burgess R. Immediate closure of traumatic upper arm and forearm injuries with the latissimus dorsi island myocutaneous pedicle flap. *Plast Reconstr Surg.* 1991;88(1):115–120.
49. Stern P, Neale H, Gregory R, Kreilein J. Latissimus dorsi musculocutaneous flap for elbow flexion. *J Hand Surg Am.* 1982;7A(1):25–30.
50. Zancolli E, Mitre H. Latissimus dorsi transfer to restore elbow flexion: an appraisal of eight cases. *J Bone Joint Surg Am.* 1973;55-A(6): 1265–1275.
51. Russell R, Pribaz J, Zook E, Leighton W, Eriksson E, Smith C. Functional evaluation of latissimus dorsi donor site. *Plast Reconstr Surg.* 1986;78(3):336–344.
52. Elhassan B, Karabekmez F, Hsu C-C, Steinmann S, Moran S. Outcome of local anconeus flap transfer to cover soft tissue defects over the posterior aspect of the elbow. *J Shoulder Elbow Surg.* 2011;20(5):807–812.
53. Lim A, Kumar V, Sebastin S, Kapickis M. Split flexor carpi ulnaris transfer: a new functioning free muscle transfer with independent dual function. *Plast Reconstr Surg.* 2006;117:1927–1932.
54. Lingaraj K, Lim A, Puhaindran M, Kumar P. The splint flexor carpi ulnaris as a local muscle flap. *Clin Orthop Relat Res.* 2006;455:262–266.
55. Stevanovic M, Sharpe F, Thommen V, Itamura J, Schnall S. Latissimus dorsi pedicle flap for coverage of soft tissue defects about the elbow. *J Shoulder Elbow Surg.* 1999;8(6):634–643.
56. Choudry U, Moran S, Li S, Khan S. Soft-tissue coverage of the elbow: an outcome analysis and reconstructive algorithm. *Plast Reconstr Surg.* 2007;119(6):1852–1857.

42B

Vascularized Free Fibula Bone Graft for Upper Extremity Reconstruction

Milan Stevanovic, MD
Frances Sharpe, MD

The introduction of vascularized bone transfer in 1975 by Taylor et al dramatically expanded the surgical armamentarium for upper extremity reconstruction.[1] Vascularized grafts provide a living piece of corticocancellous bone that has immediate structural integrity that does not decrease with time. Vascularized grafts are less likely than allograft to suffer stress fractures and are immediately alive and capable of remodeling including undergoing bone hypertrophy as a response to physiologic stress. The presence of living osteoblasts facilitates healing and increases resistance to infection.

Early work on the transfer of bone on a vascular pedicle was done in animal studies. The first studies demonstrated the viability of transferred bone over time.[2–4] Later, Brunelli et al showed significantly shorter healing times in vascularized compared with nonvascularized autografts in a rabbit model.[5]

Since the first report of a vascularized free bone transfer by Taylor et al in 1975 for the reconstruction of a tibial defect, many others have used and reported on this technique for upper extremity reconstruction in the setting of congenital, neoplastic, and traumatic cases of bone loss.[6–27] Weiland et al should be credited with the first reported use of vascularized bone grafts for reconstruction for congenital anomalies and tumor. He is also the first to report on the transfer of the epiphysis and growth plate in children.[19] In the upper extremity, Innocenti et al have mastered the use of epiphyseal transfer for the proximal humerus and distal radius.[11,28–30] The first use of an osteoseptocutaneous flap was described independently by Yoshimura et al and Chen and Wang in 1983.[31,32] Since that time, the work of many others has further elucidated the variable anatomy of the septocutaneous perforators.[33–41]

While other vascularized bone grafts have been successfully utilized, the vascularized free fibula graft has become the workhorse of upper extremity reconstruction, because of its shape, structural integrity, reliability, and limited donor-site morbidity.

ANATOMY OF THE FIBULAR DONOR SITE

The fibula is a long, straight cortical bone with a length that ranges between 22 and 27 cm. Its blood supply is from the peroneal artery through nutrient branches as well as periosteal branches (Fig. 42B-1). The diameter of the arterial pedicle ranges between 1.5 and 3.0 mm, and that of the concomitant veins between 2.0 and 4.0 mm. The pedicle length, from its branch point from the posterior tibial artery to where the artery becomes intimately adherent to the fibula, ranges between 1.0 and 4.0 cm. The pedicle can be lengthened, when necessary, by stripping the periosteum, proximal to the nutrient artery, which enters the fibula near the middiaphysis.[37] The fibula can be harvested with its proximal articular surface, and with its open physis in children. In addition, it can be transferred with adjacent muscles including the soleus or flexor hallucis muscles.[42,43] Most commonly, it is transferred as an osteoseptocutaneous flap, which provides mobility of the skin paddle allowing versatility of coverage.[44]

The dominant blood supply to the diaphysis of the fibula is from the peroneal artery with venous drainage via venae comitantes of the peroneal artery (Fig. 42B-2). Branches off of the peroneal artery enter nutrient foramen in the middle third of the fibula.[10,37,45] In children, the epiphyseal blood supply is separate from the diaphyseal circulation. Epiphyseal branches of the tibialis anterior (TA) and the descending genicular artery supply the fibular epiphysis. The TA also provides circulation in the proximal two thirds of the fibular diaphysis in children and adults. Therefore, if the epiphysis is to be transferred in a child, the fibula is harvested on the TA artery[30,46] (Fig. 42B-3).

The peroneal artery is a branch of the posterior tibial artery. However, it is not always present (<0.1% of patients) or the peroneal artery may be present as a peroneus magnus, providing distal blood flow normally provided by the anterior or posterior tibial artery.[47] In 6% of legs the anterior tibial

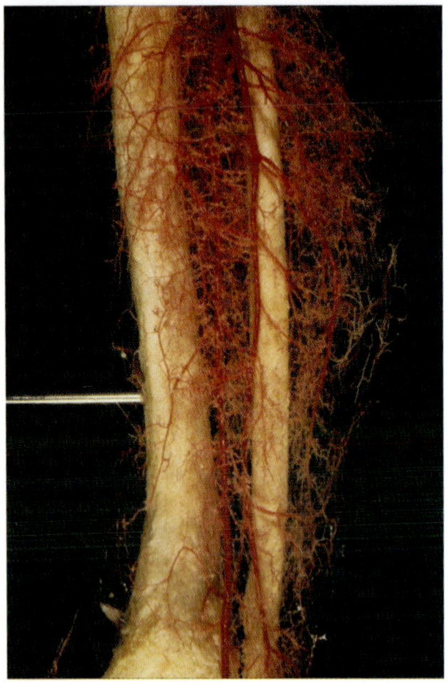

FIGURE 42B-1 Latex injection study showing the posterior aspect of the leg. The intimate relationship of the peroneal artery to the fibula is demonstrated. Multiple septocutaneous perforators are seen crossing the posterior side of the fibula. (Copyright © Milan Stevanovic, MD and Frances Sharpe, MD.)

artery is deficient in runoff and the dorsalis pedis is supplied by a perforator from the peroneal artery. In 5% of legs the posterior tibial artery is deficient and the plantar arteries branch off of the peroneal artery.[47] An important consideration when harvesting an osteoseptocutaneous fibula flap is the location of the dominant perforating branches to the skin paddle (Fig. 42B-2). The most reliable cutaneous vessels are found in the lower two thirds of the leg, and run posterior to the fibula in the posterior crural septum.[31,33,36,38–40,48]

INDICATIONS

Vascularized bone grafting is indicated in large defects of greater than 6 cm resulting from trauma, tumor, or infection. It is indicated for diaphyseal defects of the upper extremity from the clavicle to the metacarpal. It can be used for distal radial articular and proximal humeral articular reconstruction or to achieve fusion of the shoulder, elbow, or wrist. Vascularized free fibula grafting can be used to salvage failed conventional skeletal reconstruction.

For large bone defects, we find this procedure the most beneficial to the patient for speed of healing, durability, and structural integrity, and with great potential for remodeling and hypertrophy.

Candidates for reconstruction should have the medical health necessary to withstand a lengthy surgical procedure. They require a clean soft tissue bed with control of any underlying conditions such as tumor or infection. The donor site requires a normal vascular pattern of circulation to the lower extremity and no prior history of injury.

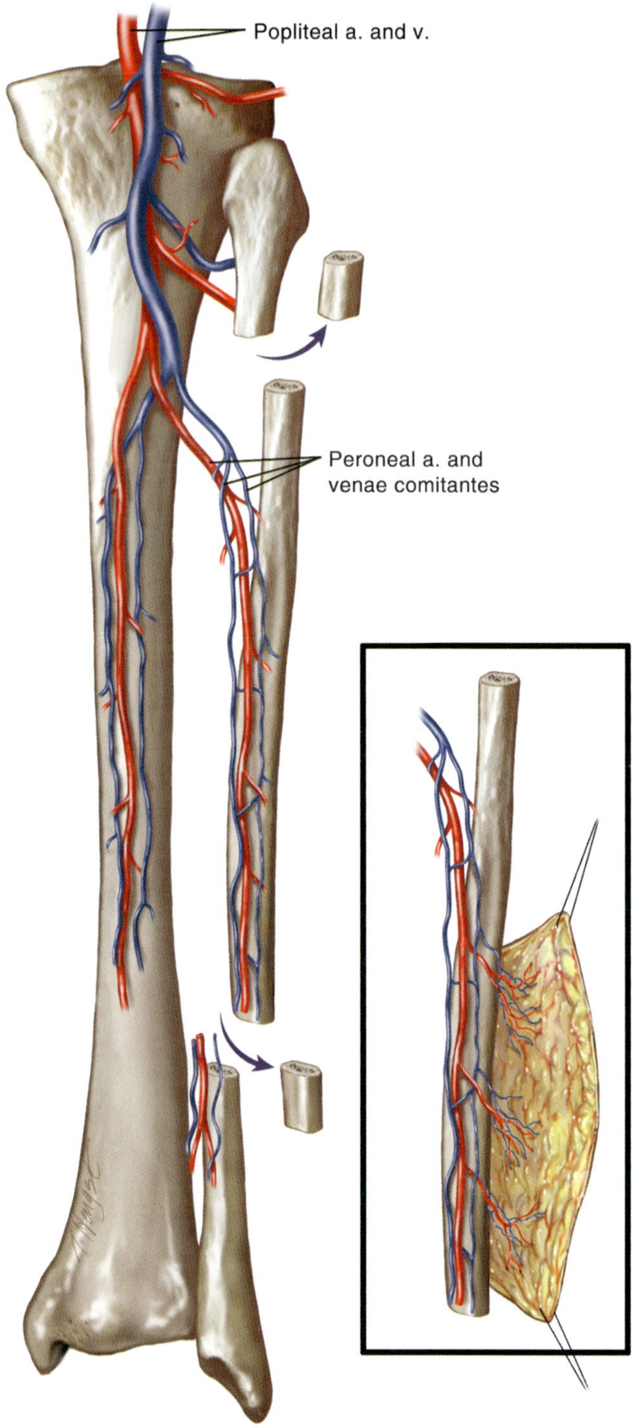

FIGURE 42B-2 Diagram showing peroneal artery circulation to the fibula. Cutout showing septocutaneous perforators to the skin paddle. (Copyright © Milan Stevanovic, MD and Frances Sharpe, MD.)

CONTRAINDICATIONS

Absolute contraindications include the absence of a peroneal artery, a peroneus magnus artery, previous donor-site trauma, active infection, active immunosuppression or radiation therapy, and lack of recipient vessels. Relative

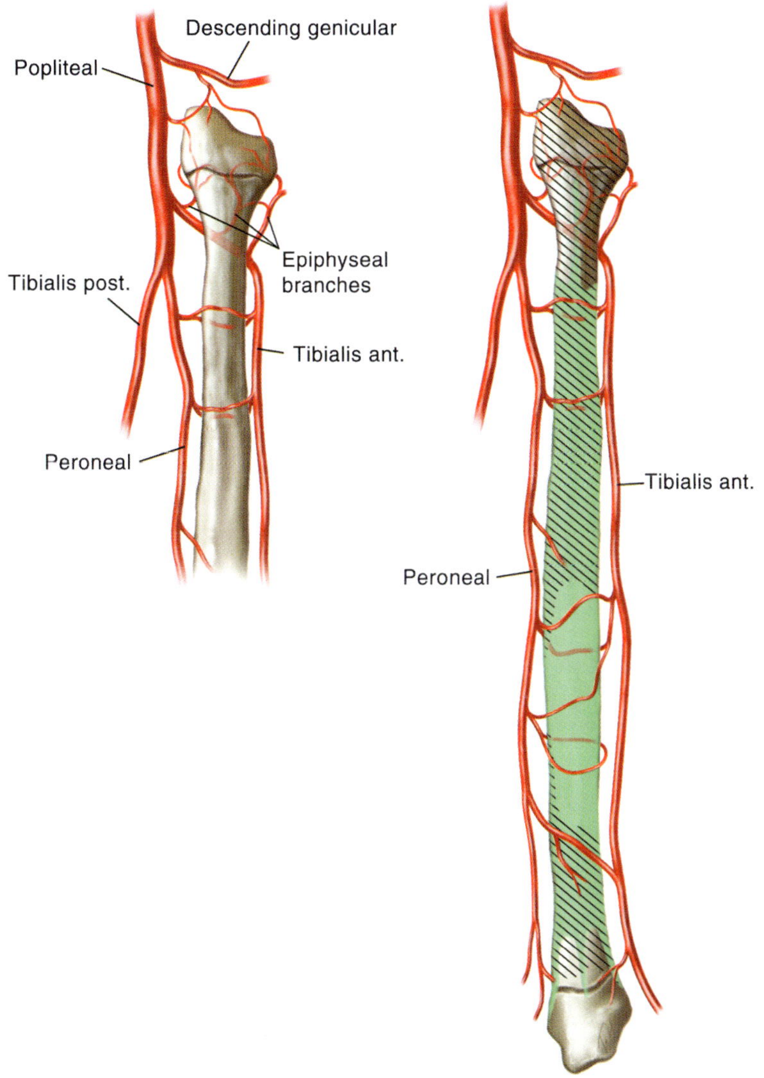

FIGURE 42B-3 The vascular supply to the fibula from the TA and peroneal arteries. The cutout shows a detailed view of circulation of the fibular epiphysis in children. The epiphysis has dual circulation from branches of the descending genicular artery (branch of the popliteal artery) and the TA artery. In children, the circulation to the epiphysis is completely independent of the peroneal artery supply to the diaphysis. Fibular circulation shown with areas supplied by peroneal artery (green) and TA circulation (hatched). Expanded view shows detailed view of pediatric epiphyseal circulation. (Copyright © Milan Stevanovic, MD and Frances Sharpe, MD.)

contraindications include smoking, medical comorbidities, and atherosclerotic vessels.

PREOPERATIVE PLANNING

When planning bone reconstruction with a vascularized free fibula, we must first establish that the patient has suitable donor- and recipient-site vascular anatomy. Conventional or magnetic resonance angiography (MRA) is used to evaluate the donor and recipient sites. Preoperative angiography is the most effective way of detecting congenital anomalies that would prevent harvest of the free fibula. In several studies, a vascular anomaly resulting in a change in the surgical plan was identified in up to 25% of patients.[47,49–51] Patients with a peroneus magnus artery, where the primary supply to the foot is from the peroneal artery, are not candidates for a vascularized free fibular graft, and another means of reconstruction must be chosen. For patients who have a peroneus magnus, clinical and Doppler examination of the pulses can provide misleading information, as the peroneus magnus often divides in the distal third of the leg into anterior and posterior tibial arteries.

In the setting of late reconstruction, where a bone defect has been present for a long period of time, a staged program of reconstruction should be used. A clean soft tissue bed is created prior to the application of the graft, and a spacer is used to create a bed for future fibular transfer. This spacer should be larger than the cross-sectional area of the planned fibula in order to prevent compression of the vascular pedicle and periosteal circulation to the fibula.

When bone reconstruction is required following infection, it is imperative that the infection be eradicated prior to bone grafting. This is accomplished with wide debridement of the infected bone, temporary spanning external fixation if necessary, systemic and/or local antibiotic delivery, and flap coverage if needed.[52]

In trauma, after provisional revascularization, bone stabilization is the first priority in reconstruction. This is followed by definitive revascularization, with immediate soft tissue reconstruction, including any necessary nerve and tendon repair or transfers. In addressing the soft tissue reconstruction, attention should be given to the importance of a vascular soft tissue envelope that is necessary for bone healing. We have found free muscle flaps to be very helpful in the reconstruction of soft tissue defects if the soft tissue defect cannot be reconstructed with an osteoseptocutaneous flap.

In general, we prefer to harvest the fibula with an osteocutaneous paddle for monitoring, and for soft tissue coverage, if needed.

SURGICAL TECHNIQUE FOR A DIAPHYSEAL GRAFT (WITH OR WITHOUT FASCIOCUTANEOUS FLAP)

A 2-team approach with 1 team preparing the recipient site and the other harvesting the contralateral fibula is the most efficient. Anesthetic support is as for other flaps with the patient maintained normothermic and normotensive with hydration sufficient to produce urine output at 80 to 100 mL/h. We prefer to use combined general and epidural anesthesia to improve perfusion of the graft, and to decrease postoperative pain.

The patient may be positioned supine, semilateral, or in the lateral decubitus position. The donor leg is draped free. A bump may be placed under the pelvis to internally rotate the leg. The bump should be removed after harvesting of the fibula to avoid prolonged compression of the sciatic nerve. After sterile preparation of the limb, a sterile tourniquet is placed about the proximal thigh.

The initial dissection is performed under tourniquet control. The skin incision is placed just posterior to the midlateral line of the leg. If an osteocutaneous flap is to be used, the skin paddle is centered over the septal perforators in the leg (Fig. 42B-4). A Doppler probe is used to identify the septal perforators on which the flap is based. The septal perforators to the skin are segmentally distributed with intervals of 3 to 5 cm along the whole length of the fibula. However, the most reliable cutaneous perforators are found in the distal two thirds of the leg and are posterior to the lateral margin of the fibula. Longer skin paddles can be harvested based on the presence of more proximal perforators (Fig. 42B-5).[10,31,33,34,38,39,41,53–55]

The fibula can be harvested from the fibular head to within 6 cm of the distal tibia-fibular syndesmosis.[56,57] The length of the harvested fibula should be 1 to 2 cm longer than the size of the defect for reconstruction of radial and ulnar defects as well as clavicular defects. For reconstruction of the humerus, an additional 2 to 4 cm of fibula should be harvested in order to seat the fibula within the medullary canal of the proximal and/or distal humerus. If the patient is skeletally immature, the distal fibular stump is fixed to the tibia with a transfixing screw to prevent mortise widening and valgus angulation of the ankle.[57]

The skin incision is placed on the lateral leg, carrying the incision to the level of the crural fascia. The fascia is sharply incised along the posterior margin of the skin paddle followed by the anterior margin. The skin paddle can then be elevated from the underlying muscle at the level of the muscle fascia, starting posterior and working toward the intermuscular septum. Careful dissection is used to identify and protect the septocutaneous and/or musculocutaneous perforators. These are usually encountered coming off of the posterior border of the fibula and penetrating through the anterior edge of the soleus, just posterior to the interval between the soleus and peroneus longus. Many times the

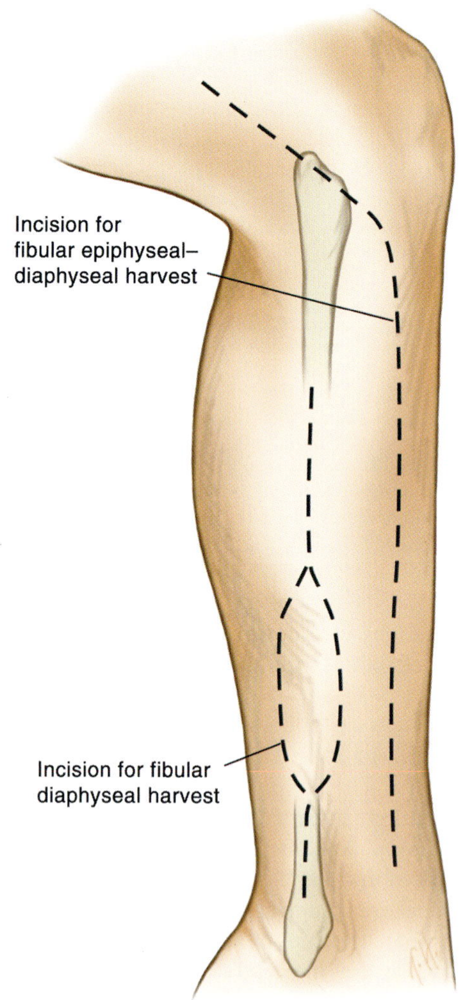

FIGURE 42B-4 Skin incisions: anterior incision for fibular epiphyseal harvest based on the tibialis anterior artery; posterior incision for fibular harvest based on the peroneal artery. (Copyright © Milan Stevanovic, MD and Frances Sharpe, MD.)

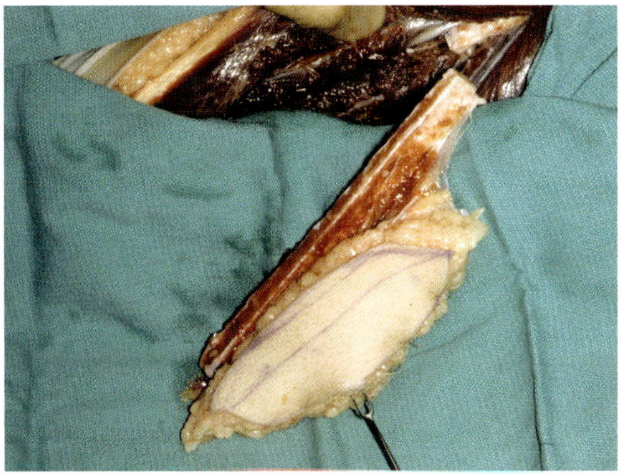

FIGURE 42B-5 Dissected fibula with skin paddle. (Copyright © Milan Stevanovic, MD and Frances Sharpe, MD.)

perforating vessels may be coming through the soleus muscle (musculocutaneous branches) (34%) or through the lateral intermuscular septum (66%).[36] If the perforating vessels are musculocutaneous, then the pedicle must be dissected through the soleus muscle or a portion of the soleus muscle containing the vessels is harvested with the skin paddle and fibula. Stay sutures should be placed throughout the dissection to hold the muscle fascia to the skin edges to prevent shearing injury to the perforating branches. The skin paddle is initially elevated from posterior. After the cutaneous perforators are identified the anterior aspect of the skin paddle can be elevated back to the lateral septum.

Next, the fibula is approached between the superficial posterior compartment (containing the soleus muscle) and the lateral compartment (containing the peroneal muscles) (Fig. 42B-6). The proximal incision is opened, incising the crural fascia and approaching the lateral edge of the fibula between the peroneus longus and soleus. Distally, the fascia is incised and the fibula is exposed along its anterior surface between peroneus longus and soleus, staying superficial to the periosteum. The exposure is continued from distal to proximal, using finger retraction to prevent injury to the deep peroneal nerve. The deep peroneal nerve is identified in the anterior compartment adjacent to the fibula in the proximal third of the dissection. It must be gently protected throughout the dissection as peroneal palsy has been described following this flap. We have had no cases of peroneal nerve palsy, since we have been using digital retraction of the anterior compartment musculature.

Exposure of the fibula is continued through an extraperiosteal dissection. It is not necessary to leave a cuff of muscle on the periosteum; however, care must be taken not to disturb the periosteum and the blood vessels running in it. Posteriorly, the soleus and flexor hallucis longus are extraperiosteally dissected from the fibula. The skin perforators penetrating through the most anterior aspect of the soleus must also be protected during this dissection. The peroneal artery and venae comitantes lie on the posterior surface of the interosseous membrane (IOM). They should not be separated from the posterior surface of the IOM.

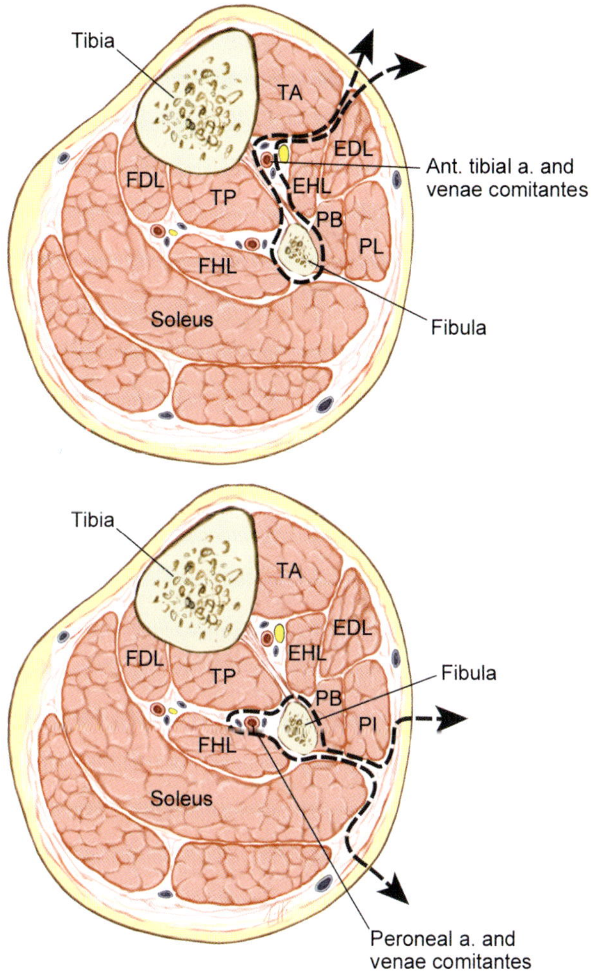

FIGURE 42B-6 The plane of dissection for the fibula harvest based on the peroneal and tibialis anterior arteries is shown in the cross-sectional diagrams. (Copyright © Milan Stevanovic, MD and Frances Sharpe, MD.)

The peroneus longus is extraperiosteally elevated off of the anterior aspect of the fibula with care taken not to injure the deep peroneal nerve that was identified at the start of the dissection. The dissection is then continued anteriorly medially elevating the extensor musculature off of the fibula and the lateral aspect of the IOM.

The IOM is perforated proximally and distally at the level required for harvesting the fibula and malleable retractors are used to protect the peroneal vessels and peroneal nerve as the fibula is cut with an oscillating or Gigli-type saw. The proximal osteotomy site should be placed proximal to where the peroneal artery lies immediately adjacent to the fibula. This is usually around 4 to 5 cm distal to the fibular head. One technique to help identify this position is the shape of the lateral aspect of the fibula. The fibula becomes more rounded rather than sharp-edged proximally, and we have found the peroneal artery is not adherent to the medial border of the fibula at this level. At the proximal and distal osteotomy sites, a 1.0-cm segment of fibula is removed. This facilitates mobilization of the fibula during the dissection of the vessels as well as facilitating ligation of the distal pedicle (Fig. 42B-2).

The peroneal vascular pedicle is ligated distally allowing the fibula to be mobilized from its bed. The fibula is controlled with a Kocher clamp placed into the distal medullary canal and the fibula is pulled laterally from its distal aspect as the IOM is carefully divided. Posteriorly, the flexor hallucis longus distally and tibialis posterior muscle proximally are dissected from the fibula and IOM. Multiple muscular branches are given off of the peroneal artery and should be ligated.

Once the fibula has been fully mobilized, the peroneal artery and accompanying vena comitantes are traced back to their junction with the posterior tibial artery. There are usually 2 concomitant veins. In order to obtain the longest possible pedicle, the more distal branching vein is ligated close to its branch point. This allows more proximal dissection of the peroneal artery and more proximal concomitant vein. The pedicle should be completely dissected and isolated with a vascular loop prior to releasing the tourniquet. The fibular graft is then placed back in its bed. The tourniquet is released and the vascularity to both the foot and the graft is checked. Usually, we wait for approximately 30 minutes, to monitor perfusion, prior to transecting the pedicle.

The fibular donor site can usually be closed primarily, although skin grafting may be necessary if a large skin paddle is used. After meticulous hemostasis is achieved, the origin of the flexor hallucis longus muscle should be sutured to the surrounding muscle (usually the deep fascia of the soleus) in order to preserve the resting length of the muscle and prevent flexion contracture of the great toe. A closed-system silastic drain is placed deep to the fascia and is left in place until there is <5 mL of drainage over a 24-hour period. To avoid the possibility of a postoperative compartment syndrome, the deep fascia should not be closed. The patient is placed into a short-leg posterior splint with a toe plate. Immobilization with a splint or cam walker is maintained for 3 weeks. Weight bearing as tolerated is begun after 2 weeks.[58]

SURGICAL TECHNIQUE FOR AN EPIPHYSEAL GRAFT

For skeletally immature patients who require reconstruction of the humeral epiphysis or distal radial epiphysis, the fibula and the proximal two thirds of the fibular diaphysis can be transferred on the TA artery. Trueta was one of the first to delineate the separate arterial supply of the diaphyseal and epiphyseal circulation. Until skeletal maturity, the fibular epiphysis is supplied through branches of the descending genicular artery and a branch of the TA artery. The proximal diaphysis receives a significant contribution to its circulation through the anterior tibial artery, allowing diaphyseal–epiphyseal transfer of the fibula based on the anterior tibial artery[30,46,59] (Fig. 42B-3).

The surgical technique for harvesting of the fibular epiphysis with proximal diaphysis was eloquently described in detail by Innocenti et al.[30] The surgical positioning and preparation is as described above. The surgical incision begins in the midlateral leg, centered over the middle of the anterior compartment. The incision curves posteriorly to cross over the proximal tip of the fibular head and extends proximally in the lateral thigh over the biceps femoris tendon (Fig. 42B-4). The deep dissection begins distally. The fascia is sharply incised at the intermuscular plane between the TA and the extensor digitorum longus (Fig. 42B-6). The common peroneal nerve is then identified proximally at the level of the fibular neck. It is mobilized from the surrounding soft tissues and protected throughout the remainder of the procedure. The dissection of the vascular pedicle begins distally, separating the deep peroneal nerve from the TA artery and concomitant veins. The TA artery and concomitant veins are mobilized along with a cuff of intermuscular septum. The IOM is divided on the tibial side of the vessels in order to preserve the periosteal branches from the TA artery to the fibular diaphysis. A muscular cuff of the EDL and PL are taken to preserve the delicate periosteal vessels. Exposure of the fibular head and the origin of the TA pedicle is done by sharply dividing the extensor digitorum longus, peroneus longus, and peroneus brevis. This is done 2 cm distal to their origin, preserving a muscular cuff that serves to protect the recurrent epiphyseal branch supplying the growth plate. The recurrent epiphyseal branch of the TA artery arises very close to the origin of the TA artery from common trunk of the popliteal artery. This is a very small and delicate artery and should not be separately isolated, but protected within this muscular cuff.

During the separation of the peroneal nerve from the TA pedicle, multiple muscular branches from the peroneal nerve are encountered and preserved throughout the dissection. These branches are sporadically encountered in the distal dissection, but more prevalent proximally. There is significant anatomic variation in the proximal motor branching of the peroneal nerve. In some circumstances, it is necessary to sacrifice 1 or more motor branches. These branches should be tagged for later neurorraphy or neurotization after the fibular dissection is completed. If it is necessary to intentionally sacrifice a motor branch, we prefer to do this close to its origin off of the deep peroneal nerve for later primary neurorraphy. Cutting the branch close to its entry into the muscle allows for retraction of the nerve into the muscle belly and inability for later primary neurorraphy.

With the anterior fibula exposed and the neurovascular dissection completed, the distal osteotomy can be performed at the required length for the planned reconstruction, incising the periosteum distal to the osteotomy site, thereby retaining an extra "cuff" of periosteum. This can provide a potential source of healing at the recipient site when using that cuff to overlap the union site. After completing the osteotomy, the proximal tibiofibular joint is opened. The lateral collateral ligament is severed as distally as possible. The tendon of the biceps femoris is divided longitudinally, taking the posterior half of the tendon with the fibula. This is later used to stabilize the fibular epiphysis at the recipient site. The anterior half of the biceps femoris tendon will be used to augment the stability of the lateral knee joint. Proximally, the branch of the descending genicular artery must be ligated. The medial collateral medial branches around the muscular cuff at the fibular

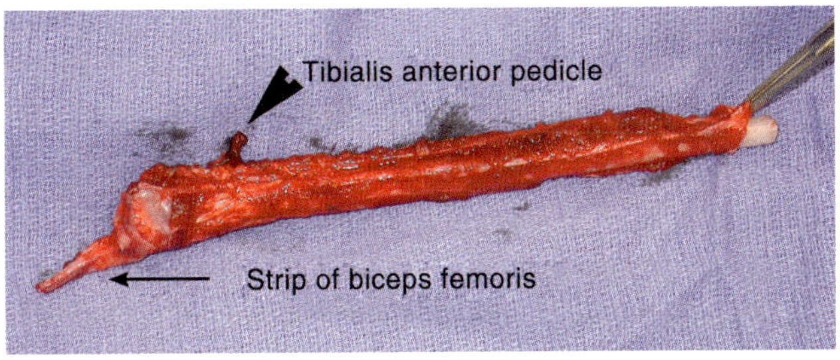

FIGURE 42B-7 Dissected fibular epiphysis and two thirds of the diaphysis on the tibialis anterior artery. (Copyright © Milan Stevanovic, MD and Frances Sharpe, MD.)

head are divided. The separation of the IOM can then be completed and the fibular head subluxed laterally. Now the origin of the TA artery can be identified in the posterior compartment. Dissection of the proximal pedicle should be completed and vessel loops placed around the isolated pedicle. The distal pedicle should then be ligated and transected at the osteotomy site. The tourniquet may then be released. Adequate perfusion should be noted either from bleeding from the muscular cuff or from the fibular diaphysis. Once the tissues have perfused, the graft may be harvested close to the branching site of the TA from the popliteal vessels (Fig. 42B-7).

Closure of the donor site requires meticulous hemostasis. Nerve branches are repaired under magnification. The preserved tendinous portion of the biceps femoris muscle should be secured through bone tunnels or suture anchors to the lateral portion of the tibia. Fascia is not closed. A drain is placed. The knee and ankle should be immobilized for approximately 3 weeks to protect the nerve repair and allow healing of the proximal anterior and lateral compartment muscles. At 3 weeks, a hinged knee brace may be used to neutralize varus stresses across the knee during healing of the repaired lateral structures. The immobilization may be discontinued at 6 weeks.

PREPARATION OF THE RECIPIENT SITE

Each recipient site presents a unique challenge related to access to recipient vessels, bone fixation, and patient rehabilitation. Preoperative planning of anticipated recipient vessels and types of fixation along with alternative options can minimize surgical time and reduce difficulties associated with these complex cases.

General guidelines for preoperative planning and site preparation are discussed above. Recipient sites require good recipient vessels with strong inflow. Ideally, a 2-team approach is taken to have 1 team preparing the recipient site and isolating the recipient vessels as the graft is being harvested. Stable fixation with plates reduces tension on the anastomotic site and promotes healing at the coaptation site. Intramedullary fixation is not used as this disrupts the endosteal blood supply and is less stable. Plates that provide 4 to 8 cortices of proximal and distal fixation and that can span the fibular graft are preferred. No periosteal stripping from the fibula is necessary below the plate. However, if the fibula is inserted into the medullary cavity, the periosteum from that portion of the fibula should be elevated off of the fibula and placed over the coaptation site. Liberal use of supplemental bone graft from the iliac crest is used at the proximal and distal sites. When the vascularized free fibula is not used as an osteofasciocutaneous flap, the outflow pressure is very low. For this reason, we recommend the anastomosis of only a single vein in order to increase the outflow pressure and improve the success of the vascular transfer. We choose the vein with the highest flow for repair and ligate the other concomitant vein. Postoperatively the skin paddle is monitored to ensure flap survival. The patient is treated similar to other free flap transfers and is kept warm and well hydrated. Anticoagulation is not routinely used in our institution.

Site-specific techniques are provided for common reconstructive sites in the upper extremity.

Site-specific Technique: Clavicle

- Indications: Relatively rare. Large clavicular defects with cosmetic deformity, function disability at the shoulder, or pain (Fig. 42B-8).
- Recipient vessels: Thoracoacromial artery and branch of the cephalic vein.
- Alternate vessels: Transverse cervical artery.
- Fixation: Precontoured plate and screws.

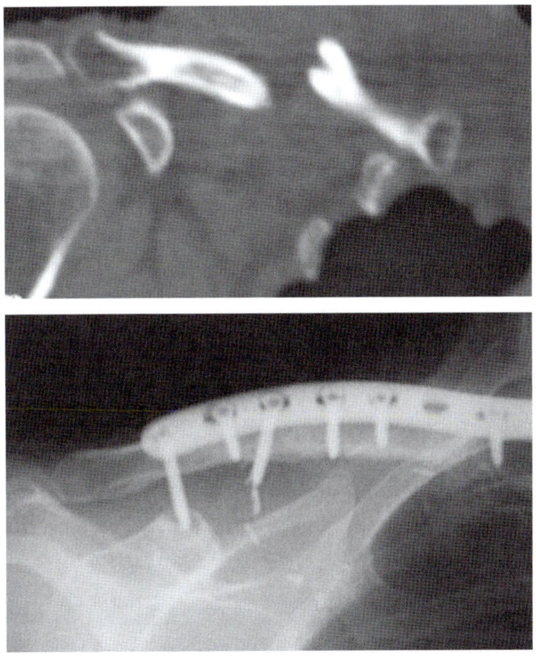

FIGURE 42B-8 Clavicular reconstruction: this 63-year-old woman developed a chronic infection of the clavicle after multiple failed fixation attempts. She developed chronic pain at the nonunion site. After radical debridement and placement of an antibiotic spacer for 6 weeks, a vascularized free fibular graft was used to bridge a 6-cm defect. Preoperative CT scan showing the atrophic nonunion site is seen above. Five-month postoperative view shows fibular healing and incorporation. (Copyright © Milan Stevanovic, MD and Frances Sharpe, MD.)

- Pearls: If necessary, the fibula can be osteotomized to reconstruct the curvature of the clavicle.
- Immobilization: Sling × 6 weeks. Codman pendulum exercises.

Site-specific Technique: Humerus

- Indications: Large defect from tumor, trauma, or infection. Can be used for humeral shaft reconstruction or primary shoulder fusion[24] (Fig. 42B-9).
- Pediatric patients: Sarcoma with need to reconstruct proximal humeral epiphysis.
- Recipient vessels: End-to-side brachial artery or profundus brachii with concomitant veins.
- Alternate vessels: Any proximal branch of the brachial artery or fibula can be rotated 180° and anastomosed to distal vessels from the brachial artery or profunda brachii or recurrent ulnar artery.
- Fixation: If possible, place fibula 2 cm inside the proximal and/or distal medullary canal. Spanning 3.5- or 4.5-mm plate. Plate is preferably placed on the medial side.
- Pearls:
  - The medial approach to the humerus provides easier access to the blood vessels, visualization and protection of the median and ulnar nerves, and low risk of radial nerve injury. Plate stabilization can be performed on the medial or anterior humerus through this approach.
  - Some authors recommend distal fixation of the fibula to the humerus. Vascular repair is facilitated by the ability to externally rotate the humerus. After completing the vascular anastomosis, proximal osteosynthesis is completed.[22]
  - Immobilization: Sling immobilization if fixation is stable. Shoulder immobilizer with abduction pillow and Desault or Velpeau bandaging are other options. Consider thoracobrachial casting if fixation is limited, especially for children requiring epiphyseal reconstruction. Casting can be performed preoperatively and 2 half shells created to facilitate postoperative placement.
  - Humeral fracture bracing should be used after 6 weeks of immobilization. Bracing should continue for activities for at least 6 months postoperatively to reduce the risk of stress fracture.[60]

Site-specific Technique: Radius and Ulna

- Indications: Large defect from tumor, trauma, or infection. Epiphyseal transfer in children for growth arrest that starts at a very young age (Fig. 42B-10).

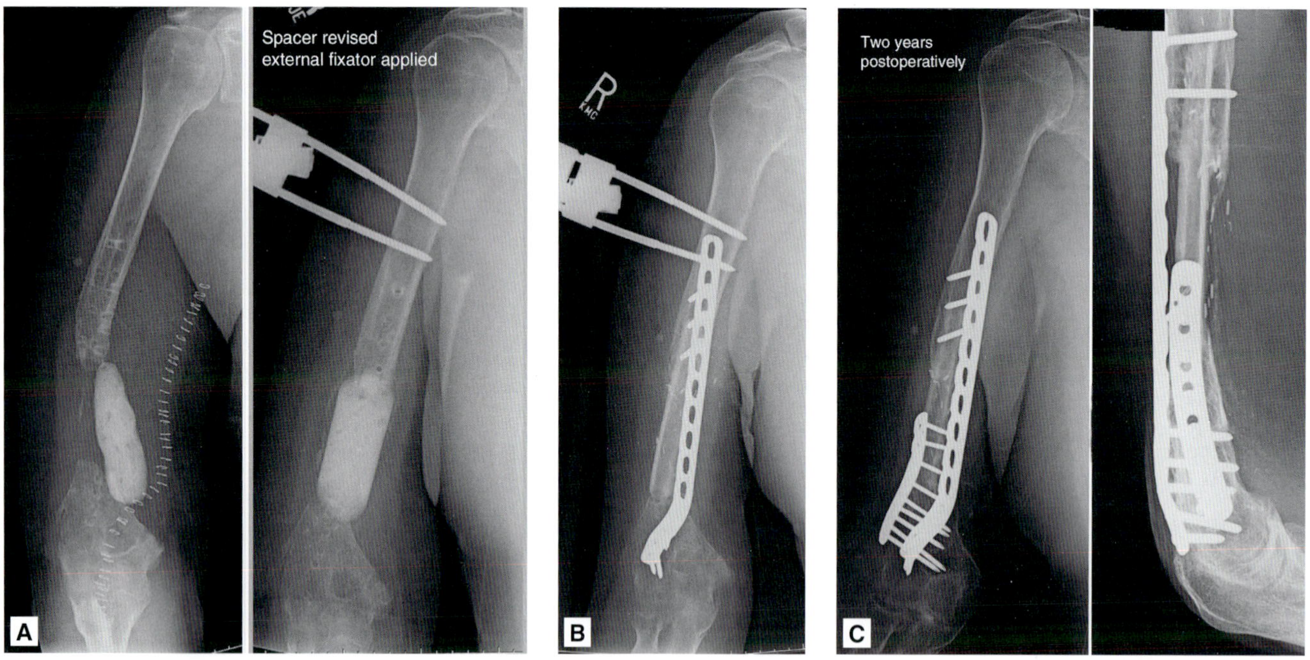

FIGURE 42B-9 Humeral reconstruction: a 42-year-old male sustained an open humerus fracture following motor cycle accident. The patient developed an infection after initial surgical stabilization and failed 5 subsequent surgical attempts to eradicate the infection. The patient presented to our clinic 2 years after injury with an open draining sinus and a bone defect filled by an antibiotic-containing cement spacer. After radical debridement and spacer replacement, a vascularized free fibula was used to reconstruct the distal half of his humerus. Additional surgery was necessary to achieve union at the distal coaptation site. Radiographically stable union was present at 6 months. However, he recovered only a limited arc of motion at the elbow (40° flexion–extension arc). **A.** Radiographs at presentation with displaced antibiotic spacer and unstable arm. At presentation, the patient had undergone 5 surgical procedures and had been on antibiotic therapy for almost 2 years. Revision debridement, antibiotic spacer, and application of external fixator were performed to prepare the soft tissue bed for reconstruction. **B.** At 4 months, there was good incorporation proximally, but limited progression of healing at the distal coaptation site. Supplemental plate stabilization across the distal site and iliac crest bone grafting was performed to achieve final union. **C.** Two-year follow-up radiographs. (Copyright © Milan Stevanovic, MD and Frances Sharpe, MD.)

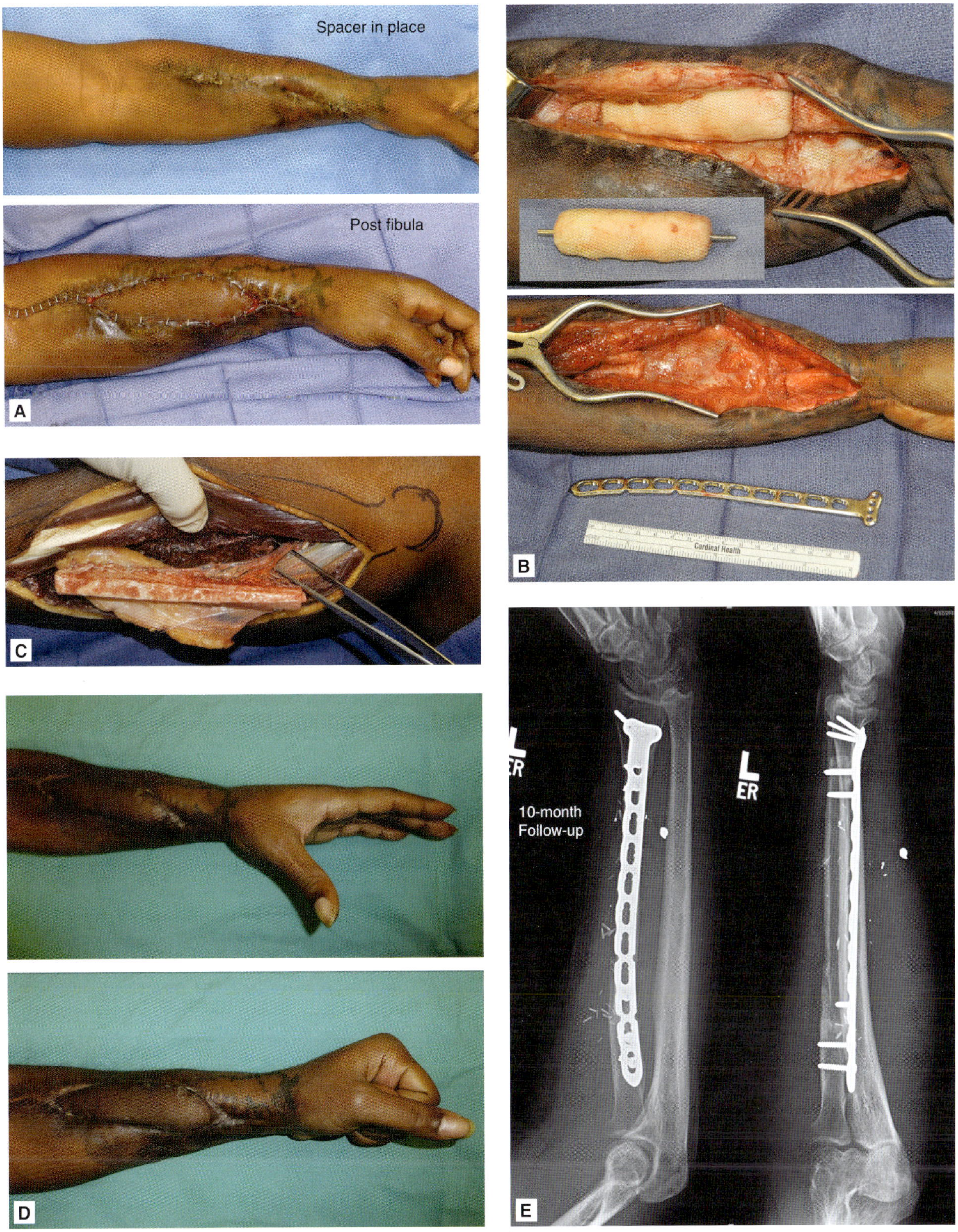

FIGURE 42B-10 Radial reconstruction. A 40-year-old patient developed an infection of the radius following radial fracture stabilization. The patient failed multiple attempts to control infection and achieve union. The infection was treated with radical debridement of the infected segment of the radius. An antibiotic-impregnated space was placed. Ten weeks later, the patient underwent radial reconstruction of a 10-cm defect using a vascularized free fibula transfer, harvested with a fasciocutaneous flap. Healing was radiographically stable by 3.5 months. **A.** Forearm appearance with spacer in place prior to reconstruction with vascularized free fibula and after free fibula. **B.** Cement spacer in place in the radius. Spacer removed and planned reconstructive plate for spanning the ~10-cm defect. **C.** Fibular harvest on peroneal pedicle. **D.** Forearm and function at 10 months. **E.** Radiographs at 10 months. (Copyright © Milan Stevanovic, MD and Frances Sharpe, MD.)

- Recipient vessels: End-to-side or end-to-end to the radial or ulnar arteries and concomitant veins. End-to-end anastomosis is preferred for osteoseptocutaneous flaps or flow-through flaps where the proximal and distal peroneal artery is anastomosed to the proximal and distal recipient vessel (radial artery).
- Alternate vessels: Anterior interosseous artery.
- Fixation: Long spanning plates when possible:
  - Precontoured plate that reproduces the radial bow for radius:
    - Long plates that provide metaphyseal fixation are available.
  - Similar for ulna:
    - Incorporation of olecranon in fixation construct as needed
- Pearls:
  - Strive for good coaptation at the proximal and distal osteosynthesis sites.
  - Iliac crest cancellous bone grafting to reduce the risk of nonunion.
- Immobilization: Long arm cast or sugar tong splint.

Site-specific Technique: Wrist Fusion

- Indications: Large defect from tumor, trauma, or infection with loss of the articular surface of the distal radius (Fig. 42B-11).
- Recipient vessels: End-to-side or end-to-end to the radial artery and concomitant vein. End-to-end anastomosis is preferred for osteoseptocutaneous flaps.
- Alternate vessels: Princeps pollicis.
- Fixation: Plate fixation to the third metacarpal distally with wrist fusion plate if available. Two plates may be necessary since fusion plates are usually not long enough to span both sites. A spanning plate that will accommodate metacarpal and radial diameters may also be used.
- Pearls:
  - A trough is created in the carpus to accommodate the fibular graft.
  - Try to achieve 15° to 20° of dorsiflexion by bending the plate.
  - If anastomosis is done to the princeps pollicis, then the fibula should be rotated 180°.
  - Iliac crest bone grafting at proximal and distal union sites.
- Above-elbow casting for 4 weeks can be converted to short arm casting through union.

Site-specific Technique: Metacarpal

- Indications: Relatively rare. We would use for first metacarpal reconstruction following tumor resection or severe trauma, especially in the setting of soft tissue loss.[61]
- Recipient vessels: Princeps pollicis and local superficial vein.
- Alternate vessels: Radial artery and concomitant vein.
- Fixation: Kirschner wires, screws, or small plates. Supplemental external fixation to radius and second metacarpal for stress neutralization.

COMPLICATIONS

Complication rates following vascularized free fibula grafting are frequent and combined donor- and recipient-site morbidity rates commonly range between 30% and 50%.[6,7,23,27,62–65]

Donor Site

Donor-site morbidity is widely reported. Most patients generally have mild complaints of aching or stiffness at the donor site.[65] As with any surgical procedure, risks related to poor wound healing, hematoma formation, and infection can occur. More serious complications are rare, but include great toe motor weakness, clawing of the great toe, subjective or objective ankle instability, valgus deformity, ankle stiffness, and transient and permanent peroneal motor and sensory deficits, and postoperative compartment syndrome.[65–71]

Shindo et al evaluated donor-site complications associated with harvesting osteoseptocutaneous flaps and identified a 7.5% incidence of major wound complications in 53 patients and a 20% incidence of minor wound complications. All major complications were seen in heavy smokers.[64]

Specific techniques to reduce donor-site complications include meticulous hemostasis at the donor site and use of drains to reduce the occurrence of postoperative hematoma formation, seroma formation, or compartment syndrome. Great toe weakness and flexion contracture can be minimized by a repair of the origin of the flexor hallucis muscle and postoperative immobilization in a splint with toe support for 3 weeks postoperatively. Instability or valgus deformity at the ankle may be reduced by syndesmotic screw placement when harvesting the fibula within 6 cm of the distal tibiofibular syndesmosis. Later stabilization creating a tibiofibular synostosis may be needed if instability persists. Peroneal nerve complications are frequently transient. Nevertheless, these can be minimized by gentle retraction and protection of the nerve during surgery.

Recipient Site

The most common recipient-site complication is a nonunion at the coaptation site(s) (12%-30%).[7,23,24,62,63,65] This is followed by stress fracture of the fibular graft (17%-20% for upper extremity reconstruction)[62,63,71] and infection (0%-10%).[25,26,63]

Stress fractures are less common in the upper extremity than in lower extremity. Stress fracture rates have been reported at a 35% incidence in lower extremity tibial reconstruction[72] compared with a 17% stress fracture rate seen in the radius and ulna[71] and a 20% rate in the humerus.[63,73] Most

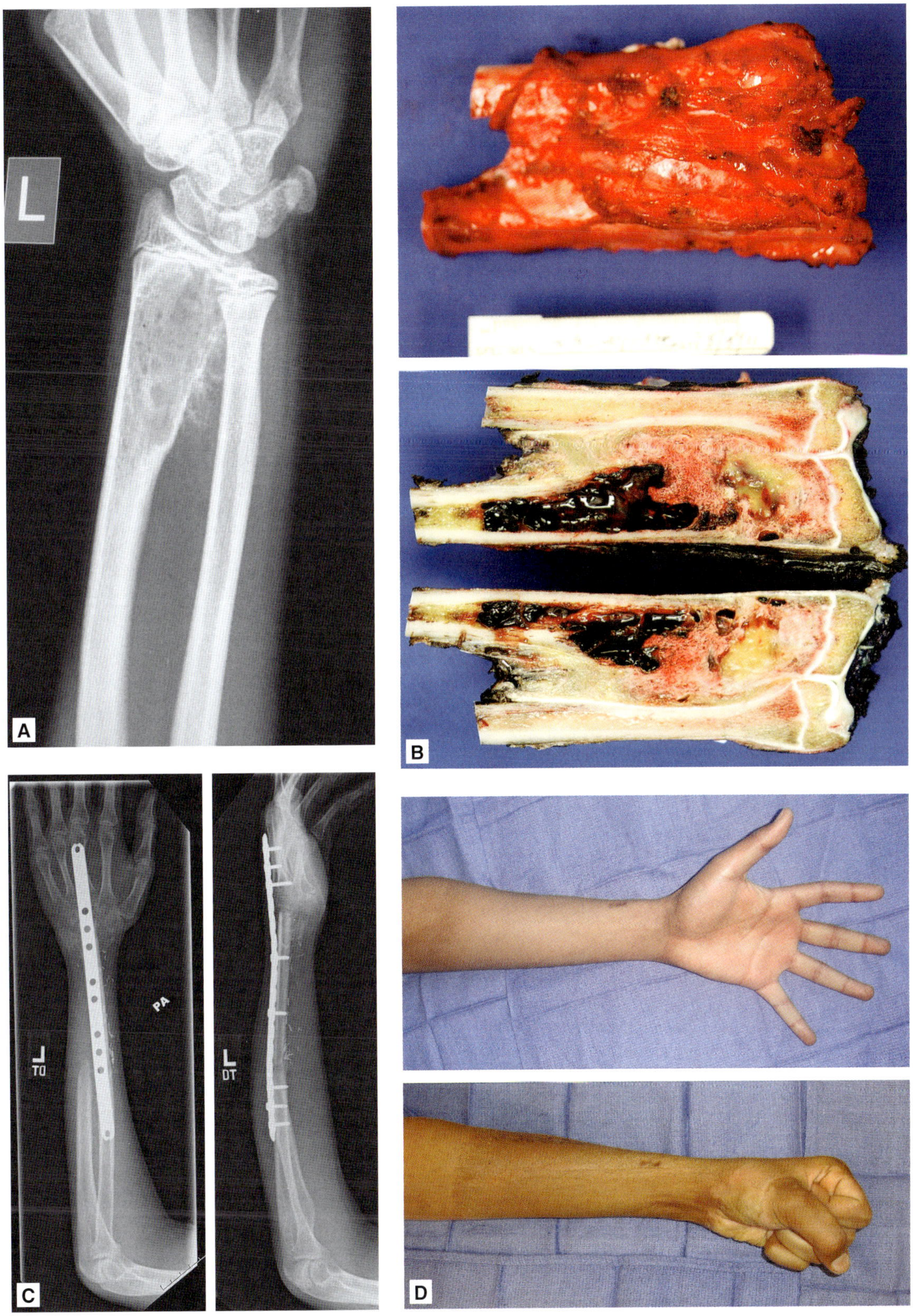

FIGURE 42B-11 Radial reconstruction and wrist fusion for osteosarcoma. A 15-year-old male diagnosed with osteosarcoma of the distal radius. The patient was treated with chemotherapy followed by radical resection of the distal radius and ulna. Radial reconstruction and wrist fusion was performed immediately at the time of resection. Radiation therapy was started after wound healing. Bone union was achieved after 9 months. **A.** Presenting PA radiograph. **B.** Resected specimen and coronal cross-section. **C.** Radiographs at 4 months postoperative. **D.** Function at 4 months postoperative. (Copyright © Milan Stevanovic, MD and Frances Sharpe, MD.)

stress fractures occurred within the first year of surgery, suggesting that external support in the form of a splint or fracture brace may be valuable during this recovery period. Partial or complete graft failure remains rare. Failure of the skin paddle is most frequently caused by venous congestion and can be salvaged nonsurgically if not severe. Failure or partial failure of the skin paddle does not always correlate with failure of the fibular graft.[27]

OUTCOMES

Successful union of the transferred vascularized fibula has been reported in several series to occur in greater than 90% of patients.[20,21,74,75] Although Weiland reported a 100% union rate for all upper extremity bone defects treated with a vascularized free fibula graft, Wood described in a larger series of patients a decrease in the union rate when including patients with defects of the humerus and clavicle. Both series had 100% union rate for forearm defects treated with vascularized bone grafts. De Boer et al noted higher union rates when the bone loss was due to trauma (95% union rate) as compared with tumor and infection (92% and 59%, respectively).[72] Many patients required secondary surgeries to achieve union at the coaptation sites.

In 1 of the largest series of vascularized bone grafts, Han et al from the Mayo Clinic reported the results of 132 patients who underwent a vascularized free fibula transfer for upper or lower extremity reconstruction. Their overall union rate was 81%. Factors that positively correlated with union included reconstruction following tumor resection and congenital anomalies with poorer outcomes following bone resection for osteomyelitis. Stable fixation at the coaptation site and supplemental bone grafting also increased union rates, as did graft vascularity.[71] Falder et al also found stable fixation at the coaptation site correlated with higher primary union rates.[62]

The time to union was variable, ranging from 4.7 to 9 months. Return to unrestricted activity was more difficult to determine. Han et al reported return to unrestricted activity for upper and lower extremity patients at 18 months.[71] Jupiter et al reported 6 of 9 patients with radial reconstructions returning to pre-injury occupation at an average of 2 years post reconstruction.[44]

Graft hypertrophy was less consistent in the upper extremity than in the lower extremity. Falder et al noted graft hypertrophy in 3/6 (50%) upper extremity reconstructions compared with 14/16 (87.5%) lower extremity reconstructions at time of final follow-up that ranged from 5 months to 14 years. They acknowledge the work of De Boer who showed that minor variations in the position of the rotation of the fibular graft can give a false impression of radiographic hypertrophy, with 10° of rotation from the neutral position increasing the radiographically measured width by as much as 20%.[62] Lazar et al compared graft hypertrophy in the upper and lower extremities in a small group of patients. They found that the graft hypertrophied similar to the lower extremity and the extent of cortical thickening increased over time.[76]

Innocenti et al reported their experience of vascularized reconstructions including the fibular epiphysis for reconstruction of the proximal humeral and distal radial epiphyses. Six patients who underwent reconstruction of the distal radius had regained approximately 70% of the range of motion of the contralateral limb at an average 3-year follow-up. There was remodeling of the distal fibular epiphysis that mimicked the normal contour of the distal radius and evidence of ongoing longitudinal growth in all surviving patients (5/6). For the humeral epiphyseal reconstructions, Onoda et al reported on 8 skeletally immature patients. The follow-up ranged from 9 months to 10 years. The grafts retained their vascularity and the epiphysis remained open radiographically and demonstrated longitudinal growth. The fibular epiphysis had remodeled to mimic the appearance of the humeral head, and patients recovered approximately 70% function of the contralateral limb.[23]

SUMMARY

Bone defects of the upper extremity managed with vascularized free fibular grafts either with or without a fasciocutaneous flap can produce excellent cosmetic and functional results with immediate structural integrity provided to the defect site. The use of a biologic solution to bone deficits also provides structural longevity unlike that provided by endoprosthetic reconstruction.

REFERENCES

1. Taylor G, Miller G, Ham F. The free vascularized bone graft. A clinical extension of microvascular techniques. *Plast Reconstr Surg.* 1975;55(5):533–544.
2. Strauch B, Murray D. Transfer of composite graft with immediate suture anastomosis of its vascular pedicle measuring less than 1 mm in external diameter using microsurgical techniques. *Plast Reconstr Surg.* 1967;40(4):325–329.
3. Strauch B, Bloomberg A, Lewin M. An experimental approach to mandibular replacement: island vascular composite rib grafts. *Br J Plast Surg.* 1971;24(4):334–341.
4. Ostrup L, Fredrickson J. Distant transfer of a free living bone graft by microvascular anastomoses. An experimental study. *Plast Reconstr Surg.* 1974;54(3):274–285.
5. Brunelli G, Guizzi P, Battison B, Vigasio A. A comparison of vascularized and non-vascularized bone transfer in rabbits: a radiographic, scintigraphic, and histologic evaluation. *J Reconstr Microsurg.* 1987;3(4):301–307.
6. Adani R, Delcroix L, Innocenti M, et al. Reconstruction of large posttraumatic skeletal defects of the forearm by vascularized free fibular graft. *Microsurgery.* 2004;24(6):423–429.
7. Adani R, Delcroix L, Tarallo L, Baccarani A, Innocenti M. Reconstruction of posttraumatic bone defects of the humerus with vascularized fibular graft. *J Shoulder Elbow Surg.* 2008;17(4):578–584.
8. Chew W, Low C, Tan S. Long-term results of free vascularized fibular graft. A clinical and radiographic evaluation. *Clin Orthop.* 1995;311:258–261.
9. del Pinal F, Innocenti M. Evolving concepts in the management of the bone gap in the upper limb. Long and small defects. *J Plast Reconstr Aesthet Surg.* 2007;60(7):776–792.
10. Gilbert A. Vascularized transfer of the fibular shaft. *Int J Microsurg.* 1979;1(2):100–102.

11. Innocenti M, Delcroix L, Balatri A. Vascularized growth plate transfer for distal radius reconstruction. *Semin Plast Surg.* 2008;22(3): 186–194.
12. Innocenti M, Delcroix L, Manfrini M, Ceruso M, Capanna R. Vascularized proximal fibular epiphyseal transfer for distal radial reconstruction. *J Bone Joint Surg Am.* 2004;86-A:1504–1511.
13. Jupiter J. Complex non-union of the humeral diaphysis. Treatment with a medial approach, an anterior plate, and a vascularized fibula graft. *J Bone Joint Surg Am.* 1990;72-A(5):701–707.
14. Mathoulin C, Gilbert A, Azze R. Congenital pseudarthrosis of the forearm: treatment of six cases with vascularized fibular graft and a review of the literature. *Microsurgery.* 1993;14(4):252–259.
15. Minami A, Kiyoshi K, Itoga H. Treatment of infected segmental defect of long bone with vascularized bone transfer. *J Reconstr Microsurg.* 1992;8(2):75–82.
16. Newington D, Sykes P. The versatility of the free fibula on the management of traumatic long bone defects. *Injury.* 1991;22(4):275–281.
17. Olekas J, Guobys A. Vascularised bone transfer for defects and pseudarthroses of forearm bones. *J Hand Surg Br.* 1991;16B(4):406–408.
18. Weiland A, Daniel R, Riley L. Application of the free vascularized bone graft in the treatment of malignant or aggressive bone tumors. *Johns Hopkins Med J.* 1977;140:85–96.
19. Weiland A, Kleinert H, Kutz J, Daniel R. Free vascularized bone grafts in surgery of the upper extremity. *J Hand Surg Am.* 1979;4(2): 129–144.
20. Weiland A, Moore J, Daniel R. Vascularized bone autografts. Experience with 41 cases. *Clin Orthop.* 1983;174:87–95.
21. Wood M. Upper extremity reconstruction by vascularized bone transfers: results and complications. *J Hand Surg Am.* 1987;12A(3): 422–427.
22. Wood M. Free vascularized fibular grafting—25 years' experience: tips, techniques and pearls. *Orthop Clin North Am.* 2007;38:1–12.
23. Onoda S, Sakuraba M, Asano T, et al. Use of vascularized free fibular head grafts for upper limb oncologic reconstruction. *Plast Reconstr Surg.* 2011;127:1244–1252.
24. Viehweger E, Gonzalez J-F, Launay F, Legre R, Jouve J-L, Bollini G. Arthrodese d' epaule avec fibula vascularisee apres resection tuborale de l'extremite superieure de l'humerus [Shoulder arthrodesis with vascularized fibular graft after tumor resection of the proximal humerus]. *Rev Chir Orthop Reparatrice Appar Mot.* 2005;91:523–529.
25. Zalavras C, Femino DT, Triche R, Zionts L, Stevanovic M. Reconstruction of large skeletal defects due to osteomyelitis with the vascularized fibular graft in children. *J Bone Joint Surg Am.* 2007;89A:2233–2240.
26. Rashid M, Hafeez S, Zia ul Islam M, et al. Limb salvage in malignant tumors of the upper limb using vascularised fibula. *J Plast Reconstr Aesthet Surg.* 2008;61:648–661.
27. Arai K, Toh S, Tsubo K, Nishikawa S, Narita S, Miura H. Complications of vascularized fibula graft for reconstruction of long bones. *Plast Reconstr Surg.* 2002;109(7):2301–2306.
28. Innocenti M, Ceruso M, Manfrini M, et al. Free vascularized growth-plate transfer after bone tumor resection in children. *J Reconstr Microsurg.* 1998;14(2):137–143.
29. Innocenti M, Delcroix L, Manfrini M, Ceruso M, Capanna R. Vascularized proximal fibular epiphyseal transfer for distal radial reconstruction. *J Bone Joint Surg Am.* 2005;87:237–246.
30. Innocenti M, Delcroix L, Romano G. Epiphyseal transplant: harvesting technique of the proximal fibula based on the anterior tibial artery. *Microsurgery.* 2005;25:284–292.
31. Chen Z-W, Wang Y. The study and clinical application of the osteocutaneous flap of the fibula. *Microsurgery.* 1983;4:11–16.
32. Yoshimura M, Shimamura K, Iwai Y, Yamauchi S, Ueno T. Free vascularized fibular transplant. A new method for monitoring circulation of the grafted fibula. *J Bone Joint Surg Am.* 1983;65-A(9):1295–1301.
33. Beppu M, Hanel D, Johnston G, Carmo J, Tsai T. The osteocutaneous fibula flap: an anatomic study. *J Reconstr Microsurg.* 1992;8(3): 215–223.
34. Cho BC, Kim SY, Park JW, Baik BS. Blood supply to osteocutaneous free fibula flap and peroneus longus muscle: prospective anatomic study and clinical applications. *Plast Reconstr Surg.* 2001;108(7): 1963–1971.
35. Futran N, Stack BJ, Payne L. Use of color Doppler flow imaging for preoperative assessment in fibular osteoseptocutaneous free tissue transfer. *Otolaryngol Head Neck Surg.* 1997;117(6):660–663.
36. Heitmann C, Khan F, Levin L. Vasculature of the peroneal artery: an anatomic study focused on the perforator vessels. *J Reconstr Microsurg.* 2003;19(3):157–162.
37. Manojlovic R. *Anatomy of the Osteoseptocutaneous Flap of Fibulae and Clinical Applications* [master's thesis]. Belgrade: University of Belgrade; 1989.
38. Ozalp T, Masquelet AC, Begue TC. Septocutaneous perforators of the peroneal artery relative to the fibula: anatomical basis of the use of pedicled fasciocutaneous flap. *Surg Radiol Anat.* 2006;28(1):54–58.
39. Papadimas D, Paraskeuopoulos T, Anagnostopoulou S. Cutaneous perforators of the peroneal artery: cadaveric study with implications in the design of the osteocutaneous free fibular flap. *Clin Anat.* 2009;22(7):826–833.
40. Schusterman M, Reece G, Miller M, Harris S. The osteocutaneous free fibula flap: is the skin paddle reliable? *Plast Reconstr Surg.* 1992;90(5):787–793.
41. Yu P, Chang EI, Hanasono MM. Design of a reliable skin paddle for the fibula osteocutaneous flap: perforator anatomy revisited. *Plast Reconstr Surg.* 2011;128(2):440–446.
42. Ruch D, Koman L. The fibula-flexor hallucis longus osteomuscular flap. *J Bone Joint Surg Br.* 1997;79-B(6):964–968.
43. Strauch B, Yu H-L, Chen Z-H, Liebling R. *Atlas of Microvascular Surgery.* New York: Thieme; 1993.
44. Jupiter J, Gerhard H, Guerrero J, Nunley J, Levin L. Treatment of segmental defects of the radius with use of vascularized osteoseptocutaneous fibular autogenous graft. *J Bone Joint Surg Am.* 1997;79-A(4):542–550.
45. McKee N, Haw P, Vettese T. Anatomic study of the nutrient foramen in the shaft of the fibula. *Clin Orthop.* 1984;184:141–144.
46. Taylor G, Wilson K, Rees M, Corlett R, Cole W. The anterior tibial vessels and their role in epiphyseal and diaphyseal transfer of the fibula: experimental study and clinical applications. *Br J Plast Surg.* 1988;41(5):451–469.
47. Manaster B, Coleman D, Bell D. Pre- and postoperative imaging of vascularized fibular grafts. *Radiology.* 1990;176(1):161–166.
48. Wei F, Chen H, Chuang C, Noordhoff M. Fibular osteoseptocutaneous flap: anatomic study and clinical application. *Plast Reconstr Surg.* 1986;78(2):191–200.
49. Blackwell K. Donor site evaluation for free flap transfer. *Am J Otolaryngol.* 1998;19(2):89–95.
50. Young D, Trablusy P, Anthony J. The need for preoperative leg angiography in fibula free flaps. *J Reconstr Microsurg.* 1994;10(5):283–287.
51. Disa J, Cordeiro P. The current role of preoperative arteriography in free fibula flaps. *Plast Reconstr Surg.* 1998;102(4):1083–1088.
52. Patzakis M, Mazur K, Wilkins J, Sherman R, Holtom P. Septopal beads and autogenous bone grafting for bone defects in patients with chronic osteomyelitis. *Clin Orthop.* 1993;295:112–118.
53. Iorio ML, Cheerharan M, Olding M. A systematic review and pooled analysis of peroneal artery perforators for fibula osteocutaneous and perforator flaps. *Plast Reconstr Surg.* 2012;130(3):600–607.
54. Schusterman MA, Reece GP, Miller MJ, Harris S. The osteocutaneous free fibula flap: is the skin paddle reliable? *Plast Reconstr Surg.* 1992;90(5):787–793.
55. Winters HA, de Jongh GJ. Reliability of the proximal skin paddle of the osteocutaneous free fibula flap: a prospective clinical study. *Plast Reconstr Surg.* 1999;103(3):846–849.
56. Gerwin M, Weiland A. Vascularized bone grafts to the upper extremity. Indications and techniques. *Hand Clin.* 1992;8(3):509–523.
57. Weiland A. Vascularized bone transfers. *Instr Course Lect.* 1984;33: 446–460.
58. Stevanovic M, Gutow A, Sharpe F. The management of bone defects of the forearm after trauma. *Hand Clin.* 1999;15:299–318.
59. Trueta J. The role of the vessels in osteogenesis. *J Bone Joint Surg Br.* 1963;45B(2):402–418.
60. Sarmiento A, Zagorski JB, Zych GA, Latta LL, Capps CA. Functional bracing for the treatment of fractures of the humeral diaphysis. *J Bone Joint Surg Am.* 2000;82(4):478–486.
61. Jones N, Dickenson B, Hansen S. Reconstruction of an entire metacarpal and metacarpophalangeal joint using a fibular osteocutaneous free flap and silicone arthroplasty. *J Hand Surg Am.* 2012;37A:310–315.
62. Falder S, Sinclair J, Rogers C, Townsend P. Long-term behaviour of the free vascularised fibula following reconstruction of large bony defects. *Br J Plast Surg.* 2003;56:571–584.

63. Eward W, Kontogeorgakos V, Levin L, Brigman B. Free vascularized fibular graft reconstruction of large skeletal defects after tumor resection. *Clin Orthop Relat Res*. 2010;468:590–598.
64. Shindo M, Fong B, Funk G, Karnell L. The fibula osteocutaneous flap in head and neck reconstruction. A critical evaluation of donor site morbidity. *Arch Otolaryngol Head Neck Surg*. 2000;126(12):1467–1472.
65. Tang C, Mahoney J, McKee M, et al. Donor site morbidity following vascularized fibular grafting. *Microsurgery*. 1998;18(6):383–386.
66. Anthony J, Rawnsley J, Benhaim P, Ritter E, Sadowsky S, Singer M. Donor leg morbidity and function after fibula free flap mandible reconstruction. *Plast Reconstr Surg*. 1995;96(1):146–152.
67. Goodacre T, Walker C, Jawad A, Jackson A, Brough M. Donor site morbidity following osteocutaneous free fibula transfer. *Br J Plast Surg*. 1990;43(4):410–412.
68. Lee E, Goh J, Helm R, Pho R. Donor site morbidity following resection of the fibula. *J Bone Joint Surg Br*. 1990;72(1):129–131.
69. Shpitzer T, Neligan P, Boyd B, Gullane P, Gur E, Freeman J. Leg morbidity and function following fibular free flap harvest. *Ann Plast Surg*. 1997;38(5):460–464.
70. Vail T, Urbaniak J. Donor-site morbidity with the use of vascularized autogenous fibular grafts. *J Bone Joint Surg Am*. 1996;78-A: 204–211.
71. Han C-S, Wood M, Bishop A, Cooney W 3rd. Vascularized bone transfer. *J Bone Joint Surg Am*. 1992;74(10):1441–1449.
72. De Boer H, Wood M, Hermans J. Reconstruction of large skeletal defects by vascularized fibula transfer. Factor that influenced the outcome of union in 62 cases. *Int Orthop*. 1990;14(2):121–128.
73. Adani R, Delcroix L, Innocenti M, Tarallo L, Baccarani A. Free fibula flap for humerus segmental reconstruction: report on 13 cases. *Chir Organi Mov*. 2008;91(1):21–26.
74. Hirayama T, Suematsu N, Inoue K, Baitoh C, Takemitsu Y. Free vascularised bone grafts in reconstruction of the upper extremity. *J Hand Surg Br*. 1985;10(2):169–175.
75. Yajimi H, Tamai S, Ono H, Kazuhisa K. Vascularized bone grafts to the upper extremities. *Plast Reconstr Surg*. 1998;101(3):727–735.
76. Lazar E, Rosenthal D, Jupiter J. Free vascularized fibular grafts: radiographic evidence of remodeling and hypertrophy. *AJR Am J Roentgenol*. 1993;161:613–615.

Nerve Compression Syndromes at the Elbow

David J. Slutsky, MD

43

PROXIMAL MEDIAN NEUROPATHY

Pronator Syndrome

Median nerve compression neuropathies in the distal arm and forearm are extremely uncommon when compared with CTS. The more proximal of the median nerve compression neuropathies is the pronator syndrome. The syndrome is classically associated with any of 4 potential areas of compression including the ligament of Struthers, the lacertus fibrosis, the aponeurotic fascia of the superficial or deep head of the pronator teres (PT), or the flexor digitorum sublimus (FDS) arch. Both carpal tunnel syndrome and anterior interosseous nerve (AIN) entrapment should be excluded.

ANATOMY

The median nerve arises from the medial and lateral cords of the brachial plexus. It contains the nerve root fibers from C6-T1. It lies lateral to the axillary artery but then crosses medial to it at the level of the coracobrachialis. At the elbow it travels behind the bicipital aponeurosis but in front of the brachialis. At distal part of the cubital fossa, the motor branches of the median nerve consistently collect into 3 fascicular groups.[1] There is an anterior group (to the PT and flexor carpi radialis [FCR]), a middle group (motor to the FDS and hand intrinsics, sensory to the thumb, index and middle fingers), and a posterior group (to the AIN branch). These branch groups can be traced proximally without harm, within the main trunk of the median nerve for 2.5 to 10 cm. The nerve and artery pass through the antecubital fossa underneath the lacertus fibrosis and give off branches to the palmaris longus (PL), FCR, flexor digitorum superficialis (FDS), and rarely the flexor digitorum profundus (FDP). The nerve then dives between the deep and superficial heads of the PT to which it supplies 1 to 4 branches. The fibrous arch of the PT lies 3 to 7.5 cm below the humeral epicondylar line. The fibrous arch of the superficialis arch lies 6.5 cm below the humeral epicondylar line. The median nerve enters the forearm deep to the fibrous arch of the FDS and emerges beneath the radial side of the muscle belly of the middle finger superficialis where it is quite superficial and near the PL tendon.

PATHOPHYSIOLOGY

The nerve may be compressed by the ligament of Struthers that may or may not be associated with a supracondylar process (1% of cases).[2] It spans the supracondylar process and medial epicondyle and creates an arcade that contains the median nerve and brachial artery. The ligament of Struthers has also been described in the absence of an associated supracondylar process. In the forearm, the median nerve can be compressed by the PT, the FDS arch, or the bicipital aponeurosis. Rare causes of compression include a persistent median artery, Gantzer muscle (accessory head of the FPL), and the palmaris profundus.[3]

HISTORY

Clinical symptoms of pronator syndrome include forearm pain as well as paresthesiae and hypoesthesia in the median nerve distribution. Symptoms are typically precipitated by activity, especially repetitive elbow flexion/extension and forearm pronation/supination. Nocturnal paresthesiae are not common unlike CTS. Numbness and tingling may also involve the thenar area supplied by the palmar cutaneous branch, which takes off proximal to the carpal transverse ligament and is not compressed in CTS.

PHYSICAL EXAM

Phalen and Durkan tests are negative unless CTS coexists. There may be a positive Tinel sign over the proximal nerve as well as a firm and tender PT and a tenderness along the median nerve in the proximal forearm. Manual compression of the median nerve over the PT for 30 seconds (ie, pronator compression test) may elicit paresthesiae in the median nerve distribution.[4] Pain or paresthesiae produced by resisted forearm supination in combination with resisted elbow flexion beyond 120° suggests compression at the bicipital aponeurosis. Paresthesiae resulting from resisted forearm pronation while the elbow is slowly extended from full flexion is indicative of compression between the 2 heads of the PT. Resisted proximal interphalangeal joint flexion of the middle finger producing paresthesiae in the radial 3 digits and/or pain over the FDS arch is consistent with entrapment under the fibrous origin of the FDS. These tests are however neither specific nor sensitive.[5]

ELECTRODIAGNOSTIC STUDIES

NCS are rarely diagnostic for pronator syndrome. There may be prolongation of the distal median sensory latencies as well as a reduced amplitude of the compound motor action potential (CMAP) to the abductor pollicis brevis. There may be slowing of forearm conduction, but this can be misleading since a reduced forearm NCV is seen up to 20% to 30% of the time when there is a markedly delayed distal median motor latency due to severe CTS. This slowing was initially thought to be due to retrograde nerve demyelination but is currently attributed to test artifact. Sequential needle stimulation of the median nerve in 1-cm increments while recording from the APB may identify an area of focal conduction block near the PT muscle. Nerve conduction studies during provocative maneuvers such as elbow flexion, forearm pronation, and middle finger flexion against resistance do not increase the yield.[6–8] The EMG however may be of some value since membrane instability may be seen in the median-innervated muscles including the PT, FCR, and FDS.

NONOPERATIVE MANAGEMENT

The hallmark of treatment consists of activity modification and NSAIDs. Steroid injections are of no benefit. Immobilization in an above-elbow splint with the elbow flexed 90° with slight forearm pronation and wrist flexion for 4 to 6 weeks may relieve pressure and traction on the median nerve. The majority of patients will respond to nonoperative therapy.

SURGICAL INDICATIONS

The diagnosis of this condition is mostly based on the exclusion of other causes. Many patients will have already undergone a carpal tunnel release. The main indication is failure to improve to conservative treatment combined with reproducible physical findings compatible with this diagnosis. A positive EMG demonstrating denervation of the proximal forearm muscles or MRI evidence of nerve compression due to an underlying tumor is another straightforward indication.

CONTRAINDICATIONS

A coexistent polyneuropathy, C6-7 radiculopathy, or a brachial plexitis (Parsonage-Turner syndrome) may mimic the physical findings and should be ruled out, since these conditions will not benefit from a median nerve decompression.

SURGICAL TECHNIQUE

The procedure is performed under tourniquet control. An anteromedial incision is made crossing the antecubital fossa, starting 5 cm above the elbow flexion crease. The medial antebrachial cutaneous nerve is isolated as it runs with the basilic vein. The median nerve is identified proximal to the elbow, next to the brachial artery, and it is traced distally, resecting the ligament of Struthers if present. The nerve is followed through the 2 heads of the PT where branches from the anterior bundle (FCR, PT fascicles) are given off. Both the superficial head of the PT and the FDS can be divided and tagged for later repair if better exposure is needed. The posterior (AIN branch) and the middle (intrinsic, sensory) bundles pass deep to the superficialis arch, which is also incised. Epineurotomy or internal neurolysis is of no benefit. Subcutaneous transposition of the median nerve is also not recommended.

POSTOPERATIVE MANAGEMENT

Postoperatively, the arm is placed in an above-elbow splint for comfort with the elbow flexed 90°, the forearm in mid-pronation, and the wrist in slight flexion. Gentle elbow range-of-motion exercises are begun after the first week unless it is necessary to protect the reattachment of the PT and/or FDS insertions. Resistive activities are avoided until 6 to 8 weeks postoperatively.

COMPLICATIONS

One main complication is failure to improve due to a misdiagnosis. Vascular injury is a significant risk and meticulous hemostasis is necessary. Injury of the proximal muscular branches ranging from neuropraxia to laceration can be minimized by careful nerve handling.

OUTCOMES

Surgical decompression generally yields good results. Olehnik et al reported improvement in 77% of their patients with 33/36 patients returning to work.[4] A clinical series by Johnson et al and Hartz et al reported improvement in 92% of patients.[7,8] Patients with normal NCS seem to fare better than patients with abnormal studies, which may be related to the severity of the compression.

Anterior Interosseous Nerve Syndrome

Isolated AIN palsy is a rare occurrence. It accounts for <1% of all upper extremity peripheral neuropathies.[2] It is still uncertain as to whether this syndrome is due to a neuritis and/or a compressive neuropathy.

ANATOMY

The AIN is the largest muscular branch that emerges from the median nerve. It innervates the FDP to the index and middle fingers, the FPL, and the pronator quadratus (PQ). The terminal portion also provides sensory innervation to the carpal joints. The AIN arises from the median nerve on the dorsoradial surface about 5 to 8 cm distal to the medial epicondyle. The AIN travels between the FDS and FDP, and then passes dorsally in the interval between the FPL and FDP, giving off 2 to 6 branches to each of these muscles. The nerve reaches the anterior surface of the interosseous membrane and travels with the anterior interosseous artery where it passes deep to the PQ that it also innervates. It ends by sending sensory afferent branches to the intercarpal, radiocarpal, and distal radioulnar joints.

PATHOPHYSIOLOGY

The AIN may be compressed by fibrous bands from the deep (most common) or superficial head of the PT, the fibrous arcade of the FDS, enlarged bursae or tumors, aberrant or thrombosed vessels, an accessory bicipital aponeurosis, and fractures of the forearm and distal humerus.

HISTORY

AIN syndrome (AINS) must be differentiated from a brachial plexus neuritis, that is, Parsonage-Turner syndrome.[9] In a brachial neuritis there is usually no history of trauma. The pain symptoms may be unrelated to the motor findings, and can appear spontaneously or following a viral illness or vaccination. By contrast, the patient with AINS will usually have a history of trauma or repetitive injury. They typically complain of vague, aching pain in the proximal forearm, which occurs at rest and is exacerbated by activity. The patient can have difficulty with writing and pinching activities, and they may have sensory abnormalities in the median nerve distribution.

PHYSICAL EXAM

AINS is characterized by loss of function of the FPL and FDP to the index and sometimes the long finger and the PQ. Sensibility is unaffected. The patient cannot make an "O" sign (Fig. 43-1A). During attempted tip pinch, the index finger extends at the distal interphalangeal joint with compensatory increased flexion at the proximal interphalangeal joint. The thumb hyperextends at the interphalangeal joint with increased flexion of the metacarpophalangeal joint. The PQ can be tested by resisted pronation with the elbow flexed to relax the PT.

AINS can be incomplete, with either weakness or absence of the FPL or FDP of the index finger alone with normal PQ function. All of the profundus tendons may be AIN innervated, with subsequent weakness of all the fingers. The hand intrinsic muscles may be affected if there is a coexisting Martin-Gruber anastomosis. This is where C8-T1 motor fibers destined for the hand intrinsics travel in the median nerve. They then cross over to the ulnar nerve, usually through connections in the AIN (91%). If the FDS is also innervated by the AIN (30%), patients may present with weakness in this muscle also.[10]

One must differentiate between AINS and rupture of the FDP or FPL, which may occur from rheumatoid arthritis, Kienböck disease, and scaphoid nonunion. The integrity of these tendons can be assessed by observing the tenodesis effect of the FPL and the index FDP that causes passive thumb IP and index DIP flexion with passive wrist extension.

ELECTRODIAGNOSTIC STUDIES

Shoulder girdle and upper limb EMG should be performed to rule out a brachial plexitis. In this case there will be membrane instability in the proximal limb muscles. The most appropriate technique involves recording the CMAP from the PQ. The active surface electrode is placed in the midline dorsally, 3 cm proximal to the ulnar styloid. The median nerve is stimulated at the cubital fossa. The mean onset latency for the PQ is 3.6 ± 0.4 milliseconds, with a side-to-side difference of 0.4 millisecond. Normal amplitudes range from 2.0 to 5.5 mV.[11] Side-to-side comparative latencies are helpful in establishing the diagnosis. EMG testing of the PQ and FPL muscles should demonstrate signs of membrane instability (Fig. 43-1B).

SURGICAL INDICATIONS

If there is no improvement either clinically or by EMG studies 4 to 6 months after onset, surgical exploration is indicated. Even though return of function has been reported up to 18 months after onset of symptoms, expectant treatment is less predictable than surgical intervention.

SURGICAL TECHNIQUE

The surgical approach for AIN palsy is essentially the same as for pronator syndrome. The procedure is performed under tourniquet control. An anteromedial incision is made crossing the antecubital fossa, starting 5 cm above the elbow flexion crease. The medial antebrachial cutaneous nerve is isolated as it runs with the basilic vein. The median nerve is identified proximal to the elbow, next to the brachial artery, and it is traced distally, resecting the ligament of Struthers if present. The nerve is followed through the 2 heads of the PT where branches from the anterior bundle (FCR, PT fascicles) are given off. Both the superficial head of the PT and the FDS can be divided and tagged for later repair if better exposure is needed. The posterior (AIN branch) and the middle (intrinsic, sensory) bundles pass deep to the superficialis arch, which is also incised. A microscopic interfascicular neurolysis of the AIN up to the elbow should be considered in cases where there is no obvious compression site since

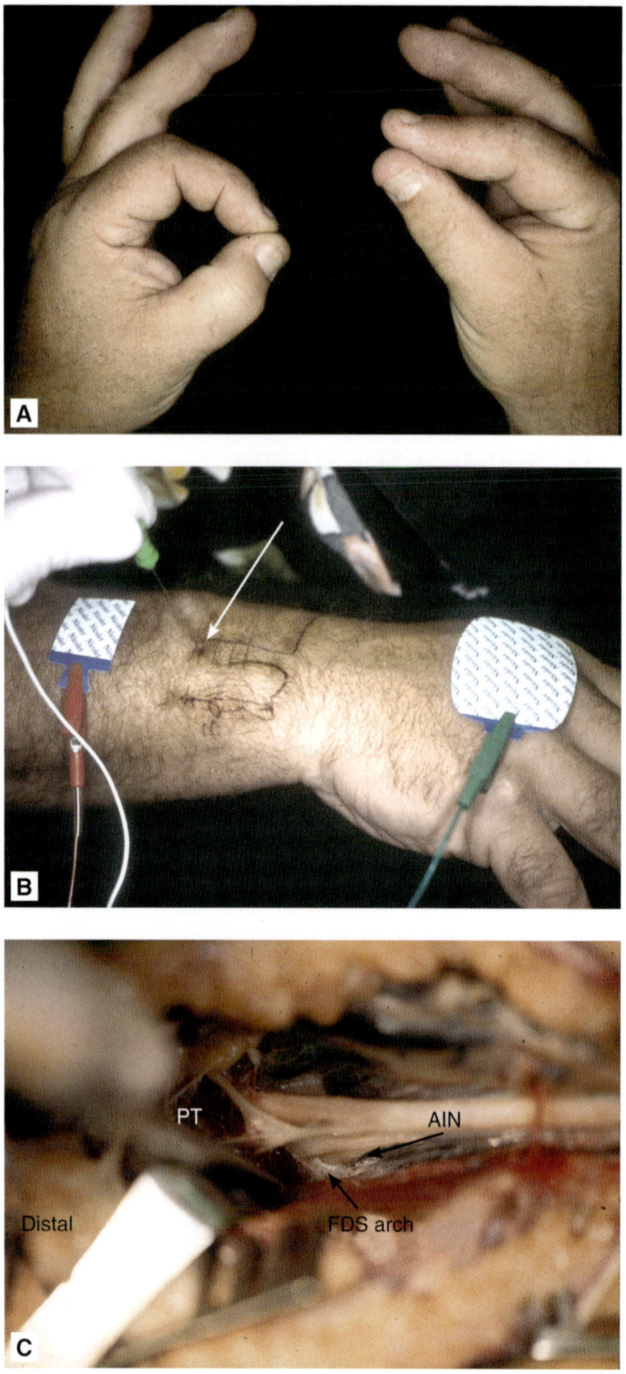

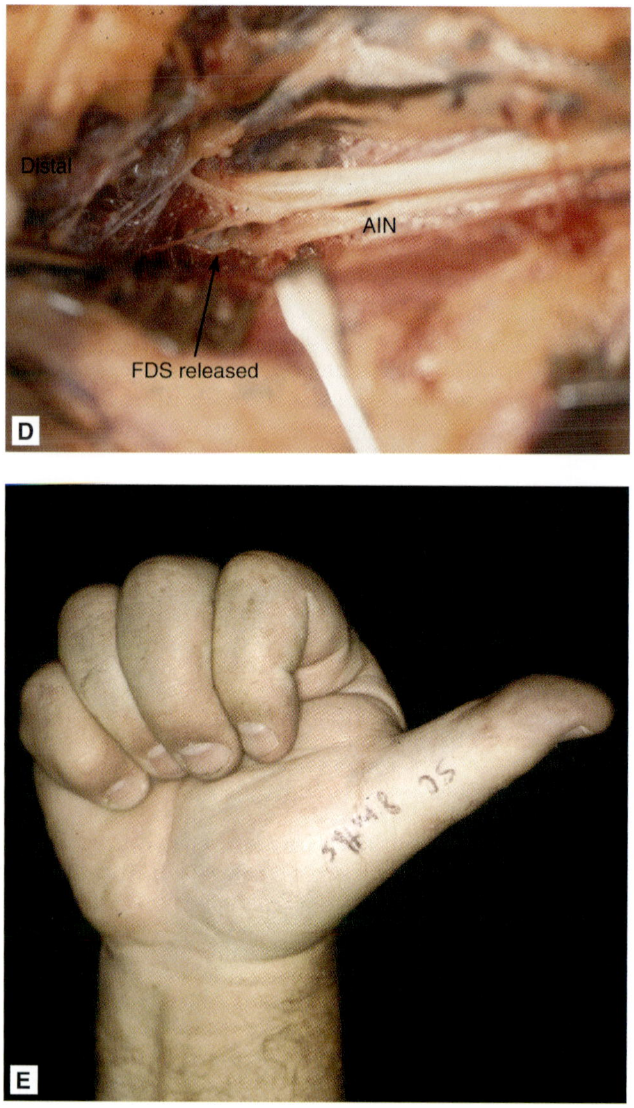

FIGURE 43-1 Anterior interosseous nerve compression. **A.** Inability to perform the "O" sign. **B.** Needle placement during EMG of the pronator quadratus. **C.** Anteromedial approach to the median nerve. Note the fibrous border of the sublimus muscle. AIN, anterior interosseous nerve; PT, pronator teres. **D.** Following release of the sublimus arch (FDS). **E.** Clinical photo at 8 months showing active flexion of the distal phalanx of the index but no active thumb interphalangeal joint flexion.

hourglass-like fascicular constrictions that are not discernible through the intact epineurium have been reported.[12]

POSTOPERATIVE MANAGEMENT

The arm is placed in a bulky, above-elbow plaster splint that maintains the elbow at 90° of flexion, the forearm in 45° of pronation, and the wrist in slight flexion for comfort.

COMPLICATIONS

The anatomy and hence the complications are virtually identical to those of pronator syndrome.

OUTCOMES

Clinical improvement may be seen for up to 1 year following surgery, but recovery is often incomplete (Fig. 43-1C-E).

Nonsurgical management is recommended for brachial plexus neuritis–induced AIN palsy.

ULNAR NEUROPATHIES

Proximal Ulnar Neuropathy

Ulnar nerve compression at the elbow is second only to median nerve compression in the carpal tunnel as the most common neuropathy in the upper limb.

ANATOMY

The ulnar nerve arises from the medial cord of the brachial plexus. It contains the nerve root fibers from C8-T1. It provides the motor supply to the hypothenar muscles, the ulnar 2 lumbricals, the interosseous muscles, the adductor pollicis, flexor carpi ulnaris (FCU), and the profundus to the ring and small fingers. Its sensory distribution includes the palmar surface of the small and the ulnar half of the ring finger as well as the dorsoulnar carpus. It lies medial to the axillary artery and continues distally to the midarm. It then passes through a fibrous canal (erroneously labeled the arcade of Struthers) from the anterior to the posterior compartments of the arm. The canal is approximately 6 cm in length with the proximal extent located approximately 10 cm from the medial epicondyle. The proximal opening of the canal is a V-shaped window made up of the medial intermuscular septum that divides the anterior and the posterior compartments of the arm and the internal brachial ligament.[13] The internal brachial ligament supports the origin of the most superficial layer of the medial head of the triceps, from the inferior border of the teres major to its fusion back to the septum. This layer appears as an oblique muscular curtain covering the medial aspect of the ulnar nerve. In 1 anatomic study, the internal brachial ligament was present in 22/30 specimens.[14] The septum makes up the anterior part of the canal; the rest is made up of deep investing fascia and epimysium of the triceps muscle. The nerve is often accompanied by the superior ulnar collateral artery. At the elbow it lies between the medial epicondyle and the olecranon where it is covered by Osborne ligament. It enters the forearm between the 2 heads of the FCU covered by a fibrous aponeurosis (the cubital tunnel). It runs deep to the FCU until the distal forearm.

PATHOPHYSIOLOGY

The ulnar nerve may be compressed anywhere from 10 cm proximal to approximately 5 cm distal to the medial epicondyle. Five potential sites for compression have been described. The most proximal site is the point at which the ulnar nerve takes a direction change as it passes through the V-shaped canal from the anterior to the posterior compartments of the arm. Hourglass indentations of the nerve were found at this point in 11/11 cadaver arms.[12] Although this has been labeled the arcade of Struthers, recent investigators have shown this to be historically incorrect.[15,16] They note that Sir John Struthers did not, in fact, describe an arcade over the ulnar nerve, but that he did describe the internal brachial ligament. Other investigators however have noted a musculotendinous arcade in 8/60 cadaver arms that could form a secondary compression site after anterior transposition of the ulnar nerve.[17] The second site is at the medial epicondyle when a cubitus valgus deformity is present. The third site is the olecranon groove, which is a fibro-osseous tunnel bounded anteriorly by the medial epicondyle, laterally by the olecranon and ulnohumeral ligament, and covered by a fibroaponeurotic band. Compression at this site can be caused by lesions within the groove such as tumors, conditions outside the groove such as external compression or anomalous muscles, and conditions that predispose the nerve to displace from the groove. The fourth site is where the nerve passes between the 2 heads of the FCU muscle. The floor of the passageway through FCU is the medial collateral ligament of the elbow and the roof is a fibrous band (Osborne ligament, the arcuate ligament) that is a continuation of the fibroaponeurotic covering of the epicondylar groove.[18] In some instances an anomalous muscle, such as the anconeus epitrochlearis, can compress the nerve (Fig. 43-2).

At the elbow the ulnar nerve contains about 20 fascicles including the motor branches to the forearm muscles. The fascicles within a nerve are not uniformly affected by compression. Those on the periphery of a nerve sustain greater injury than centrally placed fascicles. The motor fascicles to the FCU and the intrinsics are centrally located, whereas the sensory fibers are superficially located. The usual sites of compression in cubital tunnel syndrome are superficial to the nerve (Osborne ligament, arcade of Struthers).[19] The internal topography of the ulnar nerve at the elbow explains the relative sparing of the FCU and FDP since their motor fibers lay deep within the nerve.[20] The intrinsics are often uninvolved until the late stages of compression for similar

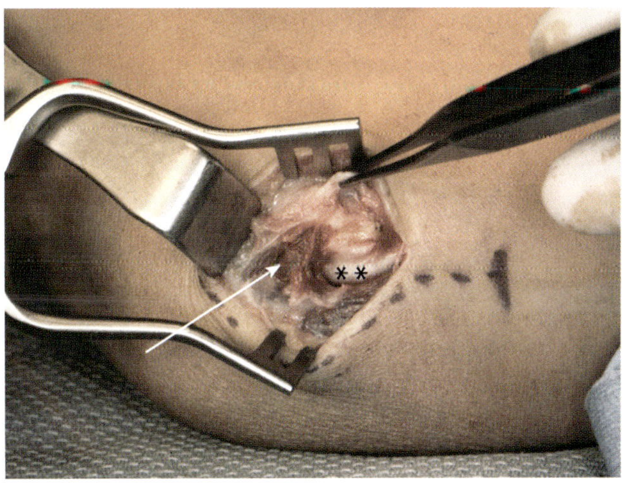

FIGURE 43-2 Anconeus epitrochlearis. Note how this anomalous muscle attaches to the fibroaponeurotic bands (forceps) that arc over the ulnar nerve (*) as it traverses the olecranon groove.

reasons, whereas the superficially located sensory fibers are more susceptible to early compression.

HISTORY

The patient presents with complaints of numbness and/or tingling in the small and/or ring finger. Symptoms can range from mild numbness in the ring and little fingers to severe pain on the medial aspect of the elbow with dysesthesias radiating distally into the hand. In chronic cases, patients may complain of a loss of dexterity with fine manipulation tasks. Symptoms are provoked by repetitive or sustained elbow flexion activities.

PHYSICAL EXAM

The ulnar nerve is palpated for enlargement or subluxation during elbow flexion. There may be a positive Tinel sign at the epicondylar groove or over the proximal FCU. An elbow flexion test is performed and consists of placing the elbow in full flexion with a hyperextended wrist, while manual pressure is applied to the nerve for 1 minute.[21] The test is considered positive when paresthesiae and/or numbness occur in the ulnar nerve distribution of the hand. False-positive results occur in approximately 10% of patients.

There may be a sensory deficit involving all or part of the ulnar nerve distribution including the dorsoulnar carpus.

When intrinsic muscle weakness is severe, there is often clawing of the ring and little fingers. One may see a positive Froment sign (flexion of the interphalangeal joint of the thumb with side pinch), a positive Jeanne's sign (hyperextension of the metacarpophalangeal joint of the thumb), and paradoxical abduction of the small finger due to a paralyzed third palmar interosseous (positive Wartenberg sign). Extrinsic weakness may involve the FDP to the little finger and ring finger. Weakness of the FCU rarely occurs.

ELECTRODIAGNOSTIC STUDIES

Ulnar Nerve Motor Studies. Ulnar motor studies are more popular than ulnar sensory studies. The distal motor latency is determined by recording from an electrode placed over the midpoint of the abductor digiti minimi (ADM) while stimulating the ulnar nerve 8 cm proximally (S1). Normal values include a DML ≤3.6 milliseconds and amplitude >4.0 MV. Alternatively, the latencies can be measured from the first dorsal interosseous (FDI), which then assesses conduction through the deep motor branch of the ulnar nerve. The FDI to ADM latency should not exceed 2.0 milliseconds. The ulnar nerve is then stimulated 4 cm distal to the medial epicondyle (S2). By subtracting the latency for S1 from S2 and measuring the intervening distance, the forearm conduction velocity is obtained. Ulnar nerve conduction across the cubital tunnel is calculated by stimulating the nerve at S3, which is 12 cm proximal to S2, and subtracting the latencies. Most labs measure conduction with the elbow flexed between 90° and 135°. Normal forearm NCV is >48 m/s. Across the cubital tunnel the NCV should be >45 m/s. More than 10 m/s of slowing between the above- and below-elbow NCV is abnormal. Amplitude drops of >20% are a more sensitive indicator of conduction block or axonal loss.

Ulnar Nerve Sensory Studies. Ring electrodes are placed on the small finger and the ulnar nerve is stimulated 14 cm proximally. Recordings are also taken from the ring finger after stimulation of both the ulnar and median nerves. This allows for comparison of the ulnar to the median SNAPs. Normal peak sensory latencies are ≤3.5 and <0.5 milliseconds median–ulnar difference. Mixed palmar orthodromic studies can be elicited by stimulating the ulnar nerve in the fourth web space and recording over the ulnar nerve at the wrist 8 cm proximally. This measures the sensory nerve conduction through Guyon canal. Normal values are <2.2 milliseconds.

Conduction velocities can be misleading if the surface measurement of the nerve is off, even by 1 cm. Testing inaccuracies also occur following ulnar nerve transposition, since the nerve no longer follows its anatomic course. With longer conduction distances an area of focal block may be missed since it tends to be averaged out. Segmental stimulation of the ulnar nerve skirts these pitfalls and is a sensitive method for determining focal conduction abnormalities. Measurement errors are minimized since the nerve is localized at each stimulation site. If the nerve is stimulated in 1-cm segments, a >0.40-millisecond jump in NCV is indicative of a focal abnormality. If the nerve is stimulated in 1-in increments, a >0.75-millisecond jump is abnormal.[22] There is a poor correlation between the area of focal conduction block and the site of entrapment at time of surgery. This is likely due to the fact that if there is a partial conduction block, it is necessary to turn up the gain on the stimulation in order to obtain a response. With increasing current, the current flow tends to arc ahead of the stimulation, resulting in depolarization ahead of the applied stimulus site.

Across-elbow sensory nerve studies have also been described.[23] The above- and below-elbow stimulation sites are the same as S2 and S3 for the motor studies, but in this case the SNAPs are recorded from ring electrodes placed on the small finger. Normal NCV values are >50 m/s. Combining ulnar motor and sensory techniques adds useful information in complex cases, where clinical exam fails to localize the lesion. Conduction to the dorsal cutaneous branch of the ulnar nerve can be measured. This test is relatively insensitive for detecting proximal ulnar nerve compression, since it is abnormal in only 55% of patients with cubital tunnel syndrome.[24]

Electromyography demonstrates axonal degeneration in muscles. Since these changes are seen in chronic neuropathies, electromyography is not as useful as conduction times for the diagnosis of early nerve compression. When muscle abnormalities are noted, they are usually initially seen in the intrinsic muscles, generally the FDI, followed in frequency by the muscles in the hypothenar eminence.

NONOPERATIVE TREATMENT

Most acute or subacute cases resolve by activity modification with avoidance of activities that require repetitive elbow flexion and avoiding external pressure from leaning on their medial elbow or forearm. Alterations can sometimes be made in the workplace such as positioning a computer keyboard so that the operator's elbows are not acutely flexed. When symptoms are severe and have persisted for weeks, temporarily immobilizing the elbow in approximately 35° of flexion and the wrist in neutral may provide relief. Patients are instructed to wear the splint day and night for 3 to 4 weeks. Nonsteroidal anti-inflammatory can be helpful, but corticosteroid injections around the nerve are ineffective.

SURGICAL INDICATIONS

Sensory loss in the ulnar nerve distribution with EMG and clinical evidence of intrinsic denervation are major indications. In these cases conservative treatment is not justified. Across-elbow motor conduction <45 m/s with a >20% drop in amplitude is another strong indication. Relative drop of >10 m/s is a softer indication that should be approached cautiously, since technical error can produce this quite easily. Focal slowing on segmental stimulation is another appropriate indication.

CONTRAINDICATIONS

Ulnar nerve symptoms due to brachial plexus compression from a Pancoast tumor or a C8-T1 radiculopathy are infrequent contraindications. Some authors maintain that normal electrodiagnostic studies are another contraindication to surgery. Patients with normal electrodiagnostic studies but appropriate signs and symptoms (McGowan Stage I: paresthesia and numbness but no weakness) however can still benefit from surgery and are appropriate candidates if conservative measures over a 3- to 6-month period have failed.[25]

SURGICAL TECHNIQUE

Surgery can be divided into 2 groups of procedures, decompression without transposition of the ulnar nerve and decompression with transposition of the nerve. The procedures are performed under axillary block or general anesthesia using a tourniquet.

SUBCUTANEOUS ANTERIOR TRANSPOSITION

A 5-cm posteromedial incision is made centered around the medial epicondyle. Branches of the medial antebrachial cutaneous nerve are identified and protected. The deep fascia overlying the proximal ulnar nerve is divided as well as any associated ligament of Struthers. The fascia over the nerve is released sequentially: first in the upper arm, followed by the fibroaponeurotic covering of the epicondylar groove, then Osborne ligament at the cubital tunnel, and, finally, the fascia where the nerve passes between the 2 heads of the FCU. A 1-cm segment of the medial intermuscular septum is resected where it attaches to the epicondyle to prevent a secondary site of compression, taking care to prevent injury to fragile veins medial to the septum. Articular branches to the elbow are divided, but motor branches to the FCU should be preserved. A vessel loop is placed around the nerve that is then gently transposed anterior to the medial epicondyle along with the superior ulnar collateral vessels. A 1 cm wide medially based flap of fascia from the common flexor origin can be turned down and sutured to the proximal skin edge to prevent posterior subluxation of the nerve. The patient uses a sling for comfort postoperatively and is started on progressive elbow extension as tolerated. These same principles can be applied to a mini incision technique (Fig. 43-3A and B).

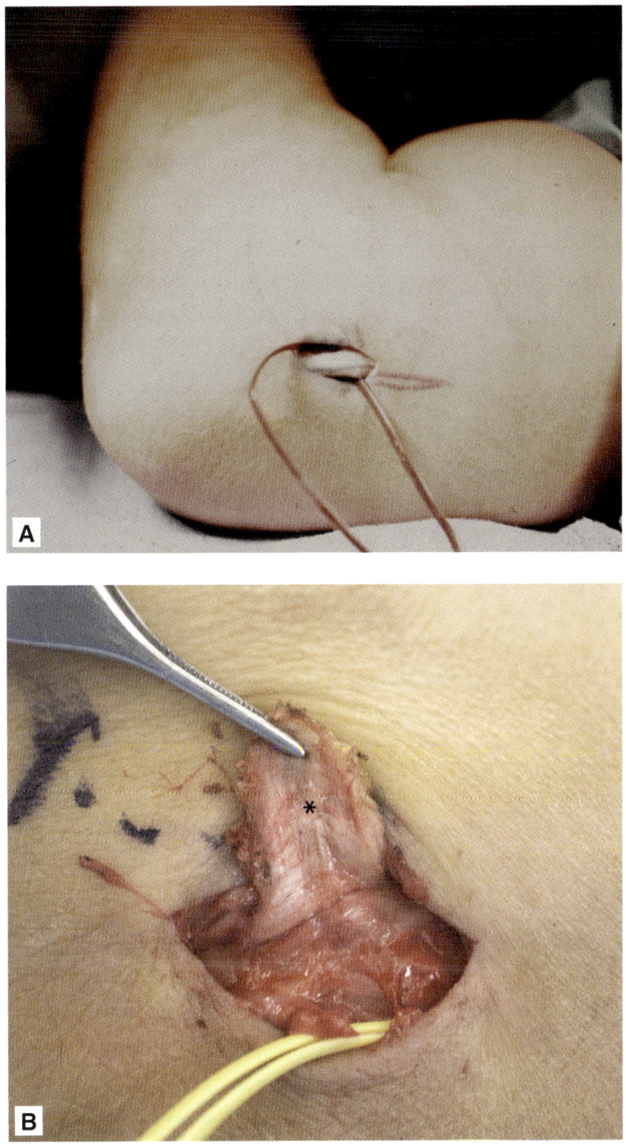

FIGURE 43-3 **A.** Mini-incision subcutaneous ulnar nerve transposition. **B.** Creation of a fascial sling to prevent posterior subluxation of the ulnar nerve after transposition.

SUBMUSCULAR TRANSPOSITION

A slightly larger incision is made and the nerve is decompressed in a similar fashion. A Z-plasty lengthening of the common flexor origin is preserved and the nerve is transposed deep to the muscle. Care must be taken to divide the fibrous attachment of the FDS to the humeral epicondyle to prevent secondary impingement while avoiding injury to the medial collateral ligament of the elbow. The ulnar nerve is now positioned onto the bed of the brachialis muscle. The flexor-pronator mass is then repaired with 2-0 nonabsorbable sutures (Fig. 43-4A-C). Postoperatively the elbow is immobilized at 90° for 4 weeks, allowing elbow flexion but no extension. The elbow is then gradually extended over the ensuring 2 to 4 weeks.

COMPLICATIONS

The most dire complication is ulnar nerve laceration. More commonly, injury to the medial antebrachial cutaneous nerve results in a tender scar and hypoesthesia along the medial forearm. Injury to the superior ulnar collateral artery or its branches is a cause of postoperative hematoma. The median nerve lies on the brachialis just behind the medial intermuscular septum and is at risk during resection of the distal septum or with aggressive retraction. Large intramuscular veins medial to the septum can also be injured during this step and are very difficult to ligate. Secondary entrapment due to creation of a fascial sling can occur with subcutaneous transpositions. Postoperative ulnar nerve subluxation due to a failure of this sling can result in painful paresthesiae with elbow flexion. Secondary impingement may also occur following a submuscular transposition due to a failure to release the deep fibers of the sublimus origin on the medial epicondyle. The ulnar collateral ligament can also be injured during this step that can lead to postoperative elbow instability.

OUTCOMES

As in CTS, the patient's clinical findings and response to conservative measures should be a major determinant in the surgical decision making. In 1 study, 92% of patients recovered grade 3 motor strength or better.[26] The results are largely determined by the preoperative degree of compression. When there are constant symptoms, demyelination is present and recovery may take 6 to 8 months. Residual sensory complaints are common. Even though intrinsic wasting rarely recovers in an adult, prevention of further denervation is crucial.

RADIAL NEUROPATHIES

Upper Arm

ANATOMY

The radial nerve arises from the posterior cord of the brachial plexus. It receives contributions from C5-C8 spinal

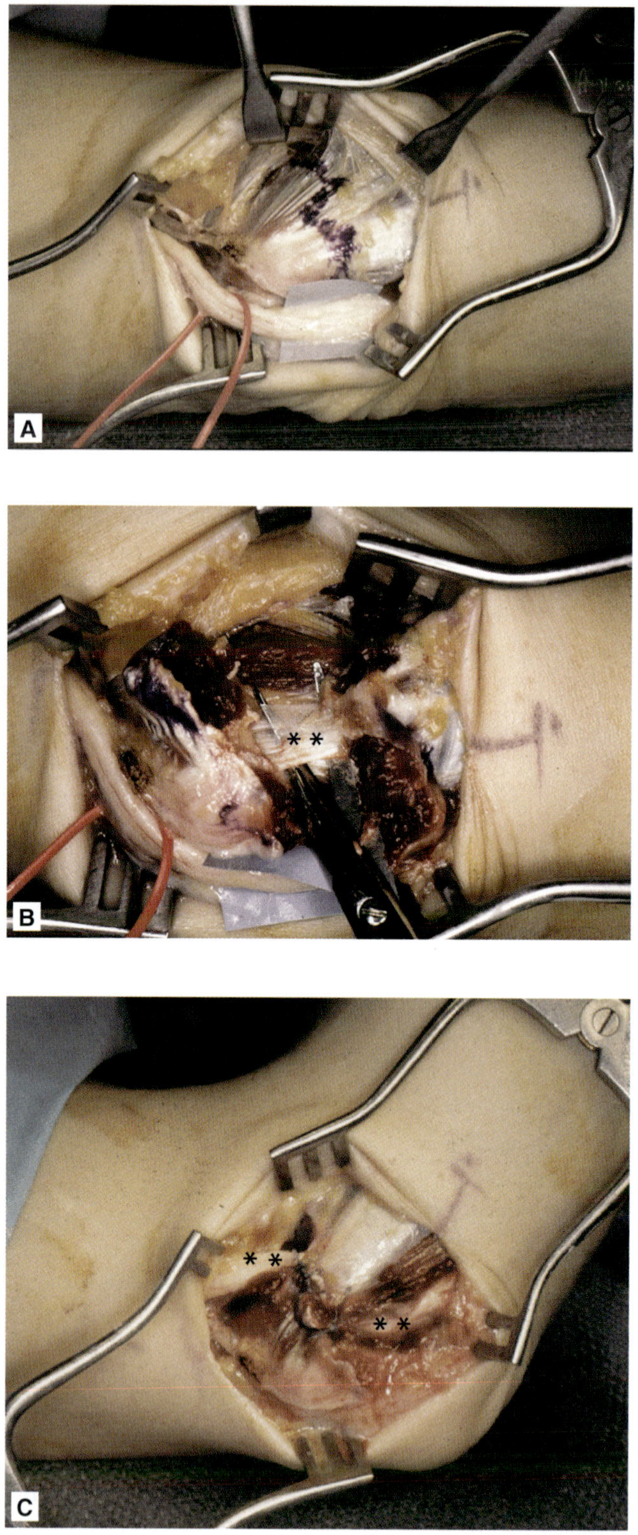

FIGURE 43-4 Submuscular ulnar nerve transposition. **A.** The ulnar nerve has been released and is being retracted by a vessel loop. The Z-plasty lengthening of the common flexor origin has been outlined. **B.** Scissors are behind the fibrous origin of the sublimus that must be released to prevent secondary ulnar nerve impingement following transposition. **C.** Course of the ulnar nerve (*) following the submuscular transposition and repair of the common flexor origin.

roots. The nerve contains approximately 16,000 myelinated fibers. It runs medial to the axillary artery. At the level of the coracobrachialis it courses posteriorly to lie in the spiral groove of the humerus. In the lower arm it pierces the lateral intermuscular septum to run between the brachialis and brachioradialis. Opposite the head of the radius there are some fibrous bands from the joint's capsule and immediately distal to this, the nerve is regularly crossed by several prominent veins, the "leash of Henry." It divides 2 cm distal to the elbow into a superficial radial sensory branch (SRN) and a deep motor branch, the posterior interosseous nerve (PIN). It gives off branches to the extensor carpi radialis longus and brevis, brachioradialis, and anconeus before giving off the PIN branch. The PIN continues on between the superficial and deep head of the supinator muscle, to exit on the dorsal forearm. After it emerges from the distal border of the supinator, the PIN sends branches to the extensor digitorum communis, extensor carpi ulnaris, extensor digiti quinti, extensor pollicis longus and brevis, and the extensor indicis proprius (EIP) in descending order, although there may be considerable variation.

HISTORY

In the arm region, the radial nerve is often injured in association with some form of unconsciousness. In a Saturday night palsy, an obtunded patient sits with their arm over a chair back or rests their head on the lateral surface of their arm. Alternatively, the radial nerve can be compressed in the groove between the brachialis and forearm muscles when 1 person rests their head on the middle third of the arm of another, that is, honeymooner's palsy.

PHYSICAL EXAM

The patient will typically present with a wrist drop and an inability to extend the fingers, thumb, or wrist. In addition, the brachioradialis will be affected along with variable involvement of the triceps. They will also have diminished sensation over the dorsum of the first web space.

ELECTRODIAGNOSTIC STUDIES

The NCS typically demonstrates the absence of the superficial radial SNAP.[26] Motor recordings are more difficult since no muscle is sufficiently isolated from other radially innervated muscles. A surface electrode over the EIP results in a volume-conducted response from the adjacent radial innervated muscles, which makes side-to-side amplitude comparisons difficult. Radial nerve recordings using needle electrodes in the EIP are more common as a result, which makes it difficult to approximate the degree of axonal loss by assessing the amplitudes. The EMG however is quite useful, and permits a relatively accurate localization of the lesion. In a spiral groove lesion, for example, all 3 heads of the triceps should be normal, with denervation of the brachioradialis and all muscles distal to it.

SURGICAL INDICATIONS

For the majority of patients, nonoperative treatment is the mainstay. A failure to improve within 6 months combined with a nonadvancing Tinel sign is an indication for exploration.

CONTRAINDICATIONS

The time for reinnervation must thus take the distance from the injury to the motor end plate into account. As a general rule, motor end plates degrade at about 1% per week, and the nerve regenerates about 1 in per month. By 12 months the nerve will have grown approximately 12 in and there will be a 50% loss of end plates; hence, the maximum length that a nerve can grow to restore motor function is approximately 13 to 18 in. For practical purposes, nerve decompression will be of no value with injuries that are more than 18 months old (>75% loss of end plates) and alternative methods should be explored.

SURGICAL TECHNIQUE

A 6- to 8-cm incision is made over the posterolateral aspect of the midhumerus. The radial nerve is identified in the spiral groove and followed distally through the intermuscular septum. Any obvious areas of nerve constriction or loss of the normal striations (bands of Fontana) should undergo an epineurolysis. The use of intraoperative nerve stimulation will help differentiate a neuroma-in-continuity from nonviable nerve tissue. In the former case an internal neurolysis is justified versus excision and grafting.

POSTOPERATIVE MANAGEMENT

Immediate elbow mobilization is instituted following nerve decompression or neurolysis. Nerve grafting may require temporary elbow splinting for 4 weeks, but it is preferable to insert a graft of sufficient length to allow early elbow extension.

COMPLICATIONS

The radial nerve is accompanied by the radial collateral artery in the spiral groove, which is at risk during decompression. Injury to the muscular branches may result in permanent denervation of 1 or more heads of the triceps. Injury to the posterior cutaneous nerve of the forearm may result in a tender scar and hypoesthesia.

Forearm

Entrapment of the PIN at the elbow can result in 2 separate clinical syndromes. Although the same nerve is compressed, the clinical presentation may be different and merely represents 2 ends of the spectrum of PIN compression. The PIN is said to be a motor nerve, but it also contains sensory nerve branches from which the pain from radial tunnel compression is derived. The different clinical presentation may reflect the internal fascicular topography of the radial nerve. Pain symptoms predominate with nerve compression secondary to superficial structures and motor paralysis occurs from compression from below due to lesions arising from the radiocapitellar joint.

PATHOPHYSIOLOGY

As it travels distally through the radial tunnel the PIN may potentially be entrapped by fibrous bands anterior to the radiocapitellar joint, the radial recurrent leash of vessels, the fibrous edge of the extensor carpi radialis brevis (ECRB), the proximal border of the supinator, that is, the arcade of Frohse, or the distal edge of the supinator muscle.

Radial Tunnel Syndrome

HISTORY

The presenting complaint in radial tunnel syndrome is proximal forearm pain often coexisting with lateral epicondylitis, without sensory or motor loss. The patient often gives a history of performing repetitive pronation/supination activities such as using a screwdriver. The symptoms of radial tunnel syndrome often coexist and overlap those of lateral epicondylitis.

PHYSICAL EXAM

A number of provocative tests have been described including resisted extension of the middle finger, which tenses the ECRB and entraps the nerve, tenderness over the supinator muscle, and pain with resisted supination. None are pathognomonic for this condition however.[26] A diagnostic local anesthetic block of the PIN that produces a temporary wrist drop is useful if the pain is completely relieved.

ELECTRODIAGNOSTIC STUDIES

Classically the NCS is normal in radial tunnel syndrome. Some authors have postulated that this syndrome reflects a dynamic entrapment of the PIN. If the ECRB develops a fibrous edge, the PIN can be entrapped by a scissoring action between this edge and the arcade of Frohse during repetitive forearm supination and pronation. This can lead to intermittent PIN compression. Differential latency testing is based on this premise.[27] Across-elbow radial motor nerve conduction is performed with the elbow extended and the forearm positioned in neutral, pronation, and supination for 30 seconds. The testing is then repeated. An abnormal latency difference of >0.30 millisecond is indicative of radial tunnel entrapment.

NONOPERATIVE MANAGEMENT

The majority of cases will resolve with activity modification. In the early stages above-elbow splinting with the elbow flexed to 90° and the forearm in supination will relieve the dynamic compression and allow the inflammatory response around the PIN to subside. PIN gliding exercises will help maintain nerve excursion and consist of simultaneous elbow extension, forearm pronation, wrist flexion, and ulnar deviation. In many instances the treatment that is instituted for a coexisting lateral epicondylitis will also resolve the symptoms of radial tunnel compression.

SURGICAL INDICATIONS

Persistent proximal forearm pain that does not resolve despite appropriate activity modification is an indication for decompression, especially if a lateral epicondylectomy has already been performed. Complete pain relief following a diagnostic PIN block is a good predictor of at least partial improvement following surgery in my experience.

CONTRAINDICATIONS

The existence of this disorder is still questioned by some authors. All efforts should be made to rule out other causes of pain such as radiocapitellar joint disorders, lateral elbow instability, and untreated lateral epicondylitis.

SURGICAL TECHNIQUE

The volar approach to the radial nerve is through an 8-cm anterolateral incision under tourniquet. The muscular fascia is divided and the intermuscular interval between the brachialis and brachioradialis is developed with blunt dissection. Recurrent branches from the radial artery must be ligated to gain access to both nerve branches. The radial nerve is identified proximal to the elbow and followed distally. At the level of the radial head the radial nerve gives off branches to the ECRB and brachioradialis that should be protected. It then divides into the superficial radial nerve branch that travels distally under the brachioradialis. The PIN continues distally crossed by the radial recurrent vessels that are ligated. The proximal border of the supinator muscle (the arcade of Frohse) is divided along with the superficial head of the supinator. The PIN disappears from view at this point as it penetrates the dorsal extensor compartment. If there is a suspicion of distal entrapment, a separate dorsal approach to the PIN is necessary. This can be accomplished by extending the incision distally and dorsally, or a separate incision is made. The PIN nerve is then approached through a dorsolateral approach, developing the plane between the ECRB and the extensor digitorum communis (Fig. 43-5A-D). At this level, the PIN contains motor fibers only; hence, separate fascicle identification is unnecessary. The distal border of the supinator is delineated and divided.

OUTCOMES

Early reports of radial tunnel decompression were generally optimistic. Beasley and coworkers reported 80% good or excellent results in their series of 109 decompressions.[28] A recent review by Sotereanos et al however found good

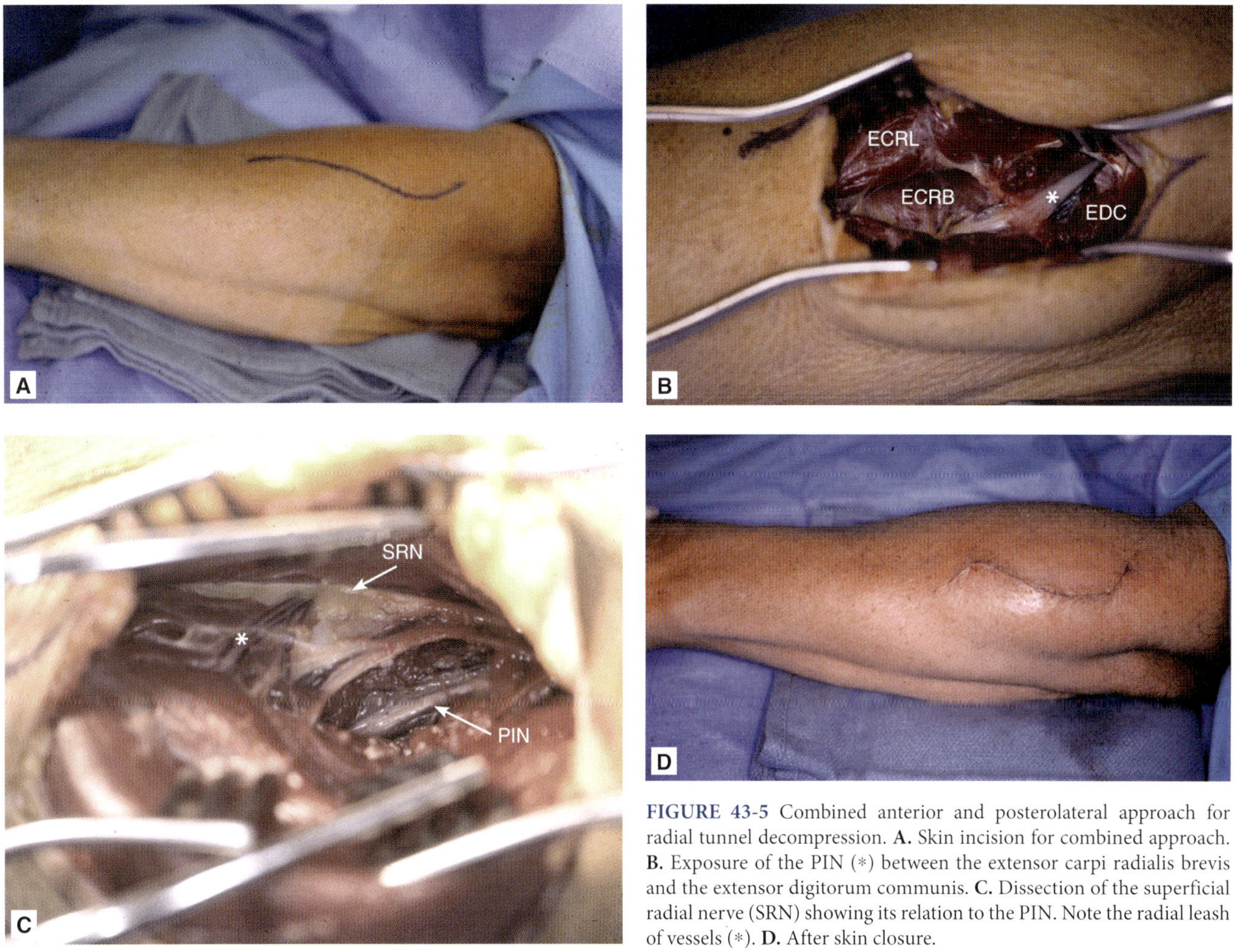

FIGURE 43-5 Combined anterior and posterolateral approach for radial tunnel decompression. **A.** Skin incision for combined approach. **B.** Exposure of the PIN (*) between the extensor carpi radialis brevis and the extensor digitorum communis. **C.** Dissection of the superficial radial nerve (SRN) showing its relation to the PIN. Note the radial leash of vessels (*). **D.** After skin closure.

results in only 11/28 patients, with many patients experiencing residual symptoms.[29] The results were worse in patients receiving workers' compensation.

COMPLICATIONS

The potential complications are similar for radial tunnel syndrome and PIN decompression. The main indication to ligate the radial leash of vessels is to prevent postoperative bleeding, since they are a rare cause of compression by themselves. The superficial radial nerve is at risk for injury through laceration or retraction. Persistent radial tunnel syndrome due to unrelieved PIN compression at the distal border of the supinator may require repeat surgery.

Posterior Interosseous Nerve Entrapment

HISTORY

In PIN syndrome the presenting symptoms are weakness and/or paralysis of the extensor muscles, which result in a wrist or finger drop. There may be a history of a fall onto an extended and pronated arm, although many cases are spontaneous, especially if due to an underlying lipoma, ganglion, or rheumatoid nodule arising from the radiocapitellar joint.

PHYSICAL EXAM

The patient will prevent with variable weakness or paralysis of the EPL, EIP, EDC, and ECU. Motor function of the ECRB/L should be preserved since they are innervated before the PIN dives between the 2 heads of the supinator muscle. The patient will hence extend their wrist in radial deviation.

ELECTRODIAGNOSTIC STUDIES

PIN lesions do not affect the superficial radial SNAP, which should be normal. The CMAP of PIN-innervated muscles may show a drop of conduction velocity or amplitude, but this is difficult to assess with surface electrodes. Needle EMG is the best technique for localization, especially with partial lesions.[19] In acute denervation decreased recruitment, increased insertional activity, and fibrillation potentials ± positive sharp waves are present. In chronic lesions seen

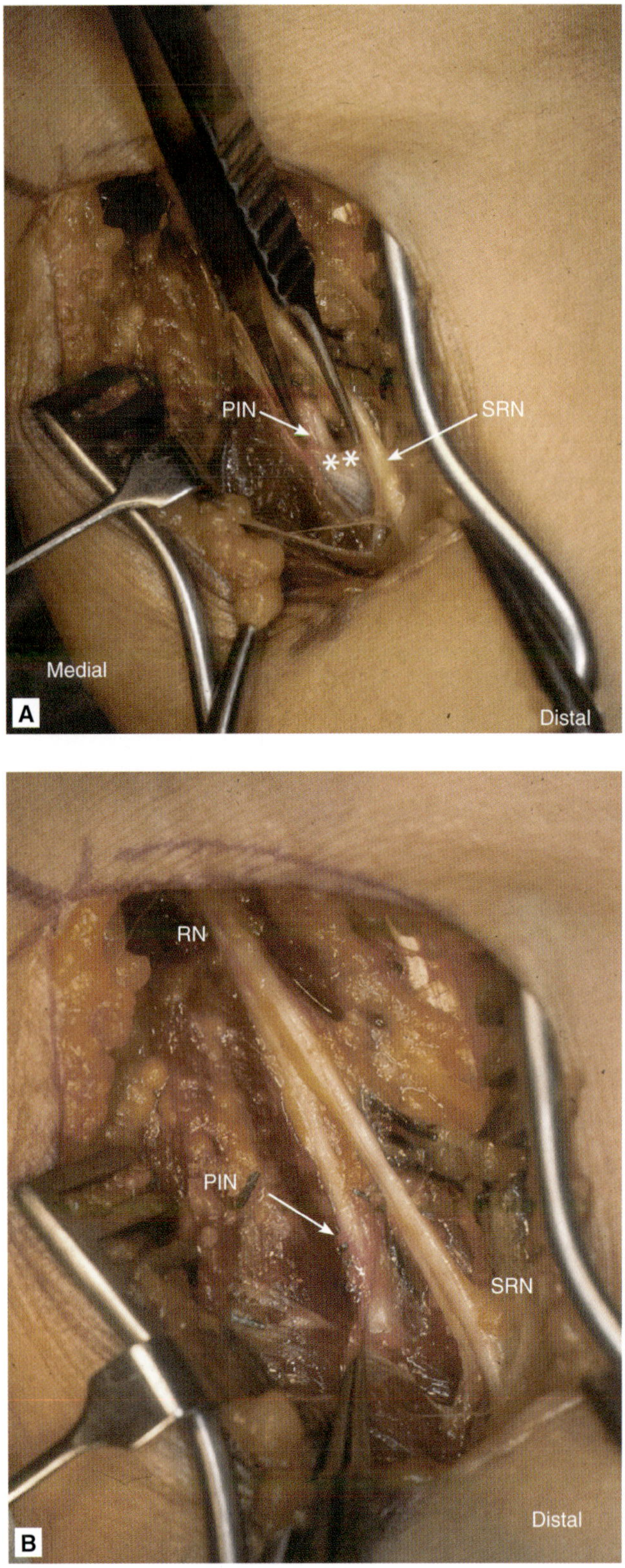

FIGURE 43-6 Anterolateral approach to PIN decompression. **A.** Anterior approach with a view of the proximal volar forearm demonstrating the arcade of Struthers (*). PIN, posterior interosseous nerve; SRN, superficial radial nerve. **B.** After release of the arcade. Note the normal appearance of the PIN. RN, radial nerve.

after 3 to 6 months, decreased recruitment may still be seen along with giant motor unit potentials and polyphasia due to peripheral axonal ingrowth.

NONOPERATIVE MANAGEMENT

Unless preoperative imaging studies reveal a mass-occupying lesion compressing the PIN, most are treated with observation and serial EMG studies. A wrist splint may be used for comfort.

SURGICAL INDICATIONS

MRI evidence of any type of mass compressing the PIN is an indication for exploration and decompression. In idiopathic cases, a failure to improve within 6 months without EMG evidence of reinnervation is an indication for exploration.

CONTRAINDICATIONS

Diffuse denervation of the upper limb muscles or any other generalized neuromuscular disorder is a contraindication to PIN decompression. A C7 radiculopathy, or extensor tendon ruptures especially in rheumatoid patients, can mimic this disorder and should be ruled out.

SURGICAL TECHNIQUE

This is identical to that of radial tunnel decompression (Fig. 43-6A and B).

POSTOPERATIVE TREATMENT

Elbow motion and PIN gliding exercises are instituted after an initial period of splinting for comfort.

OUTCOMES

Kline and coworkers reported their experience with 45 surgically treated PIN entrapments, tumors, or injuries over a 27-year period. Most muscles innervated by the PIN achieved grade 3 or better functional outcomes.[30] They generally found that the PIN entrapment or injuries responded well to PIN release and/or repair. This is most likely due to the fact that the nerve does not have far to regenerate to reach the motor end plates.

REFERENCES

1. Zhao X, Lao J, Hung LK, et al. Selective neurotization of the median nerve in the arm to treat brachial plexus palsy. An anatomic study and case report. *J Bone Joint Surg Am.* 2004;86-A:736–742.
2. Nigst H, Dick W. Syndromes of compression of the median nerve in the proximal forearm (pronator teres syndrome; anterior interosseous nerve syndrome). *Arch Orthop Trauma Surg.* 1979;93:307–312.
3. Wertsch JJ, Melvin J. Median nerve anatomy and entrapment syndromes: a review. *Arch Phys Med Rehabil.* 1982;63:623–627.
4. Olehnik WK, Manske PR, Szerzinski J. Median nerve compression in the proximal forearm. *J Hand Surg Am.* 1994;19:121–126.

5. Szabo RM, Koo JT. Compression neuropathies of the median nerve. In: Slutsky DJ, Hentz VR, eds. *Peripheral Nerve Surgery: Practical Applications in the Upper Extremity*. Philadelphia: Elsevier Inc; 2006: 219–242.
6. Werner CO, Rosen I, Thorngren KG. Clinical and neurophysiologic characteristics of the pronator syndrome. *Clin Orthop Relat Res*. 1985: 231–236.
7. Hartz CR, Linscheid RL, Gramse RR, Daube JR. The pronator teres syndrome: compressive neuropathy of the median nerve. *J Bone Joint Surg Am*. 1981;63:885–890.
8. Johnson RK, Spinner M, Shrewsbury MM. Median nerve entrapment syndrome in the proximal forearm. *J Hand Surg Am*. 1979;4:48–51.
9. Wong L, Dellon AL. Brachial neuritis presenting as anterior interosseous nerve compression—implications for diagnosis and treatment: a case report. *J Hand Surg Am*. 1997;22:536–539.
10. Srinivasan R, Rhodes J. The median-ulnar anastomosis (Martin-Gruber) in normal and congenitally abnormal fetuses. *Arch Neurol*. 1981;38:418–419.
11. Mysiew WJ, Coalchis SC. Electrophysiologic study of the anterior interosseous nerve. *Am J Phys Med Rehabil*. 1988;67:50–54.
12. Nagano A, Shibata K, Tokimura H, Yamamoto S, Tajiri Y. Spontaneous anterior interosseous nerve palsy with hourglass-like fascicular constriction within the main trunk of the median nerve. *J Hand Surg Am*. 1996;21:266–270.
13. von Schroeder HP, Scheker LR. Redefining the "arcade of Struthers". *J Hand Surg Am*. 2003;28:1018–1021.
14. Wehrli L, Oberlin C. The internal brachial ligament versus the arcade of Struthers: an anatomical study. *Plast Reconstr Surg*. 2005;115:471–477.
15. De Jesus R, Dellon AL. Historic origin of the "arcade of Struthers". *J Hand Surg Am*. 2003;28:528–531.
16. Bartels RH, Grotenhuis JA, Kauer JM. The arcade of Struthers: an anatomical study. *Acta Neurochir (Wien)*. 2003;145:295–300 [discussion 300].
17. Siqueira MG, Martins RS. The controversial arcade of Struthers. *Surg Neurol*. 2005;64(suppl 1):S1:17–S1:20 [discussion S1:20–S1:21].
18. Posner MA. Compressive ulnar neuropathies at the elbow: I. Etiology and diagnosis. *J Am Acad Orthop Surg*. 1998;6:282–288.
19. Spinner M, Spencer PS. Nerve compression lesions of the upper extremity. A clinical and experimental review. *Clin Orthop Relat Res*. 1974:46–67.
20. Campbell WW, Pridgeon RM, Riaz G, et al. Sparing of the flexor carpi ulnaris in ulnar neuropathy at the elbow. *Muscle Nerve*. 1989;12: 965–967.
21. Novak CB, Lee GW, Mackinnon SE, Lay L. Provocative testing for cubital tunnel syndrome. *J Hand Surg Am*. 1994;19:817–820.
22. Campbell WW, Pridgeon RM, Sahni KS. Short segment incremental studies in the evaluation of ulnar neuropathy at the elbow. *Muscle Nerve*. 1992;15:1050–1054.
23. Felsenthal G, Freed MJ, Kalafut R, Hilton EB. Across-elbow ulnar nerve sensory conduction technique. *Arch Phys Med Rehabil*. 1989;70: 668–672.
24. Venkatesh S, Kothari MJ, Preston DC. The limitations of the dorsal ulnar cutaneous sensory response in patients with ulnar neuropathy at the elbow. *Muscle Nerve*. 1995;18:345–347.
25. Tomaino MM, Brach PJ, Vansickle DP. The rationale for and efficacy of surgical intervention for electrodiagnostic-negative cubital tunnel syndrome. *J Hand Surg Am*. 2001;26:1077–1081.
26. Kim DH, Han K, Tiel RL, Murovic JA, Kline DG. Surgical outcomes of 654 ulnar nerve lesions. *J Neurosurg*. 2003;98:993–1004.
27. Kupfer DM, Bronson J, Lee GW, Beck J, Gillet J. Differential latency testing: a more sensitive test for radial tunnel syndrome. *J Hand Surg Am*. 1998;23:859–864.
28. Rinker B, Effron CR, Beasley RW. Proximal radial compression neuropathy. *Ann Plast Surg*. 2004;52:174–180 [discussion 81–83].
29. Sotereanos DG, Varitimidis SE, Giannakopoulos PN, Westkaemper JG. Results of surgical treatment for radial tunnel syndrome. *J Hand Surg Am*. 1999;24:566–570.
30. Kim DH, Murovic JA, Kim YY, Kline DG. Surgical treatment and outcomes in 45 cases of posterior interosseous nerve entrapments and injuries. *J Neurosurg*. 2006;104:766–777.

44

Nerve Transfer for Restoration of Elbow Flexion: The Modified Oberlin Procedure

Frances Sharpe, MD
Milan Stevanovic, MD
David J. Slutsky, MD

INTRODUCTION

Restoration of elbow flexion remains the first reconstructive priority in treating patients with injury to the upper roots of the brachial plexus (C5-C6 and C5-C6-C7). In the setting of root avulsion or an otherwise irreparable lesion, nerve transfer has been used to restore function. In 1994, Oberlin et al described the use of a fascicle of the ulnar nerve transferred to the musculocutaneous nerve (MCN) branch to the biceps brachii for reconstruction of elbow flexion. Since the introduction of this transfer, excellent functional results have been reproduced in other centers.[1,2,3,4]

INDICATIONS

Oberlin and double fascicular nerve transfers for elbow reconstruction are indicated in lesions of the brachial plexus involving C5, C6 or C5, C6, and C7 root injuries. Some global or mixed plexus injuries can be treated by this method if there is adequate clinical recovery in the lower roots. It can be used for deficits resulting from postradiation neuritis of the brachial plexus. It is indicated for nerve reconstruction in patients who present with a significant delay from their time of injury since the neurorraphy is placed close to the target muscles and for older patients who may have poor outcomes with more conventional techniques. M4 motor strength has been recovered in patients as old as 66 years of age.[4]

CONTRAINDICATIONS

The absolute contraindication for this nerve transfer is a global brachial plexus palsy with no recovery of ulnar nerve function. A relative contraindication is a global palsy that subsequently recovers lower nerve root function, since the transfer requires intact function of the C8 and T1 nerve roots. The outcomes are unpredictable after more than 1 year from injury.

A prerequisite for the transfer requires intact function of the C8 and T1 nerve roots. A preoperative clinical examination for motor strength of the flexor carpi ulnaris (FCU) and flexor carpi radialis (FCR) is imperative. Surgical alternatives to this technique should be done if a patient does not have at least a grade 4 Medical Research Council (MRC) strength in these muscles. If it is anticipated that the patient will need tendon transfers for distal hand function, using either FCU or FCR, it should be kept in mind that this nerve transfer has the potential to weaken these muscles. A preoperative EMG even in late cases may be useful to evaluate the muscle for potential for reinnervation. The absence of fibrillation potentials in a denervated muscle would suggest that the muscle has become fibrotic and is no longer capable of reinnervation.

RELEVANT ANATOMY

The MCN is the terminal branch of the lateral cord of the brachial plexus, containing donor fascicles from C5, C6, and C7 roots. The nerve leaves the lateral cord near the inferior margin of pectoralis minor and pierces the deep surface of the coracobrachialis, giving off the motor branch to this muscle as it travels through the muscle substance. It emerges from the superficial surface of the coracobrachialis muscle at an average of 7.7 cm distal to the tip of the acromion,[5,6] subsequently giving off branches to the biceps and brachialis muscles, and then terminating as the lateral antebrachial cutaneous nerve. The dominant nerve pattern to the biceps is a single muscular branch, which arises between 12 and 13 cm distal to the acromion[5] or 18 cm proximal to the medial epicondyle. This main branch quickly divides into secondary branches that then supply the short and long heads of the biceps independently. Approximately 4.5 cm distal to

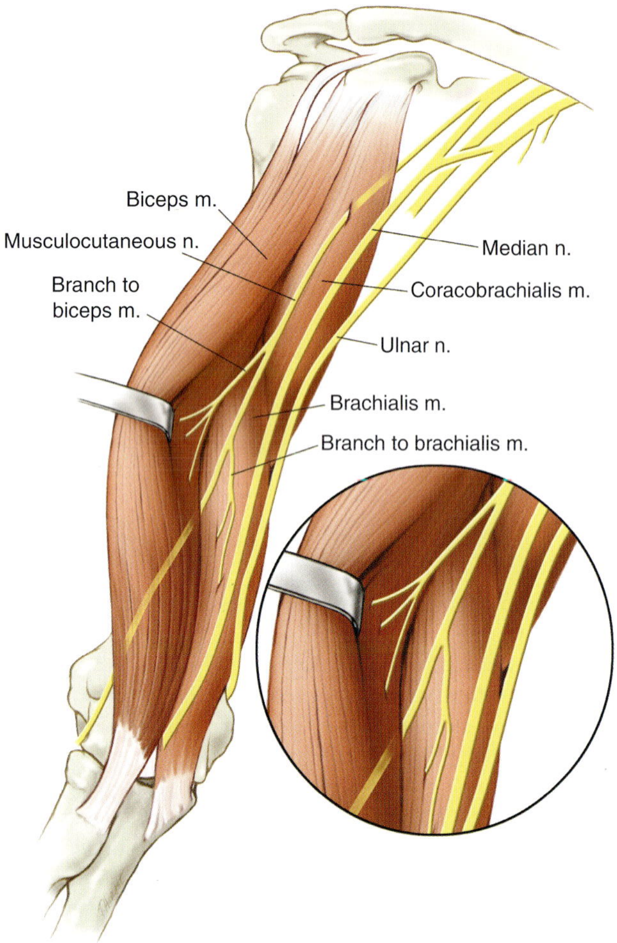

FIGURE 44-1 Anatomy of the musculocutaneous nerve and the relationships to the biceps and brachialis muscles as well as the median and ulnar nerves. (Copyright © Milan Stevanovic, MD and Frances Sharpe, MD.)

the branch to the biceps is the muscular branch to the brachialis, estimated at 17.5 to 18 cm distal to the acromion or 13.5 cm proximal to the medial epicondyle (Fig. 44-1). The internal topography of the MCN shows a consistent pattern of orientation, with the fascicle groups to the biceps, brachialis, and lateral antebrachial cutaneous nerve located from lateral to medial, respectively. The fasciculi to the biceps are grouped and can be separated proximally from their point of exit from the main nerve for a distance of 4 to 6 cm. Similarly, independent motor fascicles to the brachialis can be separated out from the MCN for an average of 5 to 9 cm proximal to the takeoff of the branch to the brachialis, with a wide range between different specimens. Variations of the branching patterns of the MCN have been described by several authors. These branching patterns to the biceps and brachialis and their relative frequencies are described in Figure 44-2. These variations may need to be accommodated in the surgical technique. Other described variations of the MCN include communicating branches between the median nerve and MCN (typically occurring proximal to the branch to the brachialis), absent MCN, and fusion with the median nerve. In most cases, when this variant is present, the motor branches to the biceps and brachialis originate from the median nerve.[7]

The internal anatomy of the proximal median and ulnar nerves allows donor fascicles to be harvested without measurable donor deficit. Despite the plexiform arrangement with multiple intrafascicular interconnections, fibers from the peripheral branches pursue a localized course in the nerve for variable, though often considerable, distances. Care is taken to harvest those motor fascicles that predominantly contribute to expendable muscle donors. Thus, in the median and ulnar nerves, we try to isolate fascicles that principally innervate the extrinsic muscle flexors, specifically fibers that are predominantly to the FCU from the ulnar nerve and to the FCR from the median nerve. Motor fascicles for the FCU should generally be anterolateral or anterocentral.[4] Motor fascicles from the median nerve are also located anteriorly, with fascicles predominantly supplying pronator teres situated anterolaterally, and FCR fascicles lying anterior and slightly medially. Deep (posterior) to the FCR fascicles are fascicles to the flexor digitorum superficialis and profundus. More posteriorly on the medial side are the fascicles that make up the anterior interosseous nerve.[8]

The biceps muscle receives its innervation from the MCN, except in cases of anatomic variations noted above. The dominant nerve root supplying the biceps is C6 with some contribution from C5. The brachialis muscle is a dually innervated muscle in more than 80% of cases, with the lateral third to half receiving innervation from the radial nerve. From the MCN, it is supplied principally by C6, and from the radial nerve, it is supplied principally by C7.

SURGICAL TECHNIQUE

The patient is placed supine on the operating table with the arm placed out on a hand table. The entire extremity and shoulder girdle should be prepped into the operative field. Clear communication with the anesthesiologist is necessary before and throughout the procedure to assure that only short-acting paralytic agents are used for the induction of anesthesia. The paralysis should resolve shortly after the start of the procedure. The dissection should be done under wide-field loupe magnification. The surgical incision on the medial side of the arm is facilitated by placing the shoulder in external rotation. The line of the incision lies between the midpoint of the axilla and the medial epicondyle, correlating with the bicipital grove. The incision starts approximately 3 fingerbreadths from the axilla (at the level of the distal edge of the insertion of the pectoralis major into the humerus) and extends to approximately 3 fingerbreadths proximal to the medial epicondyle (Fig. 44-3). If necessary, the incision can be extended proximally into the axilla and distally toward the medial epicondyle. The skin and subcutaneous tissues are dissected down to the level of the brachial fascia. This is opened in line with the skin incision on the posterior edge of

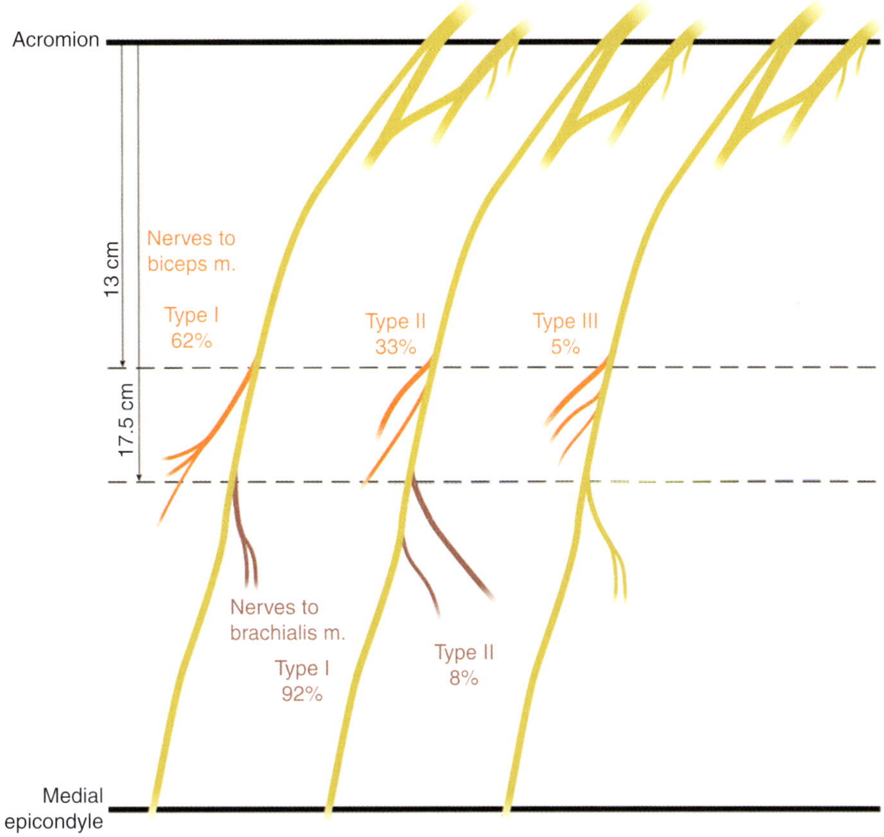

FIGURE 44-2 The most common branching patterns of the musculocutaneous nerve and the percentage of various branching patterns to the biceps and brachialis muscles. (Copyright © Milan Stevanovic, MD and Frances Sharpe, MD.)

the biceps. The ulnar and median nerves are easily identified just deep to the brachial fascia (Fig. 44-4A and B). The medial brachial and medial antebrachial nerves lie within the surgical dissection and should be protected (Fig. 44-4A). The biceps muscle is retracted laterally away from the humerus, gently lifting and rotating the biceps to be able to see the deep

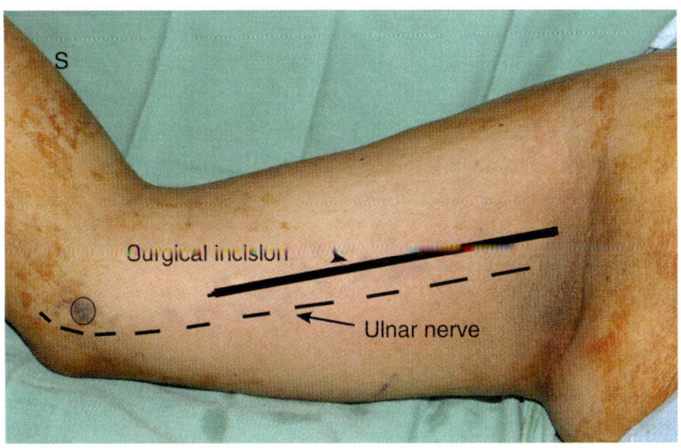

FIGURE 44-3 Surgical incision. Dotted line represents course of the ulnar nerve. (Copyright © Milan Stevanovic, MD and Frances Sharpe, MD.)

surface of its medial edge (Fig. 44-5). The MCN will lie on the deep surface of the medial edge of the biceps, and is often covered by a thin layer of fascia and fatty tissue (Fig. 44-6A and B). Careful dissection of the MCN is performed from proximal to distal, until the first motor branch to the biceps is identified. This branch usually enters the middle third of the biceps, close to one of the dominant vascular pedicles to the biceps from the brachial artery (Fig. 44-7A and B). The vascular pedicle travels more transversely than the nerve and should be preserved. Further distal dissection of the MCN is done to evaluate the pattern of innervation to the biceps. The majority of patients (62%) have a single branch from the MCN that bifurcates to separately supply the short and long heads of the biceps muscle (Type I pattern). However, a substantial percentage of patients have 2 and less commonly 3 separate branches from the MCN.

After identifying all the branches, a proximal intrafascicular dissection of the nerve should be done, separating out the fascicles to the biceps as far proximally as possible. When there is more than 1 branch to the biceps, it is sometimes possible through proximal intrafascicular dissection of the MCN to identify a single motor fascicle that can be used for neurorraphy. In cases where a single motor fasciculus cannot be identified, 2 donor motor fascicles from the ulnar nerve should be used for nerve transfer. Proximal intrafascicular

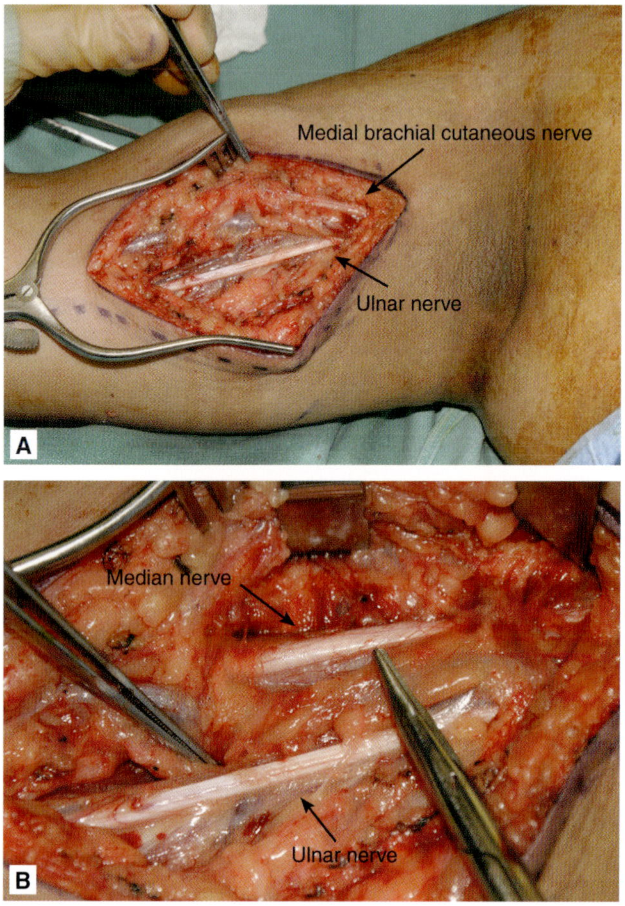

FIGURE 44-4 **A** and **B.** Identification and dissection of the median and ulnar nerves. (Copyright © Milan Stevanovic, MD and Frances Sharpe, MD.)

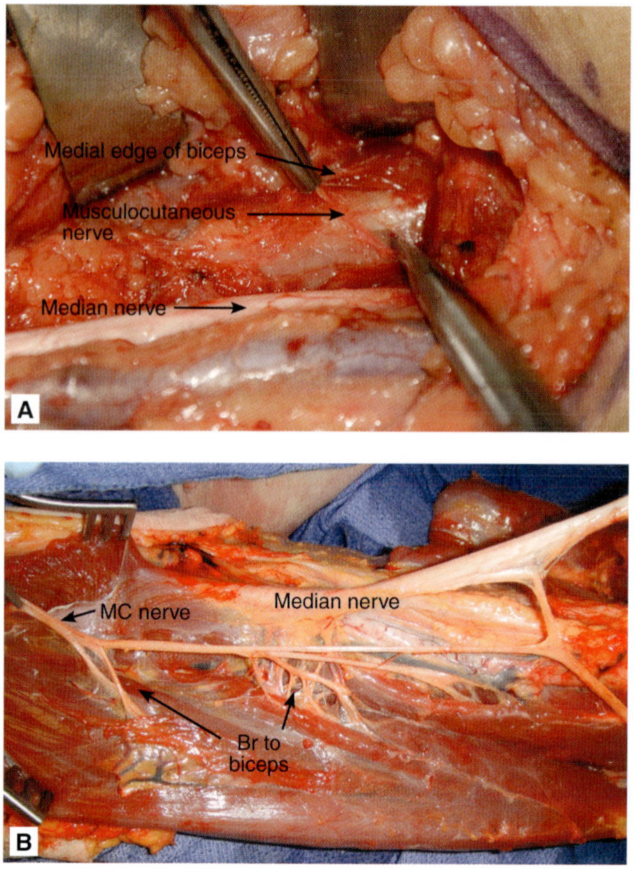

FIGURE 44-6 **A** and **B.** Location and identification of the musculocutaneous nerve on the deep surface of the medial edge of the biceps and location of biceps branches. (Copyright © Milan Stevanovic, MD and Frances Sharpe, MD.)

dissection of the MCN is carried out under loupe magnification. The dissection is carried as far proximal as the limits of intrafascicular bridging allow; usually this is 2 to 4 cm. The fascicles are divided from the main trunk of the MCN as far proximally as possible, and then they are rotated toward

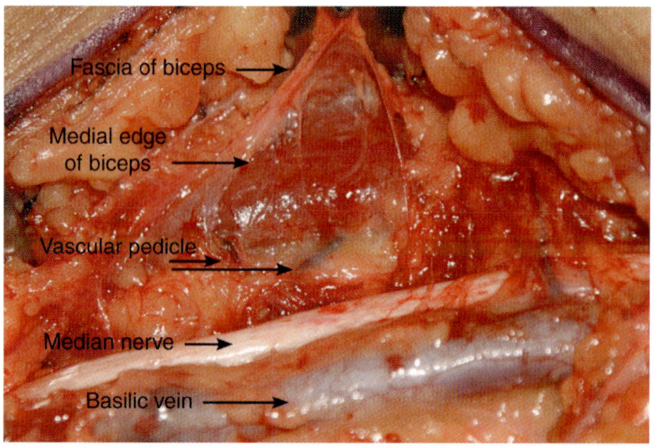

FIGURE 44-5 Elevation of the biceps muscle and identification of branches to the biceps. (Copyright © Milan Stevanovic, MD and Frances Sharpe, MD.)

the ulnar nerve. We prefer to do the intrafascicular dissection of the ulnar nerve under the operating microscope, using microsurgical dilating forceps to spread between the fascicles to help identify and protect intrafascicular connections. The dissection of the nerve is done distal to the level of the branch to the biceps, so that the harvested fascicle(s) will have sufficient length to reach the MCN branch to the biceps muscle without tension. The donor fascicle(s) are divided as far distally as possible to allow the donor fascicle to be rotated toward the recipient motor branch (Fig. 44-8A and B).

If reinnervation of the brachialis is planned, and there is adequate distal function of the median nerve–innervated muscles, then the branch of the MCN to the brachialis is identified and dissected. In most cases, the MCN branch to the brachialis is a single branch, around 4.5 cm distal to the branch to the biceps, arising from the posteromedial side of the MCN, and slightly thinner than the terminal sensory branch (the lateral antebrachial cutaneous nerve) (Fig. 44-9). Again, this branch is mobilized from the main trunk of the MCN as far proximally as possible, and then rotated toward the median nerve. Distal intrafascicular dissection of the median nerve is performed as described above for the ulnar nerve dissection (Fig. 44-10A and B). A disposable handheld

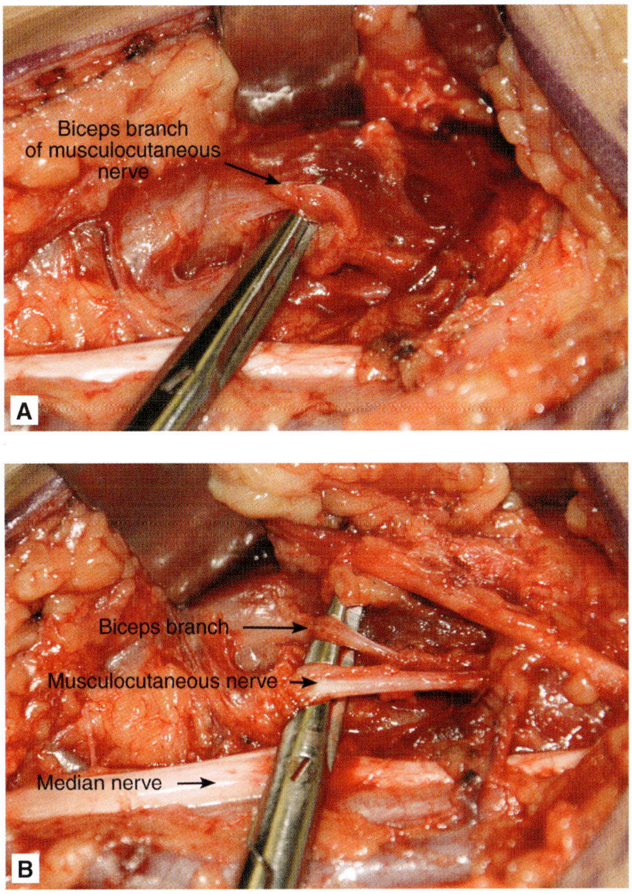

FIGURE 44-7 **A** and **B.** Separation of the biceps branch from the main trunk of the musculocutaneous nerve. (Copyright © Milan Stevanovic, MD and Frances Sharpe, MD.)

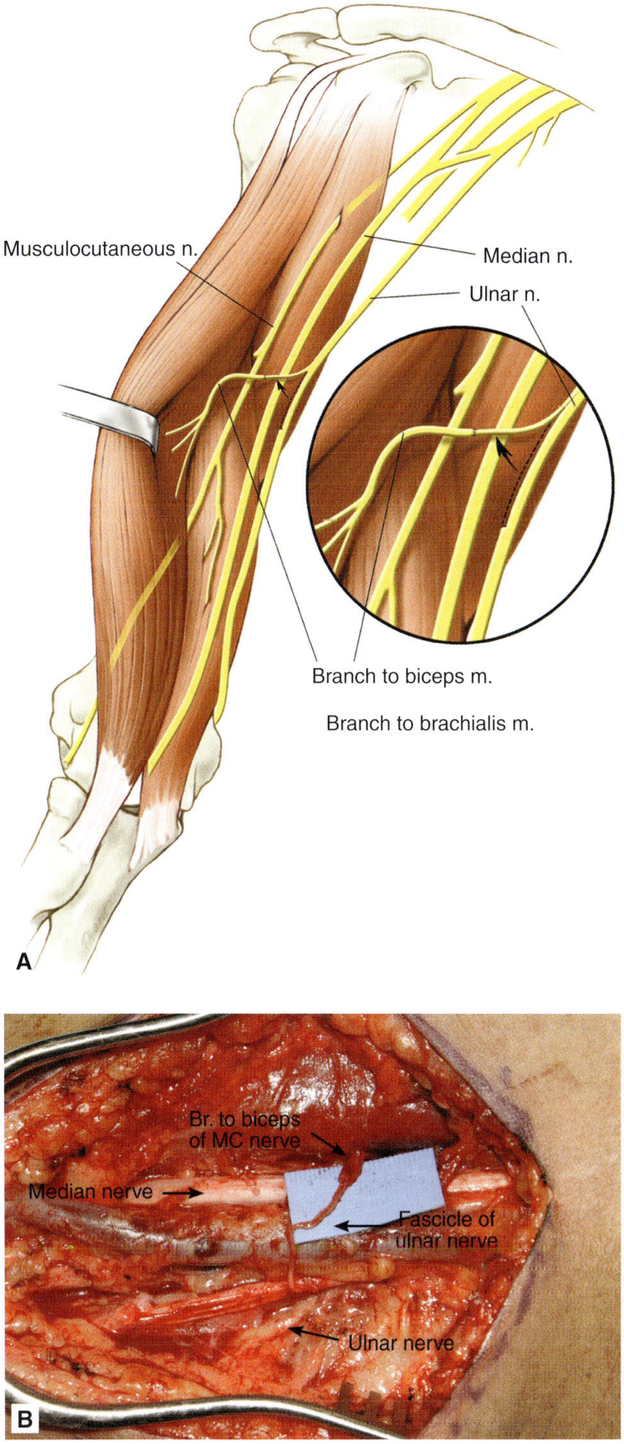

FIGURE 44-8 **A** and **B.** Donor fascicle of the ulnar nerve transferred to the biceps branch of the musculocutaneous nerve. (Copyright © Milan Stevanovic, MD and Frances Sharpe, MD.)

nerve stimulator set to the lowest setting of 0.5 Hz is used to identify the donor fascicles of the median and ulnar nerves. Alternatively, a nerve stimulator with precise variable settings used by the anesthesiologist for placement of nerve blocks can also be used. Placing the ground needle close to the neurolysed section of the donor nerve gives more precise localization of the dominant area innervated by the selected fascicle.

Intraoperative stimulation should elicit a strong motor response before proceeding with nerve transfer. In selecting donor motor fascicles from the ulnar nerve, the fascicles that produce the strongest contraction of the FCU or the flexor digitorum profundus to the ring and small fingers with stimulation are harvested. These are all C8, T1 innervated. In some circumstances, it may be better to selectively reinnervate the biceps or to use an alternative nerve transfer to reinnervate the brachialis. Similar to the principles of tendon transfer, it is preferential to select synergistic muscles for nerve transfer. Donor fascicles from the median nerve should be used with caution. The median nerve contains contributions from C5, C6, C7, C8, and T1, which means that even a clinically functioning median nerve has lost some if its nerve contributions from an upper plexus injury, particularly for C5, C6, C7 injuries. Donor fascicles from the ulnar and median nerves suitable for transfer are usually located on the anterior or anterolateral portion of the ulnar nerve and the anterior or anteromedial portion of the median nerve, as described above. One to 2 fascicles can be safely harvested from each

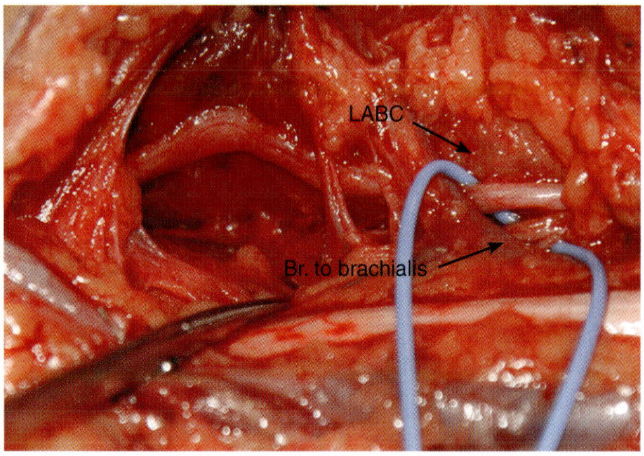

FIGURE 44-9 The branch to the brachialis lies approximately 4 to 5 cm distal to the branch to the biceps. The branch is slightly thinner than the LABC and has a posteromedial takeoff from the main trunk of the MCN. (Copyright © Milan Stevanovic, MD and Frances Sharpe, MD.)

nerve. The number of fascicles harvested is based on the size of the recipient nerve. We have not found it necessary to have an exact cross-sectional match, and prefer to have a smaller rather than larger donor fascicle. In the case where there is more than 1 motor branch to biceps, we recommend reinnervation of both branches, using 2 separate donor fascicles. Neurorraphy of the donor fascicles to the recipient branches should be done under microscopic magnification using 10-0 nylon suture on a 70- to 75-μm needle, placing 2 sutures at 180°, and augmenting the repair with fibrin glue. Meticulous hemostasis is achieved prior to wound closure.

POSTOPERATIVE REHABILITATION

The postoperative protocol following this procedure depends on whether additional procedures or nerve transfers have been performed; particularly, if the pectoralis major muscle has been detached for exploration or grafting of the infraclavicular plexus, then this repair is protected for approximately 4 weeks in a shoulder immobilizer. The immobilizer is removed only for showering and gentle circumduction exercises as well as gentle passive elbow flexion–extension exercises to prevent stiffness. If no other procedures are performed that require specific protection or rehabilitation, then the arm is immobilized in a sling. At 10 to 14 days, the sling is discontinued, but may be used on an as-needed basis for comfort. The patient is encouraged to work on regaining passive range of motion of the shoulder and elbow. A therapist is used if the patient is not able to regain passive motion independently. When there is clinical evidence of motor reinnervation, the patients are instructed in motor reeducation and strengthening. Although controversial, we prefer to use a muscle stimulator to maintain the tonicity of the biceps. We have also found it helpful to help the patient with muscle reeducation and strengthening at the first sign of reinnervation. Elbow flexion is enhanced by activation of the muscles supplied by the donor nerve. This is achieved by having the patient grip while trying to flex the elbow. Isometric strengthening by having the patient place and hold in various degrees of elbow flexion followed by light resistive strengthening continues until the patient reaches a plateau in recovery.

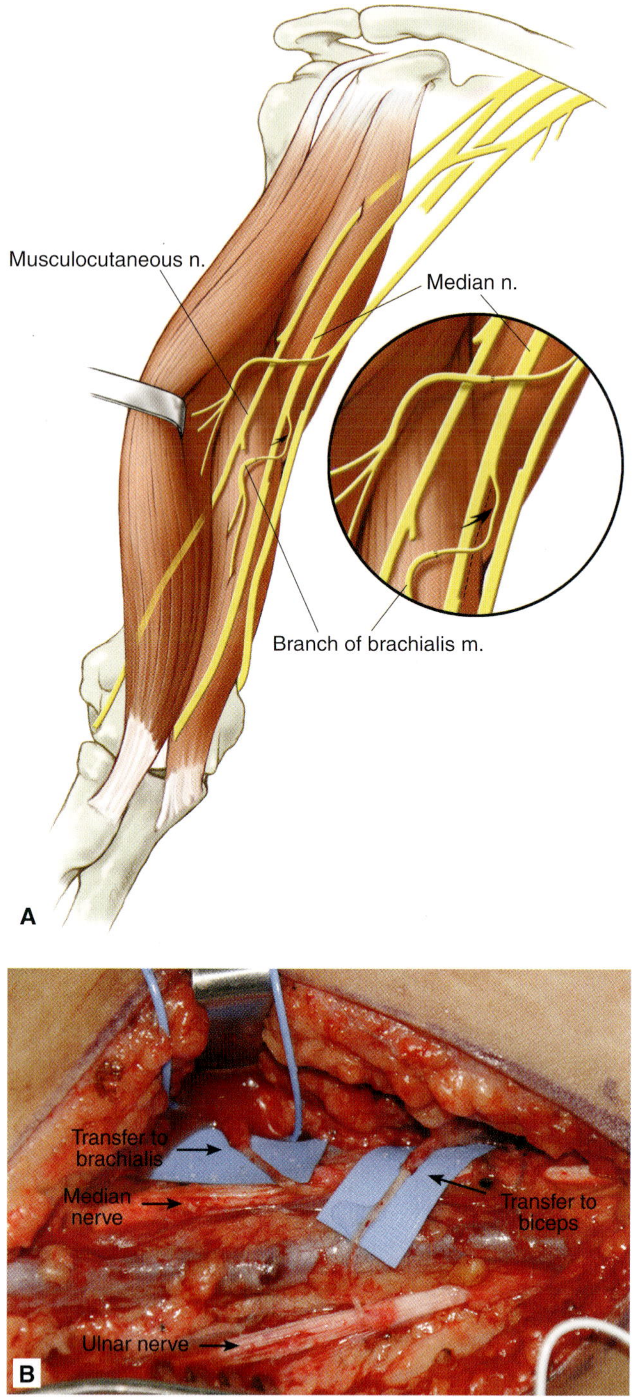

FIGURE 44-10 A and B. Double fascicular transfer. (Copyright © Milan Stevanovic, MD and Frances Sharpe, MD.)

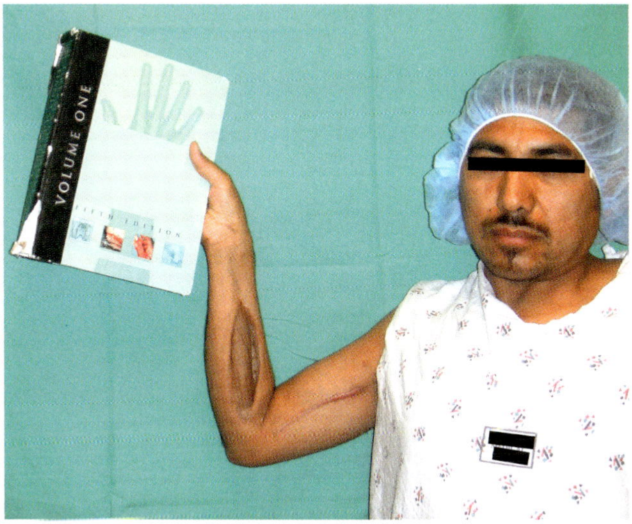

FIGURE 44-11 A 26-year-old patient who sustained a stab wound to the left supraclavicular area 11 months prior to presentation. He had isolated deficits of the upper trunk, with weak shoulder girdle function and no elbow flexion. He had had no previous treatment. A double fascicular nerve transfer was performed. Patient recovered M4 motor function at approximately 13 months from the date of transfer. (Copyright © Milan Stevanovic, MD and Frances Sharpe, MD.)

COMPLICATIONS

The harvest of fascicles from an intact functioning nerve raises the concern of causing deficits in the donor nerve distribution. To date, no long-term deficits have been reported from these techniques. Dr Oberlin has reported 2 anterior interosseous nerve palsies, which did not recover (personal communication) (Fig. 44-11). In these cases he had difficulty in identifying a donor fascicle from the median nerve that was size-matched to the branch of the MCN to the brachialis muscle. Rather than performing an intrafascicular dissection, he elected to use the "large" fascicle from the median nerve, with the resultant distal deficit.

OUTCOMES

A total of 100 cases were identified in the English literature that report outcomes for biceps reconstruction using fascicles from either the median or ulnar nerve for reinnervation of the biceps.[3,5,6,9] Eighty percent of patients recovered ≥M4 motor strength for elbow flexion, 9% recovered M3 function, and 11% had <M3 recovery. Clinical evidence of biceps reinnervation was seen at an average of 3 months (range 2-7 months). Recovery of M3 function ranged between 4 and 13 months. For those patients who recovered M4 motor function, the range of elbow flexion strength was between 0.5 and 7 kg. Factors that affected the outcome included the time from injury to surgery as well as the extent of brachial plexus injury. A low preoperative grip strength suggests a wider degree of plexus injury, despite intact function, and may help predict outcome. When C5-C6 lesions were analyzed separately from C5, C6, C7 injuries, outcomes were better in the C5-C6 group. While a delay to surgery seems to be correlated with a worse prognosis, the series reported by Teboul et al includes 2 patients operated on at 12 months following injury, both of whom recovered M4 biceps recovery.[4] Age was not correlated with poorer outcomes; however, brachial plexus injuries generally occur in a younger age group, and there were fewer patients in the age >40 group. There was a higher failure rate in part due to the longer preoperative delay to surgery (more than 2 years in 3 cases).

Double Fascicular Transfer

The double fascicular transfer as described independently by Mackinnon et al[3] and Liverneaux et al[2] refers to the use of fascicles from both the median and ulnar nerves to separately reinnervate the biceps and brachialis muscles. Initially Mackinnon reported on 8 cases where the biceps was reinnervated using the technique of Oberlin, and the brachialis was reinnervated using other nerve transfers including the medial pectoral nerve, the thoracodorsal nerve, intercostal nerves, and a triceps branch from the radial nerve. Recovery was graded as M4 in 5 patients and M4+ in 3 patients, with clinical recovery beginning at 5 months. Liverneaux et al reported their results in 10 patients. All patients recovered M4 flexion strength. The average flexion strength was 3.7 kg. This surgical option should be kept in mind since with wider plexus injuries there may not be sufficient recovery of the median nerve to allow the use of donor fascicles.

Our unpublished results in 25 patients are similar to other authors. We have used both the original Oberlin technique and the double fascicular transfer. We prefer the double fascicular transfer as long as there is good distal motor function of the hand and forearm muscles. All patients recovered grade 4 motor function, with biceps recovery occurring somewhat later than that described in other series; typically biceps contraction was noted at 5 to 6 months, and progressed to maximum recovered function at approximately 1 year (Fig. 44-11).

REFERENCES

1. Oberlin C, Beal D, Lechavengvongs S, Salon A, Dauge M, Sarcy J. Nerve transfer to the biceps muscle using a part of ulnar nerve for C5-C6 avulsion of the brachial plexus: anatomical study and report of four cases. *J Hand Surg Am*. 1994;19A(2):232–237.
2. Liverneaux P, Diaz L, Beaulieu J-Y, Durand S, Oberlin C. Preliminary results of double nerve transfer to restore elbow flexion in upper type brachial plexus palsies. *Plast Reconstr Surg*. 2006;117(3):915–919.
3. MacKinnon S, Novak C, Myckatyn T, Tung T. Results of reinnervation of the biceps and brachialis muscles with a double fascicular transfer for elbow flexion. *J Hand Surg Am*. 2005;30A(5):978–985.
4. Teboul F, Kakkar R, Ameur N, Beaulieu J-Y, Oberlin C. Transfer of fascicles from the ulnar nerve to the nerve to the biceps in the treatment of upper brachial plexus palsy. *J Bone Joint Surg Am*. 2004;86-A(7):1485–1490.
5. Chiarapattanakom P, Leechavengvongs S, Witoonchart K, Uerpairojkit C, Thuvasethakul P. Anatomy and internal topography

of the musculocutaneous nerve: the nerve to the biceps and brachialis muscle. *J Hand Surg Am.* 1998;23A(2):250–255.
6. Yang Z-X, Pho R, Kour A-K, Pereira B. The musculocutaneous nerve and its branches to the biceps and brachialis muscles. *J Hand Surg Am.* 1995;20A(4):671–675.
7. Saeed M, Rufai A. Median and musculocutaneous nerves: variant formation and distribution. *Clin Anat.* 2003;16(5):453–457.
8. Williams H, Jabaley M. The importance of internal anatomy of the peripheral nerves to nerve repair in the forearm and hand. *Hand Clin.* 1986;2(4):689–707.
9. Carlsen B, Kircher M, Spinner R, Bishop A, Shin A. Comparison of single versus double nerve transfers for elbow flexion after brachial plexus injury. *Plast Reconstr Surg.* 2011;127(1):269–276.

45

Nerve Transfers to Restore Wrist and Finger Extension

David J. Slutsky, MD

INTRODUCTION

A loss of wrist and finger extension can result from myriad causes including brachial plexus injury, radial nerve injury due to trauma, nerve tumors, compression, or idiopathic neuritis as well as posterior interosseous nerve (PIN) compression. In the latter case some radial wrist extension may be preserved. Until recently, tendon transfers have been the mainstay of treatment. Nerve transfers have long been used for brachial plexus reconstruction. The principles of nerve to nerve transfer, or neurotization, have recently been applied to peripheral nerve injuries with encouraging results. The following discussion will center on neurotization to restore wrist and finger extension.

RELEVANT ANATOMY

Radial Nerve

The radial nerve arises from the posterior cord of the brachial plexus. It receives contributions from C5-C8 spinal roots. The nerve contains approximately 16,000 myelinated fibers. It runs medial to the axillary artery, and then at the level of the coracobrachialis it courses posteriorly to lie in the spiral groove of the humerus. In the lower arm it pierces the lateral intermuscular septum to run between the brachialis and brachioradialis (BR). Opposite the head of the radius there are some fibrous bands from the joint's capsule and immediately distal to this, the nerve is regularly crossed by several prominent veins, the "leash of Henry." It divides 2 cm distal to the elbow into a superficial radial sensory branch (SRN) and a deep motor branch, the PIN. It gives off branches to the extensor carpi radialis longus (ECRL) and brevis (ECRB), BR, and anconeus before giving off the PIN branch (Fig. 45-1). The PIN continues on between the superficial and deep heads of the supinator muscle, to exit on the dorsal forearm. After it emerges from the distal border of the supinator, the PIN sends branches to the extensor digitorum communis (EDC), extensor carpi ulnaris (ECU), extensor digiti quinti, extensor pollicis longus (EPL) and brevis, and the extensor indicis proprius (EIP) in descending order, although there may be considerable variation.

In an anatomic study by Ukrit et al on 10 cadaver arms, the PIN arose from radial nerve. Its origin was 2.9 ± 0.7 cm below the interepicondylar line.[1] It contained 7447 ± 1325 myelinated axons. The ECRB branch arose from the radial nerve in 6 specimens and from the PIN in 4. The ECRB branch arose at 2.3 ± 1.5 cm below the interepicondylar line and the average length was 3.3 ± 1.6 cm. The average number of myelinated nerve fibers of the ECRB branch was 2798 ± 464.

Median Nerve

Just distal to the cubital fossa, the motor branches of the median nerve consistently collect into 3 fascicular groups (Fig. 45-2). There is an anterior group to the pronator teres (PT) and flexor carpi radialis (FCR); a middle group consisting of motor fascicles to the flexor digitorum sublimus (FDS) and the hand intrinsics, sensory fascicles to the thumb, and index and middle fingers; and a posterior group to the anterior interosseous nerve (AIN). These branch groups can be traced proximally without harm, within the main trunk of the median nerve for 2.5 to 10 cm. The nerve and artery pass through the antecubital fossa underneath the lacertus fibrosis and give off branches to the palmaris longus (PL), FCR, FDS, and rarely the flexor digitorum profundus (FDP). The nerve then dives between the deep and superficial heads of the PT to which it supplies 1 to 4 branches. The fibrous arch of the PT lies 3 to 7.5 cm below the humeral epicondylar line. The fibrous arch of the superficialis arch lies 6.5 cm below the humeral epicondylar line. The median nerve enters the forearm deep to the fibrous arch of the FDS and emerges beneath the radial side of the muscle belly of the middle finger superficialis where it is quite superficial and near the PL tendon.

In a dissection of 31 cadaver arms, Tung and Mackinnon noted that double innervation of the FDS was found in 94% of the specimens.[2] The most common branching pattern was

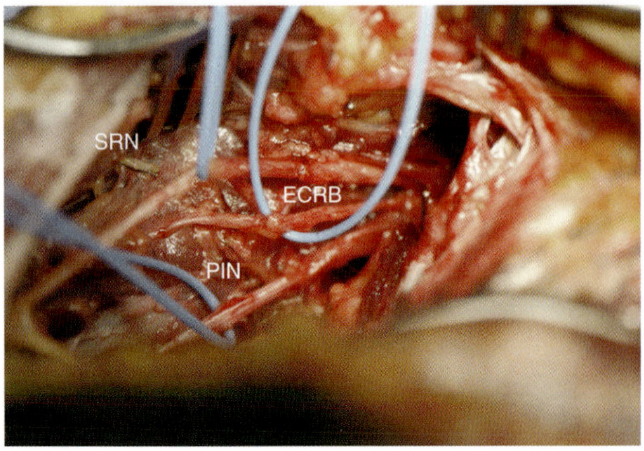

FIGURE 45-1 Exposure of the radial nerve through an anteromedial approach demonstrating the posterior interosseous nerve (PIN), the extensor carpi radialis brevis (ECRB) branch, and the superficial radial nerve (SRN) branch.

a proximal branch that also carried the branch to the PL, and a distal branch that arose from the median nerve distal to the origin of the AIN branch. The proximal branch was noted to arise 3.1 ± 1.3 cm distal to the medial epicondyle, and was 2.1 ± 0.7 cm long. The distal branch arose 7.4 ± 2.7 cm distal to the medial epicondyle, and was 2.3 ± 0.8 cm long. In the study by Ukrit et al[1] the proximal FDS branch arose 3.5 ± 0.8 cm below the interepicondylar line. The distal FDS branch arose 6.9 ± 2.2 cm below the interepicondylar line. The proximal FDS/PL branch arose 3.6 ± 1.1 cm below the interepicondylar line. The PL muscle was present in 9 specimens. The PL branch was present in 5 specimens and was combined with the proximal FDS branch in 4 specimens. It arose at 3.4 ± 1.6 cm below the interepicondylar line. The FCR branch was present in all specimens; it arose 4.6 ± 0.5 cm below the interepicondylar line. It was 4.2 ± 1.7 cm long and contained 2971 ± 345 myelinated nerve fibers, which represents approximately 39% of the axons of the PIN branch.

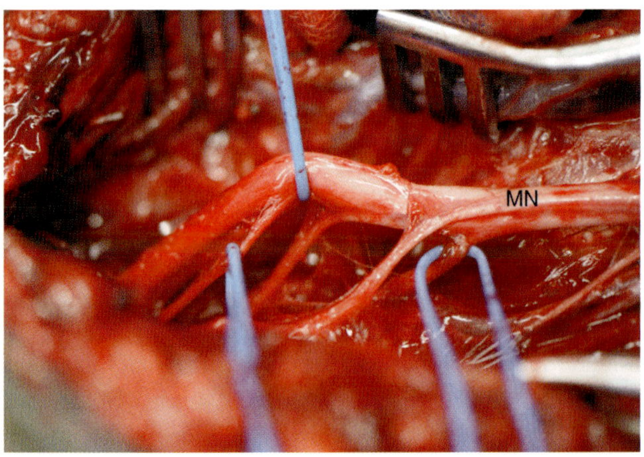

FIGURE 45-2 Exposure of the median nerve (MN) through an anteromedial approach illustrating the different fascicular groups.

The average number of myelinated nerve fibers of the proximal FDS branch was 983 ± 224, which represents approximately 35% of the axons of the ECRB branch.[1]

DIAGNOSIS

Radial Nerve Palsy in the Upper Arm

In the arm region, the radial nerve is often injured in association with some form of unconsciousness. In a Saturday night palsy, an obtunded patient sits with their arm over a chair back or rests his/her head on the lateral surface of their arm. Alternatively the radial nerve can be compressed in the groove between the brachialis and forearm muscles when 1 person rests their head on the middle third of the arm of another, that is, honeymooner's palsy. The patient will typically present with a wrist drop and an inability to extend the fingers, thumb, or wrist. In addition, the BR will be affected along with variable involvement of the triceps. They will also have diminished sensation over the dorsum of the first web space.

ELECTRODIAGNOSTIC STUDIES

The nerve conduction studies (NCS) typically demonstrate the absence of the superficial radial sensory nerve action potential (SNAP). Motor recordings are more difficult since no muscle is sufficiently isolated from other radially innervated muscles. A surface electrode over the EIP results in a volume-conducted response from the adjacent radial innervated muscles, which makes side-to-side amplitude comparisons difficult. Radial nerve recordings using needle electrodes in the EIP are more common as a result, which makes it difficult to approximate the degree of axonal loss by assessing the amplitudes. The EMG however is quite useful, and permits a relatively accurate localization of the lesion. In a spiral groove lesion, for example, all 3 heads of the triceps should be normal, with denervation of the BR and all muscles distal to it.

Posterior Interosseous Nerve Palsy

In a PIN palsy the presenting symptoms are weakness and/or paralysis of the extensor muscles, which result in a wrist or finger drop. There may be a history of a fall onto an extended and pronated arm, although many cases are spontaneous, especially if due to an underlying lipoma, ganglion, or rheumatoid nodule arising from the radiocapitellar joint. The patient will present with variable weakness or paralysis of the EPL, EIP, EDC, and ECU. Motor function of the ECRB/L should be preserved since they are innervated before the PIN dives between the 2 heads of the supinator muscle. The patient will hence extend their wrist in radial deviation. As it travels distally through the radial tunnel the PIN may potentially be entrapped by fibrous bands anterior to the radiocapitellar joint, the radial recurrent leash of vessels, the fibrous edge of the ECRB, the proximal border of the supinator, that is, the arcade of Frohse, or the distal edge of the supinator muscle.

ELECTRODIAGNOSTIC STUDIES

PIN lesions do not affect the superficial radial SNAP, which should be normal. The compound motor action potential of the PIN-innervated muscles may show a drop of conduction velocity or amplitude, but this is difficult to assess with surface electrodes. Needle EMG is the best technique for localization, especially with partial lesions. In acute denervation decreased recruitment, increased insertional activity, and fibrillation potentials ± positive sharp waves are present. In chronic lesions seen after 3 to 6 months, decreased recruitment may still be seen along with giant motor unit potentials and polyphasia due to peripheral axonal ingrowth.

INDICATIONS

The time for reinnervation must take the distance from the injury to the motor end plate into account. As a general rule, motor end plates degrade at about 1% per week. Nerve growth is limited to 1 in per month or 1 to 1.5 mm per day. By this reckoning a nerve will have regenerated 12 in at 1 year, but 50% of the end plates will be gone. The maximum length that a nerve can grow to restore motor function is hence approximately 13 to 18 in due to a critical loss of end plates. Proximal radial nerve repairs typically demonstrate superior results as compared with those for the median or ulnar nerves since they are closer to the end plate.

Nerve to nerve transfers should therefore be considered in cases of delayed treatment, where the time for nerve ingrowth would exceed this window of time for reinnervation. Proximal radial nerve injuries that are 8 to 9 months old would be an ideal indication for neurotization for this reason. Brachial plexus lesions and traction injuries that show no EMG evidence of recovery by 3 months may also be appropriate candidates.

CONTRAINDICATIONS

Contraindications include nerve palsies that may recover spontaneously such as proximal radial nerve lesions that are less than 6 months old or are best treated with conventional methods of nerve repair or graft. PIN lesions that are 12 months from the time of injury or later are a contraindication as well as concomitant median nerve injuries that would preclude use of this transfer.

SURGICAL TECHNIQUE

Harvest of the FCR and FDS Fascicles

The patient is positioned supine with the arm abducted on an arm board. The procedure is performed under tourniquet control. The tourniquet time is limited to 1 hour and must be released at least 20 minutes before stimulating the nerve. If intraoperative nerve conduction is performed, halothane and muscle relaxants are avoided since they extinguish the nerve response. The nerve should be irrigated with warm saline, since cold nerves do not conduct. A short-acting agent such as fentanyl can be used after infiltration of the wound margins with local anesthetic.

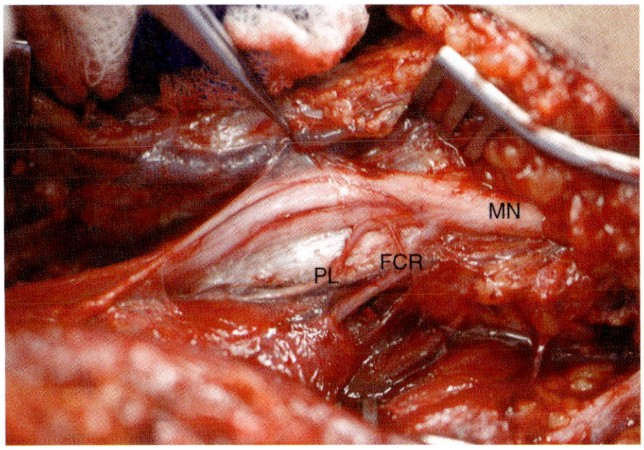

FIGURE 45-3 Dissection of the median nerve (MN) highlighting the branch to the flexor carpi radialis (FCR) and the palmaris longus (PL).

An anteromedial incision is made crossing the antecubital fossa, starting 5 cm above the elbow flexion crease. The medial antebrachial cutaneous nerve is identified next to the basilic vein and protected. Proximal to the elbow, the median nerve can be found medial to the brachial artery. The nerve is followed distally as it passes through the 2 heads of the PT. At this level the branches arising from the anterior bundle can be seen innervating the FCR and PT. The superficial head of the PT and the FDS can be divided and tagged for later repair if needed. Release of the deep head of the PT can improve the exposure. The nerve to the PT branch can be found in the proximal antecubital fossa. Distal to the antecubital crease, the branch to the FCR and PL are identified coming off the middle group of fascicles medially (Fig. 45-3).

The FDS branches arise distal to this group. They are carefully differentiated from the motor fascicles to the hand intrinsics using the handheld stimulator (Fig. 45-4). The

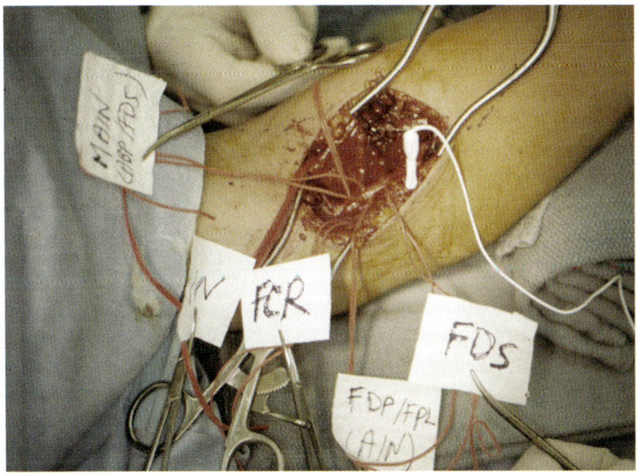

FIGURE 45-4 Intraoperative photograph depicting electrical stimulation of the median nerve to identify the individual nerve branches.

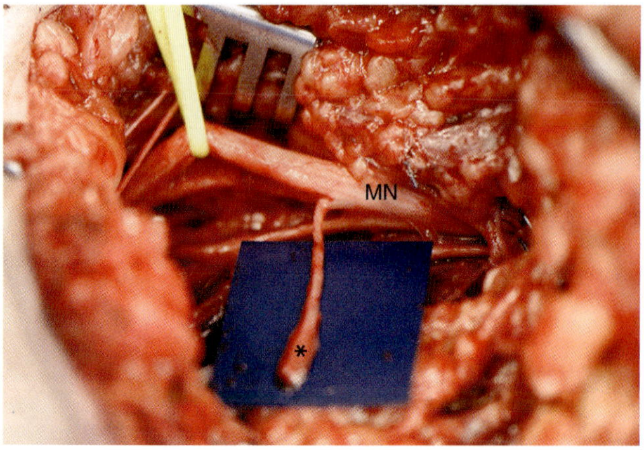

FIGURE 45-5 Division of the proximal motor branch to the flexor digitorum sublimus (FDS) arising from the median nerve (MN).

intrinsic motor fascicles and sensory fascicles travel distally in the middle group along with the posterior (AIN branch) group that passes underneath the sublimus arch. This arch is divided. The second or distal group of FDS fascicles may arise distal to the sublimus arch. At this point it is helpful to place vessel loops around the branches of interest.

A disposable 2-mA nerve stimulator is used to sequentially stimulate the branches. Careful observation of the hand will allow one to discern the individual motor branches by their corresponding muscle twitch. Once the proximal FDS branch is identified, it is divided as distal as proximal and then a proximal neurolysis is performed until an interfascicular branch is seen (Fig. 45-5).

Radial Nerve Exposure

The radial nerve is isolated through the same incision. It can be found between the BR and brachialis as it divides into the superficial sensory nerve branch and the PIN branch. The SRN is followed proximally to the main trunk of the radial nerve. The ECRB branch is found deep and radial to the SRN. In a PIN palsy with preserved radial wrist extension, the PIN is divided distal to the motor branch of the ECRB.

In proximal radial nerve injuries the ECRB branch is divided and included in the transfer. These branches are stimulated to confirm that there is total extensor muscle enervation prior to nerve division. The branch to the supinator can be divided to mobilize the nerve and to exclude axonal misdirection to the supinator muscle. An intraoperative EMG can be performed if necessary by placing the needle recording electrode in the ECRB or extensor muscle mass with the reference electrode in the subcutaneous tissue. The presence of a compound motor action potential might alter the prognosis for recovery and require modification of the procedure to a neurolysis. Alternatively, a nerve action potential can be sought by stimulating and recording across a 4-cm segment of the PIN.

Nerve Transfer

Ray and Mackinnon recommends coapting the FDS motor fascicles with the ECRB branch because this can reproduce the tenodesis effect of wrist extension with finger flexion and can facilitate motor reeducation. Similarly the FCR motor fascicles are coapted to the PIN to facilitate synergistic wrist flexion with finger extension (Fig. 45-6A-D).[3]

Further dissection of the PIN to exclude the branch to the supinator muscle also may enhance the mobilization of the nerve. In addition, removing the supinator muscle as a potential target allows all transferred axons to be directed to the primary functions of finger and wrist extension.

The redundant median nerve fascicles are harvested in close proximity to the PIN to avoid undue tension on the repair site (Fig. 45-7A and B). Mackinnon stresses the need to always section the donor nerve as distal as possible and the recipient nerve as proximal as possible to avoid tension on the coaptation site and avoid the need for a nerve graft. Coaptation of the motor fascicles proximal to the takeoff of the SRN may lead to a misdirection of fascicles down the SRN. If need be, a short nerve graft can be interposed. Similar to nerve repair, there should be <8% strain on the repair site. For practical purposes, if the repair can withstand the tension during passive elbow motion intraoperatively, then a graft is not needed.

The coaptation is performed with 9-0 nylon since the fascicles are typically 1 to 3 mm in diameter. The repair site can be augmented with fibrin glue (Fig. 45-8A-C). Recently, Mackinnon has recommended a tendon transfer of the PT to the ECRB as an internal splint to provide early wrist extension while the nerve is regenerating (Fig. 45-9).

Mackinnon has also suggested that a sensory nerve transfer of the lateral antebrachial cutaneous nerve to the SRN in the distal part of the incision can substitute the region of sensory loss over the dorsoradial hand from the SRN injury to the less essential cutaneous territory of the LABCN over the volar radial forearm (Fig. 45-10A and B).

Postoperative Rehabilitation

An above-elbow splint is applied with the elbow at 90° and the shoulder, wrist, and fingers free. Gentle elbow flexion is started after the first week followed by gradual elbow extension. Motor retraining is akin to tendon transfers. The patient is instructed in active sublimus contractions as well as active wrist flexion that will ultimately produce wrist and finger extension.

OUTCOMES

In the series of Ray and Mackinnon 17 of 19 patients had complete radial nerve palsy, whereas 2 had intact wrist extension with loss of finger and thumb extension.[3] MRC muscle strength of 0/5 to 2/5 was considered a poor outcome,

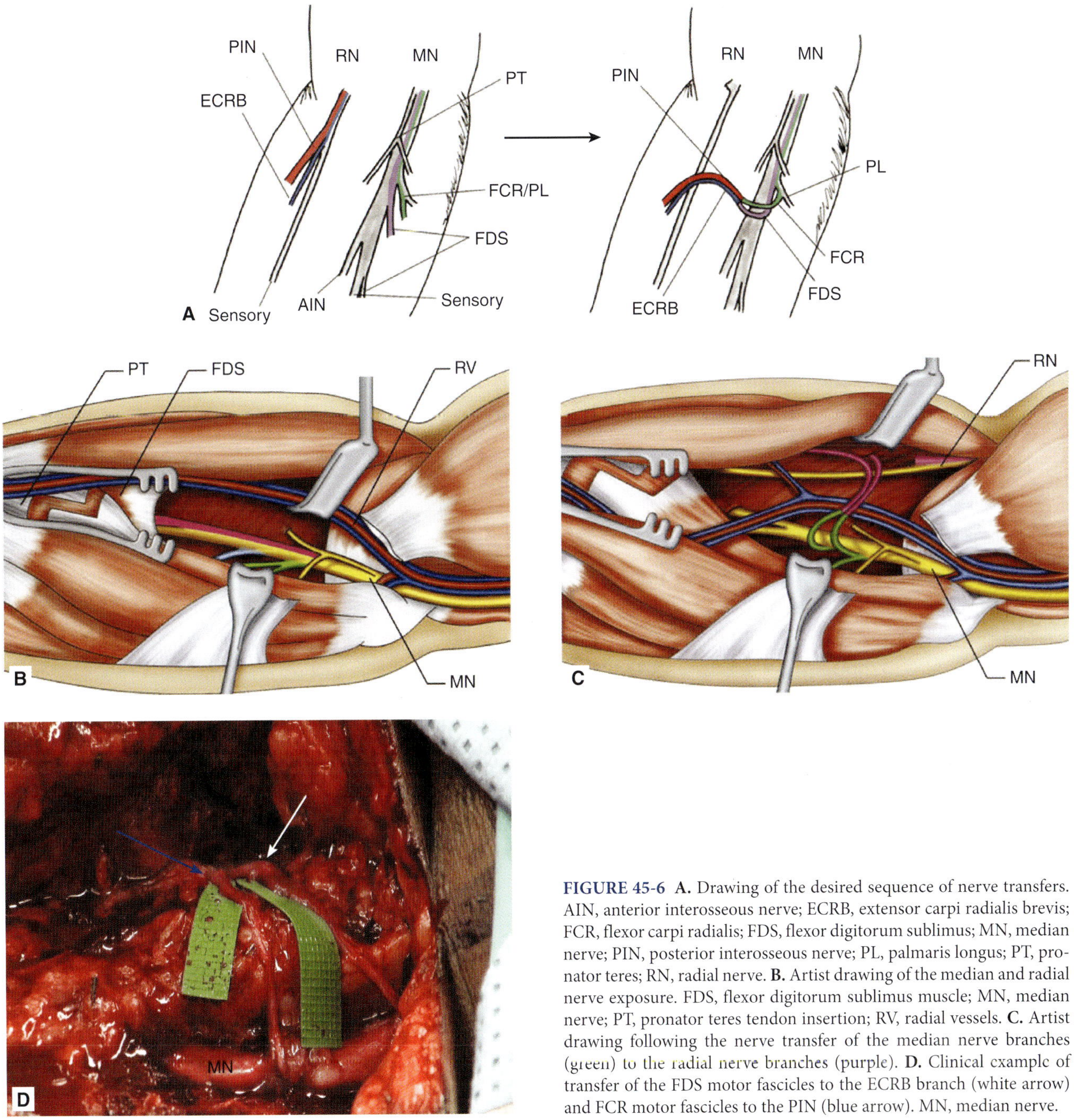

FIGURE 45-6 **A.** Drawing of the desired sequence of nerve transfers. AIN, anterior interosseous nerve; ECRB, extensor carpi radialis brevis; FCR, flexor carpi radialis; FDS, flexor digitorum sublimus; MN, median nerve; PIN, posterior interosseous nerve; PL, palmaris longus; PT, pronator teres; RN, radial nerve. **B.** Artist drawing of the median and radial nerve exposure. FDS, flexor digitorum sublimus muscle; MN, median nerve; PT, pronator teres tendon insertion; RV, radial vessels. **C.** Artist drawing following the nerve transfer of the median nerve branches (green) to the radial nerve branches (purple). **D.** Clinical example of transfer of the FDS motor fascicles to the ECRB branch (white arrow) and FCR motor fascicles to the PIN (blue arrow). MN, median nerve.

whereas an MRC grade of 3/5 was a fair result, 4/5 was a good result, and 4+/5 was an excellent outcome. The mean age of patients was 41 years (range, 17-78 years). Mean follow-up was done at 20.3 ± 5.8 months (range, 12-33). Surgery was performed at a mean of 5.7 ± 1.9 months post injury (range 3-10 months). Nine patients had a MRC grade of 4/5 wrist and finger extension: 4 of these patients had a PT to ECRB tendon transfer (Fig. 45-11). One patient obtained 5/5 wrist and finger extension along with a PT to ECRB tendon transfer. Six patients obtained 4/5 wrist extension but minimal finger extension: 3 patients had a simultaneous PT to ECRB tendon transfer. One patient with a PIN palsy obtained 4/5 finger extension. One patient with a PIN palsy obtained 3/5 finger extension and ultimately underwent a PL to EPL and FCR to EDC tendon transfer. One patient with a PIN palsy obtained 0/5 wrist and finger extension.

Ukrit et al[1] recently reported on 2 clinical cases of complete brachial plexus avulsion injuries involving C5 to C7 who underwent a neurotization of the FDS branch to the ECRB. At 24 months, both patients had regained MRC 4/5 strength in wrist extension with no loss of FDS function.

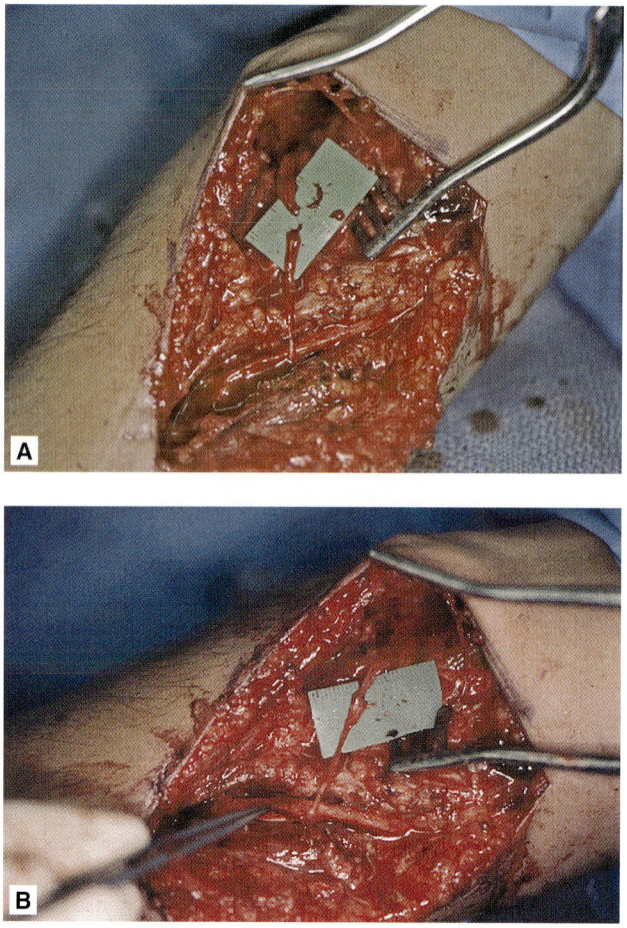

FIGURE 45-7 **A.** End-to-end transfer of FDS branch to the PIN. **B.** Following coaptation.

A number of variations have been described based on anatomic studies. These are described for completeness, but none of these transfers have enjoyed widespread clinical use however. In some instances with incomplete recovery of a high radial nerve palsy nerve and end-to-side coaptation can augment the muscle strength (Fig. 45-11A-C). Palazzi et al reported on the use of the motor branch to the brachialis muscle for neurotization of the radial nerve for a C7-C8-T1 avulsion.[4] Tubbs et al performed an anatomic study on the AIN and described a transinterosseous membrane tunneling technique for transfer to the PIN.[5]

Brown et al noted that the FCU branch of ulnar nerve can also be used, but this required a second incision.[6] Ukrit et al performed an FDS to ECRB transfer in 2 patients with a complete brachial plexus avulsion injury that involved the C5-C7 roots and obtained an MRC grade of 4/5 wrist extension at 24 months with no loss of FDS function.[1] Bertelli and Ghizoni have described the successful transfer of the supinator motor branch to the PIN in cases of C5-C6 brachial plexus injuries.[7]

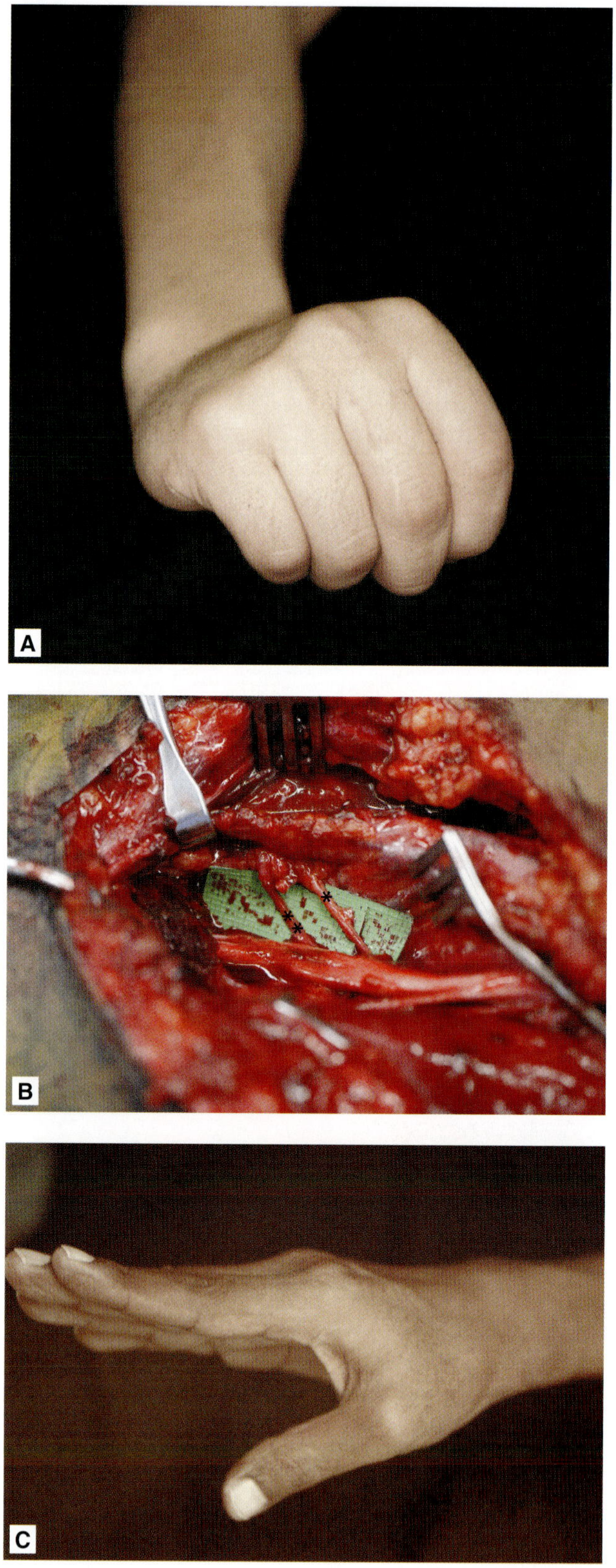

FIGURE 45-8 **A.** A 28-year-old male with a 6-month-old PIN palsy. **B.** Coaptation of the FCR branch to the PIN (single asterisk) and the FDS branch to the ECRB branch (double asterisk) in a PIN nerve palsy. **C.** Outcome at 1 year demonstrating good wrist and finger extension.

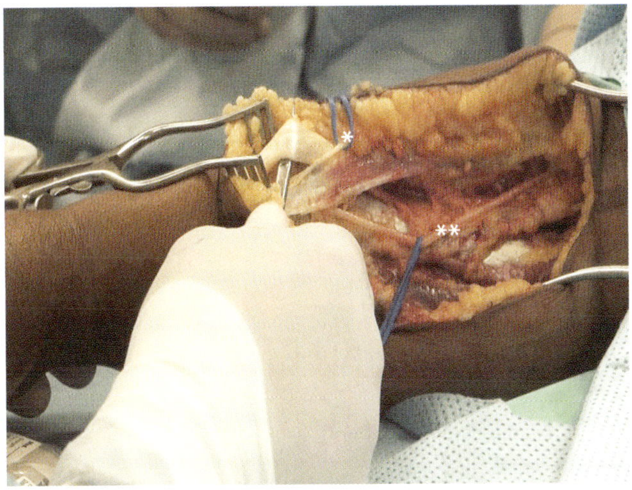

FIGURE 45-9 The extensor carpi radialis brevis tendon is isolated for an end-to-side transfer of the pronator teres.

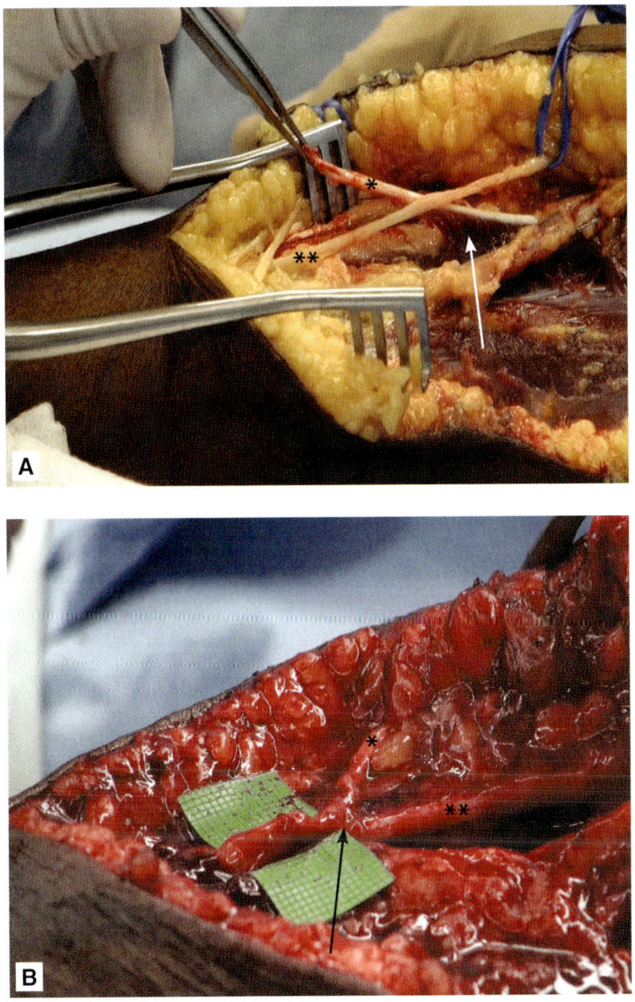

FIGURE 45-10 **A.** Sensory nerve transfer of the lateral antebrachial cutaneous nerve (*) to the superficial radial nerve (**) following a PT to ECRB transfer (arrow). **B.** Complete anastomosis (arrow).

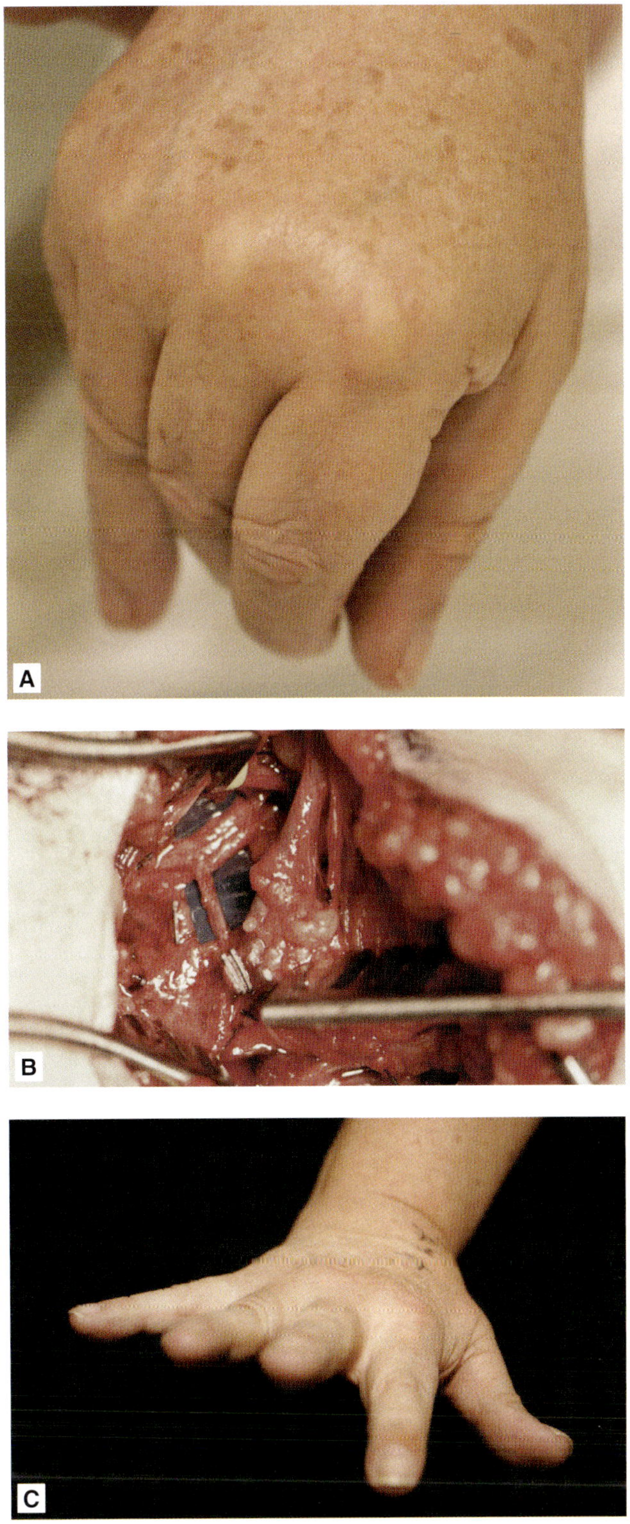

FIGURE 45-11 **A.** Recovering high radial nerve palsy in a 65-year-old female at 7 months following internal fixation of a proximal humerus fracture. Note the weak wrist extension but no finger extension. **B.** End-to-side coaptation of the FDS branch to the PIN distal to the ECRB branch. **C.** Result at 4 months following nerve transfer (11 months following palsy). Patient has regained good wrist, thumb, and finger extension save for a residual extensor lag of the index.

REFERENCES

1. Ukrit A, Leechavengvongs S, Malungpaishrope K, Uerpairojkit C, Chongthammakun S, Witoonchart K. Nerve transfer for wrist extension using nerve to flexor digitorum superficialis in cervical 5, 6, and 7 root avulsions: anatomic study and report of two cases. *J Hand Surg Am*. 2009;34:1659–1666.
2. Tung TH, Mackinnon SE. Flexor digitorum superficialis nerve transfer to restore pronation: two case reports and anatomic study. *J Hand Surg Am*. 2001;26:1065–1072.
3. Ray WZ, Mackinnon SE. Clinical outcomes following median to radial nerve transfers. *J Hand Surg Am*. 2011;36:201–208.
4. Palazzi S, Palazzi JL, Caceres JP. Neurotization with the brachialis muscle motor nerve. *Microsurgery*. 2006;26:330–333.
5. Tubbs RS, Custis JW, Salter EG, Wellons JC 3rd, Blount JP, Oakes WJ. Quantitation of and superficial surgical landmarks for the anterior interosseous nerve. *J Neurosurg*. 2006;104:787–791.
6. Brown JM, Yee A, Mackinnon SE. Distal median to ulnar nerve transfers to restore ulnar motor and sensory function within the hand: technical nuances. *Neurosurgery*. 2009;65:966–977 [discussion 977–978].
7. Bertelli JA, Ghizoni MF. Transfer of supinator motor branches to the posterior interosseous nerve in C7-T1 brachial plexus palsy. *J Neurosurg*. 2010;113:129–132.

VII

SHOULDER

46

Fractures of the Shoulder Girdle: Humeral Shaft, Humeral Head, Scapula and Glenoid, and Clavicle

Kyle Caswell, DO
Todd C. Moen, MD
Sumant "Butch" Krishnan, MD

HUMERAL SHAFT FRACTURES

Rationale and Basic Science Pertinent to the Procedure

Humeral shaft fractures represent 4% of all fractures. A bimodal pattern exists with a peak in the third decade (mostly males with severe trauma) and another peak in the seventh decade (mostly females involved in minor trauma).[1]

The blood supply to the humeral shaft is predominantly provided by the nutrient artery, a branch of the brachial artery that penetrates the proximal third of the medial humerus. The radial nerve lies adjacent to bone in the spiral groove just posterior to the deltoid tuberosity and courses posterolaterally until it exits the spiral groove on the lateral aspect of the humerus 10 to 15 cm distal to the lateral acromion. It is bounded by the lateral intermuscular septum in this area, making it susceptible to traction injury.[2]

Operative Indications

a. These include greater than 20° of anterior angulation, greater than 30° of varus angulation, and/or greater than 3 cm of shortening of the humeral shaft. Other indications include open fractures, fracture with a vascular injury, polytrauma, associated ipsilateral upper extremity injury, fractures with intra-articular extension, and morbidly obese patient who cannot fit/tolerate the functional brace. There is no specific age range and primary surgery should be accomplished within 3 weeks.

Contraindications

a. These include hemodynamic instability and sepsis. A relative contraindication would include inadequate soft tissue coverage, although this could be managed with regional and distant flap coverage.

Surgical Technique

a. General anesthesia is used with muscle relaxation. The patient is placed in a modified beach chair position. An adjustable arm holder is used for arm positioning. Instrumentation includes two 3.5-mm LCDC plates orthogonally placed (double plating). The surgical approaches include posterior, lateral, or anterolateral based on fracture location and surgeon preference. We prefer an anterolateral incision to expose and reduce the fracture and to perform a double plating technique (Fig. 46-1).
b. A 3.5-mm LCDC plate is applied laterally in order to gain compression, and then an LCDC plate is placed anteriorly for both rotational control and 90°-90° fixation that increases the rigidity of the construct. Extensive soft tissue and bone stripping in the proximal medial aspect of the humeral shaft must be avoided since the nutrient artery enters in this area.

Complications

Nonunions in nonoperatively and operatively treated humeral shaft fractures are reported to be between 2% and 12%.[3-5]

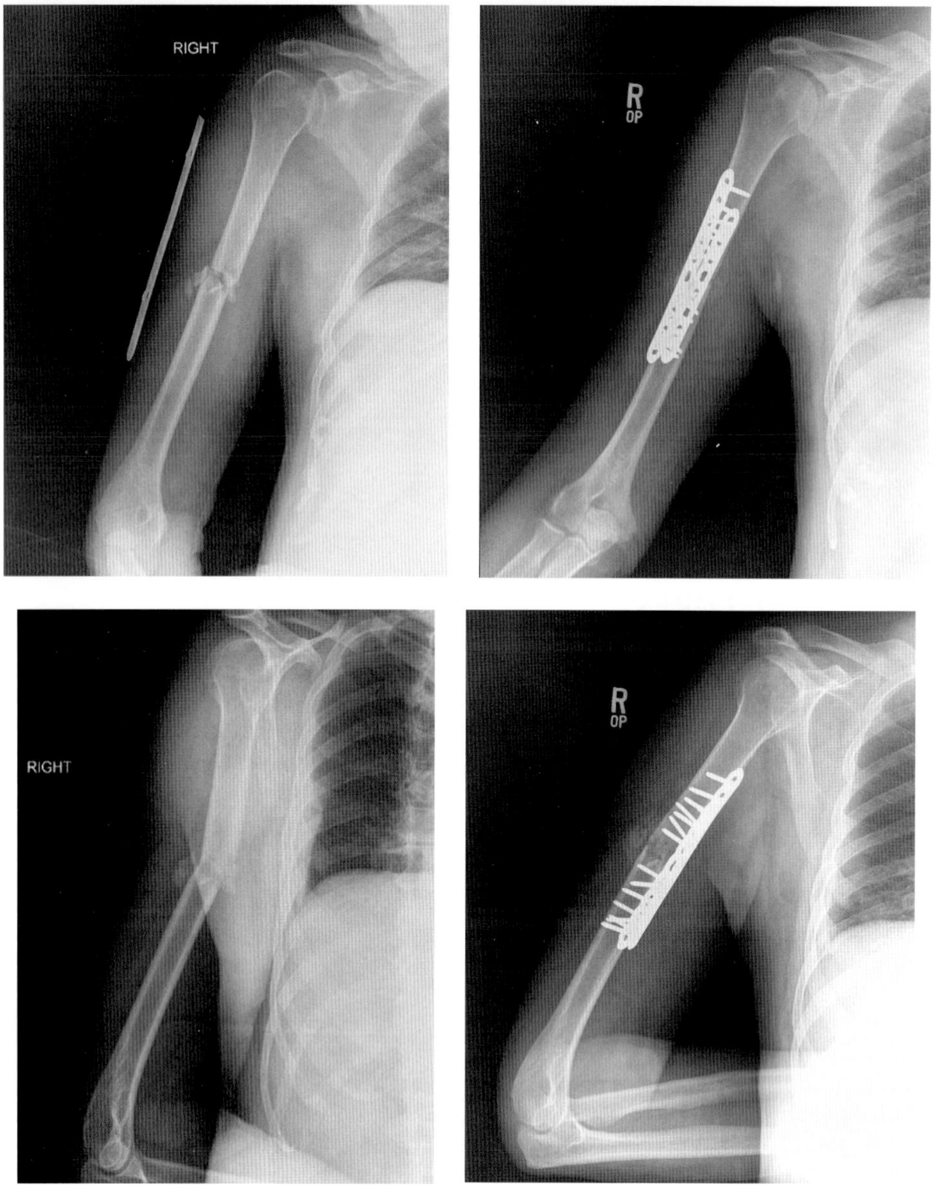

FIGURE 46-1 ORIF for humeral shaft fracture with orthogonal plating technique. (Reproduced with permission from Sumant G. Krishnan, MD.)

a. Radial nerve palsy occurs in up to 18% of closed injuries. Recovery can be expected with observation alone in 90% at 3 to 4 months after injury.[6] Due to the low probability of closed injuries and radial nerve transection and poor results of primary repair, routine exploration of the radial nerve is not recommended.[7] If there are no clinical signs of radial nerve recovery 6 weeks after injury, an EMG is performed. If muscle action potentials are present, observation of the radial nerve should be continued. If fibrillation potentials (denervation) are present, EMG and nerve conduction studies are repeated 12 weeks after injury. If nerve recovery is absent on clinical exam and EMG at 12 weeks, surgical exploration of the radial nerve is recommended.[5]

Outcomes

Functional bracing has a high success and low complication rate. Sarmiento et al found nonunion rates of 2% and 6% for closed and open fractures, respectively.[3] A recent meta-analysis found a nonunion rate of 5.5% with an average of 10.7 weeks to union.[8]

a. Compressive plating of the humeral shaft fracture has union rates of 92% to 96%. The time to union is approximately 10 to 12 weeks.[5]

b. A recent meta-analysis showed humeral nailing had higher rates of reoperation, radial nerve injury, chronic subacromial pain, and iatrogenic fracture when compared with compression plating.[9]

PROXIMAL HUMERUS FRACTURES

Rationale and Basic Science Pertinent to the Procedure

Proximal humerus fractures make up 4% to 5% of all fractures. They are the third most common fracture in the elderly. The incidence is increasing worldwide with the aging population. The most common mechanism is a simple, low-energy fall in an elderly patient.[10]

Evaluation of medical comorbidities is critical in this patient population and should thoroughly evaluate the patient for traumatic head injury, cardiac disease, cerebrovascular disease, and neurologic disease.[11] EMG evidence has shown a 67% incidence of acute neurologic injury with 58% of axillary neurapraxia and 48% incidence of suprascapular neurapraxia. Regardless of treatment, eventual functional recovery requires 12 to 18 months.[12]

The majority of patients will receive nonoperative treatment. However, some will require surgical fixation. We use an evidence-based algorithm to choose a head preserving versus head replacing procedure based on the patient's age, bone quality, fracture pattern, and timing of surgery.[13] We look at the patient's physiologic age and comorbid disease. Is the patient's bone osteoporotic or osteopenic? We also look at fracture pattern and if there are predictors of humeral head ischemia. Hertel et al described predictors of humeral head ischemia at time zero: posteromedial metaphyseal extension less than 8 mm, disruption of the medial hinge greater than 2 mm, and an anatomic neck fracture.[14] Timing of surgery affects the ability to reduce the fracture, viability of the humeral head, and ultimate functional outcome. An untreated fracture greater than 4 weeks is chronic sequela and no longer an acute fracture.[15,16]

Indications

Percutaneous pinning is our preferred method for a viable head and reducible fracture in young patients. The ideal surgical candidate is usually under 70 years of age with no cardiac history. Ideally the patient should have good bone quality with no history of smoking or diabetes.

a. Age: Under 70, no cardiac history:
   i. Any fracture pattern with a viable head (intact medial calcar) is appropriate provided that the fracture is stable after reduction in order to be a candidate for pinning. We prefer to operate within 10 days of injury.

b. Open reduction internal fixation/osteosynthesis of the tuberosities is considered for patients under 70 years old. Any fracture pattern with a viable head and inherently unstable fracture involving the medial calcar is preferably treated with a second orthogonal plate or intramedullary allograft strut to control rotation and varus deforming forces. The timing is not as critical to the outcome, but we prefer to operate within 4 weeks.

c. Hemiarthroplasty or reverse total shoulder arthroplasty with fracture stem for osteosynthesis of the greater and lesser tuberosities. This is considered at any age. We prefer to perform a reverse total shoulder arthroplasty for patients 75 years or older. This can be performed even with osteopenic bone and is indicated in any case of avascular necrosis of the humeral head based on the Hertel criteria.[14] Hertel et al found that good predictors of ischemia were the length of the metaphyseal head extension with calcar segments <8 mm, the integrity of the medial hinge, and the basic fracture pattern. Moderate and poor predictors of ischemia were fractures consisting of 4 fragments, angular displacement of the head, the amount of displacement of the tuberosities, glenohumeral dislocation, head-split components, and fractures consisting of 3 fragments. When the above criteria of anatomic neck fracture location, short calcar, and a disrupted medial hinge were combined, positive predictive values of up to 97% could be obtained. The optimal timing is 6 to 14 days after injury.

Contraindications

These include hemodynamic instability, sepsis, and severely osteopenic or osteoporotic bone.

Surgical Technique

a. Percutaneous pinning (Fig. 46-2): General anesthesia is used with muscle relaxation. The patient is in a modified beach chair position with an adjustable arm holder to facilitate AP and axillary views under fluoroscopic control.
   i. Under fluoroscopy anterior, lateral, and superior marks are made for reduction and pin placement positions. A Freer elevator is used to reduce the humeral head and tuberosities, which are then captured using percutaneously introduced 2.0-mm terminally threaded pins (Fig. 46-3). Arthroscopy-assisted percutaneous fixation of greater tuberosity fractures as well as 4-part humerus fractures has been reported.[17–19]

   The shoulder is then taken through a gentle range of motion to confirm the stability of fixation.
      1. One should be prepared to proceed with an ORIF in case the reduction does not hold or if the tuberosities are malreduced. Equipment is placed in the room for next procedure if initial plan fails.

b. Open reduction internal fixation/osteosynthesis of tuberosities (Fig. 46-4): General anesthesia is used with muscle relaxation. The patient is placed in a modified beach chair position with an adjustable arm holder to change positions during surgery. A large deltopectoral incision is made to provide access to the deltoid insertion. Up to 20% of the deltoid insertion is incised in order to expose the lateral aspect of the humerus.

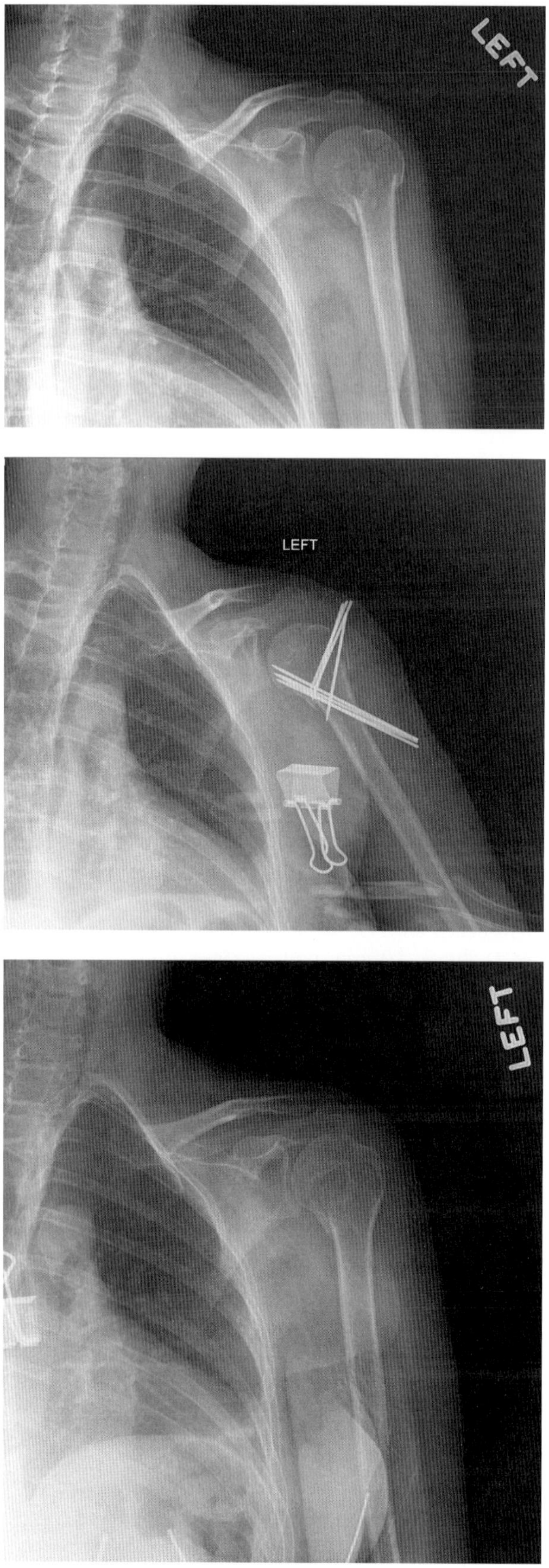

FIGURE 46-2 Percutaneous pinning proximal humerus fracture. (Reproduced with permission from Sumant G. Krishnan, MD.)

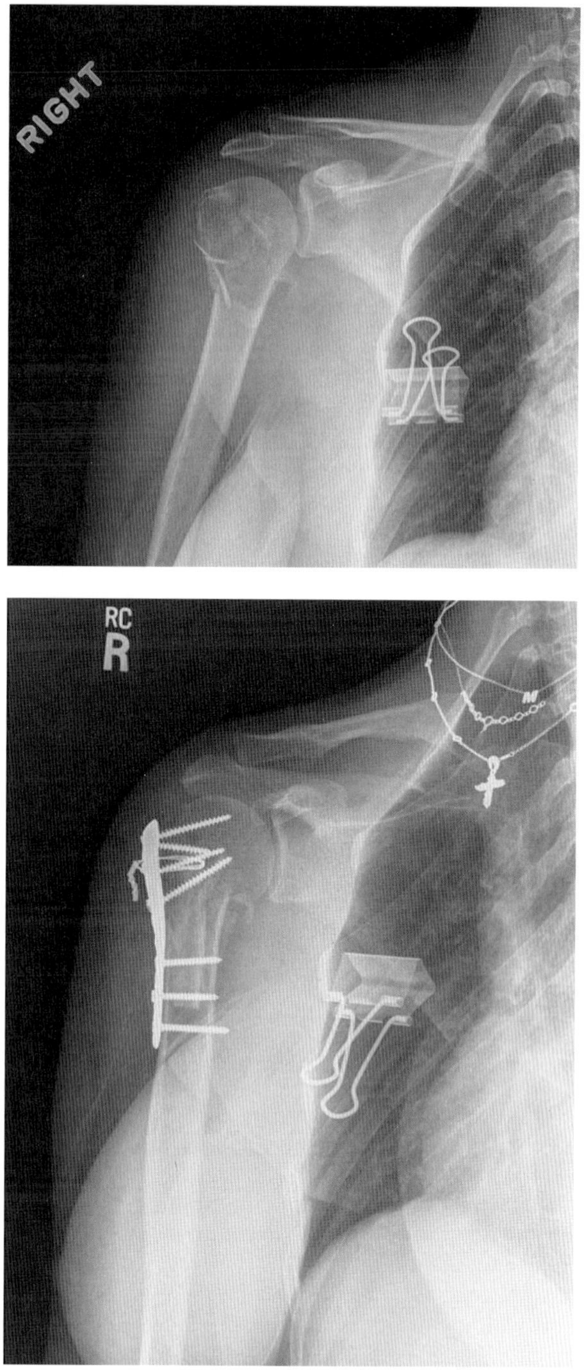

FIGURE 46-3 ORIF of proximal humerus fracture. (Reproduced with permission from Sumant G. Krishnan, MD.)

A proximal humeral locking plate may be used to reduce any varus deformity by fixing the plate to the humeral head first and then applying the metaphyseal/diaphyseal screws in a stepwise fashion.

i. If the medial calcar is significantly involved, a second orthogonally placed small fragment plate with or without an intramedullary allograft strut may be used to control rotation and the varus moment at the fracture site.

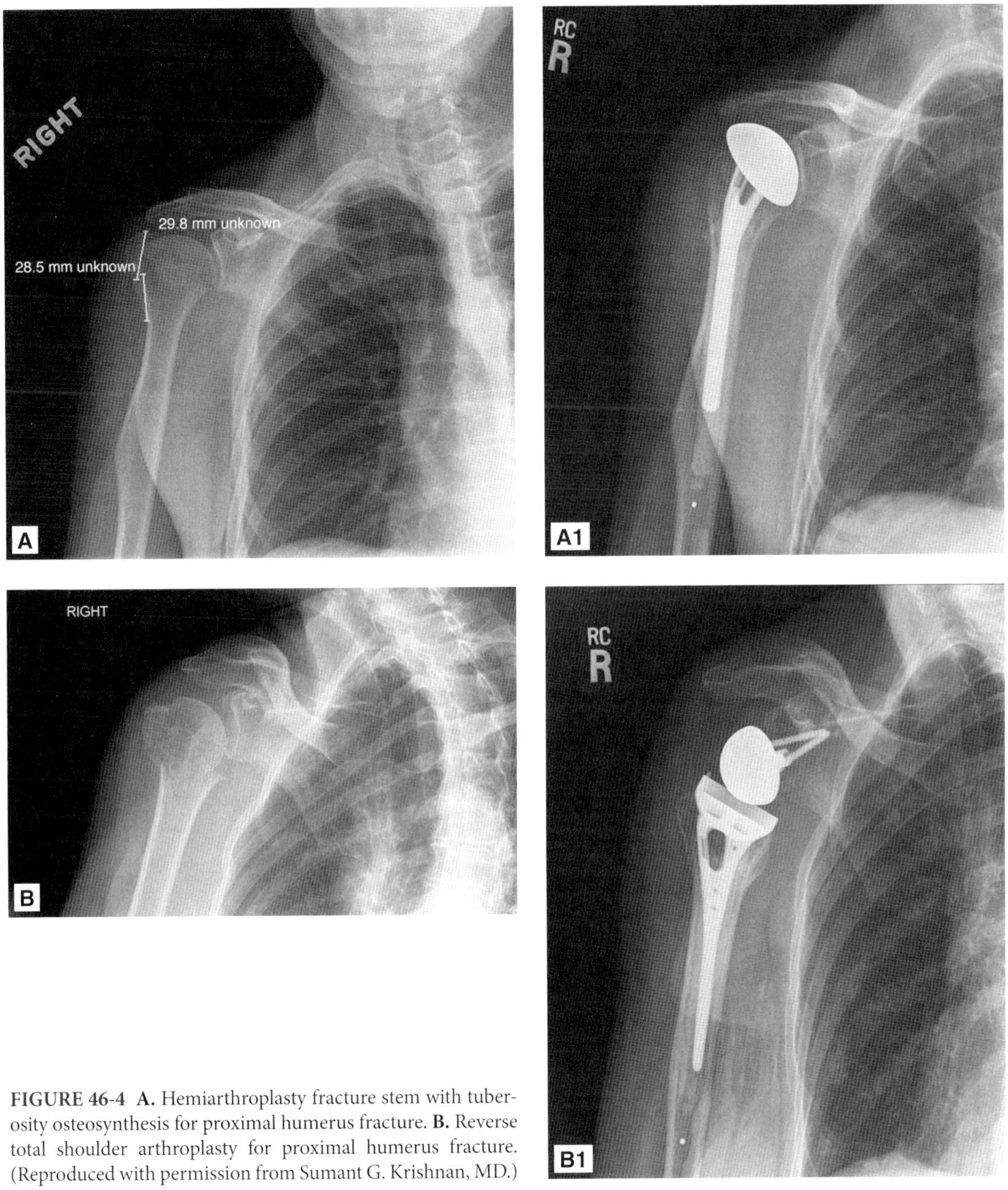

FIGURE 46-4 **A.** Hemiarthroplasty fracture stem with tuberosity osteosynthesis for proximal humerus fracture. **B.** Reverse total shoulder arthroplasty for proximal humerus fracture. (Reproduced with permission from Sumant G. Krishnan, MD.)

1. The extensile nature of the approach leads to increased soft tissue stripping that may result in an impairment of the humeral head blood supply. Adequate fixation may be difficult in osteoporotic bone.
2. Good outcomes with a low complication rate with the use of an endosteal bone strut to augment the plate fixation have recently been reported.[20]

c. Primary shoulder arthroplasty (Figs. 46-4 and 46-5):

i. General anesthesia with muscle relaxation is used. The patient is placed in a modified beach chair position with an adjustable arm holder. The fracture is exposed through a deltopectoral approach.

The use of a prosthetic jig can aid in reproducing the anatomic retroversion of 20°. The transepicondylar axis is used as a reference with the humeral head pointed toward the glenoid face and the arm in neutral rotation.

1. Preoperatively full-length scaled radiographs of injured and contralateral normal humerus with a ruler of defined length are obtained. The fractured arm is measured from the medial calcar to a defined point distally. The normal arm is measured from the superior humeral head to the same distally defined point. The difference is the amount of length that is needed to restore the normal humeral height, which restores the normal "Gothic arch" (Fig. 46-5).

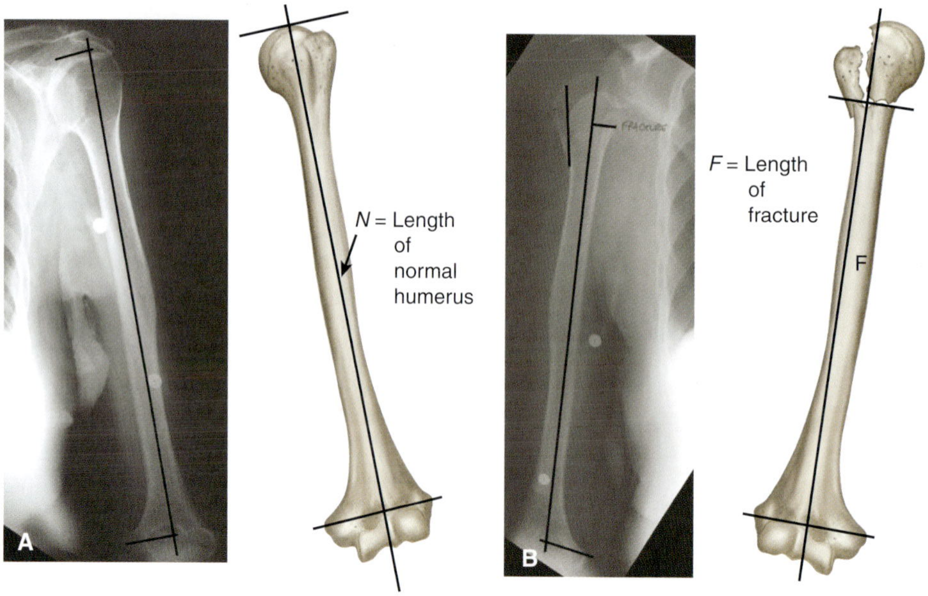

Calculations to restore gothic arch

Normal side ruler		**Fracture side ruler**	
X-ray	11.2 cm	X-ray	12.1 cm
Actual	10.0 cm	Actual	10.0 cm
Magnif.	1.12 cm	Magnif.	1.21 cm
Humeral length (*N*)		**Fx length (*F*)**	
X-ray	35.0 cm	X-ray	32.6 cm
Actual	31.3 cm	Actual	26.9 cm

Step 1. Fx to top of head: *N* – *F* = *H*

C Actual *N* (31.3 cm) minus actual *F* (26.9 cm) equals *H* (4.4 cm)

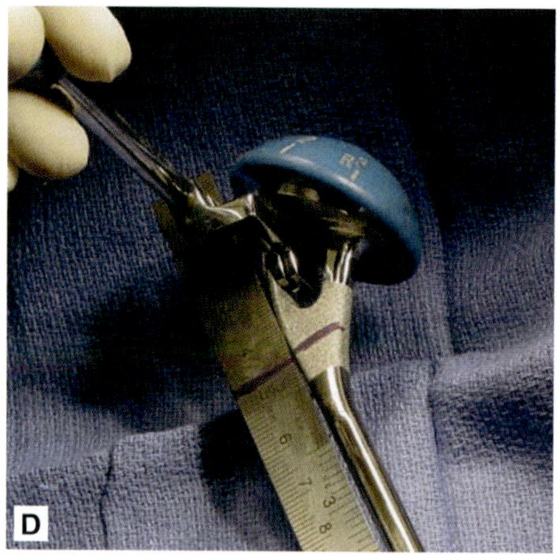

FIGURE 46-5 Calculation of humeral height for hemiarthroplasty fracture stem. (Reproduced with permission from Sumant G. Krishnan, MD.)

2. The prosthesis that is specifically designed for humeral head fractures utilizes a small proximal metaphyseal prosthetic body with a window to allow for maximal bony contact. Three structural cancellous bone graft wedges obtained from the fractured humeral head are placed (1) in the window of the fracture-specific prosthesis, (2) under the greater tuberosity at the lateral fin of the prosthesis, and (3) under the medial edge of the prosthetic head between the head and neck of the implant (Fig. 46-6A).
3. We then use 4 horizontal plane cerclage sutures passing around the prosthetic neck to bring the greater and lesser tuberosities into their correct position and 2 vertical plane tension-band sutures to bring the tuberosities into apposition with the humeral shaft (Fig. 46-6B–D).
4. Pitfalls include prosthetic malpositioning,[21] poor fixation of the tuberosities, as well as poor prosthetic design: excessive metal at the prosthetic neck level is a barrier to bone healing.
   ii. The question of whether to perform a primary reverse total shoulder versus a primary hemiarthroplasty in this situation remains unsettled.

Complications

Percutaneous pinning: Patients with tuberosity fractures have a higher rate of fixation failure following percutaneous pinning in the presence of osteoporotic bone and 4-part fractures.

There is a higher rate of avascular necrosis of the humeral head after open reduction and internal fixation.[22] Complications appear to relate to the number of screws in the humeral head, screw penetration of the humeral head articular surface, or failure of fixation with nonlocking screws in metaphyseal bone.[23]

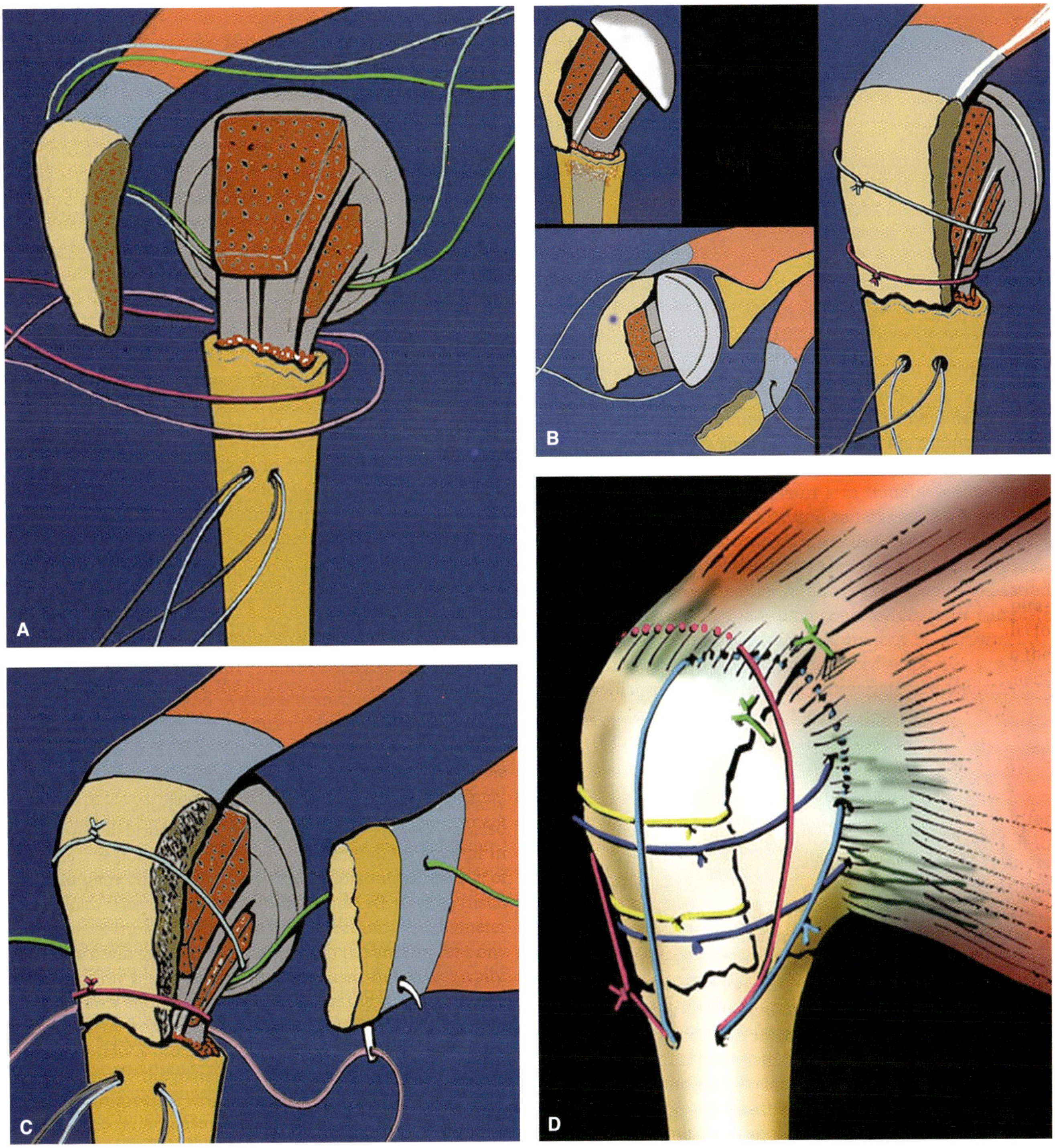

FIGURE 46-6 **A.** Bone graft placement in hemiarthroplasty fracture stem. **B–D.** Tuberosity osteosynthesis technique in hemiarthroplasty fracture stem. (Reproduced with permission from Sumant G. Krishnan, MD.)

Following a shoulder arthroplasty, prosthetic malposition leads to a proud prosthesis in the vertical plane and excessive retroversion in the horizontal plane.[21]

i. Tuberosity malposition and malunion/nonunion are detrimental to the outcomes. Passing suture through the prosthetic fin does not stabilize the tuberosities to each other or to the diaphysis. This causes tuberosity mobility/migration that progresses to failure of suture fixation.

Outcomes

Fenichel et al performed a retrospective study of 50 patients with an average age of 50 years who were treated with percutaneous pin fixation for 2- and 3-part fractures of the proximal humerus. At an average follow-up of 2.5 years (range 1-4 years) 18 (36%) obtained excellent results, 17 (34%) good results, 8 (16%) fair results, and 7 (14%) achieved only poor results. The average constant score was 81 (range 60-100). Fractures confined to the surgical or anatomic neck generally did better than those associated with a greater tuberosity fragment (average score 86 vs 78). Patients who required shaft stabilization in addition to reduction and fixation of the greater tuberosity showed a lower average score (68). There were no cases of avascular necrosis, neurovascular complications, or deep infections. A significant loss of fracture position due to failure of internal fixation occurred in 7 cases; 3 of these patients underwent revision surgery.[24]

a. Koukakis et al showed stable fixation (even in osteoporotic bone) and good to excellent functional outcomes after ORIF with a dedicated proximal humeral locking plate.[22] At follow-up 20 patients treated with a PHILOS plate had a mean constant score of 76.1% (range, 30%-100%). Krishnan et al performed a retrospective review of 58 patients treated with a conventional humeral prosthesis and then 112 patients treated with a fracture-specific humeral prosthesis. Overall, 127 of 170 (75%) greater tuberosities healed. Active anterior elevation, active external rotation, and American Shoulder and Elbow Surgeons score were better with fracture-specific stems (129.8°, 39°, and 72°, respectively) than with conventional stems (95.4°, 33.0°, and 55°, respectively). Fewer tuberosities healed with conventional stems (38 of 58, 66%) than with fracture-specific stems (89 of 112, 79%).[25]
b. Lenarz et al retrospectively reviewed 30 patients who had undergone a primary reverse total shoulder arthroplasty for displaced 3- or 4-part proximal humerus fractures. The mean age was 77 years (range, 65-94 years). At a minimum follow-up was 12 months (mean, 23 months; range, 12-36 months). The mean postoperative American Shoulder and Elbow Surgeons score was 78 (range, 36-98), the mean active forward flexion was 139° (range, 90°-180°), and the mean active external rotation was 27° (range, 0°-45°). The Mean American Shoulder and Elbow Surgeons pain score was 0.7 (range, 0-5) and the mean visual analog scale pain score was 1.1 (range, 0-5). Complications were identified in 3 of 30 patients (10%).[26]

SCAPULA AND GLENOID FRACTURES

Rationale and Basic Science Pertinent to the Procedure

Fractures of the scapula are relatively uncommon and represent only 3% to 5% of shoulder girdle fractures. They are usually the result of severe, high-energy trauma. Scapular body fractures are the most common.[27] Glenoid neck fractures are thought to occur due to direct trauma. The deforming force of this fracture is typically the long head of the triceps, which tends to displace the glenoid inferiorly and laterally. Glenoid fossa fractures result from direct impaction of the humeral head against the glenoid as a result of a medially directed force. Fractures of the coracoid process account for 2% to 5% of all scapula fractures. Direct trauma, violent musculotendinous contraction, and humeral head dislocation can cause this fracture.[28] Acromial fractures account for 8% to 10% of scapula fractures secondary to direct or indirect or stress fracture.[29]

A high index of suspicion for associated injuries should be present. Specifically, pulmonary injury, ipsilateral rib fractures, and ipsilateral upper extremity injures should be investigated.

The thickest parts of the scapular body are the scapular spine (6.6-10.3 mm) and the lateral scapular border and scapular pillar (9.2-12.5 mm). The middle third of the body is the thinnest (2.8-3.3 mm).[30]

Surgical Indications

Scapular body and glenoid neck fracture: Combined injuries (fracture of the scapula body and glenoid neck), particularly those with extensive involvement of the lateral scapular pillar, are candidates for surgery. Ada and Miller recommended glenoid neck fixation if there was 40° of angulation and greater than 1 cm of medial translation.[29] Surgery is indicated in intra-articular fractures with a glenoid articular step-off or gap greater than 2 mm. There is no age limitation if the width of the fracture fragment is greater than 21% of the overall length of the glenoid (measured from superior to inferior pole). ORIF of the glenoid fossa fracture with an open capsulolabral reconstruction is performed.[31]

a. Coracoid fractures: Operative treatment is recommended for a midprocess coracoid fracture, coracoid base fracture that includes the superior body of the scapula, and a coracoid fracture with extension into the glenoid fossa.

Acromial fractures: There is no clear consensus for operative fixation. Kuhn et al recommend ORIF for a displaced acromial fracture with loss of the subacromial space.[32]

Contraindications

a. Hemodynamic instability related to associated injuries

Surgical Technique

Scapular body and glenoid neck fracture (Fig. 46-7): General anesthesia with muscle relaxation is used. The patient is placed in the lateral decubitus position. A sterile bump is placed under the affected extremity. A basic shoulder set is shown in Figure 46-7. A 3.5-mm locking reconstruction plate is used.

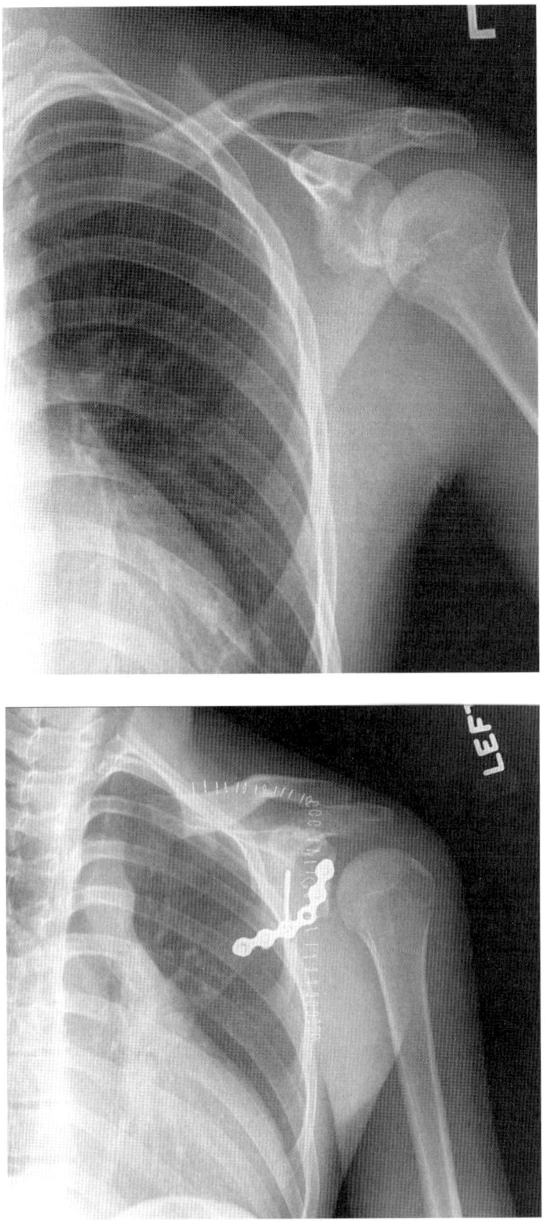

FIGURE 46-7 ORIF of glenoid neck and scapular body fracture. (Reproduced with permission from Sumant Krishnan, MD.)

1. A reverse Judet incision is the preferred approach.[33] A modified posterior subdeltoid (deltoid-sparing) approach is performed if an isolated glenoid neck fracture is present. Use of intermuscular intervals or taking down muscles from their origin on the scapula is an important element of the exposure.

   The plate can be used to reduce the glenoid neck to lateral scapular pillar. The plate is applied to the neck fossa junction, and then fastened to the lateral scapular border in a stepwise fashion. Abduction and extension of the arm relaxes the deltoid and triceps hand facilitates the reduction. Glenoid neck fractures usually result in medial translation of the glenoid. Reduction involves lateral translation of glenoid neck and fossa.
2. Fluoroscopic imaging is mandatory to confirm reduction and confirmation that screws are not intra-articular.

Intra-articular fractures of the glenoid fossa: The patient is in a modified beach chair position for anterior rim fractures. Posterior rim fractures require the patient to be in a lateral decubitus position. If an articular step-off from an impaction-type injury is present and no evidence of subluxation, a simple ORIF with small fragment screws is performed. If the anterior fossa fracture is severely comminuted, an extra-articular bone block technique (Latarjet coracoid process transfer) is performed. The coracoid is transected at its base with the conjoint tendon still intact. The posterior aspect of the coracoid is prepared with a burr. The coracoid piece is then fixed to the glenoid rim with 2 small fragment screws usually 35 to 40 mm in length. The graft is rendered extra-articular by placing suture anchors between the coracoid graft and the native glenoid. A capsule and selective ligamentous repair is then performed. A similar procedure with autograft bone can be performed for the posterior glenoid fossa fracture. For anterior rim fractures, a modified deltopectoral dissection is used. For posterior rim fractures, a posterior axillary fold subdeltoid (deltoid-sparing) approach is used. The joint is exposed through an anterior or posterior T-plasty capsular incision. The use of a Fukuda humeral head retractor aids to view the joint while placing screws.

Marginal impaction or comminution of the articular surface is often present in glenoid fossa fractures and must be reduced to prevent articular incongruity.

1. If a sizable glenoid fragment remains, this is incorporated into the reconstruction.
2. Bone grafts (coracoid if anterior and posterior iliac crest if posterior) are contoured so that they are anatomic with the glenoid surface.
3. If a bone graft is used, it must not overhang the glenoid rim laterally, or the risk of postsurgical arthrosis increases.
4. Maintaining the graft in an extra-articular or intra-articular position when repairing the capsule can be difficult.

Coracoid process fractures:

1. General anesthesia with or without muscle relaxation is used. The patient is positioned in the modified beach chair position. An arm holder is used to position the arm. A small fragment screw secures the coracoid fragment to the coracoid base.

   A deltopectoral approach is used. The musculocutaneous and suprascapular nerves around the coracoid and its base are identified and protected.
2. The conjoined tendon of the pectoralis minor is released to facilitate both the surgical exposure and an anatomic fixation of the coracoid. The tendons are then repaired.

Acromial fractures (Fig. 46-8): The patient is placed in a modified beach chair position with the arm in an adjustable arm positioning device. A saber incision and superior approach with release of the anterior deltoid provides excellent exposure. The deltoid is released as a subperiosteal sleeve

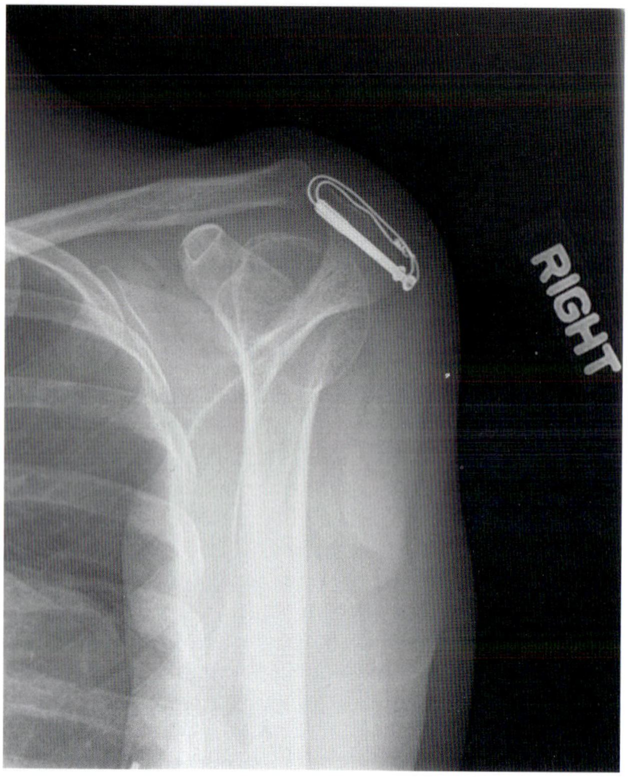

FIGURE 46-8 ORIF for acromion fracture. (*Master Skills: Fractures of the Upper Extremity*. ASSH; 2008.)

in continuity in order to provide a strong unit for repair after fixation. Release of the deltoid and retracting the humeral head with a Darrach retractor allows for excellent superior and inferior exposure of the acromion. This also allows for direct visualization of the reduction. Fixation is most commonly performed with cannulated screws, supplemented by figure-of-8 tension-band wires passed through the cannulated screws. Care should be taken to preserve an intact and thick deltotrapezial fascia for precise repair after reduction of the acromial fracture.

Outcomes

a. Kavanagh et al reported good results for 10 displaced intra-articular glenoid fractures treated with ORIF. No evidence of postoperative osteoarthritis was present at an average of 4-year follow-up. None of the patients had pain with daily use, and range of motion and strength were only mildly affected.[34] More recently Anavian et al[35] reviewed 33 patients with displaced intra-articular fractures of the glenoid who were treated surgically. The indications for operative treatment included articular fracture gap or step-off of ≥4 mm. Twenty-five patients also had extra-articular scapular involvement. A posterior approach was utilized in 21 patients, an anterior approach in 7, and a combined approach in 5. At a mean follow-up of 27 months (range, 3 months), all patients had radiographic union of the fracture. The mean DASH score was 10.8 (range, 0-42). The mean SF-36 subscores were comparable with those of the normal population. Twenty-six patients (87%) were pain-free at the time of follow-up, and 4 had mild pain with prolonged activity. Twenty-seven (90%) of 30 patients returned to their preinjury level of work and/or activities.

Complications

Heterotopic ossification: Surgical approaches that minimize soft tissue trauma decrease the incidence of heterotopic ossification, although patients with head injuries are at increased risk. Injuries to the axillary, musculocutaneous, and/or suprascapular nerves may be from the trauma or iatrogenic. Overhang of the bone graft leads to glenohumeral arthrosis.

a. Intra-articular screw placement as well as a poor reduction of the articular step-off or deformity is an additional risk.

CLAVICLE FRACTURES

Rationale and Basic Science Pertinent to the Procedure

Clavicle fractures make up 2% to 5% of all fractures in adults and 10% to 15% of all fractures in children. A bimodal population distribution is at higher risk that includes young male patients <30 years of age and elderly patients >70 years old.[36-38]

The Allman classification[39] divides this fracture into proximal third, middle third, and distal third. Middle third fractures (81%) are the most common followed by distal third fractures (15%) and proximal third (4%) occurring the least. The Neer classification of distal clavicle fractures[36] considers the location of the fracture relative to the coracoclavicular ligaments and the acromioclavicular ligament. Type I fractures are interligamentous and minimally displaced as the proximal and distal components are stabilized by the coracoclavicular ligaments. Type II fractures occur medial to the coracoclavicular ligaments and are subdivided into type IIA and type II B fracture patterns. In type IIA fractures either the conoid or the trapezoid remains attached to the distal fragment. In type IIB fractures either the conoid is torn or both ligaments are torn and the distal fracture fragment is displaced inferiorly by the downward pull of the arm. Type III fractures extend into the articular surface of the AC joint with no ligamentous injury. Medial third clavicle fractures are usually physeal fracture–dislocations. They may occur in the posterior direction.

Stanley et al found that the clavicle fails in compression. Eighty-seven percent of fractures occur from a fall onto the shoulder, 7% from a direct blow to the point of the shoulder, and 6% from a fall onto an outstretched hand.[40]

The clavicle is a "strut" connecting the appendicular skeleton to the axial skeleton. The clavicle bony morphology provides minimal ability to deform under physiologic loads. The clavicle is in close proximity to the brachial plexus and subclavian vessels.

Surgical Indications

These include middle third clavicle fractures with greater than 2 cm of shortening on an AP view of the clavicle/shoulder girdle view and 1 cm of displacement or 100% transverse displacement of fracture on clavicle uptilt view. The age range includes adolescents to adults. Ideally surgery is performed within 14 days of fracture.

a. Distal third clavicle fracture:
   1. If the conoid ligament or both the conoid and trapezoid ligaments are disrupted, surgery is indicated. Type IIB fractures are associated with delayed union and nonunion rates of up to 30% to 45%.
b. Medial third clavicle fractures: Most are managed nonoperatively. If posterior fracture–dislocation occurs and vessel or airway compromise occurs, this is a surgical indication.

Contraindications

These include hemodynamic instability due to associated injuries and sepsis.

Surgical Technique

Middle third clavicle fractures: General anesthesia with muscle relaxation is used. The patient is in a modified beach chair position.

i. The incision is inferior to the clavicle. The skin and subcutaneous tissue is reflected in a large flap. The suprascapular nerves are identified and protected. The fracture is exposed and reduced. A 3.5-mm straight locking dynamic compression plate is placed on the posterior and superior aspects of the clavicle. This provides the greatest coverage with soft tissue in order to decrease hardware irritation (Fig. 46-9).
ii. A butterfly or segmental bone fragment can be fixed and compressed into position with a #2 semiabsorbable suture racking half-hitch knot. Great care is taken not to plug while drilling the clavicle because of the proximity of the neurovascular structures.
iii. Nonoperative treatment has been the mainstay; however, this has been challenged recently. Nowak et al showed that 46% of 208 patients with a nonoperatively treated clavicle still did not consider themselves fully recovered 9 to 10 years after the injury. Fracture displacement without bony contact was most predictive of fracture sequelae and patient dissatisfaction.[41]

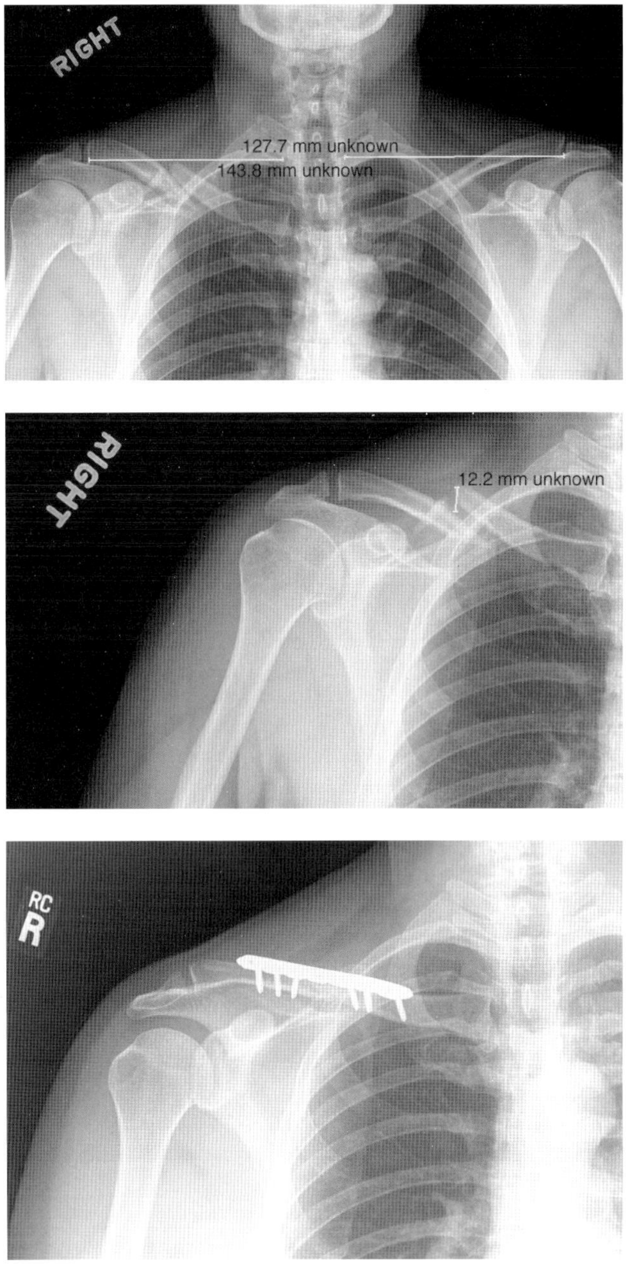

FIGURE 46-9 ORIF for middle third clavicle fracture. (Reproduced with permission from Sumant G. Krishnan, MD.)

McKee et al followed 30 clavicle fracture patients treated nonoperatively and found significant residual disability at a mean of 55 months after injury on patient and clinical outcome scores. A higher prevalence of dissatisfaction with clavicle fracture shortening greater than 2 cm was present.[42,43] Khan et al found that nonsurgical treatment of displaced shaft fractures may be associated with a higher rate of nonunion and functional deficits than previously reported.[44] The Canadian Orthopaedic Trauma Society performed a multicenter trial comparing nonsurgical treatment with primary plate fixation for displaced fractures. Better functional outcomes, lower rates of malunion and nonunion, and a shorter time to union were found in the plate group. However, the operative group had a higher complication rate of 34% and a reoperation rate of 18% mostly for hardware removal.[45]

Distal third clavicle fractures: The authors use an autograft hamstring tendon graft and three #2 semiabsorbable sutures (hold reduction until tendon reconstruction/repair heals) to "bypass" the fracture via coracoclavicular and acromioclavicular stabilization. General anesthesia is used with muscle relaxation. The patient is in a modified beach chair position. The ipsilateral leg is placed in a leg holder for semitendinosus autograft harvest. An arm holder is used for control of the arm. Equipment needed for this repair is an oscillating saw, 6-mm drill bit, hamstring harvester, Houston suture passer, vascular clamp, and three #2 semiabsorbable suture weave in a Hawkins-Warren technique.

i. A 2-in (5-cm) skin incision is placed in Langer's lines from the midportion of the ACJ directed toward the coracoid. The deltoid is split in a T-shaped fashion with the horizontal limb 2 mm anterior to the posterior edge of the clavicle and the vertical limb directed toward the coracoid. First expose the AC joint, medial acromion, posterior clavicle, and coracoid process and resect 5 mm of distal clavicle with a small sagittal saw. Three 6-mm drill holes are placed as follows: 2 holes in the lateral edge of the clavicle (1 anterior and 1 posterior) and 1 hole in the medial acromion. Nonabsorbable #2 sutures are placed in each of these 3 holes for tendon shuttling. Following tendon preparation, 3 strands of #2 semiabsorbable sutures are braided in a modified Hawkins-Warren technique. Both the semiabsorbable suture braid and autograft hamstring tendon are passed around the coracoid in a medial to lateral direction. The lateral coracoid limb of tendon/suture is passed through the anterior clavicle drill hole (deep to superficial). The suture is then separated and clamped. The tendon alone passes through the acromion drill hole (superficial to deep), and then through the posterior clavicle drill hole (deep to superficial). With a superior directed force on the arm and inferior force on the clavicle the AC joint is reduced and the suture braid is tied under maximum tension. The hamstring graft (tendon limb from medial coracoid and tendon limb from posterior clavicle drill hole) is then tied under maximal tension and reinforced with #2 nonabsorbable suture (completing the CC fixation). The remaining "tail" of the graft is tensioned maximally to the acromial tendon limb to reinforce the superior capsule of the AC joint. Finally, the graft is retensioned medially and sewn to the posterior clavicle with #2 sutures (completing the AC joint capsular reconstruction). The shoulder is placed through a full range of motion to test the graft. Routine layered closure is then performed.

ii. Practical tips: The suture weave allows for holding reduction while the tendon heals.

iii. Pitfalls: If the AC joint capsule is not reestablished with the graft, then anterior posterior stabilization of the AC joint is compromised.

iv. Controversies: A recent study by Robinson et al found a low incidence of nonunion after nonoperative treatment and a high complication rate in those treated surgically.[46] Khan et al found that displaced lateral-end fractures have a higher risk of nonunion after nonoperative treatment than do shaft fractures. However, nonunion is difficult to predict and may be asymptomatic in elderly individuals. The results of operative treatment are more unpredictable than they are for shaft fractures.[44]

Medial third clavicle fractures: Supporting evidence is limited for surgeries of this technique, and there is a lack of consensus regarding the optimal treatment of these fractures. The patient is placed in a modified beach chair position. General anesthesia with muscle relaxation is used. An adjustable arm positioner is used. A thoracic surgeon is on standby if assistance is required. Fixation methods usually involve either plate fixation (if the fragment is of sufficient length) or suture fixation of the fracture with sternoclavicular (SC) joint stabilization and/or autograft reconstruction of the SC joint after fracture reduction. An incision is made anterior to the SC joint/medial clavicle.

Complications

Nonunions/malunion: McKee et al treated symptomatic, shortened, clavicle nonunion with a clavicular osteotomy along with internal fixation and local bone graft. In their series of 15 patients they reported high satisfaction rates and 100% having improvement. Sixty-six percent of patients had complete resolution of symptoms at a mean of 20-month follow-up.[43] McKee et al found in a meta-analysis of randomized controlled trials that the nonunion rate was higher in nonoperative patients (29 of 200) compared with the operative group (3 of 212) ($P = .001$) and symptomatic malunion rate was higher in the nonoperative group (17 of 200) versus the operative group (0 of 212) ($P < .001$).[47]

a. One multicenter study (the Canadian Orthopaedic Trauma Society) noted there was a reoperation rate of 18% for hardware removal.[45] McKee et al found that irritation of soft tissue occurred due to plate prominence or pin irritation/protrusion in the posterior lateral aspect of the clavicle. The use of this intramedullary implant (Hagie pin) in this fashion was associated with a high rate of requirement for removal.[47]

b. Damage/irritation to underlying neurovascular structures may occur from the injury (3%)[44] or during surgical fixation.

c. In a recent study meta-analysis of randomized control trials, McKee et al found that 9/200 patients with midshaft clavicle fractures treated operatively had infections (6 were related to pin-tract infections and 3 were related to infections after plate fixation).[47]

Outcomes

Nonoperative treatment: Robinson et al reported significant risk factors for nonunion after nonoperative treatment of clavicles include advanced age, female sex, fracture displacement, and comminution.[46] McKee et al performed a meta-analysis of recent randomized control trials of nonoperative and operative treatment for middle third clavicle fractures. They found that operative treatment provided a significantly lower rate of nonunion and symptomatic malunion and an earlier functional return compared with nonoperative treatment.[47]

Middle third clavicle fractures: The Canadian Orthopaedic Trauma Society concluded that primary plate fixation of completely displaced midshaft clavicular fractures in active adults is an acceptable treatment method.[45]

REFERENCES

1. Rose SH, Melton LJ 3rd, Morrey BF, Ilstrup DM, Riggs BL. Epidemiologic features of humeral fractures. *Clin Orthop Relat Res*. 1982;(168):24–30.
2. Holstein A, Lewis GM. Fractures of the humerus with radial-nerve paralysis. *J Bone Joint Surg Am*. 1963;45:1382–1388.
3. Sarmiento A, Zagorski JB, Zych GA, Latta LL, Capps CA. Functional bracing for the treatment of fractures of the humeral diaphysis. *J Bone Joint Surg Am*. 2000;82(4):478–486.
4. Koch PP, Gross DF, Gerber C. The results of functional (Sarmiento) bracing of humeral shaft fractures. *J Shoulder Elbow Surg*. 2002;11(2):143–150.
5. Walker M, Palumbo B, Badman B, Brooks J, Van Gelderen J, Mighell M. Humeral shaft fractures: a review. *J Shoulder Elbow Surg*. 2011;20(5):833–844.
6. Pollock FH, Drake D, Bovill EG, Day L, Trafton PG. Treatment of radial neuropathy associated with fractures of the humerus. *J Bone Joint Surg Am*. 1981;63(2):239–243.
7. Ring D, Jupiter JB, Quintero J, Sanders RA, Marti RK. Atrophic ununited diaphyseal fractures of the humerus with a bony defect: treatment by wave-plate osteosynthesis. *J Bone Joint Surg Br*. 2000;82(6):867–871.
8. Papasoulis E, Drosos GI, Ververidis AN, Verettas DA. Functional bracing of humeral shaft fractures. A review of clinical studies. *Injury*. 2010;41(7):e21–e27.
9. Bhandari M, Devereaux PJ, McKee MD, Schemitsch EH. Compression plating versus intramedullary nailing of humeral shaft fractures—a meta-analysis. *Acta Orthop*. 2006;77(2):279–284.
10. Palvanen M, Kannus P, Niemi S, Parkkari J. Update in the epidemiology of proximal humeral fractures. *Clin Orthop Relat Res*. 2006;442:87–92.
11. Olsson C, Petersson CJ. Clinical importance of comorbidity in patients with a proximal humerus fracture. *Clin Orthop Relat Res*. 2006;442:93–99.
12. Visser CP, Coene LN, Brand R, Tavy DL. Nerve lesions in proximal humeral fractures. *J Shoulder Elbow Surg*. 2001;10(5):421–427.
13. Krishnan SG, Lin KC, Burkhead WZ. Pins, plates, and prostheses: current concepts in treatment of fractures of the proximal humerus. *Curr Opin Orthop*. 2007;18(4):380–385.
14. Hertel R, Hempfing A, Stiehler M, Leunig M. Predictors of humeral head ischemia after intracapsular fracture of the proximal humerus. *J Shoulder Elbow Surg*. 2004;13(4):427–433.
15. Boileau P, Chuinard C, Le Huec JC, Walch G, Trojani C. Proximal humerus fracture sequelae: impact of a new radiographic classification on arthroplasty. *Clin Orthop Relat Res*. 2006;442:121–130.
16. Smith AM, Mardones RM, Sperling JW, Cofield RH. Early complications of operatively treated proximal humeral fractures. *J Shoulder Elbow Surg*. 2007;16(1):14–24.
17. Dawson FA. Four-part fracture dislocation of the proximal humerus: an arthroscopic approach. *Arthroscopy*. 2003;19(6):662–666.
18. Carrera EF, Matsumoto MH, Netto NA, Faloppa F. Fixation of greater tuberosity fractures. *Arthroscopy*. 2004;20(8):e109–e111.
19. Taverna E, Sansone V, Battistella F. Arthroscopic treatment for greater tuberosity fractures: rationale and surgical technique. *Arthroscopy*. 2004;20(6):e53–e57.
20. Neviaser AS, Hettrich CM, Beamer BS, Dines JS, Lorich DG. Endosteal strut augment reduces complications associated with proximal humeral locking plates. *Clin Orthop Relat Res*. 2011;469(12):3300–3306.
21. Boileau P, Krishnan SG, Tinsi L, Walch G, Coste JS, Molé D. Tuberosity malposition and migration: reasons for poor outcomes after hemiarthroplasty for displaced fractures of the proximal humerus. *J Shoulder Elbow Surg*. 2002;11(5):401–412.
22. Koukakis A, Apostolou CD, Taneja T, Korres DS, Amini A. Fixation of proximal humerus fractures using the PHILOS plate: early experience. *Clin Orthop Relat Res*. 2006;442:115–120.
23. Moonot P, Ashwood N, Hamlet M. Early results for treatment of three- and four-part fractures of the proximal humerus using the PHILOS plate system. *J Bone Joint Surg Br*. 2007;89(9):1206–1209.
24. Fenichel I, Oran A, Burstein G, Perry Pritsch M. Percutaneous pinning using threaded pins as a treatment option for unstable two- and three-part fractures of the proximal humerus: a retrospective study. *Int Orthop*. 2006;30(3):153–157.
25. Krishnan SG, Reineck JR, Bennion PD, Feher L, Burkhead WZ Jr. Shoulder arthroplasty for fracture: does a fracture-specific stem make a difference? *Clin Orthop Relat Res*. 2011;469(12):3317–3323.
26. Lenarz C, Shishani Y, McCrum C, Nowinski RJ, Edwards TB, Gobezie R. Is reverse shoulder arthroplasty appropriate for the treatment of fractures in the older patient? Early observations. *Clin Orthop Relat Res*. 2011;469(12):3324–3331.
27. McGahan JP, Rab GT, Dublin A. Fractures of the scapula. *J Trauma*. 1980;20(10):880–883.
28. Cottias P, le Bellec Y, Jeanrot C, Imbert P, Huten D, Masmejean EH. Fractured coracoid with anterior shoulder dislocation and greater tuberosity fracture—report of a bilateral case. *Acta Orthop Scand*. 2000;71(1):95–97.
29. Ada JR, Miller ME. Scapular fractures. Analysis of 113 cases. *Clin Orthop Relat Res*. 1991;(269):174–180.
30. Burke CS, Roberts CS, Nyland JA, Radmacher PG, Acland RD, Voor MJ. Scapular thickness—implications for fracture fixation. *J Shoulder Elbow Surg*. 2006;15(5):645–648.
31. Itoi E, Lee SB, Berglund LJ, Berge GG, An KN. The effect of a glenoid defect on anteroinferior stability of the shoulder after Bankart repair: a cadaveric study. *J Bone Joint Surg Am*. 2000;82(1):35–46.
32. Kuhn JE, Blasier RB, Carpenter JE. Fractures of the acromion process: a proposed classification system. *J Orthop Trauma*. 1994;8(1):6–13.
33. Brodsky JW, Tullos HS, Gartsman GM. Simplified posterior approach to the shoulder joint. A technical note. *J Bone Joint Surg Am*. 1987;69(5):773–774.
34. Kavanagh BF, Bradway JK, Cofield RH. Open reduction and internal fixation of displaced intra-articular fractures of the glenoid fossa. *J Bone Joint Surg Am*. 1993;75(4):479–484.
35. Anavian J, Gauger EM, Schroder LK, Wijdicks CA, Cole PA. Surgical and functional outcomes after operative management of complex and displaced intra-articular glenoid fractures. *J Bone Joint Surg Am*. 2012;94(7):645–653.
36. Neer CS 2nd. Fractures of the distal third of the clavicle. *Clin Orthop Relat Res*. 1968;58:43–50.
37. Nordqvist A, Petersson CJ. Incidence and causes of shoulder girdle injuries in an urban population. *J Shoulder Elbow Surg*. 1995;4(2):107–112.
38. Postacchini F, Gumina S, De Santis P, Albo F. Epidemiology of clavicle fractures. *J Shoulder Elbow Surg*. 2002;11(5):452–456.
39. Allman FL Jr. Fractures and ligamentous injuries of the clavicle and its articulation. *J Bone Joint Surg Am*. 1967;49(4):774–784.
40. Stanley D, Trowbridge EA, Norris SH. The mechanism of clavicular fracture. A clinical and biomechanical analysis. *J Bone Joint Surg Br*. 1988;70(3):461–464.
41. Nowak J, Holgersson M, Larsson S. Can we predict long-term sequelae after fractures of the clavicle based on initial findings? A prospective study with nine to ten years of follow-up. *J Shoulder Elbow Surg*. 2004;13(5):479–486.
42. McKee MD, Wild LM, Schemitsch EH. Midshaft malunions of the clavicle. *J Bone Joint Surg Am*. 2003;85-A(5):790–797.

43. McKee M, Wild LM, Schemitsch EH. Midshaft malunions of the clavicle. Surgical technique. *J Bone Joint Surg Am.* 2004;86-A(suppl 1): 37–43.
44. Khan LA, Bradnock TJ, Scott C, Robinson CM. Fractures of the clavicle. *J Bone Joint Surg Am.* 2009;91(2):447–460.
45. Canadian Orthopaedic Trauma Society. Nonoperative treatment compared with plate fixation of displaced midshaft clavicular fractures. A multicenter, randomized clinical trial. *J Bone Joint Surg Am.* 2007;89(1):1–10.
46. Robinson CM, Court-Brown CM, McQueen MM, Wakefield AE. Estimating the risk of nonunion following nonoperative treatment of a clavicular fracture. *J Bone Joint Surg Am.* 2004;86-A(7): 1359–1365.
47. McKee RC, Whelan DB, Schemitsch EH, McKee MD. Operative versus nonoperative care of displaced midshaft clavicular fractures: a meta-analysis of randomized clinical trials. *J Bone Joint Surg Am.* 2012;94(8):675–684.

47

Shoulder Dislocation: Anterior, Posterior, Multidirectional*

Suraj S. Trivedi, MD
Lucas S. McDonald, MD, MPH&TM
Matthew T. Provencher, MD

INTRODUCTION

Due to inherent instability allowing freedom of motion, the glenohumeral joint is the most commonly dislocated joint in the human body. Shoulder dislocations follow a bimodal distribution with a peak in young adults sustaining high-energy dislocations, and a second peak in elderly adults sustaining lower-energy injuries. Age at the time of initial dislocation plays a large factor in recurrent dislocations, with younger patients being at greater risk for future episodes of instability.[1]

Shoulder dislocations can be classified according to the direction of dislocation relative to the glenoid. Anterior dislocations occur in 95% of cases, often occurring as a result of an external rotation hyperabduction injury. Posterior dislocations account for fewer than 3% of all cases and are the result of high-energy trauma or seizures.[2] Commonly associated bony injuries include an osteochondral defect secondary to impaction of the posterosuperior aspect of the humeral head (Hill-Sachs deformities) (Fig. 47-1), anterior glenoid rim fractures (bony Bankart lesions), posterior glenoid rim fractures (reverse bony Bankart lesions), and associated proximal humerus fractures.

Multiple capsular, ligamentous, and bony structures can be injured during a glenohumeral dislocation. A classic Bankart lesion is associated with a tear of the anteroinferior labrum and inferior capsule (Figs. 47-2 to 47-4). One variant of this injury is an anterior labral periosteal sleeve avulsion (ALPSA) resulting in recurrent instability when the capsule detaches from the glenoid and heals in a medially displaced position on the glenoid neck (Fig. 47-5). Other pathology may also be present in patients who sustain a shoulder dislocation including superior labrum anterior and posterior (SLAP) lesions (Fig. 47-6) and, in patients over the age of 40, rotator cuff tears. In a recent study of anterior shoulder dislocations it was noted that 10% of the patients presented with an associated SLAP lesion.[3] A less common and easily overlooked cause of shoulder instability is a humeral avulsion of the glenohumeral ligament (HAGL) resulting from capsular detachment from the humerus instead of the glenoid[3–5] (Figs. 47-7 and 47-8).

Soft tissue laxity, repetitive microtrauma, and other traumatic events[6] may result in multidirectional instability (MDI).[7] MDI is a spectrum of disease including symptomatic microinstability, voluntary positional instability, and symptomatic involuntary instability in more than 1 direction.

ANATOMY AND PATHOPHYSIOLOGY

Glenohumeral joint stability results from intricate interactions between static and dynamic shoulder stabilizers. Dynamic glenohumeral stabilizers include the rotator cuff complex, the biceps tendon, the deltoid, and the superior labrum. Static stabilizers of the shoulder include the glenoid, the labrum, the glenohumeral ligaments, and the humeral head (Fig. 47-9). Additionally, the negative intra-articular pressure maintained by an intact capsule is important for shoulder stability, especially with the arm at the side. The glenohumeral ligaments attach to the labrum and have a unique role in stabilizing the shoulder while preventing excessive translation. During normal shoulder functions, the inferior glenohumeral ligament (IGHL), middle glenohumeral ligament (MGHL), and superior glenohumeral ligament (SGHL) demonstrate a unique pattern of tension and relaxation through various shoulder positions. These ligaments tighten and loosen in a reciprocal fashion, constraining the humeral head in a load-sharing and load-bearing pattern.[6]

The IGHL consists of an anterior and a posterior band arising from the labrum, with an axillary pouch acting as a "hammock" for the humeral head.[6] The axillary pouch is interposed between the anterior and posterior bands of the IGHL, spanning the inferior two thirds of the anterior glenoid to the inferior one third of the humeral head.[4,8] The IGHL is the primary static check against anterior, posterior, and inferior translation between 45° and 90° of glenohumeral elevation.[8,9] As the IGHL

*The views expressed in this chapter are those of the authors and do not reflect the official policy or position of the Department of the Navy, Department of Defense, or US government.

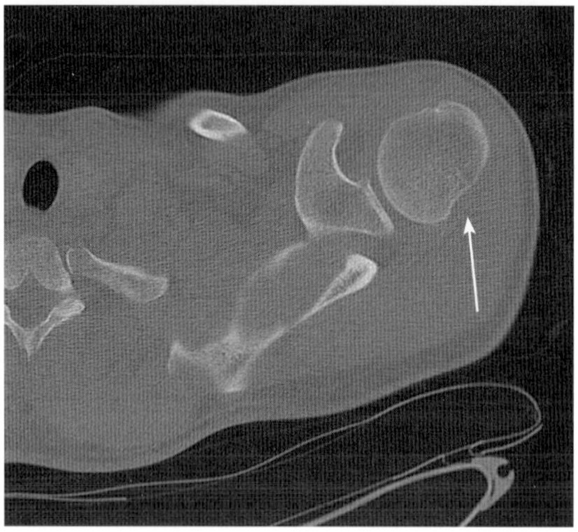

FIGURE 47-1 CT scan of a patient following recurrent glenohumeral dislocations demonstrating a Hill-Sachs lesion.

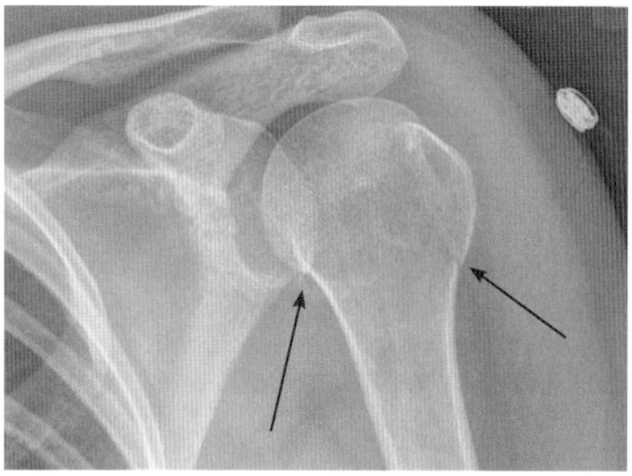

FIGURE 47-2 Radiographic anterior–posterior view demonstrating a bony Bankart lesion (inferior arrow) and a minimally displaced fracture of the greater tuberosity (lateral arrow) following an acute shoulder dislocation.

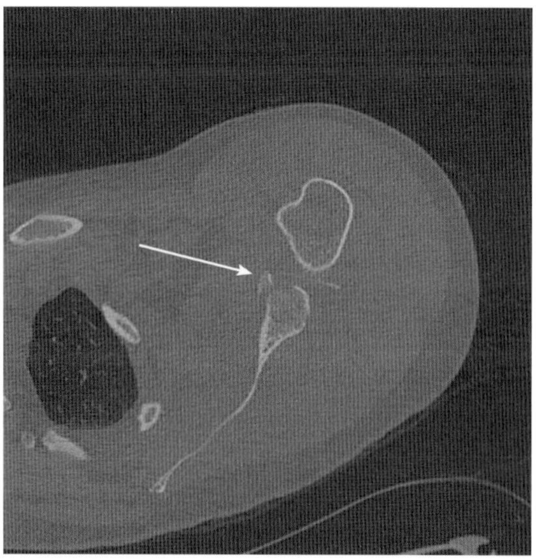

FIGURE 47-3 CT scan of the same patient from Figure 47-2 demonstrating a bony Bankart lesion.

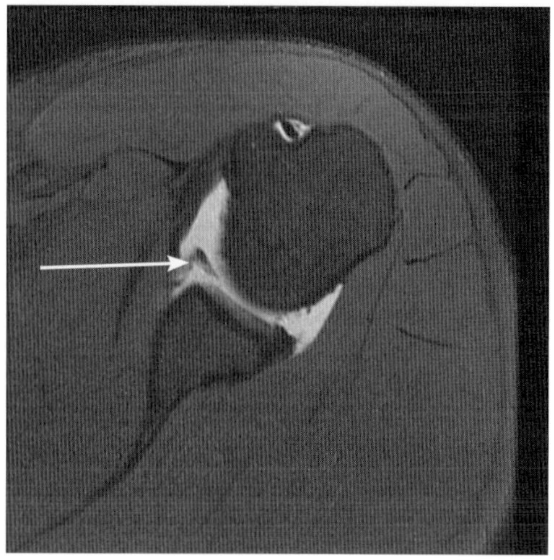

FIGURE 47-4 Axial MRA of a different patient demonstrating a Bankart lesion. The torn anterior labrum is identified by arrow.

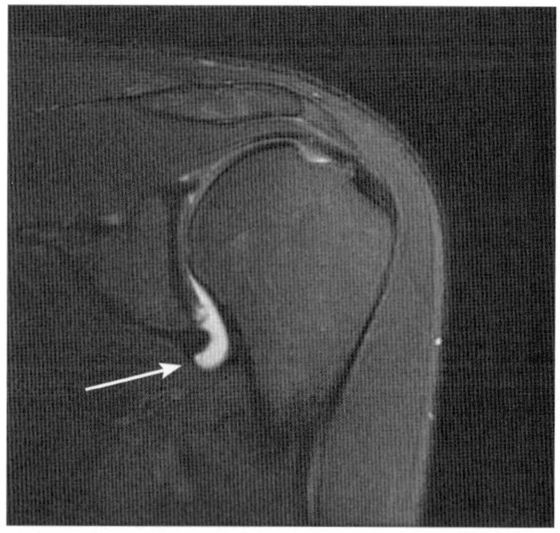

FIGURE 47-5 Coronal MRA highlighting medialization of anterior-inferior labrum in an ALPSA lesion. The arrow highlights the anterior-inferior labrum.

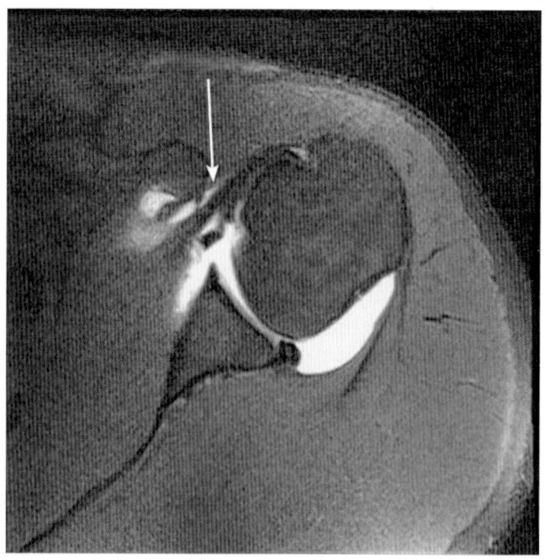

FIGURE 47-6 MRA demonstrating an anterior labral tear extending into the superior labrum with a type 3 SLAP tear.

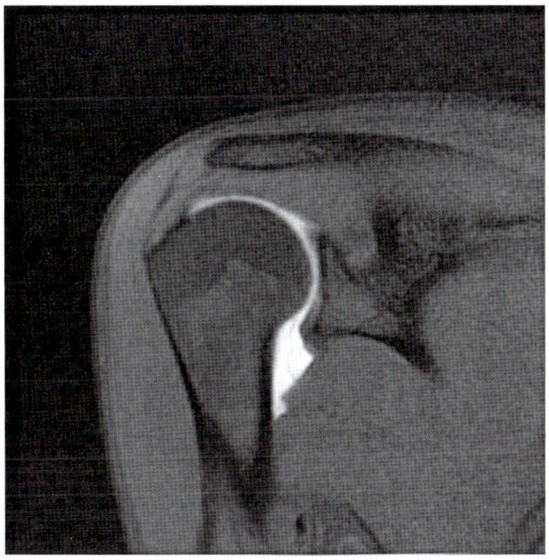

FIGURE 47-7 MRA demonstrating a lax inferior glenohumeral ligament with a marked "J-shaped" appearance with contrast extravasation about the medial humeral head characteristic of a humeral avulsion of the glenohumeral ligament (HAGL) lesion.

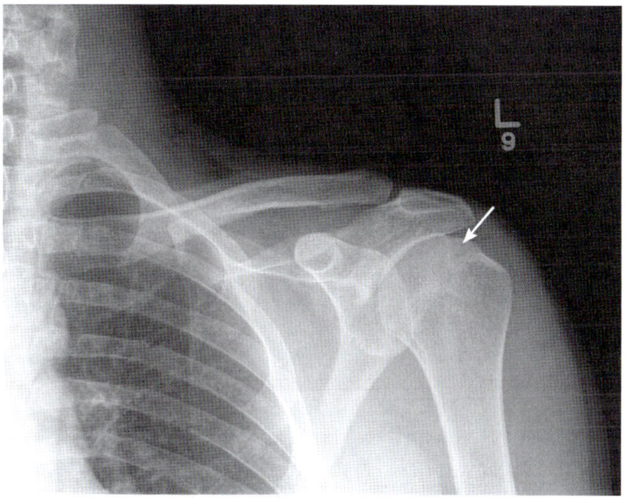

FIGURE 47-8 AP radiograph demonstrating a Hill-Sachs lesion of the left shoulder.

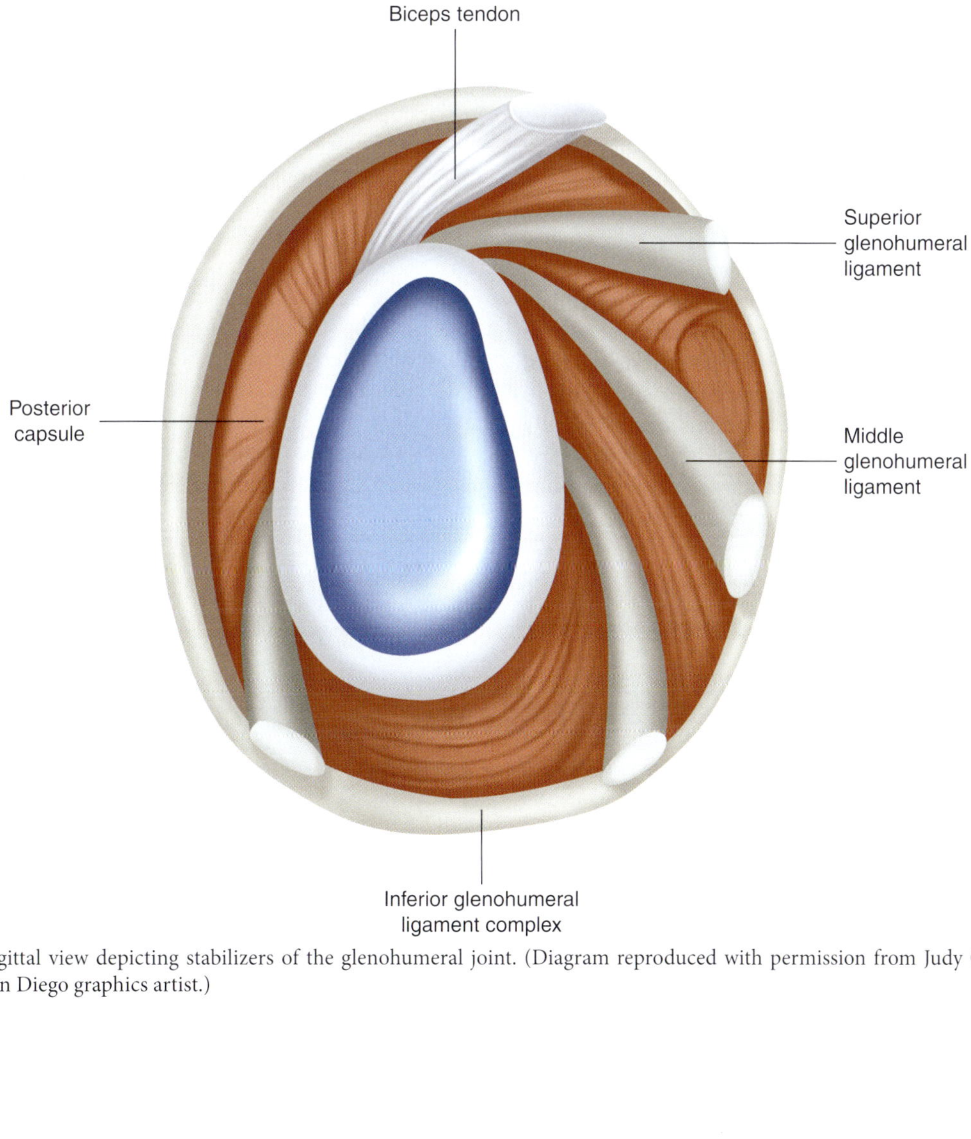

FIGURE 47-9 Sagittal view depicting stabilizers of the glenohumeral joint. (Diagram reproduced with permission from Judy Christensen, Naval Medical Center San Diego graphics artist.)

runs under the subscapularis tendon it prevents anterior, inferior, and posterior translation of the abducted arm through alternating tension in the anterior and posterior bands.[10] More specifically the anterior band of the IGHL provides resistance against anterior and inferior humeral head translation at 90° of shoulder abduction. The anterior band runs from the anterior glenoid and labrum at the 3-o'clock position, inserting on the inferior humeral neck. The posterior band of the IGHL provides posterior stability when the arm is flexed and internally rotated.[4,10,11] The posterior band runs from the posterior glenoid and labrum at the 9-o'clock position, also inserting on the inferior humeral head. Over 70 years ago, Nicola described the site of failure for the IGHL as being at the humeral insertion site in 4 of 5 acute shoulder dislocations, and in 6 of 25 recurrent glenohumeral dislocators.[12]

The SGHL and the MGHL limit anteroposterior and inferior translation in the middle and lower ranges of elevation as the arm approaches adduction.[13,14] The SGHL originates at the anterosuperior glenoid rim and labrum, merging with the biceps tendon to insert at the proximal lesser tuberosity. The SHGL, the coracohumeral ligament, and the IGHL function to limit inferior translation of the adducted shoulder acting as secondary restraints against posterior translation.[14–16] The MGHL originates at the anterosuperior glenoid rim and labrum, inferior to the SGHL, inserting just medial to the lesser tuberosity. The MGHL resists anteroposterior translation in 45° of shoulder abduction and is a secondary restraint to translation and external rotation in adduction.

A final ligamentous component to capsular stability is the region between the subscapularis and supraspinatus muscles known as the rotator interval. This triangular portion of the capsule is composed of the coracohumeral ligaments and the SGHL, serving to increase inferior stability, particularly when the arm is adducted and externally rotated.[17]

Traumatic shoulder dislocations or subluxations may cause an avulsion of the capsulolabral complex from the anterior glenoid rim, resulting in a Bankart lesion, or an avulsion of the IGHL from its humeral attachment, a HAGL lesion.[18] HAGL lesions are more likely to occur with the shoulder hyperabducted and in external rotation. Cadaveric studies by Bigliani et al demonstrated a failure of the anterior labroligamentous complex at the glenoid attachment in 40% of specimens, midsubstance tears in 35% of specimens, and at the humeral attachment in 25% of specimens.[19] Both anterior and posterior HAGL lesions are described with anterior lesions representing 93% of cases and posterior HAGL lesions representing only 7%.[20]

EXAMINATION

Patients with anterior glenohumeral dislocations often present with the arm held in an abducted and externally rotated position or adducted against the body. Posterior dislocations can be more subtle and over 50% are missed on the initial evaluation.[2] In patients with posterior dislocations, the arm is typically held in internal rotation with a block to external rotation caused by the anterior humeral head engaging the posterior glenoid rim.

Important details regarding the history of injury include the mechanism of injury, handedness, age, total number of lifetime dislocations or subluxations, sensory or motor disturbances, location of pain, ability to voluntarily dislocate the shoulder, and previous shoulder surgeries. Patients with anterior instability present with symptoms when their arm is maximally abducted and externally rotated. Symptoms of posterior instability are provoked with a flexed and internally rotated humerus.[6] In the presence of an acute dislocation, an expeditious physical examination and radiographic imaging is required to document neurovascular injuries and rule out concurrent fractures while confirming the suspected direction of the dislocation. The examination is started at the neck to assess for cervical spine pathology and range of motion. This is followed by active and passive shoulder range of motion assessing the maximum abduction, adduction, flexion, and extension. Specific tests to test the rotator cuff strength are followed by special testing for intra-articular and extra-articular shoulder pathology (Table 47-1). Specific tests include the sulcus sign, the anterior apprehension sign, glenohumeral translation, and the load and shift test. Examiners must evaluate for associated neurovascular injuries. Ligamentous laxity in joints other than the shoulder may indicate generalized

TABLE 47-1: Basic Shoulder Tests

Test	Method	Significance
Scratch test	Touch inferior and superior aspects of opposite scapula	Loss of motion indicates rotator cuff pathology[2]
Drop arm test	Arm slowly adducted from 90° abduction	Supraspinatus or teres minor pathology
Speed's test	Resisted flexion with elbow flexed to 20° and forearm supinated	Long head biceps pathology
Liftoff test	Dorsum of patient's hand is placed on lumbar spine with attempt to push off against resistance	Subscapularis pathology
Empty can test	Forward flexion of shoulder to 90° in slight abduction with thumbs pointed to ground. Pain with resisted flexion is positive	Supraspinatus pathology
External rotation test	Arms at sides with elbows flexed to 90°. Weakness or pain with resisted external rotation is positive	Infraspinatus pathology
Clunk test	Rotation of loaded shoulder from extension to forward flexion	Labral pathology[2]

TABLE 47-2: Special Tests for Multidirectional Instability

Test	Description
Apprehension test	The shoulder is placed into a position of instability, abduction and external rotation for anterior instability and flexion with internal rotation for posterior instability. If the patient senses impending dislocation, the test is positive
Relocation test	A posteriorly directed force is placed on the humeral head while abducting and externally rotating the arm. A positive test occurs if the pain and apprehension produced during the apprehension test are relieved
Load and shift test	Center the humeral head within the glenoid and translate the head anterior and posterior. Grading of the humeral head translation is relative to the glenoid rim • Grade 1: Translation to the edge of the glenoid • Grade 2: Humeral head subluxation over the glenoid rim • Grade 3: Frank dislocation without spontaneous reduction
Sulcus sign	Pull the affected adducted arm inferiorly measuring the gap between the humeral head and the inferior surface of the acromion • Grade 1: 1-cm gap • Grade 2: 2-cm gap • Grade 3: >3-cm gap

ligamentous laxity (Table 47-2). Following an anterior dislocation, inspection of the affected shoulder reveals a loss of the deltoid contour, a prominent acromion, and a palpable fullness of the humeral head below the coracoid process. The patient is usually in significant pain with the affected arm held against the body or locked in an adducted position. A closed reduction should be performed as soon as possible to avoid possible neurovascular compromise. It is important to assess the axillary, suprascapular, and long thoracic nerve function both before and after reduction. One EMG study demonstrated evidence of axonal loss in 37 out of 77 patients with axillary nerve involvement in 32 of these patients, although clinical evidence of this is much lower in actual practice.[21] Patients with recurrent instability present with a wide variety of symptoms. Patients with inferior instability often complain of pain and weakness when carrying heavy objects.

RADIOGRAPHIC IMAGING

In the case of acute dislocations, plain radiographs are required prior to reduction to assess for concurrent fractures and the direction of dislocation. These include an anterior–posterior view and adequate axillary lateral shoulder series with the possible addition of a scapular Y view. The axillary view is critical to determine the direction of dislocation as well as confirmation of a congruent glenohumeral joint post reduction. In cases of chronic or recurrent instability, radiographic images are examined for evidence of bony pathology including a Hill-Sachs lesion, a bony Bankart lesion, and attritional glenoid bone loss. The West Point view can provide a clearer picture of the glenoid rim and the Stryker notch view provides a detailed image of the humeral head to assess for Bankart lesions and Hill-Sachs deformities, respectively.[7]

Computerized tomography (CT) is an accurate method to quantify the size of an acute glenoid rim fracture as well as determine the amount of glenoid and humeral head bony injury.[22] In the setting of chronic instability, a 3-dimensional CT scan both with and without the humeral head digitally subtracted provides important information regarding any glenoid bone loss and the extent of any Hill-Sachs deformities (Fig. 47-10). Magnetic resonance imaging (MRI) and magnetic resonance arthrogram (MRA) increase the ability to detect labral, rotator cuff, cartilage, and capsular pathologies including HAGL lesions. In the acute setting, contrast is rarely required as the hemarthrosis serves as a natural contrast agent.[23]

In the setting of a posterior dislocation, the same series of plain radiographs and advanced imaging is followed. Again, the axillary view is critical to diagnose posterior dislocations.

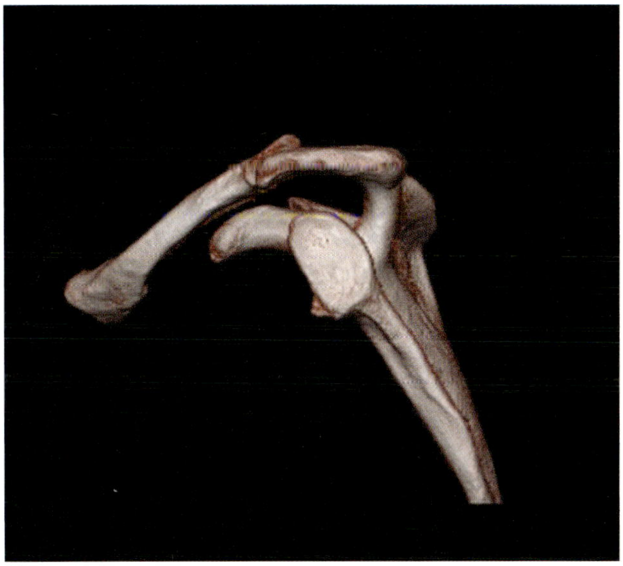

FIGURE 47-10 Three-dimensional CT scan with digital subtraction of the humerus demonstrating 20% to 25% bone loss of the glenoid surface.

Patients may present with an impaction fracture of the anterosuperior humeral head at the lesser tuberosity, known as a reverse Hill-Sachs lesion. Posterior glenoid rim defects (reverse bony Bankart lesions) and glenoid hypoplasia can also be seen on standard radiographs. Posterior labral cracks known as Kim lesions are associated with posterior shoulder instability and are visible on MRA studies.[24]

TREATMENT

In the presence of an acute dislocation, urgent reduction is performed to avoid lasting damage. Several techniques are utilized in reduction of anterior dislocations, although no studies demonstrate the superiority of 1 technique over the other. Conscious sedation is often utilized in the emergency room, although intra-articular lidocaine has been demonstrated to provide adequate pain relief with fewer complications.[25,26] In the Stimson technique the patient lays prone with the affected arm hanging off the edge of the table in traction to allow gravity traction to stretch out the deltoid spasm and reduce the joint. Alternatively the patient can be placed supine on a table with a countertraction strap around the ipsilateral chest with gentle traction applied to the affected arm in an inferior direction for reduction.[26] In an acute posterior dislocation, a reduction is achieved through disimpaction of the humeral head and maneuvering it past the posterior glenoid lip by gentle manipulation while the arm is flexed to 90° and adducted.[2,27] For fixed and chronic dislocations associated with fractures, general anesthesia with paralysis is used to reduce the shoulder with gentle lateral humeral head translation in order to prevent fracture propagation or displacement, especially in the presence of a Hill-Sachs lesion or osteopenic bone. Traditionally conservative treatment consists of shoulder immobilization in internal rotation. MRI and cadaver studies have shown better coaptation of the Bankart lesion with the arm in external rotation than in internal rotation. Itoi et al tested this theory by randomizing 198 patients to either internal rotation (94 shoulders) or external rotation (104 shoulders) for 3 weeks. At a 2-year follow-up they found the recurrent dislocation rate in the external rotation group (22 of 85; 26%) was significantly lower than that in the internal rotation group (31 of 74; 42%).[28] Although promising, this data has not been reproducible. Another study found that early mobilization and shoulder brace-wear that restricted external rotation and abduction allowed 26 out of 30 athletes to return to competitive sports following anterior dislocation.[29]

INDICATIONS FOR SURGERY

Following a reduction, the decision for further surgical treatment is based on age and activity levels. Young athletes, especially those 15 to 25 years old, and contact sports athletes have high rates of recurrent dislocation and earlier surgical repair is often indicated. Patients aged 25 to 40 have a low recurrence rate and conservative treatment is usually the best option. Studies show good results of rotator cuff repair with subacromial decompression are possible in symptomatic elderly patients failing conservative treatments.[30] Operative stabilization is considered for those with limited function secondary to instability and those who have failed an adequate trial of conservative therapy.

CONTRAINDICATIONS

The most important contraindication for arthroscopic management is the presence of significant bone loss. Glenoid bone loss of 20% or more will increase failure rates dramatically. Significant humeral head bone loss (25%-30%) also precludes arthroscopic intervention. Most authors recommend open repair of a HAGL lesion. Arthroscopic treatment for traumatic anterior shoulder instability in collision athletes is still controversial. Patients older than 40 years usually have low recurrence rates; however, they are often troubled by residual neurovascular defects and limited shoulder motion. Recurrent instability in this age group is often associated with massive rotator cuff tears.[23,26,31] In older, low-functioning patients a conservative approach to rotator cuff repairs is recommended with physical therapy and corticosteroid injection and surgical repair as needed.[32] Studies show good results of rotator cuff repair with subacromial decompression are possible in symptomatic elderly patients failing conservative treatments.[30]

ARTHROSCOPIC ANTERIOR STABILIZATION

Shoulder arthroscopy can be performed with the patient in either the beach chair or lateral decubitus position. We prefer the lateral decubitus position due to improved access to the inferior and posterior aspects of the glenohumeral joint, as documented by Seroyer et al.[33] An examination under anesthesia is performed to confirm the degree and pattern of instability. After sterile preparation the operative arm is secured at 20° of forward flexion and 50° of abduction with 10 to 15 lb of lateral balanced suspension.[34]

The arthroscopic landmarks are palpated and marked. A 3-portal technique is utilized. A standard posterior portal is established and a 4-mm arthroscope is inserted. Next, using a spinal needle for localization, an anterior-superior portal is created under direct visualization. A skin incision large enough to accommodate a 5-mm cannula is made inferior to the anterolateral aspect of the acromion. A midglenoid portal, large enough to accommodate an 8.25-mm cannula, is established superior to the subscapularis and lateral to the coracoid. Diagnostic arthroscopy is performed evaluating for pathology of the glenoid labrum, rotator cuff, or SLAP lesion or the presence of a Hill-Sachs lesion. Glenoid bone loss of greater than 6 mm from

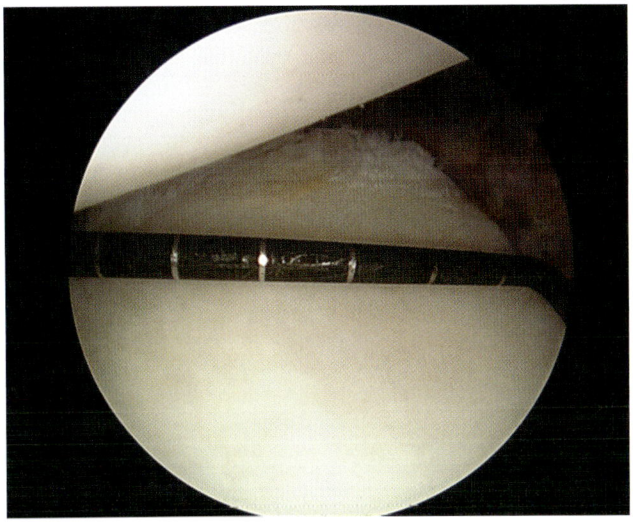

FIGURE 47-11 A graduated arthroscopic probe is used to quantify glenoid bone loss.

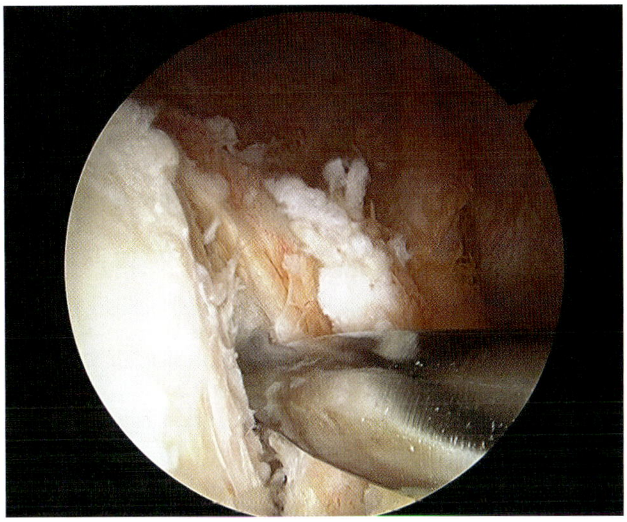

FIGURE 47-13 An arthroscopic elevator device is used to mobilize the scarred capsule and labrum.

the bare spot to the anterior glenoid should be managed with an open shoulder stabilization and bony augmentation (Fig. 47-11). MRI and MRA are poorly sensitive for evaluating capsular injuries and the diagnosis of a HAGL is must be ruled out intraoperatively.[11] If necessary, a 70° arthroscope can be utilized to evaluate the humeral bony insertions of the MGHL and IGHL[35] (Fig. 47-12).

After completion of the diagnostic arthroscopy, the involved labrum and capsule are mobilized using an arthroscopic elevator device (Fig. 47-13). There is minimal retraction following an acute dislocation, but in recurrent dislocators it is not unusual to encounter an ALSPA with the false appearance of an absent labrum after medialization and scaring to the glenoid neck (Fig. 47-14). Mobilization is sufficient when posterior fibers of the subscapularis muscle are seen. Alternatively, a probe can be used to assess the adequacy of mobilization by floating the labrum back to its anatomic position on the glenoid rim. The capsule should be gently abraded with a rasp, and the glenoid gently burred to remove enough soft tissue and bone to provide a fresh bony bed for healing (Figs. 47-15 and 47-16). In order to access the most inferior aspect of the joint, a 7-o'clock (posterolateral) portal may be utilized. The 7-o'clock portal is established under direct visualization with a spinal needle 1 cm anterior and 2 cm lateral to the standard posterior portal.[36]

Three to 4 suture anchors preloaded with a #2 stitch are usually required to secure the glenoid to the labrum. The anchors are progressively placed through the 7-o'clock or

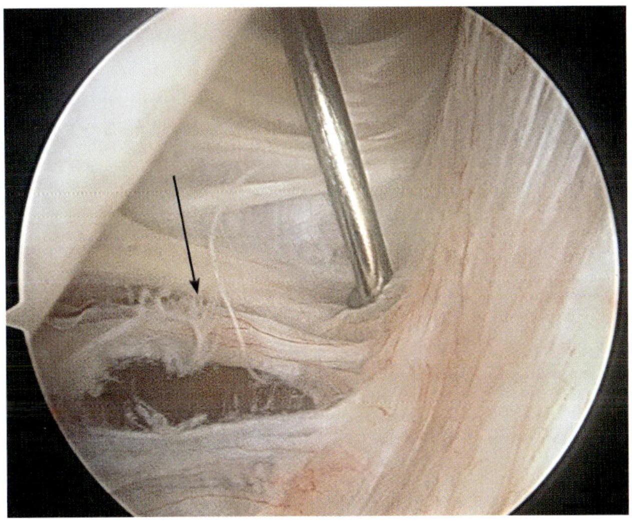

FIGURE 47-12 From a posterior portal view, the probe is brought in from an anterior-superior portal and is placed on an area of torn capsule known as humeral avulsion of the glenohumeral ligament (HAGL). The HAGL detaches off the humerus and the classic finding of a thin, strand-like anterior-inferior capsule is demonstrated here.

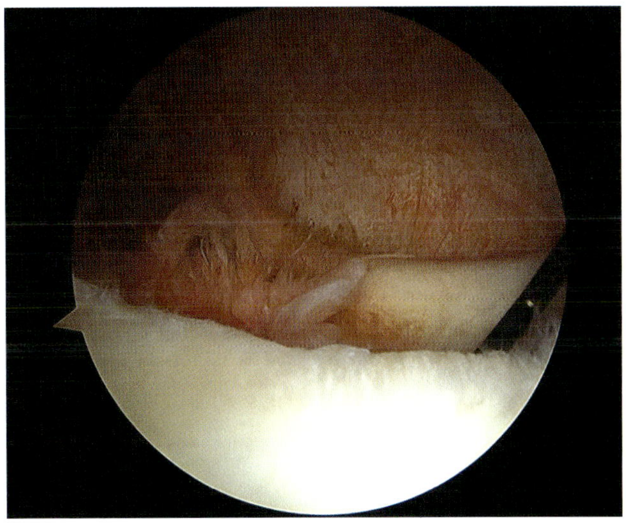

FIGURE 47-14 In this recurrent dislocator the labrum scarred medially on the glenoid neck as an ALPSA lesion. It gives the false appearance that the anterior labrum is absent.

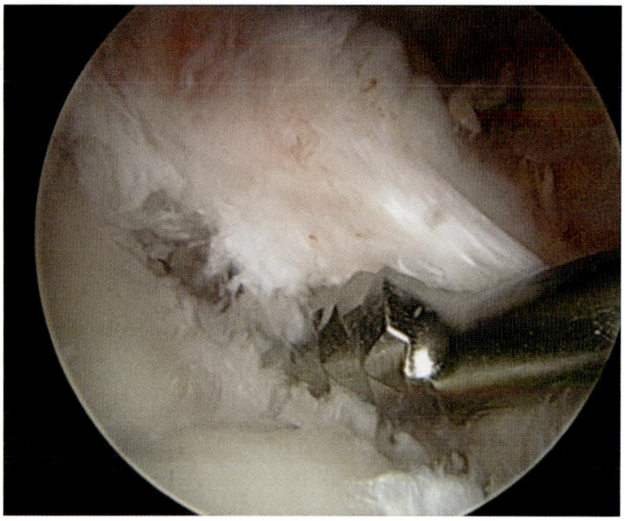

FIGURE 47-15 A footed rasp is used to debride the capsule and labrum prior to repair.

midglenoid portal starting at the inferior aspect of the lesion, just off the glenoid rim. It is critical to ensure that suture anchors are placed directly on the glenoid face to affect an appropriate labral shift (Fig. 47-17). The intent is to shift capsular tissue and the IGHL from an inferior to superior position to address the anteroinferior capsular stretch injury (Fig. 47-18). The sutures may be placed in vertical or horizontal configurations, tying the knots on the capsular side to prevent mechanical abrasion on the glenohumeral cartilage[7]. On completion the capsulolabral repair should result in an anteroinferior bumper with sufficient tension and tissue dimpling (Fig. 47-19).

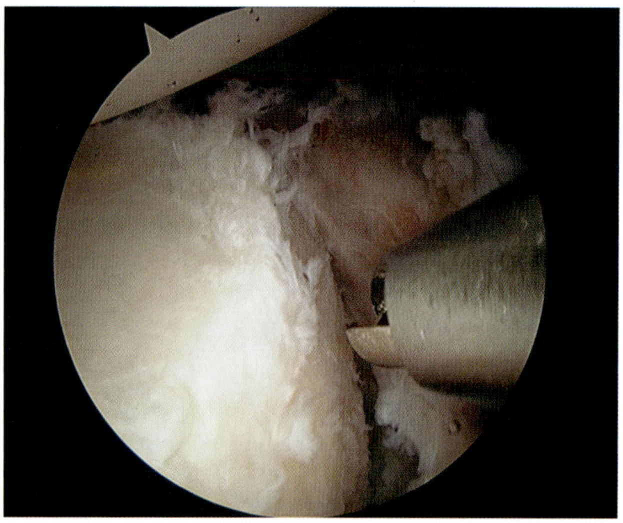

FIGURE 47-16 An arthroscopic shaver is used to debride the glenoid back to bleeding bone, taking care not to create iatrogenic glenoid bone loss.

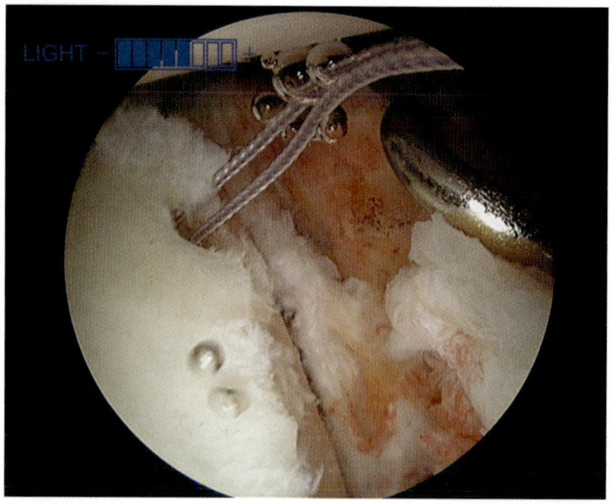

FIGURE 47-17 Proper placement of glenoid anchors on the glenoid face allows for appropriate capsulolabral shift.

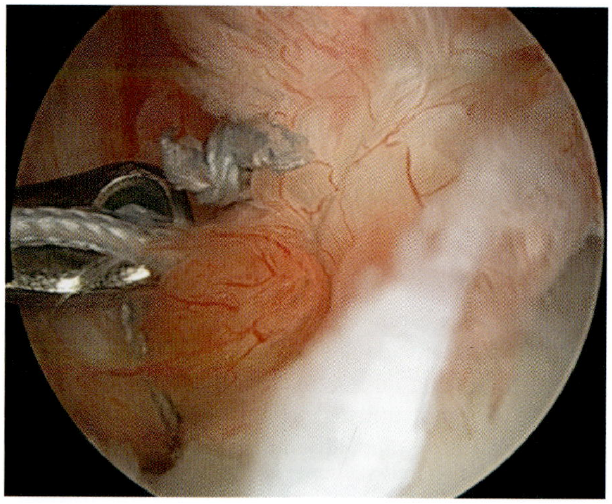

FIGURE 47-18 A suture shuttling device is used to shift capsular tissue from inferior to superior affecting an effective capsulolabral shift.

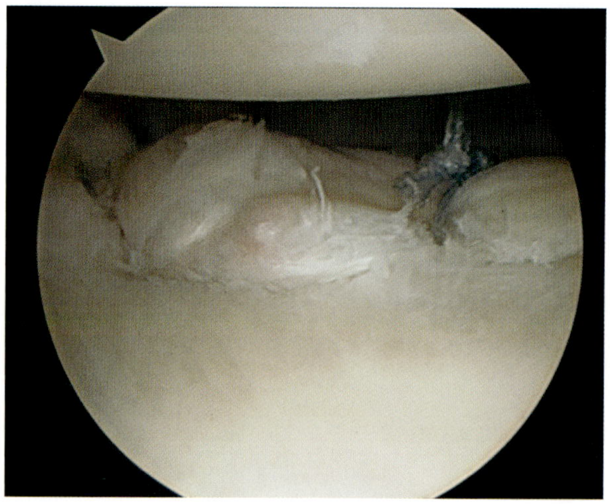

FIGURE 47-19 Sutures are placed with knots tied on the capsular side to prevent articular cartilage abrasion with recreation of an anteroinferior bumper and tissue dimpling.

OPEN ANTERIOR CAPSULORRHAPHY

Open anterior stabilization can be achieved with the patient in the beach chair position with the use of either general anesthesia or regional intrascalene block supplemented with local anesthetic to the axilla. As previously described, a physical examination under anesthesia is performed. An incision is made in the axillary fold from the inferior border of the pectoralis major tendon extending superiorly 5 cm toward the coracoid process. The dissection proceeds through the deltopectorial fascia, retracting the cephalic vein and the deltoid muscle laterally, and the pectoralis muscle medially. The clavipectoral fascia is incised lateral to the coracobrachialis–biceps tendon origin. The conjoined tendon is retracted medially taking care to avoid damaging the musculocutaneous nerve that runs deep to the conjoined tendons and medial to the coracoid.

The subscapularis tendon is identified with the shoulder in external rotation. Care is taken to identify the anterior humeral circumflex vessels at the inferior border of the subscapularis tendon. The subscapularis tendon is incised 1 cm medial to the musculotendinous junction at the uppermost portion and tagged with a #2 suture for later repair. The tendon is separated from the underlying capsule with blunt dissection, developing the plane between the capsule and tendon with an elevator medially and inferiorly. Occasionally, ligation of the 3 circumflex vessels running inferior to the subscapularis tendon is necessary. Retracting the tendon medially exposes the anterior capsule. Care must be taken to avoid damage to the axillary nerve, which resides in the inferior capsular pouch. Alternatively, the subscapularis may be split in the midportion in line with its fibers, and the capsule identified medially on the glenoid neck, just deep to the subscapularis split. This approach is technically more challenging, but may offer postoperative benefit by preserving subscapularis strength.

The patient's arm is placed in abduction and external rotation (ABER) to facilitate a capsulotomy. The anterior capsule is incised from the rotator interval to the anteroinferior capsular pouch 5 to 10 mm medial to its insertion on the humeral neck. It is important to maintain the arm in the ABER position to expose the most inferior part of the posterior capsule. The humeral head is retracted laterally with a ring retractor, and the capsule is retracted medially to inspect the labrum, the articular surfaces, and the posterior aspect of the supraspinatus tendon.

After exposure of the capsule and identification of the Bankart lesion, the torn capsulolabral complex is elevated off the glenoid rim to the level of the glenoid neck. The glenoid rim is debrided, creating a bleeding bed before the placement of suture anchors. Three to 5 anchors are usually required for an adequate repair. The capsule is shifted laterally and the sutures are passed through the capsulolabral complex anatomically securing it back to the glenoid rim.

The rotator interval and lateral capsulotomy are closed with nonabsorbable suture while maintaining the patient's arm in the ABER position. In cases of capsular redundancy, the rotator interval is closed. To accomplish this, the capsule is incised between the MGHL and IGHL, creating 2 flaps. The inferior flap is shifted superiorly before shifting the arm into 20° of abduction and 35° of external rotation. After the position change, the superior flap is shifted inferiorly and secured with suture. Finally, if the rotator interval remains lax, it is closed with suture with the arm in adduction and external rotation.

Postoperatively we immobilize patients in an abduction sling for 6 weeks. Passive pendulum exercises are instituted at postoperative day 1, followed by supervised passive range of motion in the scapular plane for 6 weeks. Aggressive external rotation at the side and in abduction is avoided for 6 weeks, through progressive stretching and full range of motion, and an active range of motion plan is emphasized from weeks 6 to 16. Participation in most sports is restricted for at least 4 months and no contact sports allowed until 6 months post surgery.

OUTCOMES

Bottoni et al randomized 24 patients to treatment with an arthroscopic tack versus immobilization.[37] At a mean follow-up of 36 months the dislocation rate was 75% in the nonoperative group versus 10% in the arthroscopically treated group. Larrain et al compared 18 patients treated with conservative measures versus 28 patients treated with an arthroscopic transglenoid suture anchor.[38] At a mean follow-up of 67 months there was a 94.4% recurrence rate in the nonoperative group compared with a recurrence rate of 3.6% in the arthroscopically stabilized group. Cho et al examined 29 athletes at a mean of 61 months following an arthroscopic Bankart suture repair.[39] The recurrence rate was 7% in the athletes who participated in a noncollision sport versus a 17% recurrence rate in athletes who participated in a collision sport.

ARTHROSCOPIC POSTERIOR STABILIZATION

Indications

A failure to respond to a well-executed physical therapy program for 6 months is an indication for surgical treatment. Similarly, if an athlete is unable to return to the preinjury level of competition, surgery can be considered. Therapy has traditionally been more effective in those patients who have an atraumatic cause, as opposed to those with generalized ligamentous laxity or who have suffered a discrete traumatic event.

Contraindications

The procedure is contraindicated in patients with a history of voluntary instability, and a noncompliant patient regarding rehabilitation.

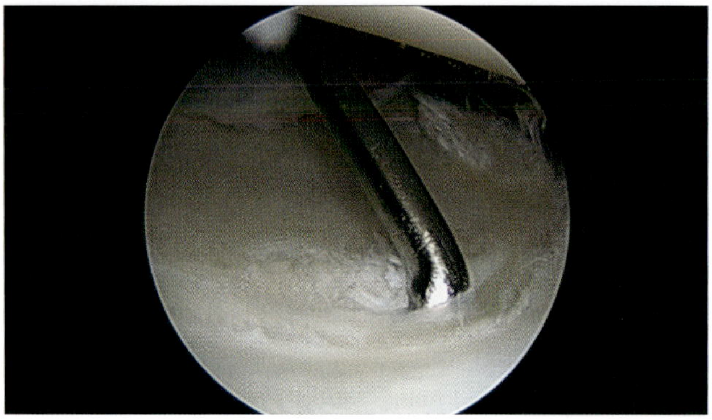

FIGURE 47-20 A posterior labral crack (Kim lesion) is identified with an arthroscopic probe.

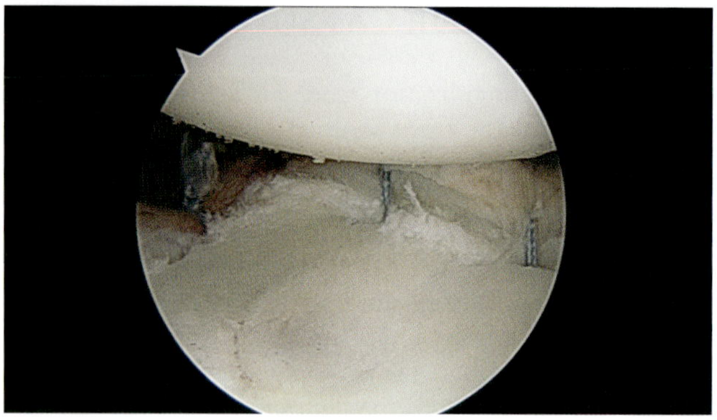

FIGURE 47-22 Completed posterior labral repair with a capsular plication and recreation of a soft tissue bumper.

Surgical Technique

An arthroscopic repair of a reverse Bankart lesion is very similar to an anterior repair. The patient is positioned in the lateral decubitus position with balanced suspension and a standard diagnostic arthroscopy is performed utilizing a 3-portal technique: a standard posterior viewing portal, an anterior-superior portal in the rotator interval, and a 7-o'clock (posterolateral) portal.[36] Although Kim et al demonstrated that the capsulorrhaphy can be performed without the use of suture anchors, a common cause of failure is not recognizing an incomplete crack of the posterior labrum.[24] For this reason the labrum should be carefully probed prior to further capsular plication and, if present, any Bankart or Kim lesions repaired with suture anchors (Fig. 47-20). Preparation of the posterior labrum and capsule is similar to that in anterior repairs (Fig. 47-21). A 1-cm capsular plication is utilized in conjunction with labral repair using 3 to 4 glenoid anchors from the 6-o'clock to the 10-o'clock position (Fig. 47-22). Following an open posterior repair patients are usually immobilized for 6 weeks, whereas those who undergo the arthroscopic procedure may begin weaning from the sling at about 4 weeks. Recommended positions for sling immobilization vary from neutral to 30° of abduction and neutral rotation.

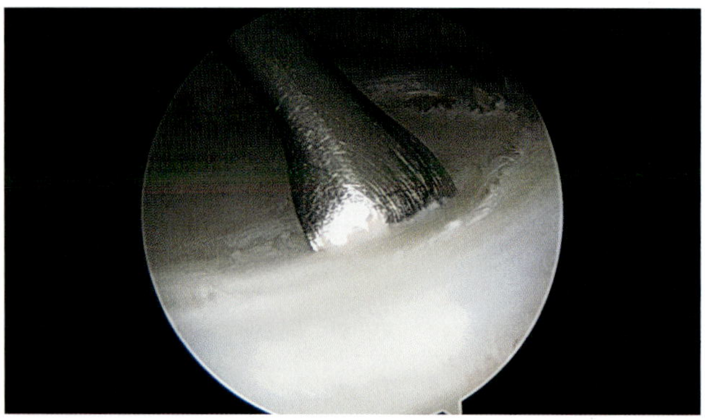

FIGURE 47-21 The posterior labrum is freed from the glenoid with an arthroscopic liberator device.

Outcomes

Williams et al reviewed their results following an isolated arthroscopic posterior capsulolabral repair with bioabsorbable tack fixation in 27 patients with symptomatic posterior capsulolabral complex detachment from the posterior glenoid rim after a distinct traumatic event, but with minimal posterior capsular laxity.[40] Ninety-three percent of patients' subjective instability and pain was eliminated, who returned to unlimited athletic activity by 6 months. Kim et al prospectively reviewed 27 athletes with traumatic unidirectional posterior instability treated with an arthroscopic posterior labral repair and capsular shift.[41] All patients had a labral lesion, and 22 also had stretching of the posterior band of the IGHL. The posterior capsule was shifted superiorly in all cases. All complete labral lesions were repaired directly and incomplete labral lesions were converted to complete tears and then repaired. The mean American Shoulder and Elbow Surgeons (ASES) Rating Scale scores improved from 51.2 to 96.2. All but 1 patient had restoration of stability and were able to return to previous athletic activities with little or no limitations.

Bradley et al reported the results of a prospective study on 91 athletes treated with an arthroscopic capsulolabral reconstruction for posterior instability.[42] At a mean follow-up of 27 months the mean ASES scores improved from 50.4 to 85.7, with 89 patients returning to sport and 67 returning to the same level as preoperative. There were 11 failures due to an undiagnosed MDI, inadequate capsular shift, and inadequate recognition of poor capsular tissue quality in those patients referred after thermal capsulorrhaphy and capsular plication performed in an isolated fashion without suture anchors.

Provencher et al reviewed 33 patients with a mean age of 25 years (range, 19-34 years) who underwent posterior arthroscopic shoulder stabilization with a mean of 3 suture anchors or a mean 5 sutures in capsulolabral plication.[43] At a mean follow-up of 39.1 months (range, 22-60 months), the mean ASES rating was 94.6, the subjective Patient Shoulder Evaluation was 20.0, and the Western Ontario Shoulder Instability Index was 389.4 (81.5% of normal). Patients with voluntary instability and prior surgery had worse outcomes. There were 7 failures, 4 for recurrent instability and 3 for symptoms of pain.

MULTIDIRECTIONAL INSTABILITY

Most patients with MDI have concomitant ligamentous laxity and should be treated without surgery. Initial treatment for these patients is aggressive physical therapy for shoulder stabilization exercises. In patients who fail therapy, or those with symptomatic involuntary instability, operative treatment can be considered.

Indications

Some typical surgical indications include a failure to respond to a well-executed physical therapy program for 6 months, psychological stability with a negative history for voluntary instability, painful instability in more than 1 direction, and a clear understanding by the patient of the necessity for postoperative immobilization and subsequent rehabilitation.

Contraindications

The procedure is contraindicated in patients with a history of voluntary instability, unidirectional instability with a labral tear, and a noncompliant patient regarding rehabilitation. Patients are again placed in the lateral decubitus position with balanced shoulder suspension following induction of anesthesia and an examination. A standard diagnostic arthroscopy is commenced and, in patients with MDI, a widened rotator interval, a patulous capsule, and a flattened labrum known as a "drive-through sign" are often present.[6]

Inferior and posteroinferior pathology are addressed before any anterior and SLAP lesions. The capsule is plicated with 3 to 5 sutures in the posteroinferior and inferior aspects of the capsulolabral complex. The goal of each stitch is to draw the capsule superiorly and medially. Anchors need to be utilized if labral pathology is present.[44] During repair it is important to place the arm in ABER with perpendicular suspension to decrease the risk of axillary nerve injury.[45] For patients presenting with a mild MDI picture, an isolated capsular shift through the rotator interval may be performed.

Since the inferior capsular shift also addresses the inferior capsule, it too must be protected during the healing phase for a minimum of 6 weeks. Conventional braces that can be removed by the patient are a poor choice of immobilization in the initial postoperative management following an inferior capsular shift. Our considerable experience suggests that if a brace can be removed, it will be removed, especially in the age group who undergo this type of procedure. Gravity is ever present and removing a brace for dressing, showering, etc, subjects the repair to inferiorly directed forces that place the capsular repair in a precarious situation. Several authors have reported on the importance of cast immobilization following inferior capsular shift.[14-16]

The capsular ligaments and tissues can certainly stretch out in the early weeks following surgical intervention, whether open or arthroscopic. Therefore, the capsular repair that involves the management of at least 3 directions of instability must be immobilized in those same 3 directions. Some authors prefer a spica cast to that of a removable brace or immobilizer. During the cast application, an assistant is holding the arm in neutral rotation to balance the anterior and posterior capsule while simultaneously holding the arm in a cephalad position to relieve inferiorly directed forces. The waist belt portion of the cast is applied and molded around the iliac crests bilaterally. The iliac crests will ultimately bear the downward force of the arm and prevent any forces on the inferior capsular repair. The arm cylinder that extends from just above the wrist to the upper arm is then applied. Lastly, the waist piece is fixed to the arm piece with a strut of casting material.

Outcomes

Treacy et al performed a retrospective study of 25 patients who underwent an arthroscopic capsular shift performed with the transglenoid technique after a failed course of physical therapy.[46] The average age was 26.4 years with 20 male and 5 female patients. All patients had a history of asymptomatic subluxation that slowly progressed to symptomatic subluxation. Eleven patients had a history of dislocation. At an average follow-up of 60 months (range, 36-80 months), the average Bankart score was 95 (range, 50-100). Eighty-eight percent of patients had a satisfactory result according to the Neer system. All but 1 patient regained full symmetric range of motion and 3 patients had episodes of recurrent instability.

More recently, Alpert et al analyzed the results of arthroscopic stabilization with labral repair in 13 patients (10 males and 3 females) with MDI and a frank labral tear, with a mean age of 27.2 years.[47] At a mean follow-up of 56 months (range, 29-72 months), 2 (15%) had recurrent instability after repair. The median scores were as follows: Western Ontario Shoulder Instability Index, 471; ASES score, 96.7; Simple Shoulder Test score, 12; visual analog pain scale, 0; and Short Form 12 mental component/physical component, 57/44. There were no differences in range of motion compared with the opposite extremity.

Complications

Complications of shoulder dislocation and surgical repair include recurrent dislocations, osteoarthritis, capsular necrosis, and neurovascular injury. Osteoarthritis is a common long-term complication following shoulder dislocation. Buscayret et al found that in 570 patients with shoulder dislocations a mean 6.5 years after surgery the incidence of glenohumeral arthritis was found to be 9.2% to 19.7%.[48] Pelet et al followed 30 shoulders over 29 years noting that 40% had arthritis suggesting that Bankart repair procedures do not prevent the development of glenohumeral degenerative arthritis.[49] Hovelius et al followed 247 patients with shoulder instability for 10 years noting that 20% developed mild osteoarthritis and 9% developed moderate to severe osteoarthritis.[50]

Recurrent instability is associated with age at first dislocation and activity level. Younger patients (aged 15-25) and those involved in contact sports are at greater risk for redislocation.[2,23,26] Hovelius et al compared operative and nonoperative treatment for glenohumeral instability and found that 50% of patients with a primary anterior dislocation treated nonoperatively had no further dislocations or had become stable over the course of 25 years.[51]

Stiffness can complicate shoulder stabilization surgery, especially when coupled with prolonged immobilization and overtensioning of the soft tissues. If a shoulder has decreased motion preoperatively, it must be restored prior to any stabilization procedure. Loss of motion is a common complication following shoulder surgery. After anterior stabilization there is a predictable loss of external rotation due to selective tightening of the anterior capsule. Although a small loss of external rotation is typically tolerated well, excessive anterior-superior capsular tightness manifested by loss of external rotation results in posterior shearing of the humeral head on the glenoid surface resulting in articular degeneration.[52]

Osteonecrosis of the humeral head has been reported following simple dislocations; however, this is more frequently encountered following injury to and surgical repair of anatomic humeral neck fracture–dislocations.[2,53] The risk of osteonecrosis increases with the degree of fracture–dislocation. Symptomatic osteonecrosis can be surgically treated with arthroplasty.

Intraoperative complications include neurovascular damage, subscapularis rupture, chondrolysis, and hardware failure. These are rare but devastating complications that can be avoided through meticulous preoperative planning and meticulous intraoperative technique. Injury to the axillary and musculocutaneous nerve can be prevented by avoiding excessive humeral distraction and careful placement of portals and capsular sutures. Thermal capsulorrhaphy has fallen out of favor to treat shoulder instability due to a high failure rate, capsular necrosis, and potential cartilage concerns including chondrolysis.

REFERENCES

1. Cutts S, Prempeh M, Drew S. Anterior shoulder dislocation. *Ann R Coll Surg Engl.* 2009;91:2–7.
2. Robinson C, Aderinto J. Posterior shoulder dislocations and fracture–dislocations. *J Bone Joint Surg Am.* 2005;87A(3):639–650.
3. Taylor D, Arciero R. Pathologic changes associated with shoulder dislocations. *Am J Sports Med.* 1997;25:306–311.
4. Burkart AC, Debski RE. Anatomy and function of the glenohumeral ligaments in anterior shoulder instability. *Clin Orthop.* 2002;(400):32–39.
5. Bach BR, Warren RF, Fronek J. Disruption of the lateral capsule of the shoulder. *J Bone Joint Surg Br.* 1988;70:274–276.
6. Bahu MJ, Trentacosta N, Vorys GC, Covey AS, Ahmad CS. Multidirectional instability: evaluation and treatment options. *Clin Sports Med.* 2008;27(4):671–689.
7. Delee J, Drez D, Miller D. *Delee & Drez's Orthopaedic Sports Medicine: Principles and Practice.* Vol. 2. 3rd ed. Philadelphia: Saunders/Elsevier; 2010.
8. Turkel SJ, Panio MW, Marshall JL, Girgis FG. Stabilizing mechanisms preventing anterior dislocation of the glenohumeral joint. *J Bone Joint Surg Am.* 1981;63(8):1208–1217.
9. Ovesen J, Nielsen S. Stability of the shoulder joint. Cadaver study of stabilizing structures. *Acta Orthop Scand.* 1985;56(2):149–151.
10. O'Brien SJ, Neves MC, Arnoczky SP, et al. The anatomy and histology of the inferior glenohumeral ligament complex of the shoulder. *Am J Sports Med.* 1990;18(5):449–456.
11. Bui-Mansfield LT, Taylor DC, Uhorchak JM, Tenuta JJ. Humeral avulsions of the glenohumeral ligament: imaging features and a review of the literature. *AJR Am J Roentgenol.* 2002;179(3):649–655.
12. Nicola T. Anterior dislocation of the shoulder. The role of the articular capsule. *J Bone Joint Surg Am.* 1942;24:614–616.
13. Warner J, Deng X, Warren R. Superior–inferior translations in the intact and vented glenohumeral joint. *J Shoulder Elbow Surg.* 1993;2:99–125.
14. Helmig P, Sojbjerg JO, Sneppen O, Loehr JF, Ostgaard SE, Suder P. Glenohumeral movement patterns after puncture of the joint capsule: an experimental study. *J Shoulder Elbow Surg.* 1993;2:209–215.
15. Harryman DT 2nd, Sidles JA, Harris SL, Matsen FA 3rd. The role of the rotator interval capsule in passive motion and stability of the shoulder. *J Bone Joint Surg Am.* 1992;74(1):53–66.
16. Harryman DT 2nd, Sidles JA, Harris SL, Matsen FA 3rd. Laxity of the normal glenohumeral joint: a quantitative in vivo assessment. *J Shoulder Elbow Surg.* 1992;1:66–67.
17. Speer KP. Anatomy and pathomechanics of shoulder instability. *Clin Sports Med.* 1995;14(4):751–760.
18. George MS, Khazzam M, Kuhn JE. Humeral avulsion of glenohumeral ligaments. *J Am Acad Orthop Surg.* 2011;19(3):127–133.
19. Bigliani LU, Pollock RG, Soslowsky LJ, Flatow EL, Pawluk RJ, Mow VC. Tensile properties of the inferior glenohumeral ligament. *J Orthop Res.* 1992;10(2):187–197.
20. Bui-Mansfield LT, Banks KP, Taylor DC. Humeral avulsion of the glenohumeral ligaments: the HAGL lesion. *Am J Sports Med.* 2007;35(11):1960–1966.
21. Visser CP, Coene LN, Brand R, Tavy DL. The incidence of nerve injury in anterior dislocation of the shoulder and its influence on functional recovery. A prospective clinical and EMG study. *J Bone Joint Surg Br.* 1999;81(4):679–685.
22. Sugaya H, Moriishi J, Dohi M, Kon Y, Tsuchiya A. Glenoid rim morphology in recurrent anterior glenohumeral instability. *J Bone Joint Surg Am.* 2003;85-A(5):878–884.
23. Arciero RA, Wheeler JH, Ryan JB, McBride JT. Arthroscopic Bankart repair versus nonoperative treatment for acute, initial anterior shoulder dislocations. *Am J Sports Med.* 1994;22(5):589–594.
24. Kim SH, Ha KI, Yoo JC, Noh KC. Kim's lesion: an incomplete and concealed avulsion of the posteroinferior labrum in posterior or multidirectional posteroinferior instability of the shoulder. *Arthroscopy.* 2004;20(7):712–720.
25. Cheok CY, Mohamad JA, Ahmad TS. Pain relief for reduction of acute anterior shoulder dislocations: a prospective randomized study comparing intravenous sedation with intra-articular lidocaine. *J Orthop Trauma.* 2011;25(1):5–10.
26. Wang RY, Arciero RA, Mazzocca AD. The recognition and treatment of first-time shoulder dislocation in active individuals. *J Orthop Sports Phys Ther.* 2009;39(2):118–123.
27. Wilson JC, McKeever FM. Traumatic posterior dislocation of the humerus. *J Bone Joint Surg Am.* 1949;31A(1):160–172.
28. Itoi E, Hatakeyama Y, Sato T, et al. Immobilization in external rotation after shoulder dislocation reduces the risk of recurrence. A randomized controlled trial. *J Bone Joint Surg Am.* 2007;89(10):2124–2131.

29. Buss DD, Lynch GP, Meyer CP, Huber SM, Freehill MQ. Nonoperative management for in-season athletes with anterior shoulder instability. *Am J Sports Med.* 2004;32(6):1430–1433.
30. Packer NP, Calvert PT, Bayley JI, Kessel L. Operative treatment of chronic ruptures of the rotator cuff of the shoulder. *J Bone Joint Surg Br.* 1983;65(2):171–175.
31. Grumet RC, Bach BR Jr, Provencher MT. Arthroscopic stabilization for first-time versus recurrent shoulder instability. *Arthroscopy.* 2010;26(2):239–248.
32. Lin JC, Weintraub N, Aragaki DR. Nonsurgical treatment for rotator cuff injury in the elderly. *J Am Med Dir Assoc.* 2008;9(9):626–632.
33. Seroyer ST, Nho SJ, Provencher MT, Romeo AA. Four-quadrant approach to capsulolabral repair: an arthroscopic road map to the glenoid. *Arthroscopy.* 2010;26(4):555–562.
34. Parameswaran AD, Provencher MT, Bach BR Jr, Verma N, Romeo AA. Humeral avulsion of the glenohumeral ligament: injury pattern and arthroscopic repair techniques. *Orthopedics.* 2008;31(8): 773–779.
35. Richards DP, Burkhart SS. Arthroscopic humeral avulsion of the glenohumeral ligaments (HAGL) repair. *Arthroscopy.* 2004;20(suppl 2): 134–141.
36. Davidson PA, Rivenburgh DW. The 7-o'clock posteroinferior portal for shoulder arthroscopy. *Am J Sports Med.* 2002;30(5):693–696.
37. Bottoni CR, Wilckens JH, DeBerardino TM, et al. A prospective, randomized evaluation of arthroscopic stabilization versus nonoperative treatment in patients with acute, traumatic, first-time shoulder dislocations. *Am J Sports Med.* 2002;30(4):576–580.
38. Larrain MV, Botto GJ, Montenegro HJ, Mauas DM. Arthroscopic repair of acute traumatic anterior shoulder dislocation in young athletes. *Arthroscopy.* 2001;17(4):373–377.
39. Cho NS, Hwang JC, Rhee YG. Arthroscopic stabilization in anterior shoulder instability: collision athletes versus noncollision athletes. *Arthroscopy.* 2006;22(9):947–953.
40. Williams RJ 3rd, Strickland S, Cohen M, Altchek DW, Warren RF. Arthroscopic repair for traumatic posterior shoulder instability. *Am J Sports Med.* 2003;31(2):203–209.
41. Kim SH, Ha KI, Park JH, et al. Arthroscopic posterior labral repair and capsular shift for traumatic unidirectional recurrent posterior subluxation of the shoulder. *J Bone Joint Surg Am.* 2003;85-A(8): 1479–1487.
42. Bradley JP, Baker CL 3rd, Kline AJ, Armfield DR, Chhabra A. Arthroscopic capsulolabral reconstruction for posterior instability of the shoulder: a prospective study of 100 shoulders. *Am J Sports Med.* 2006;34(7):1061–1071.
43. Provencher MT, Bell SJ, Menzel KA, Mologne TS. Arthroscopic treatment of posterior shoulder instability: results in 33 patients. *Am J Sports Med.* 2005;33(10):1463–1471.
44. Provencher MT, Verma N, Obopilwe E, et al. A biomechanical analysis of capsular plication versus anchor repair of the shoulder: can the labrum be used as a suture anchor? *Arthroscopy.* 2008;24:210–216.
45. Price MR, Tillett ED, Acland RD, Nettleton GS. Determining the relationship of the axillary nerve to the shoulder joint capsule from an arthroscopic perspective. *J Bone Joint Surg Am.* 2004;86-A(10): 2135–2142.
46. Treacy SH, Savoie FH 3rd, Field LD. Arthroscopic treatment of multidirectional instability. *J Shoulder Elbow Surg.* 1999;8(4):345–350.
47. Alpert JM, Verma N, Wysocki R, Yanke AB, Romeo AA. Arthroscopic treatment of multidirectional shoulder instability with minimum 270 degrees labral repair: minimum 2-year follow-up. *Arthroscopy.* 2008;24(6):704–711.
48. Buscayret F, Edwards TB, Szabo I, Adeleine P, Coudane H, Walch G. Glenohumeral arthrosis in anterior instability before and after surgical treatment: incidence and contributing factors. *Am J Sports Med.* 2004;32(5):1165–1172.
49. Pelet S, Jolles BM, Farron A. Bankart repair for recurrent anterior glenohumeral instability: results at twenty-nine years' follow-up. *J Shoulder Elbow Surg.* 2006;15(2):203–207.
50. Hovelius L, Augustini BG, Fredin H, Johansson O, Norlin R, Thorling J. Primary anterior dislocation of the shoulder in young patients. A ten-year prospective study. *J Bone Joint Surg Am.* 1996;78(11): 1677–1684.
51. Hovelius L, Olofsson A, Sandstrom B, et al. Nonoperative treatment of primary anterior shoulder dislocation in patients forty years of age and younger. A prospective twenty-five-year follow-up. *J Bone Joint Surg Am.* 2008;90(5):945–952.
52. Kang RW, Frank RM, Nho SJ, et al. Complications associated with anterior shoulder instability repair. *Arthroscopy.* 2009;25(8):909–920.
53. Hersche O, Gerber C. Iatrogenic displacement of fracture–dislocations of the shoulder. A report of seven cases. *J Bone Joint Surg Br.* 1994; 76(1):30–33.

48

Shoulder Arthroscopy: Treatment of Subacromial Impingement, Rotator Cuff Tears, and Superior Labral Anterior and Posterior Tears

Umer Dasti, MD
Craig Wright, MD
Jeffrey S. Abrams, MD

SHOULDER ARTHROSCOPY

Rationale

A recent study demonstrated that from 1996 to 2006 the number of arthroscopic rotator cuff repairs performed in the United Kingdom increased by a factor of 4, and that an arthroscopic surgical repair of patients with a first-time shoulder dislocation has doubled.[1]

Open surgical techniques have encountered certain complications that can be reduced with arthroscopic approaches. Wound infection, stiffness, and deltoid and subscapularis dehiscence have been reported after arthrotomy.[2,3]

There are many shoulder surgical procedures that are being performed arthroscopically at the present time. Each of these procedures has benefits and potential pitfalls. We will present the basic setup, indications, contraindications, and techniques as they apply to impingement, rotator cuff tears, and SLAP tears.

GENERAL SETUP AND ARTHROSCOPIC SHOULDER PORTALS

Anesthesia

Shoulder arthroscopy can be performed under general anesthesia, regional anesthesia, or a combination of both. When regional anesthesia is employed, typically in the form of a brachial plexus block, the patient can be sedated, and general anesthesia with intubation avoided. A commonly utilized block is the interscalene block, which has been shown to reduce postoperative pain and improve early recovery time compared with general anesthesia.[4] There is less of a requirement for narcotics during surgery, avoiding the potential side effects of these medications. The interscalene block is a proximal brachial plexus block, and anesthetizes the supraclavicular nerves and upper roots of the brachial plexus. This results in analgesia over the entire shoulder area. Use of ultrasound guidance allows visualization of the brachial plexus and vascular structures (Fig. 48-1). Other blocks, such as the supraclavicular, infraclavicular, and axillary blocks, may not provide adequate anesthesia, as they spare the higher brachial plexus roots.[5] Potential contraindications to the use of an interscalene block include difficult anatomy due to a short or obese neck, certain preoperative neurologic injuries, and compromised respiratory status as the interscalene block often paralyzes the phrenic nerve.

Patient Positioning

Two options exist for patient positioning during shoulder arthroscopy, the beach chair position and the lateral position. In the beach chair position, the orientation is more familiar to surgeons, arm positioning and manipulation during the procedure is less obstructed, conversion to an open surgery is easier, and the body position may be better tolerated in a minimally sedated patient (Fig. 48-2). Special anesthetic precautions are necessary when a patient is sitting to avoid unrecognized hypotension and diminished cerebral vascular blood flow. The lateral position allows for joint distraction and better access to the posterior and inferior aspects of the glenohumeral joint (Fig. 48-3). Some surgeons utilize 1 position for all cases while others change the setup depending

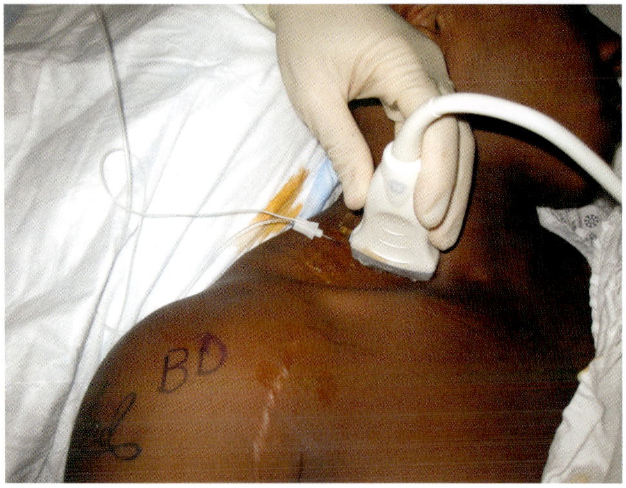

FIGURE 48-1 Ultrasound-guided interscalene block provides regional pain relief.

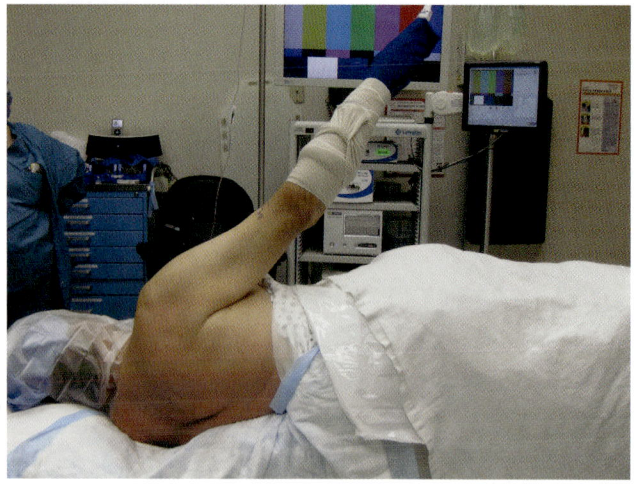

FIGURE 48-3 Lateral decubitus positioning for shoulder arthroscopy with arm suspension.

on pathology to be addressed, performing rotator cuff repair and subacromial decompressions in a beach chair position, and using the lateral position to treat articular pathology (ie, a SLAP repair). Both positions require specialized equipment to support the head, neck, trunk, and legs. The beach chair requires special table attachments, and cervical and arm support, while the lateral position requires a traction device to suspend the arm.

Equipment

The standard arthroscopic equipment includes a 4-mm 30° arthroscope and inflow/outflow ports connected to a pressure-regulating saline pump, and a variety of arthroscopic probes, punches/biters, and graspers, as well as motorized shavers, burs, and electrocautery devices. Depending on the procedure, suture anchors, suture delivery instruments, and cannulae may be required.

Portals and Relevant Anatomy

The 3 standard portals utilized for shoulder arthroscopy are the anterior, posterior, and lateral portals (Fig. 48-4). Additional small portals or punctures may be added to facilitate placement of anchors and suture management. The posterior portal is generally established first. This portal is located 1 to 2 cm inferior and 1 cm medial to the posterolateral corner of the acromion. A soft spot can usually be palpated in this area and corresponds to the posterior glenohumeral joint line. The glenohumeral joint is located with a spinal needle and then insufflated with 50 cm^3 of saline

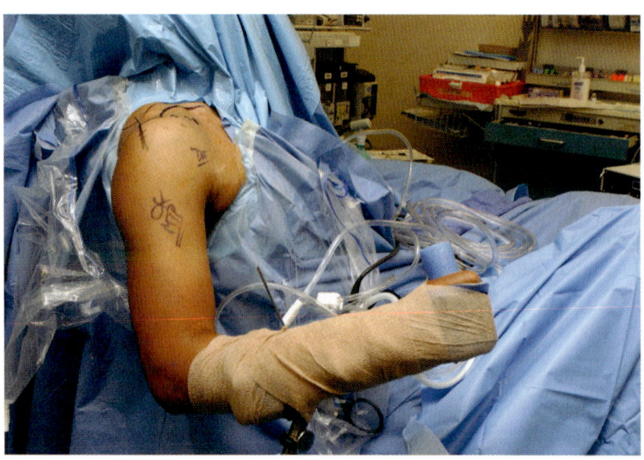

FIGURE 48-2 Beach chair positioning for shoulder arthroscopy with adjustable arm support.

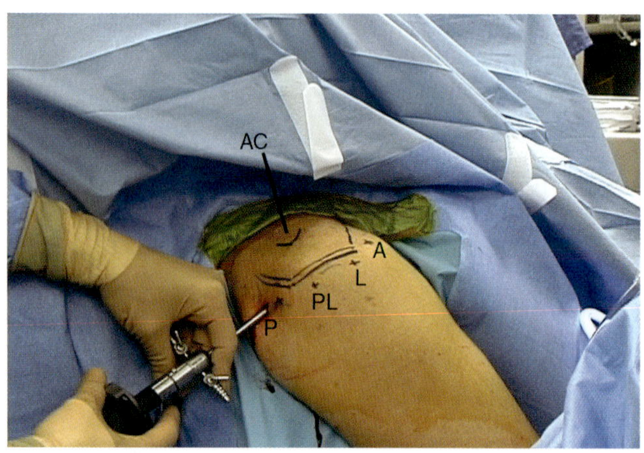

FIGURE 48-4 Right shoulder with arthroscope in the posterior viewing portal. Anterior, lateral, and posterolateral portals are marked. A, anterior; AC, acromioclavicular; L, lateral; PL, posterolateral.

prior to incising the skin, followed by introducing a blunt trocar. The trocar should be slowly advanced with a twisting motion, entering the superior aspect of the glenohumeral capsule while keeping a finger on the coracoid to aid in triangulation as the trocar is advanced toward this point. The trocar tip may encounter bone, but by gently joint distracting and rotating the humerus, the trocar can be redirected. The anterior portal is usually established with an outside-to-inside technique while inserting a spinal needle under arthroscopic control. Generally, the portal lies in line with the coracoid and the anterolateral corner of the acromion. This portal should pierce the joint capsule within the rotator cuff interval. These 2 portals are usually sufficient for most diagnostic procedures and for debridement of the glenohumeral joint. The surgeon can visualize the anterior and inferior compartments through the anterior portal. Both of these skin portals can be utilized to access the subacromial space by redirecting the arthroscope and instruments without additional incisions, but a lateral portal is often necessary as well. This portal is established approximately 3 cm lateral to the lateral aspect of the anterior third of the acromion. Care must be taken not to make this portal too close to the lateral edge of the acromion to avoid contact with bone, which may limit access to the medial aspect of the acromion and the acromioclavicular (AC) joint. Other portals have been described, such as the anterolateral portal, 5-o'clock portal, Neviaser portal, posterolateral portal, and the portal of Wilmington, which may be necessary for articular and bursal operations. The neural structures at risk during the placement of the portals include the axillary nerve, suprascapular nerve, musculocutaneous nerve, and the brachial plexus. The axillary nerve is deep to the deltoid as it courses around the humerus approximately 5 cm from the margin of the acromion. Portals placed inferiorly or medially may endanger this structure.

SUBACROMIAL IMPINGEMENT SYNDROME

Rationale and Basic Science

The subacromial impingement syndrome refers to a spectrum of conditions producing anterior and lateral shoulder pain that occur as a result of compression of the supraspinatus tendon, the subacromial bursa, and the long head of the biceps tendon from the acromion, the coracoacromial ligament, and the undersurface of the AC joint[6] during forward elevation of the arm. Controversy exists as to the pathophysiology of this condition. Some propose an "extrinsic compression" etiology due to the curvature of the acromion, the development of bony spurs on the underside of the acromion, or the development of AC joint arthritis that creates compression of the rotator cuff in an abducted or forward flexed shoulder.[7–9] Others propose "intrinsic tendon degeneration" as the first step, with superior migration of the humeral head leading to narrowing of the acromiohumeral interval. This theory suggests that the reduction of this potential space gradually leads to changes on the underside of the acromion and impingement.[10,11] In the end, both theories likely have merit, and a combination of intrinsic and extrinsic factors contributes to a self-perpetuating cycle of impingement.

Indications and Contraindications

Surgical treatment of subacromial impingement with an acromioplasty and subacromial decompression is generally indicated when a patient has failed nonoperative treatment.

Patients should have near-normal passive shoulder range of motion. A relative contraindication is a patient with radicular symptoms in the scapula and upper extremity since this may be secondary to a cervical radiculopathy, although both may coexist.

Contraindications include an active skin or deep infection, or a stiff shoulder that may be in the early phases of adhesive capsulitis. Preoperative imaging including plain x-rays and MRI can help identify the pathology and degree of cuff tendinosis (Fig. 48-5). Clear evidence of subacromial spurs combined with pathologic changes in the supraspinatus and possibly the long head of the biceps tendon supports the diagnosis. Full- or partial-thickness rotator cuff tears are common, and the surgeon should be prepared to address the tears with debridement or repair depending on the patient, location of the tear, and degree of tendinopathy. Another contraindication to decompression is incorrect preoperative diagnosis (ie, shoulder instability in a young patient).

Surgical Technique

Arthroscopic subacromial decompression is performed following a thorough diagnostic exam and treatment of any articular glenohumeral pathology. If a rotator cuff repair

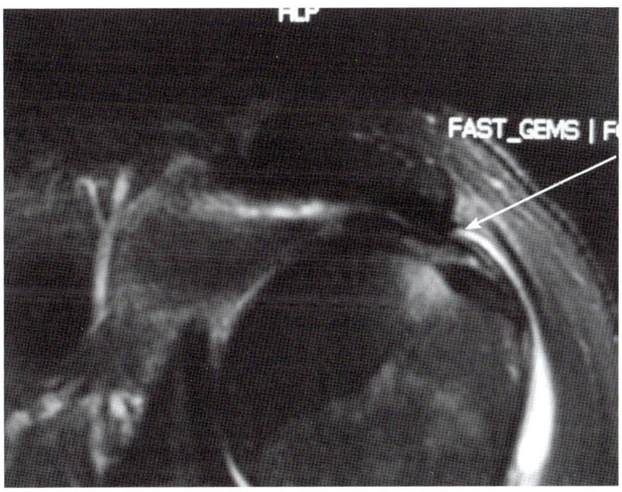

FIGURE 48-5 MRI view of patient with acromial impingement adjacent to the supraspinatus insertion.

is anticipated, the decompression is performed after determining if the rotator cuff lesion is repairable. The working portals include the anterior, posterior, and lateral portals as described above. The arthroscope is introduced into the subacromial space through the posterior portal. The camera is swept medial to lateral to visualize a space within the bursa to begin a bursectomy. The anterior portal is often used for an inflow cannula. The lateral portal is established from outside to inside after localization with a spinal needle to confirm that the planned portal location allows full access to the entire underside of the anterior acromion and the AC joint. A shaver is introduced through the lateral portal. The debridement is performed with the shaver opening always facing superiorly to avoid iatrogenic damage to the rotator cuff. The shaver and electrocautery instruments are used to define the anterior and lateral edges of the acromion. The AC joint can also be identified, and its capsule should not be violated if there is not a plan for a distal clavicle excision. An electrocautery device is used to strip periosteum and soft tissue from the undersurface of the acromion, limit bleeding, and define the bone margins. Once soft tissue has been thoroughly cleared, the shape of the acromion should be fully appreciated. A spur, hook, or prominence of the anterior aspect of the acromion can now be identified and resected using an arthroscopic bur (Fig. 48-6). The shaver

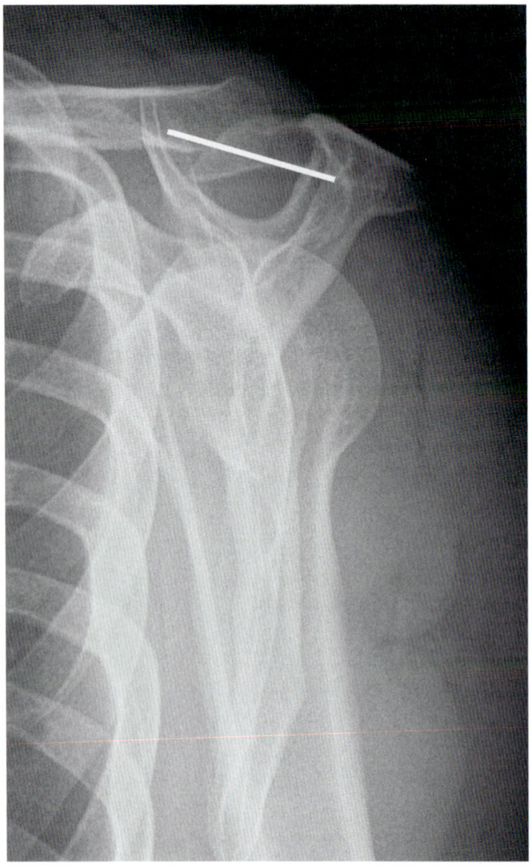

FIGURE 48-6 Lateral view of a hook-shaped acromion. Line created to determine amount of bone to resect.

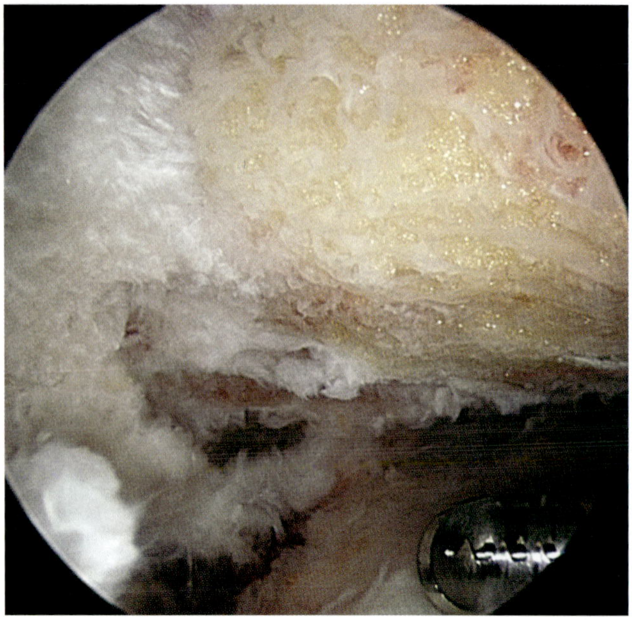

FIGURE 48-7 Arthroscopic lateral view after removal of the acromial osteophyte.

and bur are alternated using the lateral portal. The viewing portal can be switched to the lateral portal to provide a panoramic view of the profile of the acromion. The bur is placed in the posterior portal and used to create a flattened acromial undersurface. The goal is to remove bone from the anterolateral aspect of the acromion and taper the resection posteriorly and medially to achieve a smooth undersurface, flatten the acromion, and reduce any anterior extension beyond the AC joint (Fig. 48-7). The amount of bone resection should be determined by preoperative imaging studies and intraoperative evaluation. The coracoacromial ligament is often identified in the subacromial space, and the acromial attachment can be preserved with careful resection of the acromial osteophyte, especially in the setting of a large rotator cuff tear, as the coracoacromial ligament is a restraint to anterior and superior migration of the humeral head.

The AC joint may also be an independent source of pain or may contribute to impingement if large osteophytes have developed. Resection of these osteophytes and any distal clavicle excision can be performed at the same time as the subacromial decompression. For a complete resection of the distal clavicle, the anterior portal may be used for the shaver and bur while the arthroscope is in the posterior portal. The space developed between the acromion and clavicle is approximately 1 cm. The resection includes the clavicle facet of the acromion in addition to the distal clavicle (Fig. 48-8A and B). Failure to completely resect the distal clavicle may lead to continued pain, with the most common area being the posterior superior distal clavicle. To confirm a complete resection, the arthroscope may be switched to the anterior portal, and if further resection is deemed necessary, the shaver and bur are used from the posterior portal.

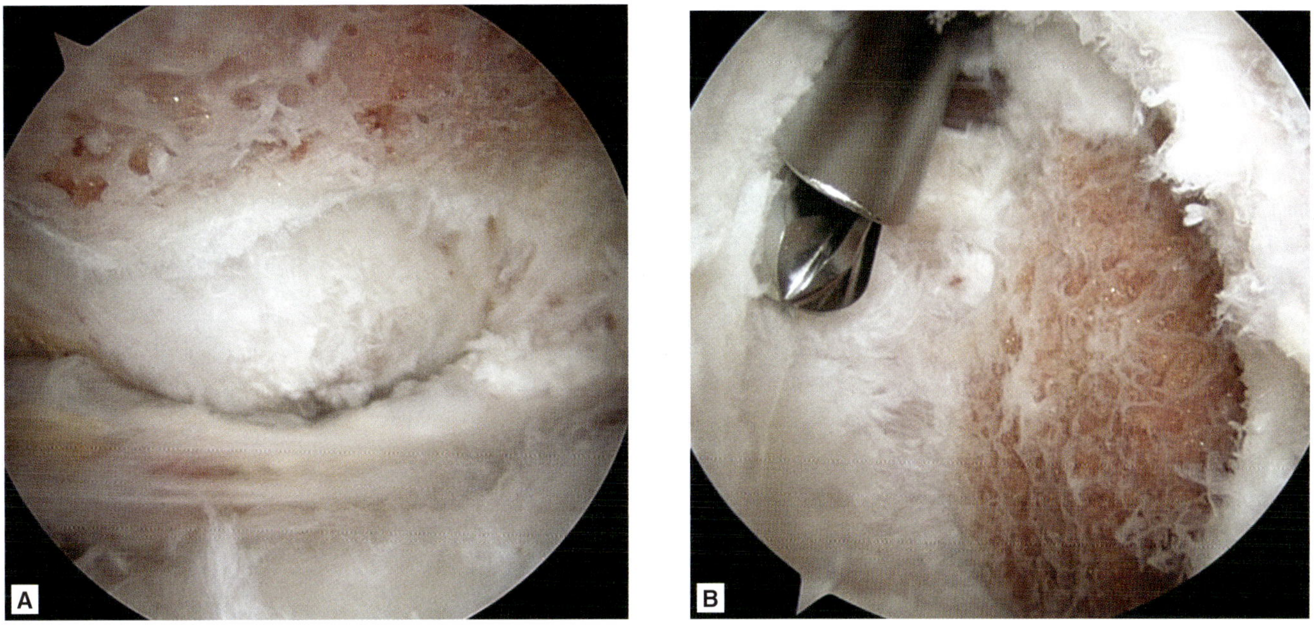

FIGURE 48-8 Acromioclavicular joint impingement. **A.** Clavicular spur impinging on supraspinatus muscle tendon junction. **B.** Resection of distal clavicle.

Preservation of the superior and posterior capsular structures and the coracoclavicular ligaments is important to the stability of the distal clavicle.

Complications

Complications during a subacromial decompression are the lowest of all arthroscopic shoulder procedures, but may occur. In general, the complication rate has been reported at 0.25% to 2%.[10] Complications include stiffness, postoperative infection, and recurrence or persistence of symptoms. Branches of the thoracoacromial artery can be lacerated and lead to significant bleeding and hematoma. The rotator cuff and structures deep to the cuff can be damaged by inadvertent shaving or use of a thermal device. Overresection or incorrect location of resection of the acromion can lead to the potential for fracture. Overresection of the distal clavicle can lead to a compromise of the capsule and stabilizing ligaments, creating instability of the AC joint (Fig. 48-9).

Outcomes

Davis et al performed a meta-analysis of arthroscopic versus open acromioplasty with minimum follow-up of 1 year. The analysis focused on 1-year clinical outcome and included a comparison of an objective 100-point score, hospital stay, time until return to work, operative time, and complications. No significant differences were found in clinical outcomes or complications for the 2 groups in the 9 studies that met their criteria. However, open acromioplasty was associated with longer hospital stays (2.3 days, $P = .05$) and a greater length in time until return to work (65.1 days) compared with the arthroscopic technique (48.6 days).[11]

Odenbring et al reviewed 24 male patients/31 shoulders, with a mean age of 49 years (range, 33-68 years) who underwent an arthroscopic acromioplasty. A group of 22 men (29 shoulders) operated on with an open acromioplasty served as controls. At 12 to 14 years the mean UCLA score was 32 points (SD, 5 points) for the patients treated with arthroscopic acromioplasty and 28 points (SD, 8 points) for those treated with open acromioplasty. The rate of change from baseline in UCLA score over time was significantly better after arthroscopic surgery than after open surgery.[12]

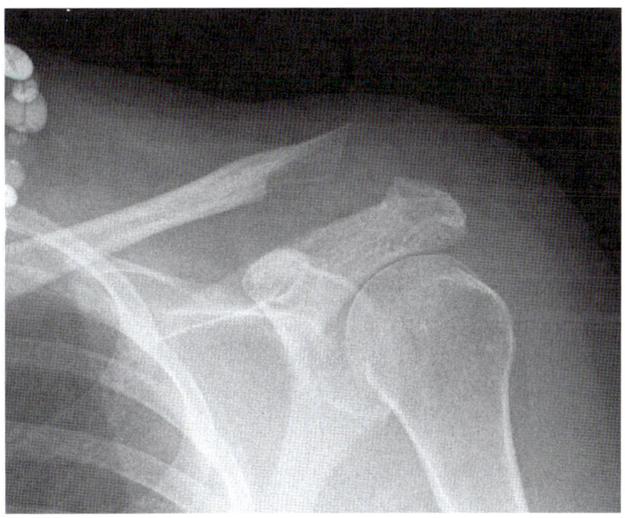

FIGURE 48-9 Resection of AC joint capsule and portions of the coracoclavicular ligaments.

Advantages of arthroscopic subacromial decompression include preservation of the deltoid and coracoacromial ligament attachments, and visualization of articular structures including the undersurface of the rotator cuff and biceps tendons. Overall, high patient satisfaction should be expected after decompression. Bengtsson et al evaluated 50 patients with a mean age of 49 (27-72) years and noted a significant improvement in both the median DASH score and the VAS at 6 months following surgery.[13]

ROTATOR CUFF TEARS

Rationale and Basic Science

Rotator cuff tendinopathy includes a spectrum of conditions ranging from tendinitis to partial- and full-thickness tears involving multiple tendons.[6] Tears can occur in many age groups, but can generally be divided into tears in younger, more active patients following an acute injury or repetitive overhead activity, tears in middle-age patients that present more insidiously and often relate to activity and subacromial space changes, and tears in the elderly resulting from gradual degeneration of the cuff. Symptoms include night pain, shoulder weakness, loss of active range of motion, and muscle atrophy. The degree of disability may not necessarily reflect the size of the tear. Patients with small symptomatic tears can be more disabled than patients with minimally symptomatic larger tears. As the number of involved tendons increases, the degree of disability increases. Multiple tendon tears can destabilize the glenohumeral articulation, leading to superior migration of the humeral head (Fig. 48-10).

Indications and Contraindications

When discussing treatment options, factors to consider are duration of symptoms, shoulder dominance, extent of disability experienced by the patient, type of tear, health of the patient, and patient activity level. An acute, full-thickness, symptomatic tear in an otherwise healthy and functional individual is an indication for surgery. In this case, surgical repair should be performed within 6 to 12 weeks following injury, as delayed treatment may lead to tendon retraction and irreversible muscle changes.[14-16] In elderly or lower-functioning patients, those with chronic tears, or those who cannot comply with the postoperative therapy protocol, nonoperative treatment is recommended as the initial treatment. Basic activities of daily living not requiring a flexed or abducted shoulder are usually well tolerated, and limited corticosteroid injections and NSAIDs often provide adequate pain control.[17]

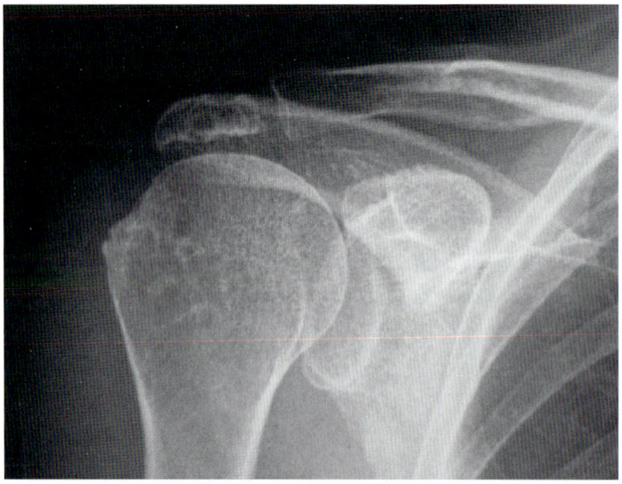

FIGURE 48-10 Superior migration of the humerus due to a large rotator cuff tear.

For most tears, a trial of conservative treatment consisting of exercise, physiotherapy, activity modification, NSAIDs, and corticosteroid injections is recommended. The 2011 AAOS Clinical Practice Guideline recommendations, however, could only find evidence to support the use of exercise and NSAIDs, and could not recommend for or against the other modalities.[18] Patients may consider the benefits of a structured physical therapy program or an independent program to improve the glenohumeral mechanics. In young patients with partial tears, surgical treatment is indicated in selected patients who have failed 12 weeks or greater of conservative management, provided they have a normal passive range of motion. In these cases, arthroscopy is performed to assess the degree of the tear, with many authors recommending debridement for minor tears less than 25% to 50% of the cuff thickness and repair for larger tears.[17] Contraindications include infection, advanced glenohumeral arthritis, fixed proximal migration of the humeral head, or advanced atrophy of the rotator cuff muscles suggestive of an irreparable tear. A relative contraindication is a patient who is unable to comply with the postoperative immobilization and rehabilitation program.

Surgical Technique

The goals of the arthroscopic rotator cuff repair should be to achieve a high initial fixation strength, to restore the anterior and posterior force couple balance, and to optimize a tendon-to-bone healing potential. Various techniques have been developed to achieve these goals, and reaching the end points requires significant skill and practice. Regardless of the chosen technique, some common underlying principles should be emphasized to optimize chances of a successful surgery.

Appropriate portal selection is essential to allow proper visualization, mobilization, and repair. The posterior portal is the primary visualization portal. Consider placing this portal or creating an additional portal more lateral to facilitate visualization. An anterior portal is then established under direct visualization. Using an outside-to-inside spinal needle technique, anterolateral and lateral working portals are established depending on the anticipated tendon repair.

Additional portals include punctures adjacent to the lateral acromion for anchors to be placed in the greater tuberosity and an anterior puncture lateral to the coracoid for lesser tuberosity anchors. Additional medial portals (ie, a Neviaser portal) in the supraspinatus fossa may facilitate instrument and suture passage.

Diagnostic glenohumeral arthroscopy is carried out to classify the shape and mobility of the tear, as well as to address intra-articular pathology. The articular surfaces of the shoulder are visualized and the biceps tendon is inspected. An articular release of the capsule will assist in tendon mobilization. A thorough bursectomy is performed with a shaver and radio-frequency device to improve visualization. The subacromial space is inspected using the posterior and lateral portals to ensure complete visualization of the tear as well as to assess for impingement (Fig. 48-11). If subacromial decompression is necessary, it is preferable to perform this prior to the repair, to create additional working space for the instruments.

The scope is rotated between the lateral and posterior portals. Grasping instruments are used to determine the repair construct based on the ability to mobilize the torn ends. The mobility of the rotator cuff is assessed in both the medial-to-lateral and anterior-to-posterior directions. Additional tissue mobilization may be required, especially for large and massive cuff tears. Acromial and subdeltoid adhesions should be thoroughly released with radio-frequency and motorized instruments. An anterior release to the base of the coracoid and a posterior release adjacent to the spine of the scapula can be performed, taking care to avoid injury to the suprascapular nerve and vascular structures. The rotator cuff margins are then gently debrided, and the greater tuberosity bone bed is prepared by removing degenerative and devitalized tissue. A tendon quality, evaluation of the fixation, and the tension of the cuff repair determine the stability of the repair. A convergence technique for "L-shaped" tears will reduce tension on the repair.[19] "L"- and "reverse-L"-shaped tears should be reapproximated with side-to-side sutures to reestablish the correct direction of muscular tendon attachment (Fig. 48-12). "U"-shaped tears may also benefit with side-to-side sutures to avoid overtensioning during reattachment to the tuberosity.

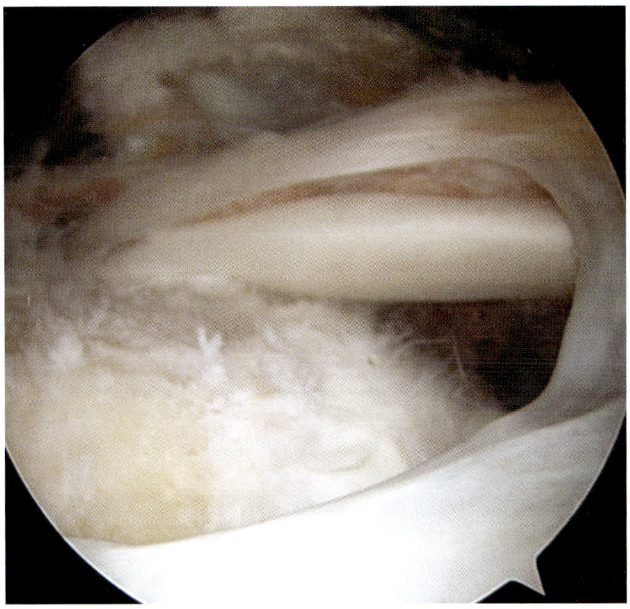

FIGURE 48-11 Posterior view of a medium size rotator cuff tear and exposed biceps tendon.

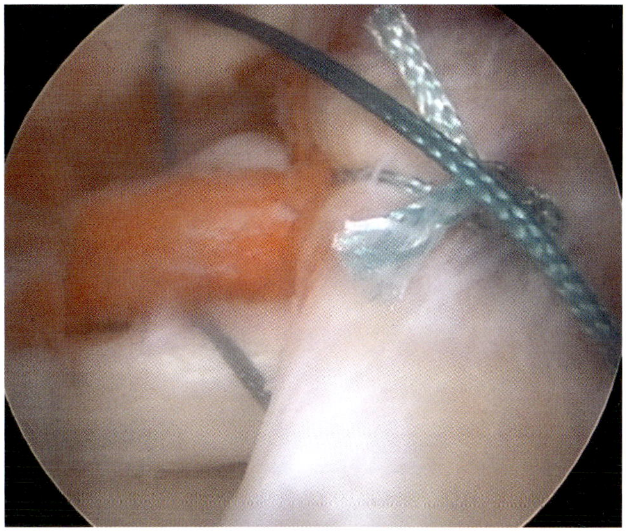

FIGURE 48-12 Margin convergence sutures of an L-shaped tear extending medial along the rotator interval.

Adequate fixation during the soft tissue repair to bone is essential to create a secure repair. The tendon–bone contact area should be maximized to promote healing. Multiple fixation points in the tissue with additional suture anchors or with double- and triple-loaded anchors will help improve initial fixation strength and repair quality, as well as reduce the risk of suture cutout through damaged tendons.[20,21] Either single- or double-row anchor constructs can be selected, depending on the mobility of the tendon. In cadaver and clinical studies, double-row constructs have been shown to be the most successful in restoring the tendon insertion footprint and have a higher load to failure, although clinical benefit has not been demonstrated.[22] There is concern of overtensioning a repair by lateralizing the tendon of a patient with a retracted tear. A combination of mattress and simple suture technique will further increase bone–tendon contact area. Anchors should be inserted such that the angle of both the suture and tendon to the anchor is $<45°$.[23] Anchors are systematically placed along the tuberosity, and sutures are passed through the free edge of the tear. The subscapularis is repaired initially due to the restricted space to work within. The posterosuperior aspect of the tear can be addressed from the posterior margin of the tear, working toward the rotator interval (Fig. 48-13). This will provide additional fixation strength to the external rotators of the shoulder and reduce the potential "dog-ear" deformity of a nonanatomical repair.

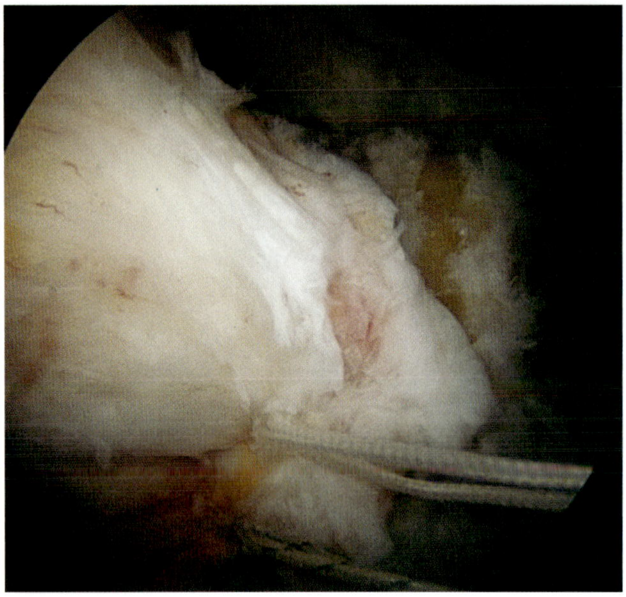

FIGURE 48-13 Infraspinatus repair right shoulder through posterior viewing portal.

Postoperatively, patients are placed in a padded sling for 6 weeks with the shoulder in slight abduction and external rotation. The patients are permitted to perform pendulum exercises, shoulder shrugs, elbow flexion and extension, and grip strengthening during the initial sling period. Formal physical therapy is delayed until 5 weeks postoperatively, at which time supine forward flexion, table slides, and gentle external rotator stretches are initiated and slowly advanced. Formal strengthening begins at 12 weeks.

Complications

Retear rates after arthroscopic repair of small- and medium-sized tears are similar to that of open repair, with most reports citing around 10% to 30% retear rate.[24] There is some evidence that retear rate for massive cuff tears may be slightly higher in the arthroscopically repaired group compared with an open repair.[25] Loosening of the suture anchors can occur, but published rates of hardware failure have been less than 1%.[26] Postoperative stiffness is a concern after any rotator cuff repair, and around 5% of patients can experience stiffness after arthroscopic repair. Most patients can be successfully managed with physiotherapy; however, arthroscopic capsular release may be needed and has been shown to be highly successful.[27] It is preferred to delay the release for 6 to 10 months to allow initial tendon healing, making the postoperative period less restrictive. Postoperative infection is uncommon and should be treated with debridement, irrigation, and removal of all accessible foreign material. Monofilament sutures can be used to maintain tendon positioning while proper antibiotic treatment is administered.

Outcomes

Multiple studies have demonstrated the efficacy of arthroscopic rotator cuff repair. Patient satisfaction responses seem to be better than actual rate of rotator cuff healing. One study demonstrated 87% good to excellent results using the UCLA score at 46 months postoperatively in 607 repairs and another reported 92% patient satisfaction at 35.8 months after surgery in 102 repairs.[28,29] In a recent study providing 5-year follow-up, the 106 patients included were found to have significant functional improvement, ASES scores went from 52.6 to 92.6, and 81.2% had a healed rotator cuff by ultrasound.[30] Persistent defects in the rotator cuff reattachment have shown to be detrimental to strength and possible progression of muscle atrophy changes, in spite of pain relief in many patients.[31]

SUPERIOR LABRUM ANTERIOR–POSTERIOR TEARS

Rationale and Basic Science

Injury to the superior aspect of the glenoid labrum (SLAP) and biceps tendon origin can result from traction injuries on the upper extremity, compressive injuries from repetitive overhead throwing activities, or torsional injuries (Fig. 48-14). Increased impaction stress on the undersurface of the cuff with the labrum during the cocking and acceleration phases of throwing creates a peel-back injury to the insertion of biceps anchor.[32] Patients with SLAP tears often have concomitant shoulder pathology, and clinical diagnosis can be difficult. Pain is the most frequent complaint; however, it is often nonspecific. The physical findings can be variable,

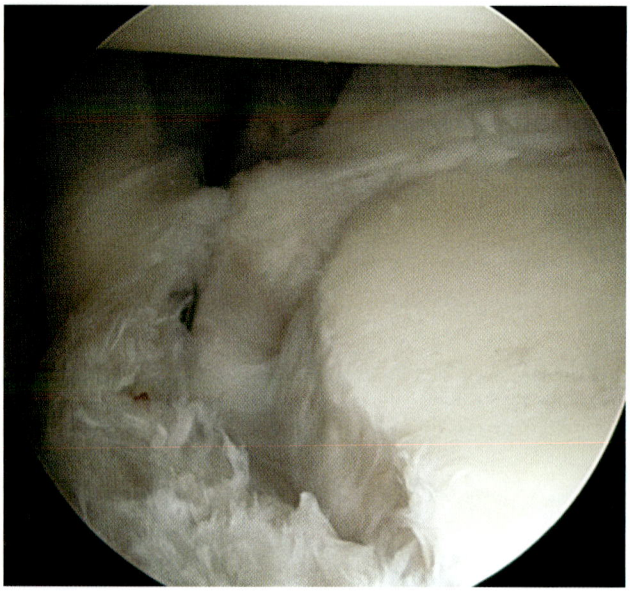

FIGURE 48-14 Superior labrum tear (SLAP II) in right shoulder with biceps anchor instability.

and advanced imaging with conventional MRI only achieves 91% specificity at best,[33] and is often lower in the community setting. Performing the MRI with articular contrast increases the diagnostic accuracy.[34] Arthroscopy remains the most sensitive and specific method of diagnosis, and should be considered after at least 3 to 6 months of conservative management in a patient with a clinically suspected SLAP tear.

Indications and Contraindications

The goals of arthroscopic treatment for SLAP tears are to relieve pain, restore the biceps anchor, and improve glenohumeral stability. Symptomatic type I SLAP lesions (superior fraying with labral and biceps anchor intact) can be treated with simple, gentle debridement. If a concomitant rotator cuff repair is being performed, especially in older patients with degenerative tears, debridement and biceps tenotomy is recommended.[35] Type II lesions (pathologic detachments of labral and biceps anchor) may destabilize the shoulder and should be considered for repair in patients with glenohumeral instability, hyperlaxity, and select overhead athletes. Type III lesions (bucket-handle type with secure biceps anchor) can be resected, or if the middle glenohumeral ligament is unstable, repaired if attached to the torn labrum. The treatment of type IV tears (bucket-handle type with extension into biceps tendon) depends on the extent of bicep involvement. Lesions involving less than 30% of bicep thickness can be debrided. Tears involving greater than 30% of biceps tendon in younger patients should be repaired if unstable, or a tenotomy or tenodesis of the biceps tendon performed, if older (Fig. 48-15). In middle-age patients with a stable shoulder, labral debridement and biceps tenodesis or tenotomy is appropriate.

Surgical Technique

A posterior articular viewing portal, an anterior interval portal, and an anterosuperior working portal that allows a 45° angle of approach to the anterosuperior corner of the glenoid are established. As the labral detachment extends posteriorly, a transrotator cuff portal, such as the portal of Wilmington, may also be needed. Diagnostic arthroscopy is carried out, and a probe is used to test the stability of the biceps anchor and superior labral attachments, keeping in mind that a normal sublabral sulcus can extend up to 5 mm medial to the articular surfaces. Other specific findings consistent with a labral tear include a displaceable biceps anchor, a positive peel-back sign, and a positive drive-through sign, which are tested for by sweeping the arthroscope from superior to inferior between the glenoid and humeral head. Next, the bone bed beneath the detached labrum on the superior neck of the glenoid is gently debrided to a bleeding bone base with a shaver.

Suture anchor fixation is the preferred method for securing the detached labrum to the glenoid. The location of the anchors often depends on the extent of the tear; however, biomechanical studies have shown that several anchor configurations with both anchors posterior, 1 anterior and 1 posterior to the biceps origin, or a multiple-stitch anchor are mechanically effective at resisting pullout.[36] The anchor is placed at the posterior edge of the biceps to avoid unintentional closure of the fovea. Once the anchor is secured to bone, a suture passer is used to thread the suture through the labrum from articular to superior margins. Mattress sutures are helpful to minimize risk of knot impingement and overconstraint of the biceps anchor (Fig. 48-16). After securing the labrum with arthroscopic knots, revisit the peel-back and drive-through test to confirm an adequate repair.

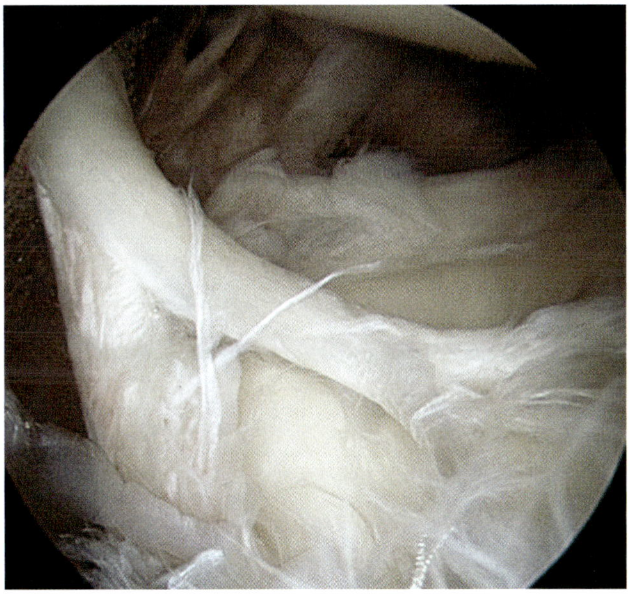

FIGURE 48-15 SLAP IV tear (right shoulder) with tear extending into the biceps tendon.

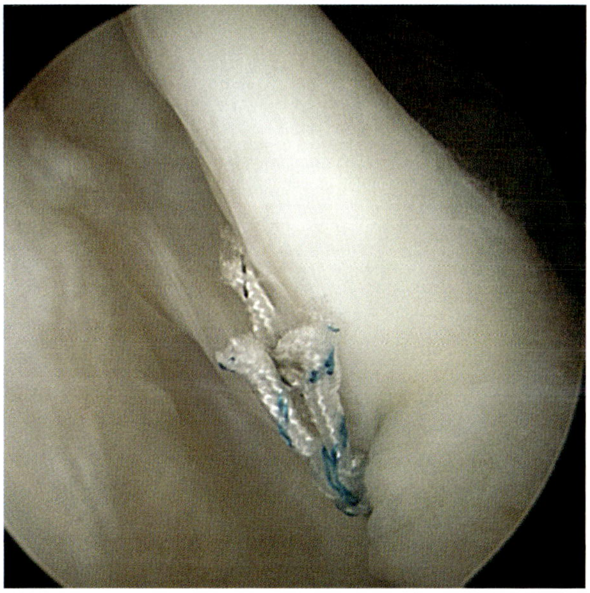

FIGURE 48-16 Mattress sutures placed through superior labral tear securing the biceps anchor to the abraded glenoid neck.

Postoperatively, the patient is placed into a padded sling with the arm at their side. Passive external rotation of the shoulder with the arm held at the side and elbow range of motion are allowed immediately. The sling is discontinued after 3 to 4 weeks, and passive elevation is initiated. From week 3 to week 6, progressive passive flexion and external rotation as tolerated are permitted. At 6 weeks, stretching and flexibility exercises are continued, and strengthening exercises for rotator cuff and scapular stabilizers are introduced. Biceps strengthening can begin at 8 weeks postoperatively. Athletes may begin an interval throwing program on level surfaces at 4 months. At 6 months, pitchers may begin throwing full speed on level ground, and at 7 months they progress to throwing off of a mound. Posteroinferior capsular stretching should be emphasized throughout the rehab process and should continue indefinitely to avoid re-injury. Avoidance of stiffness is emphasized during the rehabilitation period following repair.

Complications

Typical postoperative complications can be encountered such as infection and hematoma. Complications specific to SLAP repair include injury to glenoid chondral surface during anchor placement, anchor pullout and subsequent loose body, synovitis related to biodegradable anchors, shoulder stiffness, and failure of repair (Fig. 48-17).

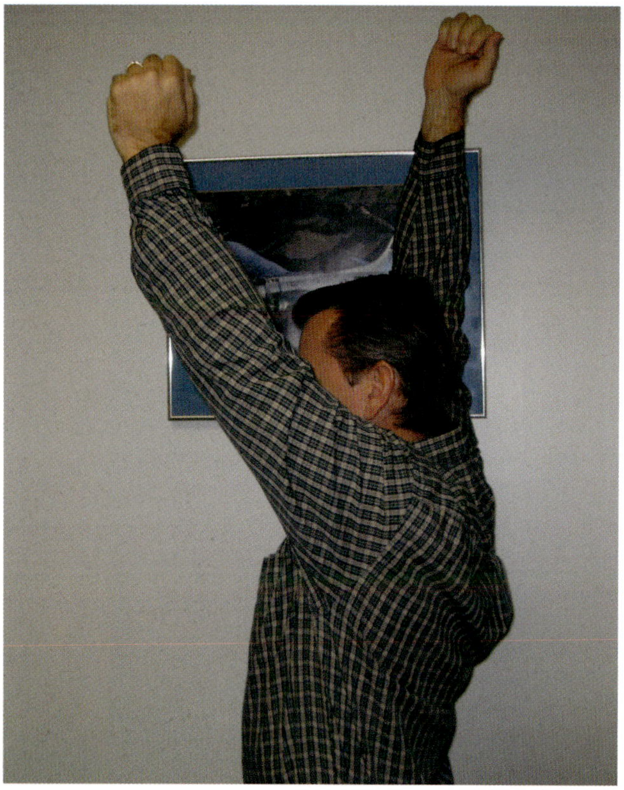

FIGURE 48-17 Postoperative stiffness in left shoulder following a SLAP repair.

Return to throwing has been a reported problem following SLAP repair due to a reduction of external rotation in the abducted shoulder.[37] The results from SLAP repair have not been as successful as many other shoulder procedures. This may be due to patient selection, overconstraint of the biceps anchor, types of demanding activities being considered after surgery, and poor vascularity in the area of potential healing. Patients need to be counseled on the potential for loss of maximum abduction and external rotation following a SLAP repair.

Outcomes

In a study looking at long-term results of simple debridement for SLAP lesions, the initial goal of pain relief was achieved in three quarters of patients during the first year after surgery. However, at 2-year follow-up, only 7% of patients remained asymptomatic. Further studies postulated that labral tears have associated occult instability and that debridement may be beneficial for short-term relief. In general, after SLAP repair in carefully selected patients, one can expect good-to-excellent pain relief and return to near-normal function. For athletes wishing to return to sports at their pre-injury level, the results are less predictable, with outcome studies varying in success rates from 22% to 84%.[37–39]

REFERENCES

1. Colvin AC, Egorova N, Harrison AK, Moskowitz A, Flatow EL. National trends in rotator cuff repair. *J Bone Joint Surg Am.* 2012;94(3): 227–233.
2. Mansat P, Cofield RH, Kersten TE, Rowland CM. Complications of rotator cuff repair. *Orthop Clin North Am.* 1997;28(2):205–213.
3. Yamaguchi K. *Complications of Rotator Cuff Repair. Techniques in Orthopaedics.* Vol. 12, No. 1. Philadelphia: Lippincott-Raven Publishers; 1997.
4. Wu CL, Rouse LM, Chen JM, Miller RJ. Comparison of postoperative pain in patients receiving interscalene block or general anesthesia for shoulder surgery. *Orthopedics.* 2002;25(1):45–48.
5. Singelyn FJ, Lhotel L, Fabre B. Pain relief after arthroscopic shoulder surgery: a comparison of intraarticular analgesia, suprascapular nerve block, and interscalene brachial plexus block. *Anesth Analg.* 2004;99(2):589–592.
6. Michener LA, McClure PW, Karduna AR. Anatomical and biomechanical mechanisms of subacromial impingement syndrome. *Clin Biomech (Bristol, Avon).* 2003;18(5):369–379.
7. Bigliani LU, Levine WN. Subacromial impingement syndrome. *J Bone Joint Surg Am.* 1997;79(12):1854–1868.
8. Neer CS II. Impingement lesions. *Clin Orthop Relat Res.* 1983;173: 70–77.
9. Vaz S, Soyer J, Pries P, Clarac JP. Subacromial impingement: influence of coracoacromial arch geometry on shoulder function. *Joint Bone Spine.* 2000;67(4):305–309.
10. Weber SC, Abrams JS, Nottage WM. Complications associated with arthroscopic shoulder surgery. *Arthroscopy.* 2002;18(2 suppl 1): 88–95.
11. Davis AD, Kakar S, Moros C, Kaye EK, Schepsis AA, Voloshin I. Arthroscopic versus open acromioplasty: a meta-analysis. *Am J Sports Med.* 2010;38(3):613–618.
12. Odenbring S, Wagner P, Atroshi I. Long-term outcomes of arthroscopic acromioplasty for chronic shoulder impingement syndrome: a prospective cohort study with a minimum of 12 years' follow-up. *Arthroscopy.* 2008;24(10):1092–1098.

13. Bengtsson M, Lunsjö K, Hermodsson Y, Nordqvist A, Abu-Zidan FM. High patient satisfaction after arthroscopic subacromial decompression for shoulder impingement: a prospective study of 50 patients. *Acta Orthop.* 2006;77(1):138–142.
14. Maman E, Harris C, White L, Tomlinson G, Shashank M, Boynton E. Treatment of symptomatic rotator cuff tears monitored by magnetic resonance imaging. *J Bone Joint Surg Am.* 2009;91:1898–1906.
15. Lahteenmaki H, Virolainen P, Hiltunen A, Heikkila J, Nelimarrka O. Results of early operative treatment of rotator cuff tears with acute symptoms. *J Shoulder Elbow Surg.* 2006;15(2):148–153.
16. Gerber C, Meyer D, Schneeberger A, Hoppeler H, von Rechenberg B. Effect of tendon release and delayed repair on the muscles of the rotator cuff: an experimental study in sheep. *J Bone Joint Surg Am.* 2004;86(9):1973–1982.
17. Fukuda H. The management of partial-thickness tears of the rotator cuff. *J Bone Joint Surg Br.* 2003;85(1):3–11.
18. Tashjian RZ. AAOS clinical practice guideline: optimizing the management of rotator cuff problems. *J Am Acad Orthop Surg.* 2011; 19(6):380–383.
19. Burkhart S, Athanasiou K, Wirth M. Margin convergence: a method of reducing strain in massive rotator cuff tears. *Arthroscopy.* 1996;12:335–338.
20. Burkhart S, Wirth M, Simonich M, Salem D, Lanctot D, Athanasiou K. Knot security in simple sliding knots and its relationship to rotator cuff repair: how secure must the knot be? *Arthroscopy.* 2000;16: 202–207.
21. Bardana D, Burks R, West J, Greis P. The effect of suture anchor design and orientation on suture abrasion: an in vitro study. *Arthroscopy.* 2003;19:274–281.
22. Lo I, Burkhart S. Double-row arthroscopic rotator cuff repair: re-establishing the footprint of the rotator cuff. *Arthroscopy.* 2003;19: 1035–1042.
23. Burkhart S. The deadman theory of suture anchors: observations along a South Texas fence line. *Arthroscopy.* 1995;11:119–123.
24. Holtby R, Misra S. Is arthroscopic rotator cuff repair superior? In: Wright JG, ed. *Evidence-based Orthopedics: The Best Answers to Clinical Questions.* Philadelphia: Elsevier; 2009:678–682.
25. Bishop J, Klepps S, Lo I, et al. Cuff integrity after arthroscopic versus open rotator cuff repair: a prospective study. *J Shoulder Elbow Surg.* 2006;15:290–299.
26. Weber S, Sager R. *All Arthroscopic Versus Mini-open in the Management of Tears of the Rotator Cuff. 68th Meeting Proceedings AAOS.* 2001;2:617.
27. Warner J, Allen A, Marks P, Wong P. Arthroscopic release of postoperative capsular contracture of the shoulder. *J Bone Joint Surg Am.* 1997;79(A)(8):1151–1158.
28. Haviv B, Dolev E, Haber M, Mayo L, Biggs D. Arthroscopic rotator cuff repair: clinical outcome of 607 patients. *Knee Surg Sports Traumatol Arthrosc.* 2010;18:1707–1711.
29. Levy O, Venkateswaran B, Even T, Ravenscroft M, Copeland S. Midterm clinical and sonographic outcome of arthroscopic repair of the rotator cuff. *J Bone Joint Surg Br.* 2008;90:1341–1347.
30. Gulotta LV, Nho SJ, Dodson CC, Adler RS, Altchek DW, MacGillivray JD. Prospective evaluation of arthroscopic rotator cuff repairs at 5 years: part I—functional outcomes and radiographic healing rates. *J Shoulder Elbow Surg.* 2011;20(6):934–940.
31. Bernhard J, Peirrmann CW, Gerber C. Clinical outcome after structural failure of rotator cuff repair. *J Bone Joint Surg Am.* 2000;82(A)(3): 304–314.
32. Burkhart S, Morgan C. The peel-back mechanism: its role in producing and extending posterior type II SLAP lesions and its effect on SLAP repair rehabilitation. *Arthroscopy.* 1999;14:637–640.
33. Jee W, McCauley T, Katz L, Matheny J, Ruwe P, Daigneault J. Superior labral anterior posterior (SLAP) lesions of the glenoid labrum: reliability and accuracy of MR arthrography for diagnosis. *Radiology.* 2001;174:1107–1114.
34. Waldt S, Burkart A, Lange P, Rummeny E, Woertler K. Diagnostic performance of MR arthrography in the assessment of superior labral anteroposterior lesions of the shoulder. *AJR Am J Roentgenol.* 2004;182:1271–1278.
35. Franceschi F, Longo U, Ruzzini L, Rizzello G, Maffulli N, Denaro V. No advantages in repairing a type II SLAP lesion when associated with rotator cuff repair in patients over 50: a randomized controlled trial. *Am J Sports Med.* 2008;36;247–253.
36. Morgan R, Kuremsky M, Peindl R, Fleischli J. A biomechanical comparison of two suture anchor configurations for the repair of type II SLAP lesions subjected to a peel-back mechanism of failure. *Arthroscopy.* 2008;24:383–388.
37. Kim S, Ha K, Kim S, Choi H. Results of arthroscopic treatment of superior labral lesions. *J Bone Joint Surg Am.* 2002;84:981–985.
38. Altchek D, Warren R. Arthroscopic labral debridement: a three-year follow-up study. *Am J Sports Med.* 1992;20:702–706.
39. Morgan C, Burkhart S, Palmeri M, Gillespie M. Type II SLAP lesions: three subtypes and their relationships to superior instability and rotator cuff tears. *Arthroscopy.* 1998;12:553–565.

49

Shoulder Arthroplasty: Humeral Head Replacement, Total Shoulder and Reverse Total Shoulder Replacement

Juan P. Simone, MD
John W. Sperling, MD

RATIONALE AND BASIC SCIENCE PERTINENT TO THE PROCEDURE

The rationale behind shoulder arthroplasty is to restore function and reduce pain in the glenohumeral joint.[1] Humeral head replacement and total shoulder arthroplasty comply with this objective by reproducing shoulder anatomy and replacing humeral or both humeral and glenoid bearing surfaces.

Reverse shoulder arthroplasty has been designed to address cuff-deficient shoulders by transferring the center of rotation of the humerus medially and downwards thereby tensioning the deltoid muscle.[2]

INDICATIONS

The ideal indications for humeral head replacement, total shoulder and reverse arthroplasty continue to evolve as surgical experience and scientific evidence show that there are often overlapping indications. The indications are individualized based on the underlying pathology, age (biological factors), and patient expectations.

One indication for shoulder replacement is that of a nonreconstructible proximal humeral fracture (4-fragment displaced fracture or humeral head-split fracture) where there is a high likelihood of failure following open reduction and internal fixation of the humeral head secondary to avascular necrosis.

The best possible outcome would be that of a hemiarthroplasty replacement as long as the tuberosities heal with correct version and humeral height restored.[3] Timing for a hemiarthroplasty for a proximal humerus fracture must be taken into consideration to avoid tuberosity reabsorption and soft tissue retraction and scarring.

Choosing between a hemiarthroplasty and a total arthroplasty will depend on glenoid wear and patient expectations in terms of restrictions as will be discussed later.

Scientific evidence is showing a trend toward reverse arthroplasty in elderly patients where the results are more predictable as tuberosity healing does not play a dramatic role in outcomes[4,5] (Fig. 49-1).

A second indication is for shoulder osteoarthritis.

While many patients with early shoulder osteoarthritis can be successfully treated with nonoperative modalities, patients with more advanced disease may require surgical intervention. Patients must accept postoperative restrictions and comply with the rehabilitation. If a patient is young or has high activity demand and does not have an arthritic glenoid, a hemiarthroplasty is a good option. Patients are counseled to expect a 70% to 80% chance of pain relief and may then resume unrestricted activity (Fig. 49-2).

The gold standard for severe osteoarthritis is total shoulder arthroplasty.[6] In our practice, we prefer to perform a total shoulder arthroplasty in patients with osteoarthritis and glenoid wear who have an intact or repairable rotator cuff tear. We counsel patients that the chance of good to excellent pain relief with total shoulder arthroplasty is greater than 90% (Fig. 49-3).

The most common reason for revision shoulder surgery in our practice is painful glenoid arthritis in a patient with a hemiarthroplasty. Although shoulder replacement for painful osteoarthritis is not an emergency procedure, patients must be aware of the fact that delayed surgery may affect ongoing glenoid wearing with increasing surgical difficulty.

A third indication is for rotator cuff arthropathy where the gold standard is now the reverse total shoulder arthroplasty. A hemiarthroplasty would be indicated in cases where glenoid bone stock or bone quality is insufficient or considered nonreconstructible to obtain adequate glenoid baseplate fixation[7] (Fig. 49-4). Until longer follow-up studies on reverse arthroplasty are published, this procedure is best reserved for patients 70 years of age or older, although a reverse total shoulder arthroplasty might be contemplated for patients in a younger age group in certain cases.

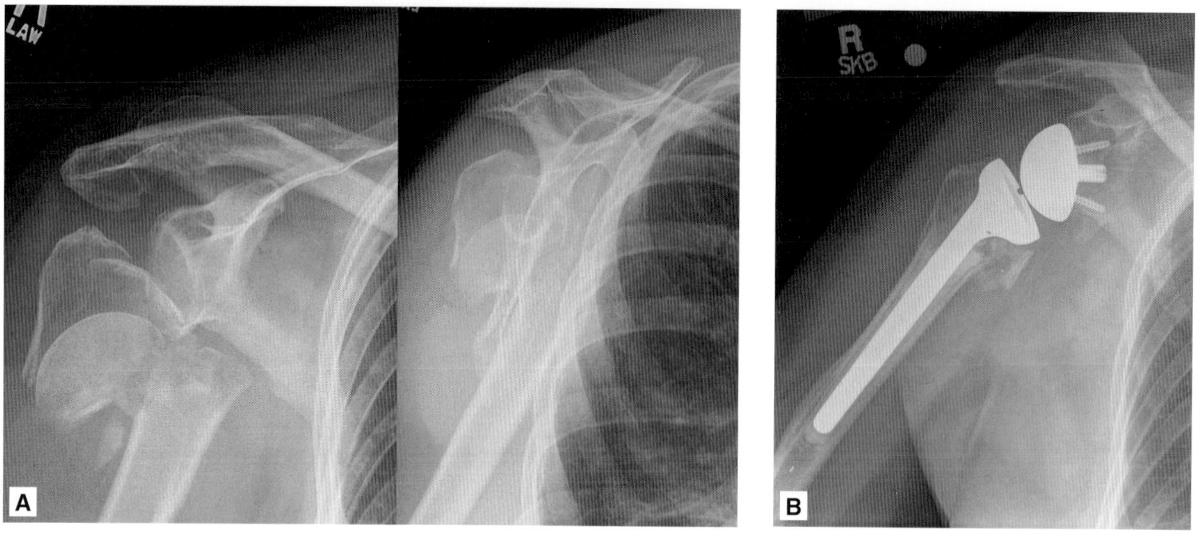

FIGURE 49-1 Four-part, head-split displaced fracture in a 71-year-old patient (**A**). Three months postoperative reverse shoulder arthroplasty with greater tuberosity healing (**B**).

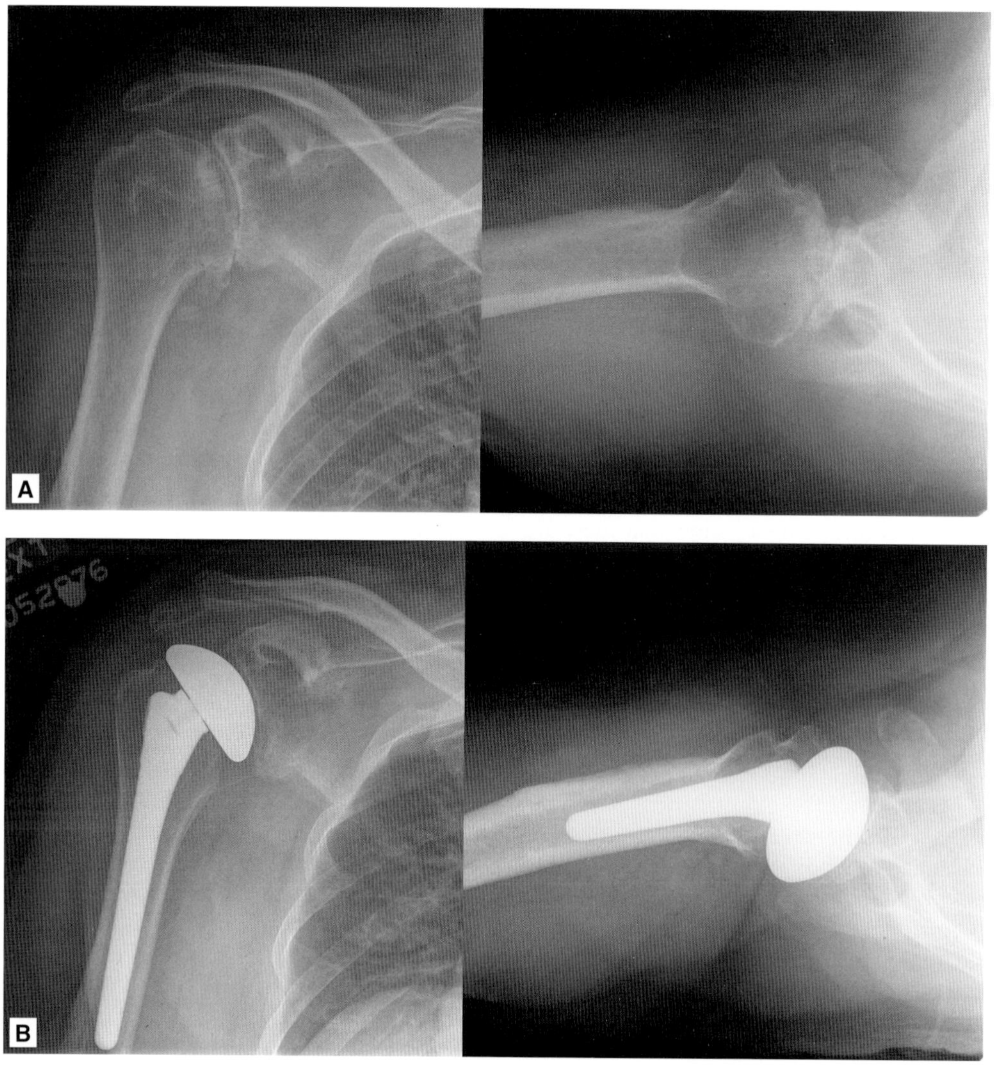

FIGURE 49-2 Primary osteoarthritis in an active 61-year-old patient (**A**). Right shoulder hemiarthroplasty for unrestricted activity (**B**).

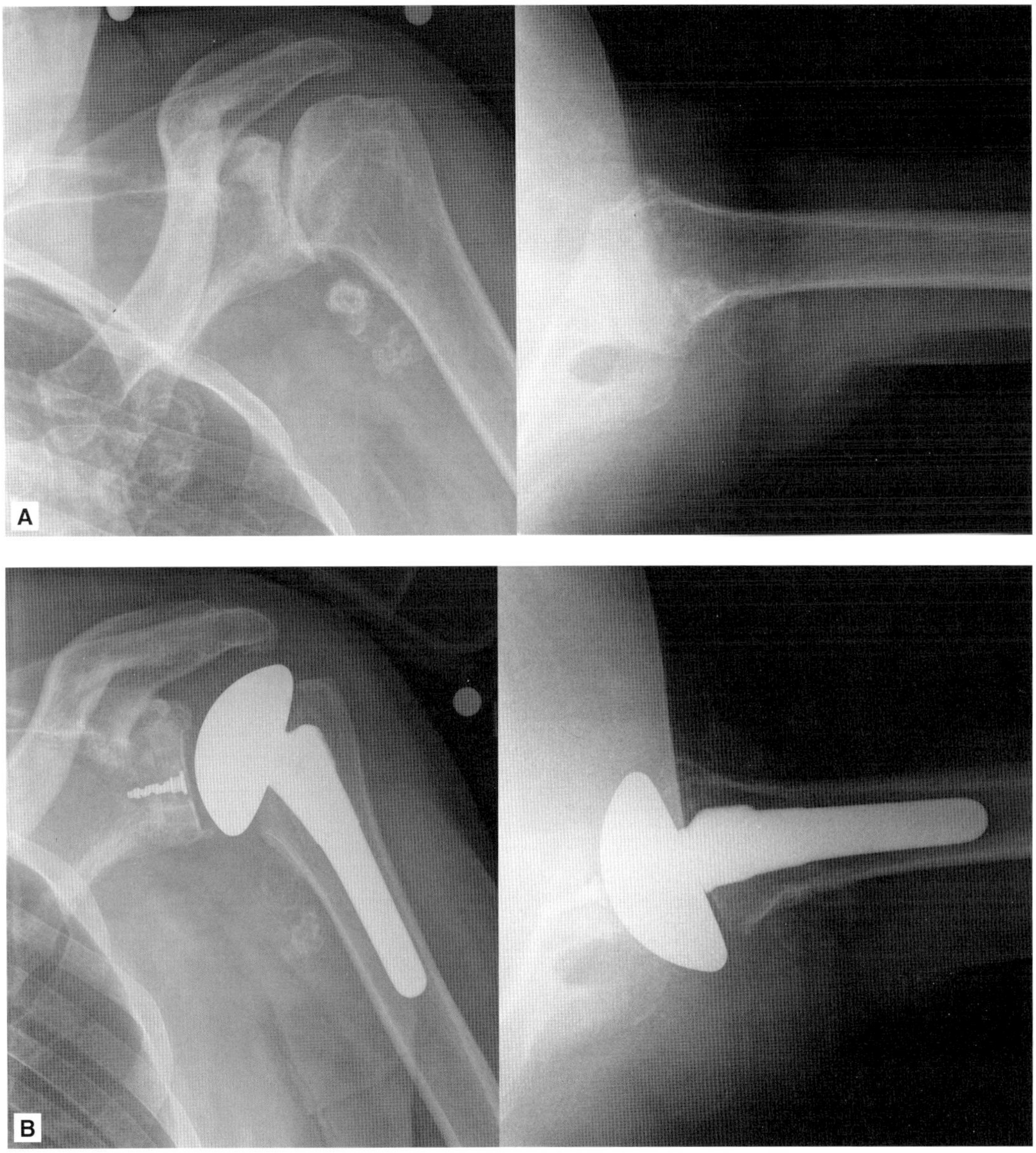

FIGURE 49-3 Primary osteoarthritis in a 67-year-old patient with a functioning rotator cuff (**A**). Total shoulder arthroplasty (**B**).

A final indication would be for revision shoulder surgeries. Choosing between the 3 different techniques will depend mainly on the status of the rotator cuff, tuberosities, and the quality of the glenoid bone stock.

CONTRAINDICATIONS

Absolute:

- Active or suspected infection
- Neurologic or mental impairment; noncompliant patients
- Severe clinical comorbidities that would not allow a surgical procedure
- Skeletal immaturity
- Deltoid dysfunction

Relative:

- Young age
- Obesity

SURGICAL TECHNIQUE

Exposure

A vertical skin incision is made on the anterior aspect of the shoulder, slightly lateral to the deltopectoral. Any previous incisions are used and revised as necessary or incorporated into a longer incision that will allow to approach the deltopectoral interval. The deltopectoral interval is most easily developed starting just distal to the clavicle.

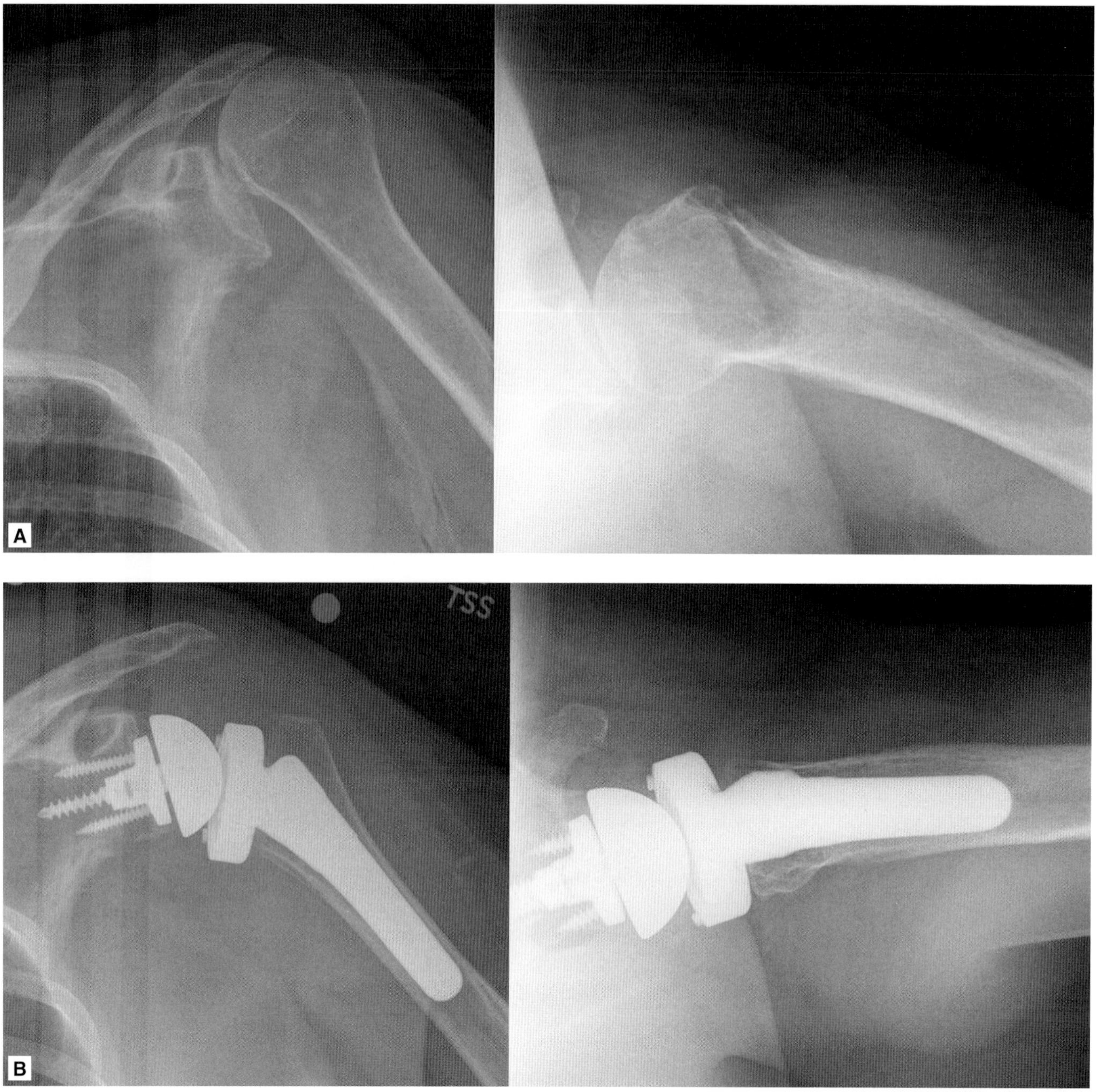

FIGURE 49-4 Rotator cuff arthropathy in a 73-year-old patient (**A**). Reverse shoulder arthroplasty (**B**).

The deltoid is retracted laterally leaving the cephalic vein medially. The anterior border of the deltoid is mobilized from the clavicle to its insertion on the humerus. The anterior portion of the deltoid insertion together with the more distal periosteum of the humerus may be elevated slightly (Fig. 49-5).

The next step is to identify the plane between the conjoined tendon and the subscapularis muscle. Dissection in this area must be done very carefully due to the close proximity of the axillary and the musculocutaneous nerve. Any scar tissue is removed from the base of the coracoid and the subacromial space. Passive shoulder range of motion is checked.

If external rotation is less than 30°, the subscapularis is incised off of bone rather than through its tendinous substance. For every 1 cm that the subscapularis is advanced medially, 20° to 30° of external rotation are gained. The rotator interval and subscapularis tendon are then incised. The inferior shoulder capsule is released from the humeral neck using cautery, proceeding from anterior to posterior with progressive external rotation of the humerus staying directly on the bone to protect the axillary nerve (Fig. 49-6).

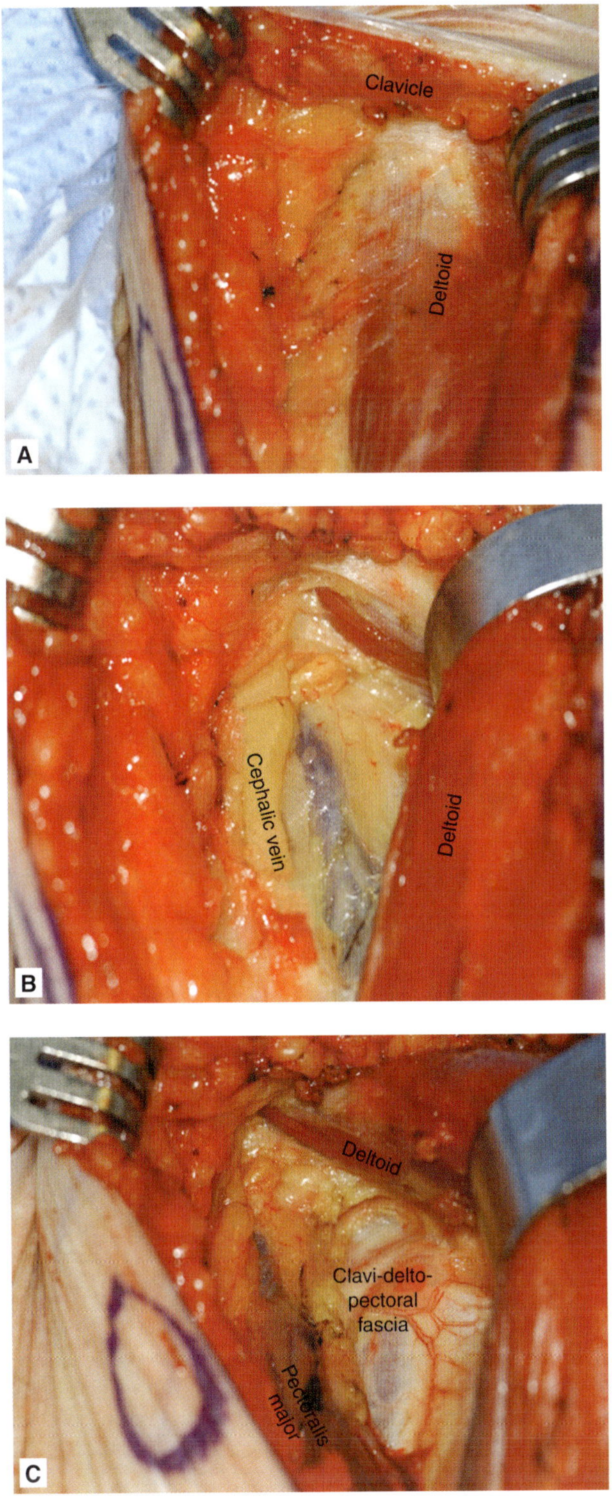

FIGURE 49-5 Deltopectoral approach.

Humeral Component

The humerus is levered forward by placing an elevator along the posterior-inferior aspect of the humeral head. The arm is then positioned in slight extension and adduction, and then progressively externally rotated. Care to limit the amount of torque placed on the humeral shaft to avoid a humeral shaft fracture must be taken. The coracoacromial arch is inspected and preserved if possible. The rotator cuff is carefully assessed, on both its outer and inner aspects, and any osteophytes are removed.

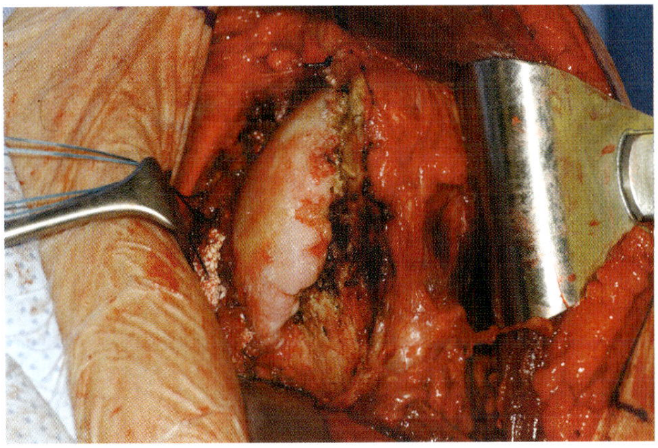

FIGURE 49-6 Subscapularis tenotomy and inferior capsular release.

An entry hole is made in the superior aspect of the humeral head. The humeral canal is then prepared with progressively larger circular reamers in 1- to 2-mm increments until resistance is encountered. A humeral resection guide is then inserted and Darrach retractors are used to protect the surrounding tissues while resecting the humeral head. We typically resect the humeral head in 30° of retroversion for both the anatomic and reverse shoulder arthroplasty. In patients with significant posterior subluxation and glenoid wear, retroversion may be slightly decreased. The cutting block is placed 1 mm above the insertion of the rotator cuff, although this may be lower for a reverse arthroplasty.

A trial component is now inserted. The selection of the head is dependent on the size of the patient, capsular laxity, and the amount of bone resection. With the arm in the neutral position (0° of external rotation and aducction), the humeral head should face directly across from the glenoid. While testing passive range of motion there should be 90° of internal rotation, elevation of 150°, and proper tension on the rotator cuff.

For tuberosity reattachment we prefer horizontal fixation with sutures through tuberosity tendons and around the neck of the implant. Vertical fixation is then achieved with the tuberosities pulled down to the metaphysis with predrilled holes and sutures (Fig. 49-7).

Glenoid Component

The key for glenoid exposure is deltoid mobilization, capsular release, humeral head resection, and osteophyte removal (Fig. 49-8).

While the trial humeral stem is kept in place, the humerus is retracted posteriorly with a Fukuda or a glenoid retractor

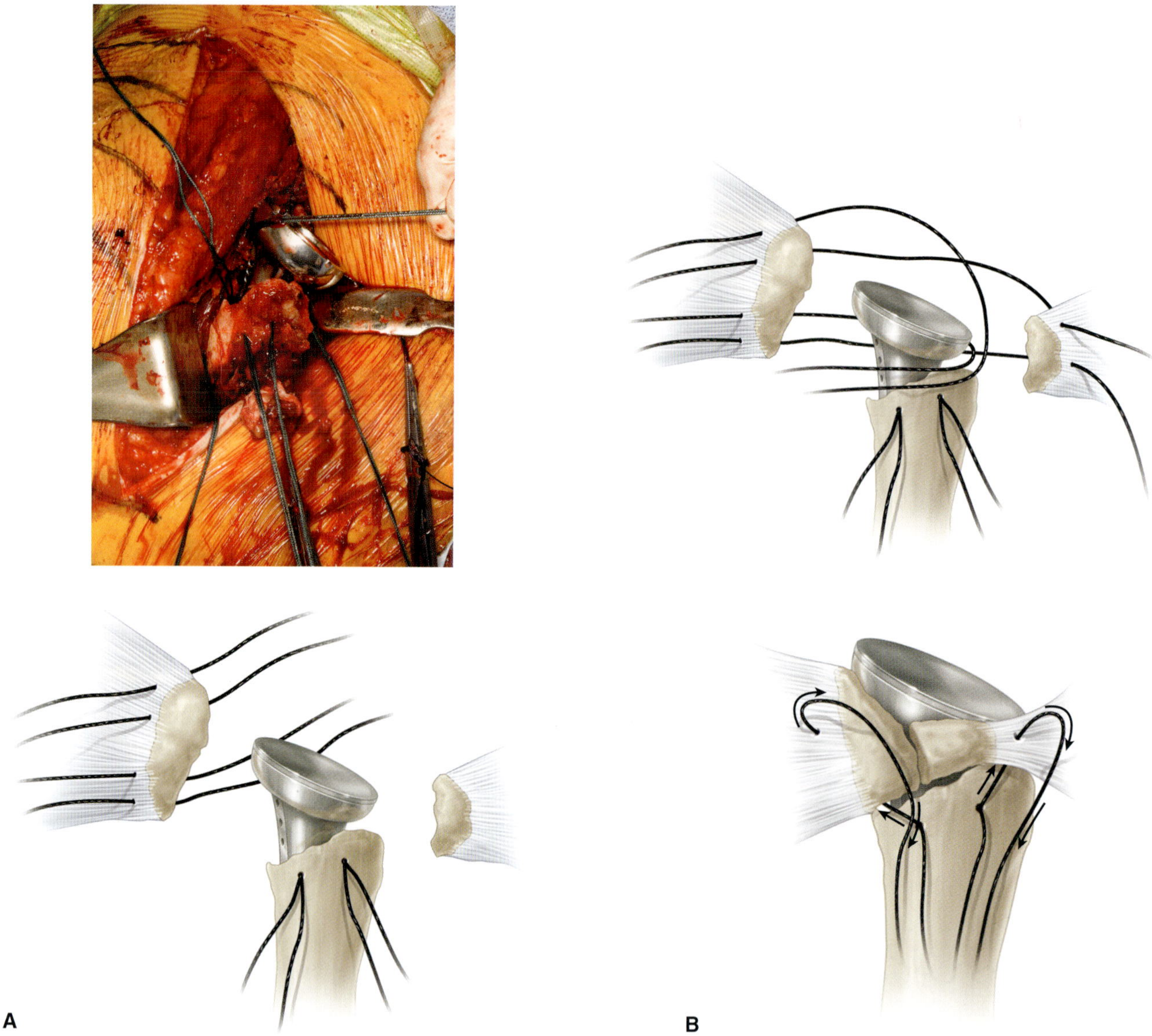

FIGURE 49-7 Tuberosity reattachment in proximal humeral fracture treated with a reverse prosthesis. Same case as in Figure 49-1. Sutures through greater tuberosity and metaphyses (**A**). Sutures from greater tuberosity go through the lesser tuberosity and around the prosthesis neck for horizontal fixation. Metaphyseal sutures are then fixed to the tuberosities for vertical fixation (**B**).

(Fig. 49-9). The arm is placed in 70° to 90° of abduction and slight flexion. The glenoid surface is then assessed for any wear or deformity. The glenoid is resurfaced unless a hemiarthroplasty is being done. A preoperative CT scan is used to determine the glenoid version and the true anatomic center of the glenoid. The labrum is removed superiorly, anteriorly, posteriorly, and inferiorly. A retractor is placed on the anterior aspect of the glenoid after any scar tissue is removed. The anterior capsule is then excised off of the glenoid rim extending from superiorly down to approximately the 4-o'clock position and extended out laterally. The inferior glenoid capsule is released while protecting the axillary nerve with a Darrach retractor.

Identifying the inferior glenoid rim is key to avoid placing the glenoid component too proximally.

A bone awl or bur is used to make a center hole. The glenoid is then prepared to accept either a pegged/keeled all-polyethylene glenoid component or the reverse shoulder prosthesis baseplate.

The glenoid is reamed down to bleeding subchondral bone below the equator of the glenoid surface while maintaining the glenoid version (Fig. 49-10).

The glenoid component can be a weak link. Thus, considerable attention to detail is taken while cementing in the glenoid component.

In the case of an anatomic arthroplasty, the columns or keel slot are undercut to facilitate locking of the cement. Pulsatile lavage is used to remove any bone debris, and then the glenoid component and the glenoid are dried. The bone

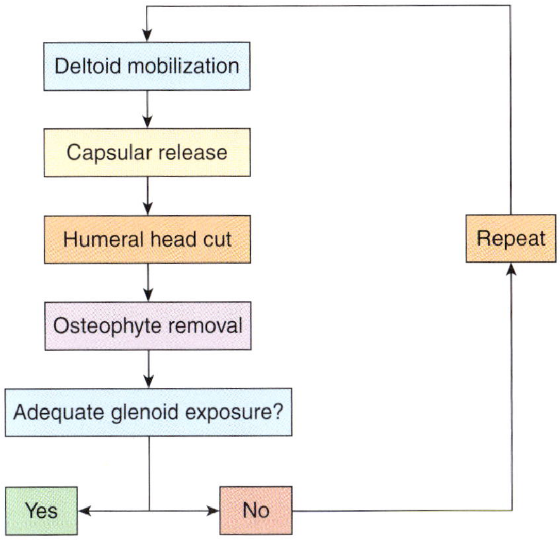

FIGURE 49-8 Glenoid exposure algorithm.

cement is compressed using vacuum mixing to enhance its strength. The cement is placed in the columns or keel slot and pressurized in 3 of 4 cycles. The glenoid is then impacted into the cement bed and held with a holding instrument while extra cement is removed. It is important during this whole process to avoid pressure on the glenoid component by the humeral head retractor.

For a reverse arthroplasty the glenosphere tilt and inferior or lateral eccentricity must be taken into consideration to avoid scapular notching (Fig. 49-11).

During the trial reductions for a hemiarthroplasty or total shoulder arthroplasty, the stability of the humerus against the glenoid is determined and the humeral head size is adjusted as necessary. A variety of offset and eccentric heads are available to aid in proper soft tissue balancing to provide stability, yet preserve motion. In osteoarthritis, the posterior

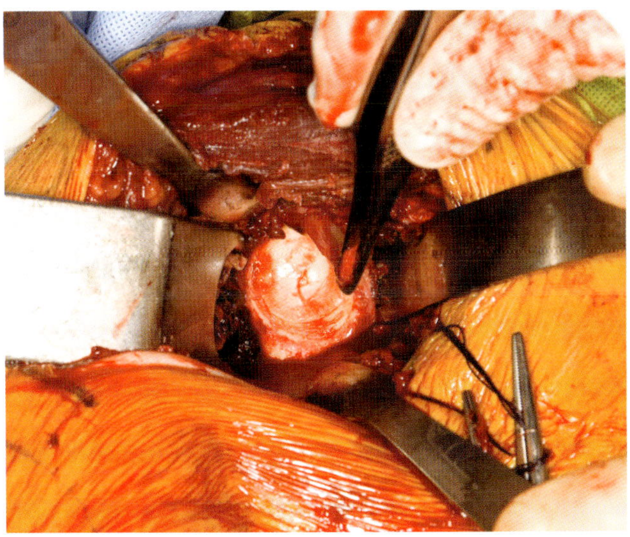

FIGURE 49-9 Glenoid exposure and labral attachments.

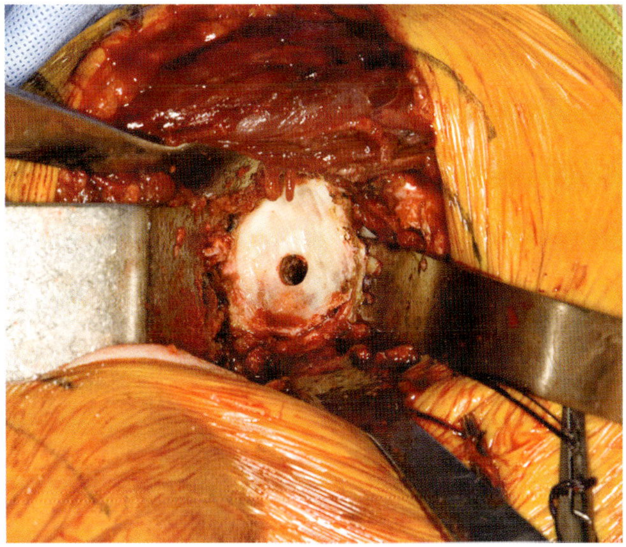

FIGURE 49-10 Center of the glenoid and bleeding subchondral bone in the inferior aspect of the glenoid.

capsule is usually lax, the anterior capsule is tight, and it is often necessary to release the inferior capsule. It might be necessary to increase the size of the humeral component to effectively tighten the posterior capsule, and lengthen the anterior shoulder capsule–subscapularis complex.

The definitive humeral component is impacted in place. If the arthrotomy was through the subscapularis tendon, it is then repaired; if the subscapularis was elevated off bone, it is reattached by placing sutures through drill holes in the humeral neck, before seating the humeral implant. It is very important to obtain a secure repair of the subscapularis tendon since this is a common site of failure. After closure of the arthrotomy, the shoulder is taken through a range of motion. The amount of humeral head translation is assessed anteriorly, posteriorly, and inferiorly, and the amount of motion obtained is recorded to provide some guidelines for postoperative mobilization.

During the trial reduction following a reverse shoulder arthroplasty, our preference is to choose a component that will restore enough soft tissue tension to provide immediate stability. If the bearing surface opens proximally during arm adduction, then further release of the inferior capsule is necessary.

Axial traction is applied to the arm to see if there is significant gapping between the glenosphere and the metaglene. We prefer less than a fingerbreadth gapping for this matter.

Arm rotation is examined to assess the version of the components[10] and finally elevation is tested for acromial impingement against the greater tuberosity. The greater tuberosity may be trimmed if necessary.

Component Choice

Our preference is to use a modular humeral component with a texturing of the stem that allows for soft tissue ingrowth proximally with a polished stem distally to

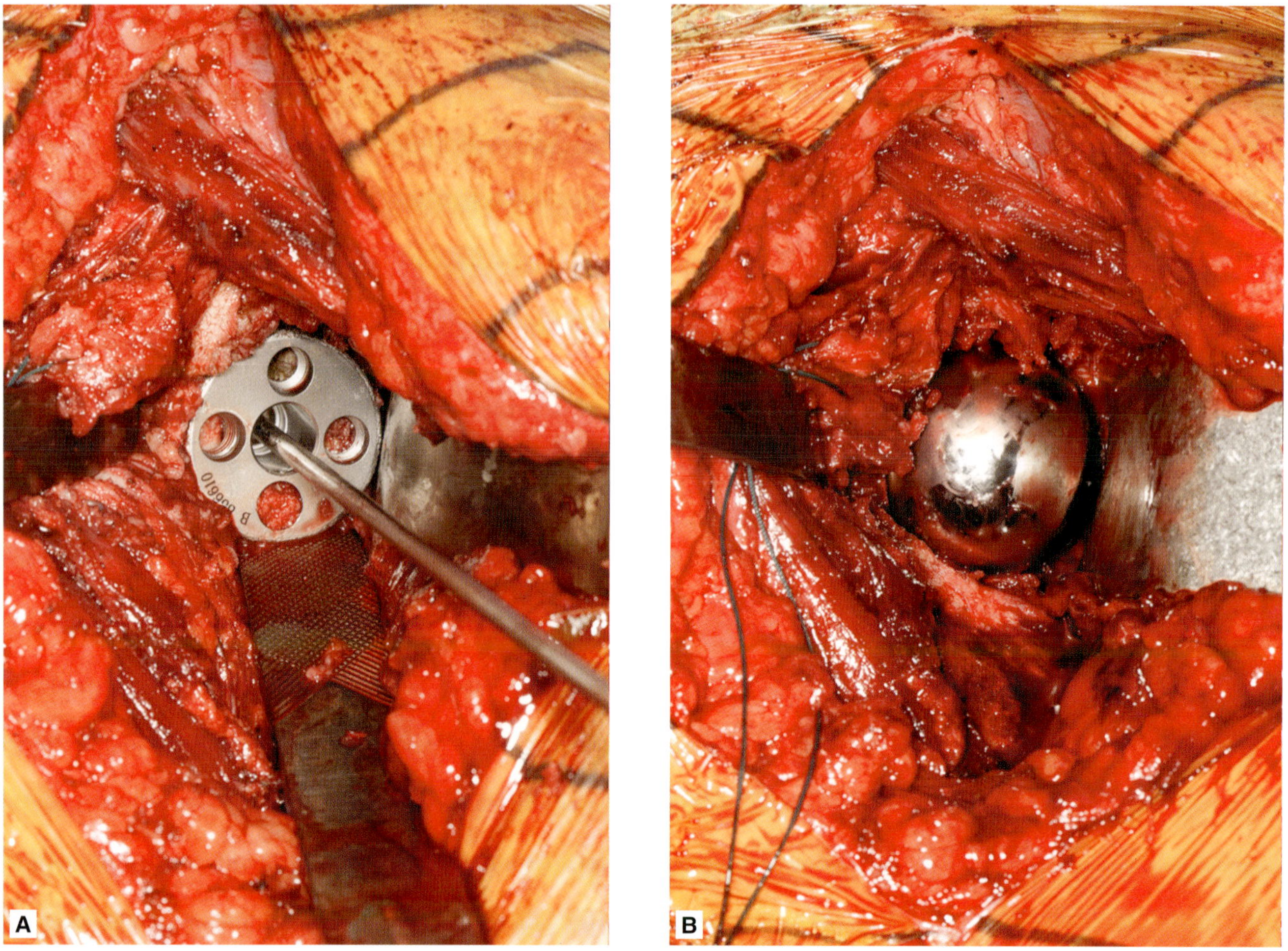

FIGURE 49-11 Baseplate position and orientation checked prior to placing central and peripheral screws (**A**). Glenosphere dialed inferiorly to prevent scapular notching (**B**).

facilitate component removal at a later time if necessary. We avoid components with texturing that extends distally along the stem since it makes component removal extremely difficult. We also prefer an all-polyethylene pegged glenoid component. For a reverse shoulder arthroplasty, we prefer to use ingrowth baseplates with a central screw and peripheral locking screws.

COMPLICATIONS

Gonzalez et al[8] reviewed the complications of 4010 unconstrained shoulder prostheses (hemiarthroplasty and total shoulder replacement) excluding fractures. The 5 most common complications in descending order were erosion of an unresurfaced glenoid (20.6%), glenoid loosening (14.3%), humeral loosening (6%), instability (4.6%), and secondary rotator cuff tear (2.7%).

In a systematic review of reverse total shoulder arthroplasties, Zumstein et al[9] reported a 44% incidence of technical problems and a 20.7% complication rate. The most common problems and complications out of 782 cases were scapular notching (35.4%), instability (4.7%), infection (3.8%), aseptic glenoid loosening (3.5%), and lucent lines around the glenoid (2.9%).

Solberg et al[10] reported a 15% incidence of greater tuberosity nonunion after hemiarthroplasty for proximal humerus fractures.

OUTCOMES

We have previously reported our experience with 57 patients who underwent a shoulder hemiarthroplasty following a proximal humerus fracture with a minimum follow-up of 5 years.[11] Eighty-four percent of the patients had no pain, mild pain, or pain only after unusual activity. Average active elevation was 100°, average external rotation 30°, and average internal rotation was to L5. According to a modified Neer result rating system, 28 patients were graded as excellent, 16 good, 2 satisfactory, and 11 unsatisfactory. Nine patients (16%) had moderate or severe pain and 2 required implant revision or removal. Two patients underwent additional surgery. Nonunion of the tuberosity occurred in 1 shoulder, malunions in 3, and resorption in 9.

Tuberosity healing was closely related to outcomes. The study data suggested that patients undergoing arthroplasty as treatment of an acute fracture of the proximal humerus may achieve satisfactory long-term pain relief; however, the result for overall shoulder motion was less predictable.

We examined 49 patients with a total of 51 humeral heads for the treatment of glenohumeral osteoarthritis, with a minimum 5-year follow-up or until the time of revision.[12] Seventeen percent of the humeral head replacements were revised. Of those revised, 90% were performed because of painful glenoid arthrosis at a mean of 7.6 years. Mean active abduction was 134°, the mean external rotation was 49°, and the median postoperative internal rotation was to L2. Overall, there was significant long-term pain relief (*P* <.0001) as well as improvement in active abduction (*P* <.0001), internal rotation (*P* <.024), and external rotation (*P* <.0001) following humeral head replacement. However, moderate pain was reported in 9 shoulders and severe pain in 7. Ten of the 51 shoulders underwent revision surgery, which was done to treat painful glenoid arthrosis in 9 of the 10. Radiographs were available for 39 shoulders, and they demonstrated an increase in glenoid erosion at a mean of 10.7 years postoperatively (*P* <.0001). Five shoulders had humeral periprosthetic lucent lines of 1.5 mm in thickness, and 3 of them had a complete line; 1 humeral component had shifted in position. According to a modification of the Neer result rating system, there were 10 excellent results, 20 satisfactory results, and 21 unsatisfactory results.

We recently published our revision and survival rates on total shoulder arthroplasty.[13] A total of 2207 patients with a mean age of 65 years underwent 2588 total shoulder arthroplasties. Osteoarthritis was the underlying diagnosis in 1640 shoulders (63%), rheumatoid arthritis in 452 (17%), and trauma in 374 (15%). A total of 212 total shoulder arthroplasties (8.2%) were revised. At 5, 10, and 20 years the survival rates were 94.2%, 90.2%, and 81.4%, respectively. Men were significantly more likely to undergo revision than women. Patients who underwent TSA with an underlying diagnosis of rotator cuff disease or tumor were significantly more likely than those with rheumatoid arthritis to undergo revision. Younger age was associated with a higher revision risk. Neither BMI nor comorbidity was associated with the risk of revision surgery.

There are few studies on long-term outcomes following a reverse total shoulder arthroplasty. Favard et al[14] reviewed 464 patients with 484 reverse total shoulder prostheses with a minimum follow-up of 2 years and 148 patients with a minimum follow-up of 5 years (mean, 7.5 years; range, 5-17 years). The mean age at the time of surgery was 73 years. Cumulative survival curves were established with end points being prosthesis revision and Constant-Murley score of less than 30 points.

Eighty-nine of 489 patients had at least 1 complication for a total of 107 complications. Survivorship free of revision was 89% at 10 years with a marked break occurring at 2 and 9 years. Survivorship to a Constant-Murley score of less than 30 was 72% at 10 years with a marked break observed at 8 years. We observed progressive radiographic changes after 5 years and an increasing frequency of large notches with long-term follow-up. They concluded that although the need for revision was relatively low at 10 years, the Constant-Murley score and radiographic changes deteriorated with time; therefore, they recommend caution when recommending a reverse shoulder arthroplasty, especially in younger patients.

REFERENCES

1. Smith KL, Matsen FA 3rd. Total shoulder arthroplasty versus hemiarthroplasty. Current trends. *Orthop Clin North Am.* 1998;29(3):491–506.
2. Walker M, Brooks J, Willis M, Frankle M. How reverse shoulder arthroplasty works. *Clin Orthop Relat Res.* 2011;469(9):2440–2451.
3. Reuther F, Mühlhäusler B, Wahl D, Nijs S. Functional outcome of shoulder hemiarthroplasty for fractures: a multicentre analysis. *Injury.* 2010;41(6):606–612.
4. Gallinet D, Clappaz P, Garbuio P, Tropet Y, Obert L. Three or four parts complex proximal humerus fractures: hemiarthroplasty versus reverse prosthesis: a comparative study of 40 cases. *Orthop Traumatol Surg Res.* 2009;95(1):48–55 [Epub February 6, 2009].
5. Lenarz C, Shishani Y, McCrum C, Nowinski RJ, Edwards TB, Gobezie R. Is reverse shoulder arthroplasty appropriate for the treatment of fractures in the older patient? Early observations. *Clin Orthop Relat Res.* 2011;469(12):3324–3331.
6. Singh JA, Sperling J, Buchbinder R, McMaken K. Surgery for shoulder osteoarthritis: a Cochrane systematic review. *J Rheumatol.* 2011;38(4):598–605.
7. Sanchez-Sotelo J. Total shoulder arthroplasty. *Open Orthop J.* 2011;5:106–114.
8. Gonzalez JF, Alami GB, Baque F, Walch G, Boileau P. Complications of unconstrained shoulder prostheses. *J Shoulder Elbow Surg.* 2011;20(4):666–682.
9. Zumstein MA, Pinedo M, Old J, Boileau P. Problems, complications, reoperations, and revisions in reverse total shoulder arthroplasty: a systematic review. *J Shoulder Elbow Surg.* 2011;20(1):146–157.
10. Solberg BD, Moon CN, Franco DP, Paiement GD. Surgical treatment of three and four-part proximal humeral fractures. *J Bone Joint Surg Am.* 2009;91(7):1689–1697.
11. Antuña SA, Sperling JW, Cofield RH. Shoulder hemiarthroplasty for acute fractures of the proximal humerus: a minimum five-year follow-up. *J Shoulder Elbow Surg.* 2008;17(2):202–209.
12. Rispoli DM, Sperling JW, Athwal GS, Schleck CD, Cofield RH. Humeral head replacement for the treatment of osteoarthritis. *J Bone Joint Surg Am.* 2006;88(12):2637–2644.
13. Singh JA, Sperling JW, Cofield RH. Revision surgery following total shoulder arthroplasty: analysis of 2588 shoulders over three decades (1976 to 2008). *J Bone Joint Surg Br.* 2011;93(11):1513–1517.
14. Favard L, Levigne C, Nerot C, Gerber C, De Wilde L, Mole D. Reverse prostheses in arthropathies with cuff tear: are survivorship and function maintained over time? *Clin Orthop Relat Res.* 2011;469(9):2469–2475.

Latissimus Dorsi Tendon Transfer for Massive Irreparable Rotator Cuff Tears

50

Guillaume Herzberg, MD, PhD

INTRODUCTION

The surgical treatment of massive irreparable rotator cuff tears is very difficult, especially for patients with painful pseudoparalysis. The use of a latissimus dorsi musculotendinous transfer (MTT) was initially reported in 1992,[1,2] and it has now become a viable treatment option.[3-9] There are however controversies regarding the technique, indications, and results of this procedure.

BIOMECHANICAL BASIS

A MTT is a procedure in which the tendon of a normal "donor" muscle with its intact blood and nerve supply is divided and reinserted into a bony part or into another tendon (with or without an intercalated tendon graft) to supplement or substitute for the action of a nonfunctioning "recipient" muscle. When dealing with a massive irreparable posterosuperior rotator cuff tear, the idea is to transfer a new structurally normal muscle with the proper vector and torque to compensate for the loss of shoulder elevation and external rotation (ER). In order for this to be successful the latissimus dorsi transfer must be strong enough and have an adequate excursion to compensate for the loss of infraspinatus and teres minor muscles. A latissimus dorsi transfer has been supplemented with a teres major transfer in some series. The transferred tendon should also have a straight line of pull, which implies that the choice of its point of fixation on the humeral head is critical.[10]

According to the Blix curve (Fig. 50-1), any tendon transfer should be set at a tension that is close to its resting length.

We dissected 13 shoulder girdle muscles in 13 fresh cadavers (ratio female/male 6/7, ages 17-89 years, average 74) with an intact rotator cuff.[11] The method of Brand and Hollister[12] was used to study each muscle or muscle belly. The potential excursion (ie, the average muscle fiber length in centimeters measured using 4.3 power magnification) and the relative tension (ie, physiologic cross-sectional area [PCSA] of each muscle expressed as a percentage within the group) was. In longitudinally arranged muscles, the fiber length was measured at the origin and the insertion and in the middle of the muscle. In pennate and multipennate muscles, the tendon was first traced back into the muscle fibers. The tendon was then cut longitudinally and spread apart so that we could measure the pennate muscle fibers from their origin to their insertion into the tendon. In multipennate muscles, measurements were made on each pennated unit and then averaged. To get a realistic PCSA, we measured the muscle fiber length taking into account the length of each pennated unit rather than measuring the whole length of the muscle. The fleshy part of each muscle was then weighed. For a given muscle, the percentage of the total weight of the 13 muscles was the mass fraction. The mass of each muscle was converted to volume according to a conversion factor of 1.02, and then divided by the mean fiber length to get the PCSA. In each cadaver, the PCSA were expressed as a percentage, providing the relative tension figures. The relative tension figures were expressed in percentages for the entire group of 13 shoulder girdle muscles. The values of the potential excursion (cm) and relative tension (%) of rotator cuff muscles, latissimus dorsi, and teres major are shown in Figures 50-2 and 50-3. Among the rotator cuff muscles, the subscapularis had the greatest relative tension (14.5%). It was well balanced by the combination of the infraspinatus and the teres minor relative tensions (12.3%). Generally speaking, it should be noted that rotator cuff muscles had a short excursion and high relative tension, whereas the latissimus dorsi and teres major muscles demonstrated larger excursions but had limited relative tension. The results of this in vitro study suggested that the teres major should be theoretically added to the latissimus dorsi transfer when dealing with a reconstruction of a massive irreparable rotator cuff tear.[13]

Another important issue is to discuss the ideal point of distal fixation of the latissimus dorsi/teres major transfer

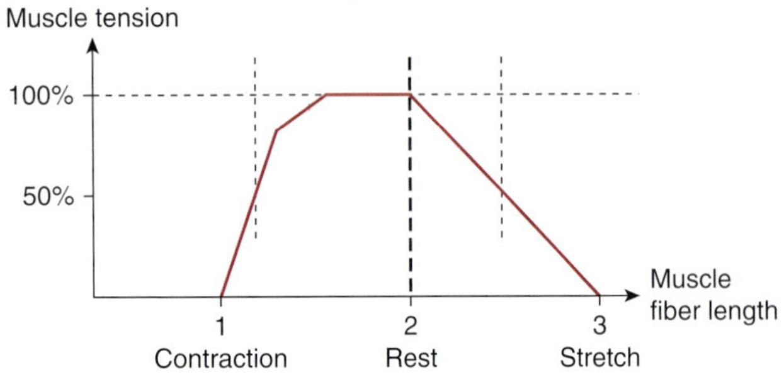

FIGURE 50-1 Blix curve, or general shape of active contraction of a muscle fiber.

on the humeral head. We investigated this by constructing a model of the relevant shoulder muscles. The right scapula and humerus were harvested from a fresh cadaver and mounted together in a frame, simulating the position of these 2 bones in the "zero" clinical position of the shoulder. Steel balls were inserted at the center of the humeral head footprint areas of the supraspinatus, infraspinatus, and teres minor.[14,15] The center areas of origin of supraspinatus, infraspinatus, teres minor, teres major, and latissimus dorsi were tagged with steel markers (Fig. 50-4). The geometric center of the humeral head was considered as the center of rotation of the simulated joint so that the generated torque could be calculated. Stereoradiography was used to obtain a 3-dimensional model of the vector forces of the normal muscle attachment and the transferred muscles that were attached to the supraspinatus, infraspinatus, or teres minor footprints.[16,17] A comparison of the vector forces with the humerus in 3 positions (neutral, 60° internal rotation, 50° ER) was performed. Each muscle vector was measured 3 times at 0° and 90° of abduction in the scapular plane. In each series, abduction/adduction and external/internal rotation moment arms were calculated by increments of 3°. The shifting of the vectors around the spherical humeral head was taken into account. Theoretical muscle forces obtained from a previous study[11] were used for muscle torque calculations. The figure used for muscle force-producing capability was 3.6 kg for 1 cm^2 of PCSA of muscle. In addition, a videotape was performed of a latissimus dorsi MTT in a fresh cadaver with fixation on either supraspinatus or infraspinatus humeral head insertions and 0° to 90° abduction motion in 50° ER or 60° internal rotation.

Theoretical values of abduction/adduction and external/internal rotation moment arms of innate infraspinatus and latissimus dorsi MTT to supraspinatus, infraspinatus, or teres minor footprints were calculated. Because of a deleterious bowstringing effect of the latissimus dorsi transfer when the humerus was in abduction with 60° internal rotation (Fig. 50-5), it was concluded that the best point of fixation was the infraspinatus footprint (Fig. 50-6). According to our results the use of this point of fixation provided a good ER torque and some abduction torque as well regardless of the position of the humerus.[16,17]

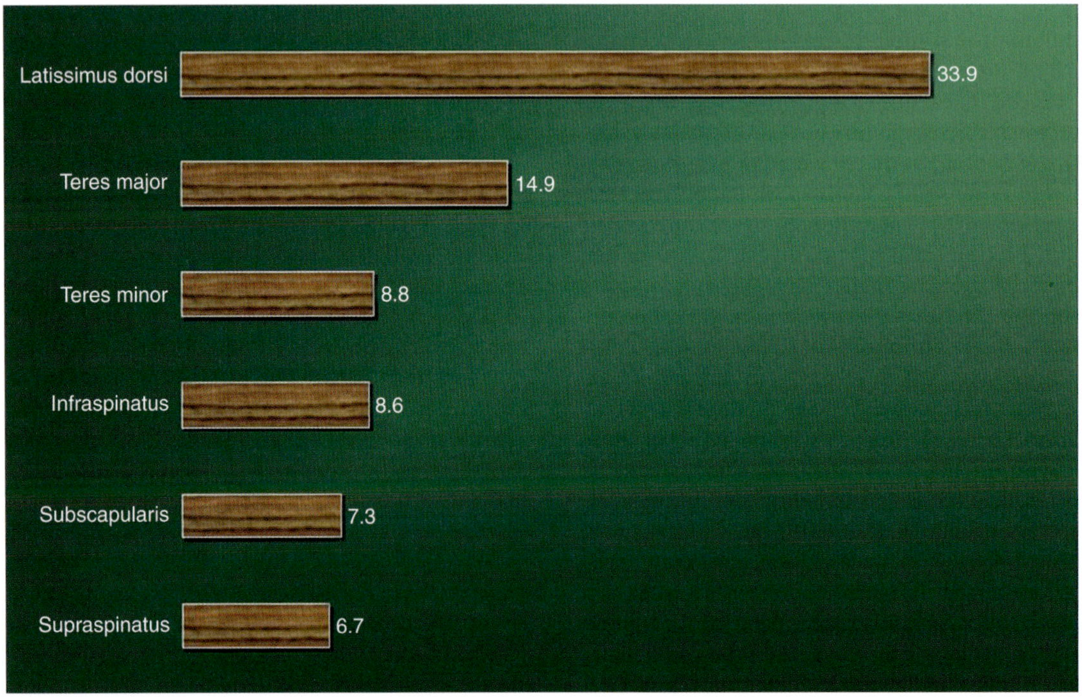

FIGURE 50-2 Distribution of potential excursion values (cm).

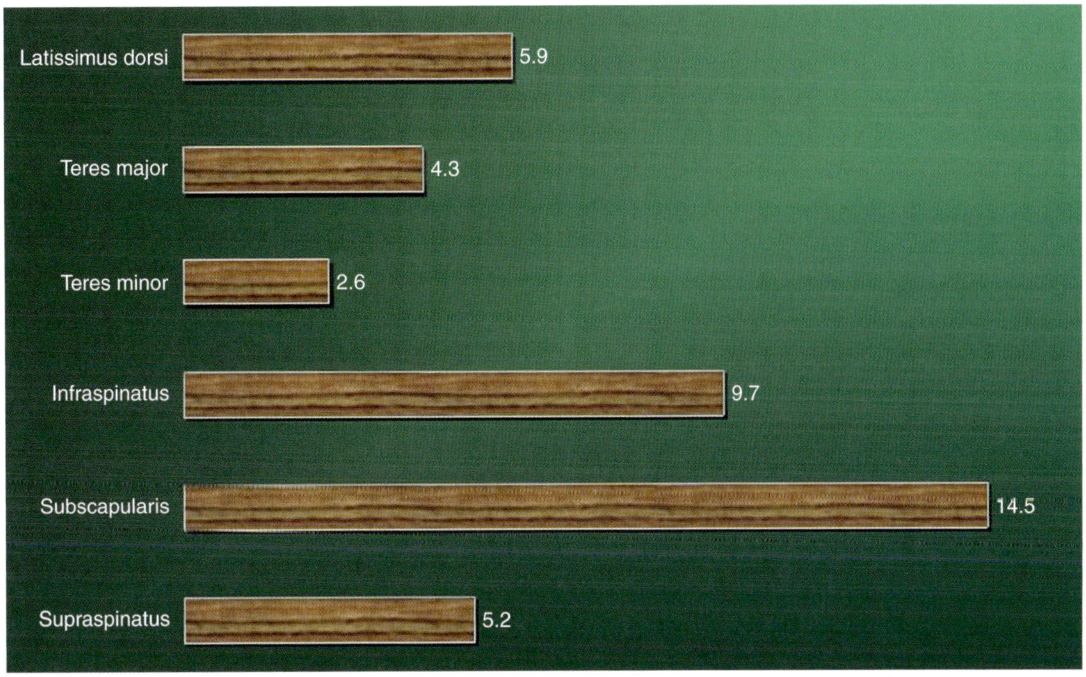

FIGURE 50-3 Distribution of relative tension values (in percentages).

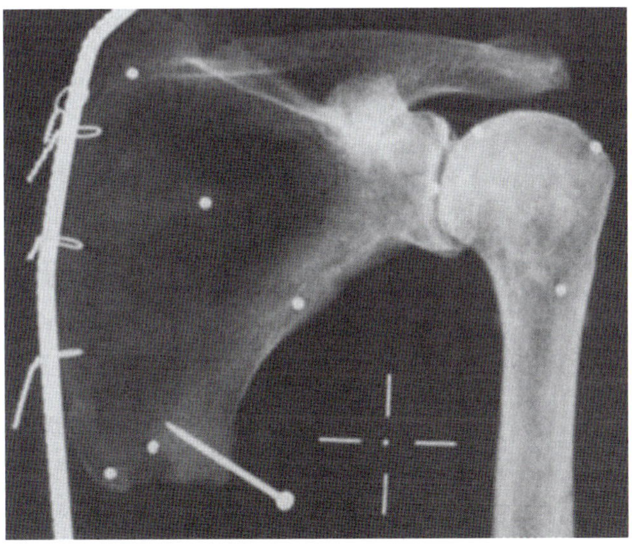

FIGURE 50-4 Scapula–humerus construct with imbedded steel balls is used to define the muscle vector forces.

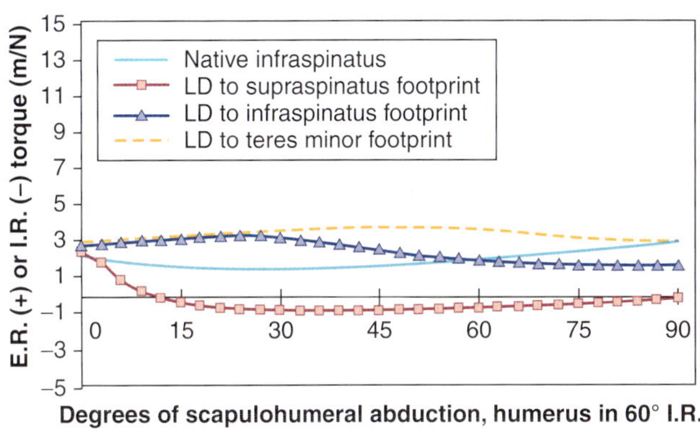

FIGURE 50-5 Comparison of latissimus dorsi transfer with fixation to the supraspinatus, infraspinatus, or teres minor footprints. With a supraspinatus insertion there is bowstringing of the tendon with the humerus in abduction and internal rotation with a deleterious effect on the internal rotation torque.

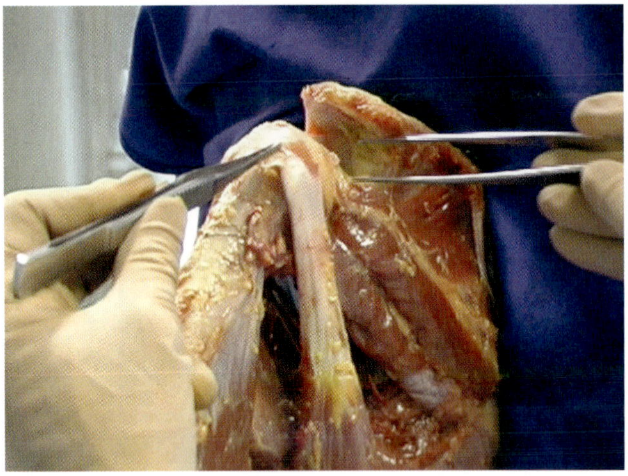

FIGURE 50-6 The best point of fixation of the latissimus dorsi transfer to humeral head is the native insertion of the infraspinatus, rather than the supraspinatus insertion.

INDICATIONS

This procedure is indicated in relatively young (about 60 years), active patients with massive irreparable posterosuperior cuff tear in the absence of advanced glenohumeral arthrosis.[17] The subscapularis muscle should be intact or reparable with no—or minor—fatty degeneration.

CONTRAINDICATIONS

This procedure is contraindicated in patients with cuff tear arthropathy or nonfunctioning deltoid muscle.

SURGICAL TECHNIQUE

The patient is placed in a beach chair position allowing about 50° of rotational motion so that the surgeon could access both the anterosuperior classic shoulder approach and a posterior axillary fold approach centered onto the humeral insertion of latissimus dorsi and teres major muscles. The anterosuperior approach is performed first. A deltoid splitting approach is used to assess the extent of the tear after thorough bursectomy and confirm its irreparability as well as the integrity or reparability of the subscapularis tendon. The long head of the biceps tendon is usually abnormal. A tenotomy of the long head followed by a tenodesis of the biceps tendon in its groove is performed using a metallic anchor. An acromioplasty is then performed. The table is now rotated to the opposite direction and a posterior approach is performed. The latissimus dorsi and teres major tendons are identified and followed to their insertions on the humerus. Care should be taken during this dissection to protect the axillary and radial nerves. The 2 tendons are detached from their humeral insertions and brought posteriorly as a unit after mobilization and protection of the neurovascular pedicles. Two Krackow stitches are placed on the tendons. The transfer is tunneled under the deltoid so as to appear in the anterosuperior operative field. The excursion and length of the transfer is checked. The transfer should reach the infraspinatus insertion without excessive tension. At this time, the posterior incision is closed, a posterior suction drain is placed, and the table is tilted back to its original classic beach chair position. The transfer is fixed to the infraspinatus insertion with transosseous sutures. The upper part of the subscapularis muscle is reattached to its original insertion. The tension of the transfer is checked in all positions of the shoulder including with the arm at the side. The anterior incision is closed over a suction drain, and the patient is placed in a soft abduction splint for 6 weeks. Early passive mobilization (40° abduction and 20° ER from the pillow position) is allowed as soon as the pain permits.

OUTCOMES

Our series consists of 16 patients (7 females) who were treated with a latissimus dorsi transfer for any massive irreparable rotator cuff tear. The average follow-up was 6 years (range, 2-17 years). The average age of these active patients was 56 years (range, 37-68 years). The duration of symptoms before surgery was 35 months. The etiology was traumatic in 50% of the cases. A total of 4 cases had undergone previous surgery. Eight patients had pseudoparalysis. The average active elevation shoulder was 91°. The average active ER was 9°. The average nonponderated Constant score for 11 patients was 26 points. The average preoperative subacromial space was 7.9 mm. A total of 12 patients had early glenohumeral arthritis, Guyette stage 1, that is, sclerosis and/or small (less than 2 mm) marginal osteophytes on only 1 side of the glenohumeral joint.[18] A total of 11 cases had massive irreparable tears of the supra and infraspinatus. In 5 cases, there was also an extension of the tear into the upper part of the subscapularis. There was fatty degeneration of Goutallier stage 3, that is, 50% fatty degeneration or worse in all patients. There was atrophy of the rotator cuff muscles in 50% of the cases. The teres minor was present in 12 of 16 shoulders. We performed 7 isolated latissimus dorsi transfers and 9 combined transfers (4 with teres major, 6 with deltoid flaps). All operations were done in the beach chair position through a double anterosuperior and posterior approach. The latissimus dorsi was transferred and fixed to the infraspinatus humeral insertion in all cases. The pain was markedly reduced at an average follow-up of 6 years (Fig. 50-7). The average improvement in the active shoulder elevation improvement was 45° (Fig. 50-8). The average improvement in the ER was 16° at the side (ER1) and 22° in abduction (ER2). The average improvement in the strength of active shoulder elevation was 2.7 kg. There was a 34-point improvement in the nonponderated Constant score. The worst results were observed in patients who had undergone

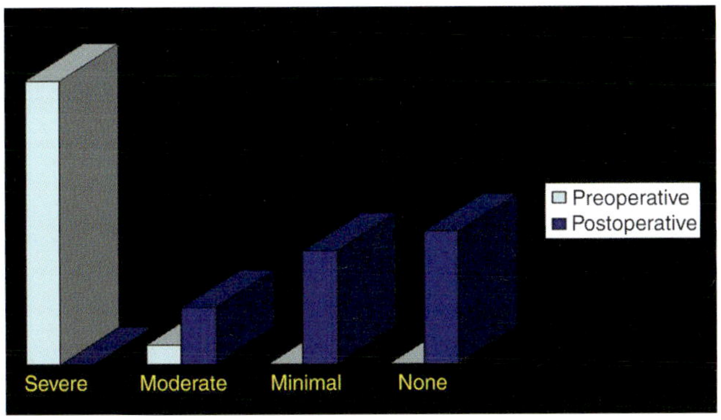

FIGURE 50-7 Pain scores.

previous surgery. Due to the limited number of patients, we were unable to clearly demonstrate the superiority of the combined latissimus dorsi/teres major transfer over the latissimus transfer alone. Our clinical experience shows that a latissimus dorsi transfer may be used in selected relatively young patients presenting with an incapacitating massive irreparable posterosuperior cuff tear. Adjuvant arthroscopy may be used in select cases.[19,20]

CASE EXAMPLE

A white-collar, 56-year-old, 90-kg male presented with a 4-year history of intractable right shoulder pain following a sudden injury while lifting a heavy object. He had pseudoparalysis of his shoulder with 70° of active elevation, zero power of shoulder elevation, and 170° passive elevation. His nonponderated Constant score was 35. The visual analog pain score was 9/10. The passive ER with the arm at the side was 30°, but the active ER was -20°. There was clinical atrophy of the infraspinatus and a positive lag sign. Internal rotation was limited to L5, but belly press test was negative indicating a functional subscapularis muscle. Standard radiographs showed signs of impingement, but the subacromial space was still acceptable (Figs. 50-9 and 50-10).

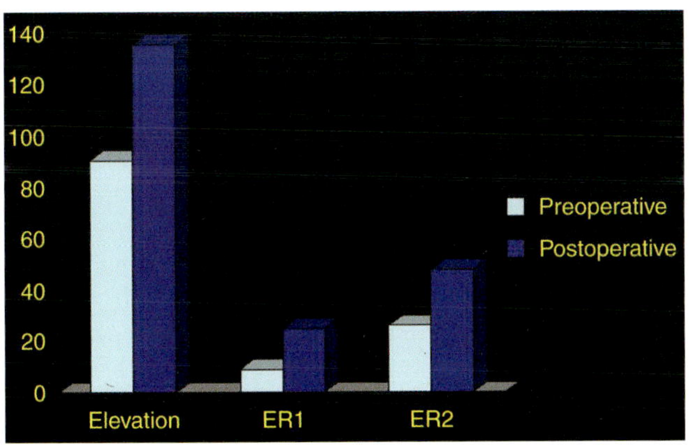

FIGURE 50-8 Active motion values.

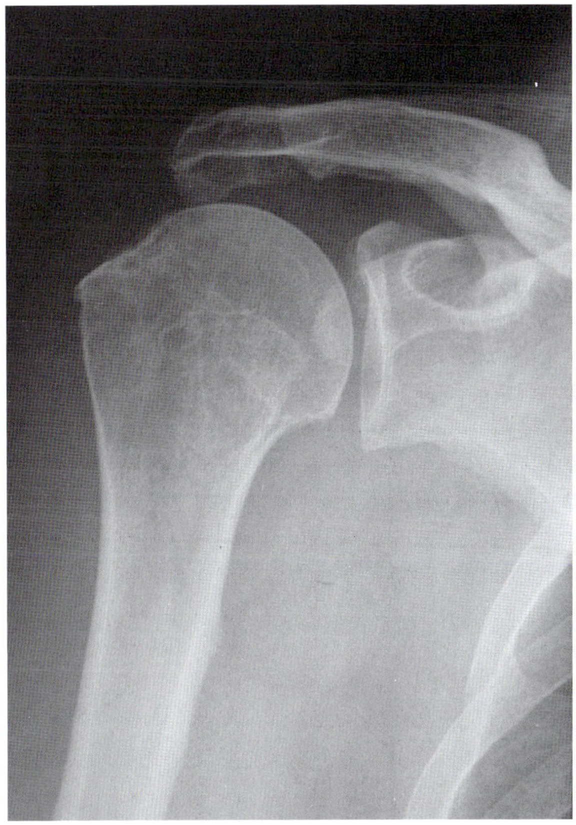

FIGURE 50-9 Clinical case: preoperative standard AP radiograph.

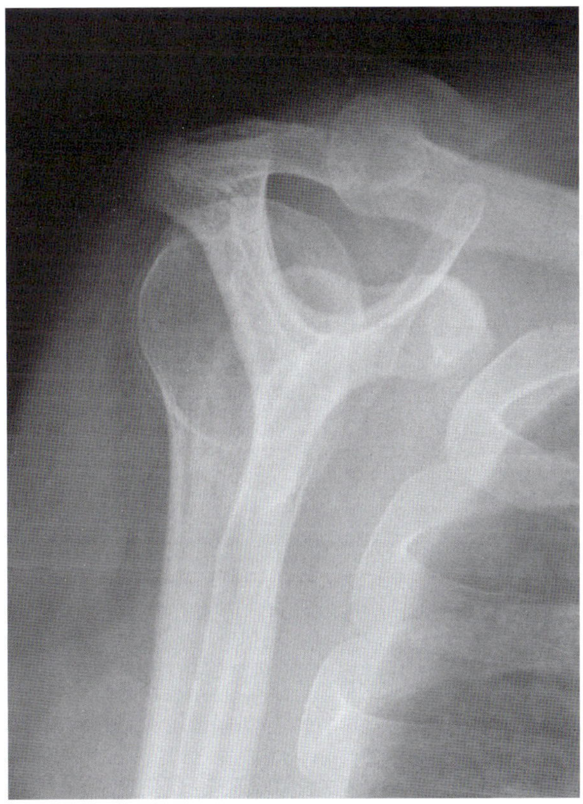

FIGURE 50-10 Clinical case: preoperative standard Y radiograph.

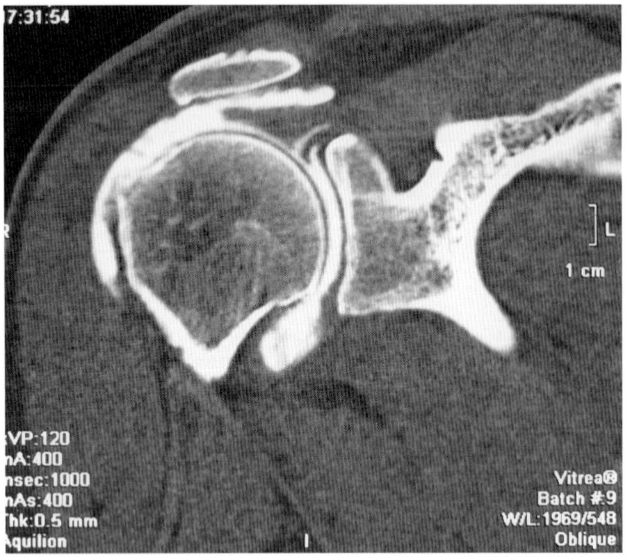

FIGURE 50-11

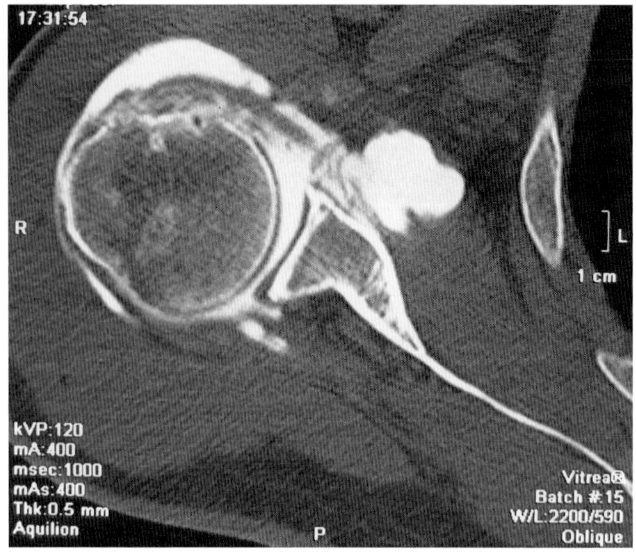

FIGURE 50-12

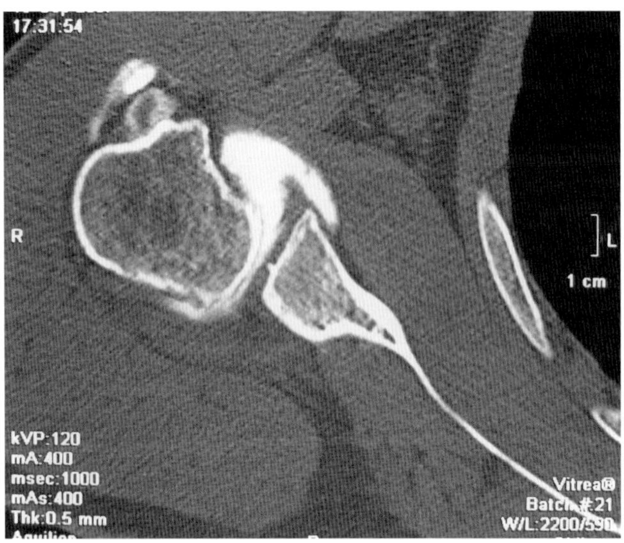

FIGURE 50-13

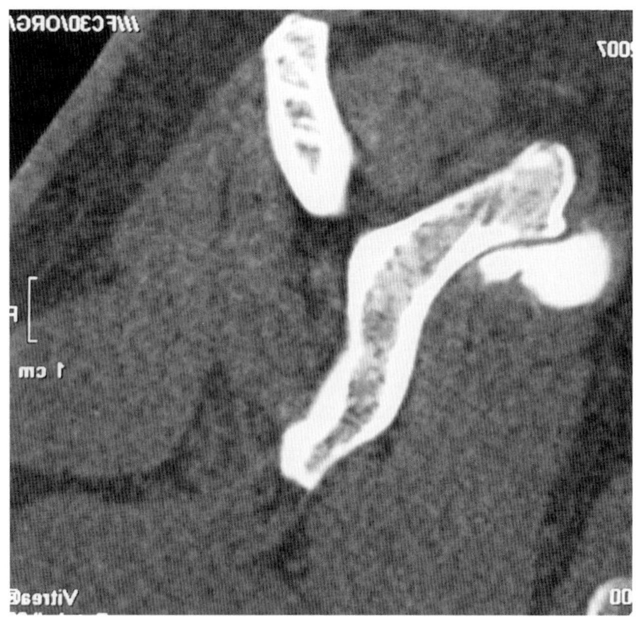

FIGURE 50-14

FIGURES 50-11 to **50-14** Clinical Case: four arthro-CT scan slices showing massive rotator cuff tear with Goutallier stage 3 infraspinatus and teres minor fatty degeneration.

Hand arthro-CT scan showed a Goutallier stage 3 infraspinatus and teres minor fatty degeneration with significant atrophy (Figs. 50-11 to 50-14). We elected to perform an open cuff reconstruction with a latissimus dorsi and teres major transfer through a double approach. Two years later, the patient was pain free. His nonponderated Constant score was 89 and his quick dash score was 14. His active shoulder elevation was 170° (Fig. 50-15), active ER at the side was 30°, and at 90° abduction ER was 70° (Figs. 50-16 and 50-17) with an M3+ power of ER strength. Standard radiographs are shown in Figures 50-18 and 50-19.

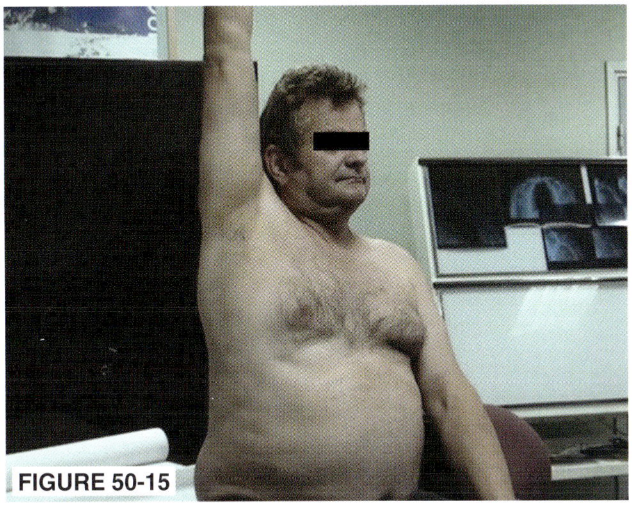
FIGURE 50-15

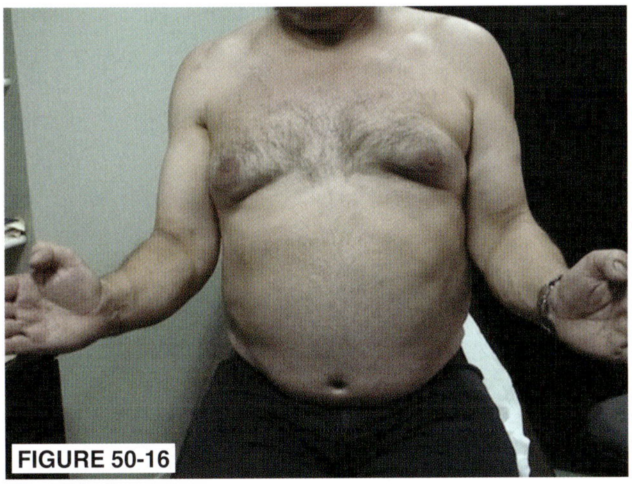
FIGURE 50-16

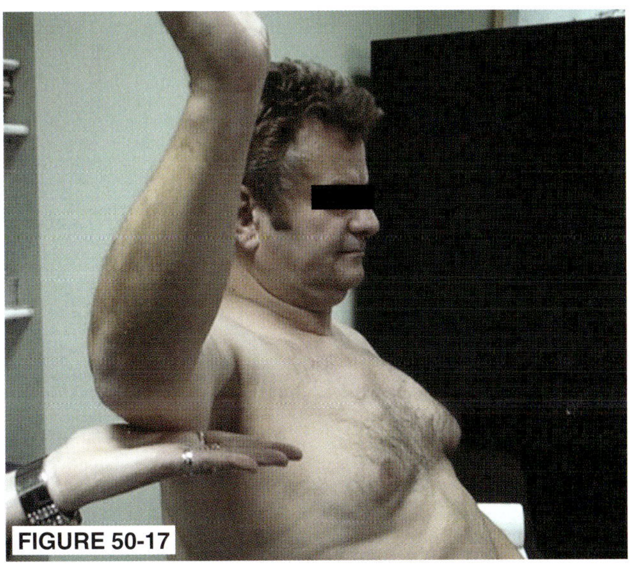
FIGURE 50-17

FIGURES 50-15 to 50-17 Clinical result at 2 years of follow-up.

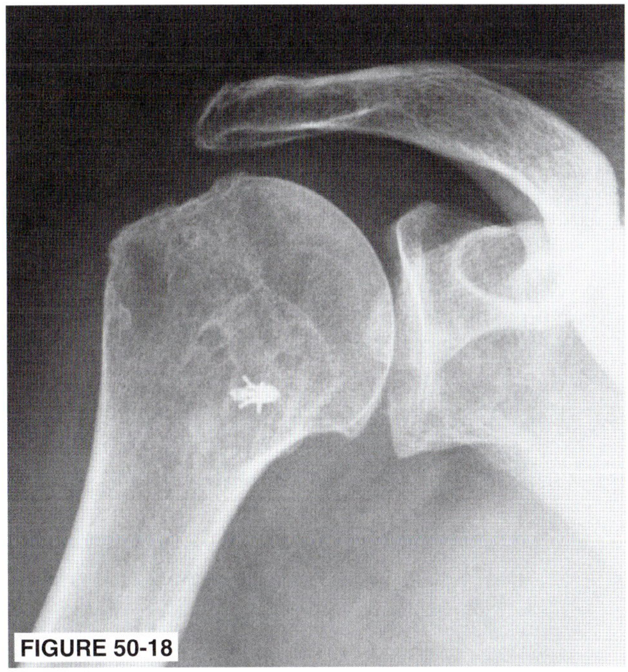
FIGURE 50-18

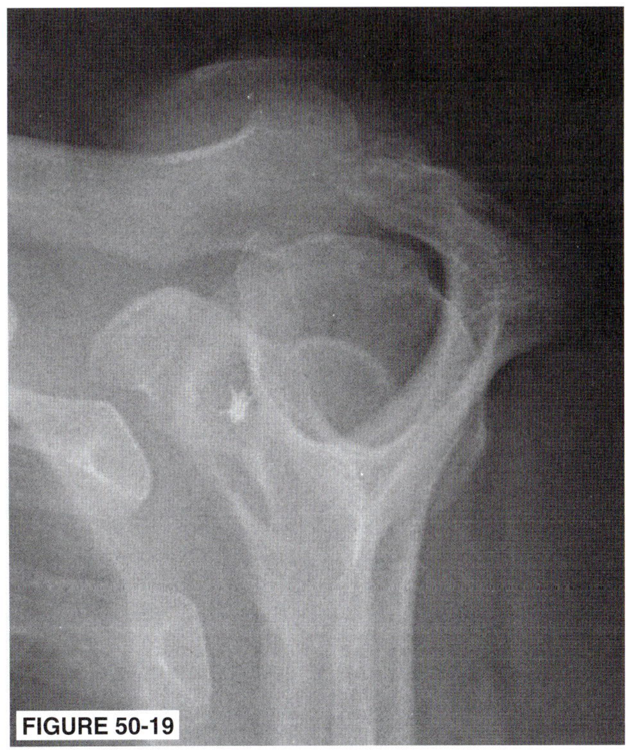
FIGURE 50-19

FIGURES 50-18 and 50-19 Standard radiographs at 2 years of follow-up.

REFERENCES

1. Gerber C. Latissimus dorsi transfer for the treatment of irreparable tears of the rotator cuff. *Clin Orthop*. 1992;275:152–160.
2. Gerber C. Latissimus dorsi transfer for the treatment of irreparable rotator cuff tears. *J Bone Joint Surg Am*. 2006;88A:113.
3. Birmingham PM, Neviaser RJ. Outcome of latissimus dorsi transfer as a salvage procedure for failed rotator cuff repair with loss of elevation. *J Shoulder Elbow Surg*. 2008;17:871–874.
4. Irlenbusch U. Latissimus dorsi transfer for irreparable rotator cuff tears: a longitudinal study. *J Shoulder Elbow Surg*. 2008;17:527–534.
5. Moursy M, Forstner R, Koller H, Resch H, Tauber M. Latissimus dorsi tendon transfer for irreparable rotator cuff tears: a modified technique to improve tendon transfer integrity. *J Bone Joint Surg Am*. 2009;91:1924.
6. Nové-Josserand L, Liotard JP, Walch G. Résutats du transfert du latissimus dorsi pour rupture non reparable de la coiffe des rotateurs. *Rev Chir Orthop Reparatrice Appar Mot*. 2009;95:125–130.
7. Tauber M, Moursy M, Forstner R, Koller H, Resch H. Latissimus dorsi tendon transfer for irreparable rotator cuff tears: a modified technique to improve tendon transfer integrity. *J Bone Joint Surg Am*. 2010;92A(suppl 1, part 2):226–239.
8. Valenti P. Résultats du transfert du Latissimus Dorsi réalisé de première intention ou après échec d'une première opération dans les ruptures irréparables de la coiffe des rotateurs. *Rev Chir Orthop Reparatrice Appar Mot*. 2010;96:176.
9. Valenti P, Kalouche I. Results of latissimus dorsi tendon transfer in primary or salvage reconstruction of massive, irreparable rotator cuff tears. In: Valenti P, ed. *Tendon Transfer for Irreparable Cuff Tear*. Paris: Springer; 2010:25–39.
10. Schoierer O, Herzberg G, Berthonnaud E, Dimnet J, Aswad R, Morin A. Anatomical basis of latissimus dorsi and teres major transfers in rotator cuff tear surgery with particular reference to the neurovascular pedicles. *Surg Radiol Anat*. 2001;23:75–80.
11. Herzberg G, Urien JP, Dimnet J. Potential excursion and relative tension of muscles in the shoulder girdle: relevance to tendon transfers. *J Shoulder Elbow Surg*. 1999;8:430–437.
12. Brand PW, Hollister A. *Clinical Mechanics of the Hand*. 2nd ed. St Louis: Mosby; 1993.
13. Berthonnaud E, Herzberg G, Schoierer O, Medda N, Dimnet J. Latissimus dorsi transfer: should we add the teres major? *Orthop Trans*. 2003.
14. Gates JJ. Influence of distinct anatomic subregions of the supraspinatus on humeral rotation. *J Orthop Res*. 2010;28:12.
15. Minagawa H, Itoi E. Humeral attachment of the supraspinatus and infraspinatus tendons: an anatomic study. *Arthroscopy*. 1998;14(3):302–306.
16. Herzberg G, Berthonnaud E, Schoierer O, Guigual V, Dimnet J, Morin A. Latissimus dorsi transfer in irreparable rotator cuff tears: what point of fixation on the humeral head? *Orthop Trans*. 2001.
17. Herzberg G, Schoierer O, Berthonnaud E, Dimnet J, Urien JP. Biomechanical analysis of tendon transfers for irreparable rotator cuff tears. In: Valenti P, ed. *Tendon Transfer for Irreparable Cuff Tear*. Paris: Springer; 2010:1–14.
18. Guyette TM, Warren RF, Craig EV, Wickiewicz TL. Results of arthroscopic SAD in patients with subacromial impingement and GH degenerative joint disease. *J Shoulder Elbow Surg*. 2002;11:299–304.
19. Kany J. Arthroscopic humeral head interference screw fixation for latissimus dorsi transfer in massive and irreparable posterosuperior cuff tear. In: Valenti P, ed. *Tendon Transfer for Irreparable Cuff Tear*. Paris: Springer; 2010:41–47.
20. Millett PJ. Arthroscopically assisted latissimus dorsi transfer for irreparable rotator cuff tears. *Tech Shoulder Elbow Surg*. 2008;9:76.

51

Pectoralis Major Tendon Repair*

Rachel M. Frank, MD
Robert A. Waltz, MD
James Richard Bailey, MD
Frank McCormick, MD
John W. McNeil II, BA
Matthew T. Provencher, MD

RATIONALE AND BASIC SCIENCE PERTINENT TO THE PROCEDURE

Anatomy

The pectoralis major muscle is a thick, pennate muscle that lies on the chest wall.[1–4] The muscle is divided into 2 portions: the clavicular and sternocostal heads (Fig. 51-1A). The clavicular head originates on the medial one half to two thirds of the clavicle. The sternocostal portion is divided into superior and inferior segments. The superior segment originates at the upper two thirds of the sternum and ribs 2 to 4 while the inferior segment originates on the distal sternum, ribs 5 and 6, and the external oblique fascia. These segments converge to form the tendon that inserts onto the lateral lip of the bicipital groove of the humerus. The tendinous footprint starts approximately 4 cm distal to the greater tuberosity on the lateral lip of the bicipital groove and measures 70 mm (proximal to distal) × 1.4 mm (medial to lateral).[5] Other studies have shown the medial to lateral insertion width measuring approximately 5 to 15 mm.[1,6] In a 3-dimensional study of the pectoralis major tendon architecture, Fung et al further defined these measurements in relationship to the tendon's anterior and posterior layers. They found the tendon's footprint to have an approximate width (proximal to distal) of 66 and 77 mm, respectfully, and thickness (anterior to posterior) of 2 mm for each.[7] The clavicular portion of the tendon inserts superficially and distally while the inferior sternocostal section is multipennated with fibers that twist 180° to insert more posteriorly and proximally on the humerus.[7] The pectoralis minor lays deep to the pectoralis major.

Innervation

The pectoralis major is primarily innervated by the lateral pectoral nerve, which is preclavicular and originates from the C5-6 nerve roots (Fig. 51-1B).[8] The nerve begins distal to the suprascapular nerve and moves inferolaterally through the clavicopectoral fascia distal to the clavicle and close to the coracoid process, directly supplying the clavicular segment of the muscle.[8] Of note, the medial pectoral nerve, which pierces through and innervates the pectoralis minor muscle, also supplies a portion of the inferior segment of the pectoralis major; however, this contribution is likely clinically irrelevant.

Blood Supply

The pectoral branch of the thoracoacromial artery contributes 60% of the pectoralis major blood supply and is not a surgical factor during repair.[9] The other 40% is supplied by the clavicular branch and the internal mammary artery (20% each).[9] The blood supply, however, is not consistent, and there are reports of contributions from the deltoid artery and the lateral thoracic artery. The internal mammary vein usually drains the medial portion of the muscle while the axillary vein drains the lateral portion of the muscle.

Function

The pectoralis major is a powerful adductor and internal rotator of the arm (Table 51-1). Due to its more

*The views expressed in this chapter are those of the authors and do not reflect the official policy or position of the Department of the Navy, Department of Defense, or US government.

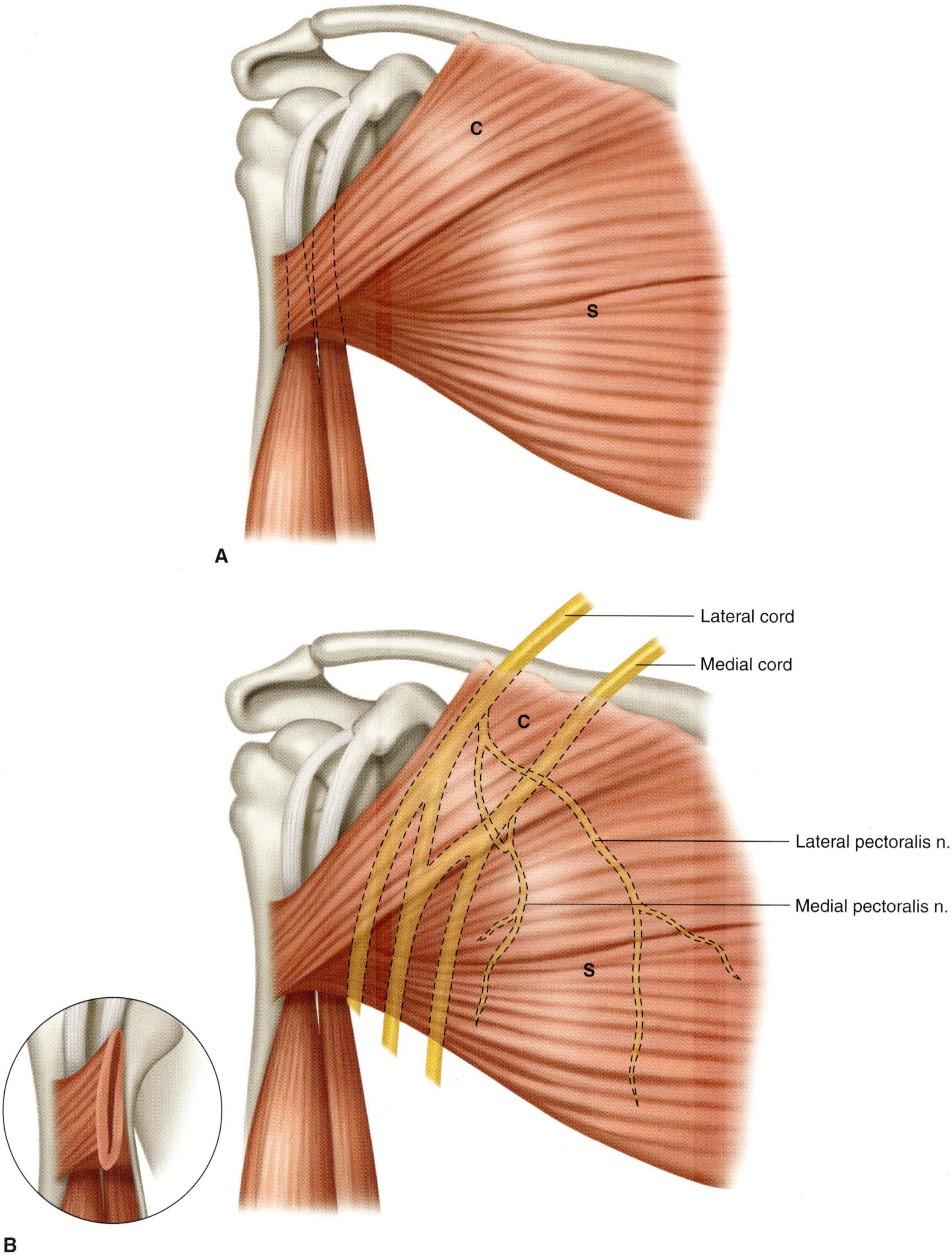

FIGURE 51-1 **A.** Anatomical representation of the 2 portions of the pectoralis major, the clavicular (C) head and sternocostal (S) head, which converge to form the tendon at the insertion point on the lateral lip of the bicipital groove of the humerus. (Redrawn with permission from Provencher et al,[12] Fig. 1.) **B.** Representation of the innervation of the pectoralis major muscle. (Redrawn with permission from Provencher et al,[12] Fig. 2.)

distal insertion on the humerus, the sternocostal head has a distinct mechanical disadvantage when the arms are in extension, such as during a bench press exercise.[1] As such, it is this portion that ruptures first, followed by the clavicular head with further tendon overload (Fig. 51-2). Of note, the pectoralis major is not necessary in normal activities of daily living; however, a fully intact muscle allows for maximal strength that is required in many high-level athletic or high-demand functional situations.[10–12]

TABLE 51-1: Function of the Pectoralis Major

Muscle Portion	Origin	Insertion	Function
Clavicular portion	Medial one half to two thirds of clavicle	Lateral lip of bicipital groove of humerus	Forward flex and adduct the arm
Sternocostal portion	Superior: originates at upper two thirds of sternum and ribs 2-4 Inferior: originates on distal sternum, ribs 5-6, and external oblique fascia	Lateral lip of bicipital groove of humerus *Note*: Inferior segment is multipennated and its fibers twist 180° to insert posteriorly and proximally on the humerus	Internally rotate and adduct the arm

MECHANISM AND PRESENTATION

Pectoralis major tears occur almost universally in males between the ages of 20 and 40.[13] The mechanism of injury involves a forceful eccentric contraction of the extended, abducted, and externally rotated humerus. The single most common activity leading to rupture of the pectoralis major tendon is the bench press exercise.[14–18] Other less common etiologies include work-related injuries and other athletic activities, including powerlifting, football, and wrestling. Risk factors for rupture include the use of anabolic steroids. Interestingly, both the dominant and nondominant shoulders are equally at risk, and bilateral ruptures have been reported.[19,20]

Patients presenting with acute pectoralis major tendon ruptures will typically report a history of bench press (or other provoking activity) followed by immediate audible pop associated with a tearing sensation near the axilla.[17,21] The patient will report immediate pain and weakness in the affected extremity. Notable findings on physical examination include swelling and ecchymosis, especially over the axilla. Patients may have thinning of or a palpable defect in the tendon; however, this can be masked by an intact fascial sheath even in the presence of a complete rupture. While patients have pain and discomfort with range of motion, one of the more specific findings on examination is loss or thinning of the anterior axillary fold (Fig. 51-3). Thus, the examiner should perform a thorough inspection of both shoulders in order to assess for asymmetry. This finding can be missed in the acute phase depending on the amount of swelling

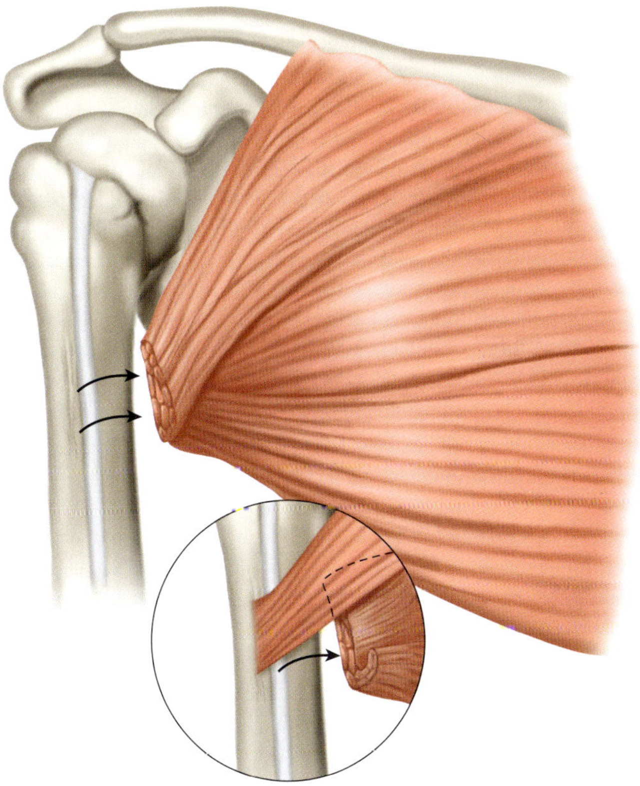

FIGURE 51-2 A representation of a rupture of both the clavicular and sternocostal portions of the pectoralis major. The inset represents only the sternocostal portion of the pectoralis major rupturing. (Reproduced with permission from Provencher et al,[12] Fig. 5.)

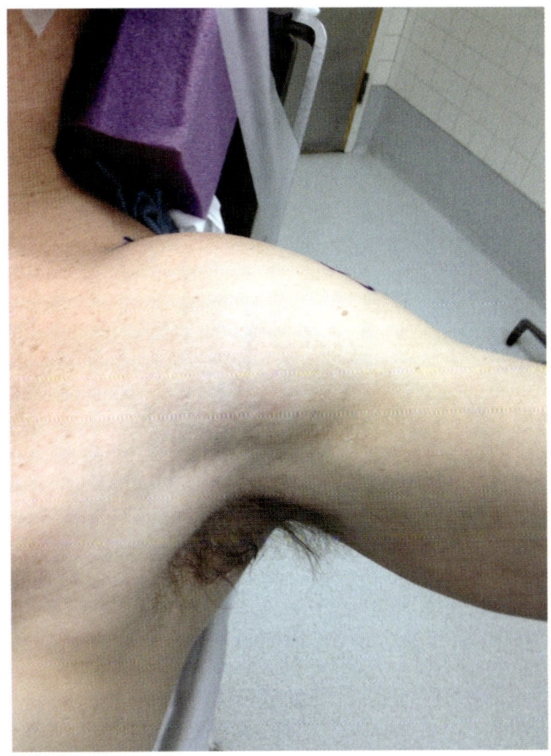

FIGURE 51-3 Photograph demonstrating loss of axillary fold due to pectoralis major tendon rupture.

present. Patients may also have a palpable bulge in the area of the rupture with adduction; however, this should not be confused for a hematoma.[12]

Imaging modalities, including radiographs, ultrasound, and magnetic resonance imaging (MRI),[22] can be performed in the patient with a suspected pectoralis major tendon rupture; however, history and physical examination are much more helpful in reaching a diagnosis.

INDICATIONS

Operative Treatment

While the pectoralis major is not needed for activities of daily living, most authors conclude surgery is indicated in all young, active patients, regardless of the chronicity of the injury.[14,23-25] A recent meta-analysis conducted by Bak et al analyzed 112 pectoralis major ruptures and found that 88% of patients treated surgically had overall excellent outcomes as compared with only 27% of patients treated nonoperatively.[26] The authors found no effect of age or tear location (humeral insertion vs musculotendinous junction) on outcomes, but did report significantly improved outcomes in patients undergoing repair within the first 8 weeks following injury as compared with more chronic repairs or with nonoperative management. Several authors have reported similar outcomes without regard to timing of surgical repair.[18,27]

Nonoperative Treatment

As mentioned, the majority of pectoralis major tendon ruptures in young, active patients warrant surgical fixation. Patients with partial tears or muscle belly ruptures, however, may be treated with an initial trial of nonoperative treatment.[18] Further, lower-demand patients may also benefit from a trial of nonoperative management.[28-31] Nonoperative treatment for pectoralis major tendon tears includes a variety of modalities as described in Table 51-2, with the mainstay of treatment being adequate rehabilitation.[21,25]

CONTRAINDICATIONS

Absolute contraindications to surgical repair of pectoralis major tendon ruptures include significant medical comorbidities and inability to comply with the required postoperative rehabilitation protocol. In terms of relative contraindications, the pectoralis major muscle is not typically utilized for normal activities of daily living, and thus one could argue surgical repair is not necessary. As such, a relative contraindication to surgery includes the desire of a patient to trial nonoperative management. However, in these situations the results are primarily unsatisfactory and the patient may eventually elect to undergo surgical repair.

TABLE 51-2: Nonoperative Treatment Modalities for Pectoralis Major Tendon Ruptures

Cold compression
Analgesics
Nonsteroidal anti-inflammatories (NSAIDs)
Sling mobilization in the adducted and internally rotated position for 1-2 weeks
Gentle passive and active ROM exercises at weeks 1-6
Gentle, controlled resistance exercises at 6 weeks
Unrestricted ROM at 8-12 weeks

SURGICAL TECHNIQUE

Relevant Surgical Anatomy

During the surgical approach, the surgeon must take care to avoid several structures. As described by Cooper et al,[32] the surgical anatomy of the shoulder can be described in 4 layers, and in surgical approaches to the pectoralis major tendon, the first 2 layers are encountered. Layer 1 is composed of the pectoralis major, the deltoid, the cephalic vein, and the overlying fascia. The superficial aspect of Layer 2 is composed of the clavicopectoral fascia, conjoined tendon, and coracoacromial ligament. The deep aspect of Layer 2 is composed of the posterior scapular fascia overlying the infraspinatus and teres minor muscle bellies, and is contiguous with the clavicopectoral fascia around the lateral aspect of the proximal humerus. Layer 2 must be retracted during surgical dissection to avoid injury to the axillary nerve. The lateral and medial pectoral nerves are typically not in danger during this approach as they enter the muscle bellies posteriorly; however, dissection medial to the coracoid should be avoided in order to prevent iatrogenic injury to these nerves.[32]

Specific surgical techniques are variable[1,20,33-45] and there is no current gold standard. The majority of techniques employ drill holes, sutures, and/or anchors to reattach the tendon to its insertion.[15,23,46-48] The technique described below is the authors' preferred technique; however, several other techniques have been reported with excellent outcomes.[12] Surgeon experience and preference, as well as patient-specific factors, play a role in the specific technique chosen.

Authors' Preferred Technique

The patient is placed in a modified beach chair position with the arm placed on padded Mayo stand or a pneumatic arm holder (Figs. 51-4 to 51-6). The humerus is abducted while the surgeon stands in the axilla that enables dissection, visualization, and repair. A palpable defect can be identified in the anterior axillary fold that is accentuated by abduction and external rotation of the shoulder. Any intact fibers of the

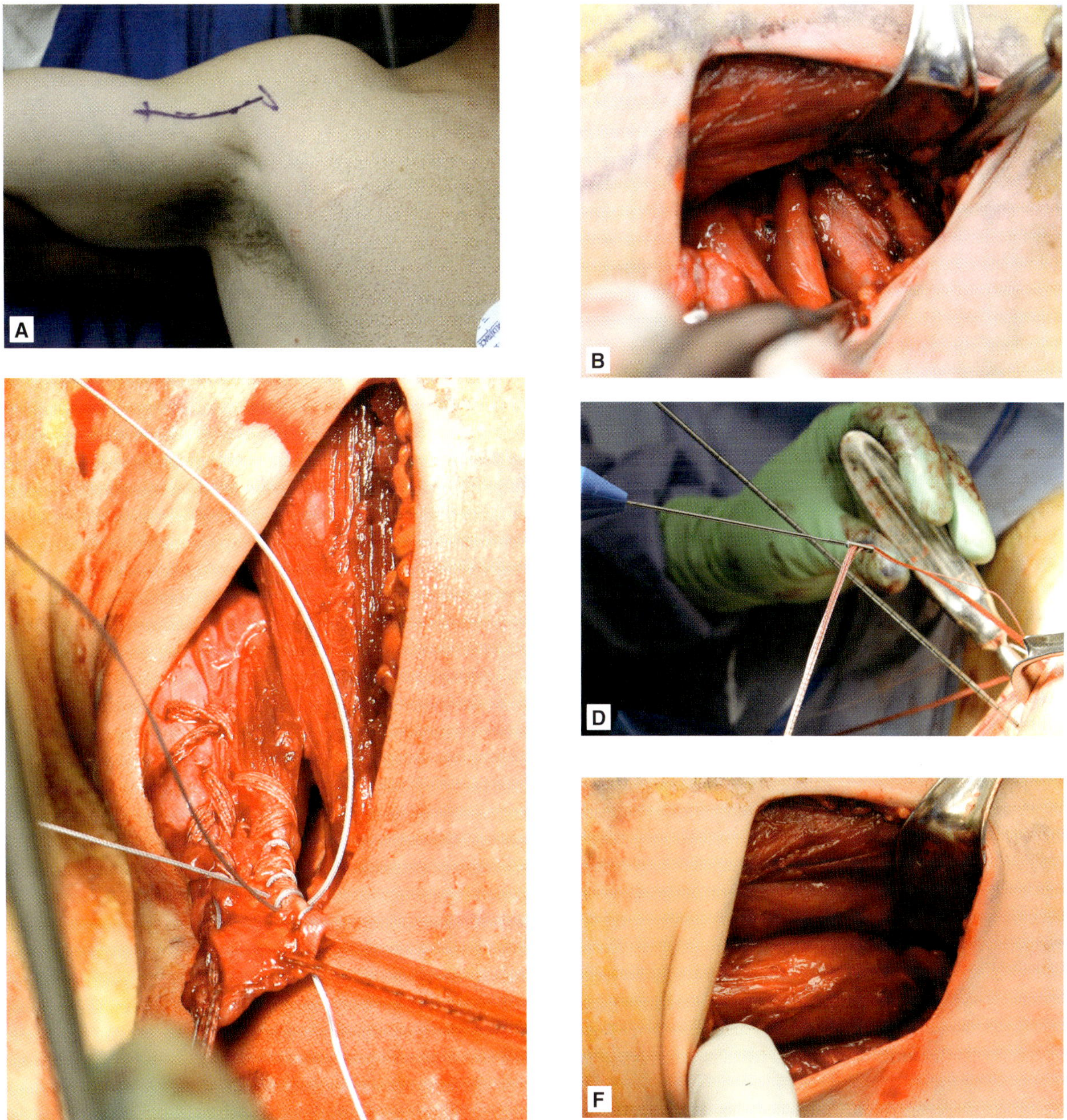

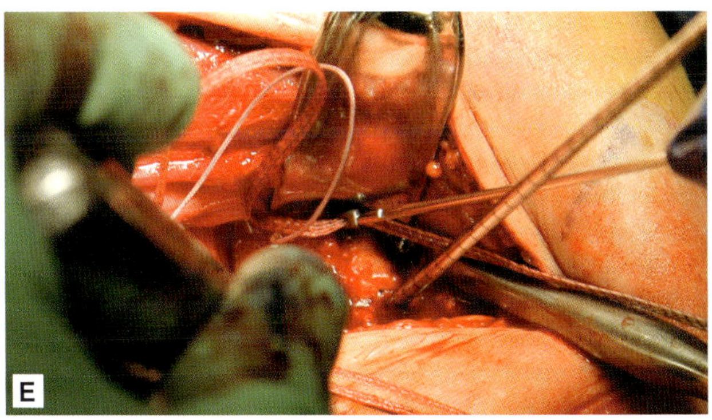

FIGURE 51-4 A. The typical incision in the deltopectoral interval and is made slightly medial. The skin is well prepared with several cleansing scrubs prior to incision. **B.** The LHB is retracted medially gently against the humerus with a blunt retractor; the attachment of the pectoralis major is just lateral to the long head of the biceps. **C.** After the torn tendon portion is identified (in this case, just the sternal head is torn), the tendon and musculotendinous junction fascia are whipstitched with a high-strength suture tape or a high-strength cylindrical suture (#5). **D.** The implants are placed into the unicortical bone tunnels, and then the sutures slid through the implants to "cinch" the tendon down anatomically to the insertion point. **E.** The tendon is "cinched" down by sliding 1 limb of the suture (the free end) through the implant and then tying. **F.** The completed repair shows the sternal head approximated directly to the anatomical insertion of the pectoralis major, and the long head of the biceps lies nicely underneath and medially without incarceration.

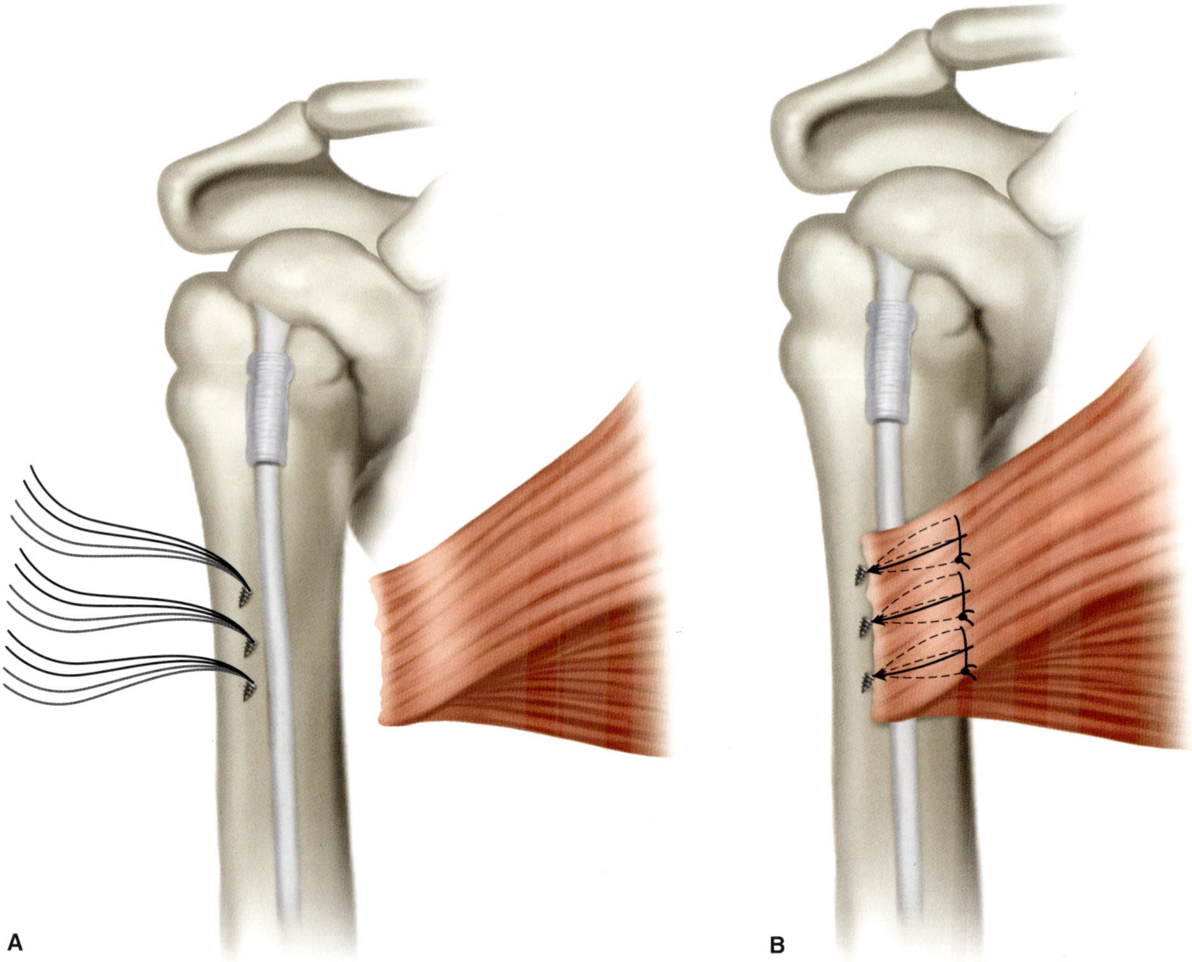

FIGURE 51-5 Surgical technique schematic. **A.** Three suture anchors are placed into the humerus in preparation for the pectoralis major reattachment. **B.** The sutures are secured medially through the tendon and tied down to reattach the pectoralis major tendon to its insertion point. (Redrawn with permission from Provencher et al,[12] Fig. 7A and B.)

tendon can be palpated and retracted. The pectoralis tendon can be identified medially on the chest wall.

The deltoid insertion and location of the coracoid are marked out. A 6- to 8-cm incision is made over the distal portion of the deltopectoral interval but slightly more medial to in the skin fold for cosmesis, but this requires a more vertical incision (Fig. 51-4A). Using either Metzenbaum scissors or electrocautery, the deltopectoral fascia is exposed, and the cephalic vein is retracted laterally. A baby Hohmann retractor is placed above the coracoid and used to retract the deltoid laterally to aid exposure. Care is taken to avoid injury to the musculocutaneous nerve, which lies medial and just deep to the conjoint tendon, approximately 5 cm inferior to the anterior tip of the coracoid. One can bluntly dissect using an index finger to separate the deltoid away from the subscapularis and distal subacromial space and the long head of the biceps is retracted medially (Fig. 51-4B). The pectoralis major inserts on the humerus just lateral to the bicipital groove. The vessels of the 3 sisters (anterior humeral circumflex artery and its 2 accompanying veins) are a visual landmark of the inferior border of the subscapularis that overlies the pectoralis major insertion. The latissimus dorsi insertion and any intact fibers of the clavicular head of the pectoralis major can also be used as a reference. The sternocostal head is the most commonly injured and can retract just medial to the axillary crease. The tendon is debrided and then mobilized until it can reach its insertion site on the humerus. If there is insufficient excursion, an Achilles tendon allograft can be used. The tendon is whipstitched with a nonabsorbable tape in a running, nonlocking fashion and a #5 nonabsorbable suture with a running Krakow stitch (Fig. 51-4C). The same construct is placed in the clavicular head if torn. The insertion site is debrided to bleeding bone with a small rongeur and rasp, staying lateral to the bicipital groove, because if the insertion site is too medial (in the biceps groove), the biceps may be incarcerated, which causes persistent pain. There

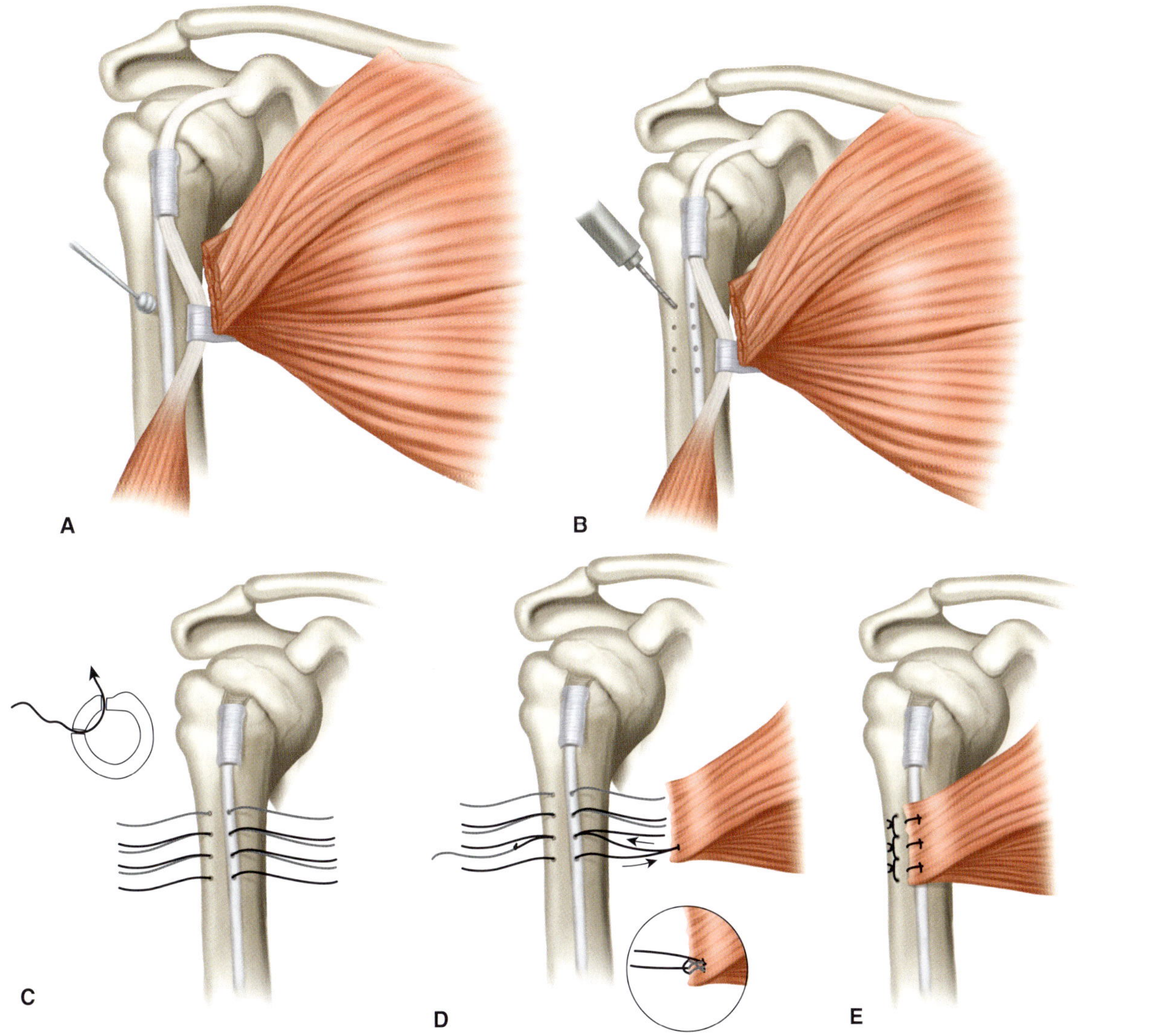

FIGURE 51-6 Surgical technique schematic. **A.** When beginning to drill the necessary bone tunnels in the humerus, the biceps tendon must be protected by pulling it just medial to the pectoralis major insertion. **B.** Two rows of between 3 and 4 drill holes, each 2 mm in diameter, are created to reattach the torn pectoralis major tendon. **C.** The No. 5 braided or No. 2 high-strength sutures are passed through each of the bone tunnels. The 2 middle bone tunnels will have a second No. 5 or No. 2 suture to assist with suture shuttling through the tunnel. **D.** Once passed through the bone tunnel, sutures are passed through the distal pectoralis major tendon with a Mason-Allen configuration. **E.** Two limbs of the suture are tied laterally for final tendon fixation. (Redrawn with permission from Provencher et al,[12] Fig. 8A-E.)

are many fixation options, including drill tunnels (3–4 tunnels spaced 1.0 cm apart, with a 2.0-mm curved drill bit), 2 to 4 suture anchors, or cortical buttons[49] (used in a unicortical fashion), at both the superior and inferior insertions of the tendon that are drilled under the anterior cortex and flipped.

The insertion of the pectoralis major is a well-defined ridge just lateral to the bicipital groove and is easily palpated and visualized, often with some amount of tendon stump remaining, especially where tears are most common inferiorly of the sternal head. One should drill lateral to the bicipital groove distal to inferior subscapularis and lateral to the bicipital groove superior to the biceps musculotendinous junction using a 3.5-mm spade tip drill over a K-wire.

The leading strands of both the superior and inferior sutures are then passed through separate pectoralis major cortical buttons. Only 1 limb of each suture is placed up and back down the tendon such that there is a free limb to tie down and "slide" through the button. We find it useful to separate these sutures or color code them, often with a marking pen at the tips. Ensure the suture is untwisted as it passes through the button fixation as this allows for sliding of the button during tendon tensioning (Fig. 51-4D and E). A 180° twist is then performed with the 2 strands of sutures, bringing the inferior portion of the sternocostal head superior and deep to the clavicular head, recreating the anatomical rotation of the tendon. The buttons are then docked intramedullary. We prefer to put the trailing suture into the hole first so the trailing suture can be toggled to seat the button on the inner cortex. The tendon is brought flush with the outer cortex of the humerus at the insertion site by pulling on the trailing sutures. The lead sutures are then tied back down onto the trailing sutures and the final repair construct is assessed.

We have found that the suture tapes have high resistance to "cutout" and pull-through in the tendon and fascia and prefer suture tapes over cylindrical sutures (Fig. 51-4F). The wound is copiously irrigated and the arm is taken through gentle abduction and external rotation is performed to assess the strength of the repair and range of motion restrictions. The wound is closed in layered fashion using absorbable skin sutures for cosmesis. A cold compress and sling are used; an abduction pillow is optional.

REHABILITATION

A sling is used for 6 weeks with pendulum exercises and passive ROM in therapy, allowing unrestricted elbow, wrist, and hand ROM. We allow shoulder flexion to 90°, abduction to 30° to 45°, and external rotation to 20° in the first 2 weeks, and then advanced as tolerated.

Phase 2:

Resistance training begins at 6 to 12 weeks postoperatively.
We recommend against heavy bench press for at least 6 months.

COMPLICATIONS

Overall, complications following pectoralis major tendon repair are rare,[50] but several have been reported. Perhaps most concerning is the potential for postoperative infection[12,51] as the axillary fold provides an environment ideal for bacterial growth given its location and ability to retain moisture. Recommended preventative measures include the use of Ioban across skin during surgery, surgical prep with alcohol and chlorhexidine, and meticulous surgical technique with respect to the soft tissue and wound closure. Another reported complication is tendon rerupture with a reported rate of 0% to 7.7%.[4,51] Recommended preventative measures include a delayed return to bench pressing and the avoidance of early heavy lifting. Intraoperatively, the repair may be made more secure with cortical fixation with suture tape medially into the fascia overlying the muscle. Other rarely reported complications include hematoma formation requiring evacuation,[51] proximal humerus shaft fracture,[46] and heterotopic ossification formation.[13] There is also a theoretical risk of pectoral denervation through aggressive dissection, retraction, and release as well as risk to the long head of the biceps tendon through dissection or abnormal pectoralis major tendon insertion during the repair.

OUTCOMES

In the authors' experience, the vast majority of young and active patients can expect very good to excellent outcomes at 6 months following surgical repair with a low risk of complications and retear (Fig. 51-7).[12] The authors do expect some residual cosmetic deformity at the anterior axillary fold coupled with scar formation; however, full strength and return to activities is often achieved. In a recent meta-analysis of 112 patients with pectoralis major tendon rupture, Bak et al[26] reported that 90% of surgically treated patients achieved an excellent outcome, while only 17% of nonoperatively treated patients achieved similar results.[26] There are a variety of surgical techniques and modifications for pectoralis major tendon repair described in the literature, all with encouraging outcomes[14-16,18,23,26,27,29,47,48,51]; however, there is currently no "gold standard" and the literature has yet to determine a clear benefit among different techniques. Schepsis et al[36] reviewed 17 patients with a mean age of 29 years at a mean follow-up of 28 months (range, 18 months to 6 years). Ten of the 17 injuries were the result of weight lifting. Thirteen patients underwent surgery within 2 weeks versus 7 chronic injuries. Four had nonoperative management. Subjectively 96% of the acute group rated their result as good as compared with 93% in the chronic group, and only 51% in the nonoperative group. Isokinetic testing showed that patients operated on acutely had the highest adduction strength (102% of the opposite side) compared with patients with chronic injuries (94%) or nonoperative treatment (71%). Garrigues et al[23] reviewed 19 patients who underwent a repair of the sternal head of the pectoralis major repair at least 6 months postoperatively. Sixteen sustained the injury while bench pressing. The average pre-injury bench press of 318 lb (range, 145-525 lb) was restored to an average of 264 lb (range, 100-500 lb) at follow-up. The average preoperative Penn Shoulder Score

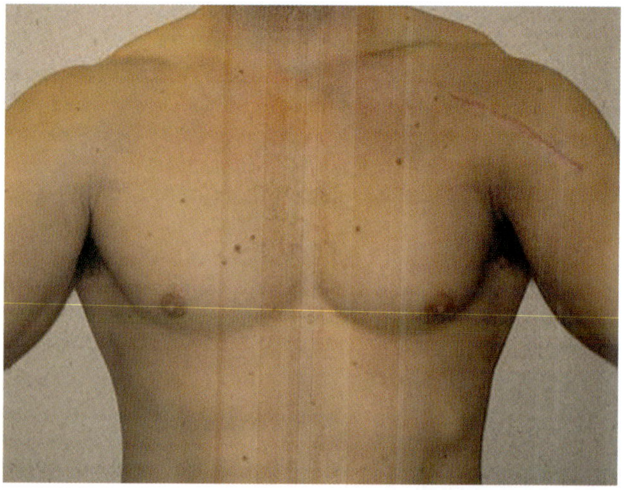

FIGURE 51-7 Final pectoralis major repair shows the healed incision and the restoration of the axillary fold. (Reproduced with permission from Provencher et al,[12] Fig. 9.)

was 60 points (range, 33-77 points), improving to 94 points (range, 64-100 points) at last follow-up. The average postoperative ASES and SANE scores were 96 points (range, 60-100 points) and 93 points (range, 50-100 points), respectively.

REFERENCES

1. Wolfe SW, Wickiewicz TL, Cavanaugh JT. Ruptures of the pectoralis major muscle. An anatomic and clinical analysis. *Am J Sports Med.* 1992;20(5):587–593.
2. Ulmer TW, Simonian PT. Muscle ruptures affecting the shoulder girdle. In: Rockwood CA, Matsen FA, III, Wirth MA, Lippitt SB, eds. *The Shoulder*. 4th ed. Philadelphia, PA: Saunders Elsevier; 2009.
3. Ianotti JP, Williams GR. *Disorders of the Shoulder: Diagnosis and Management*. Philadelphia: Lippincott Williams & Wilkins; 1999.
4. ElMaraghy AW, Devereaux MW. A systematic review and comprehensive classification of pectoralis major tears. *J Shoulder Elbow Surg.* 2012;21(3):412–422.
5. Carey P, Owens BD. Insertional footprint anatomy of the pectoralis major tendon. *Orthopedics*. 2010;33(1):23.
6. Lee J, Brookenthal KR, Ramsey ML, Kneeland JB, Herzog R. MR imaging assessment of the pectoralis major myotendinous unit: an MR imaging-anatomic correlative study with surgical correlation. *AJR Am J Roentgenol.* 2000;174(5):1371–1375.
7. Fung L, Wong B, Ravichandiran K, Agur A, Rindlisbacher T, Elmaraghy A. Three-dimensional study of pectoralis major muscle and tendon architecture. *Clin Anat.* 2009;22(4):500–508.
8. Aszmann OC, Rab M, Kamolz L, Frey M. The anatomy of the pectoral nerves and their significance in brachial plexus reconstruction. *J Hand Surg Am.* 2000;25(5):942–947.
9. Candiani P, Campigliq GL, Quattrone P, Lovaria A. Computerized angiographic study of the vascular supply of the pectoralis major muscle. *Acta Chir Plast.* 1991;33(4):185–193.
10. Guettler JH, Basamania CJ. Muscle transfers involving the shoulder. *J Surg Orthop Adv.* 2006;15(1):27–37.
11. Mosconi T, Kamath S. Bilateral asymmetric deficiency of the pectoralis major muscle. *Clin Anat.* 2003;16(4):346–349.
12. Provencher MT, Handfield K, Boniquit NT, Reiff SN, Sekiya JK, Romeo AA. Injuries to the pectoralis major muscle: diagnosis and management. *Am J Sports Med.* 2010;38(8):1693–1705.
13. Gautschi OP, Zellweger R. A complete tear of the pectoralis major muscle from a seat belt injury. *Eur J Emerg Med.* 2007;14(2):90–91.
14. de Castro Pochini A, Ejnisman B, Andreoli CV, et al. Pectoralis major muscle rupture in athletes: a prospective study. *Am J Sports Med.* 2010;38(1):92–98.
15. Antosh IJ, Grassbaugh JA, Parada SA, Arrington ED. Pectoralis major tendon repairs in the active-duty population. *Am J Orthop.* 2009;38(1):26–30.
16. Potter BK, Lehman RA Jr, Doukas WC. Pectoralis major ruptures. *Am J Orthop*. 2006;35(4):189–195.
17. Griffiths GP, Selesnick FH. Rupture of the pectoralis major muscle: diagnosis and treatment. *Phys Sportsmed.* 1997;25(8):119–125.
18. McEntire JE, Hess WE, Coleman SS. Rupture of the pectoralis major muscle. A report of eleven injuries and review of fifty-six. *J Bone Joint Surg Am.* 1972;54(5):1040–1046.
19. Valeriote J, Purchase RJ, Kelly JD. Simultaneous bilateral pectoralis major muscle rupture. *Am J Orthop.* 2005;34(6):301–302.
20. Potter BK, Lehman RA Jr, Doukas WC. Simultaneous bilateral rupture of the pectoralis major tendon. A case report. *J Bone Joint Surg Am.* 2004;86-A(7):1519–1521.
21. Butcher JD, Siekanowicz A, Pettrone F. Pectoralis major rupture: ensuring accurate diagnosis and effective rehabilitation. *Phys Sportsmed.* 1996;24(3):37–44.
22. El-Essawy MT, Al-Jassir FF, Al-Nakshabandi NA. Magnetic resonance imaging assessment of the pectoralis major muscle rupture. *Saudi Med J.* 2010;31(8):937–938.
23. Garrigues GE, Kraeutler MJ, Gillespie RJ, O'Brien DF, Lazarus MD. Repair of pectoralis major ruptures: single-surgeon case series. *Orthopedics.* 2012;35(8):e1184–e1190.
24. Aarimaa V, Rantanen J, Heikkilä J, Helttula I, Orava S. Rupture of the pectoralis major muscle. *Am J Sports Med.* 2004;32(5):1256–1262.
25. Fleury AM, Silva AC, de Castro Pochini A, Ejnisman B, Lira CA, Andrade Mdos S. Isokinetic muscle assessment after treatment of pectoralis major muscle rupture using surgical or non-surgical procedures. *Clinics (Sao Paulo).* 2011;66(2):313–320.
26. Bak K, Cameron EA, Henderson IJ. Rupture of the pectoralis major: a meta-analysis of 112 cases. *Knee Surg Sports Traumatol Arthrosc.* 2000;8(2):113–119.
27. Hanna CM, Glenny AB, Stanley SN, Caughey MA. Pectoralis major tears: comparison of surgical and conservative treatment. *Br J Sports Med.* 2001;35(3):202–206.
28. Dodds SD, Wolfe SW. Injuries to the pectoralis major. *Sports Med.* 2002;32(14):945–952.
29. Beloosesky Y, Grinblat J, Weiss A, Rosenberg PH, Weisbort M, Hendel D. Pectoralis major rupture in elderly patients: a clinical study of 13 patients. *Clin Orthop Relat Res.* 2003;(413):164–169.
30. Beloosesky Y, Hendel D, Weiss A, Rosenberg PH, Grinblat J. Rupture of the pectoralis major muscle in nursing home residents. *Am J Med.* 2001;111(3):233–235.
31. Goriganti MR, Bodack MP, Nagler W. Pectoralis major rupture during gait training: case report. *Arch Phys Med Rehabil.* 1999;80(1):115–117.
32. Cooper DE, O'Brien SJ, Warren RF. Supporting layers of the glenohumeral joint. An anatomic study. *Clin Orthop Relat Res.* 1993;(289):144–155.
33. Kingsley DM. Rupture of the pectoralis major. *J Bone Joint Surg Am.* 1946;28:644.
34. Butters AG. Traumatic rupture of the pectoralis major. *Br Med J.* 1941;2(4218):652–653.
35. Kretzler HH Jr, Richardson AB. Rupture of the pectoralis major muscle. *Am J Sports Med.* 1989;17(4):453–458.
36. Schepsis AA, Grafe MW, Jones HP, Lemos MJ. Rupture of the pectoralis major muscle. Outcome after repair of acute and chronic injuries. *Am J Sports Med.* 2000;28(1):9–15.
37. Bakalim G. Rupture of the pectoralis major muscle. A case report. *Acta Orthop Scand.* 1965;36(3):274–279.
38. Park JY, Espiniella JL. Rupture of pectoralis major muscle. A case report and review of literature. *J Bone Joint Surg Am.* 1970;52(3):577–581.
39. Mackenzie DB. Avulsion of the insertion of the pectoralis major muscle. A case report. *S Afr Med J.* 1981;60(4):147–148.
40. Egan TM, Hall H. Avulsion of the pectoralis major tendon in a weight lifter: repair using a barbed staple. *Can J Surg.* 1987;30(6):434–435.
41. Alho A. Ruptured pectoralis major tendon. A case report on delayed repair with muscle advancement. *Acta Orthop Scand.* 1994;65(6):652–653.
42. Arciero RA, Cruser DL. Pectoralis major rupture with simultaneous anterior dislocation of the shoulder. *J Shoulder Elbow Surg.* 1997;6(3):318–320.
43. Anbari A, Kelly JD 4th, Moyer RA. Delayed repair of a ruptured pectoralis major muscle. A case report. *Am J Sports Med.* 2000;28(2):254–256.
44. WarmeWJ, Whitaker DC. Pectoralis major tendon avulsion from rappelling. *Mil Med.* 2004;169(2):151–154.
45. Connell DA, Potter HG, Sherman MF, Wickiewicz TL. Injuries of the pectoralis major muscle: evaluation with MR imaging. *Radiology.* 1999;210(3):785–791.
46. Silverstein JA, Goldberg B, Wolin P. Proximal humerus shaft fracture after pectoralis major tendon rupture repair. *Orthopedics.* 2011;34(6):222.
47. He ZM, Ao YF, Wang JQ, Hu YL, Yin Y. Twelve cases of the pectoralis major muscle tendon rupture with surgical treatment—an average of 6.7-year follow-up. *Chin Med J (Engl).* 2010;123(1):57–60.
48. Hasegawa K, Schofer JM. Rupture of the pectoralis major: a case report and review. *J Emerg Med.* 2010;38(2):196–200.
49. Metzger PD, Bailey JR, Filler RD, Waltz RA, Provencher MT, Dewing CB. Pectoralis major muscle rupture repair: technique using unicortical buttons. *Arthrosc Tech.* 2012;1(1):e119–e125.
50. Petilon J, Carr DR, Sekiya JK, Unger DV. Pectoralis major muscle injuries: evaluation and management. *J Am Acad Orthop Surg.* 2005;13(1):59–68.
51. Kakwani RG, Matthews JJ, Kumar KM, Pimpalnerkar A, Mohtadi N. Rupture of the pectoralis major muscle: surgical treatment in athletes. *Int Orthop.* 2007;31(2):159–163.

52

Soft Tissue Coverage of the Shoulder

Angela Cheng, MD
Michel Saint-Cyr, MD, FRCS

INTRODUCTION

The shoulder and axillary region is a mobile area that requires durable skin flap coverage. Skin grafts often become adherent and can result in scar contractures that restrict mobility. The shoulder is also a cosmetically sensitive area that tends to be exposed and grafts can be unsightly. The ideal reconstruction is a well-contoured cutaneous flap with similar thickness to the native tissue.

Soft tissue shoulder coverage may be necessary for exposed hardware or critical structures (nerve, joint, bone, or tendon) or defects resulting from trauma, burns, infection, chronic wounds, radiation, or oncologic resection. The reconstructive options include locoregional flaps such as a pedicled flap from the torso, a reversed arm flap, and the deltoid flap or free tissue transfer. There are many regional options that need to be assessed in terms of the vascular supply and whether they have been damaged by trauma, radiation, vascular disease, or prior surgical intervention. Pedicle perforator flaps play a substantial role in reconstructing various defects in the shoulder and clavicular regions. Larger defects may require free tissue transfer and the anterior and posterior circumflex humeral vessels are commonly used recipient vessels. Computed tomographic angiography (CTA) may be helpful to identify perforator flaps or targets for free tissue transfer. The appropriate treatment option should be selected based on the defect etiology, location and size of the defect, comorbidities of the patient, and any relative/absolute contraindications.

REGIONAL FLAPS FROM THE TORSO

The regional flap options based on the posterior torso include the scapular or parascapular flap, the thoracodorsal artery perforator (TDAP) flap, muscle-sparing latissimus dorsi (msLD) or full latissimus dorsi (LD), and the trapezius flap. Each of these can provide large skin flaps with a donor site that can be closed primarily.

The scapular or parascapular flap can be harvested from the transverse and descending branches of the circumflex scapular artery that travels through the quadrangular space as defined by the triceps, teres minor, teres major muscles, and lateral scapular border. The maximal pedicle can be obtained by dissection to the origin at the subscapular artery for a length of 10 to 12 cm and a diameter of 4 mm. The scapular flap is supplied by the *transverse* branch (diameter 0.8-1.4 mm) that travels 5 to 6 cm superior and parallel to the cephalic border of the LD muscle for a pedicle length of 4 to 9 cm.[1] The parascapular flap is based on the *descending* branch that courses 6 to 8 cm medially and parallel to the lateral border of the LD muscle for a length of 3 to 7 cm and diameter of 0.8 to 1.4 mm.[2] Both flaps are drained via their respective venae comitantes and provide large skin paddles without donor-site functional morbidity. However, large flaps may require skin graft coverage of donor site unless preexpanded.

The flaps are harvested with the patient preferably in lateral decubitus and the arm fully prepped. The patient is typically under general anesthesia, but, if necessary, the procedure can be performed with sedation and local anesthetic infiltration. The quadrangular space is palpated and marked along with the origin of the circumflex scapular artery. If a scapular flap is planned, a line parallel to the superior border of the latissimus is drawn along the course of the artery extending from the posterior axillary line up to the contralateral scapula. For the parascapular flap, the arm is adducted; the flap is designed to be parallel to the lateral border of the scapula extending from the axillary crease to the 12th rib if needed. For an extended scapular flap, both branches are incorporated to maximize the amount of soft tissue that can be included in the flap for larger defects. The flap can include the teres minor, a portion of the infraspinatus, or even the subscapularis muscle. The typical dimensions of the scapular flap include a length of 18 to 20 cm, a width of 7 to 8 cm (maximal ~8 cm for primary closure), and a thickness of 2 cm, but it can be thinned down to the superficial fascia for a thickness of 8 to 9 mm.[3] The parascapular flap has similar sizes with a length of 26 cm, a width of 12 cm (maximal 10 cm for primary closure), and a thickness of 2 cm. The flap is harvested distal to proximal above the deep fascia, taking care to identify and prevent injury to the pedicle at the superior border of the teres major. For a pedicled flap, the dissection is then completed cephalad to caudal to expose the teres minor muscle and the vessels. The teres major muscle can be divided to extend the arc of rotation to reach the anterior chest. For a free flap, further length is obtained by releasing small arterial branches inside the quadrangular space to reach the subscapular artery. Delayed harvest can be used for very large flaps and the adjacent tissue can be preexpanded to permit primary closure.

The pedicled TDAP flap can cover ipsilateral defects as far distally as the elbow and distal one third of the upper arm, as well as the shoulder, neck, and upper back taking care to avoid excessive tension, compression, or kinking of the pedicle and/or perforator. The thoracodorsal artery (TDA) divides into a transverse and descending branch. The TDAP flap is primarily based on perforators arising from the descending branch since there are no perforators from the transverse branch in ~33%. The skin paddle dimension is determined by the defect and the maximal tension of the donor-site skin with an average of 11 × 25 cm but can be up to 13 × 32 cm and oriented transverse, oblique, or vertically. Primary closure is obtainable if the width is <10 cm. The pedicle is 10 to 19 cm long and 2 to 3 mm in diameter and the lateral thoracic vein can be included for extravenous outflow[4] (Fig. 52-1). The angular artery and the periosteal perforators supplying the bone and the tip of the scapula are not included in order to preserve the insertion of the serratus muscle and prevent winging. Preoperatively, the anterior border of the LD muscle is identified by having the patient forcefully adduct the upper extremity and contract the LD muscle. The flap border is marked 1 cm anterior to this point. The scapular tip and posterior axillary fold are also marked. A sterile Doppler probe is used to map the lateral perforators at ~6 to 12 cm below the posterior axillary fold and 1 to 3 cm inside the lateral free muscle border. The medial perforators are found within a 3.5-cm circumference centered at the tip of the scapular angle. The most dominant and proximal perforator will usually be found along the course of the descending branch of the TDA, which is usually 8 cm below the posterior axillary fold and 2 cm medial to the lateral border of the LD muscle. The second landmark is 4 cm below the scapular tip and 2.5 cm behind the lateral border of the LD muscle, which represents the location of the thoracodorsal neurovascular hilum. A 2-team approach is used with simultaneous flap harvest and recipient vessel preparation using loupe magnification when possible. Microsurgical instruments are needed for the anastomosis. A pinch test determines the maximal skin paddle width while permitting primary closure. The skin paddle is designed either transversely along natural resting tension lines of the upper back or obliquely following the main axis of the LD muscle fibers. The anterior border of the flap must be placed well anterior to the anterior border of the LD muscle in order to include as many potential perforators within the flap such as the descending branch of the TDA and direct cutaneous or septocutaneous branches that course along the anterior border of the LD muscle. The patient is placed in the lateral decubitus position with the arm positioned in extension and abduction on a sterile Mayo stand. The initial skin incision is anterior or lateral.

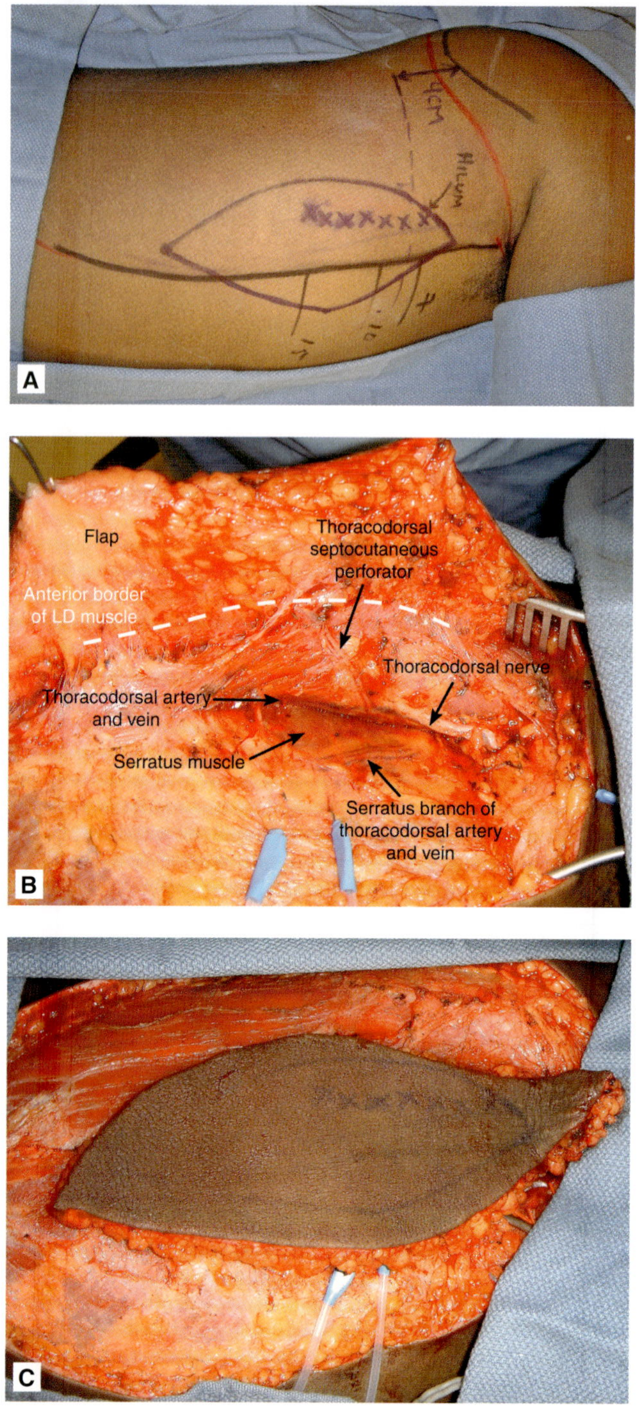

FIGURE 52-1 **A.** A patient in lateral decubitus demonstrating preoperative flap markings. **B.** Intraoperative view of dissection and anatomic landmarks. **C.** Harvested flap in situ prior to transfer.

Adjustments are made in the skin paddle design once the anterior border of the LD muscle is identified, which is always more anterior than anticipated by exam. The flap is harvested from lateral to medial in a suprafascial plane. A sensate flap can be harvested by including the posterior ramus of the lateral cutaneous branch of the intercostal nerve that is traced anteriorly between the slips of the serratus anterior muscle. Care is taken to not injure the anterior rami in order to preserve sensation to the anterior chest wall skin. The dissection proceeds anterior to posterior to avoid missing a direct cutaneous branch of the TDA or a septocutaneous perforator running along the anterior border of the LD muscle. If no cutaneous anterior perforators are encountered, then the dissection proceeds posteriorly toward the descending and transverse branches of the TDA in order to identify any suitable perforator(s). The anterior border of the LD muscle is elevated in order to identify the TDA pedicle that is traced until it enters the LD muscle, identifying any perforators within the fatty layers. The selected perforator must have a loud signal on Doppler and strong pulsation to both inspection and palpation. The Doppler is also used to confirm adequate venous outflow. If there are inadequate perforators, the flap can easily be converted to a msLD flap. The motor branches of the thoracodorsal nerve that lie deep to either the descending or transverse branches of the TDA are preserved. If the flap length is ≥20 cm, a second perforator can be included from either the descending or transverse branches of the TDA. A more distal perforator will provide better perfusion to the distal portion of the flap as compared with a more proximal one. The skin paddle axis is centered so that the perforators are within the longitudinal axis of the flap. In smaller flaps, an eccentrically placed perforator will still provide adequate perfusion. Dissection stops at the TDA and its venae comitantes or when an adequate pedicle length and vessel diameter for a microvascular anastomosis has been reached.

If adequate perforators are not located or inadvertently injured during dissection, the flap can be converted to a msLD flap with nearly identical skin paddle limits. The muscle cuff around the pedicle is typically 3 to 4 cm but can be up to 8 × 15 cm for a large defect. The descending branch of the TDA is approximately 15 cm long (range: 13-19).[5] The anterior border of the LD muscle is elevated, and the descending branch is dissected back to its origin (the bifurcation of the TDA), preserving the transverse branch. The thoracodorsal nerve is exposed, sparing the transverse branch to prevent denervation of the remaining LD muscle and ligating the descending branch. The muscle is divided 1 cm medial to the pedicle and split vertically along the fiber orientation. A cuff of muscle is harvested at the entrance of the descending branch into the LD muscle in order to capture as many perforating vessels. For a pedicled flap, the transverse branch can be divided to increase the arc of rotation. A case example is shown in Figure 52-2. For larger defects, the entire latissimus can be harvested using a cautery to detach the muscle fibers inferiorly and along midline, taking care to preserve the erector spinae muscles and lumbar fascia. This can then be rotated as a pedicled flap with or without a skin paddle as needed (Figs. 52-3 and 52-4).

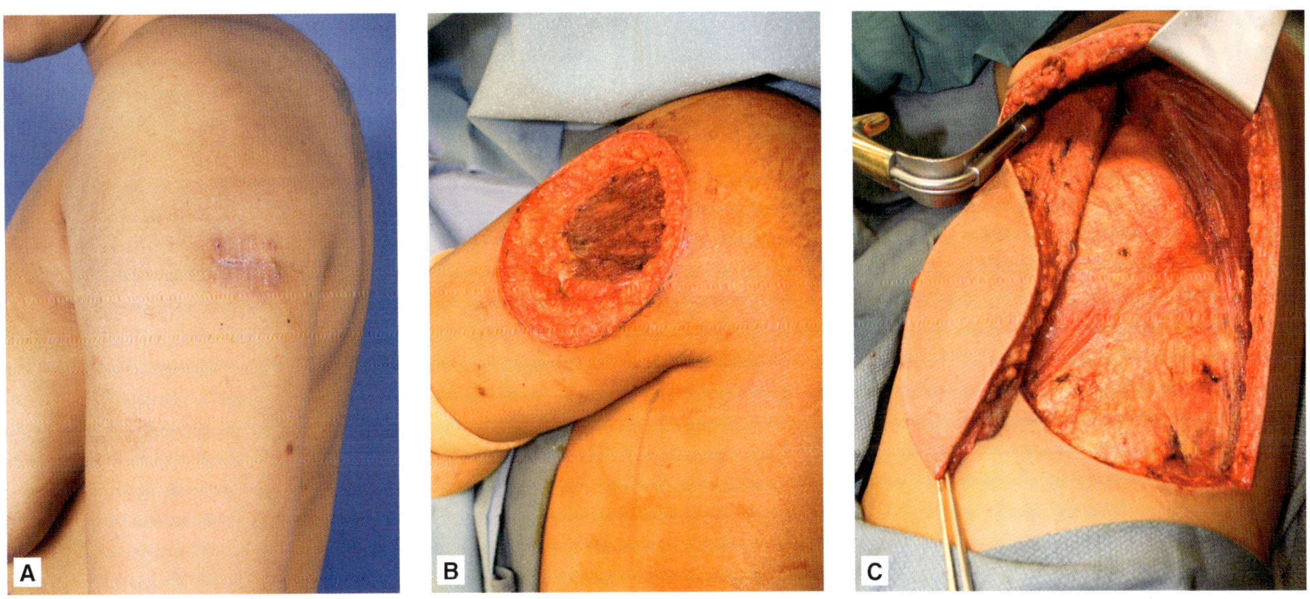

FIGURE 52-2 Case example of reconstruction of left upper arm/shoulder sarcoma defect with a pedicled descending branch muscle-sparing latissimus dorsi flap. **A.** Preoperative view of left upper arm sarcoma lesion. **B.** Intraoperative left upper arm defect following sarcoma resection. **C.** When perforators for a TDAP flap are not available or suitable, the flap can be converted to a muscle-sparing LD flap, based on either the descending or transverse branch of the thoracodorsal artery.

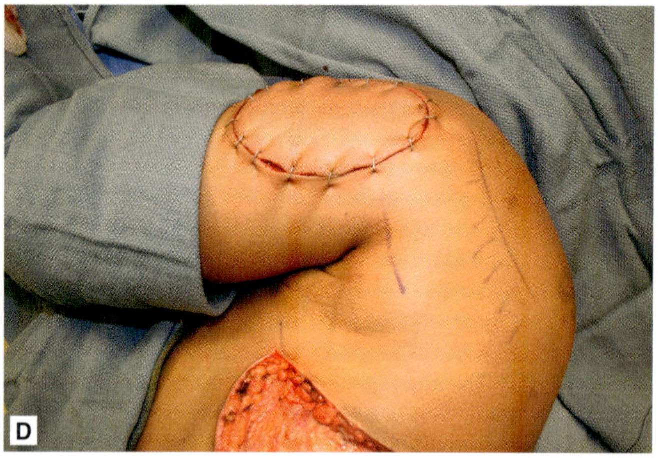

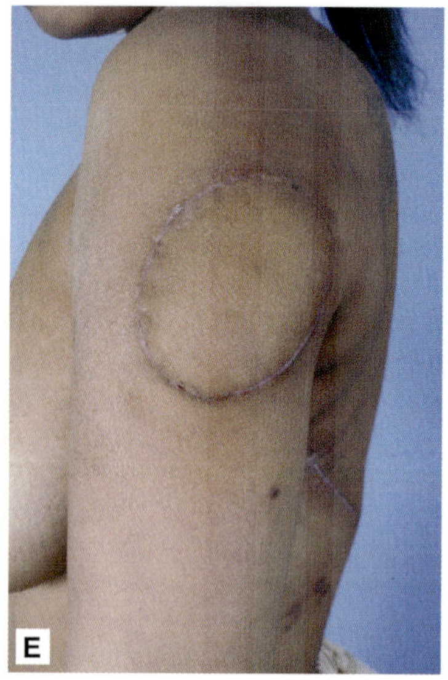

FIGURE 52-2 (*Continued*) **D.** The flap is easily rotated to the arm and shoulder to provide soft tissue coverage. **E.** Postoperative view at 6 months.

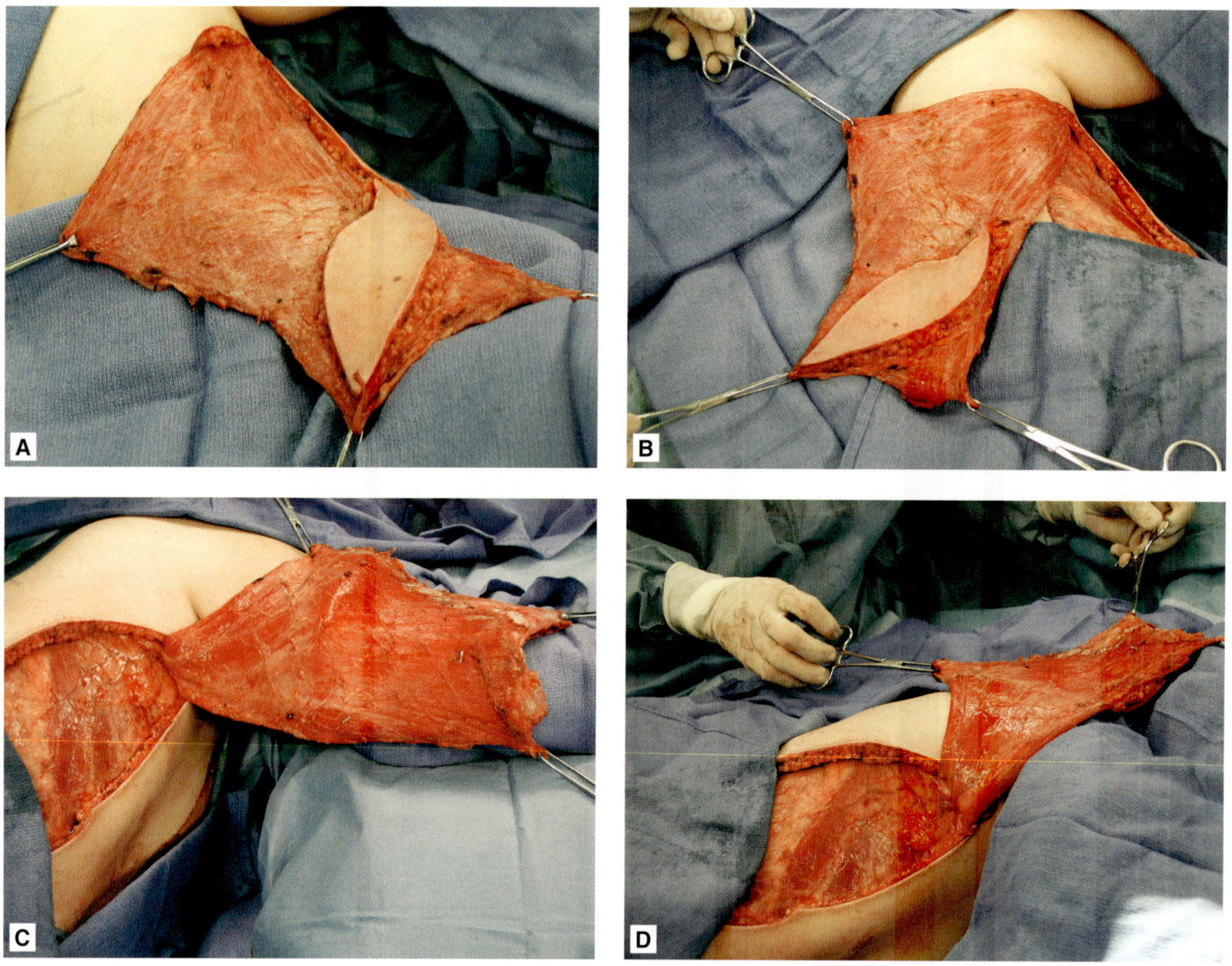

FIGURE 52-3 Intraoperative dissection of full latissimus dorsi flap. **A.** The flap is elevated with skin paddle and released medially and inferiorly. **B.** The flap is then released laterally to mobilize completely. **C.** The flap can provide a large area of coverage of either the lateral arm or shoulder (**D**).

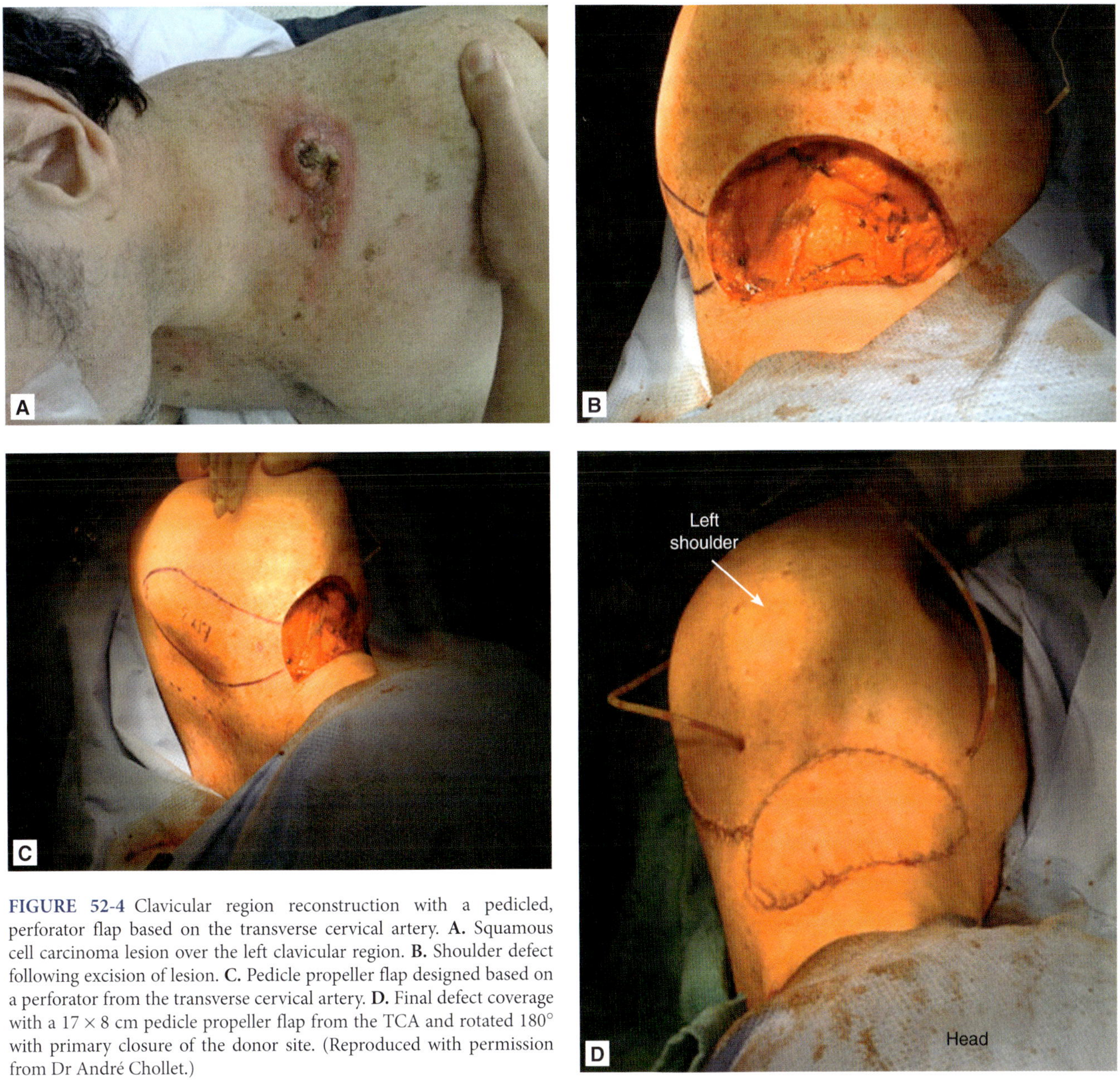

FIGURE 52-4 Clavicular region reconstruction with a pedicled, perforator flap based on the transverse cervical artery. **A.** Squamous cell carcinoma lesion over the left clavicular region. **B.** Shoulder defect following excision of lesion. **C.** Pedicle propeller flap designed based on a perforator from the transverse cervical artery. **D.** Final defect coverage with a 17 × 8 cm pedicle propeller flap from the TCA and rotated 180° with primary closure of the donor site. (Reproduced with permission from Dr André Chollet.)

Superficial Cervical Artery Flaps

The trapezius muscle is supplied by several different pedicles, the occipital artery, the superficial cervical artery (SCA), the deep branch or dorsal scapular artery (DSA), and the intercostal arteries. The trapezius has 3 parts (descending, transverse, and ascending) of which only the latter 2, based on the SCA and DSA, respectively, should be utilized to ensure shoulder function is preserved. The SCA further divides into ascending and descending branches and despite several variations in the branching patterns consistently supplies the lower trapezius muscle. The trapezius flap is drained via the SCA venae comitantes that have a variable pattern that can limit the rotation for a pedicled flap. A flap based on the SCA can be partially innervated by branches of the cervical plexus. A small segment of the scapular spine can be included, but the lateral 2 cm of the acromion must be preserved.

Preoperative markings are performed with the patient in an upright position with arms adducted to identify the scapular borders, scapular spine, acromion, posterior median, rhomboid muscles, and trapezius muscle. A Doppler probe is useful to identify and mark the course of the DSA. The flap is commonly harvested with a cuff of muscle to protect the pedicle. Both the SCA and DSA can be included to maximize perfusion, but this increases the donor-site morbidity and limits the arc of rotation. For the SCA, the skin paddle can be oriented either vertically or transversely, but the DSA flap is typically vertically oriented with a thickness of 2.5 cm.

The maximal dimensions are limited by the orientation and pedicle choice, but an 8 × 6 cm defect can be closed primarily. The patient should be under general anesthesia in either the lateral decubitus or prone position with the arm free to mobilize the scapula during the dissection.

Deltopectoral Flap

The regional skin flap options on the anterior torso are more limited. The vascular basis of the thoracoacromial artery perforator and lateral thoracic perforator flaps has been described.[6,7] However, the vascularity of this region is quite variable and caution should be exercised in harvesting these flaps. The pectoralis major muscle has a clavicular and sternocostal head supplied by the clavicular and pectoral branches of the thoracoacromial artery, respectively, as well as minor branches from the lateral thoracic, internal mammary, and intercostal arteries. The venous drainage is primarily through venae comitantes and secondary venules from the periphery. The donor-site defect can result in a distorted breast contour and functional deficits if the entire muscle is harvested. The flap may be bulky in obese patients or women with abundant overlying breast tissue for which a muscle-only flap should be considered. The patients should be carefully examined for previous chest scars as well as for the presence of the pectoralis muscle. The axis of the pedicle is marked with a line from the acromion to the xiphoid and the skin island is placed at the appropriate distance to reach the defect. Perforators are more abundant laterally that can be verified with Doppler. The skin paddle size correlates with the defect adding 10% for skin retraction after harvest. An 8 × 10 cm skin paddle can be harvested with primary closure of the donor site (thickness of 1.4 cm). The incision is extended laterally and parallel to the clavicle to preserve the deltopectoral flap territory. The skin island is incised, and then the flap is elevated laterally to identify the pectoralis muscle border that is released off the chest wall. The pedicle is identified medial to the pectoralis minor along the underside of the pectoralis major muscle that is then detached from the chest and humerus. Division of the clavicular head of the pectoralis may reduce the bulge and improve the maximal reach of the flap during insetting.

REGIONAL FLAPS FROM THE ARM

The regional flap options for shoulder and axillary reconstruction that can be harvested from the arm include the deltoid flap (posterior circumflex humeral artery), the lateral arm flap, the medial arm flap, and the posterior arm flap (perforating branch of the brachial artery).

The deltoid flap supplied by the posterior circumflex humeral artery is a reliable flap that can be used as a pedicled flap for regional reconstruction. The artery arises from the axillary or brachial artery and runs posteriorly, deep to the deltoid muscle, to anastomose with the anterior circumflex humeral artery. The posterior circumflex humeral artery supplies the deltoid muscle and overlying skin through musculocutaneous perforators. The cutaneous perforators emerge from the posterior border of the muscle and supply the skin over the posterior aspect of the shoulder. The cutaneous branch runs superiorly between the lateral head of the triceps and deltoid muscles. The deltoid flap is a reliable, well-vascularized flap. However, it tends to leave a poor donor-site scar, particularly if skin grafting is required.

The lateral arm flap can also be useful for upper arm and shoulder reconstruction. This flap is harvested based on the posterior radial collateral artery that is 6 cm in length and drainage is through the associated venae comitantes and possibly the cephalic vein if included. A preoperative evaluation for prior trauma to the humerus or previous surgical scars is critical to rule out injury to the pedicle. Imaging studies such as Doppler, angiography, or a CT angiogram (CTA) may be appropriate especially in trauma patients. The flap can be harvested with the patient in either the supine or prone position under a general anesthetic or axillary block. The skin island is centered over a line between the deltoid insertion and the lateral epicondyle. It is designed to suit the defect but can be extended distally up to 12 to 15 cm beyond the epicondyle. There is minimal donor-site morbidity and defects up to 6 to 8 cm wide can be closed primarily. Typically this is a fasciocutaneous flap, but a portion of the triceps, brachialis, or brachioradialis muscle can be included to fill deep defects. Under tourniquet control, the incision is started posteriorly and extended under the deep fascia identifying the intermuscular septum and exposing the lateral head of the triceps muscle. The dissection proceeds anteriorly to identify the perforators and expose the brachialis and brachioradialis muscles. The septum is released from the elbow to the level of the deltoid insertion. Z-plasties can be useful to avoid linear scars over the donor site near the elbow. The flap can be pedicled or harvested as a free flap, but the vessels are small (1.5 mm); they must be divided proximal to the branching of the anterior and posterior radial collateral arteries and should be marked to distinguish the artery from vein.

The medial arm flap is based on the perforator of the superior ulnar collateral artery. The flap is designed along the medial inner aspect of the arm. The perforator emerges approximately halfway along a line drawn from the anterior axillary fold to the medial epicondyle of the humerus. Medial arm flaps may be pedicled proximally or distally and may be useful for axillary reconstruction or further reconstruction of adjacent soft tissue defects. The skin is thin and pliable and the donor-site scar is excellent. The flap can be raised as a free flap as well; however, the pedicle is quite short (1-2 cm) and inconsistent. Of a historical note, this flap was originally used for cross-arm flaps. The vascular anatomy is variable and the main or dominant perforator in the region may arise from the superior ulnar collateral artery, directly from the brachial artery, or from a muscular branch to the biceps muscle.

The posterior arm flap is a useful flap based on the posterior perforator of the brachial artery, which has been described by Masquelet et al.[8] The artery supplying the flap arises from the brachial artery in 75% of cases, and from the profunda brachial artery in 25% of cases. The pedicle length is 4 to 5 cm and the diameter of the vessel at its origin is 1.5 mm. The vessel arises from the brachial artery and passes posteriorly, piercing the fibrous arcade between the long head of triceps muscle and the lateral edge of the teres major tendons. The flap may be either used as a pedicled flap for axillary reconstruction or harvested as a free flap. The flap may be harvested as an innervated flap with a branch of the radial nerve, the medial cutaneous nerve of the arm.

FREE TISSUE TRANSFER

When the soft tissue defect in the shoulder or upper arm area is particularly large, or if suitable regional skin flaps are not available, then harvest of a distant free tissue transfer becomes necessary. There are a wide variety of options depending on factors such as the size of the defect, the degree of adiposity in the patient, and the available recipient vessels. Traditional flaps such as anterior lateral thigh or radial forearm, as well as a variety of perforator flaps, can be considered based on the patient's body habitus and other comorbidities. The lateral circumflex femoral artery perforator flap (descending branch of lateral circumflex femoral artery) is a particularly useful flap for upper limb reconstruction. It is generally fairly thin and has a long pedicle length. The donor site can be closed primarily and harvest of the flap from the lower extremity allows 2 teams to operate independently. Similarly, the medial circumflex femoral artery perforator flap allows a 2-team approach with a similarly reliable flap. For particularly massive wounds, a deep inferior epigastric artery perforator flap allows the harvest and transfer of a large segment of tissue. However, the main drawback is that the tissue is usually quite bulky, which may not contour well over the shoulder area where thin skin coverage is usually required. As in other applications of microsurgery, individualized selection of the donor site provides optimal reconstruction.

REFERENCES

1. Gilbert A, Teot L. The free scapulars flap. *Plast Reconstr Surg.* 1982;69:601–604.
2. Nassif TM, Vidal L, Bovet JL, Baudet J. The parascapular flap: a new cutaneous microsurgical free flap. *Plast Reconstr Surg.* 1982;69:591–600.
3. Hamilton SG, Morrison WA. The scapular free flap. *Br J Plast Surg.* 1982;35:2–7.
4. Guerra AB, Metzinger SE, Lund KM, Cooper MM, Allen RJ, Dupin CL. The thoracodorsal artery perforator flap: clinical experience and anatomic study with emphasis on harvest techniques. *Plast Reconstr Surg.* 2004;114:32–41.
5. Colohan S, Wong C, Lakhiani C, et al. The free descending branch muscle-sparing latissimus dorsi flap: vascular anatomy and clinical applications. *Plast Reconstr Surg.* 2012;130:776e–787e.
6. Rikimaru H, Kiyokawa K, Inoue Y, Tai Y. Three-dimensional anatomical vascular distribution in the pectoralis major myocutaneous flap. *Plast Reconstr Surg.* 2005;115:1342–1352.
7. Kim JT, Ng SW, Naidu S, Kim JD, Kim YH. Lateral thoracic perforator flap: additional perforator flap option from the lateral thoracic region. *J Plast Reconstr Aesthet Surg.* 2011;64:1596–1602.
8. Masquelet AC, Rinaldi S, Mouchet A, Gilbert A. The posterior arm free flap. *Plast Reconstr Surg.* 1985;76:908–913.

53

Nerve Entrapments—Quadrilateral Space, Supraspinatus Nerve Entrapment

Timothy R. McAdams, MD

INTRODUCTION

While the true incidence of injury to the suprascapular nerve (SSN) is unclear, over the past decade clinicians have become more aware of its existence. It has been suggested that the prevalence in overhead athletes may be between 12% and 33% and between 8% and 100% in individuals with massive rotator cuff tears.[1] The mechanism of injury may result from compression, traction, friction, repetitive microtrauma, or direct injury. The common site of injury occurs at either the suprascapular or spinoglenoid notch. Most athletes are able to return to sport following nonoperative and operative treatment despite persistent atrophy, for which recovery is variable.[2] While the natural history of injury to the SSN nerve is debatable, outcomes are likely related to the specific underling etiology.

ANATOMY

The SSN's primary function is to supply motor innervation to the supraspinatus and infraspinatus muscles of the rotator cuff. Because it has sensory branches to the joint and capsule, it can also be a pain generator in the shoulder.[3,4] Pain in the posterior and lateral aspect of the shoulder due to involvement of the cutaneous sensory branches of the SSN has also been reported in some patients with nerve injury.[5–7]

The SSN originates from the upper trunk of the brachial plexus at Erb's point where it transverses the posterior cervical triangle and moves laterally to upper border of the scapula on the floor of the suprascapular fossa (Fig. 53-1). It then travels through the suprascapular notch under the transverse scapular ligament. At the suprascapular notch the nerve lies approximately 3 cm from the supraglenoid tubercle and at the spine of the scapula 1.8 to 2.1 cm medial to the posterior glenoid rim.[8,9] As the nerve exits the suprascapular notch it sends off 1 to 2 motor branches to the supraspinatus muscle. It then enters the infraspinatus fossa by way of the spinoglenoid notch. At the spinoglenoid notch it dives under the transverse scapular ligament that can vary in its presence and then divides to provide motor branches to the infraspinatus muscle. The motor branches come off approximately 2 cm medial to the posterior glenoid rim.[9]

MECHANISM OF INJURY

Suprascapular neuropathy may occur secondary to a variety of mechanisms. Because the nerve is relatively fixed at either end (Erb's point and infraspinatus muscle), wraps around the spine of scapula, and transverses 2 so-called tunnels (suprascapular and spinoglenoid notch), it is susceptible to a traction injury. Stretching of the nerve more than 6% can cause altered motor function, while more than 15% can lead to irreversible damage.[10,11] This traction phenomenon resulting in microtrauma to the nerve may be accentuated in overhead athletes.[12] In the setting of a massively retracted rotator cuff tear up to 39% of patients may have signs of a neuropathy as demonstrated by Warner et al.[9] At the suprascapular notch the nerve may be injured by compression from the overlying transverse scapular ligament. At this level both the supraspinatus and infraspinatus muscles are affected. Anatomically, both the size of the notch and the ligament can vary between individuals.[13–16] The ligament itself may be ossified or there can be an extra ligament.[17] Direct trauma from a shoulder dislocation, a fracture involving the surrounding bones, or iatrogenic damage during an arthroscopic procedure has also been reported.[18] At the spinoglenoid notch similar patterns of injury can also occur, but space-occupying lesions such as paralabral cysts and labral tears are more commonly the culprit.[2] At this level only the infraspinatus muscle is affected.

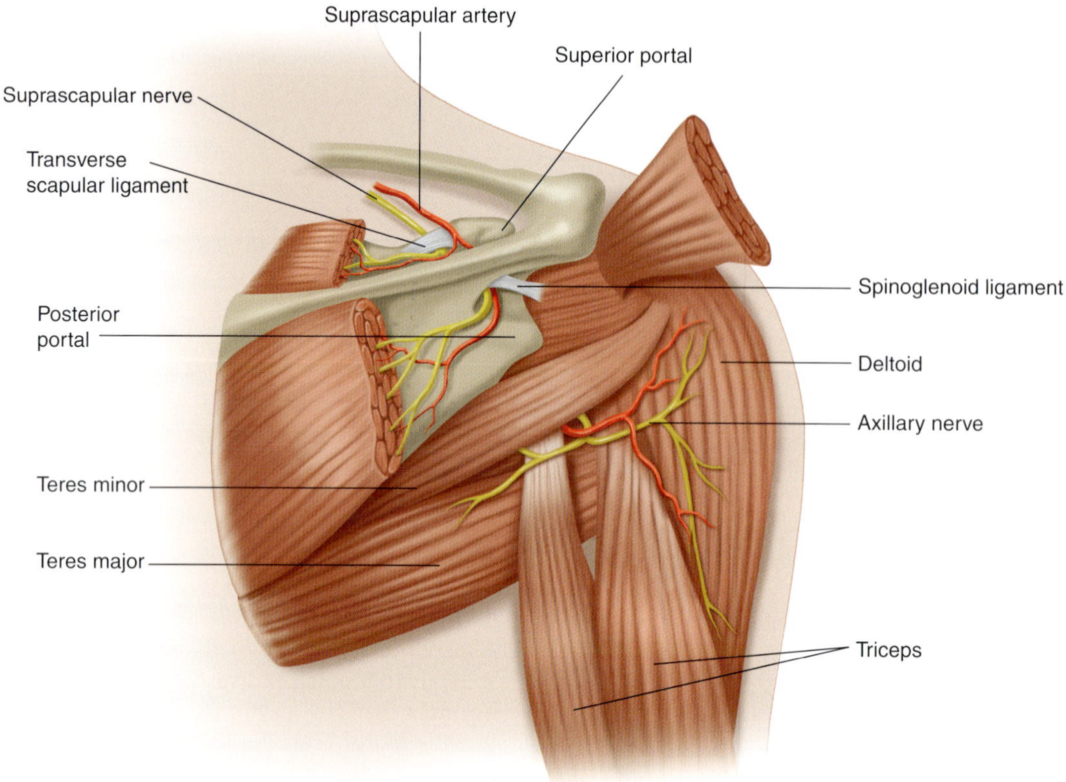

FIGURE 53-1 Anatomy of the suprascapular nerve in relation to the rotator cuff muscles and quadrilateral space, as seen from the posterior aspect of the shoulder. (Reproduced with permission from Safran.[18])

HISTORY AND PHYSICAL FINDINGS

The clinical diagnosis of SSN injury may be difficult because coexisting shoulder pathology can result in overlapping symptoms. Patients with a SSN neuropathy, most of whom are between 20 and 50 years, may present with pain, and supraspinatus and/or infraspinatus weakness and atrophy. Patients who have a more proximal level of involvement tend to present with dull, sometimes burning pain in the posterior and lateral shoulder, and a variable degree of weakness and atrophy of the supraspinatus and infraspinatus muscles. The pain may be accentuated by cross-body adduction and internal rotation that is thought to place more tension on the nerve.[13] The SSN test (Fig. 53-2) as described by Lafosse et al can be performed by laterally rotating the head away from the affected shoulder while posteriorly and inferiorly retracting the shoulder can exacerbate pain.[19] Varying degrees of scapular dyskinesis may be present. Patients who present with SSN entrapment at the level of the spinoglenoid notch may have less severe symptoms and are more likely to have varying degrees of painless wasting of infraspinatus muscle.[18] A careful evaluation for instability, labral tears, and rotator cuff pathology should be performed due to the frequent coexistence in these individuals.

Although there is no consensus for diagnostic criteria, electrophysiological studies are commonly used in the diagnosis of a SSN injury, to both establish a baseline for treatment and localize the area of entrapment. Findings include a prolonged motor latency from Erb's point to either the

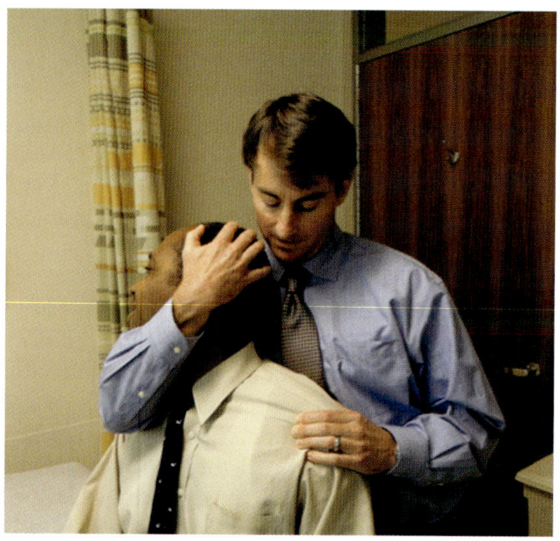

FIGURE 53-2 Suprascapular nerve compression test.

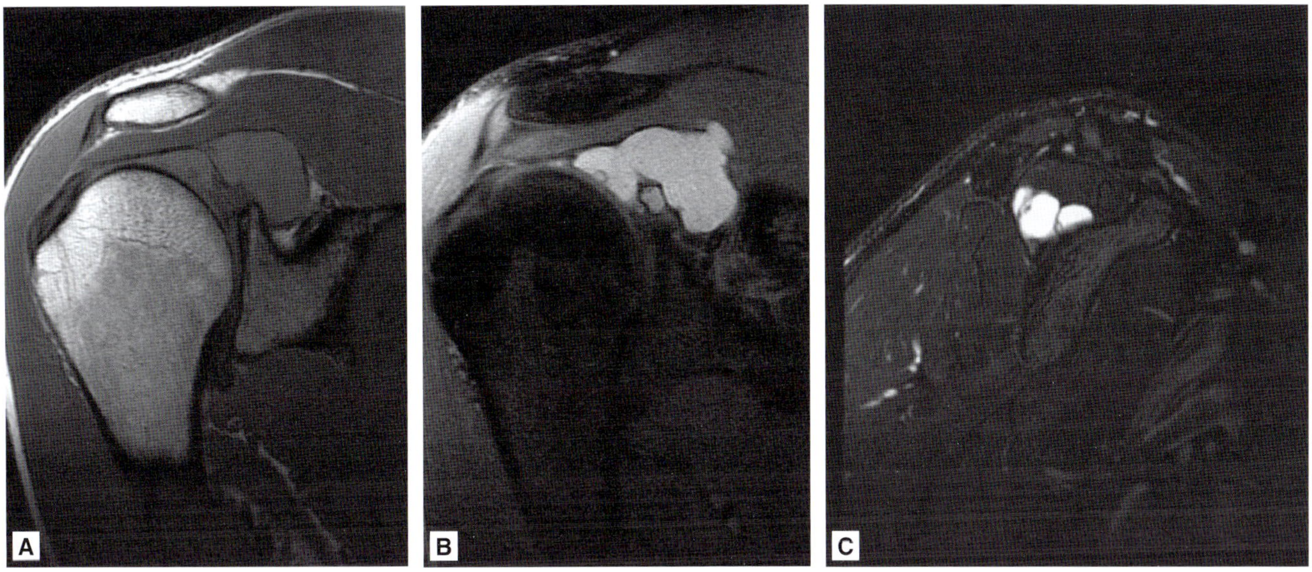

FIGURE 53-3 Coronal-oblique T1 (**A**) and T2 (**B**) and sagittal-oblique T2 (**C**) images of left shoulder paralabral cyst between the supraspinatus and infraspinatus compressing the spinoglenoid notch.

supraspinatus or infraspinatus depending on level of entrapment, and possibly denervation potentials, These studies can be normal despite SSN neuropathy as they do not detect damage to unmyelinated or thinly myelinated pain fibers and are very technique dependent.[12] Magnetic resonance imaging (MRI) can also be a very helpful diagnostic tool for discerning the degree of atrophy, the presence of edema within these muscles, the presence of space-occupying lesions, and associated rotator cuff or labral pathology[20] (Fig. 53-3A and B). Recently a report using a 3-T MRI reported that with this high-resolution scan the radiologist may be able to depict the morphologic character of the nerve with regard to alterations in caliber, contour, continuity, and signal intensity.[21] There are no studies comparing the sensitivity of electrophysiological studies with MRI and both are routinely done in clinical practice. Plain radiographs, although generally normal, may indicate a history of fracture, a small notch, or ossification of the transverse scapular ligament that can be seen on the Stryker notch view. If pain is the predominant feature, a local SSN nerve can also be used to confirm the diagnosis.[22]

SURGICAL TREATMENT

Indications: No Space-occupying Lesion

Operative management for those individuals who have no space-occupying lesion is debatable. We, and most others, proceed with operative management in those individuals who have continued pain, weakness, and/or no improvement on repeat EMG despite 6 months of conservative treatment.[18] Some feel that the patient who presents with symptoms for >6 months or evidence of atrophy warrants immediate decompression in order to avoid any possible irreversible damage.[23,24] We find it is often challenging to know the true time of onset as many "acute" atrophy changes may have been developing over a long period of time.

Space-occupying Lesion

For space-occupying lesions, which most commonly occur at the spinoglenoid notch, such as a spinoglenoid cyst, most authors recommend a more aggressive approach. The literature is consistent with the finding that up to 90% of the ganglion cysts develop in the setting of a capsulolabral tear. When this occurs, a so-called 1-way valve is established for synovial fluid.[25,26] Options for treatment include radiographic-assisted percutaneous cyst drainage, open cyst decompression, arthroscopic cyst decompression with or without labrum treatment, or nerve decompression. Percutaneous cyst drainage has been associated with a recurrence rate of approximately 50%, but is a reasonable first-line treatment option as long as there is no significant muscle atrophy.[25,27] We commonly perform image-guided aspiration using ultrasound for paralabral cysts without significant atrophy changes on MRI, especially in athletes in season, and reserve arthroscopic or open techniques if symptoms persist or the cyst recurs (Fig. 53-4A and B). Arthroscopic management has the benefit of simultaneously diagnosing and addressing intra-articular as well as any subacromial pathology with minimal morbidity. Although excellent results have been reported with open decompression, the current literature supports shoulder arthroscopy with cyst decompression and either repair or debridement of the labrum.[18,28–30]

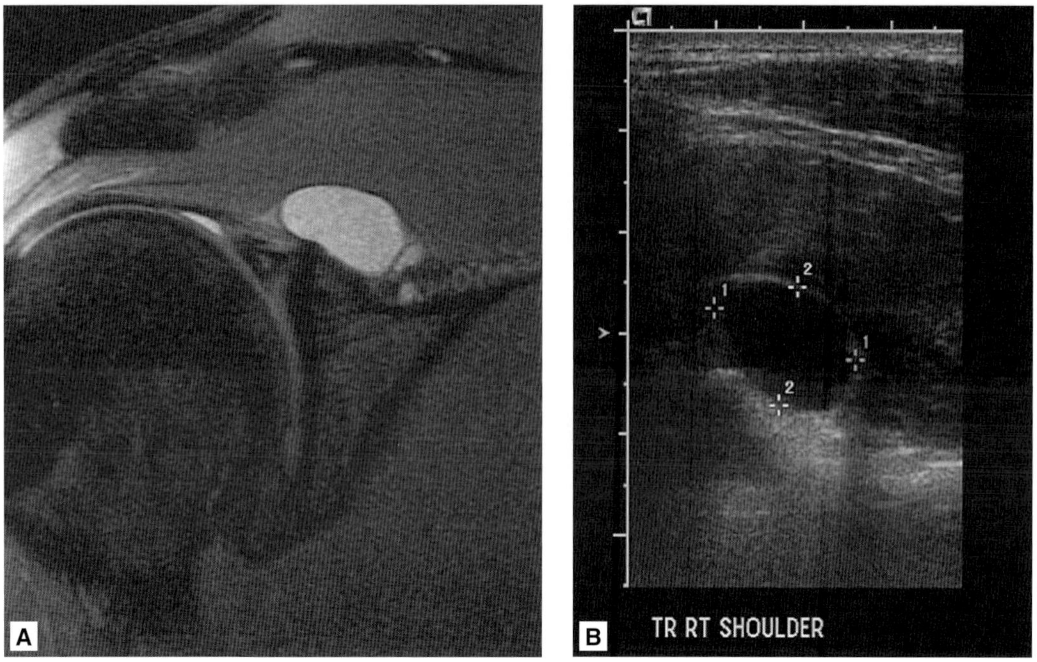

FIGURE 53-4 **A.** Coronal-oblique T2 image of paralabral cyst deep to the supraspinatus with (**B**) corresponding ultrasound image of the cyst.

CONTRAINDICATIONS

Surgery is not indicated as the initial treatment for an SSN neuropathy in the absence of a space-occupying lesion. Treatment includes a period of conservative treatment with discontinuation of aggravating overhead activities, and a shoulder rehabilitation program for rotator cuff and scapular stabilization exercises. The emphasis is placed on maintaining full glenohumeral motion and stretching the posterior capsule. Most overuse types of neuropathy will resolve within 6 to 12 months.[18] Repeat electrophysiological studies usually at 6 months are recommended to verify recovery and can help in the decision process of whether to proceed with surgical intervention.[31]

SURGICAL TECHNIQUE

The cyst can generally be decompressed through the standard portals used when addressing the labrum. A shaver can be used to release the posterior superior capsule through the glenohumeral joint and the cyst can usually be identified between the raphe of the supra and infraspinatus muscle. Some authors feel that by just repairing the labrum the 1-way valve is eliminated and the cyst will resolve over time such that decompression is not required.[26] A recent report did demonstrate increase in external rotation with arthroscopic SLAP repair and decompression of the cyst versus labral repair alone.[32] We have not found any difference in our outcomes with labrum debridement versus repair as long as the cystic lesion is adequately decompressed.

At the level of the suprascapular notch the transverse scapular ligament can be released through either an open or arthroscopically approach. A notchplasty may be required if the notch is narrow or V-shaped by removal of the medial wall. If the decision is made to perform an open procedure at this level, either a superior (difficult in big patients) or posterior approach (endangers spinal accessory nerve) can be done. Weinfeld et al[24] described the topographical landmarks prior to performing the split of fibers of the trapezius when approaching the ligament where it can be found 1.3 cm posterior to posterior border of the clavicle and 2.9 cm medial to the AC joint. In a posterior approach the trapezius is elevated off the scapula and then the suprascapular muscle can be retracted to provide visualization of the notch. These procedures can be done in beach chair or lateral decubitus position. We prefer superior approach with split of the trapezius muscle in a beach chair position under general anesthesia.

For an arthroscopic SSN decompression the patient is positioned in either lateral or beach chair position with or without traction. A standard diagnostic arthroscopy is done through a standard posterior portal. The arthoscope is redirected into the subacromial space in which a bursectomy is done. The scope is then repositioned into a standard lateral portal and a shaver or radio-frequency device is introduced via an accessory anterolateral portal. The coracoacromial ligament is exposed and traced to the base of the coracoid at which point the coracoclavicular ligaments are identified. Medial to these ligaments is the lateral margin of transverse scapular ligament. To expose this area 2 additional portals between the clavicle and scapula are recommended. An initial medial portal is placed approximately 3 cm medial to the angle created by the clavicle and scapula spine. This

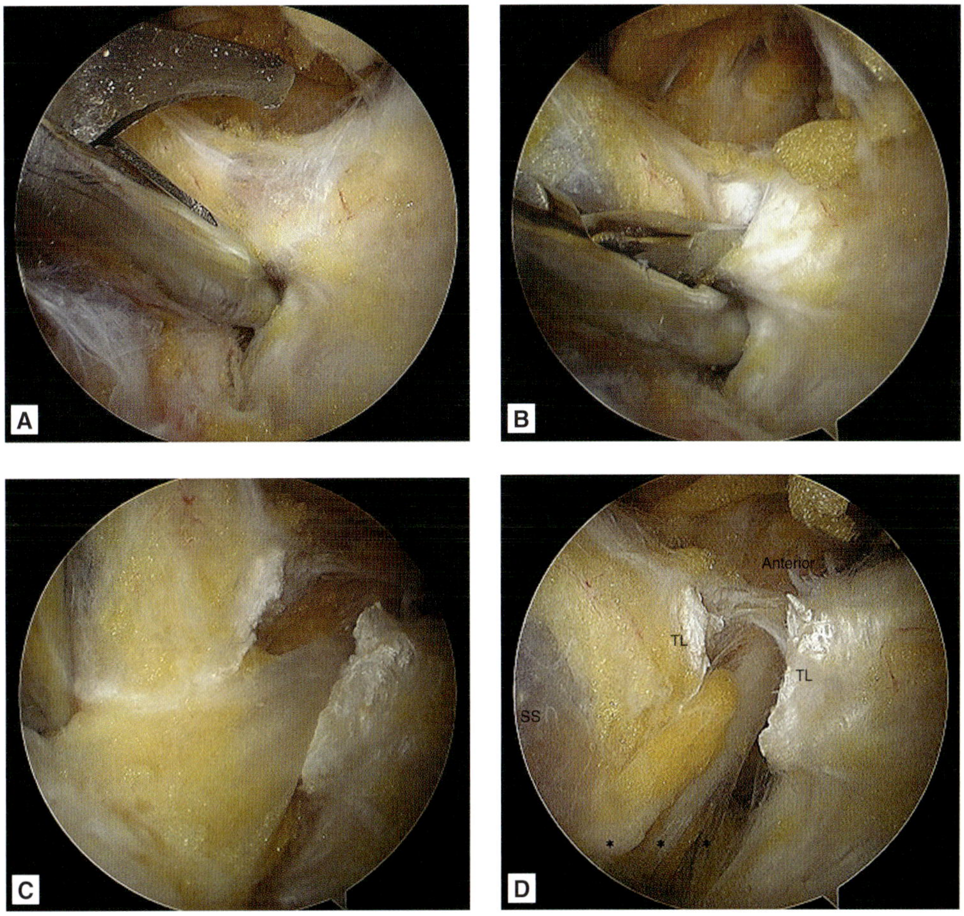

FIGURE 53-5 **A.** Arthroscopic scissors in place to resect suprascapular ligament. **B.** Arthroscopic transection of suprascapular ligament. **C.** After ligament transection. **D.** Suprascapular nerve branches (marked with asterisks) entering supraspinatus (SS). TL, transverse ligament. (Reproduced with permission from Lafosse et al.[19])

portal is used to expose the ligament as well as dissect and retract the neurovascular bundle while a second portal 5 to 10 mm medial to this portal is used to cut the ligament or notchplasty.[33,34] Another method is decompression through the subacromial space in which a single additional portal is made 2 cm medial to the Neviaser portal. Here viewing through the lateral portal a shaver removes any soft tissue and exposes the conoid ligament attachment to the coracoid. The base marks the lateral insertion of the TSL that run perpendicular to the conoid ligament. The accessory medial portal is used to retract the supraspinatus muscle so the ligament and neurovascular bundle can be identified. Several authors have described these arthroscopic techniques with good results[1,34] (Fig. 53-5A-D).

If the problem is distal at the spinoglenoid notch, the ligament is also released and in the setting of non–space-occupying lesion a notchplasty is generally combined at this level. A similar posterior approach as described above can be used in which the deltoid can be detached or retracted while the infraspinatus muscle is elevated to expose the nerve. There exists some controversy whether to decompress both notches in these patients. Arthroscopic spinoglenoid notch decompression has been described for non–space-occupying lesion but usually in association with paralabral ganglion.[28]

COMPLICATIONS

The literature regarding this topic is composed of primarily small case series such that the reported incidence of complications seems to be rare. They can include neurovascular damage, infection, and loss of motion. Nerves at risk for injury include the spinal accessory, SSN and associated branches or artery, and axillary nerve.

OUTCOMES

Westerheid et al reviewed 14 patients with SSN palsy secondary to spinoglenoid ganglion cysts.[30] The most common presenting symptoms were pain and weakness, which lasted an average of 7.5 months. Ten of 14 patients were noted on examination to have atrophy, and all 14 patients had weakness of the infraspinatus. MRI showed spinoglenoid ganglion cysts in all 14 patients, with an average cyst size of 3 cm. Labral pathology was identified intraoperatively in all 14 patients. At an average follow-up of 51 months, the average Simple Shoulder Test (SST) score was 11.5 (12 maximum), which was improved from an estimated preoperative score of 4.3. Improvement in external rotation strength was seen in 100% of patients who were examined postoperatively. No complications were reported, and there were no clinical or symptomatic recurrences.[30]

Kim et al[35] reviewed 42 patients who underwent a SSN decompression. The mean follow-up was 18 months (range, 12-48 months). Thirty-one (79%) of 39 patients with suprascapular notch SSN injuries/entrapments, excluding ganglion cysts, presented with mild-to-moderate shoulder pain and spinati weakness. Preoperatively, patients had supraspinatus function Grades 0 to 2 and infraspinatus function Grades 0 to 2. Supraspinatus function improved postoperatively to Grade 4 or better in 28 patients (90%) and to Grades 2 to 3 in 3 patients (10%). Infraspinatus function improved to better than Grade 3 in 10 patients (32%), to Grades 2 to 3 in 14 patients (45%), and to Grade 1 in 7 patients (23%). Preoperatively, 8 (21%) of 39 patients presenting with persistent severe pain had Grade 3 spinati strength. Of these 8 patients, 7 (88%) had an improvement in pain postoperatively. Strength in this group remained the same or improved to Grade 4. Postoperatively, 3 patients with ganglion cysts had good improvement in spinati function.

Shah et al reviewed 27 patients who underwent an arthroscopic SSN decompression at the suprascapular and/or spinoglenoid notch.[1] Eighty-nine percent (24/27) of patients had preoperative positive electromyography and nerve conduction EMG/NCV studies documenting SSN pathology. At an average follow-up of 22.5 months (range, 3-44), 71% (17/24) of patients reported a significant decrease in pain at an average of 9.4 weeks from surgery. Seventy-five percent (18/24) had a statistically significant improvement in the American Shoulder and Elbow Society (ASES) self-assessment scores and 71% (17/24) had a statistically significant improvement in the subjective shoulder value (SSV) scores.

QUADRILATERAL SPACE ENTRAPMENT

An infrequent but often overlooked cause of posterior shoulder pain is compression of the axillary nerve at the quadrilateral space. Injury to the axillary nerve is estimated to represent 1% of all nerve injuries and can occur from direct injury in setting of instability, iatrogenic injury during surgical exposure, proximal compression in thoracic outlet syndrome, and distal compression within the quadrilateral space.[36] The prevalence of quadrilateral space syndrome (QSS) is unclear. It was first described by Cahill and Palmer[37] in 1983 and has since been reported to occur in repetitive overhead sport athletes.[38–40] Fibrous bands are a common cause of compression of the axillary nerve at this level.[37,39]

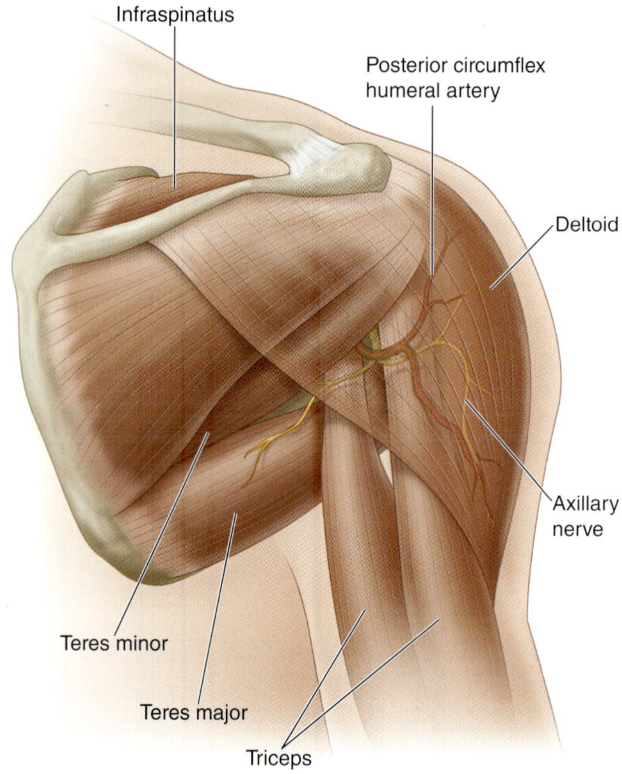

FIGURE 53-6 Quadrilateral space entrapment, posterior view of shoulder. The axillary nerve and posterior circumflex humeral artery exit between the teres minor. (Reproduced with permission from Safran.[18])

The clinical examination may be nonspecific and thus the diagnosis challenging. Many of these individuals present after having multiple surgeries prior to the correct diagnosis.[18] Careful physical examination combined by adjuvant diagnostic tests and a high index of suspicion can aid the physician in this diagnosis.

Anatomy

The axillary nerve is a branch of the posterior cord of the brachial plexus derived from the fifth and sixth cervical nerves. It travels laterally along the anterior surface of the subscapularis until it dips under the tendon to travel posteriorly adjacent to the inferomedial joint capsule. At this point it travels through the quadrilateral space accompanied by the posterior circumflex artery (Fig. 53-6). This space is bordered by the humeral shaft laterally, long head triceps medially, teres minor superiorly, and latissimus dorsi inferiorly. After transitioning through this space it wraps around the surgical neck of the humerus branching into anterior and posterior branches. This division can occur before, within, and after the quadrilateral space. Loukas et al[41] demonstrated this division occurred with the space 65% of the time and 35% after exiting. The anterior division continues to wrap around humerus while coursing on the undersurface of the deltoid to provide motor function to the anterior and medial deltoid.

The posterior branch divides into the upper lateral brachial cutaneous nerve and motor branch to the teres minor. The mean distance between the posterior lateral corner of the acromion and the point where the nerve exits the quadrilateral space is 7.8 cm (6.4-8.8 cm), while the anterior branch lies 5.55 cm (4.72-7.52) and posterior branch 4.83 cm (4.11-6.92) from the tip of humeral head.[42] This distance, as well as the size of the quadrilateral space, has been shown to change with respect to varying shoulder positions.[43] Abduction of the arm has been shown to decrease the size of the quadrangular space as well as this distance.[44]

Mechanism of Injury

QSS may be attributable to both traumatic and atraumatic causes. Potential traumatic causes include nerve stretch following a shoulder dislocation, blunt or penetrating trauma, fracture, and iatrogenic surgical injury.[45] Atraumatic causes include compression from fibrous bands,[37,39] venous dilation,[39] muscle boundary hypertrophy,[46] and paralabral cyst.[47] This syndrome may also be seen without acute injury or discrete mass in overhead athletes. It is hypothesized that repetitive microtrauma during overhead positions may have a role in some of the unexplained cases.

History and Physical Findings

This syndrome is usually seen in active individuals between 20 and 40 years of age.[48] The symptoms that occur as a result of compression of this nerve at this level can be variable. Overhead sport athletes tend to present with symptoms that are more poorly localized. These include vague posterior shoulder pain, fatigue, and a decline in performance. These symptoms tend to be aggravated with the shoulder in abduction and external rotation (ABER). Occasionally, these patients can have atrophy of the deltoid and/or teres minor, along with paresthesias over the lateral shoulder. We have found, as have others, that point tenderness in the quadrilateral space (2-3 cm distal to the standard posterior shoulder portal) is the most important clinical finding when considering a diagnosis of QSS.[18,37,39]

A variety of tests can be beneficial to diagnose QSS, as the examination may be nonspecific and the presentation unclear. We have a routine algorithm for patients who present with posterior shoulder pain. First, a history and physical examination is done taking care to delineate any signs that may point to potential causes of posterior shoulder pain such as scapular dyskinesis, labral injury, cuff injury, glenohumeral internal impingement, or SSN entrapment. Patients undergo plain x-ray films of the shoulder followed by an MRI. In this setting the radiographs are generally unremarkable. Isolated teres minor or deltoid denervation changes seen on MRI would be suggestive of QSS (Fig. 53-7). Patients who have these findings or point tenderness in the quadrilateral space then get a lidocaine block test. Five milliliters of 1% plain lidocaine is injected directly into the quadrilateral space (2-3 cm inferior to the standard posterior portal). Care must be taken not to inject into the posterior circumflex artery by standard gentle aspiration technique prior to injection. Ultrasound guidance may improve localization of the space, but we have found that a block without image guidance in the clinic is simple and predictably effective. Those patients

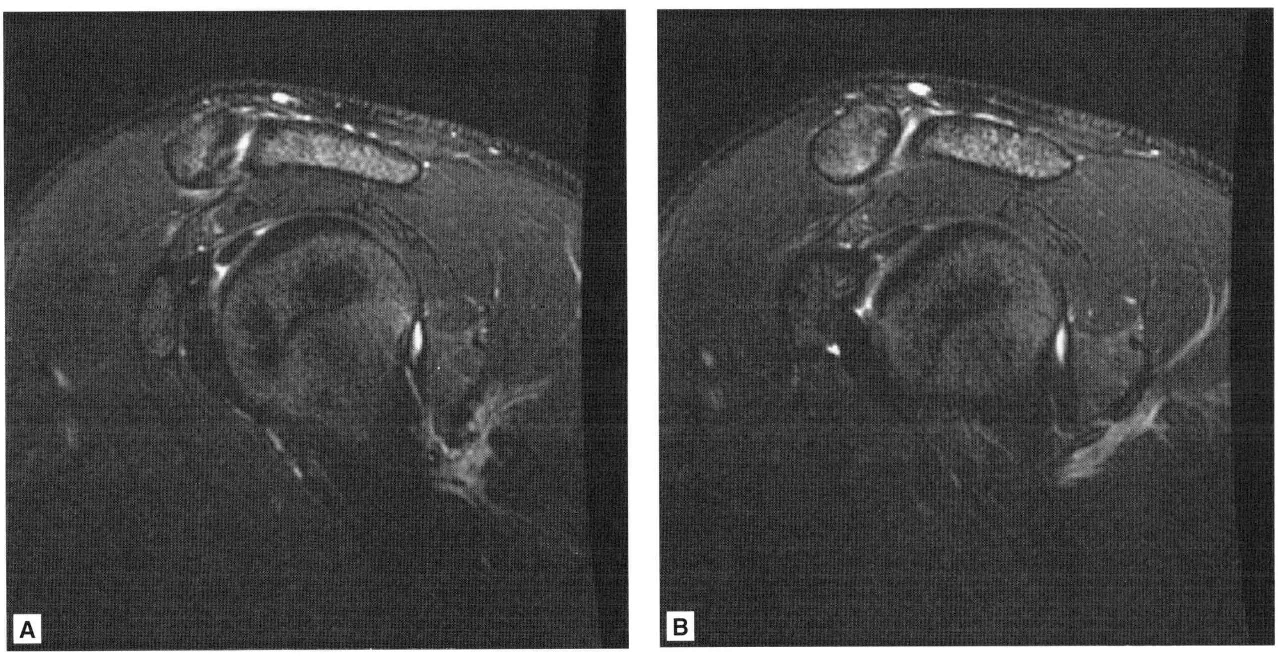

FIGURE 53-7 Sagittal-oblique T2 images (**A**, **B**) demonstrating teres minor edema consistent with compression of the axillary nerve in the quadrilateral space.

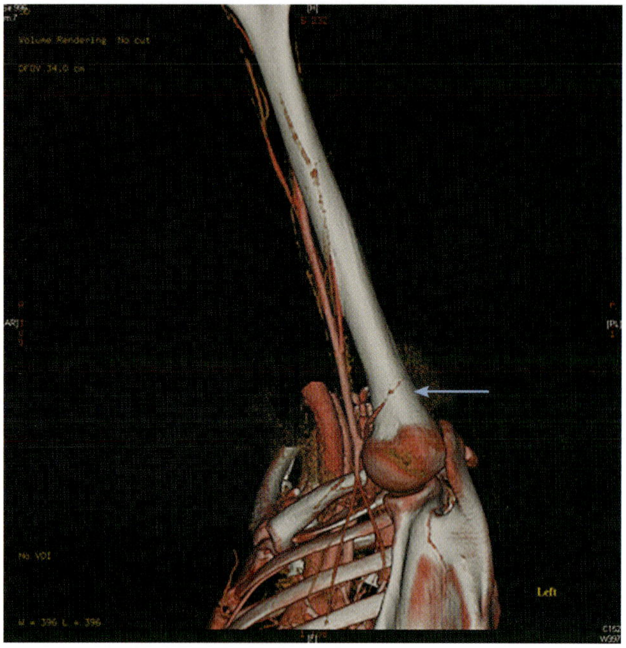

FIGURE 53-8 CT angiogram of the left shoulder in full abduction demonstrating posterior humeral circumflex compression consistent with compression of the axillary nerve in the quadrilateral space.

who have a positive block test (relief of pain) then get both an EMG and CT angiogram. Results of the EMG can help rule out SSN entrapment and provide a baseline. They may be normal in those cases that are more of a dynamic phenomenon. A CT angiogram is done in both neutral and ABER looking at compression of the posterior humeral circumflex artery due to its intimate relationship with the nerve in the quadrilateral space. However, compression in the ABER position has been shown to occur in some normal asymptomatic patients so this is used as an adjunct but does preclude the diagnosis of QSS[49] (Fig. 53-8). We have found that a positive QSS block test is the most useful diagnostic modality, and many times is the only positive test in patients who undergo decompression.

Surgical Indications

If a large compressive lesion is present, then early intervention may be warranted. For those individuals in whom the symptoms are functionally limiting and unimproved within 3 to 6 months and clinical and diagnostic tests suggest QSS, surgery is generally recommended. However, as in the case of SSN compression, by the time these patients present to an orthopedist the symptoms may have been present long enough to warrant immediate surgery and have a narrow time frame of 6 to 8 weeks prior to recommending surgery.[50]

Contraindications

Surgical treatment is not indicated for at least 6 months in the absence of a mass-occupying lesion since more than 70% tend to resolve within 6 months of conservative management.[49] Nonoperative management involves physical therapy focusing on posterior shoulder stretches, scapular stabilization exercises, and shoulder mechanics.

Surgical Technique

Although an arthroscopic approach has been recently described in the literature[50] for axillary nerve decompression at the level of the capsule, QSS is treated by an open posterior approach. We perform the surgery in the lateral decubitus position under general anesthesia. As described by Francel et al[46] a 3.5-cm incision is made longitudinally centered over the quadrilateral space (Fig. 53-9A and B). The posterior

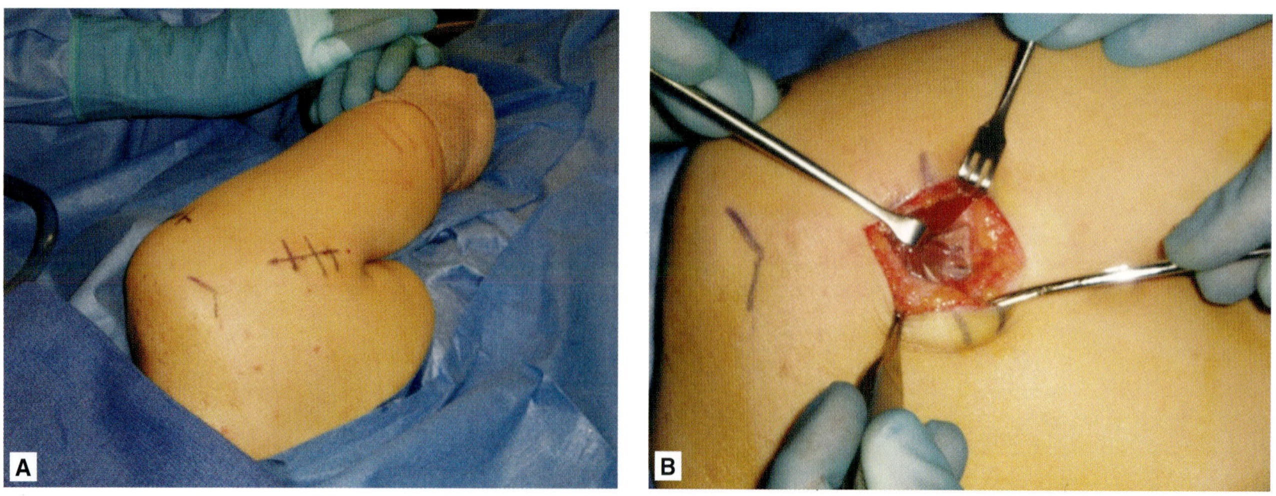

FIGURE 53-9 Intraoperative photograph of planned incision for axillary nerve decompression at the quadrilateral space (A), and visualization of the nerve exiting between the teres minor and major (B).

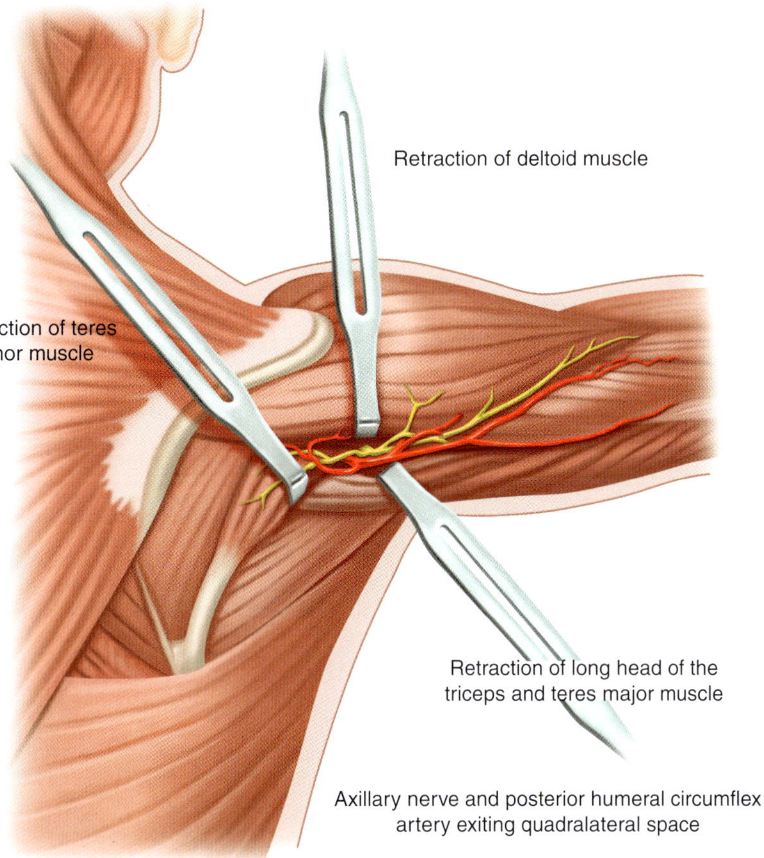

FIGURE 53-10 Surgical exposure of the quadrilateral space. The deltoid is reflected superolaterally. No deltoid fibers are split, and no part of the deltoid is detached from the acromion.

deltoid is retracted superiorly to expose this space. Gentle palpation along the humeral neck is used to verify the location with direct palpation of the axillary nerve and posterior humeral circumflex artery. The nerve is dissected free of any adhesion or underlying preidentified mass (Fig. 53-10). The shoulder is then placed in ABER to verify that nerve is free and pulse maintained. Patients are placed in a sling for comfort postoperatively for 10 to 14 days. We encourage early immediate passive range of motion to avoid new adhesions. Hyper-ABER is avoided for first 4 weeks and then at 6 weeks strengthening and sport-specific exercises are begun. Results for those who require surgery are favorable.[37,46,51]

Outcomes

In our series of 4 athletes with a mean age of 24 years, fibrous bands entrapped the axillary nerve in 3 shoulders, and venous dilation was found in the fourth shoulder. At a mean follow-up of 24.5 months all patients returned to sport at 12 weeks with complete relief of symptoms.[39] There was no loss of motion or abduction strength and patients reached maximal improvement by 4 months after surgery.

REFERENCES

1. Shah AA, Butler RB, Sung SY, Wells JH, Higgins LD, Warner JJ. Clinical outcomes of suprascapular nerve decompression. *J Shoulder Elbow Surg.* 2011;20(6):975–982.
2. Zehetgruber H, Noske H, Lang T, Wurnig C. Suprascapular nerve entrapment. A meta-analysis. *Int Orthop.* 2002;26(6):339–343.
3. Jerosch J, Saad M, Greig M, Filler T. Suprascapular nerve block as a method of preemptive pain control in shoulder surgery. *Knee Surg Sports Traumatol Arthrosc.* 2008;16(6):602–607.
4. Romeo AA, Rotenberg DD, Bach BR Jr. Suprascapular neuropathy. *J Am Acad Orthop Surg.* 1999;7(6):358–367.
5. Ajmani ML. The cutaneous branch of the human suprascapular nerve. *J Anat.* 1994;185(pt 2):439–442.
6. Horiguchi M. The cutaneous branch of some human suprascapular nerves. *J Anat.* 1980;130(pt 1):191–195.
7. Tamura A, Wakabayashi K, Onishi Y, et al. Re-evaluation and functional classification of non-synonymous single nucleotide polymorphisms of the human ATP-binding cassette transporter ABCG2. *Cancer Sci.* 2007;98(2):231–239.
8. Bigliani LU, Dalsey RM, McCann PD, April EW. An anatomical study of the suprascapular nerve. *Arthroscopy.* 1990;6(4):301–305.
9. Warner JP, Krushell RJ, Masquelet A, Gerber C. Anatomy and relationships of the suprascapular nerve: anatomical constraints to mobilization of the supraspinatus and infraspinatus muscles in the management of massive rotator-cuff tears. *J Bone Joint Surg Am.* 1992;74(1):36–45.
10. Sunderland S. The anatomy and physiology of nerve injury. *Muscle Nerve.* 1990;13(9):771–784.

11. Bora FW Jr, Pleasure DE, Didizian NA. A study of nerve regeneration and neuroma formation after nerve suture by various techniques. *J Hand Surg Am.* 1976;1(2):138–143.
12. Ringel SP, Treihaft M, Carry M, Fisher R, Jacobs P. Suprascapular neuropathy in pitchers. *Am J Sports Med.* 1990;18(1):80–86.
13. Plancher KD, Peterson RK, Johnston JC, Luke TA. The spinoglenoid ligament. Anatomy, morphology, and histological findings. *J Bone Joint Surg Am.* 2005;87(2):361–365.
14. Rengachary SS, Burr D, Lucas S, Brackett CE. Suprascapular entrapment neuropathy: a clinical, anatomical, and comparative study. Part 3: comparative study. *Neurosurgery.* 1979;5(4):452–455.
15. Rengachary SS, Burr D, Lucas S, Hassanein KM, Mohn MP, Matzke H. Suprascapular entrapment neuropathy: a clinical, anatomical, and comparative study. Part 2: anatomical study. *Neurosurgery.* 1979;5(4):447–451.
16. Rengachary SS, Neff JP, Singer PA, Brackett CE. Suprascapular entrapment neuropathy: a clinical, anatomical, and comparative study. Part 1: clinical study. *Neurosurgery.* 1979;5(4):441–446.
17. Avery BW, Pilon FM, Barclay JK. Anterior coracoscapular ligament and suprascapular nerve entrapment. *Clin Anat.* 2002;15(6):383–386.
18. Safran MR. Nerve injury about the shoulder in athletes, part 1: suprascapular nerve and axillary nerve. *Am J Sports Med.* 2004;32(3):803–819.
19. Lafosse L, Piper K, Lanz U. Arthroscopic suprascapular nerve release: indications and technique. *J Shoulder Elbow Surg.* 2011;20(2 suppl):S9–S13.
20. Hoellrich RG, Gasser SI, Morrison DS, Kurzweil PR. Electromyographic evaluation after primary repair of massive rotator cuff tears. *J Shoulder Elbow Surg.* 2005;14(3):269–272.
21. Chalian M, Faridian-Aragh N, Soldatos T, et al. High-resolution 3T MR neurography of suprascapular neuropathy. *Acad Radiol.* 2011;18(8):1049–1059.
22. Piasecki DP, Romeo AA, Bach BR Jr, Nicholson GP. Suprascapular neuropathy. *J Am Acad Orthop Surg.* 2009;17(11):665–676.
23. Post M. Diagnosis and treatment of suprascapular nerve entrapment. *Clin Orthop Relat Res.* 1999;(368):92–100.
24. Weinfeld AB, Cheng J, Nath RK, Basaran I, Yuksel E, Rose JE. Topographic mapping of the superior transverse scapular ligament: a cadaver study to facilitate suprascapular nerve decompression. *Plast Reconstr Surg.* 2002;110(3):774–779.
25. Tirman PF, Feller JF, Janzen DL, Peterfy CG, Bergman AG. Association of glenoid labral cysts with labral tears and glenohumeral instability: radiologic findings and clinical significance. *Radiology.* 1994;190(3):653–658.
26. Schroder CP, Skare O, Stiris M, Gjengedal E, Uppheim G, Brox JI. Treatment of labral tears with associated spinoglenoid cysts without cyst decompression. *J Bone Joint Surg Am.* 2008;90(3):523–530.
27. Piatt BE, Hawkins RJ, Fritz RC, Ho CP, Wolf E, Schickendantz M. Clinical evaluation and treatment of spinoglenoid notch ganglion cysts. *J Shoulder Elbow Surg.* 2002;11(6):600–604.
28. Werner CM, Nagy L, Gerber C. Combined intra- and extra-articular arthroscopic treatment of entrapment neuropathy of the infraspinatus branches of the suprascapular nerve caused by a periglenoidal ganglion cyst. *Arthroscopy.* 2007;23(3):328.e321–328.e323.
29. Tashjian RZ, Burks RT. Arthroscopic aspiration and labral repair for treatment of spinoglenoid notch cysts. *Am J Orthop.* 2009;38(2):94–96.
30. Westerheide KJ, Dopirak RM, Karzel RP, Snyder SJ. Suprascapular nerve palsy secondary to spinoglenoid cysts: results of arthroscopic treatment. *Arthroscopy.* 2006;22(7):721–727.
31. Drez D Jr. Suprascapular neuropathy in the differential diagnosis of rotator cuff injuries. *Am J Sports Med.* 1976;4(2):43–45.
32. Pillai G, Baynes JR, Gladstone J, Flatow EL. Greater strength increase with cyst decompression and SLAP repair than SLAP repair alone. *Clin Orthop Relat Res.* 2011;469(4):1056–1060.
33. Bhatia DN, de Beer JF, van Rooyen KS, du Toit DF. Arthroscopic suprascapular nerve decompression at the suprascapular notch. *Arthroscopy.* 2006;22(9):1009–1013.
34. Lafosse L, Tomasi A, Corbett S, Baier G, Willems K, Gobezie R. Arthroscopic release of suprascapular nerve entrapment at the suprascapular notch: technique and preliminary results. *Arthroscopy.* 2007;23(1):34–42.
35. Kim DH, Murovic JA, Tiel RL, Kline DG. Management and outcomes of 42 surgical suprascapular nerve injuries and entrapments. *Neurosurgery.* 2005;57(1):120–127 [discussion 120–127].
36. Pollack L, Davis L. Peripheral nerve injuries. *Am J Surg.* 1932;17:462–471.
37. Cahill BR, Palmer RE. Quadrilateral space syndrome. *J Hand Surg Am.* 1983;8(1):65–69.
38. Redler MR, Ruland LJ 3rd, McCue FC 3rd. Quadrilateral space syndrome in a throwing athlete. *Am J Sports Med.* 1986;14(6):511–513.
39. McAdams TR, Dillingham MF. Surgical decompression of the quadrilateral space in overhead athletes. *Am J Sports Med.* 2008;36(3):528–532.
40. Nuber GW, McCarthy WJ, Yao JS, Schafer MF, Suker JR. Arterial abnormalities of the shoulder in athletes. *Am J Sports Med.* 1990;18(5):514–519.
41. Loukas M, Grabska J, Tubbs RS, Apaydin N, Jordan R. Mapping the axillary nerve within the deltoid muscle. *Surg Radiol Anat.* 2009;31(1):43–47.
42. Uz A, Apaydin N, Bozkurt M, Elhan A. The anatomic branch pattern of the axillary nerve. *J Shoulder Elbow Surg.* 2007;16(2):240–244.
43. Cheung S, Fitzpatrick M, Lee TQ. Effects of shoulder position on axillary nerve positions during the split lateral deltoid approach. *J Shoulder Elbow Surg.* 2009;18(5):748–755.
44. Burkhead WZ Jr, Rockwood CA Jr. Treatment of instability of the shoulder with an exercise program. *J Bone Joint Surg Am.* 1992;74(6):890–896.
45. Millett PJ, Gaskill TR. Arthroscopic management of glenohumeral arthrosis: humeral osteoplasty, capsular release, and arthroscopic axillary nerve release as a joint-preserving approach. *Arthroscopy.* 2011;27(9):1296–1303.
46. Francel TJ, Dellon AL, Campbell JN. Quadrilateral space syndrome: diagnosis and operative decompression technique. *Plast Reconstr Surg.* 1991;87(5):911–916.
47. Sanders TG, Tirman PF. Paralabral cyst: an unusual cause of quadrilateral space syndrome. *Arthroscopy.* 1999;15(6):632–637.
48. Aval SM, Durand P Jr, Shankwiler JA. Neurovascular injuries to the athlete's shoulder: part II. *J Am Acad Orthop Surg.* 2007;15(5):281–289.
49. Robinson DJ, Marks P, Schneider-Kolsky M. Occlusion and stenosis of the posterior circumflex humeral artery: detection with ultrasound in a normal population. *J Med Imaging Radiat Oncol.* 2011;55(5):479–484.
50. Millett PJ, Gaskill TR. Arthroscopic trans-capsular axillary nerve decompression: indication and surgical technique. *Arthroscopy.* 2011;27(10):1444–1448.
51. Lester B, Jeong GK, Weiland AJ, Wickiewicz TL. Quadrilateral space syndrome: diagnosis, pathology, and treatment. *Am J Orthop.* 1999;28(12):718–722, 725.

54

Accessory to Suprascapular and Radial to Axillary Nerve Transfers for Shoulder Reconstruction with Brachial Plexus Lesions

Jayme Augusto Bertelli, MD, PhD
Marcos Flávio Ghizoni, MD, MSc
Cristiano Paulo Tacca, MD

RATIONALE AND BASIC SCIENCE

In upper-type lesions of the brachial plexus, shoulder abduction/external rotation and elbow flexion are the missing functions that require surgical reconstruction. In C5-C7 root injuries, elbow extension is preserved. Triceps palsy is observed only when the C5-C8 roots have been injured.[1] Root injury occurring proximal to the intervertebral foramen is not amenable to surgical reconstruction (ie, avulsion injury). Root lesions distal to the intervertebral foramen, at the supraclavicular level, should be grafted. In our experience, in partial palsies of the brachial plexus, avulsion of both the C5 and C6 roots is rare; it occurred in only 18% of our cases, with the C5 root available for grafting 65% of the time and both the C5 and C6 roots usable 16% of the time.[2] In terms of shoulder motion, grafting the roots of the brachial plexus to the upper trunk or a distal nerve transfer alone portends poorer results when compared against the combined procedure of root grafting plus distal nerve transfer. The problem of anatomical reconstruction with sural nerve grafts is the failure of reconstructing external rotation due to co-contractions. Distal nerve transfers address potential targets for reinnervation, but fail to address the antagonist and stabilizer muscles of a given joint/motion. For instance, elbow flexion strength is worse when ulnar nerve fascicle transfers to the biceps motor nerve are compared with ulnar nerve fascicle transfers in combination with C5 root grafting to the anterior division of the upper trunk. With the combined procedure, the repair addresses not only the biceps but also the pectoralis major. When the elbow flexes strongly against resistance, the pectoralis major co-contracts to stabilize the shoulder, thereby improving elbow flexion power. In general, 47% of patients with upper-type injuries of the brachial plexus complain about pain, which in a few cases can be ameliorated by root grafting.[3,4] Hence, if the C5 root is available for grafting, we connect it to the anterior division of the upper trunk to reinnervate the pectoralis major, coracobrachialis, brachialis, and brachioradialis. If both roots are available, the anterior portion of the roots is grafted to the anterior division, while the posterior portion is grafted to the posterior division of the upper trunk.

The supraspinatus and deltoid muscles primarily orchestrate shoulder abduction, both muscles being able to initiate abduction. Above horizontal, the pectoralis major, coracobrachialis, and biceps help to raise the arm. External rotation is primarily executed by the infraspinatus and teres minor.[5–7] To increase the likelihood of reinnervating prime abductors and external rotators, distal nerve transfers should target reinnervation of both the suprascapular and axillary nerves. In daily activities, external rotation is more important than abduction beyond horizontal. Hence, nerve transfer to the axillary nerve should not exclude the teres minor during the reinnervation process.[8] The posterior division of the axillary nerve, containing branches to the posterior deltoid and the cutaneous branch, should be excluded from reinnervation to direct regenerating axons toward the anterior division of the axillary nerve, which innervates the anterior and middle deltoid.[9] Ideally, in nerve transfer procedures, donor and recipient nerve coaptation should be close to the muscle, without using an interpositional nerve graft. These donor nerves should be "intelligent," which means easy to control voluntarily, which promotes easier muscle retraining during the postoperative period. The best nerve transfers for shoulder reconstruction are cranial nerve XI to the suprascapular nerve and the triceps branches to the axillary nerve. Any triceps branch can be used for axillary nerve neurotization. However, in brachial plexus injuries, our preference is to utilize the triceps long head or upper medial head branches, because these nerves can be dissected through an axillary approach.[9] In this regard, triceps to axillary nerve transfers can also be performed via a posterior arm approach. However, in brachial plexus injuries, the axillary approach offers advantages, because it is easier to identify the teres minor branch, and easier to concomitantly repair elbow flexion through a hidden scar. In isolated injuries of the axillary nerve, the posterior approach is preferable, because the lesion involving the axillary nerve may extend into the quadrangular space.

PREOPERATIVE EXAMINATION

The presence of a Tinel sign over the C5 root is important to document a viable root for grafting. Shoulder shrugging and scapular retraction should be tested to confirm the integrity of the entire accessory nerve. The triceps should be tested for normality. To be considered as a donor for transfer, the triceps should score at least M4, as per the British Medical Council Classification system.[10] In general, triceps strength is approximately 8 kg; however, even a muscle scoring 3 kg may be used as a donor for transfer, provided that more than 1 triceps branch is determined intraoperatively to be functional by electrical stimulation. This muscle will recover strength postoperatively.

In our opinion, electrophysiological examination and MRI have limited utility in the evaluation of brachial plexus injuries. Electrophysiological investigations cannot differentiate an axonotmetic lesion that will recuperate spontaneously from a neurotometic injury that requires surgery.[11] Moreover, even when electromyograms indicate reinnervation, the final muscle strength may be negligible.[12] Finally, imprecision in needle placement and diffuse recordings from needles are potential sources of error. Electrophysiological investigations have not influenced our surgical plans and, hence, are no longer routinely requested in our department. MRI can access the brachial plexus extradurally, but provides poor definition of the intradural portion of the C5 and C6 roots.[13] Extradural exploration of a brachial plexus lesion by MRI is of limited interest because this can be directly and more precisely explored by the surgeon with direct intraoperative electrophysiological studies. A CT tomographic myelography is our preferred method of evaluation because it can determine the intradural status of those roots that cannot be accessed during surgery without a laminectomy. For the upper roots, the accuracy of CT tomographic myelography, as demonstrated following a laminectomy, is roughly 90%.[13]

INDICATIONS

Prior to undertaking surgery, it is common practice to wait at least 3 months to see if spontaneous regeneration will take place. Preferentially, surgery should be performed within 6 months of trauma. However, good outcomes can be expected for up to 1 year. The younger the patient, the longer post injury a distal nerve transfer can be employed. Past 1 year after an accident, we avoid root grafting and perform only distal nerve transfers. We have reinnervated the biceps muscle using distal nerve transfers in young patients (ie, less than 25 years old) up to 18 months after trauma. However, in long-standing lesions, we are more reluctant to section the accessory nerve for transfer because in such circumstances we denervate the lower trapezius, which is a potential muscle for transfer for external rotation reconstruction.[14] From a practical point of view, for adults requiring shoulder reconstruction, we consider 12 months from injury to be the upper limit for nerve surgery.

CONTRAINDICATIONS

If the accessory nerve is paralyzed, it cannot be used for transfer. The site of paralysis should be determined with regards to the sternocleidomastoid muscle. In the supine position, neck flexion against resistance highlights contractions of the sternocleidomastoid muscle (Figs. 54-1 and 54-2). Patients with paralysis of the accessory nerve should have this nerve reconstructed using a platysma motor nerve transfer if the lesion is proximal to the sternocleidomastoid muscle.[15] If the lesion is distal to the sternocleidomastoid muscle, the accessory nerve should be grafted. If, during preoperative examination, shoulder shrugging is absent, but intraoperatively the nerve responds to electrical stimulation, the accessory nerve can be used for transfer because this is a regenerating nerve that will recover (Fig. 54-3). If the triceps is paralyzed or weak, there is no potential to use 1 of its branches. If completely paralyzed, elbow extension should be reconstructed.

SURGICAL TECHNIQUE

Patients are operated upon in the supine position with their head turned toward the contralateral side, while under general anesthesia without muscle relaxants. Delicate instruments are used, together with bipolar coagulation. We perform nerve coaptation using micro-instruments and 9-0 or 8-0 monofilament nylon sutures under the microscope. Sutures provide a stronger repair than fibrin glue alone.

Brachial Plexus Exploration

Before incision, a solution of adrenaline 1:200,000 is injected into the skin. The C5 and C6 roots of the brachial plexus are explored through a 6-cm long incision centered over

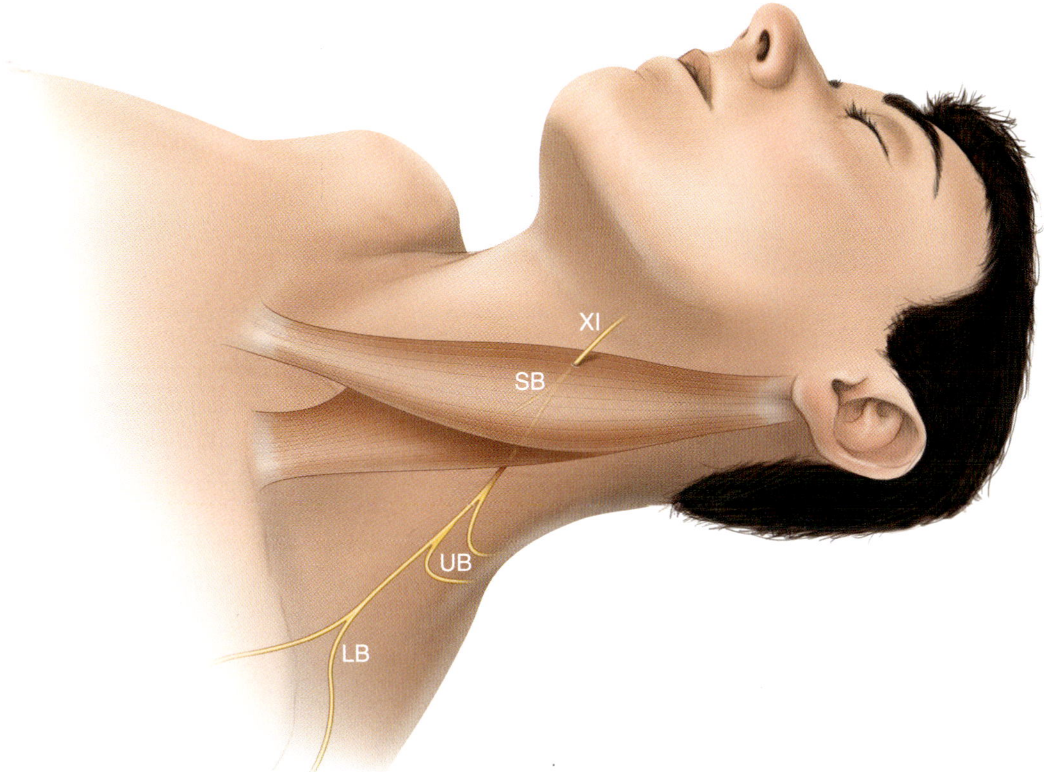

FIGURE 54-1 Schematic representation of the branches of the accessory nerve (XI). In the neck, the first branch of the accessory nerve is to the sternocleidomastoid muscle (SB). Then, after emerging beneath the SB, in the supraclavicular region the accessory nerve innervates the upper trapezius muscle and more distally innervates the middle and lower trapezius portions.

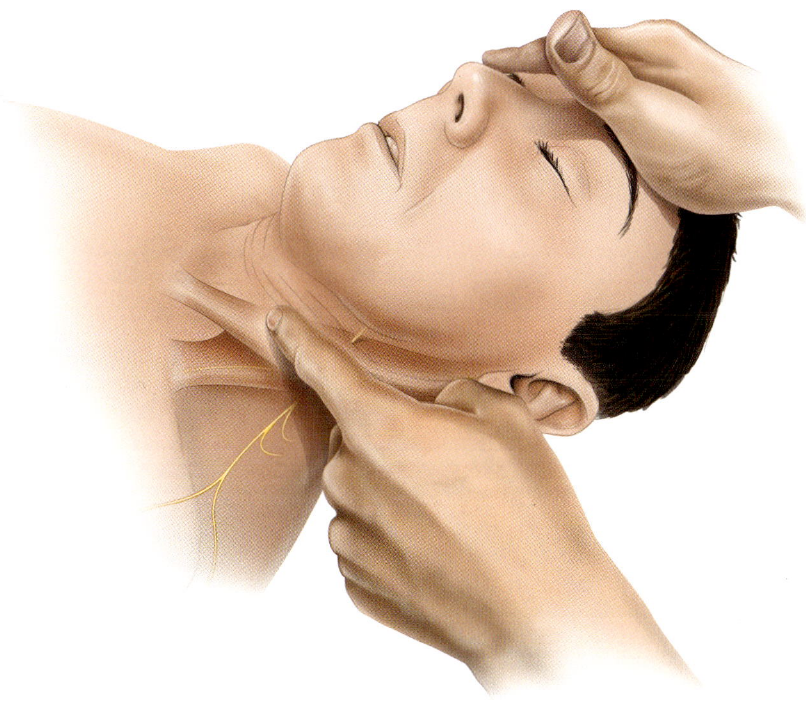

FIGURE 54-2 Clinical testing of sternocleidomastoid function by asking the patient to flex his/her neck against resistance. Contraction of the sternocleidomastoid muscle can be readily recognized.

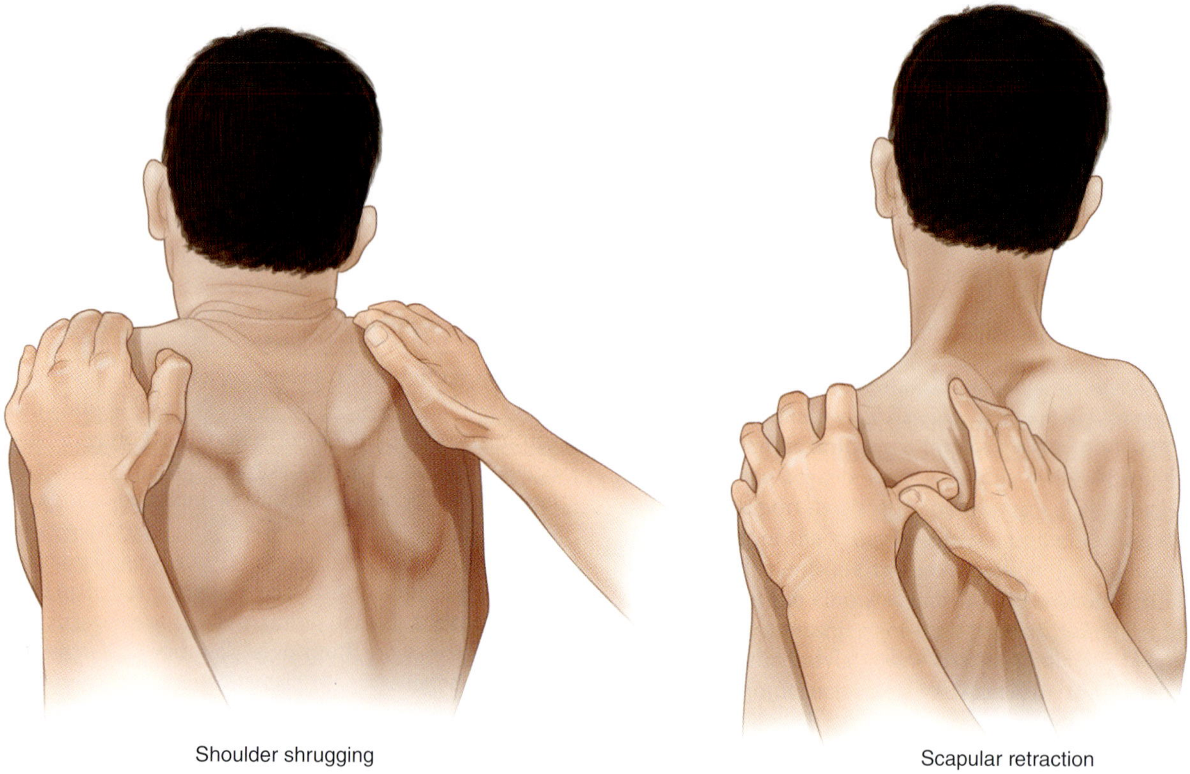

FIGURE 54-3 Clinical testing for upper trapezius function by resisting shoulder shrugging. The middle and lower trapezius portions are tested by resisting scapular retraction and palpation of the trapezius muscle.

Chassaignac tubercle (Fig. 54-4). The C5 root is dissected medial to the phrenic nerve to check for continuity and to perform nerve trimming inside a healthy zone. The root is eligible for grafting only when, after sectioning, a fascicular pattern is identified, and only after preoperative CT scans have confirmed intradural root integrity. The anterior and posterior divisions of the upper trunk are dissected through the same distal incision used to repair the suprascapular nerve (Fig. 54-2). This is a vertical incision over the trapezius muscle and the distal third of the clavicle. Sural nerves are removed and used as grafts.

Suprascapular Nerve Exposure

The lateral limit of the brachial plexus is palpated within the supraclavicular region. A point is marked at which the brachial plexus crosses the clavicle, and then a line over this point and over a point 3 cm proximal to the clavicle on the anterior margin of the trapezius muscle is drawn (Fig. 54-5). The skin is incised, the subcutaneous tissue divided, and the omohyoid muscle identified and sectioned. The lateral limit of the brachial plexus is visualized, and the suprascapular nerve is individualized as the sole branch emerging from the brachial plexus in this location (Fig. 54-6). The suprascapular nerve is dissected proximally, and then sectioned.

At the anterior margin of the trapezius muscle, the deep cervical fascia is separated from the trapezius muscle 3 to 4 cm proximal to the clavicle. The deep cervical fascia and the trapezius muscles are retracted, like book pages. The accessory nerve is individualized within the deep cervical fascia. Three to 4 cm proximal to the clavicle, the accessory nerve is more superficial and, therefore, easily recognized. Motor branches entering the trapezius muscle confirm the nerve's

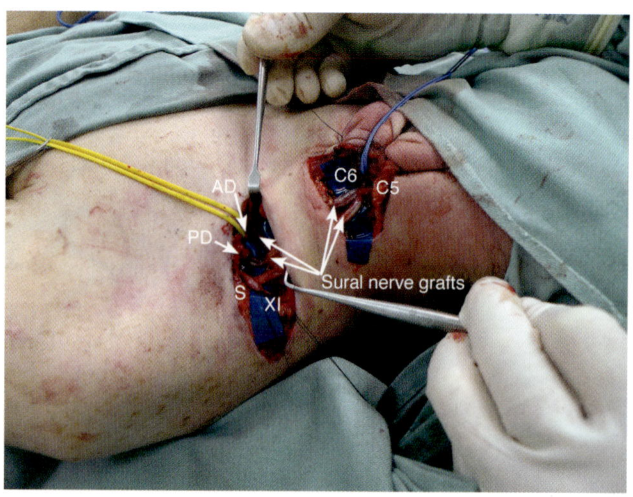

FIGURE 54-4 Reconstruction of an upper-type lesion of the left brachial plexus. Sural nerve grafts connected the C5 and C6 roots to the anterior (AD) and posterior divisions (PD) of the upper trunk. The accessory nerve (XI) was connected to the suprascapular (S) nerve.

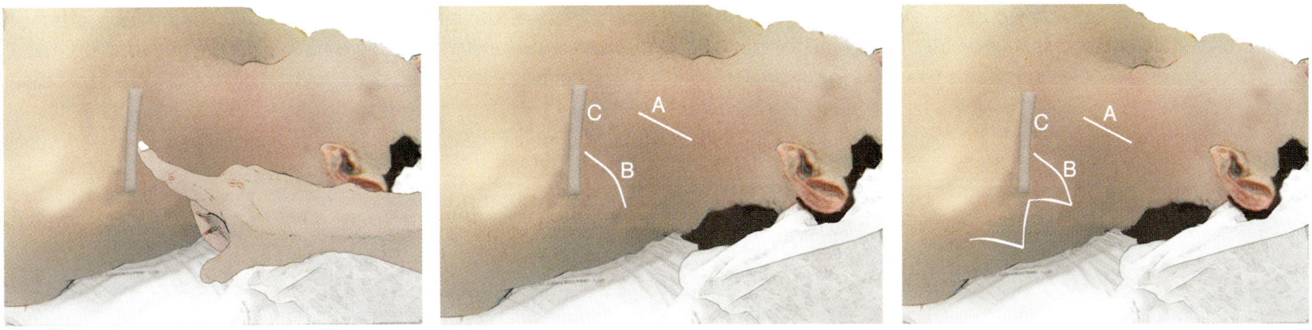

FIGURE 54-5 On the left, determination of the point at which the brachial plexus crosses the clavicle, a point used to design the incision to transfer the accessory to the suprascapular nerve. At center, design of the surgical incision to transfer the accessory to the suprascapular nerve (B). On the right, the extended incision for exposure of the suprascapular nerve. (A) Incision to explore the upper roots of the brachial plexus. (C) Clavicle.

identity. Before severing the accessory nerve, it is electrically stimulated to assess its functional integrity. The accessory nerve is divided, as distal as needed, to ensure direct coaptation to the suprascapular nerve (Fig. 54-4).

Extended Exposure of the Suprascapular Nerve

More extensive exposure to the suprascapular nerve is required under the following circumstances: (a) the suprascapular nerve cannot be identified through the proximal incision because the plexus has moved distally following traction and the nerve origin is under the clavicle; (b) the region of emergence of the suprascapular nerve is scarred following injury or previous surgery to repair a clavicular fracture; (c) a healthy distal stump of the suprascapular nerve is not obtained at its emergence from the brachial plexus; or (d) the suprascapular nerve must be evaluated to rule out a double lesion following scapular neck fracture. The patient is placed in the supine position and the head of the operating table is elevated to 45°. Supports are placed under the patient's shoulder. A zigzag incision over the anterior border of the trapezius muscle and acromion is created as a prolongation from the previous oblique incision (Fig. 54-5). The skin and subcutaneous tissue are incised, the deep cervical fascia over the trapezius muscle's anterior border divided, and the trapezius muscle is dissected off the clavicle and acromion. The suprascapular vessels are isolated; then the scapular notch is identified. For this, the surgeon's index finger is introduced to the anterior side of the scapula and moved from medial to lateral. The finger stops at the base of the coracoid process, which is the site of the scapular notch, located almost directly under the clavicle. With the help of a surgical clamp, the scapular notch is located and the suprascapular ligament divided. Alternatively, the suprascapular nerve first is identified after the suprascapular fossae and the ligament divided afterwards, or nerve coaptation is performed distal to the scapular notch (Figs. 54-7 and 54-8). Dissection of the suprascapular nerve is performed posterior to the

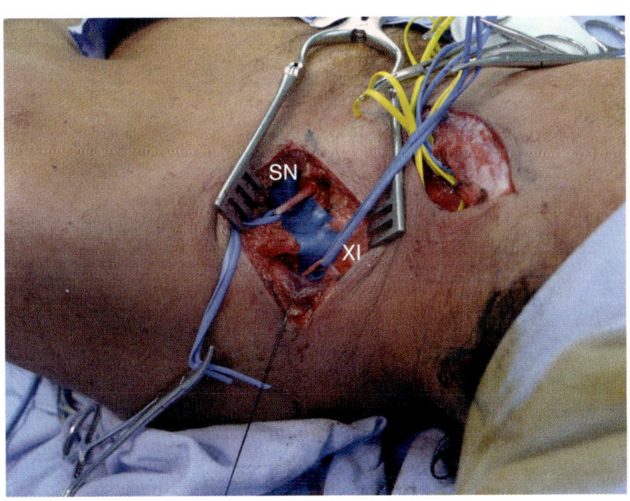

FIGURE 54-6 Intraoperative view of the suprascapular (SN) and accessory nerves (AN) dissected with an oblique supraclavicular incision.

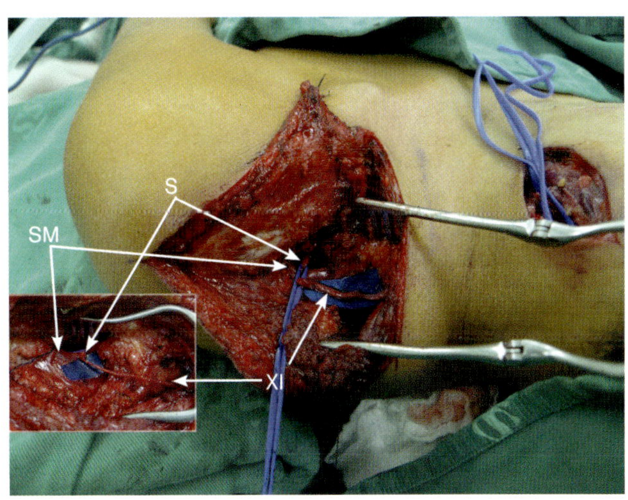

FIGURE 54-7 Intraoperative view of extended exposure of the suprascapular nerve (SN). The trapezius muscle was detached from the clavicle. In the inset, note direct coaptation of the accessory nerve (XI) with the suprascapular nerve near the supraspinatus muscle (SM) entry point.

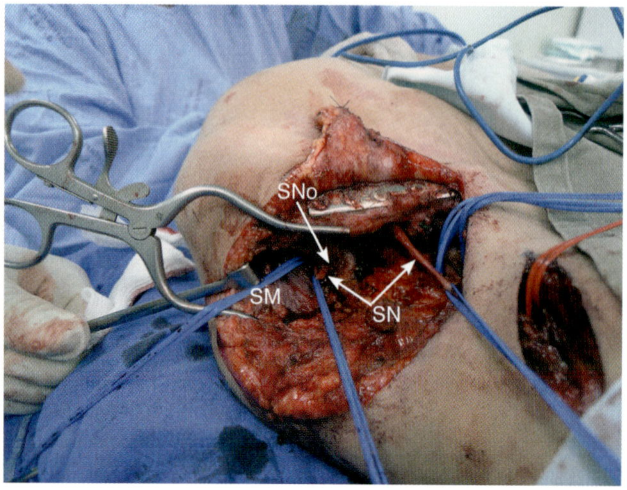

FIGURE 54-8 Intraoperative view after an extended approach to the suprascapular nerve (SN), which was injured following fracture and plating of the clavicle. SM, supraspinatus muscle; SNo, suprascapular notch.

suprascapular vessels, which are preserved. After dividing the suprascapular ligament, the branches of the suprascapular nerve are dissected and inspected for continuity. The branch for the acromioclavicular joint, which originates at the scapular notch, is divided. The suprascapular nerve is tracked proximally, and then sectioned. Frequently, the region under the clavicle is scarred and we do not dissect it, just moving directly to the suprascapular fossa. We separate the supraspinatus muscle from the scapula and identify its proximal branch, which is then followed proximally. Because the trapezius has been detached from the clavicle, the accessory nerve can be dissected very distally and, hence, the distal stump of the accessory nerve can be connected directly to the suprascapular nerve within the suprascapular fossa (Figs. 54-7 and 54-8). Finally, the trapezius muscle is reinserted with sutures.

Posterior Approach to the Suprascapular Nerve

The suprascapular and accessory nerves can be approached posteriorly after detaching the trapezius from the spine of the scapula.[16] However, we do not see any advantage to this method, which we have used in the past and since abandoned.[17] The distance from the suprascapular nerve to the surface is almost 10 cm, which makes dissection difficult. In the presence of scarring, lesions of the suprascapular vessels are possible and coagulation of these vessels may damage the suprascapular nerve. Finally, the patient generally must be positioned in a prone or lateral position, which prolongs surgery dramatically.

The extended anterior approach allows for nerve coaptation to be performed as closely as needed to the supraspinatus muscle (Fig. 54-7). Hence, there is no advantage of the posterior approach. Bhandari and Deb[18] pointed out that, after using the posterior approach, 1 advantage is greater preservation of trapezius function because more proximal branches do not need to be sectioned. After using the anterior approach, they identified muscle weakness of the trapezius in 16 of their 21 patients. When exploring the accessory nerve distally, as we proposed, via the anterior approach, all the important branches to the upper trapezius are preserved. Hence, we have never observed trapezius function downgrading in our cases. Also, even after extended exposure, upper trapezius strength is maintained after surgery.[19] Of importance is that, in 3 of their 14 patients, Bhandari and Deb[18] could not dissect the suprascapular nerve via the posterior approach, so that their patients ultimately had to be operated upon via the anterior approach. In our opinion, in the presence of fractures of the clavicle or scapula, the posterior approach is risky because of the potential for vascular injury.

Surgical Technique for Transferring the Triceps Branch to the Axillary Nerve in the Axilla

The axillary incision is V-shaped with extension over the medial arm, which allows us to reconstruct elbow flexion. The vertex of the V is positioned over the latissimus dorsi tendon (Figs. 54-9 and 54-10). After skin incision and subcutaneous division, the tendon of the latissimus dorsi muscle is located and exposed completely. After visualization of its medial margin, the humeral head is palpated and the axillary nerve identified by palpation. The posterior circumflex humeral vessels are visualized and the axillary nerve is dissected. A retractor is placed on the tendon of the latissimus

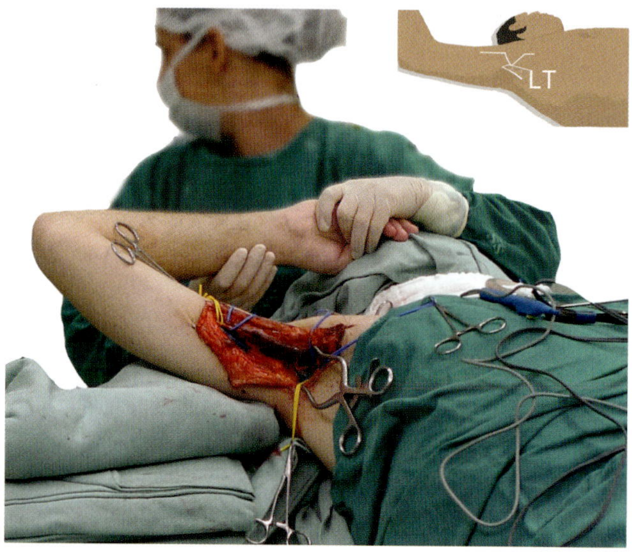

FIGURE 54-9 Incision and intraoperative view of the axillary approach for transfer of triceps motor branches to the axillary nerve. In the inset, the line drawn represents the skin incision. The vertex of the "V" incision is over the latissimus dorsi tendon (TD).

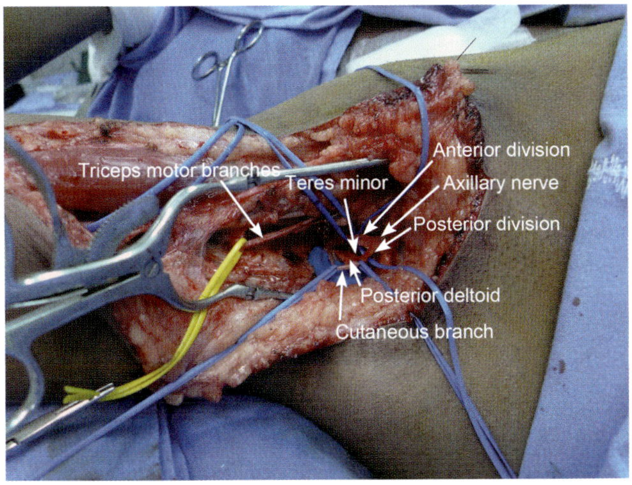

FIGURE 54-10 Intraoperative view of a triceps to axillary nerve transfer via a right axillary approach. Triceps motor branches will be sectioned distally, whereas the axillary nerve will be sectioned proximally. Triceps branches will be flipped proximally, while the axillary nerve will be flipped distally. The cutaneous branch and the posterior deltoid branches should be excluded from the reinnervation process.

dorsi tendon, which is retracted laterally, thereby exposing the quadrangular space. The anterior and posterior divisions of the axillary nerve are identified, together with the branch to the teres minor. The anterior division and the teres minor motor branches are ligatured, sectioned, and flipped distally. Anterior to the latissimus dorsi tendon, the radial nerve is identified together with the branches to the long and medial heads, which occupy an anterior and inferior position on the radial nerve. Electrical stimulation helps to identify the nerve. Alternatively, the triceps branches are identified at the muscle entry point and tracked proximally. Both the triceps long head and upper medial head motor branches are stimulated to check for integrity. If, preoperatively, the triceps strength is near normal or at least 6 to 7 kg, both branches can be used for transfer. In this situation, the trunk of the radial nerve is stimulated to check that the lower branch to the triceps medial head and anconeus muscle is functional. If triceps strength is not normal, only 1 of these branches, in general the triceps long head, is used as a donor. The triceps branches are sectioned distally and flipped proximally to be coaptated with the axillary nerve branches. After skin closure, all the incisions are infiltrated with a solution of local anesthetic for postoperative pain control. Postoperatively, only a sling is used for 1 week to 10 days.

COMPLICATIONS

We experienced no complications in our series. However, we should call attention to the possibility of hematoma formation, which should be evacuated immediately and nerve coaptation checked for any disruption. Triceps paralysis is another potential complication and the presence of innervation to the triceps medial head or lateral head should be documented before harvesting the triceps long head motor branch. This should be verified preoperatively on clinical examination and intraoperatively using direct electrical stimulation to the radial nerve, distal to the emergence of the triceps long head motor branch.

Nerve coaptation disruption is a serious complication, because it will not be detected until months later due to an absence of recovery. Hence, nerve coaptation should be tension free, and length redundant. By the end of surgery, the limb should be able to be moved freely and nerve coaptation inspected for disruption. Finally, the arm sling should not cross the operated-upon cervical lesion, because surface pressure can disrupt nerve coaptation.

OUTCOMES

We prospectively studied 37 young adults with C5-C6 brachial plexus palsy who underwent surgical repair an average of 6.3 months (±1.9 months) after trauma. The average age was 29.1 ± 14.8 years. All patients presented with palsy of shoulder abduction/external rotation, elbow flexion, and forearm supination. None of the patients presented with scapular winging. All patients had largely retained elbow extension strength and exhibited normal hand function. In 7 patients, no nerve roots were available for grafting, so reconstruction was achieved by transferring the accessory nerve to the suprascapular nerve, ulnar nerve fascicles to the biceps motor branch, and triceps branches to the axillary nerve (a triple nerve transfer). In 24 patients, C5 nerve root grafting to the anterior division of the upper trunk was combined with triple nerve transfer. In 6 patients, the C5-C6 nerve roots were grafted to the anterior and posterior divisions of the upper trunk, the accessory nerve was transferred to the suprascapular nerve, and ulnar nerve fascicles were connected to the biceps motor branch. The range of shoulder abduction/external rotation recovery and elbow flexion strength were evaluated between 24 and 26 months after surgery. Both full abduction and full external rotation of the shoulder were restored in 1 of the 7 patients in the C5 and C6 nerve root avulsion group, in 14 of 21 patients who received C5 nerve root grafting, and in 2 of 6 patients in the C5-C6 nerve root graft group. All patients recovered full range of elbow flexion and forearm supination. The average percentages of elbow flexion strength recovery, relative to the normal, contralateral side, were 27%, 43%, and 59% for the C5-C6 nerve root avulsion, C5 nerve root graft, and C5-C6 nerve root graft groups, respectively. Recovery of external rotation was greater among patients who had received a triceps to axillary nerve transfer, but there was no significant difference in the range of abduction recovered. Overall 66% of our patients recovered full abduction and external rotation, scoring M4 (Fig. 54-11). On average, the range of abduction was 143° (±40°) and external rotation was 126° (±24°).[2] At final evaluation, there was no reduction in the donor-site triceps strength compared with preoperative values and no loss in

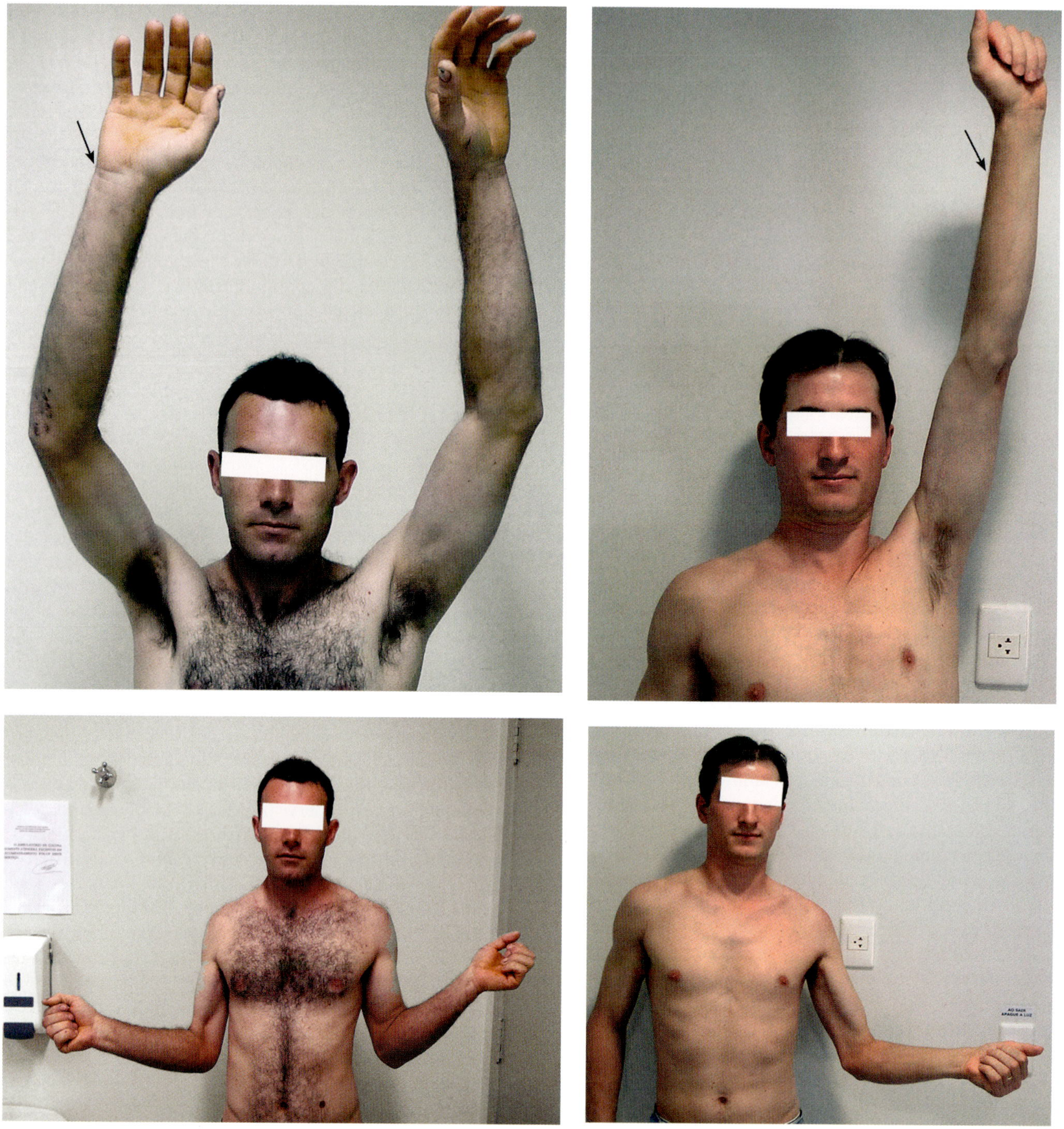

FIGURE 54-11 Postoperative results 24 months after brachial plexus grafting and shoulder motion reconstruction by accessory nerve transfer to the suprascapular nerve and triceps motor branch transfers to the axillary nerve. Fascicles of the ulnar nerve were transferred to the biceps motor branch.

pinch or grip strength. Patients with injuries that were amenable to reconstruction with both root grafting and nerve transfers had the best function. Our results call attention to the fact that not only is reinnervation of the prime movers of a given joint important, but secondary movers or joint stabilizers also may have a determining role in the success of motion, particularly if strength is required. These results suggest that the combined use of nerve transfers and root grafting may enhance outcomes in the reconstruction of C5-C6 injuries of the brachial plexus.

REFERENCES

1. Bertelli JA, Ghizoni MF. C5-8 brachial plexus root injury: the "T-1 hand". *J Neurosurg*. 2012;116:409–413.
2. Bertelli JA, Ghizoni MF. Nerve root grafting and distal nerve transfers for C5-C6 brachial plexus injuries. *J Hand Surg Am*. 2010;35A: 769–775.
3. Bertelli JA, Ghizoni MF, Loureiro Chaves DP. Sensory disturbances and pain complaints after brachial plexus root injury: a prospective study involving 150 adult patients. *Microsurgery*. 2011;31: 93–97.
4. Bertelli JA, Ghizoni MF. Pain after avulsion injuries and complete palsy of the brachial plexus: the possible role of nonavulsed roots in pain generation. *Neurosurgery*. 2008;62:1104–1113 [discussion 1113–1114].
5. Duchene de Boulogne GB. *Physiologie des mouvements*. Paris: J.-B Baillière et Fils; 1867:103.
6. Pollock LJ. Accessory muscle movements in deltoid paralysis. *JAMA*. 1922;12:526–528.
7. Babcock JL, Wray JB. Analysis of abduction in a shoulder with deltoid paralysis due to axillary nerve injury. *Clin Orthop Relat Res*. 1970;68: 116–120.
8. Bertelli JA, Ghizoni MF. Reconstruction of C5 and C6 brachial plexus avulsion injury by multiple nerve transfers: spinal accessory to suprascapular, ulnar fascicles to biceps branch, and triceps long or lateral head branch to axillary nerve. *J Hand Surg Am*. 2004;29A: 131–139.
9. Bertelli JA, Kechele PR, Santos MA, Duarte H, Ghizoni MF. Axillary nerve repair by triceps motor branch transfer through an axillary access: anatomical basis and clinical results. *J Neurosurg*. 2007;107: 370–377.
10. Hoppenfeld S. *Orthopaedic Neurology*. Philadelphia: J.B. Lippincott Company; 1977.
11. Vredeveld JW, Slooff BC, Blaauw G, Richards R. Validation of an electromyography and nerve conduction study protocol for the analysis of brachial plexus lesions in 184 consecutive patients with traumatic lesions. *J Clin Neuromuscul Dis*. 2001;2:123–128.
12. Berry H, Bril V. Axillary nerve palsy following blunt trauma to the shoulder region: a clinical and electrophysiological review. *J Neurol Neurosurg Psychiatry*. 1982;45:1027–1032.
13. Carvalho GA, Nikkhah G, Matthies C, Penkert G, Samii M. Diagnosis of root avulsions in traumatic brachial plexus injuries: value of computerized tomography myelography and magnetic resonance imaging. *J Neurosurg*. 1997;86:69–76.
14. Bertelli JA. Upper and lower trapezius muscle transfer to restore shoulder abduction and external rotation in longstanding upper type palsies of the brachial plexus in adults. *Microsurgery*. 2011;31: 263–267.
15. Bertelli JA, Ghizoni MF. Transfer of the platysma motor branch to the accessory nerve in a patient with trapezius muscle palsy and total avulsion of the brachial plexus: case report. *Neurosurgery*. 2011;68:E567–E570 [discussion E570].
16. Guan SB, Hou CL, Chen DS, Gu YD. Restoration of shoulder abduction by transfer of the spinal accessory nerve to suprascapular nerve through dorsal approach: a clinical study. *Chin Med J (Engl)*. 2006;119:707–712.
17. Bertelli JA, Ghizoni MF. Contralateral motor rootlets and ipsilateral nerve transfers in brachial plexus reconstruction. *J Neurosurg*. 2004;101:770–778.
18. Bhandari PS, Deb P. Dorsal approach in transfer of the distal spinal accessory nerve into the suprascapular nerve: histomorphometric analysis and clinical results in 14 cases of upper brachial plexus injuries. *J Hand Surg Am*. 2011;36A:1182–1190.
19. Bertelli JA, Ghizoni MF. Transfer of the accessory nerve to the suprascapular nerve in brachial plexus reconstruction. *J Hand Surg Am*. 2007;32A:989–998.

VIII

MISCELLANEOUS

55

Management of Traumatic Bone Loss in the Hand*

Elliot S. Mendelsohn, MD
Soheil Najibi, MD, PhD
David J. Slutsky, MD

In 1947, Littler described the fundamental principles of reconstruction in traumatic metacarpal bone loss: "Severe injuries of the hand are frequently complicated by massive metacarpal defects, which can be corrected only by bone-grafting ... the general principles obtaining for grafts of the larger bones are also applicable to grafts of the metacarpals."[1] In many instances, the fundamental principles of bone reconstruction can be applied to the hand. Gustilo type 3 open fractures of the hand resulting from high-energy trauma often involve segmental bone loss with extensive soft tissue damage. Freeland et al have emphasized the benefits of early bone grafting include faster bony union, less soft tissue contracture, and earlier mobilization that ultimately leads to better hand function.[2] Intramedullary nails embedded in antibiotic-impregnated cement have been commonly used for the treatment of infected tibia nonunions.[3] Antibiotic-impregnated cement spacers have been similarly used for bone defects and infected nonunions of the upper extremity.[4,5] The antibiotic-impregnated cement allows for the local delivery of a high concentration of antibiotics while maintaining a normal soft tissue tension, and creating a space that can be bone grafted. The intramedullary nail functions as a load-sharing device. This composite implant can be used on a temporary basis until definitive bone grafting and bony stabilization can be performed.

INDICATIONS

Primary bone grafting and rigid internal fixation is indicated in metacarpal and phalangeal fractures with significant bone loss such as gunshot wounds, saw injuries, severe crush injuries, and following debridement of infected bone.[2,6-10] This can also be combined with immediate soft tissue reconstruction.[11] The use of an antibiotic-impregnated cement intramedullary nail is indicated as a temporary spacer in an infected diaphyseal fracture of the metacarpal or phalanx with a significant bone defect. The cement spacer fills the dead space and creates a membrane-lined space devoid of soft tissue that can be filled with a structural bone graft and allows for elution of high concentrations of antibiotics. Those patients presenting with infected nonunions are also candidates.

CONTRAINDICATIONS

A staged reconstruction should be performed if a radical debridement and adequate soft tissue coverage of the bone cannot be achieved. Persistent infection is a contraindication to immediate bone grafting and plate fixation. Intramedullary fixation is not suitable in the face of marked rotational instability, although Bach et al have described the use of an intramedullary implant with interlocking screws for metacarpal fractures.[10] Vancomycin-impregnated cement should not be used in patients with an allergy to vancomycin.

SURGICAL TECHNIQUE

The original wound will determine the operative approach that is enlarged through extensile incisions. Care is taken to avoid crossing flexion creases at right angles. The wound is debrided starting at the periphery out of the zone of injury, to identify a clear plane between the injured and noninjured tissues. Small bony fragments that provide no structural support are excised, whereas bony fragments with viable periosteum or attached articular cartilage are left in place.[8] Traction on the finger and stretching the soft tissue out to length in the acute situation will allow one to determine the size of the bony defect. Although temporary external fixation may be used with a temporary spacer to eliminate any dead space (Fig. 55-1A-G), rigid fixation with a bridging plate is preferred. Lag screws or K-wires with tension band fixation

*Conflicts of interest and sources of funding: None of the authors have any conflicts of interest to declare relevant to this subject. There are no external sources of funding to report.

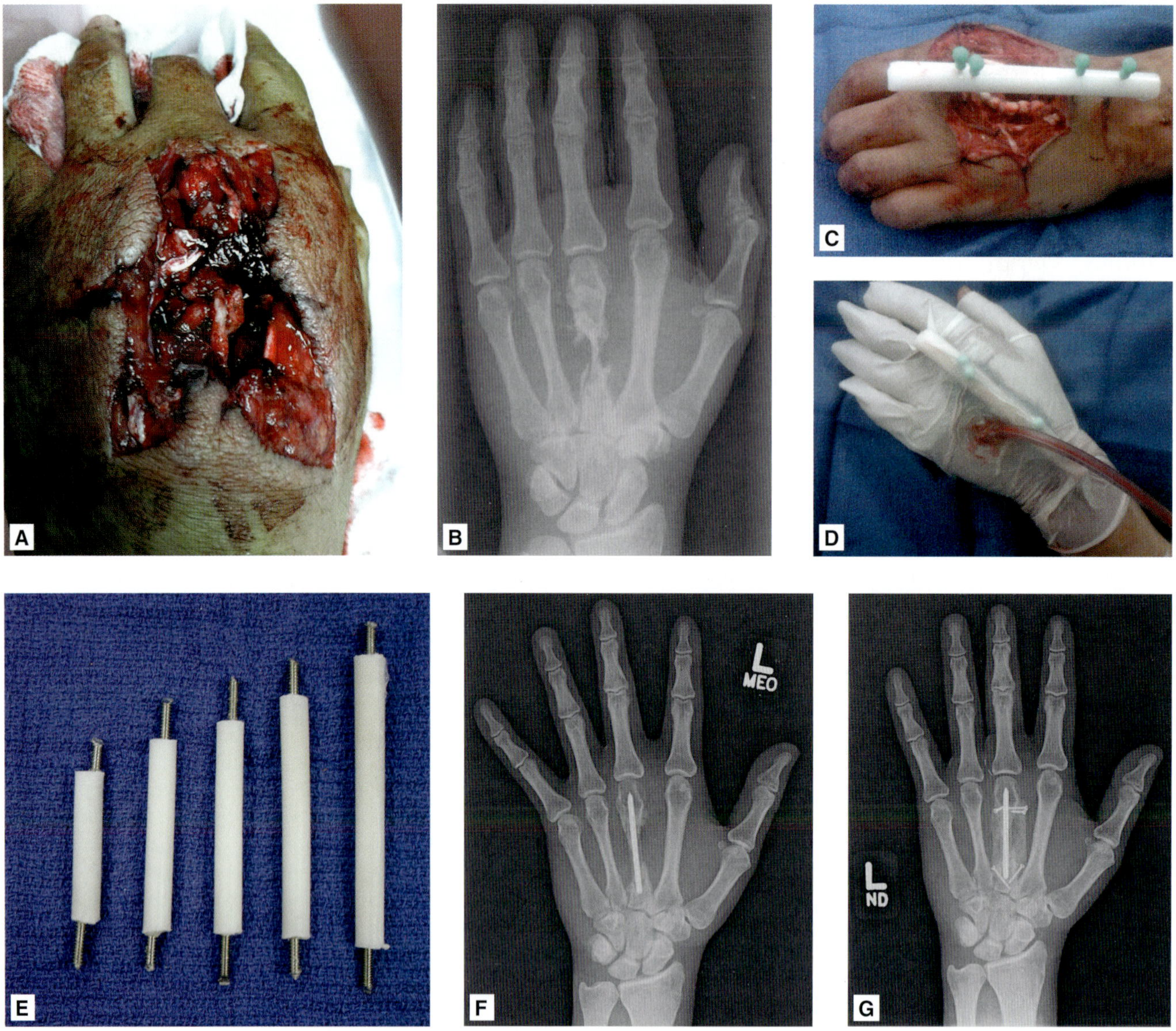

FIGURE 55-1 **A.** A 28-year-old male with low-velocity gunshot wound. **B.** A 4-cm segmental bone loss and shortening in a third metacarpal diaphyseal fracture. **C.** External fixator with antibiotic beads. **D.** VAC sponge. **E.** Antibiotic-impregnated cement intramedulllary nails. **F.** Immediate postoperative radiograph. **G.** Fracture union with antibiotic-impregnated cement nail and onlay bone graft.

should be used whenever possible to provide additional compression. Structural bone graft harvested from the iliac crest is inserted into the defect and held with cerclage wires or unicortical screws inserted through a plate (Fig. 55-2A-F). A minicondylar plate is ideally suited for periarticular fractures (Fig. 55-3A-C). Enhanced stability and bony contact can also be achieved using step-cut interlocking osteotomies between the bone graft and the recipient phalangeal or metacarpal bones, or by shaping the distal ends of the bone graft into pegs that are inserted into the intramedullary canals. Alternatively cancellous bone graft can be compacted using a 10-cm^3 syringe and inserted into the defect (Fig. 55-4A-C). A longitudinal intramedullary 0.062-in Kirschner wire may be used to provide supplementary fixation (Fig. 55-2F). Once bony fixation is achieved, any neurovascular repairs and tendon repair or tendon transfers are performed followed by immediate soft tissue coverage. Primary wound closure under minimal tension with well-vascularized tissue must be achieved in all cases. In some cases a wound VAC may be used (Fig. 55-1D) instead of pedicled flaps (Fig. 55-2E) or free tissue transfer.

A review of the literature would suggest that successful primary bone grafting requires a clean wound with a meticulous debridement, good blood supply, adequate fixation, and secure soft tissue cover.[2,6–10] If these conditions are not met, bone grafting should be staged until the soft tissue envelope is ready. Antibiotic cement spacers may be an alternative technique that can be used to maintain soft tissue tension, provide high levels of local antibiotic concentration in contaminated wound beds, and create a membrane-lined

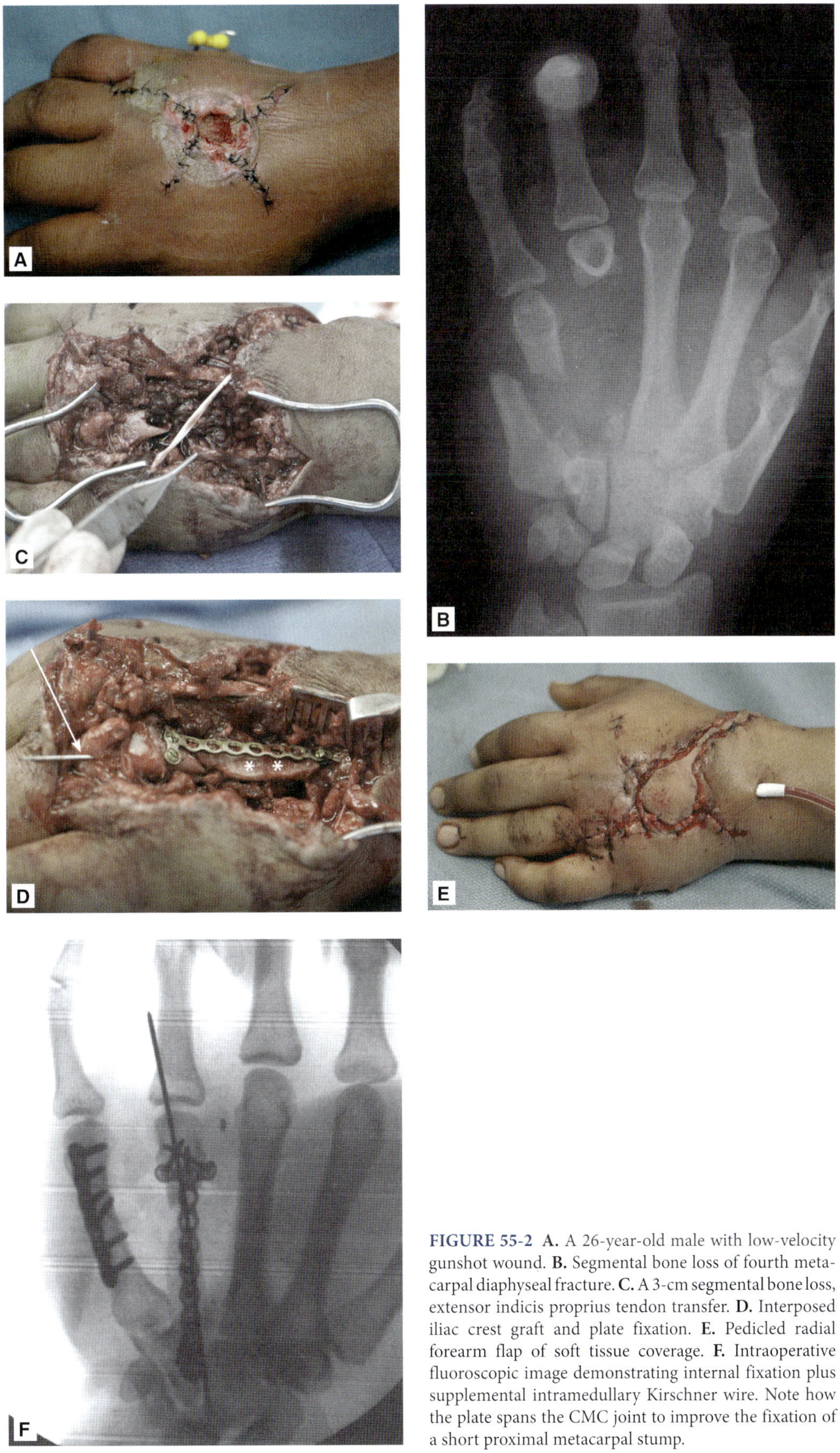

FIGURE 55-2 **A.** A 26-year-old male with low-velocity gunshot wound. **B.** Segmental bone loss of fourth metacarpal diaphyseal fracture. **C.** A 3-cm segmental bone loss, extensor indicis proprius tendon transfer. **D.** Interposed iliac crest graft and plate fixation. **E.** Pedicled radial forearm flap of soft tissue coverage. **F.** Intraoperative fluoroscopic image demonstrating internal fixation plus supplemental intramedullary Kirschner wire. Note how the plate spans the CMC joint to improve the fixation of a short proximal metacarpal stump.

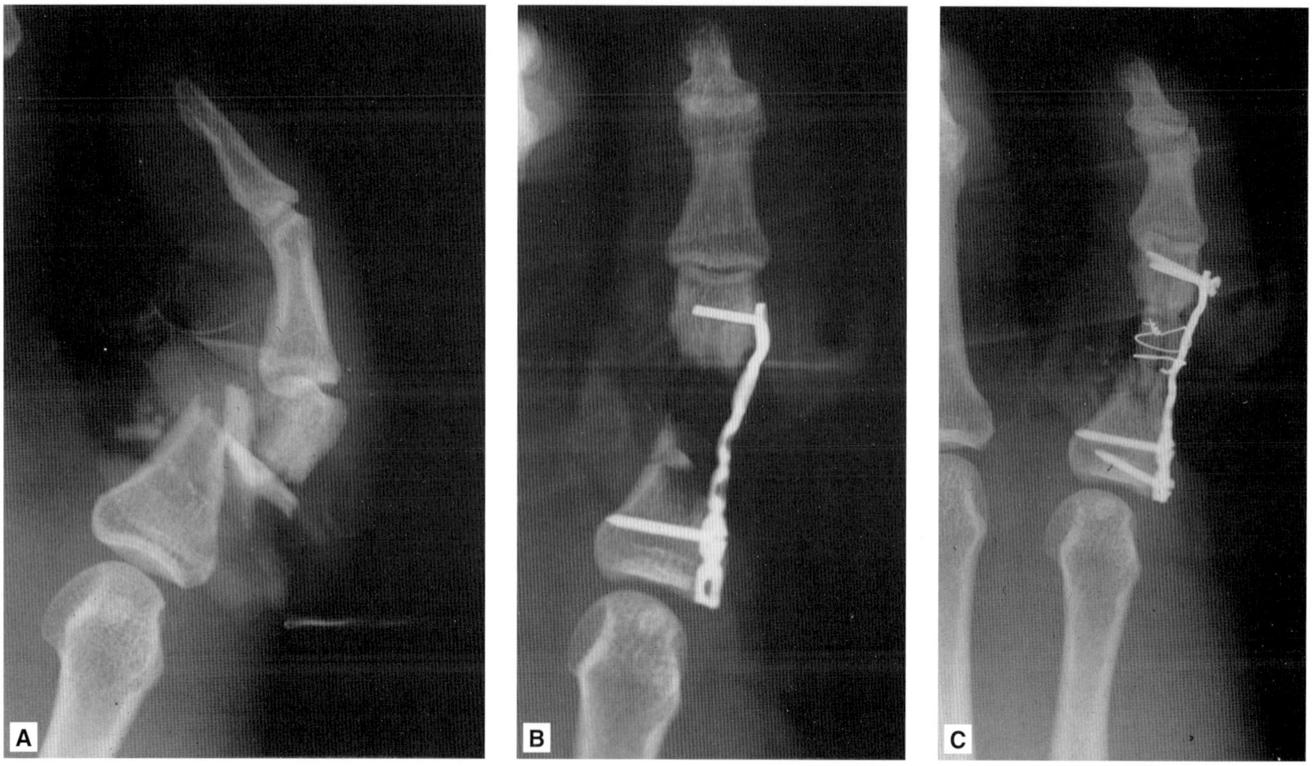

FIGURE 55-3 **A.** Crush injury of middle phalanx. **B.** Restoration of phalangeal length with a minicondylar blade plate. **C.** Interposition bone graft held with cerclage wiring and 1-mm screw.

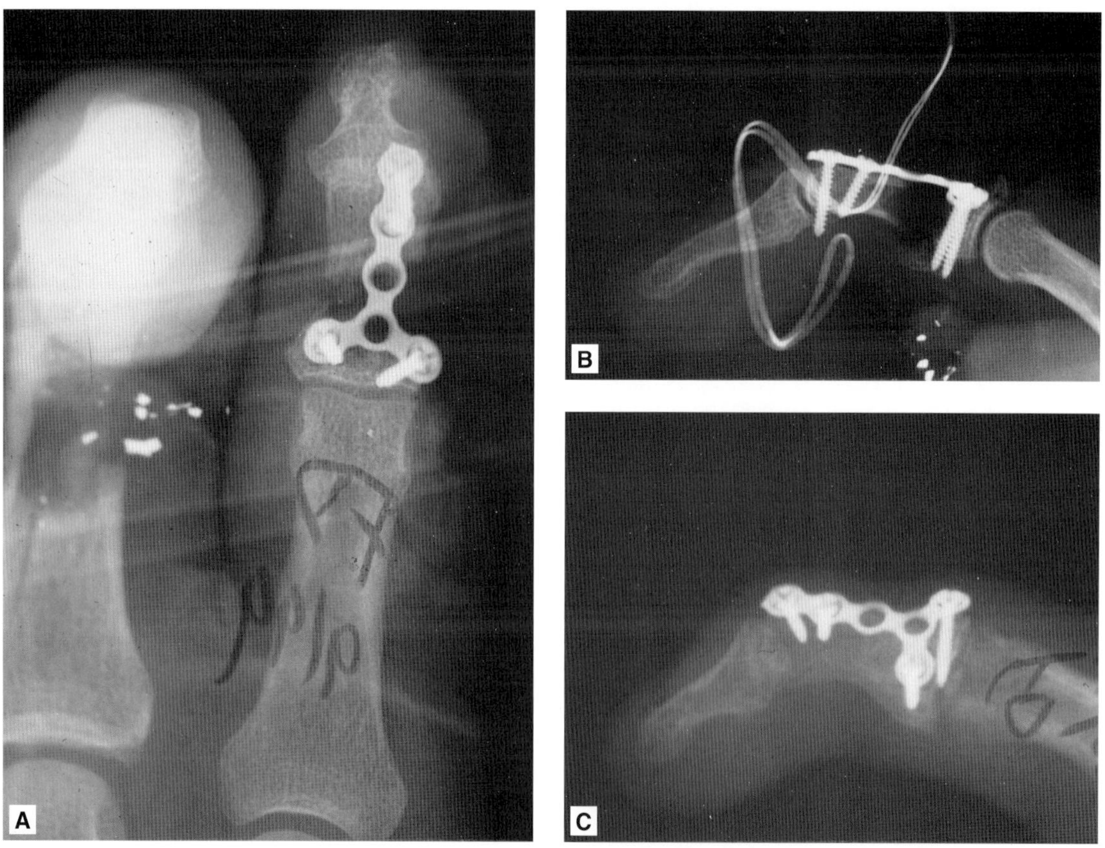

FIGURE 55-4 **A** and **B.** Loss of proximal half of middle phalanx. **C.** End result following compressed cancellous bone graft.

cavity devoid of soft tissue when grafting is deferred. In cases of infection, antibiotic cement combined with an intramedullary Steinmann pin is a useful construct that can be used as an antibacterial bone spacer. The materials required include a 28-French chest tube, a 3-mm threaded Steinmann pin, cement gun, and antibiotics. The size of the bone defect in the metacarpal is measured. A 28-French chest tube that has an inner diameter of 9.3 mm approximates the midshaft diameter of the metacarpals. The flare of the chest tube is cut off and it is cut to the appropriate length. Chest tubes and pins of various sizes are made to allow for more accurate sizing and optimal restoration of soft tissue tension in situ. One half of a package of polymethylmethacrylate (PMMA) bone cement (40 g), two 1.2-g vials of tobramycin, and two 1-g vials of vancomycin are mixed. It is important to restrict the amount of cement used to achieve the appropriate level of viscosity. The liquid monomer is added and mixed using the vacuum mixer. Often extra monomer is needed to allow adequate mixing of the Palacos bone cement (Zimmer, Warsaw, Indiana) with the antibiotic powder. This seemingly large amount of cement is necessary to allow for adequate fill of the cement gun. While the cement is still viscous, it is transferred to the cement gun. The cement is pressurized into the precut chest tube and the Steinmann pin is passed down the center of the chest tube. Once the bone cement hardens, the polyethylene chest tube is cut with a scalpel to peel it from the surface of the smooth hardened bone cement. The implants are trialed to determine the size with the most appropriate fit (Fig. 55-1E). The final antibiotic-impregnated cement nail is screwed into the distal fragment and then impacted into the proximal fragment (Fig. 55-1F).

COMPLICATIONS

Significant complications in the management of bone defects in metacarpal fractures include tendon and capsular adhesions, malunion, nonunion, and infection. The overall complication rate involving management of open fractures of the hand can be as high as 11%. In a large review of 140 open fractures, there were 15 complications (11%).[12] There were 6 infected digits, 5 nonunions (3 infected and 2 uninfected), 2 delayed unions, 1 amputation, and 1 case of reflex sympathetic dystrophy. Infection and late amputation were associated with the initial wound severity. All 4 deep infections occurred in patients with grade IIIB and IIIC open fractures. Secondary procedures in open fractures associated with significant bone loss include revision grafting, arthrodesis, and amputation. In a series of 12 patients with hand defects undergoing immediate autografting, Saint-Cyr et al described delayed amputation in 2 patients and PIP fusion in a third patient.[8]

Restoration of length is a concern when spanning large bony defects in the hand, especially with intramedullary fixation. Inadequate restoration of metacarpal lengthen will lead to an extensor lag in cadaveric studies.[13] Clinically, hyperextension at the MCP joint may compensate for small amounts of shortening. In a series of 10 metacarpal fractures treated with locked intramedullary nailing, Bach et al reported an average of 1.2 mm of shortening.[10] One patient developed an extensor lag at the MCP joint and required extensor tenolysis and capsulotomy. The use of fluoroscopy can be useful in judging restoration of metacarpal or phalangeal length intraoperatively, particularly in the application of intramedullary implants spanning large defects.

OUTCOMES

High rates of union with minimal complications have been reported in the management of bone defects in the hand, perhaps a reflection in the evolution in the timing of the bone grafting from delayed reconstruction[1,14] to "delayed primary grafting" (up to 7-10 days from the injury)[2,6,7] and "immediate grafting" (4-6 hours up to 24 hours post injury).[8,9] In one of the earliest reports, Littler recommended delayed reconstruction of metacarpals with bone graft and advised against internal fixation in the hand, relying instead on stability afforded by graft interposition.[1] Rinaldi described success with staged autografting up to 2 months delayed in 21 cases (with the exception of 1 case of immediate grafting).[14] All cases achieved union, but interpretation of the results is limited by the variety of methods of internal and external fixation and various forearm and hand bony defects as a result of trauma and tumor.

Success with early grafting in oral and maxillofacial applications prompted reports of primary grafting in hand defects. Freeland et al reported few complications with delayed primary bone grafting (performed within 10 days of the injury) in the management of hand and wrist wounds.[2] Seventeen patients had 21 bone graft operations as part of the overall delayed primary management of hand and wrist wounds. All grafts healed with the exception of 1 fibrous union at 1 bone graft juncture and few additional complications (no infections and 1 malunion). In a larger series of metacarpal fractures with bone loss due to low-velocity gunshot wounds, 40 metacarpal fractures with bone loss and/or comminution were treated with stable internal fixation supplemented with primary iliac crest bone grafting between 1 and 7 days after injury and all achieved union.[6] Similarly, in a series of 28 phalanx fractures due to low-velocity gunshot wounds, all 20 treated with internal fixation and iliac crest bone grafting within 1 week achieved union.[7] Sundine and Scheker compared a series of 7 patients who underwent staged reconstruction with 7 patients who had immediate reconstruction (within 24 hours of the initial injury) involving complex dorsal hand lesions requiring bone and tendon reconstruction and flap coverage.[11] Patients with immediate reconstruction had significantly fewer operations (2.1 compared with 5.9, $P = .002$) and a significantly faster return to maximum range of movement (214 days compared with 630 days, $P = .002$) than patients with staged reconstruction. In addition, patients undergoing immediate grafting trended toward a greater chance of returning to work (86% compared with 48.2%, $P = .3$). High rates of union have been reported in 3 cases of autografting in the hand as soon as 4 to 6 hours of injury.[9] According to Stahl et al, immediate restoration of normal bone length provides optimal circulation by improving venous and lymphatic return thereby reducing local edema of soft tissues, and eliminates dead space thereby precluding potential infection.

More recent literature substantiates the results of these earlier series with high union rates and function reported after immediate grafting. In a review of 12 type III open fractures of the hand with segmental bone loss treated with immediate bone grafting (within 24 hours of injury), Saint-Cyr et al reported a final union rate of 92%, infection rate of 0%, and mean time to return to regular work duty of 5 months and 21 days.[8] In a review of 10 metacarpal fractures with bone defects treated with locked intramedullary nailing, 9 out of 10 fractures treated with primary bone grafting achieved union.[10] The 1 nonunion was a fracture with a large bone defect that did not undergo primary grafting. After delayed grafting and revision of the internal fixation, union was achieved.

REFERENCES

1. Littler JW. Metacarpal reconstruction. *J Bone Joint Surg Am.* 1947; 29(3):723–737.
2. Freeland AE, Jabaley ME, Burkhalter WE, Chaves AM. Delayed primary bone grafting in the hand and wrist after traumatic bone loss. *J Hand Surg Am.* 1984;9A(1):22–28.
3. Thonse R, Conway J. Antibiotic cement-coated interlocking nail for the treatment of infected nonunions and segmental bone defects. *J Orthop Trauma.* 2007;21(4):258–268.
4. Allende C. Cement spacers with antibiotics for the treatment of post-traumatic infected nonunions and bone defects of the upper extremity. *Tech Hand Up Extrem Surg.* 2010;14(4):241–247.
5. Georgiadis GM, DeSilva SP. Reconstruction of skeletal defects in the forearm after trauma: treatment with cement spacer and delayed cancellous bone grafting. *J Trauma.* 1995;38(6): 910–914.
6. Gonzalez MH, McKay W, Hall RF Jr. Low-velocity gunshot wounds of the metacarpal: treatment by early stable fixation and bone grafting. *J Hand Surg Am.* 1993;18(2):267–270.
7. Gonzalez MH, Hall M, Hall RF Jr. Low-velocity gunshot wounds of the proximal phalanx: treatment by early stable fixation. *J Hand Surg Am.* 1998;23(1):150–155.
8. Saint-Cyr M, Miranda D, Gonzalez R, Gupta A. Immediate corticocancellous bone autografting in segmental bone defects of the hand. *J Hand Surg Br.* 2006;31(2):168–177.
9. Stahl S, Lerner A, Kaufman T. Immediate autografting of bone in open fractures with bone loss of the hand: a preliminary report. Case reports. *Scand J Plast Reconstr Surg Hand Surg.* 1999;33(1): 117–122.
10. Bach HG, Gonzalez MH, Hall RF Jr. Locked intramedullary nailing of metacarpal fractures secondary to gunshot wounds. *J Hand Surg Am.* 2006;31(7):1083–1087.
11. Sundine M, Scheker LR. A comparison of immediate and staged reconstruction of the dorsum of the hand. *J Hand Surg Br.* 1996; 21(2):216–221.
12. Duncan RW, Freeland AE, Jabaley ME, Meydrech EF. Open hand fractures: an analysis of the recovery of active motion and of complications. *J Hand Surg Am.* 1993;18(3):387–394.
13. Strauch RJ, Rosenwasser MP, Lunt JG. Metacarpal shaft fractures: the effect of shortening on the extensor tendon mechanism. *J Hand Surg Am.* 1998;23(3):519–523.
14. Rinaldi E. Autografts in the treatment of osseous defects in the forearm and hand. *J Hand Surg Am.* 1987;12(2):282–286.

INDEX

Page numbers followed by *f* or *t* indicate figures or tables, respectively.

F

G

H

R

S